CONTENTS

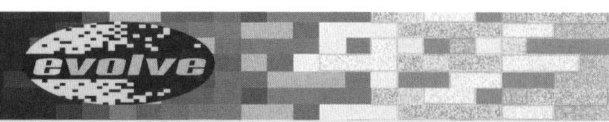

ERRATA NOTICE

Location of error: p.1003, two-thirds of the page down under the "PEDIATRIC DOSAGE (without preexisting renal/hepatic dysfunction)" heading

Currently reads: "PEDIATRIC DOSAGE (without preexisting renal/hepatic dysfunction) IV infusion: 0.05-1.5 mg/kg/day."

Should read: "PEDIATRIC DOSAGE (without preexisting renal/hepatic dysfunction) IV infusion: 0.03-0.15 mg/kg/day."

norepinephrine	oflaxacin	ondansetron	phenylephrine	piperacillin/tazobactam	potassium	procainamide	propofol	ranitidine	sodium bicarbonate	tobramycin	vancomycin	vecuronium
-	-	C	-	-	C	-	I	C	C	-	C	-
-	-	I	C	C	C	C	C	C	C	-	I	C
C	-	-	C	-	C	C	-	-	I	C	C	-
-	-	I	-	I	-	-	I	I	-	-	-	-
-	-	C	-	C	C	-	C	C	C	C	-	-
-	-	-	-	C	-	-	C	-	-	-	-	-
-	-	-	-	-	-	-	I	-	I	-	I	-
-	-	-	C	C	C	C	C	-	I	C	C	-
-	-	C	-	-	C	-	C	C	-	C	-	C
-	-	-	-	-	-	-	-	-	-	I	I	-
-	-	C	-	-	C	-	C	C	I	-	-	-
-	-	C	-	C	C	-	C	-	-	-	C	C
-	-	-	-	-	C	-	C	C	-	C	-	-
C	C	C	C	-	C	C	-	C	-	C	C	-
-	-	C	-	C	-	-	C	C	-	-	-	-
-	-	-	-	-	-	-	-	-	-	-	-	C
-	-	-	-	-	-	-	C	-	-	C	C	-
-	-	-	-	C	C	-	C	C	-	-	I	-
-	-	-	-	-	C	-	C	C	-	-	-	-
C	-	-	-	-	C	-	-	C	-	C	C	-
-	-	C	C	C	-	C	C	-	-	-	C	-
C	-	-	C	I	-	C	C	C	I	-	-	C
C	-	C	-	C	C	-	C	C	I	-	-	C
-	-	-	-	C	C	-	C	C	-	C	C	-
-	-	-	-	-	-	-	C	C	-	-	I	C
-	-	-	-	-	C	C	C	C	-	C	C	C
C	-	C	C	I	C	C	C	-	C	-	C	-
-	-	C	-	C	-	-	C	C	-	C	C	C
-	-	I	-	C	-	-	C	C	C	C	-	-
-	-	C	-	-	-	-	I	C	-	-	-	C
-	-	C	C	C	C	C	C	C	C	I	-	C
-	-	C	-	C	-	C	C	-	C	-	I	C
-	-	C	-	C	C	-	C	-	I	C	C	-

IV Compatibilities

The IV compatibility table provides data when 2 or more medications are given into a Y-site of administration. The data in this table largely represents physical incompatibilities (e.g., haze, precipitate, change in color). Therapeutic incompatibilities have not been included, so that when using the table, professional judgment should be exercised.

C = Physically compatible via Y-site administration.
I = Physically incompatible.

	amikacin	aminophylline
imipenem	-	-
insulin	-	I
labetolol	C	C
levofloxacin	C	C
lidocaine	C	C
linezolid	C	C
lorazepam	C	-
magnesium	C	-
meperidine	C	I
meropenum	-	C
methylprednisone	-	-
metoclopramide	-	-
metoprolol	-	-
metronidazole	C	C
midazolam	C	-
milrinone	C	-
morphine	C	C
multiple vitamin	-	-
nitroglycerin	-	C
nitroprusside	-	-
norepinephrine	-	-
oflaxacin	-	-
ondansetron	C	I
phenylephrine	-	C
piperacillin/tazobactam	-	C
potassium	C	C
procainamide	-	C
propofol	I	C
rantidine	C	C
sodium bicarbonate	C	C
tobramycin	-	-
vancomycin	C	I
vecuronium	-	C

amiodarone	amphotericin B	aztreonam	bumatanide	calcium chloride	calcium gluconate	cefazolin	cefepime	ceftazidime	cimetidine	ciprofloxacin	cisatracurium	clindamycin	cotrimoxazol	cyclosporine
-	-	C	-	-	-	-	-	-	-	-	C	-	-	-
C	-	C	C	-	-	C	-	-	C	-	-	-	-	-
C	-	-	-	-	C	C	-	C	C	-	-	C	C	-
-	-	-	-	-	-	-	-	-	C	-	-	C	-	-
C	-	-	-	C	C	-	-	-	C	C	C	-	-	-
-	I	C	-	-	C	C	-	C	C	-	C	C	C	C
-	-	I	C	-	-	-	-	-	C	C	C	-	-	-
-	-	C	-	I	-	C	-	-	-	I	C	-	-	C
-	-	C	C	-	-	C	-	C	C	-	C	C	C	-
-	I	-	-	-	-	-	-	-	C	-	-	-	-	-
-	C	C	-	-	C	-	-	-	C	I	-	C	-	-
C	-	C	-	-	-	-	-	-	C	C	C	C	-	-
-	-	-	-	-	-	-	-	-	-	-	-	-	-	-
C	-	I	-	-	-	-	-	C	C	C	C	C	-	C
C	-	-	I	-	C	C	-	I	C	C	C	C	-	-
-	-	-	C	C	C	C	C	C	C	C	-	C	-	-
C	-	C	C	C	-	C	-	C	C	-	C	C	C	-
-	-	-	-	-	-	-	-	-	-	-	-	-	-	-
C	-	-	-	-	-	-	-	-	-	-	C	-	-	-
-	-	-	-	C	-	-	-	-	C	-	-	-	-	-
C	-	-	-	-	-	-	-	-	-	-	C	-	-	-
-	-	-	-	-	-	-	-	-	-	-	C	-	-	-
-	I	C	-	-	-	C	-	C	C	-	C	C	-	-
C	-	-	-	-	C	-	-	-	-	-	C	-	-	-
-	I	C	C	-	C	-	-	-	C	-	-	C	-	-
C	-	C	-	-	C	C	-	C	C	C	C	-	-	-
C	-	-	-	-	C	-	-	-	-	-	C	-	-	-
-	I	C	C	I	C	C	-	C	C	C	-	C	-	C
-	I	C	-	-	-	C	-	C	-	C	C	C	-	-
I	-	C	-	I	I	-	-	I	-	-	-	-	-	-
C	-	C	-	-	C	C	I	-	-	C	C	-	-	C
C	-	-	-	I	C	-	I	-	C	-	C	-	-	C
-	-	-	-	-	-	C	-	-	C	-	-	-	C	-

linezolid	lorazepam	magnesium	meperidine	meropenem	methylprednisone	metoclopramide	metoprolol	metronidazole	midazolam	milrinone	morphine	multi-vitamin	nitroglycerin	nitropursside
C	C	C	C	-	-	-	-	C	C	C	C	-	-	-
C	-	-	I	C	-	-	-	C	-	-	C	-	C	-
-	-	-	-	-	-	C	-	C	C	-	C	-	C	-
I	-	-	-	I	C	-	-	-	-	-	-	-	-	-
C	I	C	C	-	C	C	-	I	-	-	C	-	-	-
-	C	-	C	-	-	-	-	-	I	C	C	-	-	-
-	-	I	-	-	-	-	-	-	-	C	C	-	-	C
C	-	-	-	-	C	-	-	-	C	C	-	-	-	-
C	-	C	C	-	-	-	-	-	C	C	C	-	-	-
-	-	-	-	-	-	-	-	-	-	C	-	-	-	-
C	-	-	C	-	-	-	-	C	I	C	C	-	-	-
C	C	-	C	C	C	C	-	C	C	C	C	-	-	C
-	C	I	-	-	I	C	-	C	C	C	-	-	-	-
C	C	C	C	-	-	C	-	C	C	-	C	-	C	-
C	-	-	C	-	C	C	-	C	C	C	C	-	-	-
C	-	-	C	-	-	-	-	-	-	-	C	-	-	-
C	-	C	-	-	-	-	-	C	-	-	-	-	-	-
C	C	-	C	C	-	-	-	-	-	C	C	C	-	-
C	-	-	C	C	-	-	-	-	C	C	C	-	-	-
-	C	-	C	-	-	C	-	C	-	C	C	C	C	C
C	I	-	C	C	I	-	-	-	-	-	C	-	-	-
C	-	-	C	C	-	-	-	-	-	C	C	-	C	C
C	-	-	C	C	C	-	-	-	C	C	C	-	C	C
C	-	C	-	C	C	-	-	C	-	-	C	-	-	C
-	-	-	-	-	-	-	-	-	-	C	-	C	-	C
C	-	C	-	-	-	-	-	C	C	-	C	-	C	-
C	C	C	C	-	C	C	-	-	C	-	C	-	C	C
C	C	-	C	C	-	C	-	C	C	-	C	-	C	-
C	C	-	-	C	-	I	-	-	-	I	I	-	C	C
C	C	C	C	C	-	-	-	C	C	C	C	C	-	-
C	C	C	-	C	C	-	-	C	C	C	-	-	-	C
C	C	-	-	-	-	-	-	C	-	-	C	-	-	-
C	C	C	-	-	-	-	-	C	C	-	-	-	-	-

dopamine	enalapril	epinephrine	esmolol	famotidine	fluconazole	furosemide	gentamicin	heparin	hydrocortisone	hydromorphine	imipenem	insulin	labetalol	levofloxacin	lidocaine
-	C	C	C	-	C	-	-	I	C	C	-	-	C	C	C
-	C	I	C	C	C	C	C	-	-	-	-	I	C	C	C
C	-	-	C	-	-	C	C	-	-	-	-	C	C	-	C
I	I	-	-	C	-	C	I	-	-	-	-	-	-	-	-
C	C	-	-	C	-	C	C	C	C	C	C	C	-	-	-
-	-	-	-	-	-	-	-	C	-	-	-	C	-	-	-
C	-	-	C	-	-	-	-	-	C	-	-	-	-	-	C
-	C	-	-	C	I	-	-	C	C	-	-	-	C	-	C
-	C	-	C	C	C	-	I	-	-	C	-	C	C	-	-
-	-	-	-	-	-	-	I	-	-	-	-	-	-	-	-
-	C	-	C	C	I	-	I	-	-	-	-	-	C	-	-
-	C	C	C	-	C	C	C	C	-	C	-	C	C	C	C
C	-	-	-	-	-	I	C	-	I	-	-	-	-	-	C
C	C	C	C	C	C	-	C	-	C	C	C	-	-	-	C
-	C	-	C	-	I	-	C	C	C	C	-	-	C	C	-
-	C	-	C	-	I	-	-	-	-	C	-	-	C	-	-
-	-	-	-	-	-	-	C	-	-	-	-	-	-	-	-
-	-	-	-	C	C	-	-	C	C	-	-	-	-	C	C
-	-	-	C	C	I	-	-	C	-	-	-	-	-	-	C
C	-	C	C	-	C	I	C	-	-	-	C	-	-	-	C
-	-	-	-	C	C	I	-	-	-	C	-	-	-	-	C
C	C	C	C	C	C	I	-	-	-	-	-	-	C	C	C
C	C	-	C	C	C	-	-	C	C	-	-	I	C	C	C
C	-	-	C	C	-	-	C	C	C	-	-	-	C	-	C
-	-	-	-	C	-	C	-	C	C	-	-	-	-	C	-
C	C	-	-	C	-	I	C	C	C	-	-	C	C	-	C
C	C	C	C	-	C	-	C	C	C	C	C	C	C	-	C
C	-	-	-	C	-	I	C	C	-	-	I	-	-	-	-
-	-	C	I	-	I	-	I	C	C	-	-	-	I	I	-
-	C	-	C	C	C	I	-	-	-	C	-	C	C	C	-
C	C	C	C	C	C	C	-	-	-	-	C	-	-	I	C
C	C	C	C	C	-	C	-	-	-	-	-	C	-	-	C
-	-	-	-	C	-	-	C	-	-	-	-	-	-	-	C

dexamethasone	digoxin	diltiazem	diphenhydramine	dobutamine	dopamine	enalapril	epinephrine	esmolol	famotidine	fluconazole	furosemide	gentamicin	heparin	hydrocortisone	hydromorphine
-	-	C	-	-	-	-	-	-	C	I	-	-	C	-	-
-	-	-	-	-	I	-	-	C	C	-	-	C	-	C	-
-	-	-	-	C	C	C	-	C	C	-	I	C	-	-	-
C	-	-	-	C	C	-	C	-	-	-	I	C	I	-	-
C	C	C	C	C	C	C	-	C	C	-	-	-	C	C	C
C	C	-	C	C	C	C	-	C	C	C	C	C	C	C	C
C	-	C	I	-	-	-	-	-	C	C	C	C	C	C	C
-	-	-	-	-	-	C	-	C	C	-	-	C	C	-	C
C	C	C	C	C	C	-	-	-	C	C	-	C	-	-	-
C	C	-	C	C	C	C	-	-	-	C	C	C	C	-	-
-	-	-	I	-	C	C	-	-	C	-	-	-	C	-	-
-	-	C	-	-	-	-	-	-	C	C	I	-	-	-	-
-	-	-	-	-	-	-	-	-	-	-	-	-	-	-	-
-	-	C	-	-	-	C	-	C	-	C	-	C	C	C	C
-	C	-	-	-	C	-	-	C	C	C	-	C	C	-	C
C	C	C	-	C	C	-	C	-	-	-	I	C	C	-	-
C	C	C	C	C	C	C	-	C	C	C	I	C	-	C	-
C	-	C	-	-	-	-	C	-	-	-	-	C	-	-	-
-	-	C	-	C	C	-	-	C	C	C	C	-	-	-	-
-	-	C	-	C	C	C	C	-	C	-	C	-	C	-	-
-	-	C	-	C	C	-	-	-	C	-	-	-	-	-	-
-	-	-	-	-	-	-	-	-	-	-	-	-	-	-	-
-	-	-	C	-	C	-	-	-	C	C	I	C	C	C	C
-	-	-	C	C	-	-	-	-	C	-	-	-	C	-	-
C	-	-	C	I	C	C	-	-	I	C	C	-	C	C	C
C	C	C	-	-	C	C	-	C	C	C	-	-	C	-	C
-	-	-	C	C	-	-	-	C	C	-	-	-		C	-
C	C	-	C	C	C	C	C	C	C	C	C	I	C	C	C
C	C	C	-	C	C	C	C	C	-	C	C	C	C	-	-
-	-	-	-	I	I	-	-	-	C	-	C	-	C	C	I
-	-	C	-	-	-	C	-	C	-	C	C	-	I	-	C
I	-	C	C	-	-	C	I	C	C	C	-	-	-	I	C
-	-	-	-	C	C	-	C	C	-	C	-	C	C	C	-

imipenem	insulin	labetalol	levofloxacin	lidocaine	linezolid	lorazepam	magnesium	meperidine	meropenem	methylprednisone	metoclopramide	metoprolol	metronidazole	midazolam	milrinone
-	C	-	-	-	C	I	-	I	-	-	-	-	-	I	-
C	-	I	I	-	-	-	C	C	C	-	C	-	-	C	C
-	I	-	-	C	C	-	C	C	-	-	-	-	C	C	-
-	I	-	-	C	C	C	-	-	-	-	C	-	-	-	-
-	-	C	C	-	C	-	C	C	-	C	C	-	C	-	C
C	-	C	C	C	C	-	C	C	C	C	C	-	C	C	-
I	-	C	C	-	-	C	-	-	-	-	C	-	C	-	C
-	C	C	-	-	C	-	-	C	C	-	C	-	C	-	[illegible]
I	C	C	-	C	C	-	C	-	-	C	C	C	C	C	[illegible]
-	C	-	-	-	C	-	C	-	-	-	C	-	-	-	[illegible]
-	-	-	-	-	C	-	-	C	-	-	C	-	C	-	[illegible]
-	C	-	C	C	C	-	C	C	C	C	-	-	-	-	[illegible]
-	-	-	-	-	-	-	-	C	-	-	-	-	-	-	-
-	-	C	-	-	C	C	C	C	-	C	-	-	-	C	C
I	C	C	-	-	C	-	-	C	-	-	-	-	C	-	C
I	C	-	-	C	-	C	C	-	C	C	-	-	C	C	-
-	C	C	C	C	C	C	C	I	C	C	C	C	C	C	C
-	-	-	-	-	-	-	-	-	I	-	C	-	-	-	-
-	C	C	I	C	C	-	-	-	-	-	-	-	-	C	C
-	C	C	I	C	-	-	C	-	-	-	-	-	-	C	C
-	I	C	-	-	-	-	-	-	C	-	-	-	-	C	C
-	-	-	-	-	C	-	-	-	-	-	-	-	-	-	-
C	-	-	-	-	C	-	C	C	I	-	C	-	-	C	-
-	-	-	C	C	-	-	-	-	-	-	C	-	-	-	-
-	-	-	-	-	C	C	C	C	-	C	C	-	C	-	C
-	C	C	-	C	C	C	C	C	-	-	C	-	-	C	C
-	-	-	-	C	-	-	-	-	-	-	-	-	-	-	-
C	C	C	-	-	-	C	C	C	-	I	C	-	-	-	C
-	-	C	-	C	C	C	-	C	C	C	C	-	-	C	C
-	-	I	C	-	C	-	I	I	-	-	I	-	-	-	C
-	C	C	-	-	C	-	C	C	-	-	-	-	C	C	C
-	C	C	C	-	C	C	C	C	C	-	-	-	-	C	C
-	-	-	-	-	C	C	-	-	-	-	-	-	-	C	C

	calcium gluconate	cefazolin	cefepime	ceftazidime	cimetidine	ciprofloxacin	cisatracurium	clindamycin	cotrimoxazol	cyclosporine	dexamethasone	digoxin	diltiazem	diphenhydramine	dobutamine
	C	-	-	-	C	C	C	C	-	C	C	-	C	C	-
	C	-	I	-	-	I	-	I	-	-	C	C	-	C	I
	-	I	-	-	-	-	-	C	-	-	-	-	-	-	C
	-	-	-	-	I	-	-	-	-	-	-	-	C	-	-
	C	C	-	C	C	C	C	C	C	-	C	-	C	C	C
	-	-	-	-	-	-	C	-	-	-	-	-	C	-	I
	-	-	-	-	-	-	-	-	-	-	-	-	-	-	-
	-	-	-	-	-	C	C	-	-	-	C	-	-	C	-
	-	-	-	-	-	C	-	-	-	C	C	-	C	-	-
	-	-	-	-	-	-	-	-	-	-	-	-	-	-	-
	-	-	-	-	-	C	-	C	-	-	-	-	C	-	-
	-	-	-	-	-	-	C	C	-	-	C	C	C	C	C
	C	C	-	C	-	-	C	I	-	C	I	C	C	C	C
	C	-	-	-	C	C	-	C	-	-	-	C	-	C	C
	-	-	-	C	C	I	C	-	-	C	-	-	C	-	-
	-	-	-	-	-	-	-	-	-	C	-	-	C	-	-
	-	C	-	-	-	C	-	C	C	-	-	-	-	-	-
	C	C	-	-	C	I	-	-	-	-	-	-	-	-	-
	-	-	-	-	C	C	C	-	-	-	-	-	C	-	-
	-	C	-	C	C	C	-	C	C	-	-	C	-	-	C
	C	-	-	-	C	C	C	-	-	-	-	-	-	-	-
	-	-	-	-	C	C	C	-	-	-	-	-	C	-	-
	-	-	-	-	-	C	C	-	-	-	-	-	C	-	C
	C	C	-	C	C	-	C	C	C	-	-	-	-	-	C
	-	-	-	-	C	-	C	-	-	-	-	-	C	-	C
	-	C	-	C	C	-	C	C	C	-	-	C	C	-	C
	C	C	-	C	-	-	C	-	-	-	C	C	-	C	C
	I	C	-	I	C	-	C	I	I	-	C	I	C	C	C
	-	-	-	-	C	I	-	-	-	-	-	-	I	I	I
	-	I	I	I	C	C	C	C	-	C	-	-	C	-	-
	C	-	-	-	C	-	-	C	-	-	C	C	-	-	-
	C	-	-	-	-	I	C	C	-	-	C	-	-	-	-
	-	C	-	-	C	-	C	C	C	-	-	-	-	C	-

IV Compatibilities

The IV compatibility table provides data when 2 or more medications are given into a Y-site of administration. The data in this table largely represents physical incompatibilities (e.g., haze, precipitate, change in color). Therapeutic incompatibilities have not been included, so that when using the table, professional judgment should be exercised.

C = Physically compatible via Y-site administration.
I = Physically incompatible.

	amikacin	aminophylline	amiodarone	amphotericin B	aztreonam	bumatanide
amikacin	-	C	C	I	C	-
aminophylline	C	-	I	-	C	-
amiodarone	C	I	-	-	-	-
amphotericin B	I	-	-	-	I	-
aztreonam	C	C	-	I	-	C
bumetanide	-	-	-	-	C	-
calcium chloride	C	I	-	-	-	-
calcium gluconate	C	C	-	-	C	-
cefazolin	-	-	I	-	C	-
cefepime	-	I	-	-	-	-
ceftazidime	-	-	-	-	C	-
cimetidine	C	-	-	I	C	-
ciprofloxacin	C	I	-	-	C	-
cisatracurium	C	-	-	-	C	C
clindamycin	C	I	C	-	C	-
co-trimoxazole	-	-	-	-	C	-
cyclosporine	C	-	-	-	-	-
dexamethasone	C	C	-	-	C	-
digoxin	-	C	-	-	-	-
diltiazem	C	-	-	C	C	C
diphenhydramine	C	C	-	-	C	-
dobutamine	-	I	C	-	C	I
dopamine	-	-	C	I	C	-
enalapril	C	C	-	I	C	-
epinephrine	C	I	-	-	-	-
esmolol	C	C	C	-	-	-
famotidine	-	C	-	C	C	-
fluconazole	C	C	-	-	C	-
furosemide	-	C	C	-	C	-
gentamicin	-	C	C	I	C	-
heparin	I	-	-	-	C	C
hydrocortisone	C	-	-	-	C	-
hydromorphine	C	-	-	-	C	-

morphine	multi-vitamin	nitroglycerin	nitropursside	norepinephrine	oflaxacin	ondansetron	phenylephrine	piperacillin/tazobactam	potassium	procainamide	propofol	ranitidine	sodium bicarbonate	tobramycin	vancomycin	vecuronium
-	-	-	-	-	-	C	-	-	-	-	C	-	-	-	-	-
C	-	C	C	I	-	-	-	-	C	-	C	-	-	C	C	-
C	-	C	C	C	-	-	-	-	C	-	C	C	I	C	C	-
C	-	I	I	-	-	-	C	-	-	-	-	-	C	-	C	-
C	-	C	C	-	-	-	C	-	C	C	-	C	-	-	-	-
C	-	C	-	-	C	C	-	C	C	-	-	C	C	C	C	C
C	-	-	-	-	-	-	-	C	C	-	C	C	-	-	C	C
C	-	-	C	-	-	C	-	C	C	-	C	-	I	C	C	-
I	-	-	-	-	-	C	-	C	C	-	C	C	I	C	C	-
C	I	-	-	C	-	I	-	-	-	-	-	C	-	-	C	-
C	-	-	-	-	-	-	-	C	-	-	I	C	-	-	-	-
C	C	-	-	-	-	C	C	C	C	-	C	C	I	-	-	-
C	-	-	-	-	-	-	-	-	-	-	-	-	-	-	-	-
C	-	-	-	-	-	-	-	C	-	-	-	-	-	C	-	-
C	-	C	C	C	-	C	-	-	C	-	-	C	-	C	C	C
C	-	C	C	C	-	-	-	C	C	-	C	C	C	C	C	C
-	-	-	C	C	-	C	-	C	C	-	-	C	-	C	C	C
-	-	-	-	-	-	-	-	-	-	-	-	-	-	-	-	-
-	-	-	C	-	-	-	-	-	-	-	C	C	-	-	-	C
C	-	C	-	C	-	-	-	-	C	C	C	C	-	-	-	C
C	-	-	C	-	-	-	-	-	-	-	C	C	-	-	-	-
-	-	-	-	-	-	-	-	-	C	-	C	-	C	-	-	-
C	-	-	-	-	-	-	-	C	C	-	C	C	I	-	C	-
-	-	-	-	-	-	-	-	-	-	-	-	-	-	-	C	-
C	-	-	-	-	-	C	-	-	C	-	-	C	C	-	-	-
C	-	-	C	-	C	C	-	C	-	C	C	C	C	-	-	-
-	-	-	C	-	-	-	-	-	C	-	C	C	-	-	C	-
-	-	C	C	C	C	C	-	-	C	C	-	C	C	I	C	C
C	-	C	C	C	-	C	-	C	C	C	C	-	-	-	C	C
-	-	-	-	-	C	I	-	C	C	-	C	-	-	-	I	-
C	-	-	-	-	-	-	-	-	-	-	I	-	-	-	-	-
C	-	-	-	-	-	C	C	-	-	C	C	C	I	-	-	C
C	-	C	C	-	-	-	-	-	-	-	C	C	-	-	C	-

Saunders Nursing Drug Handbook 2005

BARBARA B. HODGSON, RN, OCN
Cancer Institute
St. Joseph's Hospital
Tampa, Florida

ROBERT J. KIZIOR, BS, RPh
Education Coordinator
Department of Pharmacy
Alexian Brothers Medical Center
Elk Grove Village, Illinois

ELSEVIER
SAUNDERS

ELSEVIER
SAUNDERS

11830 Westline Industrial Drive
St. Louis, MO 63146

Saunders Nursing Drug Handbook 2005 **ISBN 0-7216-0526-5**

NOTICE

Pharmacology is an ever-changing field. Standard safety precautions must be followed, but as new research and clinical experience broaden our knowledge, changes in treatment and drug therapy may become necessary or appropriate. Readers are advised to check the most current product information provided by the manufacturer of each drug to be administered to verify the recommended dose, the method and duration of administration, and contraindications. It is the responsibility of the licensed prescriber, relying on experience and knowledge of the patient, to determine dosages and the best treatment for each individual patient. Neither the publisher nor the author assume any liability for any injury and/or damage to persons or property arising from this publication.

Previous editions copyrighted 2004, 2003, 2002, 2001, 2000, 1999, 1998, 1997, 1996, 1995, 1994, 1993.

ISSN 1098-8661

Vice President and Publishing Director, Nursing: Sally Schrefer
Editor: Sandra Clark Brown
Developmental Editor: Sophia Oh Gray
Editorial Assistant: Brooke Bagwill
Publishing Services Manager: Melissa Lastarria
Design Coordinator: Teresa McBryan
Interior Design: Paula Ruckenbrod

Printed in the United States of America.

Last digit is the print number: 9 8 7 6 5 4 3 2 1

I dedicate this work to my daughter, Lauren, a true friend, for her unconditional love; my daughter, Kathryn, always supportive, always encouraging; and my son, Keith, a source of great pride to us all.
This is also dedicated to my sons-in-law, Jim and Andy, who have added so very much to my family, and to my granddaughter, Paige Olivia, a wonder to behold.

BARBARA HODGSON

To all health care professionals, who in the expectation of little glory or material reward dedicated themselves to the art and science of healing.

ROBERT KIZIOR

AUTHOR BIOGRAPHIES

Barbara Hodgson

Born and raised in Michigan, Barbara was married and raising a young family in Chicago when she decided to fulfill a lifelong dream and become a nurse. After graduation, she started her own business as author and publisher of **Medcards, The Total Medication Reference Guide,** the first of its kind. These drug cards were designed to assist nursing students in understanding drug information to give knowledgeable care to their patients.

In 1981, she met co-author Robert (Bob) Kizior, who was teaching a pharmacology class. After class, Barbara approached him and asked if he would be interested in working on **Medcards** with her. He agreed, and together they became so successful that a few years later Barbara was able to fulfill another dream and move to Florida.

By 1987, Barbara was approached by W.B. Saunders and asked to author the **Saunders Nursing Drug Handbook.** Since then, Barbara and Bob have worked together on this handbook and on two more drug resources, the **Saunders Electronic Nursing Drug Cards** and the **Saunders Drug Handbook for Health Professions.**

Barbara specializes in oncology at the Cancer Institute, St. Joseph's Hospital, in Tampa, Florida. Barbara's daughter Lauren and her husband, Jim, are emergency nurses. Her daughter Kathryn is a research biologist. Her son, Keith, is a student and plans to become an emergency nurse.

Barbara's favorite interests are spending time with her very busy, tight-knit family and when she has a rare moment, getting her hands full of dirt working in her garden.

Robert (Bob) Kizior

Bob graduated from the University of Illinois School of Pharmacy and is licensed to practice in the state of Illinois. He has worked as a hospital pharmacist for 34 years at Alexian Brothers Medical Center in Elk Grove Village, Illinois—a suburb of Chicago. Bob is the Education Coordinator for the Department of Pharmacy, where he participates in educational programs for pharmacists, nurses, physicians, and patients. He plays a major role in conducting Drug Utilization Reviews and is a member of Infection Control Committee and Safety Champions (a committee that is focused on identifying and preventing medication errors within the medical center). His hospital experience is diverse and includes participation in clinical pharmacy initiatives on inpatient units and in the surgical pharmacy satellite. Bob is a former adjunct faculty member at William Rainey Harper Community College in Palatine, Illinois. It was there that Bob first met Barbara and commenced their long-standing professional association.

An avid fan of Big Ten college athletics, Bob also has eclectic tastes in music that range from classical, big band, rock 'n' roll, and jazz to country and western. Bob spends much of his free time reviewing the professional literature to stay current on new drug information. He and his wife, Marcia, and their two Labrador retrievers—Caty and Zak—enjoy escape weekends at their year-round lake house in central Wisconsin.

CONSULTANT REVIEWERS

Katherine B. Barbee, MSN, ANP, F-NP-C
Kaiser Permanente
Washington, District of Columbia

Marla J. DeJong, RN, MS, CCRN, CEN, Capt.
Wilford Hall Medical Center
Lackland Air Force Base, Texas

Diane M. Ford, RN, MS, CCRN
Andrews University
Berrien Springs, Michigan

Denise D. Hopkins, PharmD
Clinical Instructor of Pharmacy Practice
College of Pharmacy
University of Arkansas
Little Rock, Arkansas

Barbara D. Horton, RN, MS
Arnot Ogden Medical Center School of Nursing
Elmira, New York

Mary Beth Jenkins, RN, CCRN, CAPA
Elliott One Day Surgery Center
Manchester, New Hampshire

Kelly W. Jones, PharmD, BCPS
Associate Professor of Family Medicine
McLeod Family Medicine Center
McLeod Regional Medical Center
Florence, South Carolina

Linda Laskowski-Jones, MS, RN, CS, CCRN, CEN
Christiana Care Health Systems
Newark, Delaware

Denise Macklin, BSN, RNC, CRNI
President, Professional Learning Systems, Inc.
Marietta, Georgia

Judith L. Myers, MSN, RN
Health Sciences Center
St. Louis University School of Nursing
St. Louis, Missouri

Kimberly R. Pugh, MSEd, RN, BS
Nurse Consultant
Baltimore, Maryland

Regina T. Schiavello, BSN, RNC
Wills Eye Hospital
Philadelphia, Pennsylvania

Gregory M. Susla, PharmD, FCCM
National Institutes of Health
Bethesda, Maryland

STUDENT REVIEWER PANEL

Lisa Brown
Jackson State Community College
Jackson, Tennessee

Autumn E. Korson
Western Michigan University
Bronson School of Nursing
Kalamazoo, Michigan

Jessica K. Leet, RN, BSN
Cardinal Glennon Children's Hospital
St. Louis, Missouri

Nancy L. McCartney
Valencia Community College
Orlando, Florida

Elizabeth Taylor
Tennessee Wesleyan
College of Nursing
Fort Saunders Regional
Knoxville, Tennessee

PREFACE

Nurses face many challenges in today's environment, not the least of which is familiarity with the large number of medications available. New medications are being introduced, and new applications, dosage forms, and different routes of administration for existing medications are increasing at a rapid rate. This voluminous amount of drug information must be integrated into the patient care environment quickly.

Saunders Nursing Drug Handbook 2005 is designed as an easy-to-use source of current drug information needed by the busy nurse. What separates this book from others is that it guides the nurse through patient care to better practice, and to better care.

This handbook contains:

1. **An expanded IV Compatibility chart.** This handy trifold chart is bound into the handbook to prevent accidental loss.
2. **The Classifications section.** Presents the action and uses for some of the most common clinical and pharmacotherapeutic classes. One new class has been added in this edition—skeletal muscle relaxants. Unique to this handbook, each class provides an at-a-glance table that compares all the generic drugs within the classification according to product availability, dosages, side effects, and other characteristics. Its blue full-page color tab ensures you can't miss it!
3. **An attractive four-color atlas of medications.** Contains photographs of 160 of the most commonly used oral medications. The medications, both brand and generic, are shown in their different dosage forms. Just look for the blue full-page color tab to help you identify those medications presented to you sans prescription bottle or order! A appears in the individual drug entries when there is a corresponding illustration in the atlas.
4. **An alphabetical listing of drug and herbal entries by generic name.** Blue letter thumb tabs help you page through this section quickly. Included in this edition are full entries for 19 of the most commonly used herbs, each indicated with a blue leaf . To make scanning pages easier each new entry begins with a shaded box containing the generic name, pronunciation, trade names, fixed-combinations, and classifications.
5. **Trade name cross references** in the A to Z section of the book. Over 230 of the top trade name drugs have cross-references within the A to Z section for quick use! These entries are shaded in gray for easy identification.
6. **A comprehensive reference section.** The reference section is updated, expanded, and contains a new appendix—Spanish Phrases Often Used in Clinical Settings. The herbal therapies appendix has been expanded to include more than 53 entries. Other appendixes include vital information on poison antidotes, calculation of doses, controlled drugs, cultural aspects of drug therapy, FDA pregnancy categories, normal laboratory values, recommended childhood and adult immunizations, signs and symptoms of electrolyte imbalance, and techniques of medication administration.
7. **The New Drug Supplement.** We endeavor to include all of our drug entries in the A–Z portion of the handbook, but when the FDA releases a drug late in the

season we include its monograph here to provide you with all the most current information. Each New Drug Supplement entry includes the class, action, use, routes, dosages, and side effects of the generic drug.

8. **The indexes.** You'll find the Disorders index in the front part of the book for quick reference. This index lists common disorders and the drugs often used for treatment. The Pediatric index allows the nurse to locate drugs appropriate for the pediatric patient. Look for the full-page blue tab to locate this resource. The comprehensive index is at the back of the book on light blue pages. Undoubtedly the most comprehensive tool to help you navigate the handbook, the comprehensive index is organized by showing generic drug names in **bold,** trade names in regular type, classifications in *italics,* and the page number of the main drug entry listed first and in **bold.**
9. **A mini CD. Saunders Nursing Drug Handbook 2005** has a mini CD-ROM packaged in the back of the book. The software features 200 monographs for most commonly used medications. Users can customize and print these monographs. *New to this edition* is the addition of the Disorders index.

A DETAILED GUIDE TO THE SAUNDERS NURSING DRUG HANDBOOK

An intensive review by Consultant Reviewers and the Student Reviewer Panel helped us to revise the **Saunders Nursing Drug Handbook** so that it is most useful in educational and clinical practice. The main objective of the handbook is to provide essential drug information in a user-friendly format. The bulk of the handbook contains an alphabetical listing of drug entries by generic name.

To maintain the portability of this handbook and meet the challenge of keeping content current, we have also included additional information for some medications on an EVOLVE Internet site. EVOLVE also includes drug alerts (e.g., medications removed from the market) and drug updates (e.g., new drugs, updates on existing entries). Information is periodically added, allowing the nurse to keep abreast of current drug information. The drug entries with EVOLVE enhancement are indicated with a ⓔ next to the generic drug name.

You'll also notice that some entries for infrequently used medications are condensed to reflect only the absolutely essential points the nurse should know when called upon to administer them. These abbreviated entries always include the generic name, pronunciation, brand names, classification, action, uses, precautions, interactions, availability, indications/routes/dosage, side effects, adverse reactions/toxic effects, and nursing implications. IV drug entries also include administration/handling, IV incompatibilities, and IV compatibilities information.

We have incorporated the IV Incompatibilities heading ∅. The drugs listed in this section are not compatible with the generic drug when administered direct by IV push, via Y-site, or via IV piggyback. We have highlighted the intravenous drug information with a special heading icon and have broken it down by IV Storage, IV Reconstitution, and Rate of IV Administration. To aid in the care of volume-restricted patients, selected drug entries include a maximum concentration heading.

We revised the order of entries to follow the logical thought process that the nurse undergoes whenever a drug is ordered for a patient:

- What is the drug?
- How is the drug classified?
- What does the drug do?

- What is the drug used for?
- Under what conditions should you **not** use the drug?
- How do you administer the drug?
- How do you store the drug?
- What is the dose of the drug?
- What should you monitor the patient for once he or she has received the drug?
- What do you assess the patient for?
- What interventions should you perform?
- What should you teach the patient?

The following are included within the drug entries:

Generic Name, Pronunciation, Trade Names. Each entry begins with the generic name and pronunciation followed by the U.S. and Canadian trade names. Exclusively Canadian trade names are followed by a blue maple leaf. Trade names that were most prescribed in the year 2003 are underlined in this section.

Do Not Confuse With. Drug names that sound similar to the generic and/or brand names are listed under this heading to help you avoid potential medication errors.

Fixed-Combination Drugs. Where appropriate, fixed-combinations, or drugs made up of two or more generic medications, are listed with the generic drug.

Pharmacotherapeutic and Clinical Classification Names. Each full entry includes both the pharmacotherapeutic and clinical classifications for the generic drug. When available, the page number of the classification description in the front of the book is provided in this section as well.

Action/Therapeutic Effect. This section describes how the drug is predicted to behave, with the expected therapeutic effect under a separate heading.

Pharmacokinetics. This section includes the absorption, distribution, metabolism, excretion, and half-life of the medication. The half-life is bolded for easy access.

Uses/Unlabeled. The listing of uses for each drug includes both the FDA uses and unlabeled uses.

Precautions. This heading incorporates a discussion on when the generic drug is contraindicated or should be used with caution. The cautions warn the nurse of specific situations in which a drug should be closely monitored. **Lifespan Considerations** includes the pregnancy category and lactation data as well as age-specific information concerning children and the elderly.

Interactions. This heading enumerates drug, food, and herbal interactions with the generic drug. As the number of medications a patient receives increases, awareness of drug interactions becomes more important. Also included is information on therapeutic and toxic blood levels in addition to the altered lab values that show what effects the drug may have on lab results.

Product Availability. Each drug monograph gives the form and availability of the drug.

Administration/Handling. Instructions for administration are given for each route of administration (e.g., PO, IM, rectal). Special handling such as refrigeration is also included where applicable. **IV administration** is broken down by storage (including how long the medication is stable once reconstituted), reconstitution, and rate of administration (how fast the IV should be given).

IV Compatibilities/IV Incompatibilities ∅ give the nurse the most comprehensive compatibility information possible when administering medications by direct IV push, via a Y-site, or via IV piggyback.

Indications/Routes/Dosage. Each full entry provides specific dosing guidelines for adults, the elderly, children, and patients with renal and/or hepatic impairment. Dosages are clearly indicated for each approved indication and route.
Side Effects. Side effects are defined as those responses that are usually predictable with the drug, are **not** life-threatening, and may or may not require discontinuation of the drug. Unique to this handbook, side effects are grouped by frequency and occurrence percentages so that the nurse can focus on patient care without wading through myriad signs and symptoms of side effects.
Adverse Reactions/Toxic Effects. Adverse reactions and toxic effects are very serious and often life-threatening, undesirable responses that require prompt intervention from a health care provider.
Nursing Implications. Nursing implications are organized as care is organized. That is:

- What needs to be assessed or done before the first dose is administered? (Baseline Assessment)
- What interventions and evaluations are needed during drug therapy? (Intervention/Evaluation)
- What explicit teaching is needed for the patient and family? (Patient/Family Teaching)

Saunders Nursing Drug Handbook is an easy-to-use source of current drug information for nurses, students, and other health care providers. It is our hope that this handbook will help you provide quality care to your patients.

We welcome any comments you may have that would help us to improve future editions of the handbook. Please contact us via the publisher at *http://evolve.elsevier.com/SaundersNDH*

Barbara B. Hodgson, RN, OCN
Robert J. Kizior, BS, RPh

ACKNOWLEDGMENTS

I offer a special heartfelt thank you to my co-author, Bob Kizior, for his continuing, superb work. Without Bob's effort in this major endeavor, this book would not have reached the par excellence it has achieved. We are indebted to Sandra Brown, our nursing editor, for her consistent encouragement, and to Sophia Gray, our developmental editor, who kept such a close eye on this project, assisting our walk through the maze to final production. I thank my siblings, Milt, Bruce, Jane, Rich, Vance, and Greg, who have encouraged me through the years; Jim Witmer, BSN, CCRN, CEN for the many hours he spent assisting me in this huge endeavor and the consistent support he offered; Andrew Ross, who enlightens my family so dearly; and to Kasie Kaelin, who brightens every room she enters.

Barbara Hodgson

ILLUSTRATION CREDITS

Behrman RE (ed): *Nelson Textbook of Pediatrics,* ed 15, Philadelphia, 1996, WB Saunders.
Boothby WM, Sandiford RBL: *Boston Med Surg J* 185:337, 1921.
Kee JL, Hayes ER (eds): *Pharmacology: A Nursing Process Approach,* ed 3, Philadelphia, 2000, WB Saunders.
Lehne RA: *Pharmacology for Nursing Care,* ed 4, Philadelphia, 2000, WB Saunders.
Mosby's GenRx, ed 11, St Louis, 2001, Mosby.

BIBLIOGRAPHY

Mosby's Drug Consult, 2004, ed 14, St. Louis, 2004, Mosby.
Rakel RE, Bope ET: *Conn's Current Therapy,* Philadelphia, 2003, WB Saunders.
Trissel LA: *Handbook of Injectable Drugs,* ed 12, Bethesda, 2004, American Society of Health–System Pharmacist.
Drug Facts and Comparisons, St. Louis, 2003, Facts and Comparisons.
Lacy CF, Armstrong LL, Goldman MP, et al: *Lexi-Comp's Drug Information Handbook,* ed 11, Hudson, Ohio, 2004, Lexi-Comp.
Takemoto CR, Hodding JH, Kraus DM: *Lexi-Comp's Pediatric Dosage Handbook,* ed 10, Hudson, Ohio, 2003, Lexi-Comp.
USPDI Drug Information for the Health Care Professional, 2003.
Briggs G, Freeman R, Yaffe S: *Drugs in Pregnancy and Lactation,* ed 6, Greenwood Village, Colorado, 2003, Micromedex.

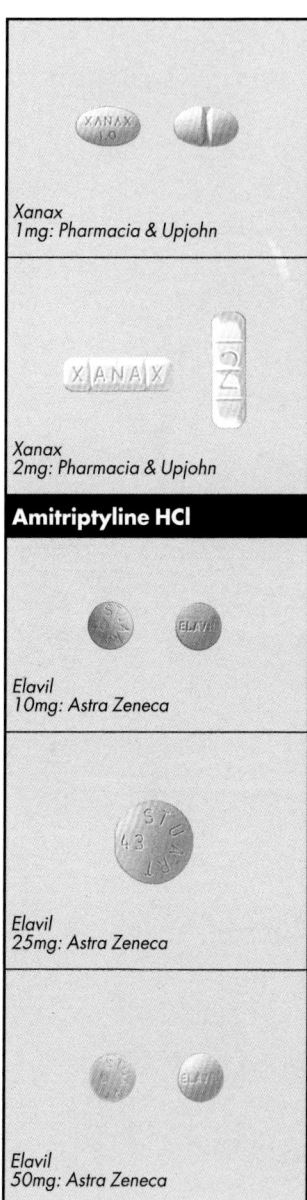

Alendronate Sodium

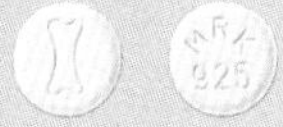

Fosamax
5mg: Merck

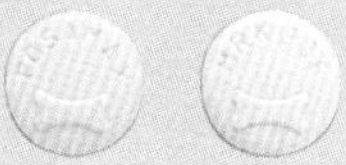

Fosamax
10mg: Merck

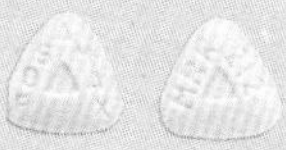

Fosamax
40mg: Merck

Alprazolam

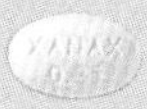

Xanax
0.25mg: Pharmacia & Upjohn

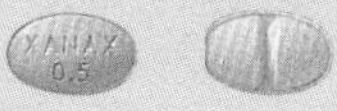

Xanax
0.5mg: Pharmacia & Upjohn

Xanax
1mg: Pharmacia & Upjohn

Xanax
2mg: Pharmacia & Upjohn

Amitriptyline HCl

Elavil
10mg: Astra Zeneca

Elavil
25mg: Astra Zeneca

Elavil
50mg: Astra Zeneca

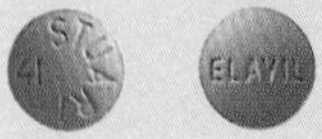

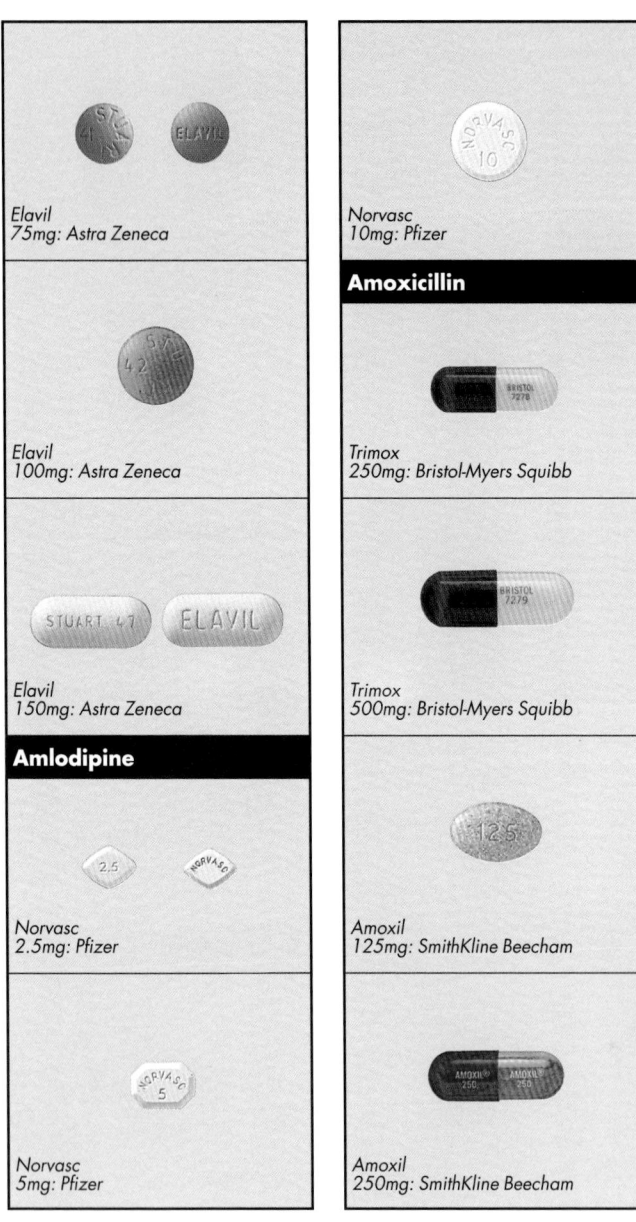

Elavil
75mg: Astra Zeneca

Elavil
100mg: Astra Zeneca

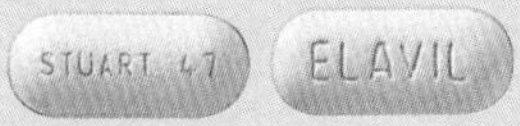

Elavil
150mg: Astra Zeneca

Amlodipine

Norvasc
2.5mg: Pfizer

Norvasc
5mg: Pfizer

Norvasc
10mg: Pfizer

Amoxicillin

Trimox
250mg: Bristol-Myers Squibb

Trimox
500mg: Bristol-Myers Squibb

Amoxil
125mg: SmithKline Beecham

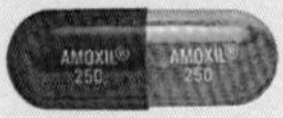

Amoxil
250mg: SmithKline Beecham

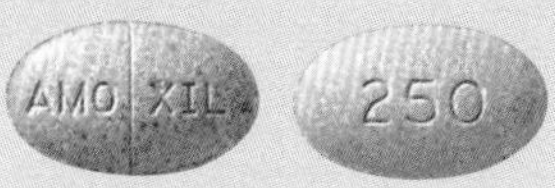

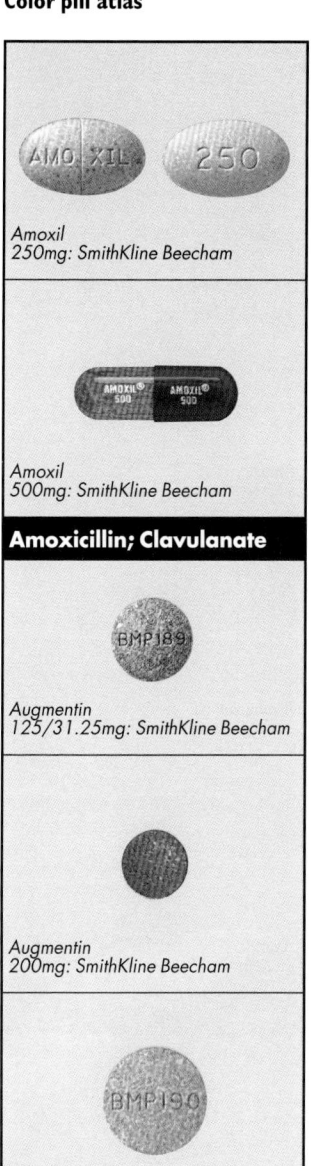

Amoxil
250mg: SmithKline Beecham

Amoxil
500mg: SmithKline Beecham

Amoxicillin; Clavulanate

Augmentin
125/31.25mg: SmithKline Beecham

Augmentin
200mg: SmithKline Beecham

Augmentin
250/62.5mg: SmithKline Beecham

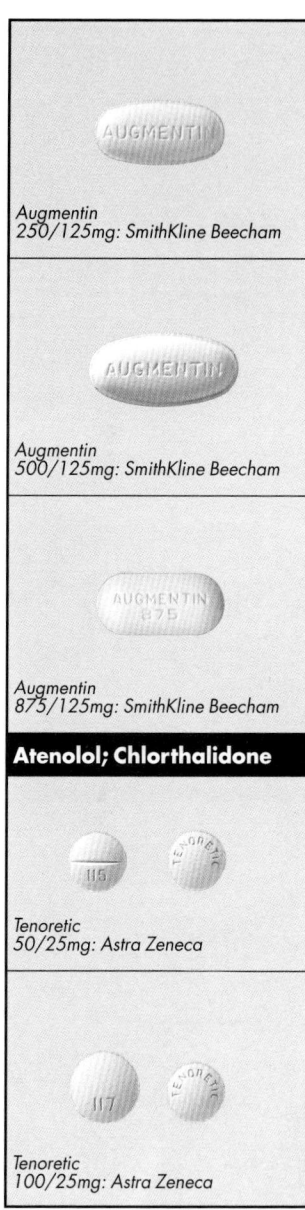

Augmentin
250/125mg: SmithKline Beecham

Augmentin
500/125mg: SmithKline Beecham

Augmentin
875/125mg: SmithKline Beecham

Atenolol; Chlorthalidone

Tenoretic
50/25mg: Astra Zeneca

Tenoretic
100/25mg: Astra Zeneca

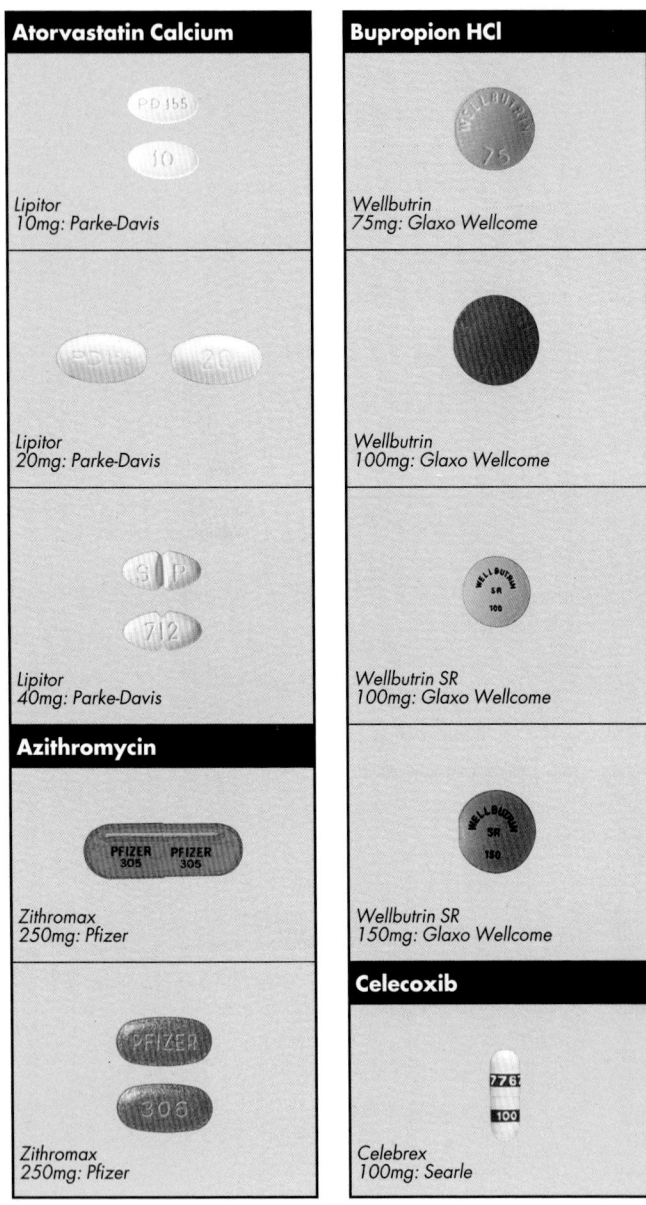

Atorvastatin Calcium

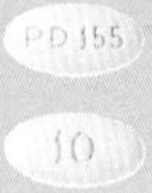

Lipitor
10mg: Parke-Davis

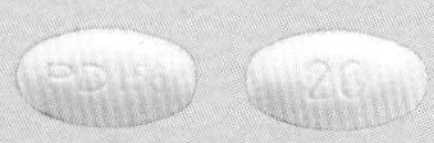

Lipitor
20mg: Parke-Davis

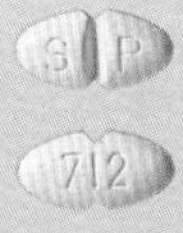

Lipitor
40mg: Parke-Davis

Azithromycin

Zithromax
250mg: Pfizer

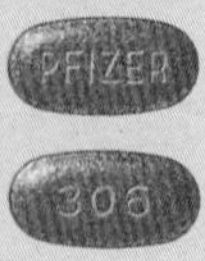

Zithromax
250mg: Pfizer

Bupropion HCl

Wellbutrin
75mg: Glaxo Wellcome

Wellbutrin
100mg: Glaxo Wellcome

Wellbutrin SR
100mg: Glaxo Wellcome

Wellbutrin SR
150mg: Glaxo Wellcome

Celecoxib

Celebrex
100mg: Searle

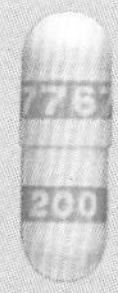

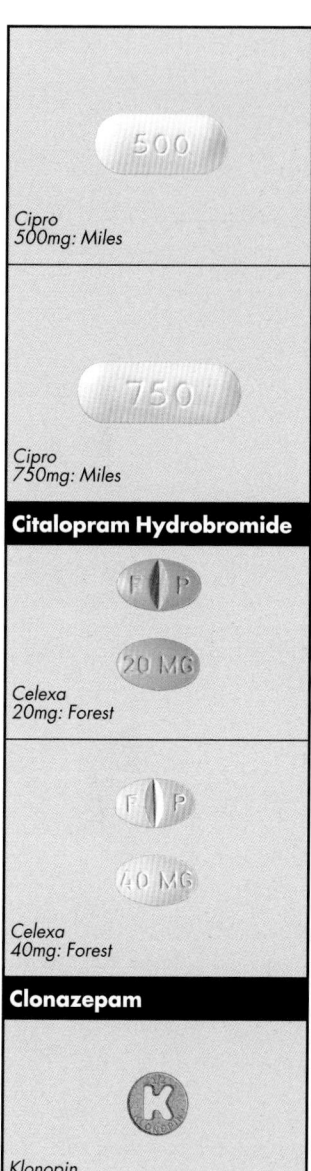

Celebrex
200mg: Searle

Cephalexin

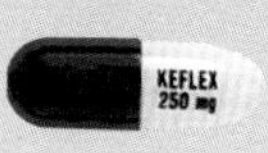

Keflex
250mg: Dista

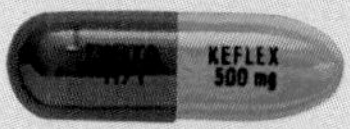

Keflex
500mg: Dista

Cetirizine

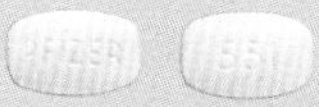

Zyrtec
10mg: Pfizer

Ciprofloxacin HCl

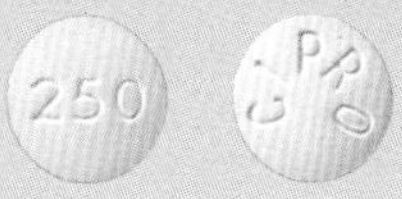

Cipro
250mg: Miles

Cipro
500mg: Miles

Cipro
750mg: Miles

Citalopram Hydrobromide

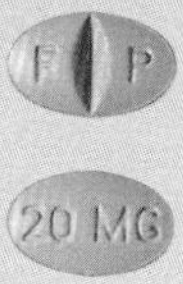

Celexa
20mg: Forest

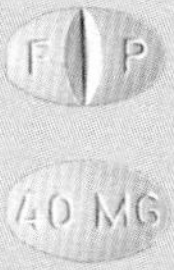

Celexa
40mg: Forest

Clonazepam

Klonopin
0.5mg: Roche

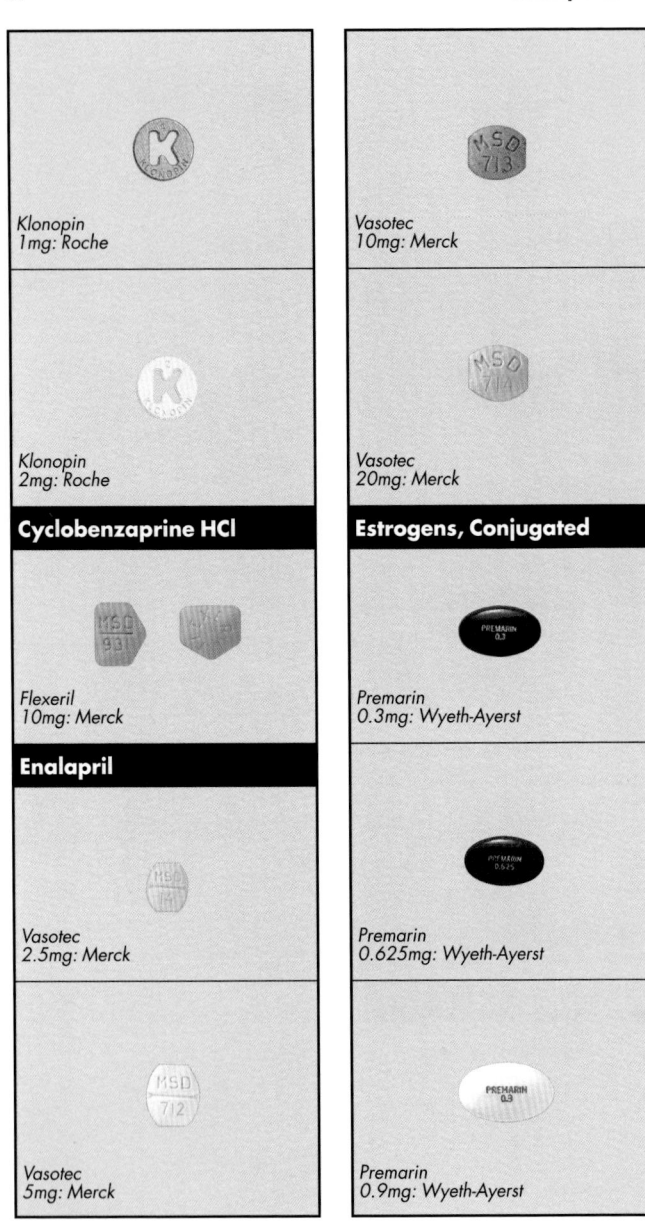

Klonopin
1mg: Roche

Klonopin
2mg: Roche

Cyclobenzaprine HCl

Flexeril
10mg: Merck

Enalapril

Vasotec
2.5mg: Merck

Vasotec
5mg: Merck

Vasotec
10mg: Merck

Vasotec
20mg: Merck

Estrogens, Conjugated

Premarin
0.3mg: Wyeth-Ayerst

Premarin
0.625mg: Wyeth-Ayerst

Premarin
0.9mg: Wyeth-Ayerst

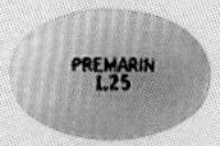

Premarin
1.25mg: Wyeth-Ayerst

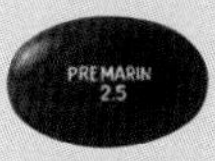

Premarin
2.5mg: Wyeth-Ayerst

Fexofenadine HCl

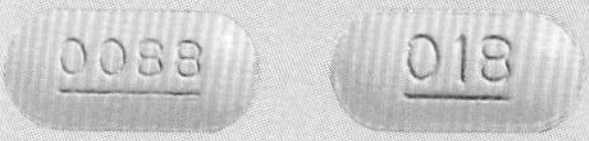

Allegra
180mg: Aventis

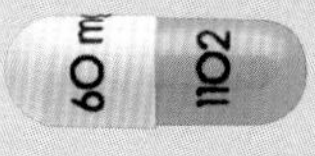

Allegra
60mg: Hoechst Marion Roussel

Fluconazole

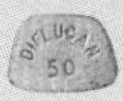

Diflucan
50mg: Roerig

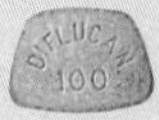

Diflucan
100mg: Roerig

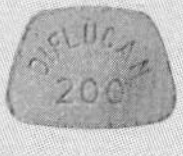

Diflucan
200mg: Roerig

Fluoxetine HCl

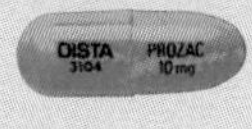

Prozac
10mg: Dista

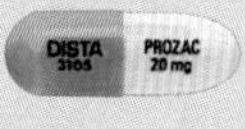

Prozac
20mg: Dista

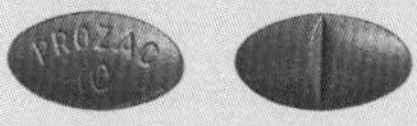

Prozac
10mg: Lilly

Furosemide

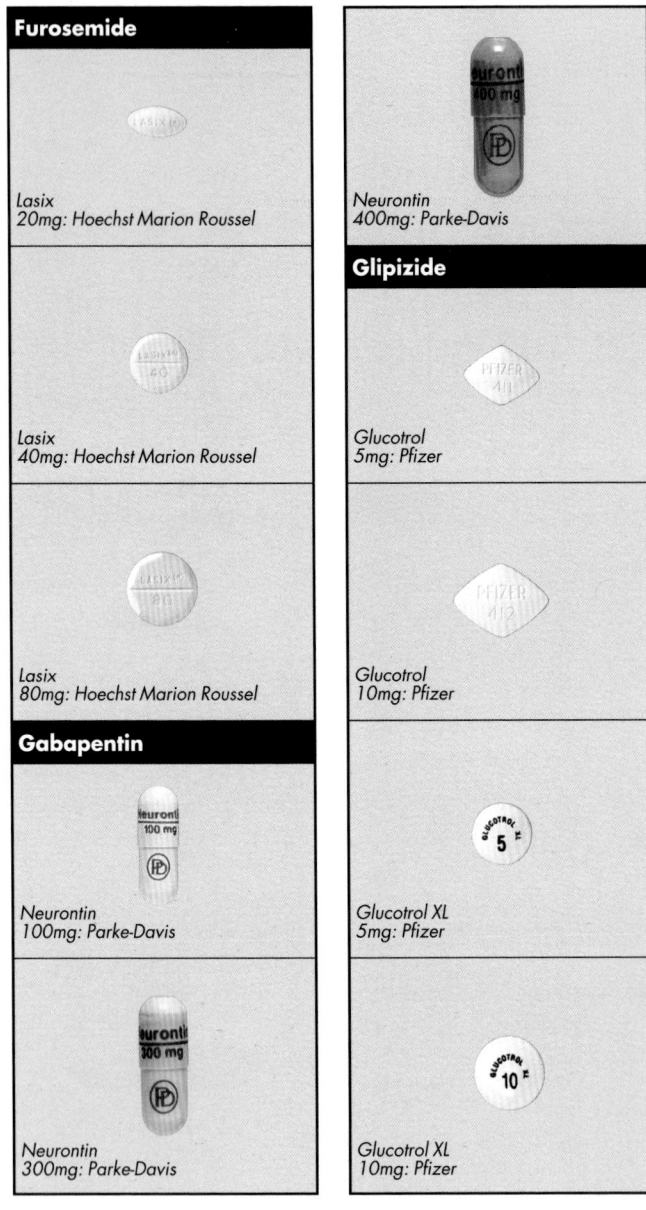

Lasix
20mg: Hoechst Marion Roussel

Lasix
40mg: Hoechst Marion Roussel

Lasix
80mg: Hoechst Marion Roussel

Gabapentin

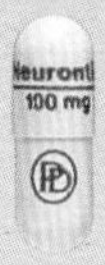

Neurontin
100mg: Parke-Davis

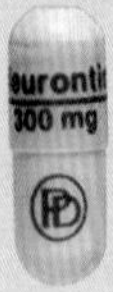

Neurontin
300mg: Parke-Davis

Neurontin
400mg: Parke-Davis

Glipizide

Glucotrol
5mg: Pfizer

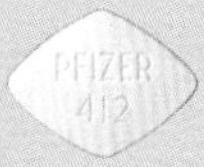

Glucotrol
10mg: Pfizer

Glucotrol XL
5mg: Pfizer

Glucotrol XL
10mg: Pfizer

Hydrochlorothiazide

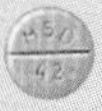

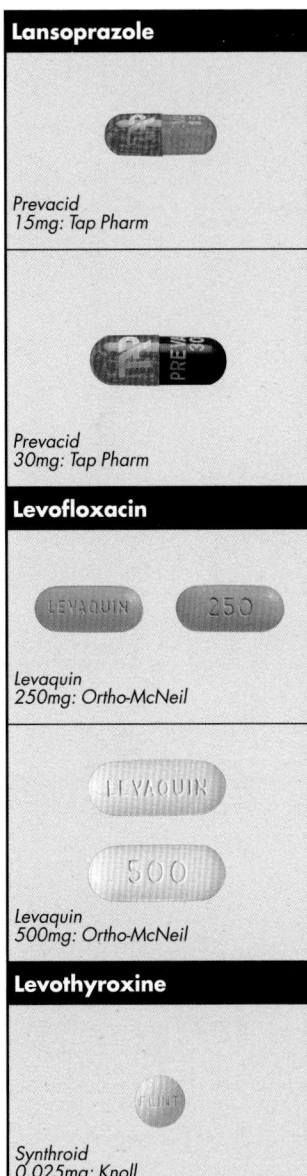

HydroDIURIL
25mg: Merck

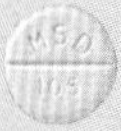

HydroDIURIL
50mg: Merck

Ibuprofen

Motrin
400mg: Pharmacia & Upjohn

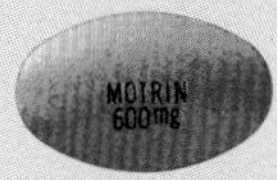

Motrin
600mg: Pharmacia & Upjohn

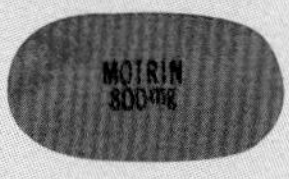

Motrin
800mg: Pharmacia & Upjohn

Lansoprazole

Prevacid
15mg: Tap Pharm

Prevacid
30mg: Tap Pharm

Levofloxacin

Levaquin
250mg: Ortho-McNeil

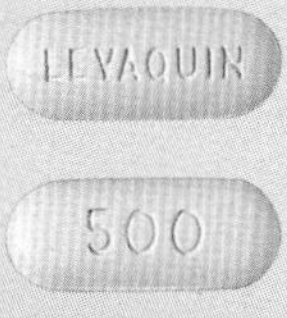

Levaquin
500mg: Ortho-McNeil

Levothyroxine

Synthroid
0.025mg: Knoll

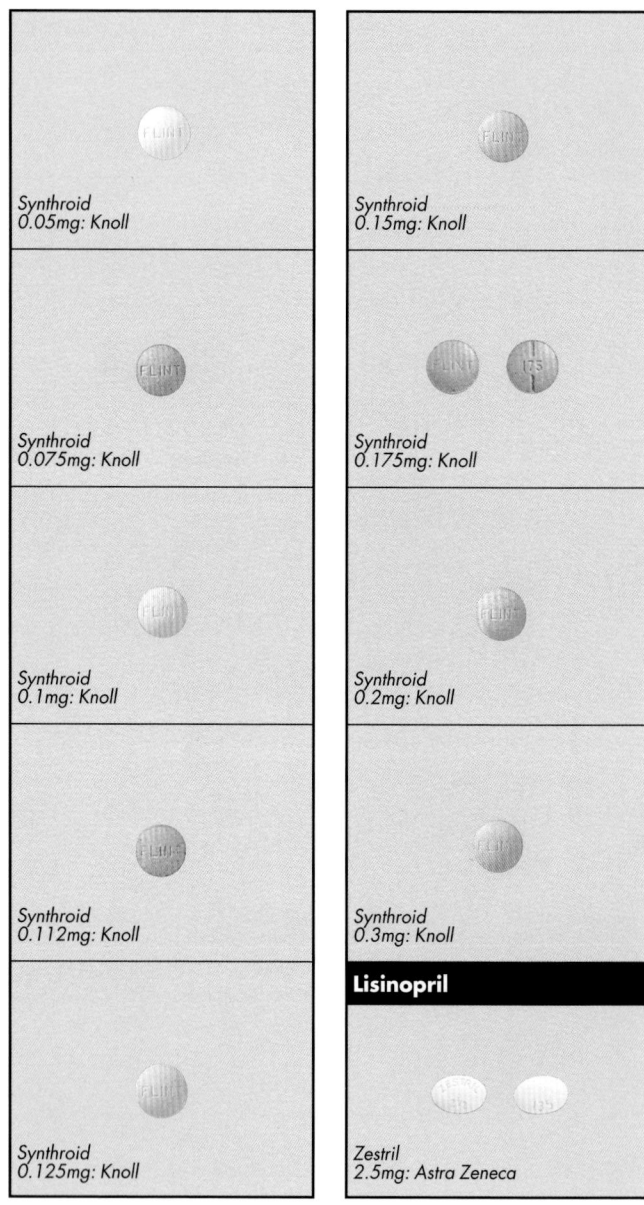

Synthroid
0.05mg: Knoll

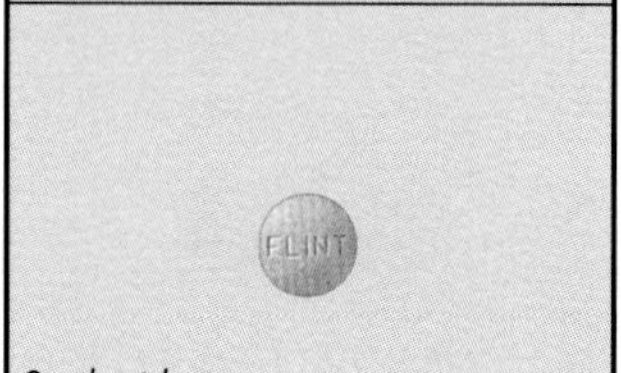

Synthroid
0.075mg: Knoll

Synthroid
0.1mg: Knoll

Synthroid
0.112mg: Knoll

Synthroid
0.125mg: Knoll

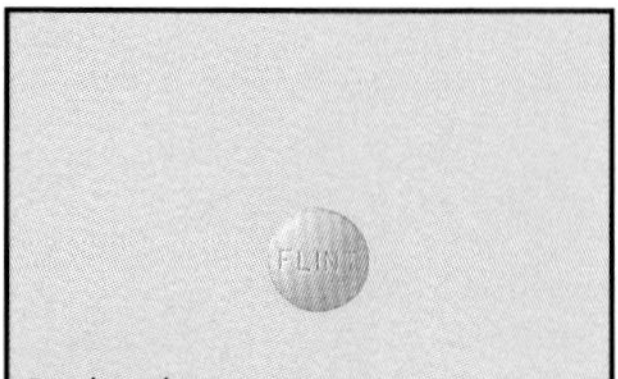

Synthroid
0.15mg: Knoll

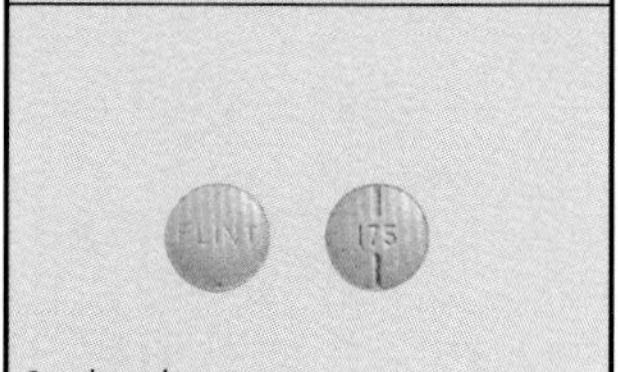

Synthroid
0.175mg: Knoll

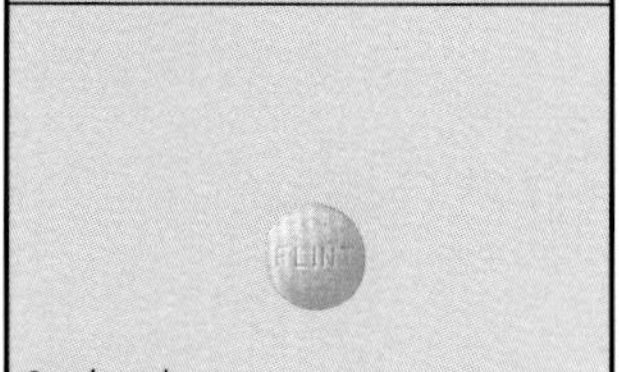

Synthroid
0.2mg: Knoll

Synthroid
0.3mg: Knoll

Lisinopril

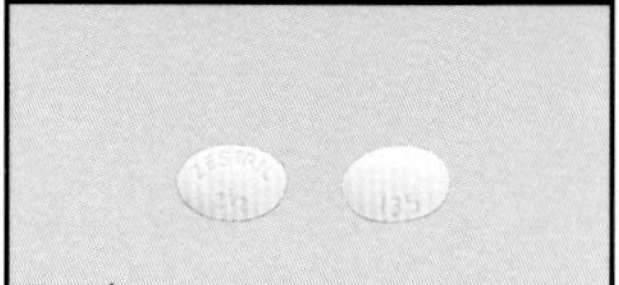

Zestril
2.5mg: Astra Zeneca

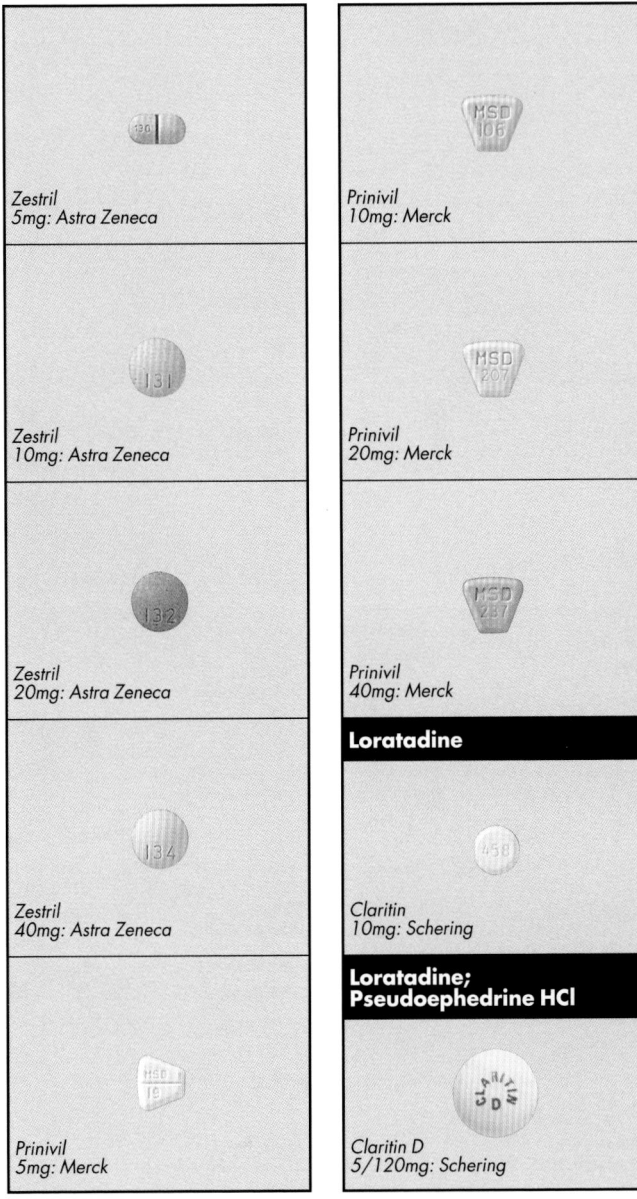

Zestril
5mg: Astra Zeneca

Zestril
10mg: Astra Zeneca

Zestril
20mg: Astra Zeneca

Zestril
40mg: Astra Zeneca

Prinivil
5mg: Merck

Prinivil
10mg: Merck

Prinivil
20mg: Merck

Prinivil
40mg: Merck

Loratadine

Claritin
10mg: Schering

Loratadine; Pseudoephedrine HCl

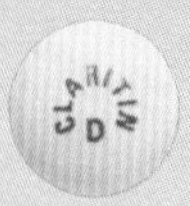

Claritin D
5/120mg: Schering

Lorazepam

Ativan
0.5mg: Wyeth-Ayerst

Ativan
1mg: Wyeth-Ayerst

Ativan
2mg: Wyeth-Ayerst

Metformin HCl

Glucophage
500mg: Lipha

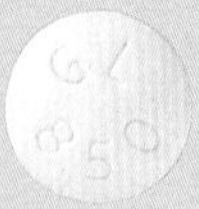

Glucophage
850mg: Lipha

Metoprolol Succinate

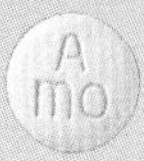

Toprol XL
50mg: Astra Zeneca

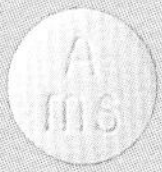

Toprol XL
100mg: Astra Zeneca

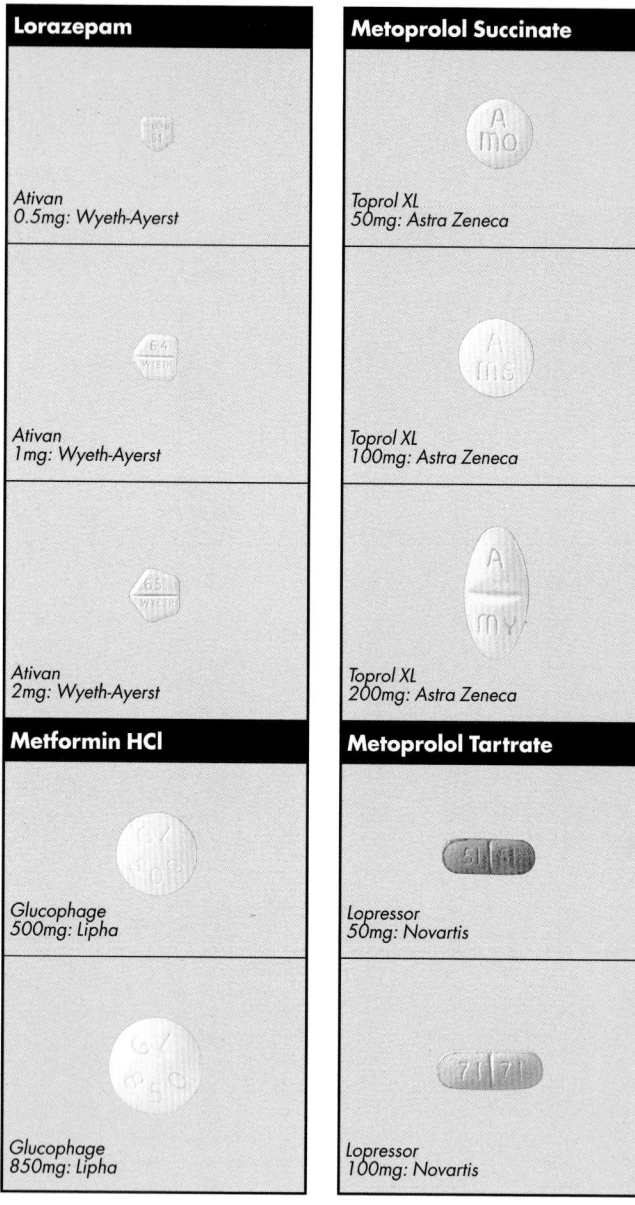

Toprol XL
200mg: Astra Zeneca

Metoprolol Tartrate

Lopressor
50mg: Novartis

Lopressor
100mg: Novartis

Montelukast Sodium

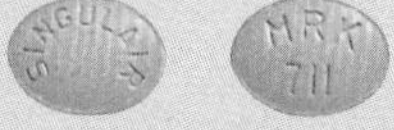

Singulair
4mg: Merck

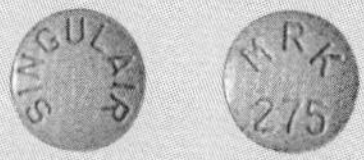

Singulair
5mg: Merck

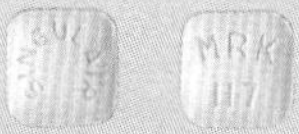

Singulair
10mg: Merck

Naproxen

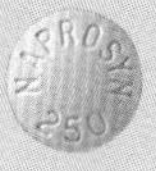

Naprosyn
250mg: Syntex

Naprosyn
375mg: Syntex

Naprosyn
500mg: Syntex

Omeprazole

Prilosec
20mg: Merck

Paroxetine HCl

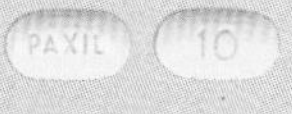

Paxil
10mg: SmithKline Beecham

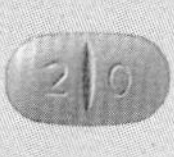

Paxil
20mg: SmithKline Beecham

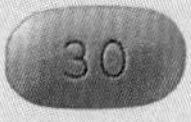

Paxil
30mg: SmithKline Beecham

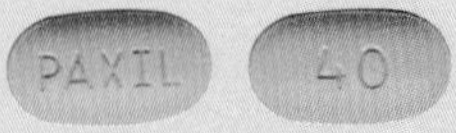

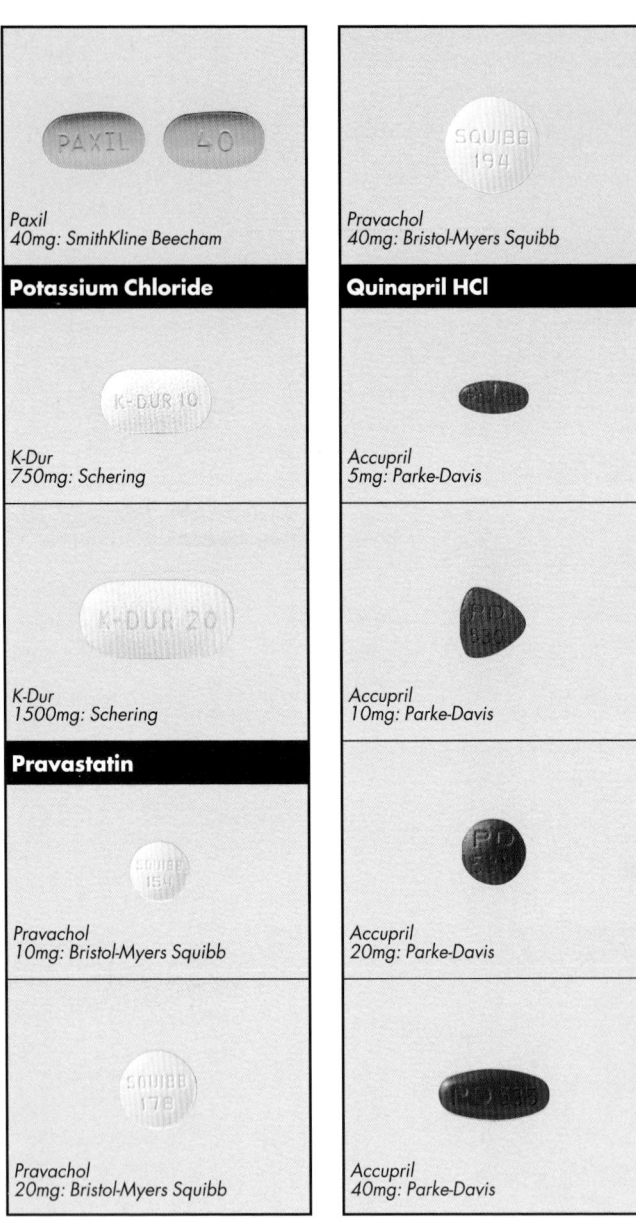

Paxil
40mg: SmithKline Beecham

Potassium Chloride

K-Dur
750mg: Schering

K-Dur
1500mg: Schering

Pravastatin

Pravachol
10mg: Bristol-Myers Squibb

Pravachol
20mg: Bristol-Myers Squibb

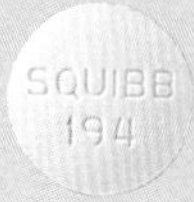

Pravachol
40mg: Bristol-Myers Squibb

Quinapril HCl

Accupril
5mg: Parke-Davis

Accupril
10mg: Parke-Davis

Accupril
20mg: Parke-Davis

Accupril
40mg: Parke-Davis

Ranitidine HCl

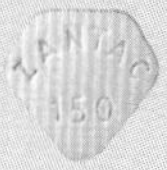

Zantac
150mg: Glaxo Wellcome

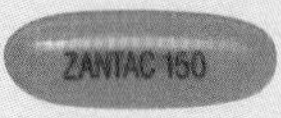

Zantac
150mg: Glaxo Wellcome

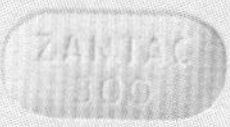

Zantac
300mg: Glaxo Wellcome

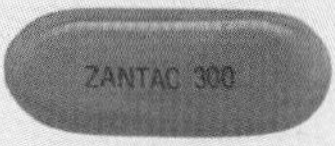

Zantac
300mg: Glaxo Wellcome

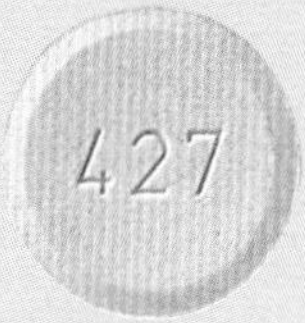

Zantac 150 Efferdose
150mg: Glaxo Wellcome

Rofecoxib

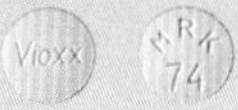

Vioxx
12.5mg: Merck

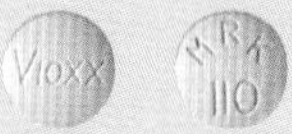

Vioxx
25mg: Merck

Sertraline HCl

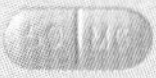

Zoloft
50mg: Roerig

Zoloft100
100mg: Roerig

Simvastatin

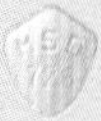

Zocor
5mg: Merck

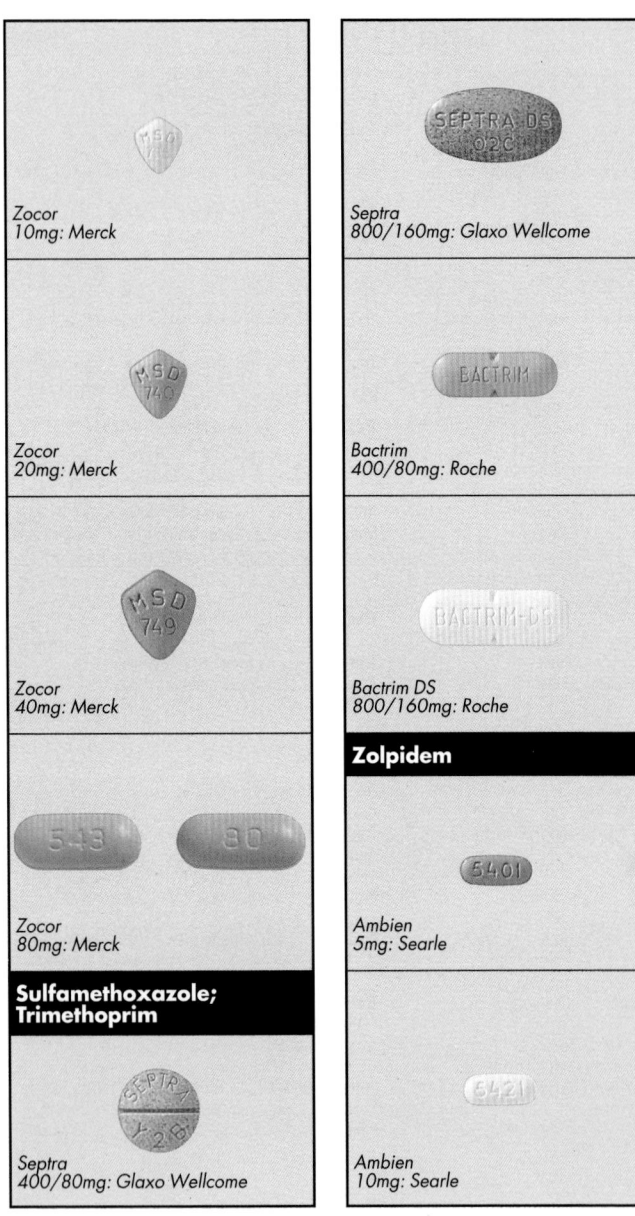

Zocor
10mg: Merck

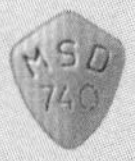

Zocor
20mg: Merck

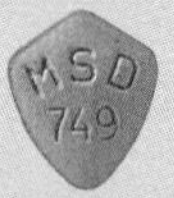

Zocor
40mg: Merck

Zocor
80mg: Merck

Sulfamethoxazole; Trimethoprim

Septra
400/80mg: Glaxo Wellcome

Septra
800/160mg: Glaxo Wellcome

Bactrim
400/80mg: Roche

Bactrim DS
800/160mg: Roche

Zolpidem

Ambien
5mg: Searle

Ambien
10mg: Searle

NEWLY APPROVED MEDICATIONS

Name	Indication
abarelix (Plenaxis)	Treatment of prostate cancer
Advate (see antihemophilic factor)	
agalsidase beta (Fabrazyme)	Enzyme for the treatment of Fabry disease
Aldurazyme (see laronidase)	
alefacept (Amevive)	Treatment of chronic plaque psoriasis
alfuzosin (UroXatral)	For symptoms of benign prostatic hyperplasia
Aloxi (see palonosetron)	
Amevive (see alefacept)	
antihemophilic factor (Advate)	For hemophilia A
aprepitant (Emend)	Treatment of nausea/vomiting associated with chemotherapy
atazanavir (Reyataz)	Treatment of HIV-1 infection
Bexxar (see tositumomab)	
Boniva (see ibandronate)	
bortezomib (Velcade)	Treatment of advanced multiple myeloma
Cialis (see tadalafil)	
Crestor (see rosuvastatin)	
Cubicin (see daptomycin)	
daptomycin (Cubicin)	Antibiotic for complicated skin infections
efalizumab (Raptiva)	Monoclonal antibody for treatment of moderate to severe psoriasis
Elestat (see epinastine)	
Emend (see aprepitant)	
emtricitabine (Emtriva)	Treatment of HIV-1 infection
Emtriva (see emtricitabine)	
enfuvirtide (Fuzeon)	Treatment of advanced HIV-1 infection
epinastine (Elestat)	An ophthalmic antihistamine for allergic conjunctivitis
Ertaczo (see sertaconazole)	
Fabrazyme (see agalsidase beta)	
Factive (see gemifloxacin)	
fosamprenavir (Lexiva)	Treatment of HIV-1 infection
Fuzeon (see enfuvirtide)	
gefitnib (Iressa)	Treatment of advanced non–small cell lung cancer
gemifloxacin (Factive)	Antibiotic for treatment of acute exacerbation of bronchitis and community acquired pneumonia
ibandronate (Boniva)	Prevention and treatment of osteoporosis
Iressa (see gefitnib)	
laronidase (Aldurazyme)	Treatment of the genetic disease MPS-1
Levitra (see vardenafil)	
Lexiva (see fosamprenavir)	
memantine (Namenda)	Treatment of moderate to severe Alzheimer's disease
miglustat (Zavesca)	Treatment of Gaucher disease
Namenda (see memantine)	
omalizumab (Xolair)	Monoclonal antibody for treatment of moderate to severe allergy related asthma

Continued

Name	Indication
palonosetron (Aloxi)	Treatment of nausea/vomiting associated with chemotherapy
pegnisomant (Somavert)	Treatment of acromegaly
Plenaxis (see abarelix)	
Raptiva (see efalizumab)	
Reyataz (see atazanavir)	
rosuvastatin (Crestor)	An HMG-CoA reductase inhibitor (statin) for the treatment of high cholesterol
sertaconazole (Ertaczo)	Antifungal for treatment of athlete's foot
Somavert (see pegvisomant)	
tadalafil (Cialis)	Treatment of erectile dysfunction
tositumomab (Bexxar)	Monoclonal antibody for refractory non-Hodgkin's lymphoma
UroXatral (see alfuzosin)	
vardenafil (Levitra)	Treatment of erectile dysfunction
Velcade (see bortezomib)	
Xolair (see omalizumab)	
Zavesca (see miglustat)	

Please note: While this book was going to press, the FDA ruled to prohibit the sale of dietary supplements containing **ephedra.** The FDA determined that ephedra presents an unreasonable risk of illness or injury and has been linked to significant adverse health effects, including heart attack and stroke.

DISORDERS INDEX

Generic names appear first, followed by brand names in parentheses.

Drug Classification Contents

Anesthetics: General

USES

IV anesthetic agents are used to induce general anesthesia. The general anesthetic state consists of unconsciousness, amnesia, analgesia, immobility, and attenuation of autonomic responses to noxious stimuli.

Volatile inhalation agents produce all the components of the anesthetic state but are administered through the lungs via an anesthesia machine. Agents for use include desflurane, sevoflurane, isoflurane, enflurane, and halothane. They are used in practice to maintain general anesthesia.

ACTION

IV anesthetic agents: Most agents produce CNS depression by action on the GABA receptor complex. GABA is the primary inhibitory neurotransmitter in the CNS. Ketamine produces dissociation between the thalamus and the limbic system.

Volatile inhalation agents: Not fully understood but may disrupt neuronal transmission throughout the CNS. These agents may either block excitatory or enhance inhibitory transmission through axons or synapses.

ANESTHETICS: GENERAL

Name	Availability	Uses	Dosage Range	Side Effects
Etomidate (Amidate)	**I:** 2 mg/ml	IV induction	0.2–0.6 mg/kg	Myoclonus, pain on injection, nausea, vomiting, respiratory depression
Ketamine (p. 602) (Ketalar)	**I:** 10 mg/ml, 50 mg/ml, 100 mg/ml	Analgesia, sedation, IV induction	1–4.5 mg/kg	Delirium, euphoria, nausea, vomiting
Methohexital (p. 688) (Brevital)	**Powder for injection:** 500 mg	IV induction, sedation	50–120 mg	Cardiovascular depression, myoclonus, nausea, vomiting, respiratory depression

Midazolam (p. 709) (Versed)	**I:** 1 mg/ml, 5 mg/ml	Anxiolytic, amnesic, sedation	1–5 mg titrated slowly	Respiratory depression
Propofol (p. 897) (Diprivan)	**I:** 10 mg/ml	Sedation IV induction Maintenance	0.5 mg/kg 2–2.5 mg/kg 100–200 mcg/kg/min	Cardiovascular depression, delirium, euphoria, pain on injection, respiratory depression
Thiopental (p. 1028) (Pentothal)	**Powder for injection:** 2.5% (25 mg/ml)	IV induction	Titrate vs. pt response. **Average:** 50–75 mg	Cardiovascular depression, nausea, vomiting, respiratory depression

I, Injection.

Anesthetics: Local

USES

Local/regional anesthesia is selective for the surgical site. Epidural, spinal (intrathecal), IV regional, peripheral nerve block, topical or local infiltration can be selected. Local anesthetics prevent the initiation of electrical impulses necessary for spinal and peripheral nerve conduction.

ACTION

Most local anesthetics fall into one of two groups: esters or amides. Both provide anesthesia and analgesia by reversibly binding to and blocking sodium (Na) channels. This slows the rate of depolarization of the nerve action potential, and propagation of the electrical impulses needed for nerve conduction is prevented.

Anesthetics: Local *(continued)*

ANESTHETICS: LOCAL

Name	Uses	Maximum Recommended Dosage (mg)	Onset/Duration	Side Effects (Most side effects are due to excessive plasma concentrations of the local anesthetic)
Esters				
Chloroprocaine (p. 215) (Nesacaine)	Local infiltrate Nerve block Spinal	600–800	Fast/Short	Excitation (e.g., convulsions) followed by depression (drowsiness to unconsciousness), bradycardia, heart block, decreased contractile force, hypotension, hypersensitivity reaction
Procaine (p. 889) (Novocain)	Local infiltrate Nerve block Spinal	400–500	Fast/Short	Same as above
Tetracaine (p. 1024) (Pontocaine)	Topical Spinal	100 (topical)	Slow/Long	Same as above
Amides				
Bupivacaine (p. 143) (Marcaine, Sensorcaine)	Local infiltrate Nerve block Epidural Spinal	175	Moderate/Long	Same as above
Etidocaine (Duranest)	Local infiltrate Nerve block Epidural	300	Fast/Long	Same as above

Levobupivacaine (p. 629) (Chirocaine)	Nerve block Epidural	—	Moderate/Long	Same as above
Lidocaine (p. 634)	Local infiltrate Nerve block Spinal Epidural Topical IV regional	300	Fast/Moderate	Same as above
Mepivacaine (p. 675) (Carbocaine, Polocaine)	Local infiltrate Nerve block Epidural	300	Moderate/ Moderate	Same as above
Ropivacaine (Naropin)	Local infiltrate Nerve block Epidural Spinal	200	Moderate/Long	Same as above

Alert: Most side effects are manifestations of excessive plasma concentrations.
Duration: *short,* <1 hr; *moderate,* 1–3 hrs; *long,* 3–12 hrs.

Angiotensin-converting enzyme (ACE) inhibitors

USES	ACTION
Treatment of hypertension (HTN), adjunctive therapy for congestive heart failure (CHF).	ACE inhibitors act primarily through suppression of the renin-angiotensin-aldosterone system. Produce a reduction in peripheral arterial resistance, an increase in cardiac output, and little or no change in heart rate.

Angiotensin-converting enzyme (ACE) inhibitors *(continued)*

ACE INHIBITORS

Name	Availability	Uses	Dosage Range (per day)	Side Effects
Benazepril (p. 112) (Lotensin)	**T:** 5 mg, 10 mg, 20 mg, 40 mg	HTN	**HTN:** 5–80 mg	Headaches, dizziness, fatigue, cough
Captopril (p. 162) (Capoten)	**T:** 12.5 mg, 25 mg, 50 mg, 100 mg	HTN CHF	**HTN:** 50–450 mg **CHF:** 12.5–450 mg	Insomnia, headaches, dizziness, fatigue, GI complaints, cough, rash
Enalapril (p. 371) (Vasotec)	**T:** 2.5 mg, 5 mg, 10 mg, 20 mg **IV:** 1.25 mg/ml	HTN CHF	**HTN:** 10–40 mg; (**IV:** 1.25 mg q6h) **CHF:** 5–20 mg	Chest pain, hypotension, headaches, fatigue, dizziness
Fosinopril (p. 472) (Monopril)	**T:** 10 mg, 20 mg, 40 mg	HTN CHF	**HTN:** 10–80 mg **CHF:** 20–40 mg	Hypotension, nausea, vomiting, cough
Lisinopril (p. 640) (Prinivil, Zestril)	**T:** 2.5 mg, 5 mg, 10 mg, 20 mg, 40 mg	HTN CHF	**HTN:** 10–40 mg **CHF:** 5–20 mg	Chest pain, hypotension, headaches, dizziness, fatigue, diarrhea
Moexipril (p. 727) (Univasc)	**T:** 7.5 mg, 15 mg	HTN	**HTN:** 7.5–30 mg	Dizziness, fatigue, diarrhea, cough
Perindopril (p. 847) (Aceon)	**T:** 2 mg, 4 mg, 6 mg	HTN	**HTN:** 4–16 mg	Hypotension, dizziness, fatigue, syncope, cough
Quinapril (p. 914) (Accupril)	**T:** 5 mg, 10 mg, 20 mg, 40 mg	HTN CHF	**HTN:** 10–80 mg **CHF:** 10–40 mg	Chest pain, hypotension, headaches, dizziness, fatigue, diarrhea, nausea, vomiting, cough
Ramipril (p. 923) (Altace)	**C:** 1.25 mg, 2.5 mg, 5 mg, 10 mg	HTN CHF	**HTN:** 2.5–20 mg **CHF:** 1.25–10 mg	Hypotension, headaches, dizziness, cough
Trandolapril (p. 1063) (Mavik)	**T:** 1 mg, 2 mg, 4 mg	HTN CHF	**HTN:** 1–4 mg **CHF:** 1–4 mg	Dizziness, dyspepsia, cough, asthenia, syncope, myalgia

C, Capsules; ***CHF,*** congestive heart failure; ***HTN,*** hypertension; ***IV,*** intravenous; ***T,*** tablets.

Angiotensin II Receptor Antagonists

USES

Treatment of hypertension (HTN) alone or in combination with other antihypertensives.

ACTION

Angiotensin II receptor antagonists (AIIRA) block vasoconstrictor and aldosterone-secreting effects on angiotensin II by selectively blocking the binding of angiotensin II to AT_1 receptors in vascular smooth muscle and adrenal gland, causing vasodilation and a decrease in aldosterone effects.

ANGIOTENSIN II RECEPTOR ANTAGONISTS

Name	Availability	Uses	Dosage Range (per day)	Side Effects
Candesartan (p. 158) (Atacand)	**T:** 4 mg, 8 mg, 16 mg, 32 mg	HTN	2–32 mg	Headaches, upper respiratory tract infections, pain, dizziness
Eprosartan (p. 388) (Teveten)	**T:** 400 mg, 600 mg	HTN	400–800 mg	Headaches, upper respiratory tract infections, myalgia
Irbesartan (p. 586) (Avapro)	**T:** 75 mg, 150 mg, 300 mg	HTN	75–300 mg	Headaches, upper respiratory tract infections
Losartan (p. 654) (Cozaar)	**T:** 25 mg, 50 mg, 100 mg	HTN	25–100 mg	Dizziness, headaches, upper respiratory tract infections, diarrhea, fatigue, cough
Olmesartan (p. 796) (Benicar)	**T:** 5 mg, 20 mg, 40 mg	HTN	20–40 mg	Headache, upper respiratory tract infection, flulike symptoms, dizziness, bronchitis, rhinitis, back pain, pharyngitis, sinusitis, diarrhea, peripheral edema
Telmisartan (p. 1010) (Micardis)	**T:** 40 mg, 80 mg	HTN	20–80 mg	Upper respiratory tract infections, dizziness, back pain, sinusitis, diarrhea
Valsartan (p. 1095) (Diovan)	**T:** 80 mg, 160 mg	HTN	80–320 mg	Dizziness, headaches, upper respiratory tract infections, diarrhea, fatigue

HTN, Hypertension; ***T,*** tablets.

Antacids

USES

Relief of symptoms associated with hyperacidity (e.g., heartburn, acid indigestion, sour stomach), hyperacidity associated with gastric/duodenal ulcers, treatment of pathologic gastric hypersecretion associated with Zollinger-Ellison syndrome, symptomatic treatment of gastroesophageal reflux disease (GERD), prevention and treatment of upper GI stress-induced ulceration and bleeding (especially in ICU).

Aluminum carbonate and hydroxide in conjunction with a low-phosphate diet to reduce elevated phosphate in pts with renal insufficiency. Calcium for calcium deficiency, magnesium for magnesium deficiency.

ACTION

Act primarily in the stomach to neutralize gastric acid (increase pH). Antacids do not have a direct effect on acid output. The ability to increase pH depends on the dose, dosage form used, presence or absence of food in the stomach, and acid-neutralizing capacity (ANC). ANC is the number of mEq of hydrochloric acid that can be neutralized by a particular weight or volume of antacid.

Reduce elevated phosphate by binding with phosphate in the intestine to form an insoluble complex, which is then eliminated.

ANTACIDS

Antacid	Brand Names	Availability	Dosage Range	Side Effects
Aluminum				
Hydroxide (p. 41)	Amphojel, Alu-Tab, Dialume	**T:** 300 mg, 500 mg, 600 mg **C:** 500 mg	500–1,500 mg 3–6 times/day	Chalky taste, mild constipation, stomach cramps *Long-term use:* Neurotoxicity in dialysis pts, hypercalcemia, osteoporosis *Large doses:* Fecal impaction, swelling of feet/legs

Calcium				
Carbonate (p. 154)	Tums, Maalox, Antacid	**T (chewable):** 500 mg, 750 mg, 1,000 mg	500–1,500 mg as needed	Chalky taste *Large doses:* Fecal impaction, swelling of feet/legs, metabolic alkalosis *Long-term use:* Difficult/painful urination
Magnesium				
Hydroxide (p. 659)	Milk of Magnesia	**T (chewable):** 311 mg **L:** 400 mg/5 ml, 800 mg/5 ml	**T:** 622–1,244 mg up to 4 times/day **L:** 2.5–7.5 ml up to 4 times/day	Chalky taste, diarrhea, laxative effect, electrolyte imbalance (dizziness, irregular heartbeat, fatigue)
Oxide (p. 659)	Mag-Ox 400, Maox 420	**T:** 400, 420, 500 mg	400–800 mg/day	Same as above

C, Capsules; ***L,*** liquid; ***S,*** suspension; ***T,*** tablets.

Antianxiety

USES

Treatment of anxiety. In addition, some benzodiazepines are used as hypnotics, anticonvulsants to prevent delirium tremors during alcohol withdrawal and as adjunctive therapy for relaxation of skeletal muscle spasms. Midazolam, a short-acting benzodiazepine, is used for preoperative sedation and relief of anxiety for short diagnostic endoscopic procedures (see individual monograph for midazolam).

Antianxiety *(continued)*

ACTION

Benzodiazepines are the largest and most frequently prescribed group of antianxiety agents. The exact mechanism is unknown but may increase the inhibiting effect of gamma-aminobutyric acid (GABA), which inhibits nerve impulse transmission by binding to specific benzodiazepine receptors in various areas of the central nervous system (CNS).

ANTIANXIETY AGENTS

Name	Availability	Uses	Dosage Range (per day)	Side Effects
Benzodiazepine				
Alprazolam (p. 35) (Xanax)	**T:** 0.25 mg, 0.5 mg, 1 mg, 2 mg **S:** 0.5 mg/5 ml, 1 mg/ml	Anxiety, panic disorder	0.75–10 mg	Drowsiness, weakness or fatigue, ataxia, slurred speech, confusion, lack of coordination, impaired memory, paradoxical agitation, dizziness, nausea
Chlordiazepoxide (p. 214) (Librium, Libritabs)	**C:** 5 mg, 10 mg, 25 mg **T:** 10 mg, 25 mg **I:** 100 mg	Anxiety, alcohol withdrawal	5–300 mg	Same as above
Clorazepate (p. 248) (Tranxene)	**C:** 3.75 mg, 7.5 mg, 15 mg **SD:** 11.25 mg, 22.5 mg	Anxiety, alcohol withdrawal, anticonvulsant	7.5–90 mg	Same as above
Diazepam (p. 314) (Valium)	**T:** 2.5 mg, 5 mg, 10 mg **S:** 5 mg/5 ml, 5 mg/ml **I:** 5 mg/ml	Anxiety, alcohol withdrawal, anticonvulsant, muscle relaxant	2–40 mg	Same as above

Lorazepam (p. 652) (Ativan)	**T**: 0.5 mg, 1 mg, 2 mg **S**: 2 mg/ml **I**: 2 mg/ml, 4 mg/ml	Anxiety	0.5–10 mg	Same as above
Oxazepam (p. 810) (Serax)	**C**: 10 mg, 15 mg, 30 mg **T**: 15 mg	Anxiety, alcohol withdrawal	30–120 mg	Same as above
Nonbenzodiazepine				
Buspirone (p. 145) (BuSpar)	**T**: 5 mg, 10 mg, 15 mg, 30 mg	Anxiety	7.5–60 mg	Dizziness, lightheadedness, headache, nausea, restlessness
Hydroxyzine (p. 541) (Atarax, Vistaril)	**T**: 10 mg, 25 mg, 50 mg, 100 mg	Anxiety, rhinitis, pruritus, urticaria, nausea or vomiting	100–400 mg	Drowsiness; dry mouth, nose, and throat
Paroxetine (p. 826) (Paxil)	**S**: 10 mg/5ml **T**: 10 mg, 20 mg, 30 mg, 40 mg **T(CR)**: 12.5 mg, 25 mg, 37.5 mg	Anxiety, depression, obsessive-compulsive disorder, panic disorder	10–50 mg	Drowsiness; dry mouth, nose, and throat; dizziness; diarrhea; increased sweating; constipation; vomiting; tremors
Trazodone (p. 1068) (Desyrel)	T: 50 mg, 100 mg, 150 mg, 300 mg	Anxiety, depression	100–400 mg	Drowsiness, dizziness, headache, dry mouth, nausea, vomiting, unpleasant taste
Venlafaxine (p. 1102) (Effexor)	**C**: 37.5 mg, 75 mg, 150 mg	Anxiety, depression	37.5–225 mg	Drowsiness, nausea, headache, dry mouth

C, Capsules; ***CR,*** controlled-release; ***I,*** injection; ***S,*** solution; ***SD,*** single dose; ***T,*** tablets.

Antiarrhythmics

USES

Prevention and treatment of cardiac arrhythmias, such as premature ventricular contractions, ventricular tachycardia, premature atrial contractions, paroxysmal atrial tachycardia, atrial fibrillation and flutter.

ACTION

The antiarrhythmics are divided into four classes based on their effects on certain ion channels and/or receptors located on the myocardial cell membrane. Class I is further divided into three subclasses (IA, IB, IC) based on electrophysiologic effects.

Class I: Block cardiac sodium channels and slow conduction velocity, prolonging refractoriness and decreasing automaticity of sodium-dependent tissue.

Class IA: Block sodium and potassium channels.

Class IB: Shorten the repolarization phase.

Class IC: No effect on repolarization phase, but slow conduction velocity.

Class II: Slow the sinus and atrioventricular (AV) nodal conduction.

Class III: Block cardiac potassium channels, prolonging the repolarization phase of electrical cells.

Class IV: Inhibit the influx calcium through its channels, causing slower conduction through the sinus and AV nodes

ANTIARRHYTHMICS

Name	Availability	Uses	Dosage Range	Side Effects
Class IA				
Disopyramide (p. 338) (Norpace SR, Norpace CR)	**C:** 100 mg, 150 mg **C(ER):** 100 mg, 150 mg	AF, WPW, PSVT, PVCs, VT	400–800 mg/day	Dry mouth, blurred vision, urinary retention, CHF, proarrhythmia

Procainamide (p. 887) (Pronestyl, Pronestyl SR, Procan-SR)	**T:** 250 mg, 375 mg, 500 mg **C:** 250 mg, 375 mg, 500 mg **T (SR):** 250 mg, 500 mg, 750 mg, 1,000 mg **I:** 100 mg/ml, 500 mg/ml	AF, WPW, PVCs, VT	**A (PO):** 250–500 mg q3h; **(ER):** 250–750 mg q6h	Hypotension, fever, agranulocytosis, SLE, headaches, proarrhythmia
Quinidine (p. 916) (Quinidex, Quinaglute)	**T:** 200 mg, 300 mg **T (ER):** 300 mg, 324 mg **I:** 80 mg/ml	AF, WPW, PVCs, VT	**A:** 200–600 mg q2–4h; **(ER):** 300–600 mg q8h	Diarrhea, hypotension, nausea, vomiting, cinchonism, fever, thrombocytopenia, proarrhythmia

Class IB

Lidocaine (p. 634) (Xylocaine)	**I:** 300 mg for IM **IV Infusion:** 2 mg/ml, 4 mg/ml	PVCs, VT, VF	**IV:** 50–100 mg bolus, then 1–4 mg/min infusion	Drowsiness, agitation, muscle twitching, seizures, paresthesias, proarrhythmia
Mexiletine (p. 707) (Mexitil)	**C:** 150 mg, 200 mg, 250 mg	PVCs, VT, VF	**A:** 600–1,200 mg/day	Drowsiness, agitation, muscle twitching, seizures, paresthesias, proarrhythmia, nausea, vomiting
Tocainide (p. 1047) (Tonocard)	**T:** 400 mg, 600 mg	PVCs, VT, VF	**A:** 1,200–1,800 mg/day	Drowsiness, agitation, muscle twitching, seizures, paresthesias, proarrhythmia, nausea, vomiting, diarrhea, agranulocytosis

(continued)

ANTIARRHYTHMICS ***(continued)***

Name	Availability	Uses	Dosage Range	Side Effects
Class IC				
Flecainide (p. 439) (Tambocor)	**T:** 50 mg, 100 mg, 150 mg	AF, PSVT, life-threatening ventricular arrhythmias	**A:** 200–400 mg/day	Dizziness, tremors, lightheadedness, flushing, blurred vision, metallic taste, proarrhythmia
Moricizine (p. 731) (Ethmozine)	**T:** 200 mg, 250 mg, 300 mg	Life-threatening ventricular arrhythmias	**A:** 600–900 mg/day	Nausea, dizziness, perioral numbness, euphoria
Propafenone (p. 896) (Rythmol)	**T:** 150 mg, 225 mg, 300 mg	PAF, WPW, life-threatening ventricular arrhythmias	**A:** 450–900 mg/day	Dizziness, blurred vision, taste disturbances, nausea, asthma worsening, proarrhythmia
Class II (Beta-Blockers)				
Acebutolol (p. 5) (Sectral)	**C:** 200 mg, 400 mg	AF, A flutter, PSVT, PVCs	**A:** 600–1,200 mg/day	Bradycardia, hypotension, depression, nightmares, fatigue, sexual dysfunction
Esmolol (p. 399) (Brevibloc)	**I:** 10 mg/ml, 250 mg/ml	AF, A flutter, PSVT, PVCs	**A:** 50–200 mcg/kg/min	Hypotension
Propranolol (p. 901) (Inderal)	**T:** 10 mg, 20 mg	AF, A flutter, PSVT, PVCs	**A:** 10–30 mg 3–4 times day	Bradycardia, hypotension, depression, nightmares, fatigue, sexual dysfunction

Class III				
Amiodarone (p. 53) (Cordarone, Pacerone)	**T:** 200 mg, 400 mg **I:** 50 mg/ml	AF, PAF, PSVT, life-threatening ventricular arrhythmias	**A (PO):** 800–1,600 mg/day for 1–3 wks, then 600–800 mg/day **(IV):** 150 mg bolus, then IV infusion	Blurred vision, photophobia, constipation, ataxia, proarrhythmia
Dofetilide (p. 346) (Tikosyn)	**C:** 125 mcg, 250 mcg, 500 mcg	AF, A flutter	**A:** Individualized	Torsades de pointes, hypotension
Ibutilide (p. 550) (Corvert)	**I:** 0.1 mg/ml	AF, A flutter	**A (>60 kg):** 1 mg over 10 min **(<60 kg):** 0.01 mg/kg over 10 min	Torsades de pointes
Sotalol (p. 983) (Betapace)	**T:** 80 mg, 120 mg, 160 mg, 240 mg	AF, PAF, PSVT, life-threatening ventricular arrhythmias	**A:** 160–640 mg/day	Fatigue, dizziness, dyspnea, bradycardia, proarrhythmia
Class IV (Calcium Channel Blockers)				
Diltiazem (p. 328) (Cardizem)	**I:** 25 mg/ml vials, **Infusion:** 1 mg/ml	AF, A flutter, PSVT	**A (IV):** 20–25 mg bolus, then infusion of 5–15 mg/hr	Hypotension, bradycardia, dizziness, headache
Verapamil (p. 1104) (Isoptin)	**I:** 5 mg/2 ml	AF, A flutter, PSVT	**A (IV):** 5–10 mg	Hypotension, bradycardia, dizziness, headaches, constipation

A, Adults; ***AF,*** atrial fibrillation; ***A flutter,*** atrial flutter; ***C,*** capsules; ***CR,*** controlled-release; ***ER,*** extended-release; ***I,*** injection; ***PAF,*** paroxysmal atrial fibrillation; ***PSVT,*** paroxysmal supraventricular tachycardia; ***PVCs,*** premature ventricular contractions; ***SLE,*** systemic lupus erythematosus; ***SR,*** sustained-release; ***T,*** tablets; ***VF,*** ventricular fibrillation; ***VT,*** ventricular tachycardia; ***WPW,*** Wolff-Parkinson-White syndrome.

Antibiotics

USES

Treatment of wide range of gram-positive or gram-negative bacterial infections; suppression of intestinal flora before surgery; control of acne; prophylactically to prevent rheumatic fever; prophylactically in high-risk situations (e.g., some surgical procedures or medical states) to prevent bacterial infection.

ACTION

Antibiotics (antimicrobial agents) are natural or synthetic compounds that have the ability to kill or suppress the growth of microorganisms.

One means of classifying antibiotics is by their antimicrobial spectrum. Narrow-spectrum agents are effective against few microorganisms (e.g., aminoglycosides are effective against gram-negative aerobes), whereas broad-spectrum agents are effective against a wide variety of microorganisms (e.g., fluoroquinolones are effective against gram-positive cocci and gram-negative bacilli).

Antimicrobial agents may also be classified based on their mechanism of action.

- Agents that inhibit cell wall synthesis or activate enzymes that disrupt cell wall, causing a weakening in the cell, cell lysis, and death. Include penicillins, cephalosporins, vancomycin, imidazole antifungal agents.
- Agents that act directly on cell wall, affecting permeability of cell membranes, causing leakage of intracellular substances. Include antifungal agents amphotericin and nystatin, polymixin, colistin.
- Agents that bind to ribosomal subunits, altering protein synthesis and eventually causing cell death. Include aminoglycosides.
- Agents that affect bacterial ribosome function, altering protein synthesis and causing slow microbial growth. Do not cause cell death. Include chloramphenicol, clindamycin, erythromycin, tetracyclines.
- Agents that inhibit nucleic acid metabolism by binding to nucleic acid or interacting with enzymes necessary for nucleic acid synthesis. Inhibit DNA or RNA synthesis. Include rifampin, metronidazole, quinolones (e.g., ciprofloxacin).
- Agents that inhibit specific metabolic steps necessary for microorganisms, causing a decrease in essential cell components or synthesis of nonfunctional analogues of normal metabolites. Include trimethoprim, sulfonamides.
- Agents that inhibit viral DNA synthesis by binding to viral enzymes necessary for DNA synthesis, preventing viral replication. Include acyclovir, vidarabine.

SELECTION OF ANTIMICROBIAL AGENTS

The goal of therapy is to produce a favorable therapeutic result by achieving antimicrobial action at the site of infection sufficient to inhibit the growth of the microorganism. The agent selected should be the most active against the most likely infecting organism, least likely to cause toxicity or allergic reaction. Factors to consider in selection of an antimicrobial agent include the following:

- Sensitivity pattern of the infecting microorganism
- Location and severity of infection (may determine route of administration)
- Pt's ability to eliminate the drug (status of renal and liver functions)
- Pt's defense mechanisms (includes both cellular and humoral immunity)
- Pt's age, whether pregnant, genetic factors, allergies, CNS disorder, preexisting medical problems

CATEGORIZATION OF ORGANISMS BY GRAM STAINING

Gram-Positive Cocci	Gram-Negative Cocci	Gram-Positive Bacilli	Gram-Negative Bacilli
Aerobic	**Aerobic**	**Aerobic**	**Aerobic**
Staphylococcus aureus	*Neisseria gonorrhoeae*	*Listeria monocytogenes*	*E. coli*
Staphylococcus epidermidis	*Neisseria meningitidis*	*Bacillus anthracis*	*Klebsiella pneumoniae*
Streptococcus pneumoniae	*Moraxella catarrhalis*	*Corynebacterium diphtheriae*	*Proteus mirabilis*
Streptococcus pyogenes		**Anaerobic**	*Serratia marcescens*
Viridans streptococci		*Clostridium difficile*	*Pseudomonas aeruginosa*
Enterococcus faecalis		*Clostridium perfringens*	*Enterobacter* spp.
Enterococcus faecium		*Clostridium tetani*	*Haemophilus influenzae*
Anaerobic		*Actinomyces* spp.	*Legionella pneumophila*
Peptostreptococcus spp.			**Anaerobic**
Peptococcus spp.			*Bacteroides fragilis*
			Fusobacterium spp.

Antibiotic: Aminoglycosides

USES

Treatment of serious infections when other less toxic agents are not effective, are contraindicated, or require adjunctive therapy (e.g., with penicillins or cephalosporins). Used primarily in the treatment of infections caused by gram-negative microorganisms, such as those caused by *Proteus, Klebsiella, Pseudomonas, Escherichia coli, Serratia,* and *Enterobacter.* Inactive against most gram-positive microorganisms. Not well absorbed systemically from GI tract (must be administered parenterally for systemic infections). Oral agents are given to suppress intestinal bacteria.

ACTION

Bactericidal. Transported across bacterial cell membrane; irreversibly binds to specific receptor proteins of bacterial ribosomes. Interfere with protein synthesis, preventing cell reproduction and eventually causing cell death.

ANTIBIOTIC: AMINOGLYCOSIDES

Name	Availability	Dosage Range	Side Effects
Amikacin (p. 45) (Amikin)	**I:** 250 mg/ml, 50 mg/ml	**A:** 15 mg/kg/day **C:** 15 mg/kg/day	Nephrotoxicity, neurotoxicity, ototoxicity (both auditory and vestibular), hypersensitivity (skin itching, redness, rash, swelling)
Gentamicin (p. 496) (Garamycin)	**I:** 40 mg/ml, 10 mg/ml	**A:** 3–5 mg/kg/day **C:** 6–7.5 mg/kg/day	Same as amikacin
Neomycin (p. 759)	**T:** 500 mg	**A:** 1 g for 3 doses as preop	Nausea, vomiting, diarrhea
Netilmicin (p. 764) (Netromycin)	**I:** 100 mg/ml	**A:** 3–6.5 mg/kg/day **C:** 5.5–8 mg/kg/day	Same as amikacin

Streptomycin **(p. 991)**	**I:** 1 g	**A:** 15 mg/kg/day **C:** 20–40 mg/kg/day **Maximum:** 1 g	Same as amikacin Peripheral neuritis (numbness), optic neuritis (any vision loss)
Tobramycin **(p. 1045)** **(Nebcin)**	**I:** 40 mg/ml, 10 mg/ml	**A:** 3–5 mg/kg/day **C:** 6–7.5 mg/kg/day	Same as amikacin

A, Adults; ***C*** *(dosage),* children; ***I,*** injection; ***T,*** tablets.

Antibiotic: Cephalosporins

USES

Broad-spectrum antibiotics, which, like penicillins, may be used in a number of diseases, including respiratory diseases, skin and soft tissue infection, bone/joint infections, GU infections, prophylactically in some surgical procedures.

First-generation cephalosporins have good activity against gram-positive organisms and moderate activity against gram-negative organisms, including *Escherichia coli, Klebsiella pneumoniae, Proteus mirabilis.*

Second-generation cephalosporins have increased activity against gram-negative organisms.

Third-generation cephalosporins are less active against gram-positive organisms but more active against the Enterobacteriaceae with some activity against *Pseudomonas aeruginosa.*

Fourth-generation cephalosporins have good activity against gram-positive organisms (e.g., *Staphylococcus aureus*) and gram-negative organisms (e.g., *Pseudomonas aeruginosa*).

ACTION

Cephalosporins inhibit cell wall synthesis or activate enzymes that disrupt cell wall, causing a weakening in the cell wall, cell lysis, and cell death. May be bacteriostatic or bactericidal. Most effective against rapidly dividing cells.

Antibiotic: Cephalosporins *(continued)*

ANTIBIOTIC: CEPHALOSPORINS

Name	Availability	Dosage Range	Side Effects
First-Generation			
Cefadroxil (p. 178) (Duricef)	**C:** 500 mg **T:** 1 g **S:** 125 mg/5 ml, 250 mg/5 ml, 500 mg/5 ml	**A:** 1–2 g/day **C:** 30 mg/kg/day	Abdominal or stomach cramps/pain, fever, nausea, vomiting, diarrhea, headaches, oral/vaginal candidiasis
Cefazolin (p. 179) (Ancef, Kefzol)	**I:** 500 mg, 1 g, 2 g	**A:** 0.75–6 g/day **C:** 25–100 mg/kg/day	Same as above
Cephalexin (p. 204) (Keftab)	**C:** 250 mg, 500 mg **T:** 250 mg, 500 mg, 1 g	**A:** 1–4 g/day **C:** 25–100 mg/kg/day	Same as above
Second-Generation			
Cefaclor (p. 176) (Ceclor)	**C:** 250 mg, 500 mg **T (ER):** 375 mg, 500 mg **S:** 125 mg/5 ml, 187 mg/5 ml, 250 mg/5 ml, 375 mg/5 ml	**A:** 250–500 mg q8h **C:** 20–40 mg/kg/day	Same as cefadroxil May have serum sickness–like reaction
Cefotetan (p. 187) (Cefotan)	**I:** 1 g, 2 g	**A:** 1–6 g/day	Same as cefadroxil May cause unusual bleeding/bruising
Cefoxitin (p. 189) (Mefoxin)	**I:** 1 g, 2 g	**A:** 3–12 g/day	Same as cefadroxil

Cefpodoxime (p. 191) **(Vantin)**	**T**: 100 mg, 200 mg **S**: 50 mg/5 ml, 100 mg/5 ml	**A**: 200–800 mg/day **C**: 10 mg/kg/day	Same as cefadroxil
Cefprozil (p. 192) **(Cefzil)**	**T**: 250 mg, 500 mg **S**: 125 mg/5 ml, 250 mg/5 ml	**A**: 0.5–1 g/day **C**: 30 mg/kg/day	Same as above
Cefuroxime (p. 201) **(Ceftin, Kefurox, Zinacef)**	**T**: 125 mg, 250 mg, 500 mg **S**: 125 mg/5 ml, 250 mg/5 ml **I**: 750 mg, 1.5 g	**A (PO)**: 0.25–1 g/day; **(IM/IV)**: 2.25–9 g/day **C (PO)**: 250–500 mg/day; **(IM/IV)**: 50–100 mg/kg/day	Same as above
Loracarbef (p. 649) **(Lorabid)**	**C**: 200 mg, 400 mg **S**: 100 mg/5 ml, 200 mg/5 ml	**A**: 200–800 mg/day **C**: 15–30 mg/kg/day	Same as above
Third-Generation			
Cefdinir (p. 181) **(Omnicef)**	**C**: 300 mg **S**: 125 mg/5 ml	**A**: 600 mg/day **C**: 14 mg/kg/day	Same as above
Cefditoren (p. 183) **(Spectracef)**	**T**: 200 mg	**A**: 400–800 mg/day	Same as above
Cefotaxime (p. 185) **(Claforan)**	**I**: 500 mg, 1 g, 2 g	**A**: 2–12 g/day **C**: 100–200 mg/kg/day	Same as above
Ceftazidime (p. 194) **(Fortaz, Tazicef, Tazidime)**	**I**: 500 mg, 1 g, 2 g	**A**: 0.5–6 g/day **C**: 90–150 mg/kg/day	Same as above
Ceftibuten (p. 196) **(Cedax)**	**C**: 400 mg **S**: 90 mg/5 ml, 180 mg/5 ml	**A**: 400 mg/day **C**: 9 mg/kg/day	Same as above

(continued)

ANTIBIOTIC: CEPHALOSPORINS ***(continued)***

Name	Availability	Dosage Range	Side Effects
Third-Generation *(continued)*			
Ceftizoxime (p. 197) (Cefizox)	**I:** 500 mg, 1 g, 2 g	**A:** 1–12 g/day **C:** 150–200 mg/kg/day	Same as above
Ceftriaxone (p. 199) (Rocephin)	**I:** 250 mg, 500 mg, 1 g, 2 g	**A:** 1–4 g/day **C:** 50–100 mg/kg/day	Same as above
Fourth-Generation			
Cefepime (p. 183) (Maxipime)	**I:** 500 mg, 1 g, 2 g	**A:** 1–6 g/day	Same as above

A, Adults; ***C,*** capsules; ***C** (dosage),* children; ***ER,*** extended-release; ***I,*** injection; ***S,*** suspension; ***T,*** tablets.

Antibiotic: Fluoroquinolones

USES

Fluoroquinolones act against a wide range of gram-negative and gram-positive organisms. They are used primarily in the treatment of lower respiratory infections, skin/skin structure infections, UTIs, and sexually transmitted diseases.

ACTION

Bactericidal. Inhibit DNA gyrase in susceptible microorganisms, interfering with bacterial DNA replication and repair.

ANTIBIOTIC: FLUOROQUINOLONES

Name	Availability	Dosage Range	Side Effects
Ciprofloxacin (p. 228) (Cipro)	**T:** 250 mg, 500 mg, 750 mg **S:** 5 g/100 ml **I:** 200 mg, 400 mg	**A (PO):** 250–750 mg q12h; **(IV):** 200–400 mg q12h	Dizziness, headaches, nervousness, drowsiness, insomnia, abdominal pain, nausea, diarrhea, vomiting, phlebitis (parenteral)
Enoxacin (p. 375) (Penetrex)	**T:** 200 mg, 400 mg	**A:** 200–400 mg q12h	Same as above
Gatifloxacin (p. 487) (Tequin)	**T:** 200 mg, 400 mg **I:** 200 mg, 400 mg	**A:** 200–400 mg q12h	Same as above
Gemifloxacin (p. 493) (Factive)	**T:** 320 mg	**A:** 320 mg/day	Same as above
Levofloxacin (p. 629) (Levaquin)	**T:** 250 mg, 500 mg, 750 mg **I:** 250 mg, 500 mg, 750 mg	**A (PO/IV):** 250–750 mg/day as single dose	Same as above
Lomefloxacin (p. 644) (Maxaquin)	**T:** 400 mg	**A:** 400 mg/day	Same as above
Moxifloxacin (p. 734) (Avelox)	**T:** 400 mg **I:** 400 mg	**A:** 400 mg/day	Same as above; may prolong QT interval
Norfloxacin (p. 785) (Noroxin)	**T:** 400 mg	**A:** 400 mg q12h	Same as above
Ofloxacin (p. 792) (Floxin)	**T:** 200 mg, 300 mg, 400 mg	**A:** 200–400 mg q12h	Same as above

A, Adults; ***I,*** injection; ***S,*** suspension; ***T,*** tablets.

Antibiotic: Macrolides

USES

Macrolides act primarily against gram-positive microorganisms and gram-negative cocci. Azithromycin and clarithromycin appear to be more potent than erythromycin. Macrolides are used in the treatment of pharyngitis/tonsillitis, sinusitis, chronic bronchitis, pneumonia, uncomplicated skin/skin structure infections.

ACTION

Bacteriostatic or bactericidal. Reversibly bind to the P site of the 50S ribosomal subunit of susceptible organisms, inhibiting RNA-dependent protein synthesis.

ANTIBIOTIC: MACROLIDES

Name	Availability	Dosage Range	Side Effects
Azithromycin (p. 102) (Zithromax)	**T**: 250 mg, 600 mg **S**: 100 mg/5 ml, 200 mg/5 ml, 1 g packet **I**: 500 mg	**A (PO)**: 500 mg once, then 250 mg days 2–5; **(IV)**: 500 mg/day **C (PO)**: 10 mg/kg once, then 5 mg/kg/day on days 2–5	**PO**: Nausea, diarrhea, vomiting, abdominal pain **IV**: Pain, redness, swelling at injection site
Clarithromycin (p. 237) (Biaxin)	**T**: 250 mg, 500 mg **T (XL)**: 500 mg **S**: 125 mg/5 ml	**A**: 250–500 mg q12h **C**: 7.5 mg/kg q12h	Headaches, loss of taste, nausea, vomiting, diarrhea, abdominal pain/discomfort
Dirithromycin (p. 337) (Dynabac)	**T**: 250 mg	**A, C (>12 yrs)**: 500 mg/day as a single daily dose	Dizziness, nausea, vomiting, diarrhea, abdominal pain, headaches, weakness

Erythromycin (p. 395) (Ery-Tab, PCE, Eryc, EES, EryPed, Erythrocin)	**T:** 200 mg, 250 mg, 333 mg, 400 mg, 500 mg **C:** 250 mg **S:** 125 mg/5 ml, 200 mg/5 ml, 250 mg/5 ml, 400 mg/5 ml, 100 mg/2.5 ml	**A (PO):** 250–500 mg q6h **C (PO):** 30–50 mg/kg/day **A, C (IV):** 15–20 mg/kg/day **Maximum:** 4 g/day	**PO:** Nausea, vomiting, diarrhea, abdominal pain **IV:** Inflammation, phlebitis at injection site

A, Adults; ***C,*** capsules; ***C*** *(dosage),* children; ***I,*** injection; ***S,*** suspension; ***T,*** tablets; ***XL,*** long acting.

Antibiotic: Penicillins

USES

Penicillins may be used to treat a large number of infections, including pneumonia and other respiratory diseases, UTIs, septicemia, meningitis, intra-abdominal infections, gonorrhea and syphilis, bone/joint infection.

Penicillins are classified based on an antimicrobial spectrum:

Natural penicillins are very active against gram-positive cocci but ineffective against most strains of *Staphylococcus aureus* (inactivated by enzyme penicillinase).

Penicillinase-resistant penicillins are effective against penicillinase-producing *Staphylococcus aureus* but are less effective against gram-positive cocci than the natural penicillins.

Broad-spectrum penicillins are effective against gram-positive cocci and some gram-negative bacteria (e.g., *Haemophilus influenzae, Escherichia coli, Proteus mirabilis*).

Extended-spectrum penicillins are effective against *Pseudomonas aeruginosa, Enterobacter, Proteus* species, *Klebsiella,* and some other gram-negative microorganisms.

ACTION

Penicillins inhibit cell wall synthesis or activate enzymes, which disrupt bacterial cell wall, causing a weakening in the cell wall, cell lysis, and cell death. May be bacteriostatic or bactericidal. Most effective against bacteria undergoing active growth and division.

Antibiotic: Penicillins *(continued)*

ANTIBIOTIC: PENICILLINS

Name	Availability	Dosage Range	Side Effects
Natural			
Penicillin G benzathine (p. 837) (Bicillin)	**I:** 600,000 units, 1.2 million units, 2.4 million units	**A:** 1.2 million units/day **C:** 0.3–1.2 million units/day	Mild diarrhea, nausea, vomiting, headaches, sore mouth/tongue, vaginal itching/discharge, allergic reaction (including anaphylaxis, skin rash, hives, itching)
Penicillin G potassium (p. 839) (Pfizerpen)	**I:** 1, 2, 3, 5 million-unit vials	**A:** 2–24 million units/day **C:** 100–250,000 units/kg/day	Same as above
Penicillin G procaine (p. 840) (Wycillin)	**I:** 600,000 units, 1.2 million units, 2.4 million units	**A, C:** 0.6–1.2 million units/day	Same as above; increased risk of mental disturbances
Penicillin V potassium (p. 841) (Pen-Vee K, V-Cillin-K)	**T:** 250 mg, 500 mg **S:** 125 mg/5 ml, 250 mg/5 ml	**A:** 0.5–2 g/day **C:** 25–50 mg/kg/day	Same as above
Penicillinase-Resistant			
Cloxacillin (p. 251) (Tegopen)	**C:** 250 mg, 500 mg **S:** 125 mg/5 ml	**A:** 1–2 g/day **C:** 50–100 mg/kg/day	Same as penicillin G benzathine; increased risk of liver toxicity
Dicloxacillin (p. 318) (Dynapen, Pathocil)	**C:** 125 mg, 250 mg, 500 mg **S:** 62.5 mg/5 ml	**A:** 1–2 g/day **C:** 12.5–25 mg/kg/day	Same as above Increased risk of liver toxicity
Nafcillin (p. 745) (Nafcil, Unipen)	**C:** 250 mg **I:** 500 mg, 1 g, 2 g	**A (PO):** 1–6 g/day; **(IV):** 2–6 g/day **C (PO):** 25–50 mg/kg/day; **(IV):** 50 mg/kg/day	Same as penicillin G benzathine; increased risk of interstitial nephritis
Oxacillin (p. 807) (Bactocill)	**C:** 250 mg, 500 mg **S:** 250 mg/5 ml **I:** 250 mg, 500 mg, 1 g, 2 g	**A (PO/IV):** 2–6 g/day **C (PO/IV):** 50–100 mg/kg/day	Same as above; increased risk of liver toxicity, interstitial nephritis

Broad-Spectrum			
Amoxicillin (p. 59) **(Amoxil, Polymox, Trimox)**	**T:** 125 mg, 250 mg, 500 mg, 875 mg **C:** 250 mg, 500 mg **S:** 50 mg/ml, 125 mg/5 ml, 250 mg/5 ml	**A:** 0.75–1.5 g/day **C:** 20–40 mg/kg/day	Same as above
Amoxicillin/clavulanate (p. 60) **(Augmentin)**	**T:** 250 mg, 500 mg, 875 mg **T (chewable):** 125 mg, 200 mg, 250 mg, 400 mg **S:** 125 mg/5 ml, 200 mg/5 ml, 250 mg/5 ml, 400 mg/5 ml	**A:** 0.75–1.5 g/day **C:** 20–40 mg/kg/day	Same as above
Ampicillin (p. 65) **(Omnipen, Polycillin, Principen)**	**C:** 250 mg, 500 mg **S:** 125 mg/5 ml, 250 mg/5 ml **I:** 125 mg, 250 mg, 500 mg, 1 g, 2 g	**A:** 1–12 g/day **C:** 50–200 mg/kg/day	Same as above
Ampicillin/sulbactam (p. 68) **(Unasyn)**	**I:** 1.5 g, 3 g	**A:** 6–12 g/day **C:** 100–200 mg/kg/day	Same as above
Extended-Spectrum			
Carbenicillin (p. 166) **(Geocillin)**	**T:** 382 mg	**A:** 382–764 mg 4 times/day	Same as above
Piperacillin/tazobactam (p. 864) **(Zosyn)**	**I:** 2.25 g, 3.375 g, 4.5 g	**A:** 2.25–4.5 g q6–8h **C:** 200–400 mg/kg/day	Same as above
Ticarcillin/clavulanate (p. 1034) **(Timentin)**	**I:** 3.1 g	**A:** 3.1 g q4–6h **C:** 200–300 mg/kg/day	Same as above

A, Adults; ***C,*** capsules; ***C (dosage),*** children; ***I,*** injection; ***S,*** suspension; ***T,*** tablets.

Anticoagulants/Antiplatelets/Thrombolytics

USES

Treatment and prevention of venous thromboembolism, acute MI, acute cerebral embolism; reduce risk of acute MI, total mortality in pts with unstable angina; occlusion of saphenous grafts following open heart surgery; embolism in select pts with atrial fibrillation, prosthetic heart valves, valvular heart disease, cardiomyopathy. Heparin also used for acute/chronic consumption coagulopathies (disseminated intravascular coagulation).

ACTION

Anticoagulants: Inhibit blood coagulation by preventing the formation of new clots and extension of existing ones. *Do not dissolve formed clots.* Anticoagulants are subdivided into two common classes: *Heparin:* Indirectly interferes with blood coagulation by blocking the conversion of prothrombin to thrombin and fibrinogen to fibrin. *Coumarin:* Acts indirectly to prevent synthesis in the liver of vitamin K–dependent clotting factors.

Antiplatelets: Interfere with platelet aggregation. Effects are irreversible for life of platelet. Medications in this group act by different mechanisms and are used in combinations to provide desired effect.

Thrombolytics: Act directly or indirectly on fibrinolytic system to dissolve clots (converting plasminogen to plasmin, an enzyme that digests fibrin clot).

ANTICOAGULANTS/ANTIPLATELETS/THROMBOLYTICS

Name	Availability	Uses	Dosage Range	Side Effects
Anticoagulants				
Dalteparin (p. 281) (Fragmin)	**I:** 2,500 international units, 5,000 international units	DVT prophylaxis, unstable angina	**DVT:** 2,500-5,000 international units/day **Angina:** 120 international units/kg q12h	Hematoma at injection site, bleeding
Enoxaparin (p. 375) (Lovenox)	**I:** 30 mg, 40 mg, 60 mg, 80 mg, 100 mg	DVT treatment/prophylaxis, DVT, unstable angina	**DVT prophylaxis:** 40 mg/day or 30 mg q12h **DVT, angina:** 1 mg/kg q12h	Same as above

Heparin (p. 522)	**I:** 5,000 units, 10,000 units, 20,000 units **Infusion**	DVT prophylaxis, thrombosis, embolism, coagulopathies	**DVT prophylaxis:** 5,000 units q8-12h **DVT, embolism:** IV bolus, then IV infusion of 20,000–40,000 units/day	Bleeding
Tinzaparin (p. 1040) (Innohep)	**I:** 20,000 international units/ml	DVT treatment	175 international units/kg once daily	Same as danaparoid
Warfarin (p. 1121) (Coumadin)	**T:** 1 mg, 2 mg, 2.5 mg, 3 mg, 4 mg, 5 mg, 6 mg, 7.5 mg, 10 mg	Thromboembolic complications with AF, PE, DVT	Initially, 5–10 mg, then 2–10 mg/day	Same as heparin

Antiplatelets

Abciximab (p. 2) (ReoPro)	**I:** 2 m/ml	ACS	IV bolus of 0.25 mg/kg, then 10 mcg/min	Bleeding, hypotension
Anagrelide (p. 71) (Agrylin)	**C:** 0.5 mg, 1 mg	Thrombocythemia	2–10 mg/day	Abdominal pain, weakness, dizziness, shortness of breath
Aspirin (p. 86)	**T:** 80 mg, 160 mg, 325 mg	Atherosclerotic events	81–325 mg/day	GI irritation
Clopidogrel (p. 247) (Plavix)	**T:** 75 mg	Atherosclerotic events	75 mg/day	Pain, dizziness, heartburn, headaches, flulike symptoms
Dipyridamole (p. 336) (Persantine)	**T:** 25 mg, 50 mg, 75 mg	Thromboembolic complications	75–100 mg 4 times/day	Abdominal discomfort, diarrhea, dizziness, headaches
Eptifibatide (p. 389) (Integrilin)	**I:** 0.75 mg/ml, 2 mg/ml	ACS	IV bolus of 180 mcg/kg, then 2 mcg/kg/min	Same as abciximab
Ticlopidine (p. 1036) (Ticlid)	**T:** 250 mg	Stroke	250 mg 2 times/day	Skin rash, abdominal pain, diarrhea, nausea, indigestion

(continued)

ANTICOAGULANTS/ANTIPLATELETS/THROMBOLYTICS *(continued)*

Name	Availability	Uses	Dosage Range	Side Effects
Tirofiban (p. 1042) (Aggrastat)	**I:** 50 mcg/ml, 250 mcg/ml	ACS	IV bolus of 0.4 mcg/kg/min, then 0.1 mcg/kg/min	Same as abciximab
Treprostinil (p. 1069) (Remodulin)	**I:** 1 mg/ml, 2.5 mg/ml, 5 mg/ml, 10 mg/ml	Pulmonary arterial HTN	0.625–1.25 ng/kg/min	Pain at injection site, headache, diarrhea, nausea, rash, jaw pain, dizziness
Thrombolytics				
Alteplase (p. 38) (Activase)	**I:** 50 mg, 100 mg	AMI, acute ischemic stroke, PE	**IV:** 100 mg over 3 hrs (PE over 2 hrs)	Same as abciximab
Reteplase (p. 931) (Retavase)	**I:** 10 units	AMI	**IV:** 10 units q30min 2 times	Same as above
Streptokinase (p. 989)	**I:** 250,000 units, 500,000 units, 1.5 million units	AMI, PE, arterial thrombus	**AMI:** 1.5 million units over 60 min **PE, arterial thrombus:** 250,000-unit bolus, then 100,000 units/hr	Same as above
Tenecteplase (p. 1014) (TNKase)	**I:** 50 mg	AMI	Based on pt weight. **Maximum:** 50 mg	Same as above

ACS, Acute coronary syndrome; ***AF,*** atrial fibrillation; ***AMI,*** acute myocardial infarction; ***C,*** capsules; ***DVT,*** deep vein thrombosis; ***HTN,*** hypertension; ***I,*** injection; ***PE,*** pulmonary embolism; ***T,*** tablets.

Anticonvulsants

USES

Anticonvulsants are used to treat seizures. Seizures can be divided into two broad categories: partial seizures and generalized seizures. Partial seizures begin focally in the cerebral cortex, undergoing limited spread. Simple partial seizures do not involve loss of consciousness but may evolve secondarily into generalized seizures. Complex partial seizures involve impairment of consciousness. Generalized seizures may be convulsive or nonconvulsive and usually produce immediate loss of consciousness.

ACTION

Anticonvulsants can prevent or reduce excessive discharge of neurons with seizure foci or decrease the spread of excitation from seizure foci to normal neurons. The exact mechanism is unknown but may be due to (1) suppressing sodium influx; (2) suppressing calcium influx; or (3) increasing the action of GABA, which inhibits neurotransmitters throughout the brain.

ANTICONVULSANTS

Name	Availability	Uses	Dosage Range	Side Effects
Barbiturates				
Phenobarbital (p. 849)	**T:** 30 mg, 60 mg, 100 mg **I:** 65 mg, 130 mg	Tonic-clonic, partial, status epilepticus	**A (PO):** 100–300 mg/day; **(IM/IV):** 200–600 mg **C (PO):** 3–5 mg/kg/day; **(IM/IV):** 100–400 mg	CNS depression, sedation, paradoxical excitement and hyperactivity, rash
Primidone (p. 884) (Mysoline)	**T:** 50 mg, 250 mg **S:** 250 mg/5 ml	Complex, partial, akinetic, tonic-clonic	**A:** 750–2,000 mg/day **C:** 10–25 mg/kg/day	CNS depression, sedation, paradoxical excitement and hyperactivity, rash, dizziness, ataxia

(continued)

ANTICONVULSANTS ***(continued)***

Name	Availability	Uses	Dosage Range	Side Effects
Benzodiazepines				
Clonazepam (p. 243) (Klonopin)	**T:** 0.5 mg, 1 mg, 2 mg	Petit mal, akinetic, myoclonic, absence seizure	**A:** 1.5–20 mg/day	CNS depression, sedation, ataxia, confusion, depression
Diazepam (p. 314) (Valium)	**T:** 2 mg, 5 mg, 10 mg **I:** 5 mg/ml **R:** 2.5 mg, 5 mg, 10 mg, 20 mg	Adjunctive therapy status epilepticus	**A (PO):** 4–40 mg/day; **(IM/IV):** 5–30 mg **C (PO):** 3–10 mg/day; **(IM/IV):** 1–10 mg	CNS depression, sedation, confusion, depression, respiratory suppression
Hydantoins				
Fosphenytoin (p. 474) (Cerebyx)	**I:** 50 mg PE/ml	Status epilepticus, seizures occurring during neurosurgery	**A:** 15–20 mg PE/kg bolus, then 4–6 mg PE/kg/day maintenance	Burning, itching, paresthesia, nystagmus, ataxia
Phenytoin (p. 855) (Dilantin)	**C:** 100 mg **T (chewable):** 50 mg **S:** 125 mg/5 ml **I:** 50 mg/ml	Tonic-clonic psychomotor seizures	**A (PO):** 300–600 mg/day; **(IV):** 150–250 mg **C (PO):** 4–8 mg/kg/day; **(IV):** 10–15 mg/kg	Nystagmus, ataxia, hypertrichosis, gingival hyperplasia, rash, osteomalacia, lymphadenopathy
Miscellaneous				
Carbamazepine (p. 164) (Tegretol)	**S:** 100 mg/5 ml **T (chewable):** 100 mg **T:** 200 mg **T (ER):** 100 mg, 200 mg, 400 mg **C (ER):** 200 mg, 300 mg	Complex partial, tonic-clonic, mixed seizures, trigeminal neuralgia	**A:** 800–1,200 mg/day **C:** 400–800 mg/day	Dizziness, diplopia, leukopenia

Gabapentin (p. 480) (Neurontin)	**C**: 100 mg, 300 mg, 400 mg	Partial seizures with and without secondary generalization	**A**: 900–1,800 mg/day	CNS depression, fatigue, somnolence, dizziness, ataxia
Lamotrigine (p. 614) (Lamictal)	**T**: 25 mg, 100 mg, 150 mg, 200 mg	Partial seizures	**A**: 100–500 mg/day	Dizziness, ataxia, somnolence, diplopia, nausea, rash
Levetiracetam (p. 628) (Keppra)	**T**: 250 mg, 500 mg, 750 mg	Partial-onset seizures	**A**: 1,000–3,000 mg/day	Asthenia, dizziness, flulike symptoms, headache, rhinitis, somnolence
Oxcarbazepine (p. 812) (Trileptal)	**T**: 150 mg, 300 mg, 600 mg	Partial seizures	**A**: 900–1,800 mg/day	Drowsiness, dizziness, blurred vision
Tiagabine (p. 1033) (Gabitril)	**T**: 4 mg, 12 mg, 16 mg, 20 mg	Partial seizures	**A**: Initially, 4 mg up to 56 mg **C**: Initially, 4 mg up to 32 mg	Dizziness, asthenia, nervousness, tremors, abdominal pain
Topiramate (p. 1053) (Topamax)	**T**: 25 mg, 100 mg, 200 mg	Partial seizures	**A**: 25–400 mg/day **C**: 1–9 mg/kg/day	Difficulty concentrating, speech problems, fatigue
Valproic acid (p. 1092) (Depakene, Depakote)	**C**: 250 mg **S**: 250 mg/5 ml **Sprinkles**: 125 mg **T**: 125 mg, 250 mg, 500 mg **T (ER)**: 500 mg **I**: 100 mg/ml	Complex partial seizures, absence seizures	**A, C**: 15–60 mg/kg/day	Nausea, vomiting, tremors, thrombocytopenia, hair loss, liver dysfunction
Zonisamide (p. 1138) (Zonegran)	**C**: 100 mg	Partial seizures	**A**: 500 mg/day	Somnolence, dizziness, anorexia, headaches, nausea

A, Adults; ***C,*** capsules; ***C** (dosage),* children; ***ER,*** extended-release; ***I,*** injection; ***PE,*** phenytoin sodium equivalents; ***R,*** rectal; ***S,*** suspension; ***T,*** tablets.

Antidepressants

USES

Used primarily for the treatment of depression. Imipramine is also used for childhood enuresis. Clomipramine is used only for obsessive-compulsive disorder (OCD). Monoamine oxidase inhibitors (MAOIs) are rarely used as initial therapy except for pts unresponsive to other therapy or when other therapy is contraindicated.

ACTION

Antidepressants are classified as tricyclic, MAOIs, or second-generation antidepressants (further subdivided into selective serotonin reuptake inhibitors [SSRIs] and atypical antidepressants). Depression may be due to reduced functioning of monoamine neurotransmitters (e.g., norepinephrine, serotonin [5-HT], dopamine) in the CNS (decreased amount and/or decreased effects at the receptor sites).

Antidepressants block metabolism, increase amount/effects of monoamine neurotransmitters, and act at receptor sites (change responsiveness/sensitivities of both presynaptic and postsynaptic receptor sites).

ANTIDEPRESSANTS

Name	Availability	Uses	Dosage Range (per day)	Side Effects
Tricyclics				
Amitriptyline (p. 55) (Elavil)	**T:** 10 mg, 25 mg, 59 mg, 75 mg, 100 mg, 150 mg	Depression	40–300 mg	Drowsiness, blurred vision, constipation, confusion, postural hypotension, conduction defects, weight gain, seizure tendency
Clomipramine (p. 242) (Anafranil)	**C:** 25 mg, 50 mg, 75 mg	OCD	25–250 mg	Same as above
Desipramine (p. 297) (Norpramin, Pertofrane)	**T:** 10 mg, 25 mg, 50 mg, 75 mg, 100 mg, 150 mg	Depression	25–100 mg	Same as above

Doxepin (p. 354) (Sinequan)	**C:** 10 mg, 25 mg, 50 mg, 75 mg, 100 mg, 150 mg **OC:** 10 mg/ml	Depression	25–300 mg	Same as above
Imipramine (p. 559) (Janimine, Tofranil)	**T:** 10 mg, 25 mg, 50 mg **C:** 75 mg, 100 mg, 125 mg, 150 mg	Depression, enuresis	30–300 mg	Same as above
Nortriptyline (p. 786) (Aventyl, Pamelor)	**C:** 10 mg, 25 mg, 50 mg, 75 mg **S:** 10 mg/5 ml	Depression	25–100 mg	Same as above
Protriptyline (p. 906) (Vivactil)	**T:** 5 mg, 10 mg	Depression	15–60 mg	Same as above
Monoamine Oxidase Inhibitors				
Phenelzine (p. 848) (Nardil)	**T:** 15 mg	Depression	15–90 mg	Sedation, hypertensive crisis, weight gain, orthostatic hypotension
Tranylcypromine (p. 1065) (Parnate)	**T:** 10 mg	Depression	30–60 mg	Same as above
Selective Serotonin Reuptake Inhibitors				
Citalopram (p. 233) (Celexa)	**T:** 20 mg, 40 mg **S:** 10 mg/5 ml	Depression	25–60 mg	Insomnia or sedation, nausea, agitation, headaches
Escitalopram (p. 398) (Lexapro)	**T:** 5 mg, 10 mg, 20 mg	Depression	10–20 mg	Insomnia or sedation, nausea, agitation, headache
Fluoxetine (p. 452) (Prozac)	**C:** 10 mg, 20 mg, 40 mg **T:** 10 mg **S:** 20 mg/5 ml	Depression, OCD, bulimia	10–80 mg	Akathisia, sexual dysfunction, skin rash, hives, itching, decreased appetite, asthenia, diarrhea, drowsiness, headache, increased sweating, insomnia, nausea, tremors

(continued)

ANTIDEPRESSANTS ***(continued)***

Name	Availability	Uses	Dosage Range (per day)	Side Effects
Selective Serotonin Reuptake Inhibitors ***(continued)***				
Fluvoxamine (p. 464) (Luvox)	**T**: 25 mg, 50 mg, 100 mg	OCD	100–300 mg	Sexual dysfunction, fatigue, constipation, dizziness, drowsiness, headache, insomnia, nausea, vomiting
Paroxetine (p. 826) (Paxil)	**T**: 10 mg, 20 mg, 30 mg, 40 mg **S**: 10 mg/5 ml	Depression, OCD, panic attack, social anxiety disorder	20–50 mg	Asthenia, constipation, diarrhea, sweating, insomnia, nausea, sexual dysfunction, tremor, vomiting, urinary frequency or retention
Sertraline (p. 966) (Zoloft)	**T**: 25 mg, 50 mg, 100 mg **S**: 20 mg/ml	Depression, OCD, panic attack	50–200 mg	Sexual dysfunction, dizziness, drowsiness, anorexia, diarrhea, nausea, dry mouth, stomach cramps, decreased weight, headache, increased sweating, tremor, insomnia
Atypical				
Bupropion (p. 143) (Wellbutrin)	**T**: 75 mg, 100 mg **SR**: 100 mg, 150 mg	Depression	150–450 mg	Insomnia, irritability, seizures
Mirtazapine (p. 719) (Remeron)	**T**: 15 mg, 30 mg, 45 mg	Depression	15–45 mg	Sedation, dry mouth, weight gain, agranulocytosis, liver toxicity
Nefazodone (p. 756) (Serzone)	**T**: 50 mg, 100 mg, 150 mg, 200 mg, 250 mg	Depression	200–600 mg	Sedation, orthostatic hypotension, nausea
Trazodone (p. 1068) (Desyrel)	**T**: 50 mg, 100 mg, 150 mg, 300 mg	Depression	50–600 mg	Sedation, orthostatic hypotension, priapism
Venlafaxine (p. 1102) (Effexor)	**T**: 25 mg, 37.5 mg, 50 mg, 75 mg, 100 mg **T (ER)**: 37.5 mg, 75 mg, 150 mg	Depression, anxiety	75–375 mg	Increased blood pressure, agitation, sedation, insomnia, nausea

C, Capsules; ***ER***, extended-release; ***OC***, oral concentrate; ***OCD***, obsessive-compulsive disorder; ***S***, suspension; ***SR***, sustained-release; ***T***, tablets.

Antidiabetics

USES	ACTION
Insulin: Treatment of insulin-dependent diabetes (type 1) and non–insulin-dependent diabetes (type 2). Also used in acute situations such as ketoacidosis, severe infections, major surgery in otherwise non–insulin-dependent diabetics. Administered to pts receiving parenteral nutrition. Drug of choice during pregnancy.	*Insulin:* A hormone synthesized and secreted by beta cells of Langerhans' islet in the pancreas. Controls storage and utilization of glucose, amino acids, and fatty acids by activated transport systems/enzymes. Inhibits breakdown of glycogen, fat, protein. Insulin lowers blood glucose by inhibiting glycogenolysis and gluconeogenesis in liver; stimulates glucose uptake by muscle, adipose tissue. Activity of insulin is initiated by binding to cell surface receptors.
Sulfonylureas: Control hyperglycemia in type 2 diabetes not controlled by weight and diet alone. Chlorpropamide also used in adjunctive treatment of neurogenic diabetes insipidus.	*Sulfonylureas:* Stimulate release of insulin from beta cells; increase sensitivity of insulin to peripheral tissue. Endogenous insulin must be present for oral hypoglycemics to be effective.
Alpha-glucosidase inhibitors: Adjunct to diet to lower blood glucose in pts with type 2 diabetes mellitus whose hyperglycemia cannot be managed by diet alone.	*Alpha-glucosidase inhibitors:* Work locally in small intestine, slowing carbohydrate breakdown and glucose absorption.
Biguanides: Adjunct to diet to lower blood glucose in pts with type 2 diabetes mellitus whose hyperglycemia cannot be managed by diet alone.	*Biguanides:* Decrease hepatic glucose output; enhance peripheral glucose uptake.
Thiazolinediones: Adjunct in pts with type 2 diabetes currently on insulin therapy.	*Thiazolinediones:* Decrease insulin resistance.

Antidiabetics *(continued)*

ANTIDIABETICS

Insulin

Name	Onset (hrs)	Peak (hrs)	Duration (hrs)	Side Effects
Rapid Acting				
Insulin aspart (p. 569) (Novolog)	½	1–3	3–5	Hypoglycemia, weight gain, lipodystrophy, local skin reactions
Lispro (p. 569) (Humalog)	¼	½–1½	4–5	Same as above
Regular (p. 569) (Humulin R, Novolin R)	½–1	2–4	5–7	Same as above
Intermediate Acting				
NPH (p. 569) (Humulin N, Novolin N)	2–4	6–14	14–18	Same as above
Long Acting				
Glargine (p. 569) (Lantus)	4	—	24+	Same as above

Oral Agents

Name	Availability	Dosage Range	Side Effects
Sulfonylureas			
Acetohexamide (p. 10) (Dymelor)	**T:** 250 mg, 500 mg	0.25–1.5 g/day	Hypoglycemia, weight gain, skin rash, hemolytic anemia, GI upset, cholestasis
Chlorpropamide (p. 219) (Diabinese)	**T:** 100 mg, 250 mg	100–500 mg/day	Same as above
Glimepiride (p. 503) (Amaryl)	**T:** 1 mg, 2 mg, 4 mg	1–8 mg/day	Same as above
Glipizide (p. 505) (Glucotrol)	**T:** 5 mg, 10 mg **T (XL):** 5 mg	**T:** 2.5–40 mg/day **XL:** 5–20 mg/day	Same as above
Glyburide (p. 509) (DiaBeta, Micronase)	**T:** 1.25 mg, 2.5 mg, 5 mg **PT:** 1.5 mg, 3 mg	**T:** 1.25–20 mg/day **PT:** 1–12 mg/day	Same as above
Tolazamide (p. 1048) (Tolinase)	**T:** 100 mg, 250 mg, 500 mg	0.2–1 g/day	Same as above
Tolbutamide (p. 1049) (Orinase)	**T:** 250 mg, 500 mg	0.5–3 g/day	Same as above
Alpha Glucosidase Inhibitors			
Acarbose (p. 4) (Precose)	**T:** 25 mg, 50 mg, 100 mg	75–300 mg/day	GI flatulence, diarrhea
Miglitol (p. 713) (Glyset)	**T:** 25 mg, 50 mg, 100 mg	75–300 mg/day	Same as above

(continued)

ANTIDIABETICS *(continued)*

ORAL AGENTS *(continued)*

Name	Availability	Dosage Range	Side Effects
Biguanides			
Metformin (p. 683) (Glucophage)	**T:** 500 mg, 850 mg **XR:** 500 mg	**T:** 0.5–2.5 g/day **XR:** 1,500–2,000 mg/day	Nausea, vomiting, diarrhea, loss of appetite, metallic taste, metabolic acidosis (rare)
Meglitinides			
Nateglinide (p. 754) (Starlix)	**T:** 60 mg, 120 mg	60–120 mg 3 times/day	Hypoglycemia, weight gain
Repaglinide (p. 928) (Prandin)	**T:** 0.5 mg, 1 mg, 2 mg	0.5–1 mg with each meal (**Maximum:** 16 mg/day)	Same as above
Thiazolidinediones			
Pioglitazone (p. 863) (Actos)	**T:** 15 mg, 30 mg, 45 mg	15–45 mg/day	Mild anemia, mild to moderate edema, weight gain
Rosiglitazone (p. 952) (Avandia)	**T:** 2 mg, 4 mg, 8 mg	4–8 mg/day	Same as above

PT, Prestab; ***T,*** tablets; ***XL,*** extended-release; ***XR,*** extended-release.

Antidiarrheals

USES	ACTION	
Acute diarrhea, chronic diarrhea of inflammatory bowel disease, reduction of fluid from ileostomies.	*Systemic agents:* Act at smooth muscle receptors (enteric), disrupting peristaltic movements, decreasing GI motility, increasing transit time of intestinal contents.	*Local agents:* Adsorb toxic substances and fluids to large surface areas of particles in the preparation. Some of these agents coat and protect irritated intestinal walls. May have local anti-inflammatory action.

ANTIDIARRHEALS

Name	Availability	Type	Dosage Range
Bismuth subsalicylate (p. 125) **(Pepto-Bismol)**	**T:** 262 mg **C:** 262 mg **L:** 130 mg/15 ml, 262 mg/15 ml, 524 mg/15 ml	Local	**A:** 2 **T** or 30 ml **C (9–12 yrs):** 1 **T** or 15 ml **C (6–8 yrs):** ⅔ **T** or 10 ml **C (3–5 yrs):** ⅓ **T** or 5 ml
Diphenoxylate (with atropine) (p. 334) **(Lomotil)**	**T:** 2.5 mg **L:** 2.5 mg/5 ml	Systemic	**A:** 5 mg 4 times/day **C:** 0.3–0.4 mg/kg/day in 4 divided doses **(L)**
Kaolin (with pectin) (p. 600) **(Kaopectate)**	**Suspension**	Local	**A:** 60–120 ml after each bowel movement **C (6–12 yrs):** 30–60 ml **C (3–5 yrs):** 15–30 ml
Loperamide (p. 646) **(Imodium)**	**C:** 2 mg **T:** 2 mg **L:** 1 mg/5 ml, 1 mg/ml	Systemic	**A:** Initially, 4 mg; 16 mg/day maximum **C (9–12 yrs):** 2 mg 3 times/day **(6–8 yrs):** 2 mg 2 times/day **(2–5 yrs):** 1 mg 3 times/day **(L)**

A, Adults; ***C,*** capsules; ***C (dosage),*** children; ***L,*** liquid; ***T,*** tablets.

Antifungals: Topical

USES

Treatment of tinea infections, cutaneous candidiasis (moniliasis) due to *Candida albicans.*

ACTION

Exact mechanism unknown. May deplete essential intracellular components by inhibiting transport of potassium, other ions into cells; alter membrane permeability, resulting in loss of potassium, other cellular components.

ANTIFUNGALS: TOPICAL

Name	Availability	Dosage Range	Side Effects
Butenafine (p. 148) (Mentax)	**C**: 1%	2 times/day	Burning, stinging, itching, contact dermatitis, erythema
Ciclopirox (p. 223) (Loprox)	**C**: 1% **L**: 1%	2 times/day	Irritation, pruritus, redness
Clioquinol (Vioform)	**C**: 3% **O**: 3%	2–3 times/day	Irritation, stinging, swelling
Clotrimazole (p. 249) (Lotrimin, Mycelex)	**C**: 1% **L**: 1% **S**: 1%	2 times/day	Erythema, stinging, blistering, edema, itching
Econazole (Spectazole)	**C**: 1%	1–2 times/day	Burning, stinging, irritation, erythema
Ketoconazole (p. 604) (Nizoral)	**C**: 2%	1–2 times/day	Irritation, itching, stinging
Miconazole (p. 708) (Micatin, Monistat)	**C**: 2% **P**: 2%	2 times/day	Irritation, burning, allergic contact dermatitis

Nystatin (p. 788) (Mycostatin, Nilstat)	**C**: 100,000 g **O**: 100,000 g **P**: 100,000 g	2–3 times/day	Irritation
Oxiconazole (p. 813) (Oxistat)	**C**: 1% **L**: 1%	1–2 times/day	Pruritus, burning, stinging, irritation, pain, tingling
Terbinafine (p. 1018) (Lamisil)	**C**: 1% **G**: 10 mg	1–2 times/day	Irritation, burning, itching, dryness
Tolnaftate (p. 1051) (Tinactin)	**C**: 1% **G**: 1% **S**: 1%	2 times/day	Mild irritation
Triacetin (Fungoid)	**C**: 1% **S**: 1%	3 times/day	Irritation
Undecylenic acid (Desenex, Cruex, Caldesene)	**C, O, P**	As needed	None significant

C, Cream; ***G,*** gel; ***L,*** lotion; ***O,*** ointment; ***P,*** powder; ***S,*** solution.

Antiglaucoma Agents

USES

Reduction of elevated intraocular pressure (IOP) in pts with open-angle glaucoma and ocular hypertension.

ACTION

Medications that decrease IOP by increasing outflow of aqueous humor:

- *Miotics (direct acting):* Cholinergic agents or miotics stimulate ciliary muscles, leading to increases in contraction of the iris sphincter muscle.

Antiglaucoma Agents (continued)

ACTION (cont.)

- *Miotics (indirect acting):* Primarily inhibit cholinesterase, allowing accumulation of acetylcholine, prolonging parasympathetic activity.
- *Sympathomimetics:* Increase both the rate of fluid flow out of the eye and decrease the rate of aqueous humor production.

Medications that decrease IOP by decreasing aqueous humor production:

- *Alpha$_2$-agonists:* Activate receptors in ciliary body, inhibiting aqueous secretion and increasing uveoscleral aqueous outflow.
- *Beta-blockers:* Reduce production of aqueous humor.
- *Carbonic anhydrase inhibitors:* Reduce fluid flow into the eye by inhibiting enzyme carbonic anhydrase.
- *Prostaglandins:* Increase outflow of aqueous fluid through uveoscleral route.

ANTIGLAUCOMA AGENTS

Name	Availability	Dosage Range	Side Effects
Miotics			
Carbachol (p. 164) (Isopto-Carbachol)	**S:** 0.75%, 1.5%, 2.25%, 3%	1 drop 2 times/day	Ciliary or accommodative spasm, blurred vision, reduced night vision, sweating, increased salivation, urinary frequency, nausea, diarrhea
Echothiophate (p. 367) (Phospholine Iodide)	**S:** 0.03%, 0.06%, 0.125%, 0.25%	1 drop 2 times/day	Headaches, accommodative spasm, sweating, vomiting, nausea, diarrhea, tachycardia
Physostigmine (p. 860) (Eserine)	**O:** 0.25%	Apply up to 3 times/day	Blurred vision, eye pain
Pilocarpine (p. 861) (Isopto, Carpine)	**S:** 0.25%, 0.5%, 1%, 2%, 3%, 4%, 5%, 6%, 8%, 10%	1–2 drops 3–4 times/day	Same as carbachol

Sympathomimetics			
Dipivefrin (p. 336) (Propine)	**S:** 0.1%	1 drop q12h	Ocular congestion, burning, stinging
Epinephrine (p. 379) (Epifrin, Epinal)	**S:** 0.5%, 1%, 2%	1 drop 1–2 times/day	Mydriasis, blurred vision, tachycardia, hypertension, tremors, headaches, anxiety
Alpha$_2$-Agonists			
Apraclonidine (p. 76) (Iopidine)	**S:** 0.5%	1–2 drops 3 times/day	Ocular allergic-like reactions, hypersensitivity reaction, change in visual activity, lethargy
Brimonidine (p. 138) (Alphagan)	**S:** 0.2%	1–2 drops 2–3 times/day	Ocular allergy, headaches, drowsiness, fatigue
Prostaglandins			
Bimatoprost (p. 124) (Lumigan)	**S:** 0.03%	1 drop daily in evening	Ocular hyperemia, eyelash growth, pruritus
Latanoprost (p. 619) (Xalatan)	**S:** 0.005%	1 drop daily in evening	Burning, stinging, iris pigmentation
Travoprost (p. 1068) (Travatan)	**S:** 0.004%	1 drop daily in evening	Ocular hyperemia, eye discomfort, foreign body sensation, pain, pruritus
Unoprostone (Rescula)	**S:** 0.15%	1 drop 2 times/day	Iris pigmentations
Beta-Blockers			
Betaxolol (p. 119) (Betoptic)	**Suspension:** 0.25% **S:** 0.5%	1–2 drops 1–2 times/day	Transient irritation, burning, tearing, blurred vision
Carteolol (p. 172) (Ocupress)	**S:** 1%	1 drop 2 times/day	Mild, transient ocular stinging, burning, discomfort

(continued)

ANTIGLAUCOMA AGENTS ***(continued)***

Name	Availability	Dosage Range	Side Effects
Beta-Blockers ***(continued)***			
Levobetaxolol (Betaxon)	**S:** 0.5%	1 drop 2 times/day	Transient irritation, burning, tearing, blurred vision
Levobunolol (p. 629) (Betagan)	**S:** 0.25%, 0.5%	1 drop 1–2 times/day	Local discomfort, conjunctivitis, brow ache, tearing, blurred vision, headache, anxiety
Metipranolol (p. 698) (OptiPranolol)	**S:** 0.3%	1 drop 2 times/day	Transient irritation, burning, stinging, blurred vision
Timolol (p. 1038) (Timoptic)	**S:** 0.25%, 0.5% **G:** 0.25%, 0.5%	**S:** 1 drop 2 times/day **G:** 1 drop daily	Same as above
Carbonic Anhydrase Inhibitors			
Acetazolamide (p. 9) (Diamox)	**T:** 125 mg, 250 mg **C:** 500 mg	0.25–1 g/day	Diarrhea, loss of appetite, metallic taste, nausea, tingling in hands/fingers
Brinzolamide (p. 138) (Azopt)	**Suspension:** 1%	1 drop 3 times/day	Blurred vision, bitter taste
Dorzolamide (p. 353) (Trusopt)	**S:** 2%	1 drop 2–3 times/day	Burning, stinging, blurred vision, bitter taste

C, Capsules; ***G,*** gel; ***O,*** ointment; ***S,*** solution; ***T,*** tablets.

Antihistamines

USES

Symptomatic relief of upper respiratory allergic disorders. Allergic reactions associated with other drugs respond to antihistamines, as do blood transfusion reactions. Used as a second-choice drug in treatment of angioneurotic edema. Effective in treatment of acute urticaria and other dermatologic conditions. May also be used for preop sedation, Parkinson's disease, and motion sickness.

ACTION

Antihistamines (H_1 antagonists) inhibit vasoconstrictor effects and vasodilator effects on endothelial cells of histamine. They block increased capillary permeability, formation of edema/wheal caused by histamine. Many antihistamines can bind to receptors in CNS, causing primarily depression (decreased alertness, slowed reaction times, somnolence) but also stimulation (restlessness, nervousness, inability to sleep). Some may counter motion sickness.

ANTIHISTAMINES

Name	Availability	Dosage Range	Side Effects
Azatadine (Optimine)	**T:** 1 mg	**A:** 1–2 mg q12h **C:** 0.05 mg/kg/day	Dry mouth, urinary retention, blurred vision, sedation, dizziness, paradoxical excitement
Brompheniramine (p. 140) (Dimetane)	**T:** 4 mg **T (SR):** 4 mg, 6 mg **S:** 2 mg/5 ml	**A:** 4–8 mg q4–6h or **T (SR):** 8–12 mg q12–24h **C:** 0.5 mg/kg/day	Dry mouth, urinary retention, blurred vision
Cetirizine (p. 206) (Zyrtec)	**T:** 5 mg, 10 mg **S:** 5 mg/5 ml	**A:** 5–10 mg/day **C (6–12 yrs):** 5–10 mg/day **C (2–5 yrs):** 2.5–5 mg/day	Minimal CNS and anticholinergic side effects

(continued)

ANTIHISTAMINES *(continued)*

Name	Availability	Dosage Range	Side Effects
Chlorpheniramine (p. 217) (Chlor-Trimeton)	**T**: 4 mg **T (chewable)**: 2 mg **T (SR)**: 8 mg, 12 mg **S**: 2 mg/5 ml	**A**: 2–4 mg q4–6h or **SR**: 8–12 mg q12–24h **C**: 0.35 mg/kg/day	Same as brompheniramine
Clemastine (p. 238) (Tavist)	**T**: 1.34 mg, 2.68 mg **S**: 0.67 mg/5 ml	**A**: 1.34–2.68 mg q8–12h **C (6–12 yrs)**: 0.67–1.34 mg q8–12h	Same as azatadine
Cyproheptadine (p. 275) (Periactin)	**T**: 4 mg **S**: 2 mg/5 ml	**A**: 4 mg q8h **C**: 0.25 mg/kg/day	Same as azatadine
Dexchlorpheniramine (Polaramine)	**T**: 2 mg **S**: 2 mg/5 ml	**A**: 2 mg q4–6h **C**: 0.5–1 mg q4–6h	Same as brompheniramine
Dimenhydrinate (p. 330) (Dramamine)	**T**: 50 mg **L**: 12.5 mg/5 ml	**A**: 50–100 mg q4–6h **C**: 12.5–50 mg q6–8h	Same as azatadine
Diphenhydramine (p. 332) (Benadryl)	**T**: 25 mg, 50 mg **C**: 25 mg, 50 mg **L**: 6.25 mg/5 ml, 12.5 mg/5 ml	**A**: 25–50 mg q6–8h **C (6–11 yrs)**: 12.5–25 mg q4–6h **(2–5 yrs)**: 6.25 mg q4–6h	Same as azatadine
Fexofenadine (p. 434) (Allegra)	**T**: 30 mg, 60 mg, 180 mg	**A**: 60 mg q12h or 180 mg/day; **C (6–11 yrs)**: 30 mg q12h	Same as cetirizine
Hydroxyzine (p. 541) (Atarax, Vistaril)	**T**: 10 mg, 25 mg, 50 mg, 100 mg **C**: 25 mg, 50 mg, 100 mg **S**: 10 mg/5 ml, 25 mg/5 ml	**A**: 25 mg q6–8h **C**: 2 mg/kg/day	Same as azatadine

Loratadine (p. 651) **(Claritin)**	**T**: 10 mg **S**: 1 mg/ml	**A**: 10 mg/day **C (6–12 yrs)**: 10 mg/day	Same as cetirizine
Promethazine (p. 894) **(Phenergan)**	**T**: 12.5 mg, 25 mg, 50 mg **S**: 6.25 mg/5 ml, 25 mg/5 ml	**A**: 25 mg at bedtime or 12.5 mg q8h **C**: 0.5 mg/kg at bedtime or 0.1 mg/kg q6–8h	Same as azatadine

A, Adults; ***C,*** capsules; ***C (dosage),*** children; ***L,*** liquid; ***S,*** syrup; ***SR,*** sustained-release; ***T,*** tablets.

Antihyperlipidemics

USES	ACTION
Cholesterol management.	*Bile acid sequestrants:* Bind bile acids in the intestine; prevent active transport and reabsorption and enhance bile acid excretion. Depletion of hepatic bile acid results in the increased conversion of cholesterol to bile acids. *HMG-CoA reductase inhibitors (statins):* Inhibit HMG-CoA reductase, the last regulated step in the synthesis of cholesterol. Cholesterol synthesis in the liver is reduced. *Niacin (nicotinic acid):* Reduces hepatic synthesis of triglycerides and secretion of VLDL by inhibiting the mobilization of free fatty acids from peripheral tissues. *Fibric acid:* Increases the oxidation of fatty acids in the liver, resulting in reduced secretion of triglyceride-rich lipoproteins and increases lipoprotein lipase activity and fatty acid uptake. *Cholesterol absorption inhibitor:* Acts in the gut wall to prevent cholesterol absorption through the intestinal villi.

Antihyperlipidemics *(continued)*

ANTIHYPERLIPIDEMICS

Name	Availability	Primary Effect	Dosage Range (per day)	Side Effects
Bile Acid Sequestrants				
Cholestipol (Colestid)	**T:** 1 g **G:** 5 g	Decreases LDL	**T:** 2–16 g **G:** 5–30 g	GI complaints (constipation, bloating, abdominal pain, gas), reduced absorption of other drugs
Cholestyramine (p. 221) (Questran, Prevalite)	**P:** 4 g	Decreases LDL	4–8 g	Same as cholestipol
Colesevelam (p. 256) (Welchol)	**T:** 625 mg	Decreases LDL	4–6 **T**	Same as cholestipol
HMG-CoA Reductase Inhibitors (Statins)				
Atorvastatin (p. 93) (Lipitor)	**T:** 10 mg, 20 mg, 40 mg, 80 mg	Decreases LDL, TG Increases HDL	10–80 mg	Headaches, dizziness, nausea, vomiting, diarrhea, myalgia, increased LFTs, rhabdomyolysis
Fluvastatin (p. 462) (Lescol)	**C:** 20 mg, 40 mg **T (ER):** 80 mg	Decreases LDL, TG Increases HDL	20–80 mg	Same as above
Lovastatin (p. 656) (Mevacor)	**T:** 10 mg, 20 mg, 40 mg	Decreases LDL, TG Increases HDL	10–80 mg	Same as above
Pravastatin (p. 878) (Pravachol)	**T:** 10 mg, 20 mg, 40 mg	Decreases LDL, TG Increases HDL	10–40 mg	Same as above

Rosuvastatin (p. 953) (Crestor)	**T:** 5 mg, 10 mg, 20 mg, 40 mg	Decreases LDL, TG Increases HDL	5–40 mg	Same as above
Simvastatin (p. 971) (Zocor)	**T:** 5 mg, 10 mg, 20 mg, 40 mg, 80 mg	Decreases LDL, TG Increases HDL	5–80 mg	Same as above
Niacin				
Nicotinic acid (p. 765) *Crystalline* (Niacor)	**T:** 500 mg	Decreases LDL, TG Increases HDL	Up to 6 g	Flushing, liver toxicity, increased glucose, GI complaints, gout
Nicotinic acid (p. 765) *Long-acting* (Niaspan)	**T (ER):** 500 mg, 750 mg, 1,000 mg	Decreases LDL, TG Increases HDL	Up to 2,000 mg	Same as above
Fibric Acid				
Fenofibrate (p. 425) (Tricor)	**C:** 67 mg, 134 mg, 200 mg	Decreases TG	67–200 mg	Diarrhea, nausea, constipation, abdominal pain, back pain, headaches
Gemfibrozil (p. 492) (Lopid)	**T:** 600 mg	Decreases TG	1,200 mg	Dyspepsia, abdominal pain, diarrhea, nausea, vomiting, fatigue
Cholesterol Absorption Inhibitor				
Ezetimibe (p. 419) (Zetia)	**T:** 10 mg	Decreases LDL, TG	10 mg	Headache, viral infection, arthralgia, upper respiratory tract infections

C, Capsules; ***ER,*** extended-release; ***G,*** granules; ***HDL,*** high-density lipoprotein; ***LDL,*** low-density lipoprotein; ***LFTs,*** liver function tests; ***P,*** powder; ***T,*** tablets; ***TG,*** triglycerides.

Antihypertensives

USES

Treatment of mild to severe hypertension.

ACTION

Many groups of medications are used in the treatment of hypertension. In addition to the alpha-adrenergic central agonists, peripheral antagonists, and vasodilators listed in the following table, refer to the classifications of diuretics, beta-adrenergic blockers, calcium channel blockers, and ACE inhibitors or to individual drug monographs.

Alpha-agonists (central action): Stimulate alpha$_2$-adrenergic receptors in the cardiovascular centers of the CNS, reducing sympathetic outflow and producing an antihypertensive effect.

Alpha-antagonists (peripheral action): Block alpha$_1$-adrenergic receptors in arterioles and veins, inhibiting vasoconstriction and decreasing peripheral vascular resistance, causing a fall in B/P.

Vasodilators: Directly relax arteriolar smooth muscle, decreasing vascular resistance. Exact mechanism unknown.

ANTIHYPERTENSIVES

Name	Availability	Dosage Range	Side Effects
Alpha-Agonists: Central Action			
Clonidine (p. 245) (Catapres)	**T:** 0.1 mg, 0.2 mg, 0.3 mg **P:** 0.1 mg/hr, 0.2 mg/hr, 0.3 mg/hr	**PO:** 0.2–0.8 mg/day **Topical:** 0.1–0.6 mg/wk	Sedation, dry mouth, constipation, sexual dysfunction, bradycardia
Guanabenz (p. 519) (Wytensin)	**T:** 4 mg, 8 mg	**PO:** 8–32 mg/day	Same as above
Guanfacine (p. 519) (Tenex)	**T:** 1 mg, 2 mg	**PO:** 1–3 mg/day	Same as above
Methyldopa (p. 692) (Aldomet)	**T:** 125 mg, 250 mg, 500 mg	**PO:** 0.5–3 g/day	Same as above Forgetfulness, depression, nasal stuffiness

Alpha-Agonists: Peripheral Action			
Doxazosin (p. 353) (Cardura)	**T:** 1 mg, 2 mg, 4 mg, 8 mg	**PO:** 2–16 mg/day	Dizziness, vertigo, headaches
Prazosin (p. 879) (Minipress)	**C:** 1 mg, 2 mg, 5 mg	**PO:** 6–20 mg/day	Dizziness, lightheadedness, headaches, drowsiness
Terazosin (p. 1016) (Hytrin)	**C:** 1 mg, 2 mg, 5 mg, 10 mg	**PO:** 1–20 mg/day	Dizziness, headaches, asthenia
Vasodilators			
Hydralazine (p. 527) (Apresoline)	**T:** 10 mg, 25 mg, 50 mg, 100 mg	**PO:** 40–300 mg/day	Anorexia, nausea, diarrhea, vomiting, headaches, palpitations
Minoxidil (p. 717) (Loniten)	**T:** 2.5 mg, 10 mg	**PO:** 10–40 mg/day	Fast/irregular heartbeat, hypertrichosis, swelling of feet/legs

C, Capsules; ***P,*** patch; ***T,*** tablets.

Antimigraine (Triptans)

USES

Treatment of migraine headaches with or without aura in adults ≥18 yrs.

ACTION

Triptans are selective agonists of the serotonin (5-HT) receptor that inhibit neuropeptide release and vasodilation, causing vasoconstriction.

Antimigraine (Triptans) *(continued)*

TRIPTANS

Name	Availability	Dosage Range	Contraindications	Side Effects
Almotriptan (p. 32) (Axert)	**T:** 6.25 mg, 12.5 mg	6.25–12.5 mg; may repeat in >2 hrs	Ischemic heart disease, angina pectoris, arrhythmias, previous MI, uncontrolled hypertension	Drowsiness, dizziness, fatigue, hot flashes, chest tightness, tingling in extremities, nausea, vomiting
Eletriptan (p. 369) (Relpax)	**T:** 20 mg, 40 mg	**A:** 20–40 mg. May repeat in >2 hrs	Same as above	Asthenia, nausea, dizziness, somnolence
Frovatriptan (p. 476) (Frovan)	**T:** 2.5 mg	2.5 mg; may repeat in >2 hrs; no more than 3 **T**/day	Same as above	Hot/cold sensations, dizziness, fatigue, headache, chest pain, skeletal pain, dry mouth, dyspepsia, flushing
Naratriptan (p. 753) (Amerge)	**T:** 1 mg, 2.5 mg	2.5 mg; may repeat once >4 hrs	Same as above	Atypical sensations, pain, nausea
Rizatriptan (p. 948) (Maxalt, Maxalt-MLT)	**T:** 5 mg, 10 mg **DT:** 5 mg, 10 mg	5 or 10 mg; may repeat in >2 hrs	Same as above	Atypical sensations, pain, nausea, dizziness, somnolence, asthenia, fatigue
Sumatriptan (p. 999) (Imitrex)	**T:** 25 mg, 50 mg **NS:** 5 mg, 20 mg **I:** 6 mg	**PO:** 25–100 mg; may repeat q2h **NS:** 5–20 mg; may repeat in >2 hrs **Subcutaneous:** 6 mg; may repeat in >1 hr	Ischemic heart disease, angina pectoris, arrhythmias, previous MI, uncontrolled hypertension	*Oral:* Atypical sensations, pain, malaise, fatigue *Injection:* Atypical sensations, flushing, chest discomfort, injection site reaction, dizziness, vertigo *Nasal:* Discomfort, nausea, vomiting, altered taste

Zolmitriptan (p. 1136) (Zomig)	**T:** 2.5 mg, 5 mg **DT:** 2.5 mg, 5 mg	2.5–5 mg; may repeat in >2 hrs	Same as above	Atypical sensations, pain, nausea, dizziness, asthenia, somnolence

DT, Disintegrating tablets; ***I,*** injection; ***NS,*** nasal spray; ***T,*** tablets.

Antipsychotics

USES

Antipsychotics are primarily used in managing psychotic illness (esp. in pts with increased psychomotor activity). They are also used to treat the manic phase of bipolar disorder, behavioral problems in children, nausea and vomiting, intractable hiccups, anxiety and agitation, as adjunct in treatment of tetanus, and to potentiate effects of narcotics.

ACTION

Effects of these agents occur at all levels of the CNS. Antipsychotic mechanism unknown but may antagonize dopamine action as a neurotransmitter in basal ganglia and limbic system. Antipsychotics may block postsynaptic dopamine receptors, inhibit dopamine release, increase dopamine turnover. These medications can be divided into the phenothiazines and nonphenothiazines (miscellaneous). In addition to their use in symptomatic treatment of psychiatric illness, some have antiemetic, antinausea, antihistamine, anticholinergic, and/or sedative effects.

ANTIPSYCHOTICS

			Relative Side Effects Profile			
Name	Availability	Dosage	EPS	Anticholinergic	Sedation	Hypotension
Aripiprazole (p. 79) (Abilify)	**T:** 5 mg, 10 mg, 15 mg	15–30 mg/day	Low	Low	Low	Low

(continued)

ANTIPSYCHOTICS *(continued)*

Name	Availability	Dosage	Relative Side Effects Profile			
			EPS	Anticholinergic	Sedation	Hypotension
Chlorpromazine (p. 217) (Thorazine)	**T:** 10 mg, 25 mg, 50 mg, 100 mg, 200 mg **SR:** 30 mg, 75 mg, 100 mg **OC:** 30 mg/ml, 100 mg/ml	50–2,000 mg/day	Moderate	Moderate	High	High
Clozapine (p. 251) (Clozaril)	**T:** 25 mg, 100 mg	75–900 mg/day	Rare	High	High	High
Fluphenazine (p. 455) (Prolixin)	**T:** 1 mg, 2.5 mg, 5 mg, 10 mg **I:** 25 mg/ml **OC:** 5 mg/ml	**PO:** 2–40 mg/day **I:** 12.5–75 mg q2wks	High	Low	Low	Low
Haloperidol (p. 519) (Haldol)	**T:** 0.5 mg, 1 mg, 2 mg, 5 mg, 10 mg, 20 mg **I:** 5 mg/ml **OC:** 2 mg/ml	2–40 mg/day	High	Low	Low	Low
Loxapine (p. 657) (Loxitane)	**C:** 5 mg, 10 mg, 25 mg, 50 mg **OC:** 25 mg/ml **I:** 50 mg/ml	20–250 mg/day	High	Low	Moderate	Moderate
Mesoridazine (p. 680) (Serentil)	**T:** 10 mg, 25 mg, 50 mg, 100 mg **I:** 25 mg/ml **OC:** 25 mg/ml	100–400 mg/day	Low	High	High	High
Olanzapine (p. 795) (Zyprexa)	**T:** 2.5 mg, 5 mg, 7.5 mg, 10 mg, 15 mg, 20 mg **DT:** 5 mg, 10 mg	10–20 mg/day	Low	Low	Moderate	Low

Quetiapine (p. 913) (Seroquel)	**T:** 25 mg, 100 mg, 200 mg, 300 mg	100–800 mg/day	Rare	Low	Moderate	Moderate
Risperidone (p. 942) (Risperdal)	**T:** 0.25 mg, 0.5 mg, 1 mg, 2 mg, 3 mg, 4 mg **OC:** 1 mg/ml	2–6 mg/day	Low	Low	Low	Moderate
Thioridazine (p. 1028) (Mellaril)	**T:** 10 mg, 15 mg, 25 mg, 50 mg, 100 mg, 150 mg, 200 mg **OC:** 30 mg/ml, 100 mg/ml	50–800 mg/day	Low	High	High	High
Thiothixene (p. 1031) (Navane)	**C:** 1 mg, 2 mg, 5 mg	5–60 mg/day	High	Low	Low	Low
Trifluoperazine (p. 1078) (Stelazine)	**T:** 1 mg, 2 mg, 5 mg, 10 mg **I:** 5 mg/ml **OC:** 2 mg/ml	5–80 mg/day	High	Low	Low	Low
Ziprasidone (p. 1133) (Geodon)	**C:** 20 mg, 40 mg, 60 mg, 80 mg **I:** 20 mg	40–160 mg/day	Low	Low	Low to moderate	Low to moderate

C, Capsules; ***DT,*** disintegrating tablets; ***EPS,*** extrapyramidal symptoms; ***I,*** injection; ***OC,*** oral concentrate; ***SR,*** sustained-release; ***T,*** tablets.

Antivirals

USES

Treatment of HIV infection. Treatment of CMV retinitis in pts with AIDS, acute herpes zoster (shingles), genital herpes (recurrent), mucosal and cutaneous herpes simplex virus, chickenpox, and influenza A viral illness.

ACTION

Effective antivirals must inhibit virus-specific nucleic acid/protein synthesis. Possible mechanisms of action of antivirals used for non-HIV infection may include interference with viral DNA synthesis and viral replication, inactivation of viral DNA polymerases, incorporation and termination of the growing viral DNA chain, prevention of release of viral nucleic acid into the host cell, or interference with viral penetration into cells.

Antivirals *(continued)*

ANTIVIRALS

Name	Availability	Uses	Side Effects
Abacavir (p. 1) (Ziagen)	**T:** 300 mg **OS:** 20 mg/ml	HIV infection	Nausea, vomiting, loss of appetite, diarrhea, headaches, fatigue
Acyclovir (p. 12) (Zovirax)	**T:** 400 mg, 800 mg **C:** 200 mg **I:** 50 mg/ml	Mucosal/cutaneous HSV-1 and HSV-2, varicella-zoster (shingles), genital herpes, herpes simplex, encephalitis, chickenpox	Malaise, anorexia, nausea, vomiting, lightheadedness
Adefovir (p. 15) (Hepsera)	**T:** 10 mg	Chronic hepatitis B	Asthenia, headache, abdominal pain, nausea, diarrhea, flatulence, dyspepsia
Amantadine (p. 42) (Symmetrel)	**C:** 100 mg **S:** 50 mg/5 ml	Influenza A	Anxiety, dizziness, lightheadedness, headaches, nausea, loss of appetite
Amprenavir (p. 69) (Agenerase)	**C:** 50 mg, 150 mg **OS:** 15 mg/ml	HIV infection	Hyperglycemia, rash, abdominal pain, nausea, vomiting, diarrhea
Cidofovir (p. 223) (Vistide)	**I:** 75 mg/ml	CMV retinitis	Decreased urination, fever, chills, diarrhea, nausea, vomiting, headaches, loss of appetite
Delavirdine (p. 293) (Rescriptor)	**T:** 100 mg, 200 mg	HIV infection	Diarrhea, fatigue, rash, headaches, nausea
Didanosine (p. 320) (Videx)	**T:** 25 mg, 50 mg, 100 mg, 150 mg, 200 mg **C:** 125 mg, 200 mg **Powder for suspension:** 100 mg, 167 mg, 250 mg	HIV infection	Peripheral neuropathy, anxiety, headaches, rash, nausea, diarrhea, dry mouth

Efavirenz (p. 367) (Sustiva)	**C:** 50 mg, 100 mg, 200 mg	HIV infection	Diarrhea, dizziness, headaches, insomnia, nausea, vomiting, drowsiness
Famciclovir (p. 420) (Famvir)	**T:** 125 mg, 250 mg, 500 mg	Herpes zoster, genital herpes	Headaches
Foscarnet (p. 469) (Foscavir)	**I:** 24 mg/ml	CMV retinitis, HSV infections	Decreased urination, abdominal pain, nausea, vomiting, dizziness, fatigue, headaches
Ganciclovir (p. 483) (Cytovene)	**C:** 250 mg, 500 mg **I:** 500 mg	CMV retinitis, CMV disease	Sore throat, fever, unusual bleeding/bruising
Indinavir (p. 564) (Crixivan)	**C:** 200 mg, 400 mg	HIV infection	Blood in urine, weakness, nausea, vomiting, diarrhea, headaches, insomnia, altered taste
Lamivudine (p. 613) (Epivir)	**T:** 100 mg, 150 mg **OS:** 5 mg/ml, 10 mg/ml	HIV infection	Nausea, vomiting, stomach pain, tingling, numbness
Lopinavir/ritonavir (p. 648) (Kaletra)	**C:** 133/33 mg **OS:** 80/20 mg	HIV infection	Diarrhea, nausea
Nelfinavir (p. 758) (Viracept)	**T:** 250 mg **Powder:** 50 mg/g	HIV infection	Diarrhea
Oseltamivir (p. 806) (Tamiflu)	**C:** 75 mg **S:** 12 mg/ml	Influenza	Diarrhea, nausea, vomiting
Ribavirin (p. 934) (Virazole)	**Aerosol:** 6 g	Lowers respiratory infections in infants, children due to respiratory syncytial virus (RSV)	Anemia
Ritonavir (p. 944) (Norvir)	**C:** 100 mg **OS:** 80 mg/ml	HIV infection	Weakness, diarrhea, nausea, decreased appetite, vomiting, altered taste

(continued)

ANTIVIRALS ***(continued)***

Name	Availability	Uses	Side Effects
Saquinavir (p. 958) (Invirase)	**C:** 200 mg	HIV infection	Weakness, diarrhea, nausea, mouth ulcers, abdominal pain
Stavudine (p. 986) (Zerit)	**C:** 15 mg, 20 mg, 30 mg, 40 mg **OS:** 1 mg/ml	HIV infection	Numbness in hands/feet, decreased appetite, chills, fever, rash
Tenofovir (p. 1015) (Viread)	**T:** 300 mg	HIV infection	Diarrhea, nausea, pharyngitis, headaches
Valacyclovir (p. 1087) (Valtrex)	**T:** 500 mg	Herpes zoster, genital herpes	Headaches, nausea
Valganciclovir (p. 1091) (Valcyte)	**T:** 450 mg	CMV retinitis	Anemia, abdominal pain, diarrhea, headaches, nausea, vomiting, numbness in hands/feet
Zalcitabine (p. 1125) (Hivid)	**T:** 0.375 mg, 0.75 mg	HIV infection	Numbness in arms/feet/legs, joint pain, rash, nausea, vomiting
Zanamivir (p. 1128) (Relenza)	**Inhalation:** 5 mg	Influenza	Cough, diarrhea, dizziness, headaches, nausea, vomiting
Zidovudine (p. 1129) (Retrovir)	**T:** 300 mg **C:** 100 mg **S:** 50 mg/5 ml	HIV infection	Unusual tiredness, fever, chills, headaches, nausea, muscle pain

C, Capsules; ***I,*** injection; ***OS,*** oral solution; ***S,*** syrup; ***T,*** tablets.

Beta-Adrenergic Blockers

USES

Management of hypertension, angina pectoris, arrhythmias, hypertrophic subaortic stenosis, migraine headaches, MI (prevention), glaucoma.

ACTION

Beta-adrenergic blockers competitively block $beta_1$-adrenergic receptors, located primarily in myocardium, and $beta_2$-adrenergic receptors, located primarily in bronchial and vascular smooth muscle. By occupying beta-receptor sites, these agents prevent naturally occurring or administered epinephrine/norepinephrine from exerting their effects. The results are basically opposite to those of sympathetic stimulation.

Effects of $beta_1$-blockade include slowing heart rate, decreasing cardiac output and contractility; effects of $beta_2$-blockade include bronchoconstriction, increased airway resistance in pts with asthma or chronic obstructive pulmonary disease (COPD). Beta-blockers can affect cardiac rhythm/automaticity (decrease sinus rate, SA/AV conduction; increase refractory period in AV node). Decrease systolic and diastolic B/P; exact mechanism unknown but may block peripheral receptors, decrease sympathetic outflow from CNS, or decrease renin release from kidney. All beta-blockers mask tachycardia that occurs with hypoglycemia. When applied to the eye, reduce intraocular pressure and aqueous production.

BETA-ADRENERGIC BLOCKERS

Name	Availability	Selectivity	Dosage Range	Side Effects
Acebutolol (p. 5) (Sectral)	**C:** 200 mg, 400 mg	$Beta_1$	200–1,200 mg/day	Lightheadedness, fatigue, weakness, decreased sexual ability, trouble sleeping
Atenolol (p. 89) (Tenormin)	**T:** 25 mg, 50 mg, 100 mg	$Beta_1$	50–100 mg/day	Same as above
Betaxolol (p. 119) (Kerlone)	**T:** 10 mg, 20 mg	$Beta_1$	10–20 mg/day	Same as above

(continued)

BETA-ADRENERGIC BLOCKERS ***(continued)***

Name	Availability	Selectivity	Dosage Range	Side Effects
Bisoprolol (p. 126) (Zebeta)	**T:** 5 mg, 10 mg	$Beta_1$	2.5–20 mg/day	Same as above
Carteolol (p. 172) (Cartrol)	**T:** 2.5 mg, 5 mg	$Beta_1$, $beta_2$	2.5–10 mg/day	Same as above
Carvedilol (p. 172) (Coreg)	**T:** 3.125 mg, 6.25 mg, 12.5 mg, 25 mg	$Beta_1$, $beta_2$, $alpha_1$	12.5–50 mg/day	Same as above
Esmolol (p. 399) (Brevibloc)	**I:** 10 mg/ml, 250 mcg/ml	$Beta_1$	50–200 mcg/kg/min	Same as above
Metoprolol (p. 702) (Lopressor)	**T:** 50 mg, 100 mg/ml **I:** 1 mg/ml	$Beta_1$	50–450 mg/day	Same as above, increased risk of CNS effects
Nadolol (p. 742) (Corgard)	**T:** 20 mg, 40 mg, 80 mg, 120 mg, 160 mg	$Beta_1$, $beta_2$	40–320 mg/day	Same as above
Penbutolol (p. 835) (Levatol)	**T:** 20 mg	$Beta_1$, $beta_2$	10–40 mg/day	Same as above
Pindolol (p. 863) (Visken)	**T:** 5 mg, 10 mg	$Beta_1$, $beta_2$	10–60 mg/day	Same as above
Propranolol (p. 901) (Inderal)	**T:** 10 mg, 20 mg, 40 mg, 60 mg, 80 mg, 90 mg **C (SR):** 60 mg, 80 mg, 120 mg, 160 mg **S:** 4 mg/ml, 8 mg/ml **I:** 1 mg/ml	$Beta_1$, $beta_2$	80–320 mg/day	Same as above, increased risk of CNS effects

Sotalol (p. 983) (Betapace)	**T:** 80 mg, 120 mg, 160 mg, 240 mg	$Beta_1$, $beta_2$	160–640 mg/day	Same as above
Timolol (p. 1038) (Blocadren)	**T:** 5 mg, 10 mg, 20 mg	$Beta_1$, $beta_2$	10–60 mg/day	Same as above

C, Capsules; ***I,*** injection; ***S,*** solution; ***SR,*** sustained-release; ***T,*** tablets.

Bronchodilators

USES	ACTION
Relief of bronchospasm occurring during anesthesia and in bronchial asthma, bronchitis, emphysema.	*Inhaled corticosteroids:* Exact mechanism unknown. May act as anti-inflammatories, decrease mucus secretion. *$Beta_2$-adrenergic agonists:* Stimulate beta-receptors in lung, relax bronchial smooth muscle, increase vital capacity, decrease airway resistance. *Anticholinergics:* Inhibit cholinergic receptors on bronchial smooth muscle (block acetylcholine action). *Leukotriene modifiers:* Decrease effect of leukotrienes, which increase migration of eosinophils, producing mucus/edema of airway wall, causing bronchoconstriction. *Methylxanthines:* Directly relax smooth muscle of bronchial airway, pulmonary blood vessels (relieve bronchospasm, increase vital capacity). Increase cyclic 3,5-adenosine monophosphate.

Bronchodilators *(continued)*

BRONCHODILATORS

Name	Availability	Dosage Range	Side Effects
Beta-Agonists			
Albuterol (p. 21) **(Proventil, Ventolin, Ventolin Rotacaps, Volmax, Accuneb)**	**T:** 2 mg, 4 mg **T (SR):** 4 mg, 8 mg **S:** 2 mg/5 ml **MDI (Neb):** 0.5%, 2.5 mg/3 ml, 1.25 mg/3 ml, 0.63 mg/3 ml	**A, C (MDI):** 2 puffs q4–6h as needed **A, C (Rotacaps):** 1–2 caps q4–6h as needed **A (Neb):** 2.5 mg q4–6h as needed **C (Neb):** 0.1–0.15 mg/kg q4–6h as needed **A [T (SR)]:** 4–8 mg q12h **C [T (SR)]:** 4 mg q12h	Tremors, tachycardia, palpitations, hypokalemia
Formoterol (p. 468) **(Foradil)**	**C:** 12 mcg	**A:** 1 capsule q12h	Same as above
Levalbuterol (p. 627) **(Xopenex)**	**Neb:** 0.63 mg/3 ml, 1.25 mg/3 ml	**A:** 0.63 mg q6–8h as needed	Same as above
Metaproterenol (p. 681) **(Alupent, Metaprel)**	**MDI (Neb):** 5% **S:** 10 mg/5 ml **T:** 10 mg, 20 mg		Same as above
Piruterol **(Maxair)**	**MDI**	**A, C:** 2 puffs q4–6h as needed	Same as above

Salmeterol (p. 955) **(Serevent)**	**MDI** **C:** 50 mcg	**A (MDI):** 2 puffs q12h **C:** 1–2 puffs q12h **A, C (C):** 1 inhalation q12h	Same as above
Terbutaline (p. 1019) **(Brethine, Bricanyl)**	**MDI** **T:** 2.5 mg, 5 mg	**A:** 2.5 mg 3–4 times/day **C:** 0.05 mg/kg/dose 3 times/day	Same as above
Inhaled Anti-Inflammatory Agents			
Beclomethasone (p. 111) **(Beclovent, Vanceril, Qvar)**	**MDI**	1–2 inhalations 2–4 times/day	Oropharyngeal candidiasis, dysphonia, hoarseness, cough
Budesonide (p. 140) **(Pulmicort)**	**MDI** **Neb**	**MDI (A):** 1–4 inhalations 2 times/day **D (>6 yrs):** 1–2 inhalations 2 times/day	Same as above
Cromolyn (p. 266) **(Intal)**	**MDI** **Neb**	**MDI: C (>5 yrs):** 2 inhalations up to 4 times/day **Neb: C (>2 yrs):** 20 mg 4 times/day	Cough, urticaria, bronchospasm
Flunisolide (p. 447) **(AeroBid)**	**MDI**	**A:** 2–4 inhalations 2 times/day **C (6–15 yrs):** 1–2 inhalations 2 times/day	Same as beclomethasone
Fluticasone (p. 460) **(Flovent)**	**MDI** **Rotadisk**	**MDI: A, C (>12 yrs):** 2 inhalations 2 times/day **Rotadisk: A, C (>4 yrs):** 1 inhalation 2 times/day	Same as beclomethasone
Nedocromil (p. 756) **(Tilade)**	**MDI**	**A, C (>6 yrs):** 2 inhalations 4 times/day	Unpleasant taste, headaches, nausea
Triamcinolone (p. 1073) **(Azmacort)**	**MDI**	**A:** 2 inhalations 3–4 times/day or 4–8 inhalations 2 times/day **C:** 1–2 inhalations 3–4 times/day or 2–6 inhalations 2 times/day	Same as beclomethasone

(continued)

BRONCHODILATORS ***(continued)***

Name	Availability	Dosage Range	Side Effects
Leukotriene Modifiers			
Montelukast (p. 730) (Singulair)	**T:** 4 mg, 5 mg, 10 mg	**A:** 10 mg/day **C (6–14 yrs):** 5 mg/day **C (2–5 yrs):** 4 mg/day	Dyspepsia, increased liver function tests
Zafirlukast (p. 1124) (Accolate)	**T:** 10 mg, 20 mg	**A, C (≥12 yrs):** 20 mg 2 times/day **C (5–11 yrs):** 10 mg 2 times/day	Same as above
Zileuton (p. 1131) (Zyflo)	**T:** 600 mg	**A:** 600 mg 4 times/day	Same as above

A, Adults; ***C,*** capsules; ***C (dosage),*** children; ***MDI,*** metered dose inhaler; ***Neb,*** nebulization; ***S,*** syrups; ***SR,*** sustained-release; ***T,*** tablet.

Calcium Channel Blockers

USES

Treatment of essential hypertension, treatment of and prophylaxis of angina pectoris (including vasospastic, chronic stable, unstable), prevention/control of supraventricular tachyarrhythmias, prevention of neurologic damage due to subarachnoid hemorrhage.

ACTION

Calcium channel blockers inhibit the flow of extracellular Ca^{2+} ions across cell membranes of cardiac cells, vascular tissue. They relax arterial smooth muscle, depress the rate of sinus node pacemaker, slow AV conduction, decrease heart rate, produce negative inotropic effect (rarely seen clinically due to reflex response). Calcium channel blockers decrease coronary vascular resistance, increase coronary blood flow, reduce myocardial oxygen demand. Degree of action varies with individual agent.

CALCIUM CHANNEL BLOCKERS

Name	Availability	Dosage Range	Side Effects
Amlodipine (p. 57) (Norvasc)	**T:** 2.5 mg, 5 mg, 10 mg	2.5–10 mg/day	Abdominal pain, flushing, headaches
Diltiazem (p. 328) (Cardizem)	**T:** 30 mg, 60 mg, 90 mg **T (SR):** 120 mg, 180 mg, 240 mg **C (SR):** 60 mg, 90 mg, 120 mg, 180 mg, 240 mg, 300 mg, 360 mg **I:** 5 mg/ml	**PO:** 120–360 mg/day **I:** 20–25 mg IV bolus, then 5–15 mg/hr infusion	Dizziness, drowsiness
Felodipine (p. 423) (Plendil)	**T:** 2.5 mg, 5 mg, 10 mg	5–10 mg/day	Peripheral edema, headaches
Isradipine (p. 597) (DynaCirc)	**T:** 5 mg, 10 mg **C:** 2.5 mg, 5 mg	5–20 mg/day	Headaches
Nicardipine (p. 767) (Cardene)	**C:** 20 mg, 30 mg **C (ER):** 30 mg, 45 mg, 60 mg **I:** 2.5 mg/ml	**PO:** 60–120 mg/day	Flushing, feeling of warmth
Nifedipine (p. 771) (Adalat, Procardia)	**C:** 10 mg, 20 mg **T (ER):** 30 mg, 60 mg, 90 mg	30–120 mg/day	Peripheral edema, dizziness, flushed face, headaches, nausea
Nimodipine (p. 773) (Nimotop)	**C:** 30 mg	60 mg q4h for 21 days	Nausea
Verapamil (p. 1104) (Calan, Isoptin)	**T:** 40 mg, 80 mg, 120 mg **T (SR):** 120 mg, 180 mg, 240 mg	120–480 mg/day	Constipation, nausea

C, Capsules; ***ER,*** extended-release; ***I,*** injection; ***SR,*** sustained-release; ***T,*** tablets.

Cancer Chemotherapeutic Agents

USES

Treatment of a variety of cancers; may be palliative or curative. Treatment of choice in hematologic cancers. Often used as adjunctive therapy (e.g., with surgery or irradiation); most effective when tumor mass has been removed or reduced by radiation. Often used in combinations to increase therapeutic results, decrease toxic effects. Certain agents may be used in nonmalignant conditions; polycythemia vera, psoriasis, rheumatoid arthritis, or immunosuppression in organ transplantation (used only in select cases that are severe and unresponsive to other forms of therapy). Refer to individual monographs.

ACTION

Most antineoplastics inhibit cell replication by interfering with the supply of nutrients or genetic components of the cell (DNA or RNA). Some antineoplastics, referred to as *cell cycle–specific* (CCS), are particularly effective during a specific phase of cell reproduction (e.g., antimetabolites and plant alkaloids). Other antineoplastics, referred to as *cell cycle–nonspecific,* act independently of a specific phase of cell division (e.g., alkylating agents and antibiotics). Some hormones are also classified as antineoplastics. Although not cytotoxic, they act to depress cancer growth by altering the hormone environment. In addition, there are a number of miscellaneous agents acting through different mechanisms.

CANCER CHEMOTHERAPEUTIC AGENTS

Name	Availability	Side Effects
Abarelix (p. 1196) (Plenaxis)	**I:** 100 mg	Fatigue, headache, nausea, abdominal pain, hot flushes, menstrual disorders
Aldesleukin (p. 23) (Proleukin)	**I:** 22 million units **Powder**	Hypotension, sinus tachycardia, nausea, vomiting, diarrhea, renal impairment, anemia, rash, fatigue, agitation, pulmonary congestion, dyspnea, fever, chills, oliguria, weight gain, dizziness

Alemtuzumab (p. 24) (Campath)	**I:** 30 mg/3 ml	Rigors, fever, fatigue, hypotension, neutropenia, anemia, sepsis, dyspnea, bronchitis, pneumonia, urticaria
Alitretinoin (p. 29) (Panretin)	**Gel:** 0.1%	Burning, pain, edema, dermatitis, rash, skin disorders
Altretamine (p. 40) (Hexalen)	**C:** 50 mg	Nausea, vomiting, myelosuppression, peripheral neuropathy, altered mood, ataxia, dizziness, nervousness, vertigo
Aminoglutethimide (Cytadren)	**T:** 250 mg	Orthostatic hypotension, hypothyroidism, vomiting, anorexia, rash, drowsiness, headaches, fever, myalgia
Anastrozole (p. 73) (Arimidex)	**T:** 1 mg	Peripheral edema, chest pain, nausea, vomiting, diarrhea, constipation, abdominal pain, anorexia, pharyngitis, vaginal hemorrhage, anemia, leukopenia, rash, weight gain, sweating, increased appetite, pain, headaches, dizziness, depression, paresthesias, hot flashes, increased cough, dry mouth, asthenia, dyspnea, phlebitis
Arsenic trioxide (p. 80) (Trisenox)	**I:** 10 mg/ml	AV block, GI hemorrhage, hypertension, hypoglycemia, hypokalemia, hypomagnesemia, neutropenia, oliguria, prolonged QT interval, seizures, sepsis, thrombocytopenia
Asparaginase (p. 84) (Elspar)	**I:** 10,000 units	Anorexia, nausea, vomiting, liver toxicity, pancreatitis, nephrotoxicity, clotting factor abnormalities, malaise, confusion, lethargy, EEG changes, respiratory distress, fever, hyperglycemia, depression, stomatitis, allergic reactions, drowsiness
BCG (p. 110) (Tice BCG, TheraCys)	**I:** 50 mg, 81 mg	Nausea, vomiting, anorexia, diarrhea, dysuria, hematuria, cystitis, urinary urgency, anemia, malaise, fever, chills
Bexarotene (p. 121) (Targretin)	**C:** 75 mg **Gel:** 1%	Anemia, dermatitis, fever, hypercholesterolemia, infection, leukopenia, peripheral edema
Bicalutamide (p. 123) (Casodex)	**T:** 50 mg	Gynecomastia, hot flashes, breast pain, nausea, diarrhea, constipation, nocturia, impotence, pain, muscle pain, asthenia, abdominal pain

(continued)

CANCER CHEMOTHERAPEUTIC AGENTS *(continued)*

Name	Availability	Side Effects
Bleomycin (p. 130) (Blenoxane)	**I:** 15 units, 30 units	Nausea, vomiting, anorexia, stomatitis, hyperpigmentation, nail changes, alopecia, pruritus, hyperkeratosis, urticaria, pneumonitis progression to fibrosis, decreased weight, rash
Bortezomib (p. 132) (Velcade)	**I:** 3.5 mg	Anxiety, dizziness, headache, insomnia, peripheral neuropathy, pruritus, rash, abdominal pain, decreased appetite, constipation, diarrhea, dyspepsia, nausea, vomiting, arthralgia, dyspnea, asthenia, edema, pain
Busulfan (p. 146) (Myleran)	**T:** 2 mg	Nausea, vomiting, hyperuricemia, myelosuppression, skin hyperpigmentation, alopecia, anorexia, decreased weight, diarrhea, stomatitis
Capecitabine (p. 160) (Xeloda)	**T:** 150 mg, 300 mg	Nausea, vomiting, diarrhea, stomatitis, bone marrow depression, hand-and-foot syndrome, dermatitis, fatigue, anorexia
Carboplatin (p. 168) (Paraplatin)	**I:** 50 mg, 150 mg, 450 mg	Nausea, vomiting, nephrotoxicity, bone marrow suppression, alopecia, peripheral neuropathy, hypersensitivity, ototoxicity, asthenia, diarrhea, constipation
Carmustine (p. 170) (BiCNU)	**I:** 100 mg	Anorexia, nausea, vomiting, bone marrow depression, pulmonary fibrosis, pain at injection site, diarrhea, skin discoloration
Chlorambucil (p. 211) (Leukeran)	**T:** 2 mg	Bone marrow suppression, dermatitis, nausea, vomiting, liver toxicity, anorexia, diarrhea, abdominal discomfort, rash
Cisplatin (p. 231) (Platinol)	**I:** 50 mg, 100 mg	Nausea, vomiting, nephrotoxicity, bone marrow depression, neuropathies, ototoxicity, anaphylactic-like reactions, hyperuricemia, hypomagnesemia, hypophosphatemia, hypokalemia, hypocalcemia, pain at injection site
Cladribine (p. 235) (Leustatin)	**I:** 1 mg/ml	Nausea, vomiting, diarrhea, bone marrow depression, chills, fatigue, rash, fever, headaches, anorexia, diaphoresis
Cyclophosphamide (p. 270) (Cytoxan)	**I:** 100 mg, 200 mg, 500 mg, 1 g, 2 g **T:** 25 mg, 50 mg	Nausea, vomiting, hemorrhagic cystitis, bone marrow depression, alopecia, interstitial pulmonary fibrosis, amenorrhea, azoospermia, diarrhea, darkening skin/fingernails, headaches, diaphoresis

Cytarabine (p. 276) (Cytosar, Ara-C)	**I:** 100 mg, 500 mg, 1 g, 2 g	Anorexia, nausea, vomiting, stomatitis, esophagitis, diarrhea, bone marrow depression, alopecia, rash, fever, neuropathies, abdominal pain
Dacarbazine (p. 278) (DTIC)	**I:** 200 mg	Nausea, vomiting, anorexia, liver necrosis, bone marrow depression, alopecia, rash, facial flushing, photosensitivity, flulike syndrome, confusion, blurred vision
Daunorubicin (p. 289) (Cerubidine)	**I:** 20 mg	CHF, nausea, vomiting, stomatitis, mucositis, diarrhea, red urine, bone marrow depression, alopecia, fever, chills, abdominal pain
Daunorubicin (p. 289) (DaunoXome)	**I:** 50 mg	Nausea, diarrhea, abdominal pain, anorexia, vomiting, stomatitis, myelosuppression, rigors, back pain, headaches, neuropathy, depression, dyspnea, fatigue, fever, cough, allergic reactions, sweating
Denileukin (p. 295) (Ontak)	**I:** 300 mcg/2 ml	Hypersensitivity reaction, back pain, dyspnea, rash, chest pain, tachycardia, asthenia, flulike syndrome, chills, nausea, vomiting, infection
Docetaxel (p. 342) (Taxotere)	**I:** 20 mg, 80 mg	Hypotension, nausea, vomiting, diarrhea, mucositis, bone marrow suppression, rash, paresthesia, hypersensitivity, fluid retention, alopecia, asthenia, stomatitis, fever
Doxorubicin (p. 356) (Adriamycin)	**I:** 10 mg, 20 mg, 50 mg, 75 mg, 150 mg, 200 mg	Cardiotoxicity, including CHF; arrhythmias, nausea, vomiting, stomatitis, esophagitis, GI ulceration, diarrhea, anorexia, red urine, bone marrow depression, alopecia, hyperpigmentation of nail beds and skin, local inflammation at injection site, rash, fever, chills, urticaria, lacrimation, conjunctivitis
Doxorubicin (p. 356) (Doxil)	**I:** 20 mg, 50 mg	Neutropenia, palmoplantar erythrodysesthesia syndrome, cardiomyopathy, CHF
Epirubicin (p. 381) (Ellence)	**I:** 2 mg/ml	Anemia, leukopenia, neutropenia, infection, mucositis

(continued)

CANCER CHEMOTHERAPEUTIC AGENTS *(continued)*

Name	Availability	Side Effects
Estramustine (p. 405) (Emcyt)	**C:** 140 mg	Increased risk of thrombosis, gynecomastia, nausea, vomiting, diarrhea, thrombocytopenia, peripheral edema
Etoposide (p. 415) (VePesid)	**I:** 20 mg/ml **C:** 50 mg	Nausea, vomiting, anorexia, bone marrow depression, alopecia, diarrhea, somnolence, peripheral neuropathies
Exemestane (p. 417) (Aromasin)	**T:** 25 mg	Dyspnea, edema, hypertension, mental depression
Fludarabine (p. 442) (Fludara)	**I:** 50 mg	Nausea, diarrhea, stomatitis, bleeding, anemia, bone marrow depression, skin rash, weakness, confusion, visual disturbances, peripheral neuropathy, coma, pneumonia, peripheral edema, anorexia
Fluorouracil (p. 450)	**I:** 50 mg/ml **Cream:** 1%, 5% **Solution:** 1%, 2%, 5%	Nausea, vomiting, stomatitis, GI ulceration, diarrhea, anorexia, bone marrow depression, alopecia, skin hyperpigmentation, nail changes, headaches, drowsiness, blurred vision, fever
Flutamide (p. 459) (Eulexin)	**C:** 125 mg	Hot flashes, nausea, vomiting, diarrhea, hepatitis, impotence, decreased libido, rash, anorexia
Fulvestrant (p. 477) (Faslodex)	**I:** 250 mg/5 ml, 125 mg/2.5 ml syringes	Asthenia, pain, headache, injection site pain, flulike symptoms, fever, nausea, vomiting, constipation, anorexia, diarrhea, peripheral edema, dizziness, depression, anxiety, rash, increased cough, UTI
Gefitinib (p. 489) (Iressa)	**T:** 250 mg	Diarrhea, rash, acne, nausea, dry skin, vomiting, pruritus, anorexia
Gemcitabine (p. 490) (Gemzar)	**I:** 200 mg, 1 g	Increased LFTs, nausea, vomiting, diarrhea, stomatitis, hematuria, myelosuppression, rash, mild paresthesias, dyspnea, fever, edema, flulike symptoms, constipation

Gemtuzumab (p. 495) (Mylotarg)	**I:** 5 mg/20 ml	Anemia, hematuria, liver toxicity, pneumonia, herpes simplex, nausea, vomiting, dyspnea, headaches, hypotension, hypoxia, mucositis, myelosuppression, peripheral edema, tachycardia, thrombocytopenia
Goserelin (p. 514) (Zoladex)	**I:** 3.6 mg, 10.8 mg	Hot flashes, sexual dysfunction, decreased erections, gynecomastia, breast swelling, lethargy, pain, lower urinary tract symptoms, headaches, nausea, depression, sweating
Hydroxyurea (p. 540) (Hydrea)	**C:** 500 mg	Anorexia, nausea, vomiting, stomatitis, diarrhea, constipation, bone marrow depression, fever, chills, malaise
Ibritumomab (p. 546) (Zevalin)	Injection kit	Neutropenia, thrombocytopenia, anemia, infection, asthenia, abdominal pain, fever, pain, headache, nausea, peripheral edema, allergic reaction, GI hemorrhage, apnea
Idarubicin (p. 551) (Idamycin PFS)	**I:** 5 mg, 10 mg, 20 mg	CHF, arrhythmias, nausea, vomiting, stomatitis, bone marrow depression, alopecia, rash, urticaria, hyperuricemia, abdominal pain, diarrhea, esophagitis, anorexia
Ifosfamide (p. 553) (Ifex)	**I:** 1 g, 3 g	Nausea, vomiting, hemorrhagic cystitis, bone marrow depression, alopecia, lethargy, somnolence, confusion, hallucinations, hematuria
Imatinib (p. 555) (Gleevec)	**C:** 100 mg	Nausea, fluid retention, hemorrhage, musculoskeletal pain, arthralgia, weight gain, pyrexia, abdominal pain, dyspnea, pneumonia
Interferon alfa-2a (p. 572) (Roferon-A)	**I:** 3 million U, 6 million U, 9 million U, 18 million U	Anorexia, nausea, diarrhea, bone marrow depression, pruritus, myalgia, dizziness, headaches, paresthesias, numbness, fatigue, fever, chills, dyspnea, flulike symptoms, vomiting, coughing, altered taste
Interferon alfa-2b (p. 573) (Intron-A)	**I:** 3 million U, 5 million U, 10 million U, 18 million U, 25 million U, 50 million U	Mild hypotension, hypertension, tachycardia with high fever, nausea, diarrhea, altered taste, weight loss, thrombocytopenia, bone marrow depression, rash, pruritus, myalgia, arthralgia associated with flulike syndromes
Irinotecan (p. 587) (Camptosar)	**I:** 40 mg, 100 mg	Diarrhea, nausea, vomiting, abdominal cramping, anorexia, stomatitis, increased SGOT (AST), severe myelosuppression, alopecia, sweating, rash, decreased weight, dehydration, increased alkaline phosphatase, headaches, insomnia, dizziness, dyspnea, cough, asthenia, rhinitis, fever, pain, back pain, chills

(continued)

CANCER CHEMOTHERAPEUTIC AGENTS *(continued)*

Name	Availability	Side Effects
Letrozole (p. 622) (Femara)	**T:** 2.5 mg	Hypertension, nausea, vomiting, constipation, diarrhea, abdominal pain, anorexia, rash, pruritus, musculoskeletal pain, back pain, arm/leg pain, arthralgia, fatigue, headaches, dyspnea, coughing, hot flashes
Leuprolide (p. 625) (Lupron)	**I:** 3.75 mg, 5 mg, 7.5 mg, 11.25 mg, 15 mg, 22.5 mg, 30 mg	Hot flashes, gynecomastia, nausea, vomiting, constipation, anorexia, dizziness, headaches, insomnia, paresthesias, bone pain
Lomustine (p. 645) (CeeNU)	**C:** 10 mg, 40 mg, 100 mg	Anorexia, nausea, vomiting, stomatitis, liver toxicity, nephrotoxicity, bone marrow depression, alopecia, confusion, slurred speech
Mechlorethamine (p. 664) (Mustargen)	**I:** 10 mg/ml	Severe nausea and vomiting, metallic taste, diarrhea, bone marrow depression, alopecia, phlebitis, vertigo, tinnitus, hyperuricemia, infertility, azoospermia, anorexia, headaches, drowsiness, fever
Megestrol (p. 667) (Megace)	**T:** 20 mg, 40 mg **Suspension:** 40 mg/ml	Deep vein thrombosis, Cushing-like syndrome, alopecia, carpal tunnel syndrome, weight gain, nausea
Melphalan (p. 670) (Alkeran)	**T:** 2 mg	Anorexia, nausea, vomiting, bone marrow depression, diarrhea, stomatitis
Mercaptopurine (p. 676) (Purinethol)	**T:** 50 mg	Anorexia, nausea, vomiting, stomatitis, liver toxicity, bone marrow depression, hyperuricemia, diarrhea, rash
Methotrexate (p. 688)	**T:** 2.5 mg, 5 mg, 7.5 mg, 10 mg, 15 mg **I:** 5 mg, 50 mg, 100 mg, 200 mg, 250 mg	Nausea, vomiting, stomatitis, GI ulceration, diarrhea, liver toxicity, renal failure, cystitis, bone marrow suppression, alopecia, urticaria, acne, photosensitivity, interstitial pneumonitis, fever, malaise, chills, anorexia
Mitomycin-C (p. 722) (Mutamycin)	**I:** 20 mg, 40 mg	Anorexia, nausea, vomiting, stomatitis, diarrhea, renal toxicity, bone marrow depression, alopecia, pruritus, fever, hemolytic uremic syndrome, weakness
Mitotane (p. 724) (Lysodren)	**T:** 500 mg	Anorexia, nausea, vomiting, diarrhea, skin rashes, depression, lethargy, somnolence, dizziness, adrenal insufficiency, blurred vision, decreased hearing

Mitoxantrone (p. 724) (Novantrone)	**I:** 20 mg, 25 mg, 30 mg	CHF, tachycardia, EKG changes, chest pain, nausea, vomiting, stomatitis, mucositis, myelosuppression, rash, alopecia, urine color change to bluish green, phlebitis, diarrhea, cough, headaches, fever
Nilutamide (p. 772) (Nilandron)	**T:** 50 mg	Hypertension, angina, hot flashes, nausea, anorexia, increased liver enzymes, dizziness, dyspnea, visual disturbances, impaired adaptation to dark, constipation, loss of libido
Oxaliplatin (p. 807) (Eloxatin)	**I:** 50 mg, 100 mg	Fatigue, neuropathy, abdominal pain, dyspnea, diarrhea, nausea, vomiting, anorexia, fever, edema, chest pain, anemia, thrombocytopenia, thromboembolism, altered LFTs
Paclitaxel (p. 818) (Taxol)	**I:** 30 mg, 100 mg	Hypertension, bradycardia, EKG changes, nausea, vomiting, diarrhea, mucositis, bone marrow depression, alopecia, peripheral neuropathies, hypersensitivity reaction, athralgia, myalgia
Pegaspargase (p. 828) (Oncaspar)	**I:** 750 IU/ml	Hypotension, anorexia, nausea, vomiting, liver toxicity, pancreatitis, depression of clotting factors, malaise, confusion, lethargy, EEG changes, respiratory distress, hypersensitivity reaction, fever, hyperglycemia, stomatitis
Pentostatin (p. 844) (Nipent)	**I:** 10 mg	Nausea, vomiting, liver disorder, elevated LFTs, leukopenia, anemia, thrombocytopenia, rash, fever, upper respiratory infection, fatigue, hematuria, headaches, myalgia, arthralgia, diarrhea, anorexia
Plicamycin (p. 868) (Mithracin)	**I:** 2.5 mg	Anorexia, nausea, vomiting, stomatitis, diarrhea, clotting factor disorders, facial flushing, mental depression, confusion, fever, hypocalcemia, hypophosphatemia, hypokalemia, headaches, dizziness, rash
Procarbazine (p. 889) (Matulane)	**C:** 50 mg	Nausea, vomiting, stomatitis, diarrhea, constipation, bone marrow depression, pruritus, hyperpigmentation, alopecia, myalgia, paresthesias, confusion, lethargy, mental depression, fever, liver toxicity, arthralgia, respiratory disorders
Rituximab (p. 945) (Rituxan)	**I:** 100 mg, 500 mg	Hypotension, arrhythmias, peripheral edema, nausea, vomiting, abdominal pain, leukopenia, thrombocytopenia, neutropenia, rash, pruritus, urticaria, angioedema, myalgia, headaches, dizziness, throat irritation, rhinitis, bronchospasm, hypersensitivity reaction
Streptozocin (p. 991) (Zanosar)	**I:** 1 g	May lead to insulin-dependent diabetes, nausea, vomiting, nephrotoxicity, renal tubular acidosis, bone marrow depression, lethargy, diarrhea, confusion, depression

(continued)

CANCER CHEMOTHERAPEUTIC AGENTS *(continued)*

Name	Availability	Side Effects
Tamoxifen (p. 1005) (Nolvadex)	**T:** 10 mg, 20 mg	Skin rash, nausea, vomiting, anorexia, menstrual irregularities, hot flashes, pruritus, vaginal discharge or bleeding, bone marrow depression, headaches, tumor or bone pain, ophthalmic changes, weight gain, confusion
Temozolomide (p. 1012) (Temodar)	**C:** 5 mg, 20 mg, 100 mg, 250 mg	Amnesia, fever, infection, leukopenia, neutropenia, peripheral edema, seizures, thrombocytopenia
Teniposide (p. 1015) (Vumon)	**I:** 50 mg/5 ml	Hypotension with rapid infusion, diarrhea, nausea, vomiting, mucositis, bone marrow depression, alopecia, anemia, rash, hypersensitivity reaction
Thioguanine (p. 1028)	**T:** 40 mg	Anorexia, stomatitis, bone marrow depression, hyperuricemia, nausea, vomiting, diarrhea
Thiotepa (p. 1030)	**I:** 15 mg	Anorexia, nausea, vomiting, mucositis, bone marrow depression, amenorrhea, reduced spermatogenesis, fever, hypersensitivity reactions, pain at injection site, headaches, dizziness, alopecia
Topotecan (p. 1054) (Hycamtin)	**I:** 4 mg	Nausea, vomiting, diarrhea, constipation, abdominal pain, stomatitis, anorexia, neutropenia, leukopenia, thrombocytopenia, anemia, alopecia, headaches, dyspnea, paresthesia
Toremifene (p. 1056) (Fareston)	**T:** 60 mg	Elevated LFTs, nausea, vomiting, constipation, skin discoloration, dermatitis, dizziness, hot flashes, sweating, vaginal discharge or bleeding, ocular changes, cataracts, anxiety
Tositumomab (p. 1059) (Bexxar)	**I:** 14 mg/ml	Headache, rash, pruritus, abdominal pain, anorexia, diarrhea, nausea, vomiting, arthralgia, myalgia, cough, dyspnea, asthenia, chills, fever, infection

Trastuzumab (p. 1066) (Herceptin)	**I:** 440 mg	CHF, S_3 gallop, nausea, vomiting, diarrhea, abdominal pain, anorexia, rash, peripheral edema, back or bone pain, asthenia, headaches, insomnia, dizziness, cough, dyspnea, rhinitis, pharyngitis
Tretinoin (p. 1070) (Vesanoid)	**C:** 10 mg	Flushing, nausea, vomiting, diarrhea, constipation, dyspepsia, mucositis, leukocytosis, dry skin/mucous membranes, rash, itching, alopecia, dizziness, anxiety, insomnia, headaches, depression, confusion, intracranial hypertension, agitation, dyspnea, shivering, fever, visual changes, earaches, hearing loss, bone pain, myalgia, arthralgia
Valrubicin (p. 1094) (Valstar)	**I:** 200 mg/5 ml	Dysuria, hematuria, urinary frequency/incontinence, red urine, urinary urgency
Vinblastine (p. 1107) (Velban)	**I:** 10 mg	Nausea, vomiting, stomatitis, constipation, bone marrow depression, alopecia, peripheral neuropathy, loss of deep tendon refluxes, paresthesias, diarrhea
Vincristine (p. 1109) (Oncovin)	**I:** 1 mg, 2 mg, 3 mg	Nausea, vomiting, stomatitis, constipation, pharyngitis, polyuria, bone marrow depression, alopecia, numbness, paresthesias, peripheral neuropathy, loss of deep tendon reflexes, headaches, abdominal pain
Vinorelbine (p. 1111) (Navelbine)	**I:** 10 mg, 50 mg	Elevated LFTs, nausea, vomiting, constipation, ileus, anorexia, stomatitis, bone marrow suppression, alopecia, vein discoloration, venous pain, phlebitis, interstitial pulmonary changes, asthenia, fatigue, diarrhea, peripheral neuropathy, loss of deep tendon reflexes

C, Capsules; ***I,*** injection; ***T,*** tablets.

Cardiac Glycosides (Inotropic Agents)

USES

CHF, atrial fibrillation, atrial flutter, paroxysmal atrial tachycardia, treatment of cardiogenic shock with pulmonary edema.

ACTION

Direct action on myocardium causes increased force of contraction, resulting in increased stroke volume and cardiac output. Depression of SA node, decreased conduction time through AV node, and decreased electrical impulses due to vagal stimulation slow heart rate. Improved myocardial contractility is probably due to improved transport of calcium, sodium, and potassium ions across cell membranes.

CARDIAC GLYCOSIDES (INOTROPIC AGENTS)

Name	Availability	Dosage Range	Side Effects
Digoxin (p. 324) (Lanoxin)	**C:** 0.05 mg, 0.1 mg, 0.2 mg **T:** 0.125 mg, 0.25 mg **E:** 0.05 mg/ml **I:** 0.1 mg/ml, 0.25 mg/ml	**PO/IV:** 0.125–0.375 mg/day	Arrhythmias, blurred vision, confusion, hallucinations, nausea, vomiting, diarrhea, abdominal pain
Inamrinone	**I:** 5 mg/ml	**IV:** 0.75 mg/kg bolus, then 5–10 mcg/kg/min infusion	Arrhythmias, hypotension
Milrinone (p. 715) (Primacor)	**I:** 1 mg/ml	**IV:** 50 mcg/kg bolus, then 0.375–0.75 mcg/kg/min infusion	Arrhythmias, hypotension, headaches

C, Capsules; ***E,*** elixir; ***I,*** injection; ***T,*** tablets.

Cholinergic Agonists/Anticholinesterase

USES

Paralytic ileus and atony of urinary bladder. Myasthenia gravis (weakness, marked fatigue of skeletal muscle). Terminates, reverses effects of neuromuscular blocking agents.

ACTION

Cholinergic agonists: Referred to as *muscarinics* or *parasympathetics* and consist of two basic drug groups: choline esters and cholinomimetic alkaloids. Primary action mimics actions of acetylcholine at postganglionic parasympathetic nerves. Primary properties include the following: *Cardiovascular system:* Vasodilation; decreased cardiac rate; decreased conduction in SA, AV nodes; decreased force of myocardial contraction. *Gastrointestinal:* Increased tone, motility of GI smooth muscle, increased secretory activity of GI tract. *Urinary tract:* Increased contraction of detrusor muscle of urinary bladder, resulting in micturition. *Eye:* Miosis, contraction of ciliary muscle.

Anticholinesterase (anti-ChE), also known as *cholinesterase inhibitors:* Inactivates cholinesterase, which prevents acetylcholine breakdown, causing acetylcholine to accumulate at cholinergic receptor sites. These agents can be considered indirect-acting cholinergic agonists. Primary properties include action of cholinergic agonists just noted. *Skeletal neuromuscular junction:* Effects are dose dependent. At therapeutic doses, increases force of skeletal muscle contraction; at toxic doses, reduces muscle strength.

CHOLINERGIC AGONISTS/ANTICHOLINESTERASE

Name	Availability	Uses	Dosage Range	Side Effects
Bethanechol (p. 120) (Urecholine)	**T:** 5 mg, 10 mg, 25 mg, 50 mg **I:** 5 mg/ml	Nonobstructive urinary retention	**PO:** 10–50 mg 3–4 times/day **Subcutaneous:** 2.5–5 mg 3–4 times/day	Increased urinary frequency, salivation, belching, nausea, dizziness

(continued)

CHOLINERGIC AGONISTS/ANTICHOLINESTERASE ***(continued)***

Name	Availability	Uses	Dosage Range	Side Effects
Edrophonium (Tensilon)	**I:** 10 mg/ml	Diagnosis of myasthenia gravis, reverses tubocurarine	**IV:** 10 mg over 30 sec up to 40 mg	Bradycardia, nausea, vomiting, diarrhea, urinary frequency
Neostigmine (p. 761) (Prostigmin)	**T:** 15 mg **I:** 0.25 mg/ml, 0.5 mg/ml, 1 mg/ml	Symptomatic control of myasthenia gravis, neuromuscular blocker	**PO:** 15–365 mg/day **Subcutaneous, IM:** 0.5 mg **IV:** 0.5–2 mg	Diarrhea, increased sweating, nausea, vomiting, stomach cramps
Pyridostigmine (p. 910) (Mestinon)	**T:** 60 mg **T (ER):** 180 mg **S:** 60 mg/5 ml **I:** 5 mg/ml	Treats myasthenia gravis, reverses tubocurarine	**PO:** 60–1,500 mg/day **IM:** 0.5–1.5 mg/kg **IV:** 0.1–0.25 mg/kg	Diarrhea, increased sweating, nausea, vomiting, stomach cramps

ER, Extended release; ***I,*** injection; ***S,*** suspension; ***T,*** tablets.

Corticosteroids

USES

Replacement therapy in adrenal insufficiency, including Addison's disease. Symptomatic treatment of multiorgan disease/conditions. Rheumatoid arthritis, osteoarthritis, severe psoriasis, ulcerative colitis, lupus erythematosus, anaphylactic shock, status asthmaticus, organ transplant.

ACTION

Suppress migration of polymorphonuclear leukocytes (PML) and reverse increased capillary permeability by their anti-inflammatory effect. Suppress immune system by decreasing activity of lymphatic system.

CORTICOSTEROIDS

Name	Availability	Route of Administration	Side Effects
Beclomethasone (p. 111) (Beclovent, Beconase, Vanceril, Vancenase)	**Inhalation** **Nasal:** 42 mcg/spray, 84 mcg/spray	Inhalation, intranasal	**I:** Cough, dry mouth/throat, headaches, throat irritation **Nasal:** Headaches, sore throat, sores inside nose
Betamethasone (p. 117) (Celestone, Diprosone)	**I:** 4 mg/ml	IV, intralesional, intra-articular	Nausea, vomiting, increased appetite, weight gain, trouble sleeping
Budesonide (p. 140) (Rhinocort, Pulmicort)	**Nasal:** 32 mcg/spray	Intranasal	**Nasal:** Headaches, sore throat, sores inside nose
Cortisone (p. 261) (Cortone)	**T:** 5 mg, 10 mg, 25 mg	PO	Same as betamethasone
Dexamethasone (p. 303) (Decadron)	**T:** 0.5 mg, 1 mg, 4 mg, 6 mg **OS:** 0.5 mg/5 ml **I:** 4 mg/ml	PO, parenteral	Same as betamethasone
Fludrocortisone (p. 444) (Florinef)	**T:** 0.1 mg	PO	Same as betamethasone
Flunisolide (p. 447) (AeroBid, Nasalide)	**Inhalation, nasal:** 25 mcg/spray	Inhalation, intranasal	Same as beclomethasone
Fluticasone (p. 460) (Flonase, Flovent)	**Inhalation:** 44 mcg, 110 mg/220 mcg **Nasal:** 50 mg, 100 mcg	Inhalation, intranasal	Same as beclomethasone
Hydrocortisone (p. 533) (Cortef, Solu-Cortef)	**T:** 5 mg, 10 mg, 25 mg **I:** 100 mg, 250 mg, 500 mg, 1 g	PO, parenteral	Same as betamethasone
Methylprednisolone (p. 696) (Solu-Medrol)	**T:** 4 mg **I:** 40 mg, 125 mg, 500 mg, 1 g, 2 g	PO, parenteral	Same as betamethasone

(continued)

CORTICOSTEROIDS *(continued)*

Name	Availability	Route of Administration	Side Effects
Prednisolone (p. 881) (Prelone)	**T:** 5 mg **OS:** 5 mg/5 ml, 15 mg/5 ml	PO	Same as betamethasone
Prednisone (p. 882) (Deltasone)	**T:** 1 mg, 2.5 mg, 5 mg, 10 mg, 20 mg, 50 mg	PO	Same as betamethasone
Triamcinolone (p. 1073) (Azmacort, Kenalog)	**T:** 4 mg, 8 mg **Inhalation:** 100 mcg	PO, inhalation	Same as betamethasone **I:** Cough, dry mouth/throat, headaches, throat irritation

I, Injection; ***OS,*** oral suspension; ***T,*** tablets.

Corticosteroids: Topical

USES

Provide relief of inflammation/pruritus associated with corticosteroid-responsive disorders (e.g., contact dermatitis, eczema, insect bite reactions, first- and second-degree localized burns/sunburn).

ACTION

Diffuse across cell membranes, form complexes with cytoplasm. Complexes stimulate protein synthesis of inhibitory enzymes responsible for anti-inflammatory effects (e.g., inhibit edema, erythema, pruritus, capillary dilation, phagocytic activity).

Topical corticosteroids can be classified based on potency:

Low potency: Modest anti-inflammatory effect, safest for chronic application, facial and intertriginous application, with occlusion, for infants/young children.

Medium potency: For moderate inflammatory conditions (e.g., chronic eczematous dermatoses). May use for facial and intertriginous application for only limited time.

High potency: For more severe inflammatory conditions (e.g., lichen simplex chronicus, psoriasis). May use for facial and intertriginous application for short time only. Used in areas of thickened skin due to chronic conditions.

Very high potency: Alternative to systemic therapy for local effect (e.g., chronic lesions caused by psoriasis). Increased risk of skin atrophy. Used for short periods on small areas. Avoid occlusive dressings.

CORTICOSTEROIDS: TOPICAL

Name	Availability	Potency	Side Effects
Alclometasone (p. 23) (Aclovate)	**C, O:** 0.05%	Low	Burning, stinging, irritation, itching, rash

(continued)

CORTICOSTEROIDS: TOPICAL *(continued)*

Name	Availability	Potency	Side Effects
Amcinonide (p. 44) **(Cyclocort)**	**C, O, L:** 0.1%	High	Same as above
Betamethasone dipropionate (p. 117) **(Diprosone)**	**C, O, G, L:** 0.05%	High	Same as above
Betamethasone valerate (p. 117) **(Valisone)**	**C:** 0.01%, 0.05%, 0.1% **O:** 0.1% **L:** 0.1%	High	Same as above
Clobetasol (p. 242) **(Temovate)**	**C, O:** 0.05%	High	Same as above
Desonide (p. 303) **(Tridesilon)**	**C, O, L:** 0.05%	Low	Same as above
Desoximetasone (p. 303) **(Topicort)**	**C:** 0.25%, 0.5% **O:** 0.25% **G:** 0.05%	High	Same as above
Dexamethasone (p. 303) **(Decadron)**	**C:** 0.1%	Medium	Same as above
Fluocinonide (p. 449) **(Lidex)**	**C, O, G:** 0.05%	High	Same as above
Fluocinolone (p. 449) **(Synalar)**	**C:** 0.01%, 0.025%, 0.2% **O:** 0.025%	High	Same as above
Flurandrenolide (p. 456) **(Cordran)**	**C, O, L:** 0.025%, 0.05%	Medium	Same as above
Fluticasone (p. 460) **(Cutivate)**	**C:** 0.05% **O:** 0.005%	Medium	Same as above

Halobetasol (p. 519) (Ultravate)	**C, O:** 0.05%	High	Same as above
Hydrocortisone (p. 533) (Cort-Dome, Hytone)	**C, O:** 0.5%, 1%, 2.5%	Medium	Same as above
Mometasone (p. 729) (Elocon)	**C, O, L:** 0.1%	Medium	Same as above
Prednicarbate (p. 881) (Dermatop)	**C:** 0.1%	—	Same as above
Triamcinolone (p. 1073) (Aristocort, Kenalog)	**C, O, L:** 0.025%, 0.1%, 0.5%	Medium	Same as above

C, Cream; ***G,*** gel; ***L,*** lotion; ***O,*** ointment.

Diuretics

USES

Thiazides: Management of edema resulting from a number of causes (e.g., CHF, hepatic cirrhosis); hypertension either alone or in combination with other antihypertensives.

Loop: Management of edema associated with CHF, cirrhosis of the liver, and renal disease. Furosemide used in treatment of hypertension alone or in combination with other antihypertensives.

Potassium-sparing: Adjunctive treatment with thiazides, loop diuretics in treatment of CHF and hypertension.

Diuretics *(continued)*

ACTION

Diuretics act to increase the excretion of water/sodium and other electrolytes via the kidneys. Exact mechanism of antihypertensive effect unknown; may be due to reduced plasma volume or decreased peripheral vascular resistance. Subclassifications of diuretics are based on their mechanism and site of action.

Thiazides: Act at the cortical diluting segment of nephron, block reabsorption of Na, Cl, and water; promote excretion of Na, Cl, K, and water.

Loop: Act primarily at the thick ascending limb of Henle's loop to inhibit Na, Cl, and water absorption.

Potassium-sparing: Spironolactone blocks aldosterone action on distal nephron (causes K retention, Na excretion). Triamterene, amiloride act on distal nephron, decreasing Na reuptake, reducing K secretion.

DIURETICS

Name	Availability	Dosage Range	Side Effects
Thiazides			
Chlorothiazide (p. 217) **(Diuril)**	**T:** 250 mg, 500 mg **S:** 250 mg/5 ml **I:** 500 mg	5–20 mg/day	Confusion, fatigue, muscle cramps, upset stomach
Chlorthalidone (p. 219) **(Hygroton)**	**T:** 15 mg, 25 mg, 50 mg, 100 mg	25–200 mg/day	Same as above
Hydrochlorothiazide (p. 529) **(HydroDIURIL)**	**T:** 25 mg, 50 mg, 100 mg **C:** 12.5 mg **Solution:** 50 mg/15 ml	25–100 mg/day	Same as above
Indapamide (p. 562) **(Lozol)**	**T:** 1.25 mg, 2.5 mg	2.5–5 mg/day	Same as above

Metolazone (p. 701) (Diulo, Zaroxolyn)	**T:** 2.5 mg, 5 mg, 10 mg	2.5–10 mg/day	Same as above
Loop			
Bumetanide (p. 141) (Bumex)	**T:** 0.5 mg, 1 mg, 2 mg **I:** 0.25 mg/ml	5–10 mg/day	Orthostatic hypotension
Ethacrynic acid (p. 409) (Edecrin)	**T:** 25 mg, 50 mg **I:** 50-mg vial	50–200 mg/day	Same as above
Furosemide (p. 478) (Lasix)	**T:** 20 mg, 40 mg, 80 mg **OS:** 10 mg/ml, 40 mg/5 ml **I:** 10 mg/ml	**HTN:** 40–80 mg/day **Edema:** Up to 600 mg/day	Same as above
Torsemide (p. 1058) (Demadex)	**T:** 5 mg, 10 mg, 20 mg, 100 mg **I:** 10 mg/ml	**Edema:** 10–200 mg/day **HTN:** 5–10 mg/day	Constipation, dizziness, headaches, stomach upset
Potassium-Sparing			
Amiloride (p. 48) (Midamor)	**T:** 5 mg	5–20 mg/day	Hyperkalemia
Spironolactone (p. 984) (Aldactone)	**T:** 25 mg, 50 mg, 100 mg	25–100 mg/day	Hyperkalemia, nausea, vomiting, cramps, diarrhea
Triamterene (p. 1075) (Dyrenium)	**C:** 50 mg, 100 mg	Up to 300 mg/day	Same as amiloride

C, Capsules; ***HTN,*** hypertension; ***I,*** injection; ***OS,*** oral solution; ***S,*** suspension; ***T,*** tablets.

Fertility Agents

Infertility is defined as a decreased ability to reproduce as opposed to *sterility*, the inability to reproduce. Infertility may be due to reproduction dysfunction of the male, female, or both.

Female infertility can be due to disruption of any phase of the reproductive process. The most critical phases include follicular maturation, ovulation, transport of the ovum through the fallopian tubes, fertilization of the ovum, nidation, and growth/development of the conceptus. Causes of infertility include the following:

Anovulation, failure of follicular maturation: Absence of adequate hormonal stimulation; ovarian follicles do not ripen, and ovulation will not occur.

Unfavorable cervical mucus: Normally the cervical glands secrete large volumes of thin, watery mucus, but if the mucus is unfavorable (scant, thick, or sticky), sperm is unable to pass through to the uterus.

Hyperprolactinemia: Excessive prolactin secretion may cause amenorrhea, galactorrhea, and infertility.

Luteal phase defect: Progesterone secretion by the corpus luteum is insufficient to maintain endometrial integrity.

Endometriosis: Endometrial tissue is implanted in abnormal locations (e.g., uterine wall, ovary, extragenital sites).

Androgen excess: May decrease fertility (the most common condition is polycystic ovary).

Male infertility is due to decreased density or motility of sperm or semen of abnormal volume or quality. The most obvious manifestation of male infertility is impotence (inability to achieve erection). Whereas in female infertility an identifiable endocrine disorder can be found, most cases of male infertility are not associated with an identifiable endocrine disorder.

MEDICATIONS TO INDUCE OVULATION

Name	Category	Availability	Uses	Side Effects
Cetrorelix (p. 207) (Cetrotide)	GnRH antagonist	**I:** 0.25 mg, 3 mg	Inhibition of premature LH surges in women undergoing ovarian hyperstimulation	**OHSS:** Abdominal pain, indigestion, bloating, decreased urine, nausea, vomiting, diarrhea, rapid weight gain, shortness of breath, swelling of lower legs, headaches, pain/redness at injection site

Chorionic gonadotropin (p. 222) (APL, Pregnyl, Profasi, Profasi HP)	Gonadotropin	**I:** 5,000 U, 10,000 U, 20,000 U	In conjunction with clomiphene, human menotropins, or urofollitropin to stimulate ovulation	**OHSS:** Abdominal pain, indigestion, bloating, decreased urine, nausea, vomiting, diarrhea, rapid weight gain, shortness of breath, swelling of lower legs, ovarian enlargement, ovarian cyst formation
Clomiphene (Clomid, Milophene, Serophene)	Antiestrogen	**T:** 50 mg	Anovulation, oligo-ovulation with intact pituitary/ovarian response and endogenous estrogen	Ovarian cyst formation, ovarian enlargement, visual disturbances, premenstrual syndrome, hot flashes
Follitropin alpha (p. 466) (Gonal-F)	Gonadotropin	**I:** 37.5 IU FSH, 75 IU FSH, 150 IU FSH	In conjunction with hCG to stimulate ovarian follicular development in pts with ovulatory dysfunction not due to primary ovarian failure (e.g., anovulation, oligo-ovulation)	**OHSS:** Abdominal pain, indigestion, bloating, decreased urine, nausea, vomiting, diarrhea, rapid weight gain, shortness of breath, swelling of lower legs, flulike symptoms, upper respiratory tract infections, bleeding between menstrual periods, ovarian enlargement, ovarian cysts, acne, breast pain/tenderness
Follitropin beta (Follistem)	Gonadotropin	**I:** 75 IU FSH	Same as above	**OHSS:** Abdominal pain, indigestion, bloating, decreased urine, nausea, vomiting, diarrhea, rapid weight gain, shortness of breath, swelling of lower legs, flulike symptoms, breast tenderness, dry skin, rash, dizziness, fever, headaches, unusual tiredness
Ganirelex (p. 486) (Antagon)	GnRH antagonist	**I:** 250 mcg/0.5 ml	Inhibition of premature LH surges in women undergoing ovarian hyperstimulation	Same as cetrorelix
Goserelin (p. 514) (Zoladex)	GnRH agonist	**Implant:** 3.6 mg	Endometriosis, adjunct to menotropins/hCG for ovulation induction	Hot flashes, amenorrhea, blurred vision, edema, headaches, nausea, vomiting, breast tenderness, weight gain

(continued)

MEDICATIONS TO INDUCE OVULATION *(continued)*

Name	Category	Availability	Uses	Side Effects
Leuprolide (p. 625) (Lupron)	GnRH agonist	5 mg/ml for SC injection	Endometriosis, adjunct to menotropins/hCG for ovulation induction	Same as goserelin
Menotropins (p. 673) (Humegon, Pergonal)	Gonadotropin	**FSH:** 75 U, 150 U **LH activity:** 75 U, 150 U	In conjunction with hCG for ovulation stimulation in pts with ovulatory dysfunction due to primary ovarian failure	Same as chorionic gonadotropin
Nafarelin (p. 744) (Synarel)	GnRH agonist	**Nasal Spray:** 2 mg/ml	Same as leuprolide	Loss of bone mineral density, breast enlargement, bleeding between regular menstrual periods, acne, mood swings, seborrhea, hot flashes
Urofollitropoin (Fertinex, Metrodin)	Gonadotropin	**FSH activity:** 75 U, 150 U	In conjunction with hCG for ovulation stimulation in pts with polycystic ovary syndrome who have elevated LH/FSH ratio and have failed clomiphene therapy	Same as chorionic gonadotropin

FSH, Follicle-stimulating hormone; ***hCG,*** human chorionic gonadotropin; ***GnRH,*** gonadotropin-releasing hormone; ***I,*** injection; ***LH,*** luteinizing hormone; ***OHSS,*** ovarian hyperstimulation syndrome; ***T,*** tablets.

H_2 Antagonists

USES

Short-term treatment of duodenal ulcer (DU), active benign gastric ulcer (GU); maintenance therapy of DU; pathologic hypersecretory conditions (e.g., Zollinger-Ellison syndrome); gastroesophageal reflux disease (GERD); and prevention of upper GI bleeding in critically ill pts.

ACTION

Inhibit gastric acid secretion by interfering with histamine at the histamine H_2 receptors in parietal cells. Also inhibit acid secretion caused by gastrin. Inhibition occurs with basal (fasting), nocturnal, food-stimulated, or fundic distention secretion. H_2 antagonists decrease both the volume and H_2 concentration of gastric juices.

H_2 ANTAGONISTS

Name	Availability	Dosage Range	Side Effects
Cimetidine (p. 226) (Tagamet)	**T:** 200 mg, 300 mg, 400 mg, 800 mg **L:** 300 mg/5 ml **I:** 150 mg/ml	**Treatment of DU:** 800 mg/at bedtime, 400 mg 2 times/day or 300 mg 4 times/day **Maintenance of DU:** 400 mg/at bedtime **Treatment of GU:** 800 mg/at bedtime or 300 mg 4 times/day **GERD:** 1,600 mg/day **Hypersecretory:** 1,200–2,400 mg/day	Headaches, fatigue, dizziness, confusion, diarrhea, gynecomastia

(continued)

H_2 ANTAGONISTS ***(continued)***

Name	Availability	Dosage Range	Side Effects
Famotidine (p. 421) (Pepcid)	**T**: 10 mg, 20 mg, 40 mg **T (chewable)**: 10 mg **DT**: 20 mg, 40 mg **Gelcap**: 10 mg **OS**: 40 mg/5 ml **I**: 10 mg/ml	**Treatment of DU**: 40 mg/day **Maintenance of DU**: 20 mg/day **Treatment of GU**: 40 mg/day **GERD**: 40–80 mg/day **Hypersecretory**: 80–640 mg/day	Headaches, dizziness, diarrhea, constipation, abdominal pain, tinnitus
Nizatidine (p. 782) (Axid)	**T**: 75 mg **C**: 150 mg, 300 mg	**Treatment of DU**: 300 mg/day **Maintenance of DU**: 150 mg/day	Fatigue, urticaria, abdominal pain, constipation, nausea
Ranitidine (p. 925) (Zantac)	**T**: 75 mg, 150 mg, 300 mg **C**: 150 mg, 300 mg **Syrup**: 15 mg/ml **Granules**: 150 mg **I**: 0.5 mg/ml, 25 mg/ml	**Treatment of DU**: 300 mg/day **Maintenance of DU**: 150 mg/day **Treatment of GU**: 300 mg/day **GERD**: 300 mg/day **Hypersecretory**: 0.3–6 g/day	Blurred vision, constipation, nausea, abdominal pain

C, Capsules; ***DT,*** disintegrating tablets; ***I,*** injection; ***L,*** liquid; ***OS,*** oral suspension; ***T,*** tablets.

Hematinic Preparations

USES

Prevention or treatment of iron deficiency resulting from improper diet, pregnancy, impairment of absorption, or prolonged blood loss.

ACTION

Iron supplements are provided to ensure adequate supplies for the formation of hemoglobin, which is needed for erythropoiesis and O_2 transport.

HEMATINIC (IRON) PREPARATIONS

Name	Availability	Elemental Iron	Side Effects
Ferrous fumarate (p. 431) **(Femiron, Ircon, Feostat, Vitron C)**	**T**: 63 mg, 200 mg, 324 mg **S**: 100 mg/5 ml **D**: 45 mg/0.6 ml	33	Constipation, nausea, vomiting, diarrhea, abdominal pain/cramping
Ferrous gluconate (p. 431) **(Fergon)**	**T**: 240 mg, 325 mg	12	Same as above
Ferrous sulfate (p. 431) **(Fer-Iron, Fer-In-Sol, Feosol)**	**T**: 325 mg **Syrup**: 90 mg/5 ml **E**: 220 mg/5 ml **D**: 75 mg/0.6 ml	20	Same as above
Ferrous sulfate exsiccated (p. 431) **(Slow-Fe, Feosol, Feratab)**	**T**: 187 mg, 200 mg **T (SR)**: 160 mg **C (ER)**: 160 mg	30	Same as above

C, Caplets; ***D,*** drops; ***E,*** elixir; ***ER,*** extended-release; ***S,*** suspension; ***SR,*** sustained-release; ***T,*** tablets.

Hormones

Functions of the body are regulated by two major control systems: the nervous system and the endocrine (hormone) system. Together they maintain homeostasis and control different metabolic functions in the body.

Hormones are concerned with control of different metabolic functions in the body (e.g., rates of chemical reactions in cells, transporting substances through cell membranes, cellular metabolism [growth/secretions]). By definition, a hormone is a chemical substance secreted into body fluids by cells and has control over other cells in the body. Hormones can be local or general:

- *Local hormones* have specific local effects (e.g., acetylcholine, which is secreted at parasympathetic and skeletal nerve endings).

Hormones *(continued)*

ACTION

- *General hormones* are mostly secreted by specific endocrine glands (e.g., epinephrine/norepinephrine are secreted by the adrenal medulla in response to sympathetic stimulation), transported in the blood to all parts of the body, causing many different reactions.

Some general hormones affect all or almost all cells of the body (e.g., thyroid hormone from the thyroid gland increases the rate of most chemical reactions in almost all cells of the body); other general hormones affect only specific tissue (e.g., ovarian hormones are specific to female sex organs and secondary sexual characteristics of the female).

Endocrine hormones almost never directly act intracellularly affecting chemical reactions. They first combine with hormone receptors either on the cell surface or inside the cell (cell cytoplasm or nucleus). The combination of hormone and receptors alters the function of the receptor, and the receptor is the direct cause of the hormone effects. Altered receptor function may include the following: *Altered cell permeability,* which causes a change in protein structure of the receptor, usually opening or closing a channel for one or more ions. The movement of these ions causes the effect of the hormone. *Activation of intracellular enzymes* immediately inside the cell membrane (e.g., hormone combines with receptor that then becomes the activated enzyme adenyl cyclase, which causes formation of cAMP).

Alert: cAMP has effects inside the cell. It is not the hormone but cAMP that causes these effects.

Regulation of hormone secretion is controlled by an internal control system, the negative feedback system:

- Endocrine gland oversecretes.
- Hormone exerts more and more of its effect.
- Target organ performs its function.
- Too much function in turn feeds back to endocrine gland to decrease secretory rate.

The endocrine system contains many glands and hormones. A summary of the important glands and their hormones secreted are as follows:

The pituitary gland (hypophysis) is a small gland found in the sella turcica at the base of the brain. The pituitary is divided into two portions physiologically: the anterior pituitary (adenohypophysis) and the posterior pituitary (neurohypophysis). Six important hormones are secreted from the anterior pituitary and two from the posterior pituitary.

Anterior pituitary hormones:

- Growth hormone
- Adrenocorticotropin (corticotropin)
- Thyroid-stimulating hormone (thyrotropin)
- Follicle-stimulating hormone (FSH)
- Luteinizing hormone (LH)

ACTION *(cont.)*

- Prolactin

Posterior pituitary hormones:

- Antidiuretic hormone (vasopressin)
- Oxytocin

Almost all secretions of the pituitary hormones are controlled by hormonal or nervous signals from the hypothalamus. The hypothalamus is a center of information concerned with the well-being of the body, which in turn is used to control secretions of the important pituitary hormones just listed. Secretions from the posterior pituitary are controlled by nerve signals originating in the hypothalamus; anterior pituitary hormones are controlled by hormones secreted within the hypothalamus. These hormones are as follows:

- Thyrotropin-releasing hormone (TRH) releasing thyroid-stimulating hormone
- Corticotropin-releasing hormone (CRH) releasing adrenocorticotropin
- Growth hormone-releasing hormone (GHRH) releasing growth hormone and growth hormone inhibitory hormone (GHIH) (same as somatostatin)
- Gonadotropin-releasing hormone (GnRH) releasing the two gonadotropic hormones LH and FSH
- Prolactin inhibitory factor (PIF) causing inhibition of prolactin and prolactin-releasing factor

ANTERIOR PITUITARY HORMONES

All anterior pituitary hormones (except growth hormone) have as their principal effect stimulating target glands.

Growth Hormone (GH)

Growth hormone affects almost all tissues of the body. GH (somatopropin) causes growth in almost all tissues of the body (increases cell size, increases mitosis with increased number of cells, and differentiates certain types of cells). Metabolic effects include increased rate of protein synthesis, mobilization of fatty acids from adipose tissue, decreased rate of glucose utilization.

Thyroid-Stimulating Hormone (TSH)

Thyroid-stimulating hormone controls secretion of the thyroid hormones. The thyroid gland is located immediately below the larynx on either side of and anterior to the trachea and secretes two significant hormones, thyroxine (T_4) and triiodothyroxine (T_3), which have a profound effect on increasing the metabolic rate of the body. The thyroid gland also secretes calcitonin, an important hormone for calcium metabolism. Calcitonin promotes deposition of calcium in the bones, which decreases calcium concentration in the extracellular fluid.

Adrenocorticotropin

Adrenocorticotropin causes the adrenal cortex to secrete adrenocortical hormones. The adrenal glands lie at the superior poles of the two kidneys. Each gland is composed of two distinct parts: the adrenal medulla and the cortex. The adrenal medulla, related to the sympathetic nervous system, secretes the hormones epinephrine and norepinephrine. When stimulated, they cause constriction of blood vessels, increased activity of the heart, inhibitory effects on the GI tract, and dilation of the pupils. The adrenal cortex secretes corticosteroids, of which there are two major types: mineralocorticoids and glucocorticoids. Aldosterone, the princi-

Hormones *(continued)*

ACTION *(cont.)*

pal mineralocorticoid, primarily affects electrolytes of the extracellular fluids. Cortisol, the principal glucocorticoid, affects glucose, protein, and fat metabolism.

Luteinizing Hormone (LH)

Luteinizing hormone plays an important role in ovulation and causes secretion of female sex hormones by the ovaries and testosterone by the testes.

Follicle-Stimulating Hormone (FSH)

Follicle-stimulating hormone causes growth of follicles in the ovaries before ovulation and promotes formation of sperm in the testes.

Ovarian sex hormones are estrogens and progestins. Estradiol is the most important estrogen; progesterone is the most important progestin.

Estrogens mainly promote proliferation and growth of specific cells in the body and are responsible for development of most of the secondary sex characteristics. Primarily cause cellular proliferation and growth of tissues of sex organs/other tissue related to reproduction. Ovaries, fallopian tubes, uterus, vagina increase in size. Estrogen initiates growth of breast and milk-producing apparatus, external appearance.

Progesterone stimulates secretion of the uterine endometrium during the latter half of the female sexual cycle, preparing the uterus for implantation of the fertilized ovum. Decreases the frequency of uterine contractions (helps prevent expulsion of the implanted ovum). Progesterone promotes development of breasts, causing alveolar cells to proliferate, enlarge, and become secretory in nature.

Testosterone is secreted by the testes and formed by the interstitial cells of Leydig. Testosterone production increases under the stimulus of the anterior pituitary gonadotropic hormones. It is responsible for distinguishing characteristics of the masculine body (stimulates the growth of male sex organs and promotes the development of male secondary sex characteristics, e.g., distribution of body hair, effect on voice, protein formation, and muscular development).

Prolactin

Prolactin promotes the development of breasts and secretion of milk.

POSTERIOR PITUITARY HORMONES

Antidiuretic Hormone (ADH) (vasopressin)

Antidiuretic hormone can cause antidiuresis (decreased excretion of water by the kidneys). In the presence of ADH the permeability of the renal-collecting ducts and tubules to water increases, which allows water to be absorbed, conserving water in the body. ADH in higher concentrations is a very potent vasoconstrictor, constricting arterioles everywhere in the body, increasing B/P.

Oxytocin

Oxytocin contracts the uterus during the birthing process, esp. toward the end of the pregnancy, helping expel the baby. Oxytocin also contracts myoepithelial cells in the breasts, causing milk to be expressed from the alveoli into the ducts so that the baby can obtain it by suckling.

ACTION *(cont.)*

PANCREAS

The pancreas is composed of two tissue types: *acini* (secrete digestive juices in the duodenum) and *islets of Langerhans* (secrete insulin/glucagon directly into the blood). The islets of Langerhans contain three cells: alpha, beta, and delta. Alpha cells secrete glucagon, beta cells secrete insulin, and delta cells secrete somatostatin.

Insulin promotes glucose entry into most cells, thus controlling the rate of metabolism of most carbohydrates. Insulin also affects fat metabolism.

Glucagon effects are opposite those of insulin, the most important of which is increasing blood glucose concentration by releasing it from the liver into the circulating body fluids.

Somatostatin (same chemical as secreted by the hypothalamus) has multiple inhibitory effects: depresses secretion of insulin and glucagon, decreases GI motility, decreases secretions/absorption of the GI tract.

Human Immunodeficiency Virus (HIV) Infection

USES

Antiretroviral agents are used in the treatment of HIV infection.

ACTION

There are currently five classes of antiretroviral agents used in the treatment of HIV disease. *Nucleoside reverse transcriptase inhibitors (NRTIs)* compete with natural substrates for formation of proviral DNA by reverse transcriptase inhibiting viral replication. *Nucleotide reverse transcriptase inhibitors* (NtRTIs) inhibit reverse transcriptase by competing with the natural substrate deoxyadenosine triphosphate and by DNA chain termination. *Nonnucleoside reverse transcriptase inhibitors (NNRTIs)* directly bind to reverse transcriptase and blocks the RNA-dependent and DNA-dependent DNA polymerase activities by causing a disruption of the enzyme's catalytic site. *Protease inhibitors (PIs)* bind to the active site of HIV-1 protease and prevent the processing of viral gag and gag-pol polyprotein precursors resulting in immature, noninfectious viral particles. Fusion inhibitors interfere with the entry of HIV-1 into cells by inhibiting fusion of viral and cellular membranes.

Human Immunodeficiency Virus (HIV) Infection *(continued)*

ANTIRETROVIRAL AGENTS FOR TREATMENT OF HIV INFECTION

Name	Availability	Dosage Range	Side Effects
Nucleoside Analogues			
Abacavir (p. 1) (Ziagen)	**T:** 300 mg **OS:** 20 mg/ml	**A:** 300 mg 2 times/day	Nausea, vomiting, malaise, rash, fever, headaches, asthenia, fatigue
Didanosine (p. 320) (Videx)	**T:** 25 mg, 50 mg, 100 mg, 150 mg, 200 mg **C:** 125 mg, 200 mg, 250 mg, 400 mg **OS:** 100 mg, 167 mg, 250 mg	**T (>60 kg):** 200 mg 2 times/day; **(<60 kg):** 125 mg 2 times/day **OS (>60 kg):** 250 mg 2 times/day; **(<60 kg):** 167 mg 2 times/day	Peripheral neuropathy, pancreatitis, diarrhea, nausea, vomiting, headaches, insomnia, rash, hepatitis, seizures
Emtricitabine (p. 370) (Emtriva)	**C:** 200 mg	**A:** 200 mg/day	Headache, insomnia, depression, diarrhea, nausea, vomiting, rhinitis, asthenia, rash
Lamivudine (p. 613) (Epivir)	**T:** 100 mg, 150 mg **OS:** 5 mg/ml, 10 mg/ml	**A:** 150 mg 2 times/day **C:** 4 mg/kg 2 times/day	Diarrhea, malaise, fatigue, headaches, nausea, vomiting, abdominal pain, peripheral neuropathy, arthralgia, myalgia, skin rash
Stavudine (p. 986) (Zerit)	**C:** 15 mg, 20 mg, 30 mg, 40 mg **OS:** 1 mg/ml	**A:** 40 mg 2 times/day (20 mg 2 times/day if peripheral neuropathy occurs)	Peripheral neuropathy, anemia, leukopenia, neutropenia
Zalcitabine (p. 1125) (Hivid)	**T:** 0.375 mg, 0.75 mg	**A (>60 kg):** 0.75 mg 3 times/day; **(<60 kg):** 0.375 mg 3 times/day	Peripheral neuropathy, stomatitis, granulocytopenia, leukopenia

Zidovudine (p. 1129) (Retrovir)	**C:** 100 mg **T:** 300 mg **Syrup:** 50 mg/5 ml, 10 mg/ml	**A:** 500–600 mg/day (100 mg 5 times/day or 300 mg 2 times/day)	Anemia, granulocytopenia, myopathy, nausea, malaise, fatigue, insomnia
Zidovudine/lamivudine (AZT/3TC) (p. 1129) (Combivir)	**C:** 300 mg AZT/150 mg 3TC	**A:** 1 capsule 2 times/day	Bone marrow suppression, peripheral neuropathy, pancreatitis
Zidovudine/lamivudine/abacavir (AZT/3TC/ABC) (p. 1129) (Trizivir)	**C:** 300 mg AZT/150 mg 3TC/300 mg ABC	**A:** 1 capsule 2 times/day	Bone marrow suppression, peripheral neuropathy, anaphylactic reaction
Nucleotide Analogues			
Tenofovir (p. 1015) (Viread)	**T:** 300 mg	**A:** 300 mg/day	Nausea, vomiting, diarrhea
Nonnucleoside Analogues			
Delavirdine (p. 293) (Rescriptor)	**T:** 100 mg, 200 mg	**A:** 200 mg 3 times/day for 14 days, then 400 mg 3 times/day	Rash, nausea, headaches, elevations in liver function tests
Efavirenz (p. 367) (Sustiva)	**C:** 50 mg, 100 mg, 200 mg	**A:** 600 mg/day **C:** 200–600 mg/day based on weight	Headaches, dizziness, insomnia, fatigue, rash, nightmares
Nevirapine (p. 764) (Viramune)	**T:** 200 mg	**A:** 200 mg/day for 14 days, then 200 mg 2 times/day	Rash, nausea, fatigue, fever, headaches, abnormal LFTs
Protease Inhibitors			
Amprenavir (p. 69) (Agenerase)	**C:** 50 mg, 150 mg **OS:** 15 mg/ml	**A:** 1,200 mg 2 times/day **C (4–16 yrs, <50 kg):** 20 mg/kg 2 times/day or 15 mg/kg 3 times/day	Rash, diarrhea, headaches, nausea, vomiting, numbness, abdominal pain, fatigue

(continued)

ANTIRETROVIRAL AGENTS FOR TREATMENT OF HIV INFECTION ***(continued)***

Name	Availability	Dosage Range	Side Effects
Protease Inhibitors *(continued)*			
Atazanavir (p. 88) (Reyataz)	**C:** 100 mg, 150 mg, 200 mg	**A:** 400 mg/day	Headache, diarrhea, abdominal pain, nausea, rash
Fosamprenavir (p. 1198) (Lexiva)	**T:** 700 mg	**A:** 1,400–2,800 mg/day	Headache, fatigue, rash, nausea, diarrhea, vomiting, abdominal pain
Indinavir (p. 564) (Crixivan)	**C:** 200 mg, 400 mg	**A:** 800 mg q8h	Nephrolithiasis, hyperbilirubinemia, abdominal pain, asthenia, fatigue, flank pain, nausea, vomiting, diarrhea, headaches, insomnia, dizziness, altered taste
Lopinavir/ritonavir (p. 648) (Kaletra)	**C:** 133/33 mg **OS:** 80/20 mg	**A:** 400/100 mg/day **C (4–12 yrs):** 10–13 mg/kg 2 times/day	Diarrhea, nausea, vomiting, abdominal pain, headaches, rash
Nelfinavir (p. 758) (Viracept)	**T:** 250 mg **Oral Powder:** 50 mg/g	**A:** 750 mg q8h **C:** 20–25 mg/kg q8h	Diarrhea, fatigue, asthenia, headaches, hypertension, decreased ability to concentrate
Ritonavir (p. 944) (Norvir)	**C:** 100 mg **OS:** 80 mg/ml	**A:** Titrate up to 600 mg 2 times/day	Nausea, vomiting, diarrhea, altered taste sensation, fatigue, elevated LFTs and triglyceride levels
Saquinavir (p. 958) (Fortovase)	**C:** 200 mg	**A:** 1,200 mg 3 times/day	Diarrhea, elevations in LFTs, hypertriglycerides, cholesterol, abnormal fat accumulation, hyperglycemia
Saquinavir (p. 958) (Invirase)	**C:** 200 mg	**A:** 600 mg 3 times/day	Diarrhea, elevations in LFTs, hypertriglycerides, cholesterol, abnormal fat accumulation, hyperglycemia

Fusion Inhibitors

Enfuvirtide (p. 374) (Fuzeon)	**I:** 108 mg (90 mg when reconstituted)	**Subcutaneous:** 90 mg 2 times/day	Insomnia, depression, peripheral neuropathy, decreased appetite, constipation, asthenia, cough

A, Adults; ***C,*** capsules; ***C (dosage),*** children; ***I,*** injection; ***OS,*** oral solution; ***T,*** tablets.

Immunosuppressive agents

USES	ACTION
Improvement of both short- and long-term allograft survivals.	*Basiliximab:* An interleukin-2 (IL-2) receptor antagonist inhibiting IL-2 binding. This prevents activation of lymphocytes and the response of the immune system to antigens is impaired. *Cyclosporine:* Inhibits production and release of IL-2. *Daclizumab:* An IL-2 receptor antagonist inhibiting IL-2 binding. *Mycophenolate:* A prodrug that reversibly binds and inhibits inosine monophosphate dehydrogenase (IMPD), resulting in inhibition of purine nucleotide synthesis, inhibiting DNA and RNA synthesis and subsequent synthesis of T and B cells. *Sirolimus:* Inhibits IL-2–stimulated T-lymphocyte activation and proliferation, which may occur through formation of a complex. *Tacrolimus:* Inhibits IL-2–stimulated T-lymphocyte activation and proliferation, which may occur through formation of a complex.

IMMUNOSUPPRESSIVES

Name	Availability	Dosage	Side Effects
Basiliximab (p. 108) (Simulect)	**I:** 20 mg	20 mg for 2 doses	Abdominal pain, asthenia, cough, dizziness, dyspnea, dysuria, edema, hypertension, infection, tremor
Cyclosporine (p. 272) (Neoral, Sandimmune)	**C:** 25 mg, 50 mg, 100 mg **S:** 100 mg/ml **I:** 50 mg/ml	7–10 mg/kg/day	Hypertension, hyperkalemia, nephrotoxicity, coarsening of facial features, hirsutism, gingival hyperplasia, nausea, vomiting, diarrhea, liver toxicity, hyperuricemia, hypertriglycerides/cholesterol, tremors, parasthesia, seizures, risk of infection/malignancy
Daclizumab (p. 280) (Zenapax)	**I:** 25 mg/5 ml	1 mg/kg (**Maximum:** 100 mg)	Dyspnea, fever, hypertension, nausea, peripheral edema, tachycardia, tremor, vomiting, weakness, wound infection
Mycophenolate (p. 739) (CellCept)	**C:** 250 mg **I:** 500 mg **S:** 200 mg/ml **T:** 500 mg	1 g 2 times/day	Diarrhea, vomiting, leukopenia, neutropenia, infections
Sirolimus (p. 973) (Rapamune)	**S:** 1 mg/ml **T:** 1 mg	2–10 mg/day	Dyspnea, leukopenia, thrombocytopenia, hyperlipidemia, abdominal pain, acne, arthralgia, fever, diarrhea, constipation, headache, vomiting, weight gain
Tacrolimus (p. 1002) (Prograf)	**C:** 0.5 mg, 1 mg, 5 mg **I:** 5 mg/ml	0.1–0.15 mg/kg/day	Nephrotoxicity, neurotoxicity, hyperglycemia, nausea, vomiting, photophobia, infections, hypertension, hyperlipidemia

C, Capsules; ***I,*** injection; ***S,*** oral solution or suspension; ***T,*** tablets.

Laxatives

USES

Short-term treatment of constipation; colon evacuation before rectal/bowel examination; prevention of straining (e.g., after anorectal surgery, MI); to reduce painful elimination (e.g., episiotomy, hemorrhoids, anorectal lesions); modification of effluent from ileostomy, colostomy; prevention of fecal impaction; removal of ingested poisons.

ACTION

Laxatives ease or stimulate defecation. Mechanisms by which this is accomplished include (1) attracting, retaining fluid in colonic contents due to hydrophilic or osmotic properties; (2) acting directly or indirectly on mucosa to decrease absorption of water and NaCl; or (3) increasing intestinal motility, decreasing absorption of water and NaCl by virtue of decreased transit time.

Bulk-forming: Act primarily in small/large intestine. Retain water in stool, may bind water, ions in colonic lumen (soften feces, increase bulk); may increase colonic bacteria growth (increases fecal mass). Produce soft stool in 1–3 days.

Lubricant: Mineral oil is the only agent in this group. Promotes stool passage by coating the fecal surface with an oil layer that retains fecal fluid and prevents absorption of fecal water by the colon.

Hyperosmotic agents: Acts in colon. Similar to saline laxatives. Osmotic action may be enhanced in distal ileum/colon by bacterial metabolism to lactate, other organic acids. This decrease in pH increases motility, secretion. Produces soft stool in 1–3 days.

Saline: Acts in small/large intestine, colon (sodium phosphate). Poorly, slowly absorbed; causes hormone cholecystokinin release from duodenum (stimulates fluid secretion, motility); possesses osmotic properties; produces watery stool in 2–6 hrs (small doses produce semifluid stool in 6–12 hrs).

Stimulant: Acts in colon. Enhances accumulation of water/electrolytes in colonic lumen, enhances intestinal motility. May act directly on intestinal mucosa. Produces semifluid stool in 6–12 hrs.

Alert: Bisacodyl suppository acts in 15–60 min.

Surfactants: Act in small/large intestine. Hydrate and soften stools by their surfactant action, facilitating penetration of fat and water into stool. Produce soft stool in 1–3 days.

LAXATIVES

Name	Onset of Action	Uses
Bulk-forming		
Methylcellulose (p. 691) (Citrucel)	12–24 hrs up to 3 days	First line for postpartum women; elderly; pts with diverticulosis, irritable bowel syndrome, hemorrhoids Safe for chronic use
Polycarbophil (p. 870) (Fibercon, Mitrolan)	Same as above	Same as above
Psyllium (p. 907) (Metamucil, Konsyl)	Same as above	Same as above
Surfactant		
Docusate calcium (p. 345) (Surfak)	Same as above	Same as above
Docusate potassium (p. 345) (Dialose)	Same as above	Same as above
Docusate sodium (p. 345) (Colace)	1–3 days	Aids in passage of hard, painful feces Prevents straining
Lubricant		
Mineral oil (Kondremul)	6–8 hrs	Prevents straining
Saline		
Magnesium citrate (p. 659) (Citro-Nesia)	30 min to 3 hrs	Bowel evacuation for colonic procedures/exams, fecal impaction, hepatic coma

Magnesium hydroxide (p. 659)	Same as above	Same as above
Sodium phosphate (Fleets Phospho-Soda)	5–15 min	Same as above
Hyperosmotic		
Glycerin	<30 min	Short-term relief of constipation
Lactulose (p. 611) (Chronulac)	1–3 days	Hepatic comas
Polyethylene glycol-electrolyte solution (p. 871) (GoLYTELY)	30–60 min	Bowel evacuation for colonic procedures/exams
Stimulant		
Bisacodyl (p. 124) (Dulcolax)	**PO:** 6–12 hrs **Rectal:** 15–60 min	Same as above
Casanthranol *(in Peri-Colace)*	6–12 hrs	Same as above
Cascara sagrada (p. 174)	6–12 hrs	Bowel evacuation for colonic procedures/exams
Castor oil	6–12 hrs	Same as above
Senna (p. 964) (Senokot)	6–12 hrs	Same as above

Neuromuscular Blockers

USES

Adjuvant in surgical anesthesia to obtain relaxation of skeletal muscle (esp. abdominal wall) for surgery (allows lighter level of anesthesia; valuable in orthopedic procedures). Neuromuscular blocking agents of short duration often used to facilitate intubation with endotracheal tube; facilitate laryngoscopy, bronchoscopy, and esophagoscopy in combination with general anesthetics. Provide muscle relaxation in pts undergoing mechanical ventilation, muscle relaxation in diagnosis of myasthenia gravis. Prevent convulsive movements during electroconvulsive therapy.

ACTION

Paralysis results from the blocking of the normal neuromuscular transmission. Succinylcholine, a depolarizing agent, attaches to the acetylcholine (ACh) receptor on the motor end plate, causing depolarization. It prevents the binding of ACh to the receptor. Nondepolarizing agents also bind to the receptor at the motor end plate but competitively block ACh from attaching to the receptor. These agents also block presynaptic channels that cause the release of ACh.

NEUROMUSCULAR BLOCKERS

Name	Class	Intubation Dose	ICU Dose	Side Effects
Atracurium (p. 95) (Tracrium)	Short	0.4–0.5 mg/kg	0.4–0.5 mg/kg bolus, then 4–12 mcg/kg/min	Flushed skin, hives
Cisatracurium (p. 231) (Nimbex)	Intermediate	0.15–2 mg/kg	0.10–0.2 mg/kg bolus, then 2.5–3 mcg/kg/min	Skin rash, flushing
Doxacurium (p. 353) (Nuromax)	Long	0.05 mg/kg	0.025–0.05 mg/kg bolus, then 0.3–0.5 mg/kg/min	Injection site reaction, urticaria
Mivacurium (p. 725) (Mivacron)	Short	0.15–0.2 mg/kg	0.15–0.25 mg/kg bolus, then 9–10 mcg/kg/min	Flushing, hypotension, dizziness, muscle spasm

Pancuronium (p. 825) (Pavulon)	Long	0.06–0.1 mg/kg	0.05–0.1 mg/kg bolus, then 1–2 mcg/kg/hr	Increased B/P, increased salivation, pruritus
Rocuronium (p. 949) (Zemuron)	Intermediate	0.45–1.2 mg/kg	0.15–0.25 mg/kg bolus, then 10–12 mcg/kg/min	Pain at injection site, hypertension or hypotension
Succinylcholine (p. 993) (Anectine, Quelicin)	Ultrashort	1–2 mg/kg	NA	Increased intraocular pressure, postop muscle pain, weakness, increased salivation, bradycardia, cardiac arrhythmias
Tubocurarine (p. 1086)	Intermediate	0.5–0.6 mg/kg	NA	Decreased B/P
Vecuronium (p. 1102) (Norcuron)	Intermediate	0.08–0.1 mg/kg	0.08–0.1 mg/kg bolus, then 0.8–1.2 mcg/kg/min	Skeletal muscle weakness with prolonged use

Nitrates

USES

Sublingual: Acute relief of angina pectoris.

Oral, topical: Long-term prophylactic treatment of angina pectoris.

Intravenous: Adjunctive treatment in CHF associated with acute MI. Produce controlled hypotension during surgical procedures; control B/P in perioperative hypertension, angina unresponsive to organic nitrates or beta-blockers.

ACTION

Relax most smooth muscles, including arteries and veins. Effect is primarily on veins (decrease left/right ventricular end-diastolic pressure). In angina, nitrates decrease myocardial work and O_2 requirements (decrease preload by venodilation and afterload by arteriodilation). Nitrates also appear to redistribute blood flow to ischemic myocardial areas, improving perfusion without increase in coronary blood flow.

Nitrates *(continued)*

NITRATES

Name	Availability	Dosage Range	Side Effects
Isosorbide (p. 594) (Isordil, Sorbitrate)	**T**: 5 mg, 10 mg, 20 mg, 30 mg, 40 mg **T (ER)**: 30 mg, 40 mg, 60 mg, 120 mg **SL**: 2.5 mg, 5 mg **T (chewable)**: 5 mg, 10 mg **C (SR)**: 40 mg	**SL**: 2.5–10 mg q2–3h **PO**: 10–40 mg q6h **PO (SR)**: 40–80 mg q8–12h	Flushing, headaches, nausea, vomiting, orthostatic hypotension, restlessness, tachycardia
Nitroglycerin (p. 777) (Minitran, Nitro-Bid, Nitrodisc, Nitro-Dur, Nitroglyn, Nitrostat, Transderm-Nitro)	**SL**: 0.4 mg **T (SR)**: 2.6 mg, 6.5 mg, 9 mg **C (SR)**: 2.5 mg, 6.5 mg, 9 mg, 13 mg **Topical**: 2% ointment **Trans**: 0.1 mg/hr, 0.2 mg/hr, 0.3 mg/hr, 0.4 mg/hr, 0.6 mg/hr, 0.8 mg/hr **I**: 0.5 mg/ml, 5 mg/ml **Infusion**: 100 mcg/ml, 200 mcg/ml	**SL**: 0.4 mg up to 3 times q15min **SR**: 2.5–26 mg 3–4 times/day **Trans**: 0.1–0.8 mg/hr **T**: 1–2 inches up to 4–5 inches q4h	Same as above

C, Capsules; ***ER,*** extended-release; ***I,*** injection; ***SL,*** sublingual; ***SR,*** sustained-release; ***T,*** tablets; ***Trans,*** transdermal.

Nonsteroidal Anti-Inflammatory Drugs (NSAIDs)

USES

Provide symptomatic relief from *pain/inflammation* in the treatment of musculoskeletal disorders (e.g., rheumatoid arthritis, osteoarthritis, ankylosing spondylitis); *analgesic* for low to moderate pain; *reduction in fever* (many agents not suited for routine/prolonged therapy due to toxicity). By virtue of its action on platelet function, aspirin is used in treatment or prophylaxis of diseases associated with hypercoagulability (reduces risk of stroke/heart attack).

ACTION

Exact mechanism for anti-inflammatory, analgesic, antipyretic effects unknown. Inhibition of enzyme cyclooxygenase, the enzyme responsible for prostaglandin synthesis, appears to be a major mechanism of action. May inhibit other mediators of inflammation (e.g., leukotrienes). Direct action on hypothalamus heat-regulating center may contribute to antipyretic effect.

NSAIDs

Name	Availability	Dosage Range	Side Effects
Aspirin (p. 86)	**T:** 81 mg, 160 mg, 325 mg **Supplement:** 300 mg, 600 mg	**P (A):** 325–650 mg q4h as needed **C:** Up to 60–80 mg/kg/day **Arthritis:** 3.2–6 g/day **JRA:** 60–110 mg/kg/day **RF (A):** 5–8 g/day **C:** 75–100 mg/kg/day **TIA:** 1,300 mg/day **MI:** 81–325 mg/day	GI upset, dizziness, headaches

(continued)

NSAIDs *(continued)*

Name	Availability	Dosage Range	Side Effects
Celecoxib (p. 203) (Celebrex)	**C:** 100 mg, 200 mg	**OA:** 200 mg/day **RA:** 100–200 mg 2 times/day **FAP:** 400 mg 2 times/day	Diarrhea, back pain, dizziness, heartburn, headaches, nausea, stomach pain
Diclofenac (p. 316) (Voltaren)	**T:** 25 mg, 50 mg, 75 mg, 100 mg	**Arthritis:** 100–200 mg/day	Indigestion, constipation, diarrhea, nausea, headaches, fluid retention, abdominal cramps
Diflunisal (p. 322) (Dolobid)	**T:** 250 mg, 500 mg	**Arthritis:** 0.5–1 g/day **P:** 0.5 g q8–12h	Headaches, abdominal cramps, indigestion, diarrhea, nausea
Etodolac (p. 413) (Lodine)	**T:** 400 mg, 500 mg **T (ER):** 400 mg, 500 mg, 600 mg **C:** 200 mg, 300 mg	**Arthritis:** 600–800 mg/day **P:** 200–400 mg q6–8h	Indigestion, dizziness, headaches, bloated feeling, diarrhea, nausea, weakness, abdominal cramps
Fenoprofen (p. 427) (Nalfon)	**C:** 200 mg, 300 mg **T:** 600 mg	**Arthritis:** 300–600 mg 3–4 times/day **P:** 200 mg q4–6h as needed	Nausea, indigestion, nervousness, constipation, shortness of breath, heartburn
Flurbiprofen (p. 458) (Ansaid)	**T:** 50 mg, 100 mg	**Arthritis:** 200–300 mg/day	Indigestion, nausea, fluid retention, headaches, abdominal cramps, diarrhea
Ibuprofen (p. 548) (Motrin, Advil)	**T:** 100 mg, 200 mg, 400 mg, 600 mg, 800 mg **T (chewable):** 50 mg, 100 mg **C:** 200 mg **S:** 100 mg/5 ml, 100 mg/2.5 ml **Drops:** 40 mg/ml	**Arthritis:** 1.2–3.2 g/day **P:** 400 mg q4–6h as needed **Fever:** 200 mg q4–6h as needed **JA:** 30–40 mg/kg/day	Dizziness, abdominal cramps, stomach pain, heartburn, nausea
Indomethacin (p. 565) (Indocin)	**C:** 25 mg, 50 mg **C (SR):** 75 mg **S:** 25 mg/5 ml **Supplement:** 50 mg	**Arthritis:** 50–200 mg/day **Bursitis/tendonitis:** 75–150 mg/day **GA:** 150 mg/day	Fluid retention, dizziness, headaches, abdominal pain, indigestion, nausea
Ketoprofen (p. 605) (Orudis)	**T:** 12.5 mg **C:** 25 mg, 50 mg, 75 mg **C (ER):** 100 mg, 150 mg, 200 mg	**Arthritis:** 150–300 mg/day **P:** 25–50 mg q6–8h as needed	Headaches, nervousness, abdominal pain, bloated feeling, constipation, diarrhea, nausea

Ketorolac (p. 607) **(Toradol)**	**T:** 10 mg **I:** 15 mg/ml, 30 mg/ml	**P (PO):** 10 mg q4–6h as needed; **(IM/IV):** 60–120 mg/day	Fluid retention, abdominal pain, diarrhea, dizziness, headaches, nausea
Meloxicam (p. 669) **(Mobic)**	**C:** 7.5 mg	**Arthritis:** 7.5–15 mg/day	Heartburn, indigestion, nausea, diarrhea, headaches
Nabumetone (p. 741) **(Relafen)**	**T:** 500 mg, 750 mg	**Arthritis:** 1–2 g/day	Fluid retention, dizziness, headaches, abdominal pain, constipation, diarrhea, nausea
Naproxen (p. 751) **(Anaprox, Naprosyn)**	**T:** 200 mg, 250 mg, 375 mg, 500 mg **T (CR):** 375 mg **S:** 125 mg/5 ml	**Arthritis:** 250–550 mg/day **P:** 250 mg q6–8h **JA:** 10 mg/kg/day **GA:** 750 mg once, then 250 mg q8h	Tinnitus, fluid retention, shortness of breath, dizziness, drowsiness, headaches, abdominal pain, constipation, heartburn, nausea
Oxaprozin (p. 809) **(Daypro)**	**C:** 600 mg	**Arthritis:** 600–1,800 mg/day	Constipation, diarrhea, nausea, indigestion
Piroxicam (p. 866) **(Feldene)**	**C:** 10 mg, 20 mg	**Arthritis:** 20 mg/day	Abdominal pain, stomach pain, nausea
Rofecoxib (p. 949) **(Vioxx)**	**T:** 12.5 mg, 25 mg, 50 mg	**OA:** 12.5–25 mg/day **P:** 25–50 mg/day	Weakness, diarrhea, dizziness, nausea, fluid retention, stomach pain
Sulindac (p. 997) **(Clinoril)**	**T:** 150 mg, 200 mg	**Arthritis:** 300 mg/day **GA:** 400 mg/day	Dizziness, abdominal pain, constipation, diarrhea, nausea
Tolmetin (p. 1050) **(Tolectin)**	**T:** 200 mg, 600 mg **C:** 400 mg	**Arthritis:** 600–1,800 mg/day **JA:** 15–30 mg/kg/day	Fluid retention, dizziness, headaches, weakness, abdominal pain, diarrhea, indigestion, nausea, vomiting
Valdecoxib (p. 1088) **(Bextra)**	**T:** 10 mg, 20 mg	**Arthritis:** 10 mg/day **Primary dysmenorrhea:** 20 mg 2 times/day	Dyspepsia, nausea, headaches

A, Adults; ***C,*** capsules; ***C (dosage), children;*** ***CR,*** controlled-release; ***ER,*** extended-release; ***FAP,*** familial adenomatous polyposis; ***GA,*** gouty arthritis; ***I,*** injection; ***JA,*** juvenile arthritis; ***JRA,*** juvenile rheumatoid arthritis; ***MI,*** myocardial infarction; ***OA,*** osteoarthritis; ***P,*** pain; ***RA,*** rheumatoid arthritis; ***RF,*** rheumatic fever; ***S,*** suspension; ***T,*** tablets; ***TIA,*** transient ischemic attack.

Nutrition: Enteral

	INDICATIONS	ROUTES OF ENTERAL NUTRITION DELIVERY
Enteral nutrition (EN), also known as *tube feedings,* provides food/nutrients via the GI tract using special formulas, delivery techniques, and equipment. All routes of EN consist of a tube through which liquid formula is infused.	Tube feedings are used in pts with major trauma, burns; those undergoing radiation and/or chemotherapy; pts with liver failure, severe renal impairment, physical or neurologic impairment; preop and postop to promote anabolism; prevention of cachexia, malnutrition.	**NASOGASTRIC (NG):** **INDICATIONS:** Most common for short-term feeding in pts unable or unwilling to consume adequate nutrition by mouth. Requires at least a partially functioning GI tract. **ADVANTAGES:** Does not require surgical intervention and is fairly easily inserted. Allows full use of digestive tract. Decreases chance hyperosmolar solutions may cause distention, nausea, vomiting. **DISADVANTAGES:** Temporary. May be easily pulled out during routine nursing care. Has potential for pulmonary aspiration of gastric contents, risk of reflux esophagitis, regurgitation. **NASODUODENAL (ND), NASOJEJUNAL (NJ):** **INDICATIONS:** Pts unable or unwilling to consume adequate nutrition by mouth. Requires at least a partially functioning GI tract. **ADVANTAGES:** Does not require surgical intervention and is fairly easily inserted. Preferred for pts at risk of aspiration. Valuable for pts with gastroparesis.

ROUTES OF ENTERAL NUTRITION DELIVERY *(cont.)*

DISADVANTAGES: Temporary. May be pulled out during routine nursing care. May be dislodged by coughing, vomiting. Small lumen size increases risk of clogging when medication is given through them, more susceptible to rupturing when using infusion device. Must be radiographed for placement, frequently extubated.

Gastrostomy:

INDICATIONS: Pts with esophageal obstruction or impaired swallowing; pts in whom NG, ND, or NJ not feasible; or, when long-term feeding indicated. **ADVANTAGES:** Permanent feeding access. Tubing has larger bore, allowing noncontinuous (bolus) feeding (300–400 ml over 30–60 min q3–6h). May be inserted endoscopically using local anesthetic (procedure called *percutaneous endoscopic gastrostomy* [PEG]). **DISADVANTAGES:** Requires surgery; may be inserted in conjunction with other surgery or endoscopically (see **ADVANTAGES**). Stoma care required. Tube may be inadvertently dislodged. Risk of aspiration, peritonitis, cellulitis, leakage of gastric contents.

Jejunostomy:

INDICATIONS: Pts with stomach or duodenal obstruction, impaired gastric motility; pts in whom NG, ND, or NJ not feasible; or when long-term feeding indicated. **ADVANTAGES:** Allows early postop feeding (small bowel function is least affected by surgery). Risk of aspiration reduced. Rarely pulled out inadvertently. **DISADVANTAGES:** Requires surgery (laparotomy). Stoma care required. Risk of intraperitoneal leakage. Can be dislodged easily.

INITIATING ENTERAL NUTRITION

With continuous feeding, initiation of isotonic (about 300 mOsm/L) or moderately hypertonic feeding (up to 495 mOsm/L) can be given full strength, usually at a slow rate (30–50 ml/hr) and gradually increased (25 ml/hr q6–24h). Formulas with osmolality of >500 mOsm/L are generally started at half strength and gradually increased in rate, then concentration. Tolerance is increased if the rate and concentration are not increased simultaneously.

Nutrition: Enteral *(continued)*

SELECTION OF FORMULAS

Protein: Has many important physiologic roles and is the primary source of nitrogen in the body. Provides 4 kcal/g protein. Sources of protein in enteral feedings: sodium caseinate, calcium caseinate, soy protein, dipeptides.

Carbohydrate (CHO): Provides energy for the body and heat to maintain body temperature. Provides 3.4 kcal/g carbohydrate. Sources of CHO in enteral feedings: corn syrup, cornstarch, maltodextrin, lactose, sucrose, glucose.

Fat: Provides concentrated source of energy. Referred to as ***kilocalorie dense*** or ***protein sparing.*** Provides 9 kcal/g fat. Sources of fat in enteral feedings: corn oil, safflower oil, medium-chain triglycerides.

Electrolytes, vitamins, trace elements: Contained in formulas (not found in specialized products for renal and hepatic insufficiency).

All products containing protein, fat, carbohydrate, vitamin, electrolytes, trace elements are nutritionally complete and designed to be used by pts for long periods.

COMPLICATIONS

MECHANICAL: Usually associated with some aspect of the feeding tube.

Aspiration pneumonia: Caused by delayed gastric emptying, gastroparesis, gastroesophageal reflux, or decreased gag reflex. May be prevented or treated by reducing infusion rate, using lower fat formula, feeding beyond pylorus, checking residuals, using small-bore feeding tubes, elevating head of bed 30°–45° during and for 30–60 min after intermittent feeding, and regularly checking tube placement.

Esophageal, mucosal, pharyngeal irritation, otitis: Caused by using large-bore NG tube. Prevented by use of small bore whenever possible.

Irritation, leakage at ostomy site: Caused by drainage of digestive juices from site. Prevented by close attention to skin/stoma care.

Tube, lumen obstruction: Caused by thickened formula residue, formation of formula-medication complexes. Prevented by frequently irrigating tube with clear water (also before and after giving

COMPLICATIONS (cont.)

formulas/medication), avoiding instilling medication if possible.

GASTROINTESTINAL: Usually associated with formula, rate of delivery, unsanitary handling of solutions or delivery system.

Diarrhea: Caused by low-residue formulas, rapid delivery, use of hyperosmolar formula, hypoalbuminemia, malabsorption, microbial contamination, or rapid GI transit time. Prevented by using fiber-supplemented formulas, decreasing rate of delivery, using dilute formula and gradually increasing strength.

Cramping, gas, abdominal distention: Caused by nutrient malabsorption, rapid delivery of refrigerated formula. Prevented by delivering formula by continuous methods, giving formulas at room temperature, decreasing rate of delivery.

Nausea, vomiting: Caused by rapid delivery of formula, gastric retention. Prevented by reducing rate of delivery, using dilute formulas, selecting low-fat formulas.

Constipation: Caused by inadequate fluid intake, reduced bulk, inactivity. Prevented by supplementing fluid intake, using fiber-supplemented formula, encouraging ambulation.

METABOLIC: Fluid/electrolyte status should be monitored. Refer to monitoring section. In addition, the very young and very old are at greater risk in developing complications such as dehydration or overhydration.

MONITORING

Daily: Estimate nutrient intake, fluid intake/output, weight of pt, clinical observations.

Weekly: Electrolytes (potassium, sodium, magnesium, calcium, phosphorus), blood glucose, BUN, creatinine, liver function tests (e.g., SGOT [AST], alkaline phosphatase), 24-hr urea and creatinine excretion, total iron-binding capacity (TIBC) or serum transferrin, triglycerides, cholesterol.

Monthly: Serum albumin.

Other: Urine glucose, acetone (when blood glucose >250), vital signs (temperature, respirations, pulse, B/P) q8h.

Nutrition: Parenteral

	INDICATIONS	COMPONENTS OF PN
Parenteral nutrition (PN), also known as *total parenteral nutrition* (TPN) or *hyperalimentation* (HAL), provides required nutrients to pts by IV route of administration. The goal of PN is to maintain or restore nutritional status caused by disease, injury, or inability to consume nutrients by other means.	Conditions when pt is unable to use alimentary tract via oral, gastrostomy, or jejunostomy routes. Impaired absorption of protein caused by obstruction, inflammation, or antineoplastic therapy. Bowel rest necessary because of GI surgery or ileus, fistulas, or anastomotic leaks. Conditions with increased metabolic requirements (e.g., burns, infection, trauma). Preserve tissue reserves as in acute renal failure. Inadequate nutrition from tube feeding methods.	To meet IV nutritional requirements, six essential categories in PN are needed for tissue synthesis and energy balance. *Protein:* In the form of crystalline amino acids (CAA), primarily used for protein synthesis. Several products are designed to meet specific needs for pts with renal failure (e.g., NephrAmine), liver disease (e.g., HepatAmine), stress/trauma (e.g., Aminosyn HBC), use in neonates and pediatrics (e.g., Aminosyn PF, TrophAmine). Calories: 4 kcal/g protein. *Energy:* In the form of dextrose, available in concentrations of 5%–70%. Dextrose <10% may be given peripherally; concentrations >10% must be given centrally. Calories: 3.4 kcal/g dextrose. *IV fat emulsion:* Available in the form of 10% and 20% concentrations. Provides a concentrated source of energy/calories (9 kcal/g fat) and is a source of essential fatty acids. May be administered peripherally or centrally.

COMPONENTS OF PN *(cont.)*

Electrolytes: Major electrolytes (calcium, magnesium, potassium, sodium; also acetate, chloride, phosphate). Doses of electrolytes are individualized, based on many factors (e.g., kidney and/or liver function, fluid status).

Vitamins: Essential components in maintaining metabolism and cellular function; widely used in PN.

Trace elements: Necessary in long-term PN administration. Trace elements include zinc, copper, chromium, manganese, selenium, molybdenum, and iodine.

Miscellaneous: Additives include insulin, albumin, heparin, and histamine$_2$ blockers (e.g., cimetidine, ranitidine, famotidine). Other medication may be included, but compatibility for admixture should be checked on an individual basis.

ROUTE OF ADMINISTRATION

PN is administered via either peripheral or central vein.

Peripheral: Usually involves 2–3 L/day of 5%–10% dextrose with 3%–5% amino acid solution along with IV fat emulsion. Electrolytes, vitamins, trace elements are added according to pt needs. Peripheral solutions provide about 2,000 kcal/day and 60–90 g protein/day. **ADVANTAGES:** Lower risks vs. central mode of administration. **DISADVANTAGES:** Peripheral veins may not be suitable (esp. in pts with illness of long duration); more susceptible to phlebitis (due to osmolalities >600 mOsm/L); veins may be viable only 1–2 wks; large volumes of fluid are needed to meet nutritional requirements, which may be contraindicated in many pts.

Central: Usually utilizes hypertonic dextrose (concentration range of 15%–35%) and amino acid solution of 3%–7% with IV fat emulsion. Electrolytes, vitamins, trace elements are added according to pt needs. Central solutions provide 2,000–4,000 kcal/day. Must be given through large central vein with high blood flow, allowing rapid dilution, avoiding phlebitis/thrombosis (usually through percutaneous insertion of catheter into subclavian vein then advancement of catheter to superior vena cava). **ADVANTAGES:** Allows more alternatives/flexibility in establishing regimens; allows ability to provide full nutritional requirements without need of daily fat emulsion; useful in pts who are fluid restricted (increased concentration), those needing large nutritional requirements (e.g., trauma, malignancy), or those for whom PN indicated >7–10 days. **DISADVANTAGES:** Risk with insertion, use, maintenance of central line; increased risk of infection, catheter-induced trauma, and metabolic changes.

Nutrition: Parenteral *(continued)*

MONITORING

May vary slightly from institution to institution.

Baseline: CBC, platelet count, prothrombin time, weight, body length/head circumference (in infants), electrolytes, glucose, BUN, creatinine, uric acid, total protein, cholesterol, triglycerides, bilirubin, alkaline phosphatase, LDH, SGOT (AST), albumin, other tests as needed.

Daily: Weight, vital signs (TPR), nutritional intake (kcal, protein, fat), electrolytes (potassium, sodium chloride), glucose (serum, urine), acetone, BUN, osmolarity, other tests as needed.

2–3 times/wk: CBC, coagulation studies (PT, PTT), creatinine, calcium, magnesium, phosphorus, acid-base status, other tests as needed.

Weekly: Nitrogen balance, total protein, albumin, prealbumin, transferrin, liver function tests (SGOT [AST], SGPT [ALT]), alkaline phosphatase, LDH, bilirubin, Hgb, uric acid, cholesterol, triglycerides, other tests as needed.

COMPLICATIONS

Mechanical: Malfunction in system for IV delivery (e.g., pump failure; problems with lines, tubing, administration sets, catheter). Pneumothorax, catheter misdirection, arterial puncture, bleeding, hematoma formation may occur with catheter placement.

Infectious: Infections (pts often more susceptible to infections), catheter sepsis (e.g., fever, shaking chills, glucose intolerance) where no other site of infection is identified.

Metabolic: Includes hyperglycemia, elevated cholesterol and triglycerides, abnormal LFTs.

Fluid, electrolyte, acid-base disturbances: May alter potassium, sodium, phosphate, magnesium levels.

Nutritional: Clinical effects seen may be due to lack of adequate vitamins, trace elements, essential fatty acids.

Obesity Management

USES

Noradrenergic agents: Short-term treatment of obesity.

Orlistat, sibutramine: Long-term treatment of obesity.

ACTIONS

Noradrenergic agents (benzphetamine, diethylpropion, phendimetrazine, phentermine): Activate central beta-receptors in the hypothalamus.

Orlistat: Inhibits pancreatic lipase, resulting in decreased fat absorption. In addition, inhibits digestion of dietary triglycerides, decreases absorption of cholesterol and fat-soluble vitamins.

Sibutramine: A serotonin, dopamine, and norepinephrine reuptake inhibitor that stimulates thermogenesis.

ANOREXANTS

Name	Availability	Dosage	Side Effects
Benzphetamine (Didrex)	**T:** 50 mg	25–50 mg 1–3 times/day	Headache, insomnia, nervousness, irritability, dry mouth, constipation, euphoria, palpitations, hypertension
Diethylpropion (Tenuate)	**T:** 25 mg, 75 mg	25 mg 3 times/day or 75 mg sustained-release once daily	Headache, insomnia, nervousness, irritability, dry mouth, constipation, euphoria, palpitations, hypertension
Orlistat (p. 805) (Xenical)	**C:** 120 mg	120 mg 3 times/day before meals	Flatulence, rectal incontinence, oily stools
Phendimetrazine (Bontril)	**C:** 105 mg **T:** 35 mg	17.5–70 mg 2–3 times/day or 105 mg sustained-release once daily	Headache, insomnia, nervousness, irritability, dry mouth, constipation, euphoria, palpitations, hypertension
Phentermine (Ionamin)	**C:** 15 mg, 30 mg, 37.5 mg	18.75–37.5 mg once daily	Headache, insomnia, nervousness, irritability, dry mouth, constipation, euphoria, palpitations, hypertension
Sibutramine (p. 968) (Meridia)	**C:** 5 mg, 10 mg, 15 mg	10 mg initially, then increase to 15 mg/day or decrease to 5 mg/day	Increased B/P, heart rate, headache, dry mouth, loss of appetite, insomnia, constipation

C, Capsules; ***T,*** tablets.

Opioid Analgesics

USES

Relief of moderate to severe pain associated with surgical procedures, MI, burns, cancer, or other conditions. May be used as an adjunct to anesthesia, either as a preop medication or intraoperatively as a supplement to anesthesia. Also used for obstetric analgesia. Codeine and hydrocodone have an antitussive effect. Opium tinctures, such as paregoric, are used for severe diarrhea. Methadone relieves severe pain but is used primarily as part of heroin detoxification.

ACTION

Opioids refer to all drugs having actions similar to morphine and to receptors combining with these agents. Major effects are on the CNS (produce analgesia, drowsiness, mood changes, mental clouding, analgesia without loss of consciousness, nausea and vomiting) and GI tract (decrease HCl secretion; diminish biliary, pancreatic, and intestinal secretions; diminish propulsive peristalsis). Also affects respiration (depressed) and cardiovascular system (peripheral vasodilation, decrease peripheral resistance, inhibit baroreceptor reflexes).

OPIOID ANALGESICS

Names	Availability	Analgesic Effect: Onset (min)	Analgesic Effect: Peak (min)	Analgesic Effect: Duration (hrs)	Dosage Range
Butorphanol (p. 149) (Stadol)	**I:** 1 mg/ml, 2 mg/ml	**IM:** 10–30 **IV:** 2–3	**IM:** 30–60 **IV:** 30	**IM:** 3–4 **IV:** 2–4	**IM:** 1–4 mg q3–4h **IV:** 0.5–2 mg q3–4h
Codeine (p. 253)	**I:** 30 mg, 60 mg **T:** 30 mg, 60 mg	**IM:** 10–30 **PO:** 30–45	**IM:** 30–60 **PO:** 60–120	**IM/PO:** 4–6	**IM/PO (A):** 15–60 mg q4–6h; **(C):** 0.5 mg/kg q4–6h
Fentanyl (p. 429) (Sublimaze)	**I:** 50 mcg/ml	**IM:** 7–15 **IV:** 1–2	**IM:** 20–30 **IV:** 3–5	**IM:** 1–2 **IV:** 0.5–1	**IM:** 50–100 mcg q1–2h
Hydrocodone (p. 531)	Combination oral	10–30	30–60	4–6	5–10 mg q4–6h

Hydromorphone (p. 536) (Dilaudid)	**T**: 1 mg, 2 mg, 3 mg, 4 mg, 8 mg **S**: 3 mg **I**: 1 mg/ml, 2 mg/ml, 3 mg/ml, 4 mg/ml, 10 mg/ml	**PO**: 30 **IM**: 15 **IV**: 10–15	**PO**: 90–120 **IM**: 30–60 **IV**: 15–30	**PO**: 4–5 **IM**: 4–5 **IV**: 4	**PO**: 1–4 mg q3–6h **IM**: 1–4 mg q3–6h **IV**: 0.5–1 mg q3h **ER**: 3 mg q4–8h
Levorphanol (p. 631) (Levo-Dromoran)	**T**: 2 mg **I**: 2 mg/ml	**PO**: 10–60 **IM**: —	**PO**: 90–120 **IM**: 60	4–5	**PO**: 2–4 mg q4h **IM**: 2–3 mg q4h
Meperidine (p. 673) (Demerol)	**T**: 50 mg, 100 mg **I**: 25 mg/ml, 50 mg/ml, 75 mg/ml, 100 mg/ml	**PO**: 15 **IM**: 10–15 **IV**: 1	**PO**: 60–90 **IM**: 30–60 **IV**: 5–7	2–4	**PO/IM (A)**: 50–150 mg q3–4h **(C)**: 1–1.8 mg/kg q3–4h
Methadone (p. 685) (Dolophine)	**T**: 5 mg, 10 mg **OS**: 5 mg/5 ml, 10 mg/5 ml **I**: 10 mg/ml	**PO**: 30–60 **IM**: 10–20 **IV**: —	**PO**: 90–120 **IM**: 60–120 **IV**: 15–30	**PO**: 4–6 **IM**: 4–5 **IV**: 3–4	**IM/PO**: 2.5–10 mg q3–4h
Morphine (p. 731) (Roxanol, MS Contin)	**T (ER)**: 15 mg, 30 mg, 60 mg, 100 mg, 200 mg **OS**: 10 mg/5 ml, 20 mg/5 ml, 20 mg/ml **I**: 4 mg/ml, 10 mg/ml, 15 mg/ml	**PO**: 30–60 **IM**: 10–30 **IV**: —	**PO**: 90 **IM**: 30–60 **IV**: 20	**PO**: 4 **IM/IV**: 4–5	**PO**: 10–30 mg q4h **IM**: 5–20 mg q4h **IV**: 0.05–0.1 mg/kg q4h
Nalbuphine (p. 746) (Nubain)	**I**: 10 mg/ml, 20 mg/ml	**IM**: 2–15 **IV**: 2–3	**IM**: 60 **IV**: 30	**IM**: 3–6 **IV**: 3–4	**IM/IV**: 10–20 mg q3–6h
Oxycodone (p. 814) (Roxicodone)	**T**: 15 mg, 30 mg **OS**: 5 mg/5 ml, 20 mg/ml **T (ER)**: 10 mg, 20 mg, 40 mg, 80 mg, 160 mg	30	60	3–4	5–15 mg or 5 ml q4–6h **(ER)**: q12h (dose titrated)
Propoxyphene (p. 899) (Darvon)	**T**: 100 mg	15–60	60–120	4–6	**PO**: 100 mg q4–6h

A, Adults; ***C (dosage),*** children; ***ER,*** extended-release; ***I,*** injection; ***OS,*** oral solution; ***S,*** supplement; ***T,*** tablets.

Opioid Antagonists

USES

Primarily used to reverse respiratory depression induced by narcotic overdosage. Naloxone is the drug of choice for reversal of respiratory depression.

ACTION

Prevents/reverses effects of mu (μ) receptor opioid agonists (e.g., increases respiration, reverses sedative effect).

OPIOID ANTAGONISTS

Name	Availability	Dosage Range	Side Effects
Nalmefene (Revex)	**I:** 100 mcg/ml, 1 mg/ml	**IV/IM/Subcutaneous:** Titrated individually	Nausea, vomiting, tachycardia, hypertension
Naloxone (p. 748) (Narcan)	**I:** 0.02 mg/ml, 0.4 mg/ml, 1 mg/ml	**IV/IM/Subcutaneous (A):** 0.4–2 mg May repeat at 2- to 3-min intervals; **(C):** 0.01 mg/kg May give subsequent doses of 0.1 mg/kg	Same as above
Naltrexone (Depade, ReVia)	**T:** 50 mg	**PO:** 50 mg/day or 100 mg every other day or 150 mg every third day	Abdominal pain, anxiety, diarrhea, tachycardia, increased sweating, loss of appetite, nausea

A, Adults; ***C*** *(dosage),* children; ***I,*** injection, ***T,*** tablets.

Oral Contraceptives

ACTION

Combination oral contraceptives decrease fertility primarily by inhibition of ovulation. In addition, they can promote thickening of the cervical mucus, thereby creating a physical barrier for the passage of sperm. Also, they can modify the endometrium, making it less favorable for nidation.

CLASSIFICATION

Oral contraceptives either contain both an estrogen and a progestin (combination oral contraceptives) or contain only a progestin (progestin-only oral contraceptives). The combination oral contraceptives have four subgroups:

Monophasic: Daily estrogen and progestin dosage remains constant.

Biphasic: Estrogen remains constant, but the progestin dosage increases during the second half of the cycle.

Triphasic: Progestin changes for each phase of the cycle.

Estrophasic: Progestin remains constant, and the estrogen dose gradually increases through the monthly cycle.

ORAL CONTRACEPTIVES

Brand Names	Estrogen (mcg)	Progestin (mg)	Brand Names	Estrogen (mcg)	Progestin (mg)
Monophasic			**Monophasic**		
Genora 1/50	50 mestranol	1 norethindrone	**Modicon**		
Nelova 1/50M			**Nelova 0.5/35E**		
Norethin 1/50M			**Ovcon-35**	35 ethinyl estradiol	0.4 norethindrone
Norinyl 1+ 50			**Ortho-Cyclen**	35 ethinyl estradiol	0.25 norgestimate
Ortho-Novum 1/50			**Demulen 1/35**	35 ethinyl estradiol	1 ethynodiol diacetate
Ovcon-50	50 ethinyl estradiol	1 norethindrone	**Loestrin 21 1.5/30**	30 ethinyl estradiol	1.5 norethindrone acetate

(continued)

ORAL CONTRACEPTIVES *(continued)*

Brand Names	Estrogen (mcg)	Progestin (mg)	Brand Names	Estrogen (mcg)	Progestin (mg)
Monophasic			**Monophasic**		
Demulen 1/50	50 ethinyl estradiol	1 ethynodiol diacetate	**Loestrin Fe 1.5/30**		
Ovral	50 ethinyl estradiol	0.5 norgestrel	**Lo/Ovral**	30 ethinyl estradiol	0.3 norgestrel
Genora 1/35	35 ethinyl estradiol	1 norethindrone	**Desogen**	30 ethinyl estradiol	0.15 desogestrel
Nelova 1/35E			**Ortho-Cept**		
Norethin 1/35E			**Levlen**	30 ethinyl estradiol	0.15 levonorgestrel
Norinyl 1+35			**Levora**		
Ortho-Novum 1/35			**Nordette**		
Brevicon	35 ethinyl estradiol	0.5 norethindrone	**Loestrin 21 1/20**	20 ethinyl estradiol	1 norethindrone acetate
Genora 0.5/35			**Yasmin**	30 ethinyl estradiol	3 drospirenone
Ortho Evra	0.02 ethinyl estradiol	0.15 norelgestromin			
NuvaRing	2.7 ethinyl estradiol	11.7 etonogestrel			

	Phase 1	Phase 2	
Biphasic			
Jenest-28	0.5 mg norethindrone 35 mcg ethinyl estradiol	1 mg norethindrone 35 mcg ethinyl estradiol	
Nelova 10/11	0.5 mg norethindrone 35 mcg ethinyl estradiol	1 mg norethindrone 35 mcg ethinyl estradiol	
Ortho-Novum 10/11	0.5 mg norethindrone 35 mcg ethinyl estradiol	1 mg norethindrone 35 mcg ethinyl estradiol	

	Phase 1	Phase 2	Phase 3
Triphasic			
Estrostep	1 mg norethindrone 20 mcg ethinyl estradiol	1 mg norethindrone 30 mcg ethinyl estradiol	1 mg norethindrone 35 mcg ethinyl estradiol
Ortho-Novum 7/7/7	0.5 mg norethindrone 35 mcg ethinyl estradiol	0.75 mg norethindrone 35 mcg ethinyl estradiol	1 mg norethindrone 35 mcg ethinyl estradiol
Ortho Tri-Cyclen	0.18 mg norgestimate 35 mcg ethinyl estradiol	0.215 mg norgestimate 35 mcg ethinyl estradiol	0.25 mg norgestimate 35 mcg ethinyl estradiol
Tri-Levlen Triphasil	0.05 mg levonorgestrel 30 mcg ethinyl estradiol	0.075 mg levonorgestrel 40 mcg ethinyl estradiol	0.125 mg levonorgestrel 30 mcg ethinyl estradiol
Tri-Norinyl	0.5 mg norethindrone 35 mcg ethinyl estradiol	1 mg norethindrone 35 mcg ethinyl estradiol	0.5 mg norethindrone 35 mcg ethinyl estradiol
Progestin Only			
Micronor Nor Q D	0.35 mg norethindrone		
Ovrette	0.075 mg norgestrel		

(continued)

NEW CONTRACEPTIVE OPTIONS

Name	Ingredients	Cycle Duration
Oral Contraceptive		
Micrette, Kariva	20 mcg ethinyl estradiol 0.15 mg desogestrel 10 mcg placebo, ethinyl estradiol	28-day cycle (21 days active, 2 days placebo, 5 days ethinyl estradiol 10 mcg)
Nortrel 7/7/7	35 mcg ethinyl estradiol norethindrone 0.5 mg (7 days), 0.75 mg (7 days), 1 mg (7 days), 7 days placebo	28-day cycle (21 days active; 7 days placebo)
Ortho Tri-Cyclen Lo	25 mcg ethinyl estradiol 180 mcg norgestimate (7 days); 215 mcg (7 days), 250 mcg (7 days), 7 days placebo	28-day cycle (21 days active; 7 days placebo)
Yasmin 28	30 mcg ethinyl estradiol 3 mg drospirenone	28-day cycle (21 days active; 7 days placebo)

Name	Ingredients	Cycle Duration
Extended Contraceptive Regimen		
Seasonale	30 mcg ethinyl estradiol 150 mcg levonorgestrel	91-day cycle (84 days active; 7 days placebo)

Name	Ingredients	Cycle Duration
Intrauterine System		
Mirena	52 mg levonorgestrel; total releasing 20 mcg/day	Device inserted into uterus once every 5 years

Name	Ingredients	Cycle Duration
Vaginal Ring		
Nuva-Ring	15 mcg ethinyl estradiol 120 mcg/day etonogestrel	28-day cycle; self-inserted vaginal ring releasing active for 21 days

Name	Ingredients	Cycle Duration
Transdermal Patch		
Ortho-Evra	20 mcg ethinyl estradiol 150 mcg norelgestromin released per day	28-day cycle patch applied once per wk for 3 wks in the 4-wk cycle

Name	Ingredients	Cycle Duration
Injectable		
Lunelle	5 mg ethinyl cypionate 25 mg medroxyprogesterone	28-day cycle administered IM once q28days

Oxytocics

USES

To induce, augment labor when maternal or fetal medical need exists; control of postpartum hemorrhage; cause uterine contraction after cesarean section or during other uterine surgery; induce therapeutic abortion.

ACTION

Oxytocics (Pitocin) stimulate frequency/force of contraction of uterine smooth muscle. Responsiveness of uterus increases closer to term. Stimulates breast (contracting of myoepithelial cells surrounding mammary gland) to release milk.

See Oxytocin individual monograph

Proton Pump Inhibitors

USES

Treatment of various gastric disorders, including gastric and duodenal ulcers, GERD, pathologic hypersecretory conditions.

ACTION

Suppress gastric acid secretion by specific inhibition of the hydrogen-potassium-adenosine triphosphatase (H^+/K^+ ATPase) enzyme system, which transports the acid at the gastric parietal cells. These agents do not have anticholinergic or histamine receptor antagonistic properties.

PROTON PUMP INHIBITORS

Name	Availability	Dosage Range (per day)	Side Effects
Esomeprazole (p. 401) (Nexium)	**C:** 20 mg, 40 mg	20–40 mg	Headaches, diarrhea, abdominal pain, nausea
Lansoprazole (p. 616) (Prevacid)	**C:** 15 mg, 30 mg	15–30 mg	Diarrhea, skin rash, itching, headaches
Omeprazole (p. 800) (Prilosec)	**C:** 10 mg, 20 mg, 40 mg	20–40 mg	Headaches, diarrhea, abdominal pain, nausea
Pantoprazole (p. 825) (Protonix)	**T:** 20 mg, 40 mg **I:** 40 mg	40 mg	Diarrhea, headaches
Rabeprazole (p. 921) (Aciphex)	**T:** 20 mg	20 mg	Headaches

C, Capsules; ***I,*** injection; ***T,*** tablets.

Sedative-Hypnotics

USES

Treatment of insomnia (e.g., difficulty falling asleep initially, frequent awakening, awakening too early).

ACTION

Sedatives decrease activity, moderate excitement, and have calming effects. Hypnotics produce drowsiness, enhance onset/maintenance of sleep (resembling natural sleep). Benzodiazepines are the most widely used agents (largely replace barbiturates): greater safety, lower incidence of drug dependence. Benzodiazepines potentiate gamma-aminobutyric acid, which inhibits impulse transmission in the CNS reticular formation in brain. Benzodiazepines decrease sleep latency, number of awakenings, and time spent in awake stage of sleep; increase total sleep time. Schedule IV drugs.

Name	Availability	Dosage Range	Side Effects
Benzodiazepines			
Estazolam (p. 402) (ProSom)	**T:** 1 mg, 2 mg	**A:** 1–2 mg **E:** 0.5–1 mg	Daytime sedation, memory and psychomotor impairment, tolerance, withdrawal reactions, rebound insomnia, dependence
Flurazepam (p. 456) (Dalmane)	**C:** 15 mg, 30 mg	**A/E:** 15–30 mg	Same as above
Quazepam (p. 913) (Doral)	**T:** 7.5 mg, 15 mg	**A:** 7.5–15 mg **E:** 7.5 mg	Same as above
Temazepam (p. 1011) (Restoril)	**C:** 7.5 mg, 15 mg, 30 mg	**A:** 15–30 mg **E:** 7.5–15 mg	Same as above
Triazolam (p. 1077) (Halcion)	**T:** 0.125 mg, 0.25 mg	**A:** 0.125–0.25 mg **E:** 0.125 mg	Same as above

(continued)

Sedative-Hypnotics *(continued)*

Name	Availability	Dosage Range	Side Effects
Nonbenzodiazepines			
Zaleplon (p. 1127) (Sonata)	**C:** 5 mg, 10 mg	**A:** 5–10 mg **E:** 5 mg	Headaches, dizziness, myalgia, somnolence, asthenia, abdominal pain
Zolpidem (p. 1137) (Ambien)	**T:** 5 mg, 10 mg	**A:** 10 mg **E:** 5 mg	Dizziness, daytime drowsiness, headaches, confusion, depression, hangover, asthenia

A, Adults; ***C,*** capsules; ***E,*** elderly; ***T,*** tablets.

Skeletal Muscle Relaxants

USES

Central acting muscle relaxants: Adjunct to rest, physical therapy for relief of discomfort associated with acute, painful musculoskeletal disorders, i.e., local spasms from muscle injury.

Baclofen, dantrolene, diazepam: Treatment of spasticity characterized by heightened muscle tone, spasm, loss of dexterity caused by multiple sclerosis, cerebral palsy, spinal cord lesions, stroke.

ACTION

Central acting muscle relaxants: Exact mechanism unknown. May act in CNS at various levels to depress polysynaptic reflexes; sedative effect may be responsible for relaxation of muscle spasm.

Baclofen, diazepam: May mimic actions of gamma-aminobutyric acid on spinal neurons; does not directly affect skeletal muscles.

Dantrolene: Acts directly on skeletal muscle, relieving spasticity.

SKELETAL MUSCLE RELAXANTS

Name	Availability	Dosage Range	Side Effects
Baclofen (p. 107) (Lioresal)	**T:** 10 mg, 20 mg	**A:** 40–80 mg/day	Drowsiness, dizziness, weakness, confusion, nausea
Carisoprodol (p. 170) (Rela)	**T:** 350 mg	**A:** 350 mg 4 times/day	Drowsiness
Chlorzoxazone (p. 220) (Parafon Forte DSC)	**T:** 250 mg, 500 mg **Caplets:** 250 mg, 500 mg	**A:** 250–750 mg 3–4 times/day **C:** 125–500 mg 3–4 times/day	Drowsiness, dizziness
Cyclobenzaprine (p. 269) (Flexeril)	**T:** 10 mg	**A:** 10 mg 3 times/day	Drowsiness, dizziness, dry mouth, blurred vision

(continued)

SKELETAL MUSCLE RELAXANTS *(continued)*

Name	Availability	Dosage Range	Side Effects
Dantrolene (p. 284) (Dantrium)	**C:** 25 mg, 50 mg, 100 mg	**A:** 25 mg/day increased slowly to 400 mg/day or less	Drowsiness, dizziness, fatigue, diarrhea
Diazepam (p. 314) (Valium)	**T:** 2 mg, 5 mg, 10 mg	**A:** 2–10 mg 3–4 times/day **E:** 2–2.5 mg initially **C:** 1–2.5 mg 3–4 times/day	Ataxia, dizziness, drowsiness, slurred speech
Methocarbamol (p. 688) (Robaxin)	**T:** 500 mg, 750 mg	**A:** 500–1,000 mg 4 times/day	Altered vision, drowsiness, dizziness
Orphenadrine (p. 806) (Norflex)	**T:** 100 mg	**A:** 100 mg 2 times/day	Drowsiness
Tizanidine (p. 1043) (Zanaflex)	**T:** 2 mg, 4 mg	**A:** 4–8 mg/dose; 24–36 mg/day	Drowsiness, dizziness, weakness, dry mouth, heartburn

A, Adults; ***C,*** capsules; ***C (dosage),*** children; ***E,*** elderly; ***T,*** tablets.

Sympathomimetics

USES

Stimulation of alpha$_1$-receptors: Induce vasoconstriction primarily in skin and mucous membranes; nasal decongestion; combine with local anesthetics to delay anesthetic absorption; increases B/P in certain hypotensive states; produce mydriasis, facilitating eye exams, ocular surgery.

Stimulation of beta$_1$-receptors: Treatment of cardiac arrest, heart failure, shock, AV block.

Stimulation of beta$_2$-receptors: Treatment of asthma.

Stimulation of dopamine receptors: Treatment of shock.

ACTION

The sympathetic nervous system (SNS) is involved in maintaining homeostasis (involved in regulation of heart rate, force of cardiac contractions, B/P, bronchial airway tone, carbohydrate, fatty acid metabolism). The SNS is mediated by neurotransmitters (primarily norepinephrine, epinephrine, and dopamine), which act on adrenergic receptors. These receptors include beta$_1$, beta$_2$, alpha$_1$, alpha$_2$, and dopaminergic. Sympathomimetics differ widely in their actions based on their specificity to affect these receptors.

- *Alpha$_1$:* Causes mydriasis, constriction of arterioles, veins.
- *Alpha$_2$:* Inhibits transmitter release.
- *Beta$_1$:* Increases rate, force of contraction, conduction velocity of heart; releases renin from kidney.
- *Beta$_2$:* Dilates arterioles, bronchi, relaxes uterus.
- *Dopaminergic:* Dilates kidney vasculature.

SYMPATHOMIMETICS

Name	Availability	Receptor Specificity	Uses	Dosage Range
Dobutamine (p. 340) (Dobutrex)	**I:** 12.5 mg/ml, 500 mg/250 ml	Beta$_1$, beta$_2$, alpha$_1$	Inotropic support in cardiac decompensation	**IV infusion:** 2.5–10 mcg/kg/min
Dopamine (p. 351) (Intropin)	**I:** 40 mg, 80 mg, 160-ml vials, 800 mcg/ml, 1,600 mcg/ml	Beta$_1$, alpha$_1$, dopaminergic	Vasopressor, cardiac stimulant	**Dopaminergic:** 0.5–3 mcg/kg/min **Beta$_1$:** 2–10 mcg/kg/min **Alpha$_1$:** >10 mcg/kg/min

(continued)

SYMPATHOMIMETICS *(continued)*

Name	Availability	Receptor Specificity	Uses	Dosage Range
Epinephrine (p. 379) (Adrenalin)	**I:** 0.1 mg/ml, 1 mg/ml	$Beta_1$, $beta_2$, $alpha_1$	Cardiac arrest, anaphylactic shock	**Vasopressor:** 1–10 mcg/min **Cardiac arrest:** 1 mg q3–5min during resuscitation
Norepinephrine (p. 783) (Levophed)	**I:** 1 mg/ml	$Beta_1$, $alpha_1$	Vasopressor	**IV:** 0.5–1 mcg/min up to 2–12 mcg/min
Phenylephrine (p. 853) (Neo-Synephrine)	**I:** 10 mg/ml	$Alpha_1$	Vasopressor	**IV:** Initially, 10–180 mcg/min, then 40–60 mcg/min

I, Injection.

Thyroid

USES

Treatment of primary or secondary hypothyroidism, myxedema, cretinism, or simple goiter.

ACTION

Thyroid hormone (thyroxine [T_4] and triiodothyronine [T_3]) are essential for normal growth, development, and energy metabolism. *Promotes growth/development:* Controls DNA transcription and protein synthesis. Necessary in development of nervous system. *Stimulates energy use:* Increases basal metabolic rate (increases O_2 consumption, heat production). *Cardiovascular:* Stimulates heart by increased rate, force of contraction, cardiac output.

Thyroid *(continued)*

THYROID

Name	Availability	Dosage Average	Side Effects
Levothyroxine (p. 632) (Levoxyl, Synthroid)	**T:** 25 mcg, 50 mcg, 75 mcg, 88 mcg, 100 mcg, 112 mcg, 150 mcg, 175 mcg, 200 mcg, 300 mcg	75–100 mcg/day	Weight loss, palpitations, increased appetite, tremors, nervousness, tachycardia, increased B/P, headaches, insomnia, menstrual irregularities
Liothyronine (p. 638) (Cytomel)	**T:** 5 mcg, 25 mcg, 50 mcg	25–50 mcg/day	Same as above
Liotrix (Thyrolar)	**T:** ¼ grain, ½ grain, 1 grain, 2 grains, 3 grains	½–1 grain/day	Same as above
Thyroid (p. 1033)	**T:** 15 mg, 30 mg, 60 mg, 90 mg, 120 mg, 180 mg, 240 mg, 300 mg	60–120 mg/day	Same as above

T, Tablets.

Vitamins

INTRODUCTION

Vitamins are organic substances required for growth, reproduction, and maintenance of health and are obtained from food or supplementation in small quantities (vitamins cannot be synthesized by the body or the rate of synthesis is too slow/inadequate to meet metabolic needs). Vitamins are essential for energy transformation and regulation of metabolic processes. They are catalysts for all reactions using proteins, fats, carbohydrates for energy, growth, and cell maintenance.

WATER SOLUBLE

Water-soluble vitamins include vitamin C (ascorbic acid), B_1 (thiamine), B_2 (riboflavin), B_3 (niacin), B_5 (pantothenic acid), B_6 (pyridoxine), folic acid, B_{12} (cyanocobalamin). Water-soluble vitamins act as coenzymes for almost every cellular reaction in the body. B-complex vitamins differ from one another in both structure and function but are grouped together because they first were isolated from the same source (yeast and liver).

FAT SOLUBLE

Fat-soluble vitamins include vitamins A, D, E, and K. They are soluble in lipids and are usually absorbed into the lymphatic system of the small intestine and then into the general circulation. Absorption is facilitated by bile. These vitamins are stored in the body tissue when excessive quantities are consumed. May be toxic when taken in large doses (see sections on individual vitamins).

VITAMINS

Name	Uses	RDA	Side Effects
Vitamin A (p. 1114)	Required for normal growth, bone development, vision, reproduction, maintenance of epithelial tissue	**M:** 1,000 mcg **F:** 800 mcg	**High dosages:** Liver toxicity, cheilitis, facial dermatitis, photosensitivity, mucosal dryness
Vitamin B_1 (Thiamine) (p. 1027)	Important in red blood cell formation, carbohydrate metabolism, neurologic function, myocardial contractility, growth, energy production	**M:** 1.5 mg **F:** 1.1 mg	**Large parenteral doses:** May cause pain on injection

Vitamin B_2 (Riboflavin)	Necessary for function of coenzymes in oxidation-reduction reactions, essential for normal cellular growth, assists in absorption of iron and pyridoxine	**M:** 1.7 mg **F:** 1.3 mg	Orange-yellow discoloration in urine
Vitamin B_3 (Niacin) (p. 765)	Coenzyme for many oxidation-reduction reactions	**M:** 19 mg **F:** 15 mg	**High dosage (>500 mg):** Nausea, vomiting, diarrhea, gastritis, liver toxicity, skin rash, facial flushing, headaches
Vitamin B_5 (Pantothenic acid)	Precursor to coenzyme A, important in synthesis of cholesterol, hormones, fatty acids	**M:** 4–7 mg **F:** 4–7 mg	Occasional GI problems (e.g., diarrhea)
Vitamin B_6 (Pyridoxine) (p. 911)	Enzyme cofactor for amino acid metabolism, essential for erythrocyte production, Hgb synthesis	**M:** 2 mg **F:** 1.6 mg	**High dosages:** May cause sensory neuropathy
Vitamin B_{12} (Cyanocobalamin) (p. 268)	Coenzyme in cells, including bone marrow, CNS, and GI tract, necessary for lipid metabolism, formation of myelin	**M:** 2 mcg **F:** 2 mcg	Skin rash, diarrhea, pain at injection site
Vitamin C (Ascorbic acid) (p. 82)	Cofactor in various reactions Necessary for collagen formation, acts as an antioxidant	**M:** 60 mg **F:** 60 mg (increased with smoking, pregnancy, lactation)	**High dosages:** May cause calcium oxalate crystalluria, esophagitis, diarrhea
Vitamin D (Calciferol) (p. 1115)	Necessary for proper formation of bone, calcium, mineral homeostasis; regulation of parathyroid hormone, calcitonin, phosphate	**M:** 200–400 units **F:** 200–400 units	Hypercalcemia, kidney stones, renal failure, hypertension, psychosis, diarrhea, nausea, vomiting, anorexia, fatigue, headaches, mental changes
Vitamin E (Tocopherol) (p. 1117)	Antioxidant	**M:** 10 mg **F:** 8 mg	**High dosages:** GI complaints, malaise, headache

F, Females; ***M,*** males.

abacavir

ah-bah-**kay**-veer
(Ziagen)

FIXED-COMBINATION(S)

Trizivir: abacavir/lamivudine/zidovudine: 300 mg/150 mg/300 mg.

CLASSIFICATION

PHARMACOTHERAPEUTIC: Antiretroviral agent. **CLINICAL:** Antiviral (see pp. 58C, 98C).

ACTION

Inhibits activity of HIV-1 reverse transcriptase by competing with natural substrate dGTP and by its incorporation into viral DNA. **Therapeutic Effect:** Inhibits viral DNA growth.

PHARMACOKINETICS

Rapidly, extensively absorbed following PO administration. Protein binding: 50%. Widely distributed, including CSF and erythrocytes. Metabolized in liver to inactive metabolites. Primarily excreted in urine. Unknown if removed by hemodialysis. **Half-life:** 1.5 hrs.

USES

Treatment of HIV infection, in combination with other agents.

PRECAUTIONS

CONTRAINDICATIONS: Hypersensitivity to any component. **CAUTIONS:** Liver disease.

LIFESPAN CONSIDERATIONS: Pregnancy/lactation: Unknown if excreted in breast milk. Do not breast-feed while taking abacavir (may increase potential for HIV transmission, adverse effects). **Pregnancy Category C. Children:** No safety issues noted in those 3 mos–13 yrs. **Elderly:** No information available.

INTERACTIONS

DRUG: Alcohol may increase concentration and half-life. **HERBAL: St. John's wort** may decrease concentration, effect. **FOOD:** None known. **LAB VALUES:** May increase SGOT (AST), SGPT (ALT), GGT, blood glucose, triglycerides.

AVAILABILITY (Rx)

TABLETS: 300 mg. **ORAL SOLUTION:** 20 mg/ml.

ADMINISTRATION/HANDLING

PO

- May give without regard to food.
- Oral solution may be refrigerated. Do not freeze.

INDICATIONS/ROUTES/DOSAGE

HIV (in combination)

PO: ADULTS: 300 mg 2 times/day. CHILDREN 3 MOS–16 YRS: 8 mg/kg 2 times/day. **Maximum:** 300 mg 2 times/day.

SIDE EFFECTS

ADULT: **FREQUENT:** Nausea (47%), nausea with vomiting (16%), diarrhea (12%), decreased appetite (11%). **OCCASIONAL (7%):** Insomnia.

CHILDREN: **FREQUENT:** Nausea with vomiting (39%), fever (19%), headache, diarrhea (16%), rash (11%). **OCCASIONAL:** Decreased appetite (9%).

ADVERSE REACTIONS/ TOXIC EFFECTS

Hypersensitivity reaction (may be life threatening). Symptoms include fever, rash, fatigue, intractable nausea and vomiting, severe diarrhea, abdominal pain, cough, pharyngitis, dyspnea. May include life-threatening hypotension. Lactic acidosis, severe hepatomegaly may occur.

NURSING IMPLICATIONS

BASELINE ASSESSMENT

Question for possibility of pregnancy. Obtain baseline laboratory testing, esp. liver function tests, before beginning therapy and at periodic intervals during therapy. Offer emotional support.

INTERVENTION/EVALUATION

Assess for nausea, vomiting. Determine pattern of bowel activity and stool consistency. Assess eating pattern; monitor for weight loss. Monitor lab values carefully, particularly liver function.

PATIENT/FAMILY TEACHING

Do not take any medications, including OTC drugs, without consulting physician. Small, frequent meals may offset anorexia, nausea. Abacavir is not a cure for HIV infection, nor does it reduce risk of transmission to others.

abciximab

ab-**six**-ih-mab
(c7E3 Fab, ReoPro)

CLASSIFICATION

PHARMACOTHERAPEUTIC: Glycoprotein IIb/IIIa receptor inhibitor. **CLINICAL:** Antiplatelet; antithrombotic (see p. 29C).

ACTION

Produces rapid inhibition of platelet aggregation by preventing the binding of fibrinogen to GP IIb/IIIa receptor sites on platelets. **Therapeutic Effect:** Prevents closure of treated coronary arteries. Prevents acute cardiac ischemic complications.

PHARMACOKINETICS

Rapidly cleared from plasma with an initial-phase half-life of <10 min and a second-phase half-life of 30 min. Platelet function generally returns within 48 hrs.

USES

Adjunct to aspirin and heparin therapy to prevent cardiac ischemic complications in pts undergoing percutaneous coronary intervention (PCI) and those with unstable angina not responding to conventional medical therapy when PCI is planned within 24 hrs.

PRECAUTIONS

CONTRAINDICATIONS: Active internal bleeding, recent (≤6 wks) GI or GU bleeding, history of CVA <2 yrs or CVA with residual neurologic defect, oral anticoagulants <7 days unless prothrombin time <1.2 × control, thrombocytopenia (<100,000 cells/mcl), recent surgery or trauma (≤6 wks), intracranial neoplasm, arteriovenous malformation or aneurysm, severe uncontrolled hypertension, history of vasculitis, prior IV dextran use before or during PTCA. **CAUTIONS:** Pts who weigh <75 kg; those >65 yrs; those with history of GI disease; those receiving thrombolytics, heparin, aspirin, PTCA <12 hrs of onset of symptoms for acute MI, prolonged PTCA (>70 min), failed PTCA.

LIFESPAN CONSIDERATIONS: Pregnancy/lactation: Unknown if distributed in breast milk. **Pregnancy Category C. Children:** Safety and efficacy not established. **Elderly:** Major bleeding risk increased.

INTERACTIONS

DRUG: Anticoagulants, heparin may increase risk of hemorrhage. **Platelet aggregation inhibitors (e.g., aspirin, dextran, thrombolytic agents)** may increase risk of bleeding. **HERBAL:** None known. **FOOD:** None known. **LAB**

VALUES: Increases clotting time (ACT), prothrombin time (PT), activated partial thromboplastin time (aPTT); decreases platelet count.

AVAILABILITY (Rx)

INJECTION: 2 mg/ml (5-ml vials).

ADMINISTRATION/HANDLING

IV

Storage • Store vials in refrigerator. Solution appears clear, colorless. Do not shake. Discard any unused portion left in vial or if preparation contains *any* opaque particles.

Reconstitution • Use 0.2- to 0.22-micron filter; filtering may be done during preparation or at administration. • Bolus dose may be given undiluted. • Withdraw desired dose and further dilute in 250 ml of 0.9% NaCl or D_5W (e.g., 10 mg in 250 ml equals concentration of 40 mcg/ml).

Rate of administration • See Indications/Routes/Dosage.

Administration precautions • Give in separate IV line; do not add any other medication to infusion. • For bolus injection and continuous infusion, use sterile, nonpyrogenic, low protein-binding 0.2- or 0.22-micron filter. • While vascular sheath is in position, maintain pt on complete bed rest with head of bed elevated at 30°. • Maintain affected limb in straight position. • After sheath removal, apply femoral pressure for 30 min, either manually or mechanically, then apply pressure dressing.

∅ IV INCOMPATIBILITY

Administer in separate line; no other medication should be added to infusion solution.

INDICATIONS/ROUTES/DOSAGE

PERCUTANEOUS CORONARY INTERVENTION (PCI)

IV bolus: ADULTS: 0.25 mg/kg given 10–60 min before angioplasty or atherectomy, then 12-hr IV infusion of 0.125 mcg/kg/min. **Maximum:** 10 mcg/min.

PCI (unstable angina)

IV bolus: ADULTS: 0.25 mg/kg, followed by 18- to 24-hr infusion of 10 mcg/min, end 1 hr after procedure.

SIDE EFFECTS

FREQUENT: Nausea (16%), hypotension (12%). **OCCASIONAL (9%):** Vomiting. **RARE (3%):** Bradycardia, abnormal thinking, dizziness, pain, peripheral edema, urinary tract infection.

ADVERSE REACTIONS/ TOXIC EFFECTS

Major bleeding complications may occur; stop infusion immediately. Hypersensitivity reaction may occur. Atrial fibrillation/flutter, pulmonary edema, complete AV block occur occasionally.

NURSING IMPLICATIONS

BASELINE ASSESSMENT

Heparin should be discontinued 4 hrs prior to arterial sheath removal. Maintain pt on bed rest for 6–8 hrs following sheath removal or drug discontinua-tion, whichever is later. Check platelet count, PT, aPTT prior to med infusion (assess for preexisting blood abnormalities), 2–4 hrs following treatment and at 24 hrs or prior to discharge, whichever is first. Check insertion site, distal pulse of affected limb while femoral artery sheath is in place, and then routinely for 6 hrs following femoral artery sheath removal. Minimize need for numerous injection sites, blood draws, intubations, catheters.

INTERVENTION/EVALUATION

Stop abciximab and/or heparin infusion if any serious bleeding occurs that is uncontrolled by pressure. Assess skin for bruises, petechiae, particularly femoral arterial access, also catheter insertion, arterial and venous puncture, cutdown, needle site, GI sites. Handle pt carefully and as infrequently as possible to prevent bleeding. Do not obtain B/P in lower extremities (possible deep vein thrombi). Assess for decrease in B/P, increase in pulse rate, complaint of abdominal/back pain, severe headache, evidence of hemorrhage, ACT, PT, aPTT, platelet count. Question for increase in discharge during menses. Assess urine output for hematuria. Monitor for any occurring hematoma. Use care in removing any dressing, tape.

Abilify

see aripiprazole

acarbose

ah-**car**-bose
(Prandase, Precose)
Do not confuse with PreCare.

CLASSIFICATION

PHARMACOTHERAPEUTIC: Alpha glucosidase inhibitor. **CLINICAL:** Antidiabetic: Oral (see p. 39C).

ACTION

Delays glucose absorption and digestion of carbohydrates. **Therapeutic Effect:** Results in smaller rise in blood glucose concentration after meals, lowers postprandial hyperglycemia.

USES

Adjunctive therapy to diet in treatment of pts with type 2 diabetes. May be used alone or in combination with other antidiabetic agents.

PRECAUTIONS

CONTRAINDICATIONS: Significant renal dysfunction (serum creatinine >2 mg/dl), hypersensitivity to drug, diabetic ketoacidosis or cirrhosis, inflammatory bowel disease, colonic ulceration, partial intestinal obstruction or predisposition to intestinal obstruction, chronic intestinal diseases associated with marked disorders of digestion or absorption, conditions that may deteriorate as result of increased gas formation in the intestine. **CAUTIONS:** Fever, infection, surgery, trauma (may cause loss of glycemic control). **Pregnancy Category B.**

INTERACTIONS

DRUG: **Digestive enzymes, intestinal absorbents (e.g., charcoal)** reduce acarbose effect. Do not use concurrently. **HERBAL:** None known. **FOOD:** None known. **LAB VALUES:** May increase serum transaminase levels.

AVAILABILITY (Rx)

TABLETS: 25 mg, 50 mg, 100 mg.

ADMINISTRATION/HANDLING

PO

- Give with the first bite of each main meal.

INDICATIONS/ROUTES/DOSAGE

DIABETES MELLITUS

PO: ADULTS, ELDERLY: Initially, 25 mg 3 times/day at the start (with first bite) of each main meal. Increase at 4- to 8-wk intervals. **Maximum: <60 kg:** 50 mg 3 times/day; **>60 kg:** 100 mg 3 times/day.

SIDE EFFECTS

FREQUENT: Transient GI disturbances: flatulence (77%), diarrhea (33%), abdominal pain (21%). Symptoms tend to diminish in frequency and intensity over time.

ADVERSE REACTIONS/ TOXIC EFFECTS

None known.

NURSING IMPLICATIONS

BASELINE ASSESSMENT

Check blood glucose level. Discuss lifestyle to determine extent of learning, emotional needs.

INTERVENTION/EVALUATION

Monitor blood glucose, glycosylated hemoglobin, transaminase values, and food intake. Assess for hypoglycemia (cool wet skin, tremors, dizziness, anxiety, headache, tachycardia, numbness in mouth, hunger, diplopia) or hyperglycemia (polyuria, polyphagia, polydipsia, nausea, vomiting, dim vision, fatigue, deep rapid breathing). Be alert to conditions that alter glucose requirements: fever, increased activity or stress, surgical procedure.

PATIENT/FAMILY TEACHING

Do not skip or delay meals. Check with physician when glucose demands are altered (e.g., fever, infection, trauma, stress, heavy physical activity). Avoid alcoholic beverages. Weight control, exercise, hygiene (including foot care), and nonsmoking are an essential part of therapy.

Accupril

see quinapril

acebutolol

ah-see-**beaut**-oh-lol
(Monitan ♣, Novo-Acebutolol ♣, Rhotral ♣, Sectral)

Do not confuse with Factrel, Septra.

◆ CLASSIFICATION

PHARMACOTHERAPEUTIC: Beta$_1$-adrenergic blocker. **CLINICAL:** Antihypertensive, antiarrhythmic (see pp. 14C, 61C).

ACTION

Competitively blocks beta$_1$-adrenergic receptors in cardiac tissue. Reduces rate of spontaneous firing of sinus pacemaker, AV conduction. **Therapeutic Effect:** Slows sinus heart rate, decreases cardiac output, decreases B/P, exhibits antiarrhythmic activity.

PHARMACOKINETICS

Onset	Peak	Duration
PO (hypotensive)		
1–1.5 hrs	2–8 hrs	24 hrs
PO (antiarrhythmic)		
1 hr	4–6 hrs	10 hrs

Well absorbed from GI tract. Protein binding: 26%. Undergoes extensive first-pass liver metabolism to active metabolite. Eliminated via bile, secreted into GI tract via intestine, excreted in urine. Removed by hemodialysis. **Half-life:** 3–4 hrs; metabolite: 8–13 hrs.

USES

Management of mild to moderate hypertension. Used alone or in combination with other antihypertensives. Management of cardiac arrhythmias (primarily PVCs). **Unlabeled:** Treatment of chronic angina pectoris, hypertrophic cardiomyopathy, myocardial infarction, pheochromocytoma, tremors, anxiety, thyrotoxicosis, syndrome of mitral valve prolapse.

PRECAUTIONS

CONTRAINDICATIONS: Overt cardiac failure, cardiogenic shock, heart block greater than first degree, severe bradycardia. **CAUTIONS:** Impaired renal or hepatic function, peripheral vascular disease, hyperthyroidism, diabetes, inadequate cardiac function, bronchospastic disease.

LIFESPAN CONSIDERATIONS: Pregnancy/lactation: Readily crosses placenta; distributed in breast milk. May produce bradycardia, apnea, hypoglycemia, hypothermia during delivery, low birth-weight infants. **Pregnancy Category B** (**D** if used in second or third trimester). **Children:** No age-related precautions noted. Dosage not established. **Elderly:** Age-related peripheral vascular disease requires caution.

INTERACTIONS

DRUG: Diuretics, other **hypotensives** may increase hypotensive effect; **sympathomimetics, xanthines** may mutually inhibit effects; may mask symptoms of hypoglycemia, prolong hypoglycemic effect of **insulin, oral hypoglycemics. HERBAL:** None known. **FOOD:** None known. **LAB VALUES:** May increase ANA titer, SGOT (AST), SGPT (ALT), alkaline phosphatase, LDH, bilirubin, BUN, creatinine, potassium, uric acid, lipoproteins, triglycerides.

AVAILABILITY (Rx)

CAPSULES: 200 mg, 400 mg.

ADMINISTRATION/HANDLING

PO

- May be given without regard to meals.

INDICATIONS/ROUTES/DOSAGE

MILD TO MODERATE HYPERTENSION

PO: ADULTS: Initially, 400 mg/day in 1–2 divided doses. MAINTENANCE: 400–800 mg/day. RANGE: ADULTS: Up to 1,200 mg/day in 2 divided doses.

VENTRICULAR ARRHYTHMIAS

PO: ADULTS: Initially, 200 mg q12h. Increase gradually up to 600–1,200 mg/day in 2 divided doses.

USUAL ELDERLY DOSAGE

PO: Initially, 200–400 mg/day. **Maximum:** 800 mg/day.

DOSAGE IN RENAL IMPAIRMENT

Creatinine Clearance	% of Normal Dosage
<50 ml/min	50
<25 ml/min	25

SIDE EFFECTS

Generally well tolerated, with mild and transient effects. **FREQUENT:** Hypotension manifested as dizziness, nausea, diaphoresis, headache, cold extremities, fatigue, constipation/diarrhea. **OCCASIONAL:** Insomnia, flatulence, urinary frequency, impotence or decreased libido. **RARE:** Rash, arthralgia, myalgia, confusion (esp. elderly), change in taste.

ADVERSE REACTIONS/ TOXIC EFFECTS

Overdosage may produce profound bradycardia, hypotension. Abrupt withdrawal may result in sweating, palpitations, headache, tremulousness. May precipitate CHF, MI in pts with cardiac disease; thyroid storm in those with thyrotoxicosis; peripheral ischemia in those with existing peripheral vascular disease. Hypoglycemia may occur in previously controlled diabetics. Thrombocytopenia (unusual bruising, bleeding) occurs rarely.

NURSING IMPLICATIONS

BASELINE ASSESSMENT

Assess B/P, apical pulse immediately prior to drug administration. (If pulse is ≤60/min or systolic B/P is <90 mm Hg, withhold medication, contact physician.)

INTERVENTION/EVALUATION

Monitor B/P for hypotension, respiration for shortness of breath. Assess pulse for quality, rate, rhythm. Monitor EKG for cardiac arrhythmias, shortening of QT interval, prolongation of PR interval. Assess frequency, consistency of stools. Assess for evidence of CHF: dyspnea (particularly on exertion or lying down), night cough, peripheral edema, distended neck veins, decreased urine output, weight gain. Assess for nausea, diaphoresis, headache, fatigue.

PATIENT/FAMILY TEACHING

Do not abruptly discontinue medication. Compliance with therapy regimen is essential to control hypertension, arrhythmias. Report shortness of breath, excessive fatigue, weight gain, prolonged dizziness or headache. Do not use nasal decongestants, OTC cold preparations (stimulants) without physician approval. Restrict salt, alcohol intake.

acetaminophen

ah-see-tah-**min**-oh-fen

(Abenol ✦, Apo-Acetaminophen ✦, Atasol ✦, Feverall, Tempra, Tylenol)

Do not confuse with Fiorinal, Hycodan, Indocin, Percodan, Tuinal.

FIXED-COMBINATION(S)

Anexsia: acetaminophen/hydrocodone: 500 mg/5 mg, 650 mg/7.5 mg, 660 mg/10 mg. **Capital with Codeine, Tylenol with Codeine:** acetaminophen/codeine: 120 mg/12 mg per 5 ml. **Darvocet-N:** acetaminophen/propoxyphene: 325 mg/50 mg, 650 mg/100 mg. **Fioricet:** acetaminophen/caffeine/butalbital: 325 mg/40 mg/50 mg. **Lortab:** acetaminophen/hydrocodone: 500 mg/2.5 mg; 500 mg/5 mg; 500 mg/7.5 mg. **Lortab Elixir:** acetaminophen/hydrocodone: 167 mg/2.5 mg per 5 ml. **Norco:** acetaminophen/hydrocodone: 325 mg/10 mg. **Percocet, Roxicet:** acetaminophen/oxycodone: 325 mg/5 mg. **Tylenol with Codeine:** acetaminophen/codeine: 300 mg/15 mg, 300 mg/30 mg, 300 mg/60 mg. **Tylox:** acetaminophen/oxycodone: 500 mg/5 mg. **Ultracet:** acetaminophen/tramadol: 325 mg/37.5 mg. **Vicodin:** acetaminophen/hydrocodone: 500 mg/5 mg. **Vicodin ES:** acetaminophen/hydrocodone: 750 mg/7.5 mg. **Vicodin HP:** acetaminophen/hydrocodone: 660 mg/10 mg. **Zydone:** acetaminophen/hydrocodone: 400 mg/5 mg; 400 mg/7.5 mg; 400 mg/10 mg.

◆CLASSIFICATION

PHARMACOTHERAPEUTIC: Central analgesic. **CLINICAL:** Non-narcotic analgesic, antipyretic.

ACTION

Exact mechanism unknown, but appears to inhibit prostaglandin synthesis in CNS and, to a lesser extent, by blocking pain impulse through peripheral action. Acts centrally on hypothalamic heat-regulating center, producing peripheral vasodilation (skin erythema, sweating, heat loss). **Therapeutic Effect:** Results in antipyresis. Produces analgesic effect.

PHARMACOKINETICS

Onset	Peak	Duration
PO		
15–30 min	1–1.5 hrs	4–6 hrs

Rapidly, completely absorbed from GI tract; rectal absorption variable. Protein binding: 20%–50%. Widely distributed to most body tissues. Metabolized in liver; excreted in urine. Removed by hemodialysis. **Half-life:** 1–4 hrs (half-life increased in hepatic disease, elderly, neonates; decreased in children).

USES

Relief of mild to moderate pain, fever.

PRECAUTIONS

CONTRAINDICATIONS: Active alcoholism, liver disease, or viral hepatitis (increases risk hepatotoxicity). **CAUTIONS:** Sensitivity to acetaminophen, severe impaired renal function, phenylketonuria, G6PD deficiency.

LIFESPAN CONSIDERATIONS: Pregnancy/lactation: Crosses placenta; distributed in breast milk. Routinely used in all stages of pregnancy, appears safe for short-term use. **Pregnancy Category B. Children/elderly:** No age-related precautions noted.

INTERACTIONS

DRUG: **Alcohol** (chronic use), **liver enzymes inducers (e.g., cimetidine), hepatotoxic medications (e.g., phenytoin)** may increase risk of hepatotoxicity with prolonged high dose or single toxic dose. May increase risk of bleeding with **warfarin** with regular use. **HERBAL:** None known. **FOOD:** None known. **LAB VALUES:** May increase SGOT (AST), SGPT (ALT), bilirubin, prothrombin levels (may indicate hepatotoxicity). Therapeutic blood serum level: 10–30 mcg/ml; toxic blood serum level: >200 mcg/ml.

AVAILABILITY (OTC)

CAPSULES: 80 mg, 160 mg, 325 mg, 500 mg. **DROPS:** 100 mg/ml. **ELIXIR:** 100 mg/ml, 130 mg/5 ml, 160 mg/5 ml, 500 mg/5 ml. **LIQUID:** 32 mg/ml, 100 mg/ml, 160 mg/5 ml. **SUPPOSITORY:** 80 mg, 120 mg, 325 mg, 650 mg. **SUSPENSION:** 100 mg/ml, 160 mg/5 ml. **SYRUP:** 160 mg/5 ml. **TABLETS:** 80 mg, 160 mg, 325 mg, 500 mg, 650 mg. **TABLETS (chewable):** 80 mg, 160 mg. **TABLETS (controlled release):** 650 mg.

ADMINISTRATION/HANDLING

PO

- Give without regard to meals.
- Tablets may be crushed.

RECTAL

- Moisten suppository with cold water before inserting well up into rectum.

INDICATIONS/ROUTES/DOSAGE

ANALGESIA, ANTIPYRESIS

Alert: Children may repeat doses 4–5 times/day; maximum of 5 doses/24 hrs.

PO: ADULTS, ELDERLY: 325–650 mg q4–6h or 1 g 3–4 times/day. **Maximum:** 4 g/day. CHILDREN: 10–15 mg/kg/dose q4–6h as needed. **Maximum:** 5 doses/24 hrs. NEONATES: 10–15 mg/kg/dose q6–8h as needed.

Rectal: ADULTS: 650 mg q4–6h. **Maximum:** 6 doses/24 hrs. CHILDREN: 10–20 mg/kg/dose q4–6h as needed. NEONATES: 10–15 mg/kg/dose q6–8h as needed.

DOSAGE IN RENAL IMPAIRMENT

Creatinine Clearance	Frequency
10–50 ml/min	q6h
<10 ml/min	q8h

SIDE EFFECTS

Well tolerated. **RARE:** Hypersensitivity reaction.

ADVERSE REACTIONS/ TOXIC EFFECTS

EARLY SIGNS OF ACETAMINOPHEN TOXICITY: Anorexia, nausea, diaphoresis, generalized weakness within first 12–24 hrs. **LATER SIGNS OF TOXICITY:** Vomiting, right upper quadrant tenderness, elevated liver function tests within 48–72 hrs after ingestion. **ANTIDOTE:** Acetylcysteine.

NURSING IMPLICATIONS

BASELINE ASSESSMENT

If given for analgesia, assess onset, type, location, duration of pain. Effect of medication is reduced if full pain response recurs prior to next dose. **Fixed-Combination:** Obtain vital signs before giving medication. If respirations are ≤12/min (≤20/min in children), withhold medication, contact physician.

INTERVENTION/EVALUATION

Assess for clinical improvement and relief of pain, fever. Therapeutic blood serum level: 10–30 mcg/ml; toxic serum level: >200 mcg/ml.

PATIENT/FAMILY TEACHING

Consult physician for use in children <2 yrs; oral use >5 days (children), >10 days (adults), or fever >3 days. Severe/recurrent pain or high/continuous fever may indicate serious illness.

acetazolamide

ah-seat-ah-**zole**-ah-myd
(Apo-Acetazolamide ✤, Diamox)

Do not confuse with acetohexamide, Trimox.

◆CLASSIFICATION

PHARMACOTHERAPEUTIC: Carbonic anhydrase inhibitor. **CLINICAL:** Antiglaucoma, anticonvulsant, diuretic, urinary alkalinizer (see p. 46C).

ACTION

Reduces formation of hydrogen and bicarbonate ions by inhibiting the enzyme carbonic anhydrase. **Therapeutic Effect:** Increases excretion of sodium, potassium, bicarbonate, and water in kidney; decreases formation of aqueous humor in eye; retards abnormal discharge from CNS neurons.

USES

Decreases intraocular pressure in treating glaucoma, diuretic, adjunct in treatment of refractory seizure disorders, prevents acute altitude sickness. **Unlabeled:** Lowers intraocular pressure in treatment of malignant glaucoma, treatment of toxicity of weakly acidic medications, prevents uric acid/renal calculi by alkalinizing the urine.

PRECAUTIONS

CONTRAINDICATIONS: Hypersensitivity to sulfonamides, severe renal disease, adrenal insufficiency, hypochloremic acidosis. **CAUTIONS:** History of hypercalcemia, diabetes mellitus, gout, concurrent digoxin therapy, obstructive pulmonary disease. **Pregnancy Category C.**

INTERACTIONS

DRUG: May increase **digoxin** levels (due to hypokalemia). May increase effects/toxicity of **amphetamines;** may decrease effects of **methenamine. HERBAL:** None known. **FOOD:** None known. **LAB VALUES:** May increase ammonia, bilirubin, glucose, chloride, uric acid, calcium; may decrease bicarbonate, potassium.

AVAILABILITY (Rx)

CAPSULES (sustained-release): 500 mg. **TABLETS:** 125 mg, 250 mg. **INJECTION:** 500 mg.

INDICATIONS/ROUTES/DOSAGE

GLAUCOMA

PO: ADULTS, ELDERLY: 250 mg 1–4 times/day. **Extended-release:** 500 mg 2 times/day. CHILDREN: 8–30 mg/kg/day in divided doses q8h.

IV: ADULTS, ELDERLY: 250–500 mg; may repeat in 2–4 hrs, then continue with oral therapy. CHILDREN: 5–10 mg/kg q6h. **Maximum:** 1 g/day.

EPILEPSY

PO: ADULTS, ELDERLY, CHILDREN: 375–1,000 mg/day in up to 4 divided doses.

EDEMA

PO: ADULTS: 250–375 mg/day. CHILDREN: 5 mg/kg/dose once daily.

ALTITUDE SICKNESS

PO: ADULTS, ELDERLY: 250 mg 2–4 times/day. If possible, begin 24–48 hrs prior to ascent; continue for at least 48 hrs at high altitude as needed to control symptoms.

SIDE EFFECTS

FREQUENT: Unusually tired/weak; diarrhea; increased urination/frequency; decreased appetite/weight; altered taste (metallic); nausea; vomiting; numbness in extremities, lips, mouth. **OCCASIONAL:** Depression, drowsiness. **RARE:** Headache, photosensitivity, confusion, tinnitus, severe muscle weakness, loss of taste.

ADVERSE REACTIONS/ TOXIC EFFECTS

Long-term therapy may result in acidotic state. Nephrotoxicity/hepatotoxicity occurs occasionally, manifested as dark urine/stools, pain in lower back, jaundice, dysuria, crystalluria, renal colic/calculi. Bone marrow depression may be manifested as aplastic anemia, thrombocytopenia, thrombocytopenic purpura, leukopenia, agranulocytosis, hemolytic anemia.

NURSING IMPLICATIONS

BASELINE ASSESSMENT

Glaucoma: Assess affected pupil for dilation, response to light. **Epilepsy:** Obtain history of seizure disorder (length, intensity, duration of seizure, presence of aura, LOC).

INTERVENTION/EVALUATION

Monitor for acidosis (headache, lethargy progressing to drowsiness, CNS depression, Kussmaul's respiration).

PATIENT/FAMILY TEACHING

Report presence of tingling or tremor in hands or feet, unusual bleeding/bruising, unexplained fever, sore throat, flank pain.

acetohexamide

(Dymelor)

See Classification section under: Antidiabetics (p. 39C)

acetylcysteine (*N*-acetylcysteine)

ah-sea-tyl-**sis**-teen

(Mucomyst, Parvolex)

Do not confuse with acetylcholine.

CLASSIFICATION

PHARMACOTHERAPEUTIC: Respiratory inhalant, intratracheal. **CLINICAL:** Mucolytic, antidote.

ACTION

Splits linkage of mucoproteins. **Therapeutic Effect:** Reduces viscosity of pulmonary secretions, facilitates removal by coughing, postural drainage, mechanical means. Protects against acetaminophen overdose–induced liver toxicity.

USES

Adjunctive treatment for abnormally viscid mucous secretions present in acute and chronic bronchopulmonary disease and pulmonary complication of cystic fibrosis, tracheostomy care; treatment of acetaminophen overdose. **Unlabeled:** Prevention of renal damage from dyes given during certain diagnostic tests (e.g., CT scans).

PRECAUTIONS

CONTRAINDICATIONS: None known. **CAUTIONS:** Bronchial asthma, elderly, debilitated with severe respiratory insufficiency. **Pregnancy Category B.**

INTERACTIONS

DRUG: None known. **HERBAL:** None known. **FOOD:** None known. **LAB VALUES:** None known.

AVAILABILITY (Rx)

SOLUTION: 10%, 20%.

INDICATIONS/ROUTES/DOSAGE

BRONCHOPULMONARY, TRACHEOSTOMY

Nebulization: ADULTS, ELDERLY, CHILDREN: (20% SOLUTION): 3–5 ml 3–4 times daily. RANGE: 1–10 ml q2–6h. ADULTS, ELDERLY, CHILDREN: (10% SOLUTION): 6–10 ml 3–4 times daily. RANGE: 2–20 ml q2–6h. INFANTS: 1–2 ml (20%) or 2–4 ml (10%) 3–4 times daily.

Intratracheal instillation: ADULTS, CHILDREN: 1–2 ml of 10%–20% solution instilled into tracheostomy q1–4h.

ACETAMINOPHEN OVERDOSE

Oral solution (5%): ADULTS, ELDERLY, CHILDREN: Loading dose of 140 mg/kg, followed in 4 hrs by maintenance dose of 70 mg/kg q4h for 17 additional doses (unless acetaminophen assay reveals nontoxic level).

PREVENTION OF RENAL DAMAGE

PO: ADULTS, ELDERLY: 600 mg 2 times daily for 4 doses starting the day before the procedure.

SIDE EFFECTS

FREQUENT: Inhalation: Stickiness on face, transient unpleasant odor. **OCCASIONAL: Inhalation:** Increased bronchial secretions, irritated throat, nausea, vomiting, rhinorrhea. **RARE: Inhalation:** Skin rash. **Oral:** Facial edema, bronchospasm, wheezing.

ADVERSE REACTIONS/ TOXIC EFFECTS

Large dosage may produce severe nausea, vomiting.

NURSING IMPLICATIONS

BASELINE ASSESSMENT

Mucolytic: Assess pretreatment respirations for rate, depth, rhythm.

INTERVENTION/EVALUATION

If bronchospasm occurs, treatment should be discontinued and physician notified; bronchodilator may be added to therapy. Monitor rate, depth, rhythm, type of respiration (abdominal, thoracic). Check sputum for color, consistency, amount.

PATIENT/FAMILY TEACHING

A slight, disagreeable odor from solution may be noticed during initial administration but disappears quickly. Explain importance of adequate hydration. Teach proper coughing and deep breathing.

Actiq

see fentanyl

Actos

see pioglitazone

acyclovir

aye-**sigh**-klo-veer
(Avirax, Zovirax)

Do not confuse with Zostrix.

CLASSIFICATION

PHARMACOTHERAPEUTIC: Synthetic nucleoside. **CLINICAL:** Antiviral (see p. 58C).

ACTION

Converted to acyclovir triphosphate, becoming part of DNA chain. **Therapeutic Effect:** Interferes with DNA synthesis and viral replication. Virustatic.

PHARMACOKINETICS

Poorly absorbed from GI tract; minimal absorption following topical application. Protein binding: 9%–36%. Widely distributed. Partially metabolized in liver. Excreted primarily in urine. Removed by hemodialysis. **Half-life:** 2.5 hrs (increased in impaired renal function).

USES

Treatment of herpes zoster (shingles), varicella-zoster (chickenpox), herpes simplex encephalitis, neonatal simplex. Treatment of initial and recurrent episodes of genital herpes, mucocutaneous herpes simplex. **Topical:** Initial episodes of genital herpes, immunocompromised pts with limited nonthreatening herpes simplex infections. **Cream:** Cold sores. **Unlabeled:** Herpes simplex ocular infections, infectious mononucleosis.

PRECAUTIONS

CONTRAINDICATIONS: Acyclovir reconstituted with bacteriostatic water containing benzyl alcohol should not be used in neonates. **CAUTIONS:** Renal or hepatic impairment, dehydration, fluid/electrolyte imbalance, concurrent use of nephrotoxic agents, neurologic abnormalities.

LIFESPAN CONSIDERATIONS: Pregnancy/lactation: Crosses placenta; distributed in breast milk. **Pregnancy Category B. Children:** Safety and efficacy in children <2 yrs not established (<1 yr for IV use). **Elderly:** Age-related decrease in renal function may require decreased dosage.

INTERACTIONS

DRUG: Probenecid may increase half-life. **Nephrotoxic medications (e.g., aminoglycosides)** may increase nephrotoxicity. **HERBAL:** None known. **FOOD:** None known. **LAB VALUES:** May increase BUN, serum creatinine concentrations.

AVAILABILITY (Rx)

TABLETS: 400 mg, 800 mg. **CAPSULES:** 200 mg. **ORAL SUSPENSION:** 200 mg/5 ml. **POWDER FOR INJECTION:** 500 mg, 1,000 mg. **OINTMENT:** 5%. **CREAM:** 5%.

ADMINISTRATION/HANDLING

PO

• May give without regard to food. • Do not crush or break capsules. • Store capsules at room temperature.

TOPICAL

• Avoid eye contact. • Use finger cot or rubber glove to prevent autoinoculation.

IV

Storage • Store vials at room temperature. • Solutions of 50 mg/ml stable for 12 hrs at room temperature; may form precipitate when refrigerated. Potency not affected by precipitate and redissolution. • IV infusion (piggyback) stable for 24 hrs at room temperature. Yellow discoloration does not affect potency.

Reconstitution • Add 10 ml Sterile Water for Injection to each 500-mg vial (50 mg/ml). Do not use bacteriostatic water for injection containing benzyl alcohol or parabens (will cause precipitate). • Shake well until solution clear. • Further dilute with at least 100 ml D_5W or 0.9% NaCl. Final concentration should be ≤7 mg/ml.

Rate of administration • Infuse over at least 1 hr (renal tubular damage may occur with too rapid rate). • Maintain adequate hydration during infusion and for 2 hrs following IV administration.

∅ IV INCOMPATIBILITIES

Aztreonam (Azactam), cefepime (Maxipime), diltiazem (Cardizem), dobutamine (Dobutrex), dopamine (Intropin), levofloxacin (Levaquin), meropenem (Merrem IV), ondansetron (Zofran), piperacillin/tazobactam (Zosyn).

IV COMPATIBILITIES

Allopurinol (Alloprim), amikacin (Amikin), ampicillin, cefazolin (Ancef), cefotaxime (Claforan), ceftazidime (Fortaz), ceftriaxone (Rocephin), cimetidine (Tagamet), clindamycin (Cleocin), famotidine (Pepcid), fluconazole (Diflucan), gentamicin, heparin, hydromorphone (Dilaudid), imipenem (Primaxin), lorazepam (Ativan), magnesium sulfate, methylprednisolone (SoluMedrol), metoclopramide (Reglan), metronidazole (Flagyl), morphine, multivitamins, potassium chloride, propofol (Diprivan), ranitidine (Zantac), trimethoprim/sulfamethoxazole (Bactrim, Septra), vancomycin.

INDICATIONS/ROUTES/DOSAGE

HERPES SIMPLEX

IV: ADULTS, ELDERLY, CHILDREN >12 YRS: 5 mg/kg/dose q8h for 5–10 days.

GENITAL HERPES

PO: ADULTS, ELDERLY, CHILDREN >12 YRS: 200 mg q4h (5 times/day) for 10 days (initial episode) or 5 days (recurrent episode).

VARICELLA-ZOSTER (chickenpox)

IV: ADULTS, ELDERLY, CHILDREN >12 YRS: 10 mg/kg/dose q8h for 7 days.

PO: ADULTS, ELDERLY 600–800 mg/dose q4h (5 times/day) for 7–10 days **or** 1,000 mg q6h for 5 days. CHILDREN: 10–20 mg/kg/dose (**Maximum:** 800 mg) 4 times/day for 5 days.

HERPES ZOSTER (shingles)

IV: ADULTS, CHILDREN: 10 mg/kg/dose q8h. ELDERLY: 7.5 mg/kg/dose.

PO: ADULTS: 800 mg q4h (5 times/day) for 7–10 days. CHILDREN: 250–600 mg/m^2/dose 4–5 times/day for 7–10 days.

USUAL TOPICAL DOSAGE

Topical: ADULTS, ELDERLY: 3–6 times/day for 7 days.

DOSAGE IN RENAL IMPAIRMENT

Dose and/or frequency is modified based on severity of infection, degree of renal impairment.

PO: Creatinine clearance of ≤10 ml/1.73 m^2: 200 mg q12h.

IV

Creatinine Clearance (ml/min)	Dosage Percent	Dosage Interval
>50	100	8 hrs
26–50	100	12 hrs
10–25	100	24 hrs
<10	50	24 hrs

SIDE EFFECTS

FREQUENT: **Parenteral (7%–9%):** Phlebitis/inflammation at IV site, nausea, vomiting. **Topical (28%):** Burning, stinging. OCCASIONAL: **Parenteral (3%):** Itching, rash, hives. **PO (6%–12%):** Malaise, nausea, headache. **Topical (4%):** Itching. RARE: **Parenteral (1%–2%):**

Confusion, hallucinations, seizures, tremors. **Topical (<1%):** Skin rash. **PO (1%–3%):** Vomiting, rash, diarrhea, headache.

ADVERSE REACTIONS/ TOXIC EFFECTS

Rapid parenteral administration, excessively high doses, or fluid/electrolyte imbalance may produce renal failure (abdominal pain, decreased urination, decreased appetite, increased thirst, nausea, vomiting). Toxicity not reported with oral or topical use.

NURSING IMPLICATIONS

BASELINE ASSESSMENT

Question for history of allergies, particularly to acyclovir. Assess herpes simplex lesions before treatment to compare baseline with treatment effect.

INTERVENTION/EVALUATION

Assess IV site for phlebitis (heat, pain, red streaking over vein). Evaluate cutaneous lesions. Ensure adequate ventilation. Manage chickenpox and disseminated herpes zoster with strict isolation. Provide analgesics and comfort measures; esp. exhausting to elderly. Encourage fluids.

PATIENT/FAMILY TEACHING

Drink adequate fluids. Do not touch lesions with fingers to prevent spreading infection to new site. **Genital Herpes:** Continue therapy for full length of treatment. Space doses evenly. Use finger cot or rubber glove to apply topical ointment. Avoid sexual intercourse during duration of lesions to prevent infecting partner. Acyclovir does not cure herpes. Pap smear should be done at least annually due to increased risk of cancer of cervix in women with genital herpes.

Adalat

see nifedipine

adalimumab

ah-dah-**lim**-you-mab
(Humira)

◆ CLASSIFICATION

PHARMACOTHERAPEUTIC: Monoclonal antibody. **CLINICAL:** Rheumatoid arthritis agent.

ACTION

Binds specifically to tumor necrosis factor (TNF) alpha cell, blocking its action with the cell surface of TNF receptors. **Therapeutic Effect:** Reduces inflammation, tenderness; swelling of joints slows or prevents progressive destruction of joints in those with rheumatoid arthritis.

PHARMACOKINETICS

Half-life: 10–20 days.

USES

Reduces signs, symptoms, progression of structural damage in adults with moderate to severe rheumatoid arthritis unresponsive to other disease-modifying antirheumatic drugs.

PRECAUTIONS

CONTRAINDICATIONS: Active infections. **CAUTIONS:** History of sensitivity to monoclonal antibodies, cardiovascular disease, pregnancy, preexisting or recent onset CNS demyelinating disorders, elderly.

LIFESPAN CONSIDERATIONS: Pregnancy/lactation: Unknown if excreted in breast milk. **Pregnancy Category B. Children:** Safety and efficacy not established. **Elderly:** Cautious use due to increased risk of serious infection and malignancy.

INTERACTIONS

DRUG: Methotrexate reduces absorption of adalimumab by 29%–40% (but no adjustment to drug dose is necessary if given concurrently with methotrexate). **HERBAL:** None known. **FOOD:** None known. **LAB VALUES:** May increase alkaline phosphatase, cholesterol, lipid profile.

AVAILABILITY (Rx)

INJECTION: Syringe: 40 mg/0.8 ml.

ADMINISTRATION/HANDLING

SUBCUTANEOUS

- Refrigerate. Do not freeze. Discard unused portion. Rotate injection sites. Give new injection at least 1 inch from an old site and never into area where skin is tender, bruised, red, or hard.

INDICATIONS/ROUTES/DOSAGE

RHEUMATOID ARTHRITIS

Subcutaneous: ADULTS, ELDERLY: 40 mg every other week.

SIDE EFFECTS

FREQUENT (20%): Injection site reactions (erythema, itching, pain, swelling). **OCCASIONAL (9%–12%):** Headache, rash, sinusitis, nausea. **RARE (5%–7%):** Abdominal pain, back pain, hypertension.

ADVERSE REACTIONS/ TOXIC EFFECTS

Infection consisting primarily of upper respiratory tract infections, bronchitis, and urinary tract infections occur rarely. More serious infection as pneumonia, hypersensitivity reaction, tuberculosis, cellulitis, pyelonephritis, septic arthritis also rarely occur.

NURSING IMPLICATIONS

BASELINE ASSESSMENT

Assess onset, type, location, duration of pain or inflammation. Inspect appearance of affected joints for immobility, deformities, skin condition. If pt is to self-administer, instruct subcutaneous injection technique, including areas of the body acceptable for injection sites.

INTERVENTION/EVALUATION

Monitor lab values, particularly alkaline phosphatase. Assess for therapeutic response: relief of pain, stiffness, swelling, increased joint mobility, reduced joint tenderness, improved grip strength.

PATIENT/FAMILY TEACHING

Injection site reaction generally occurs in first month of treatment and decreases in frequency during continued therapy. Do not receive live vaccines during treatment.

adefovir dipivoxil

add-eh-**foe**-vur

(Hepsera)

CLASSIFICATION

PHARMACOTHERAPEUTIC: Antiviral. **CLINICAL:** Hepatitis B agent.

ACTION

Inhibits DNA polymerase, an enzyme, causing DNA chain termination after its incorporation into viral DNA. **Therapeutic Effect:** Prevents DNA cell replication.

PHARMACOKINETICS

Following oral administration, binds to proteins. Excreted in the urine. **Half-life:** 7 hrs (half-life increased with impaired renal function).

USES

Treatment of chronic hepatitis B in adults with evidence of active viral replication and evidence of persistent elevations of SGOT (AST) or SGPT (ALT) or active disease.

PRECAUTIONS

CONTRAINDICATIONS: None known. **CAUTIONS:** Patients with known risk factors for liver disease, impaired renal function, elderly. **Pregnancy Category C.**

INTERACTIONS

DRUG: Ibuprofen increases adefovir plasma concentration. **HERBAL:** None known. **FOOD:** None known. **LAB VALUES:** May increase SGPT (ALT), SGOT (AST), serum creatinine, amylase.

AVAILABILITY (Rx)

TABLETS: 10 mg.

ADMINISTRATION/HANDLING

PO

- Give without regard to food.

INDICATION/DOSAGE/ROUTES

CHRONIC HEPATITIS B, NORMAL RENAL FUNCTION

PO: ADULTS, ELDERLY: 10 mg once daily. IMPAIRED RENAL FUNCTION, CREATININE CLEARANCE ≥50 ML/MIN: 10 mg q24h; CREATININE CLEARANCE 20–49 ML/MIN: 10 mg q48h; CREATININE CLEARANCE 10–19 ML/MIN: 10 mg q72h; HEMODIALYSIS: 10 mg q7days following dialysis.

SIDE EFFECTS

FREQUENT (13%): Asthenia (loss of strength, energy). **OCCASIONAL (4%–9%):** Headache, abdominal pain, nausea, flatulence. **RARE (3%):** Diarrhea, dyspepsia (heartburn, epigastric discomfort).

ADVERSE REACTIONS/ TOXIC EFFECTS

Nephrotoxicity characterized by increased serum creatinine and decreased serum phosphorus is treatment-limiting toxicity of drug therapy. Lactic acidosis, severe hepatomegaly may occur rarely, particularly found in women.

NURSING IMPLICATIONS

BASELINE ASSESSMENT

Obtain baseline renal function lab values before therapy begins and routinely thereafter. For those with preexisting renal insufficiency or during treatment, may require dose adjustment. HIV antibody testing should be performed before therapy begins (unrecognized or untreated HIV infection may result in emergency of HIV resistance).

INTERVENTION/EVALUATION

Monitor I&O, serum creatinine. Closely monitor for adverse reactions in those taking other medications that are excreted renally or with other drugs known to affect renal function.

adenosine

ah-**den**-oh-seen
(Adenocard)

CLASSIFICATION

PHARMACOTHERAPEUTIC: Cardiac agent, diagnostic aid. **CLINICAL:** Antiarrhythmic.

ACTION

Slows impulse formation in SA node, slows conduction time through AV node. **Therapeutic Effect:** Depresses left ventricular function and restores normal sinus rhythm.

USES

Treatment of paroxysmal supraventricular tachycardia, including those associated with accessory bypass tracts (Wolff-Parkinson-White syndrome). Adjunct in diagnosis in myocardial perfusion imaging or stress echocardiography.

PRECAUTIONS

CONTRAINDICATIONS: Second- or third-degree AV block or sick sinus syndrome (with functioning pacemaker), atrial flutter or fibrillation, ventricular tachycardia. **CAUTIONS:** Heart block, arrhythmias at time of conversion, asthma, hepatic/renal failure. **Pregnancy Category C.**

INTERACTIONS

DRUG: Methylxanthines (e.g., caffeine, theophylline) may decrease effect. **Dipyridamole** may increase effect. **Carbamazepine** may increase degree of heart block caused by adenosine. **HERBAL:** None known. **FOOD:** None known. **LAB VALUES:** None known.

AVAILABILITY (Rx)

INJECTION: 3 mg/ml in 6-mg and 12-mg syringes.

ADMINISTRATION/HANDLING

IV

Storage • Store at room temperature. Solution appears clear. • Crystallization occurs if refrigerated; if crystallization occurs, dissolve crystals by warming to room temperature. Discard unused portion.

Rate of administration • Administer very rapidly (over 1–2 sec) undiluted directly into vein, or if using IV line, use closest port to insertion site. If IV line is infusing any fluid other than 0.9% NaCl, flush line first. • After rapid bolus injection, follow with rapid 0.9% NaCl flush.

∅ IV INCOMPATIBILITIES

Any other drug or solution other than 0.9% NaCl or D_5W.

INDICATIONS/ROUTES/DOSAGE

USUAL DOSAGE

Rapid IV bolus: ADULTS, ELDERLY: Initially, 6 mg (over 1–2 sec). If first dose does not convert within 1–2 min, give 12 mg; may repeat 12-mg dose in 1–2 min if no response has occurred. CHILDREN: Initially, 0.1 mg/kg (maximum 6 mg) if ineffective may give 0.2 mg/kg (maximum 12 mg).

DIAGNOSTIC TESTING

IV infusion: ADULTS: 140 mcg/kg/min for 6 min.

SIDE EFFECTS

FREQUENT (12%–18%): Facial flushing, shortness of breath/dyspnea. **OCCASIONAL (2%–7%):** Headache, nausea, lightheadedness, chest pressure. **RARE (≤1%):** Numbness/tingling in arms, dizziness, sweating, hypotension, palpitations, chest/jaw/neck pain.

ADVERSE REACTIONS/ TOXIC EFFECTS

May produce short-lasting heart block.

NURSING IMPLICATIONS

BASELINE ASSESSMENT

Identify arrhythmia per cardiac monitor and apical pulse.

INTERVENTION/EVALUATION

Assess cardiac performance per continuous EKG. Monitor B/P, apical pulse (rate, rhythm, quality), and respirations. Monitor I&O; assess for fluid retention. Check electrolytes.

Advair

see fluticasone

A

agalsidase beta

ah-**gull**-sigh-dase
(Fabrazyme)

◆ **CLASSIFICATION**

PHARMACOTHERAPEUTIC: Enzyme.
CLINICAL: Fabry disease agent.

ACTION

Fabry disease is an X-linked genetic disorder. Agalsidase beta catalyzes the hydrolysis of glycosphingolipid metabolism, reducing the deposits in capillary endothelium of the kidney and other cell types. **Therapeutic Effect:** Provides an exogenous source of alpha-galactosidase A, an enzyme, missing in those with Fabry disease.

USES

Treatment of Fabry disease.

PRECAUTIONS

CONTRAINDICATIONS: None known. **CAUTIONS:** Moderate to severe hypertension, renal impairment, febrile pts, compromised cardiac function. **Pregnancy Category B.**

INTERACTIONS

DRUG: None known. **HERBAL:** None known. **FOOD:** None known. **LAB VALUES:** None known.

ADMINISTRATION/HANDLING

IV

Storage • Store vials in refrigerator. Use reconstituted and diluted solution immediately; if not possible, solution is stable for 24 hrs if refrigerated.

Reconstitution • Allow vial to reach room temperature prior to reconstitution (about 30 min). Reconstitute each vial by slowly injecting 7.2 ml Sterile Water for Injection. Roll and tilt gently. Prior to adding reconstituted solution to 500 ml 0.9% NaCl, remove an equal volume from the 500-ml infusion bag, and then add to 500 ml 0.9% NaCl infusion bag.

Rate of administration • Give no more than 0.25 mg/min (15 mg/hr). May slow infusion rate if infusion-related reaction occurs. If no reaction, infusion rate may be increased in increments to 0.05–0.08 mg/min (increments of 3–5 mg/hr).

IV INCOMPATIBILITY

Do not mix with any other medications.

AVAILABILITY (Rx)

POWDER FOR INJECTION: 37 mg (5 mg/ml when reconstituted).

INDICATIONS/ ROUTES/DOSAGE

FABRY DISEASE

IV infusion: ADULTS, ELDERLY: 1 mg/kg infused every 2 wks.

SIDE EFFECTS

Alert: Pretreat with antipyretics prior to infusion.

COMMON (45%–52%): Rigors, fever, headache. **FREQUENT (21%–38%):** Rhinitis, nausea, anxiety, pharyngitis, edema, skeletal pain. **OCCASIONAL (10%–17%):** Temperature change sensation, hypotension, pallor, paresthesia, pruritus, urticaria, bronchitis. **RARE (7%):** Bronchitis, depression, arthralgia, dyspepsia (epigastric discomfort, heartburn), laryngitis, sinusitis.

ADVERSE REACTON/TOXIC EFFECTS

Frequently occurring serious infusion reactions include tachycardia, hypertension, throat tightness, chest pain, dyspnea, vomiting, lip edema, rash. Other adverse events characterized by bradycardia, arrhythmias, vertigo, nephritic syndrome, stroke, cardiac arrest.

NURSING IMPLICATIONS

BASELINE ASSESSMENT

Give antipyretics prior to IV infusion.

INTERVENTION/EVALUATION

Monitor for infusion reaction. If reaction occurs, decrease infusion rate or temporarily stop infusion. Additional antipyretics, antihistamines, steroids may alleviate these symptoms. Closely monitor those with compromised cardiac function (increased risk of severe complications from infusion reactions).

PATIENT/FAMILY TEACHING

Inform pts a registry has been established to better understand Fabry disease and to evaluate long-term treatment effects of agalsidase.

Aggrenox

see dipyridamole or aspirin

albumin, human

al-**byew**-min
(Albuminar, Albutein, Buminate, Plasbumin)

CLASSIFICATION

PHARMACOTHERAPEUTIC: Plasma protein fraction. **CLINICAL:** Blood derivative.

ACTION

Blood volume expander. **Therapeutic Effect:** Provides temporary increase in blood volume, reduces hemoconcentration and blood viscosity.

PHARMACOKINETICS

Onset	Peak	Duration
IV		
15 min	—	—

Distributed throughout extracellular water. Onset of action: 15 min provided patient is well hydrated. **Half-life:** 15–20 days.

USES

Treatment of hypovolemia, plasma volume expansion and maintenance of cardiac output in treatment of shock or impending shock, hypoproteinemia resulting in edema or decreased intravascular volume (e.g., acute nephrotic syndrome, premature neonates).

PRECAUTIONS

CONTRAINDICATIONS: Severe anemia, cardiac failure, history of allergic reaction to albumin, hypervolemia, pulmonary edema, no albumin deficiency. **CAUTIONS:** Hypertension, normal serum albumin concentration, low cardiac reserve, pulmonary disease, hepatic or renal failure.

LIFESPAN CONSIDERATIONS: Pregnancy/lactation: Unknown if drug crosses placenta or is distributed in breast milk. **Pregnancy Category C. Children/elderly:** No age-related precautions noted.

INTERACTIONS

DRUG: None known. **HERBAL:** None known. **FOOD:** None known. **LAB VALUES:** May increase serum alkaline phosphatase concentrations.

AVAILABILITY (Rx)

INJECTION: 5%, 25%.

ADMINISTRATION/HANDLING

IV

Storage • Store at room temperature. Appears as clear, brownish, odorless, moderate viscous fluid. • Do not use if solution has been frozen, appears turbid, or contains sediment, or if not used within 4 hrs of opening vial.

Reconstitution • 5% solution may be made from 25% solution by adding 1 volume 25% to 4 volumes 0.9% NaCl or D_5W (NaCl preferred). Do not use sterile water for injection (life-threatening hemolysis, acute renal failure can result).

Rate of administration • Give by IV infusion. Rate is variable, depends on use, blood volume, concentration of solute. • 5%: usually given at 5–10 ml/min; 25%: usually at 2–3 ml/min. • 5% administered undiluted; 25% may be administered undiluted or diluted with 0.9% NaCl or D_5W. NaCl preferred. • May give without regard to pt blood group or Rh factor.

⊘ IV INCOMPATIBILITIES

Midazolam (Versed), vancomycin (Vancocin), verapamil (Isoptin).

IV COMPATIBILITIES

Diltiazem (Cardizem), lorazepam (Ativan).

INDICATIONS/ROUTES/DOSAGE

Alert: Dosage based on pt's condition; duration of administration based on pt's response.

HYPOVOLEMIA

IV: ADULTS, ELDERLY: Initially, 25 g, may repeat in 15–30 min. **Maximum:** 250 g within 48 hrs. CHILDREN: 0.5–1 g/kg/dose (10–20 ml/kg/dose of 5% albumin) **Maximum:** 6 g/kg/day.

HYPOPROTEINEMIA

IV: ADULTS, ELDERLY, CHILDREN: 0.5–1 g/kg/dose (10–20 ml/kg/dose of 5% albumin) repeat in 1–2 days.

BURNS

IV: ADULTS, ELDERLY, CHILDREN: Initially, begin with administration of large volumes of crystalloid injection to maintain plasma volume. After 24 hrs, an initial dose of 25 g with dosage adjusted to maintain plasma albumin concentration of 2–2.5 g/100 ml.

CARDIOPULMONARY BYPASS

IV: ADULTS, ELDERLY: 5% OR 25%: With crystalloid to maintain plasma albumin concentration of 2.5 g/100 ml.

ACUTE NEPHROSIS, NEPHROTIC SYNDROME

IV: ADULTS, ELDERLY: 25 g of 25% injection, with diuretic once a day for 7–10 days.

RENAL DIALYSIS

IV: ADULTS, ELDERLY: 25%: 100 ml (25 g).

HYPERBILIRUBINEMIA, ERYTHROBLASTOSIS FETALIS

IV: INFANTS: 1 g/kg 1–2 hrs before transfusion.

SIDE EFFECTS

OCCASIONAL: Hypotension. **RARE:** High dose, repeated therapy may result in altered vital signs; chills, fever, increased salivation, nausea, vomiting, urticaria, tachycardia.

ADVERSE REACTIONS/ TOXIC EFFECTS

Fluid overload (headache, weakness, blurred vision, behavioral changes, incoordination, isolated muscle twitching) and CHF (rapid breathing, rales, wheezing, coughing, increased B/P, distended neck veins) may occur.

NURSING IMPLICATIONS

BASELINE ASSESSMENT

Obtain B/P, pulse, respirations immediately prior to administration. There should be adequate hydration before albumin is administered.

INTERVENTION/EVALUATION

Monitor B/P for hypotension/hypertension. Assess frequently for evidence of fluid overload, pulmonary edema (see Adverse Reaction/Toxic Effects).

Check skin for flushing, urticaria. Monitor I&O ratio (watch for decreased output). Assess for therapeutic response (increased B/P, decreased edema).

albuterol

ale-**beut**-er-all

(Novosalmol✦, Proventil, Ventolin, Volmax, Vospire ER)

Do not confuse with atenolol, Prinivil.

FIXED-COMBINATION(S)

Combivent: albuterol/ipratropium (a bronchodilator): 103 mcg/18 mcg per actuation. **Duoneb:** albuterol/ipratropium 3 mg/0.5 mg.

CLASSIFICATION

PHARMACOTHERAPEUTIC: Sympathomimetic (adrenergic agonist). **CLINICAL:** Bronchodilator (see p. 64C).

ACTION

Stimulates $beta_2$-adrenergic receptors in the lungs, resulting in relaxation of bronchial smooth muscle. **Therapeutic Effect:** Relieves bronchospasm, reduces airway resistance.

PHARMACOKINETICS

Onset	Peak	Duration
PO		
15–30 min	2–3 hrs	4–6 hrs
PO extended-release		
30 min	2–4 hrs	12 hrs
Inhalation		
5–15 min	0.5–2 hrs	2–5 hrs

Rapidly, well absorbed from GI tract; gradual absorption from bronchi following inhalation. Metabolized in liver. Primarily excreted in urine. **Half-life:** Oral: 2.7–5 hrs; inhalation: 3.8 hrs.

USES

Relief of bronchospasm due to reversible obstructive airway disease, exercise-induced bronchospasm.

PRECAUTIONS

CONTRAINDICATIONS: History of hypersensitivity to sympathomimetics. **CAUTIONS:** Hypertension, cardiovascular disease, hyperthyroidism, diabetes mellitus.

LIFESPAN CONSIDERATIONS: Pregnancy/lactation: Appears to cross placenta; unknown if distributed in breast milk. May inhibit uterine contractility. **Pregnancy Category C. Children:** Safety and efficacy not established in children <2 yrs (syrup) or <6 yrs (tablets). **Elderly:** May be more sensitive to tremor or tachycardia due to age-related increased sympathetic sensitivity.

INTERACTIONS

DRUG: Beta-adrenergic blocking agents (beta-blockers) antagonize effects. May increase risk of arrhythmias with **digoxin. MAOIs, tricyclic antidepressants** may potentiate cardiovascular effects. **HERBAL:** None known. **FOOD:** None known. **LAB VALUES:** May decrease serum potassium levels, increase glucose levels.

AVAILABILITY (Rx)

TABLETS: 2 mg, 4 mg. **TABLETS (extended-release):** 4 mg, 8 mg. **SYRUP:** 2 mg/5 ml. **AEROSOL:** Metered dose inhaler. **SOLUTION FOR INHALATION:** 0.83 mg/ml, 5 mg/ml. **CAPSULES FOR INHALATION:** 200 mcg.

ADMINISTRATION/HANDLING

PO

• Do not crush or break extended-release tablets. • May give without regard to food.

INHALATION

• Shake container well, exhale completely through mouth; place mouthpiece into mouth and close lips, holding inhaler upright. • Inhale deeply through mouth while fully depressing the top of canister. Hold breath as long as possible before exhaling slowly. • Wait 2 min before inhaling second dose (allows for deeper bronchial penetration). • Rinse mouth with water immediately after inhalation (prevents mouth/throat dryness).

NEBULIZATION

• Dilute 0.5 ml of 0.5% solution to final volume of 3 ml with 0.9% NaCl to provide 2.5 mg. • Administer over 5–15 min. • Nebulizer should be used with compressed air or O_2 at rate of 6–10 L/min.

INDICATIONS/ROUTES/DOSAGE

BRONCHOSPASM

PO: ADULTS: 2–4 mg 3–4 times/day. **Maximum:** 8 mg 4 times/day. **Sustained-release:** 1–2 tabs q12h. ELDERLY: 2 mg 3–4 times/day. **Maximum:** 8 mg 4 times/day. CHILDREN 6–12 YRS: 2 mg 3–4 times/day. **Repeatabs:** 4 mg 2 times/day. CHILDREN 2–6 YRS: 0.1–0.2 mg/kg 3–4 times/day. **Maximum:** 4 mg 3 times/day.

Inhalation: ADULTS, ELDERLY, CHILDREN >12 YRS: METERED DOSE INHALER: 1–2 inhalations q4–6h. **Maximum:** 12 inhalations/day. CHILDREN <12 YRS: 1–2 inhalations 4 times/day.

Nebulization: ADULTS, ELDERLY: 2.5–10 mg q1–4h as needed or continuous infusion of 10–15 mg/hr. CHILDREN: 0.15–0.3 mg/hr (**Maximum:** 10 mg) q1–4h as needed or continuous infusion of 0.5 mg/kg/hr.

EXERCISE-INDUCED BRONCHOSPASM

Inhalation: ADULTS, ELDERLY, CHILDREN >12 YRS: 2 inhalations 30 min before exercise.

SIDE EFFECTS

FREQUENT: Headache (27%); nausea (15%); restlessness, nervousness, trembling (20%); dizziness (<7%); throat dryness/irritation, pharyngitis (<6%); B/P changes/hypertension (3%–5%); heartburn, transient wheezing (<5%). **OCCASIONAL (2%–3%):** Insomnia, weakness, unusual/bad taste or taste/smell change. **Inhalation:** Dry, irritated mouth or throat; coughing; bronchial irritation. **RARE:** Drowsiness, diarrhea, dry mouth, flushing, sweating, anorexia.

ADVERSE REACTIONS/ TOXIC EFFECTS

Excessive sympathomimetic stimulation may produce palpitations, extrasystoles, tachycardia, chest pain, slight increase in B/P followed by substantial decrease, chills, sweating, blanching of skin. Too frequent or excessive use may lead to loss of bronchodilating effectiveness and/or severe, paradoxical bronchoconstriction.

NURSING IMPLICATIONS

BASELINE ASSESSMENT

Offer emotional support (high incidence of anxiety due to difficulty in breathing and sympathomimetic response to drug).

INTERVENTION/EVALUATION

Monitor rate, depth, rhythm, type of respiration; quality and rate of pulse; EKG; serum potassium, ABG determinations. Assess lung sounds for wheezing (bronchoconstriction) and rales.

PATIENT/FAMILY TEACHING

Instruct on proper use of inhaler. Increase fluid intake (decreases lung secretion viscosity). Do not take more than 2 inhalations at any one time (excessive use may produce paradoxical bronchoconstriction or a decreased bronchodilating effect). Rinsing mouth with water immediately after inhalation may prevent mouth/throat dryness. Avoid excessive use of caffeine derivatives (chocolate, coffee, tea, cola, cocoa).

alclometasone

(Aclovate)
See Classification section under: Corticosteroids: topical (p. 83C)

aldesleukin

all-des-**lyew**-kin
(Interleukin-2, IL-2, Proleukin)
See Interleukin-2, pp. 68C, 581

alefacept

ale-fah-cept
(Amevive)

◆ CLASSIFICATION

PHARMACOTHERAPEUTIC: Immunologic agent. **CLINICAL:** Immunosuppressive.

ACTION

Interferes with lymphocyte activation by binding to the lymphocyte antigen, inhibiting interaction of T lymphocytes. **Therapeutic Effect:** Reduces the number of circulating total lymphocytes, predominant in psoriatic lesions.

PHARMACOKINETICS

Half-life: 270 hrs.

USES

Treatment of adults with moderate to severe chronic plaque psoriasis who are candidates for systemic therapy or phototherapy.

PRECAUTIONS

CONTRAINDICATIONS: History of systemic malignancy, concurrent immunosuppressive agents or phototherapy. **CAUTIONS:** Those at high risk for malignancy, chronic infections, history of recurrent infection, elderly.

LIFESPAN CONSIDERATIONS: Pregnancy/lactation: Unknown if drug crosses placenta or is distributed in breast milk. **Pregnancy Category B. Children:** Safety and efficacy not established. **Elderly:** Cautious use due to higher incidence of infections and certain malignancies.

INTERACTIONS

DRUG: None known. **HERBAL:** None known. **FOOD:** None known. **LAB VALUES:** Decreases T lymphocyte levels. May increase serum transaminase.

AVAILABILITY (Rx)

POWDER FOR INJECTION: 7.5 mg, 15 mg.

ADMINISTRATION/HANDLING

IM/IV

Storage • Store unopened vials at room temperature. Following reconstitution, use immediately, or if refrigerated, within 4 hrs. Discard unused portion within 4 hrs of reconstitution. Reconstituted solution should be clear and colorless to slightly yellow. Do not use if discolored or cloudy or if undissolved material remains.

IM/IV

Alert: For both IM/IV administration, withdraw 0.6 ml of the supplied diluent and with the needle pointed at the sidewall of the vial, slowly inject the diluent into the vial of alefacept. Although some foaming will occur, avoid excessive foaming by not shaking or vigorously agitating the vial, but swirl gently to dissolve.

IM

Reconstitution • Reconstitute 15 mg with 0.6 ml of supplied diluent (Sterile Water for Injection); 0.5 mg of reconstituted solution contains 15 mg alefacept. Inject the full 0.5 ml of solution. Use a different IM site for each new injection. Give new injections at least 1 inch from the old site. Avoid areas where the skin is tender, bruised, red, or hard.

IV

Reconstitution • Reconstitute 7.5 mg with 0.6 ml of supplied diluent (Sterile Water for Injection); 0.5 mg of reconstituted solution contains 7.5 mg alefacept.

Rate of administration • Prepare 2 syringes with 3 ml 0.9% NaCl for pre- and postadministration flush. Prime the winged infusion set with 3 ml 0.9% NaCl and insert the set into the vein. Attach the medication-filled syringe to the infusion set and give over no more than 5 sec. Flush with 3 ml 0.9% NaCl.

IV INCOMPATIBILITY

Do not mix with any other medications. Do not reconstitute with other diluents other than that supplied by the manufacturer.

INDICATIONS/ROUTES/DOSAGE

Alert: May re-treat for an additional 12 wks if a minimum of a 12-wk interval has passed since previous course of therapy and CD4+ T lymphocyte counts are within normal limits.

PLAQUE PSORIASIS

IM: ADULTS, ELDERLY: 15 mg once weekly for 12 wks.

IV: ADULTS, ELDERLY: 7.5 mg once weekly for 12 wks.

SIDE EFFECTS

FREQUENT (16%): Injection site reactions with IM administration (pain, inflammation). **OCCASIONAL (5%):** Chills. **RARE (≤2%):** Pharyngitis, dizziness, cough, nausea, myalgia, injection site pain/inflammation.

ADVERSE REACTIONS/ TOXIC EFFECTS

Lymphopenia, malignancies, serious infections requiring hospitalization (cellulites, abscess, pneumonia, postoperative wound infection), hypersensitivity reactions occur rarely. Coronary artery disorder, myocardial infarction occur in <1%.

NURSING IMPLICATIONS

BASELINE ASSESSMENT

Obtain baseline CD4+ T lymphocyte levels prior to treatment and weekly during the 12-wk dosing period.

INTERVENTION/EVALUATION

Closely monitor CD4+ T lymphocyte levels. Withhold dose if CD4+ T lymphocyte levels are below 250 cells/mcl. If the levels remain below 250 cells/mcl for 1 mo, discontinue treatment.

PATIENT/FAMILY TEACHING

Regular monitoring of WBC count during therapy is necessary. Promptly report any signs of infection or evidence of malignancy.

alemtuzumab

al-lem-**two**-zoo-mab
(Campath)

CLASSIFICATION

PHARMACOTHERAPEUTIC: Monoclonal antibody. **CLINICAL:** Antineoplastic (see p. 69C).

ACTION

Binds to CD52, a cell surface glycoprotein, found on surface of all B and T lymphocytes, most monocytes, macrophages, NK cells, and granulocytes. **Therapeutic Effect:** Produces cytotoxicity, reduces tumor size.

PHARMACOKINETICS

Half-life: About 12 days. Peak and trough levels rise during first few wks of therapy, approach steady state by about wk 6.

USES

Treatment of B-cell chronic lymphocytic leukemia (B-CLL) in pts who have been treated with alkylating agents and who have failed fludarabine (Fludara) therapy.

PRECAUTIONS

CONTRAINDICATIONS: Active systemic infections, immunosuppression, known hypersensitivity or anaphylactic reaction. **CAUTIONS:** None known.

LIFESPAN CONSIDERATIONS: Pregnancy/lactation: Has potential to cause fetal B and T lymphocyte depletion. Discontinue breast-feeding during treatment and for ≥3 mos after last dose. **Pregnancy Category C. Children:** Safety and efficacy not established. **Elderly:** No age-related precautions noted.

INTERACTIONS

DRUG: None known. **HERBAL:** None known. **FOOD:** None known. **LAB VALUES:** May decrease white blood cell count, Hgb, platelet count.

AVAILABILITY (Rx)

SOLUTION FOR INJECTION: 30 mg/3 ml.

ADMINISTRATION/HANDLING

IV

Storage

Alert: Do not give by IV push or bolus. • Prior to dilution, refrigerate ampoules. Do not freeze. • Use within 8 hrs after dilution. Diluted solution may be stored at room temperature or refrigerated. • Discard if particulate matter is present or if solution is discolored.

Reconstitution • Withdraw needed amount from ampoule into a syringe. • Using a low-protein binding, nonfiber-releasing 5-micron filter, inject into 100 ml 0.9% NaCl or D_5W. • Invert bag to mix; do not shake.

Rate of administration • Give the 100 ml solution as a 2-hr IV infusion.

∅ IV INCOMPATIBILITY

Do not mix with any other medications.

INDICATIONS/ROUTES/DOSAGE

Alert: Pretreatment with 650 mg acetaminophen and 50 mg diphenhydramine before each infusion may prevent infusion-related side effects.

CHRONIC LYMPHOCYTIC LEUKEMIA (B-CLL)

IV infusion: ADULTS, ELDERLY: Initially, 3 mg/day given as a 2-hr infusion. When the 3-mg daily dose is tolerated (low grade or no infusion-related toxicities), increase daily dose to 10 mg. When the 10 mg/day dose is tolerated, maintenance dose of 30 mg/day may be initiated. MAINTENANCE DOSE: 30 mg/day 3 times/wk on alternate days (Mon., Wed., Fri. or Tues., Thurs., Sat.) for ≤12 wks (increase to 30 mg/day is usually achieved in 3–7 days).

SIDE EFFECTS

FREQUENT: Rigors (86%); fever (85%); nausea (54%); vomiting (41%); rash (40%); fatigue (34%); hypotension (32%); urticaria (30%); pruritus, skeletal pain, headache (24%); diarrhea (22%); anorexia (20%). **OCCASIONAL (<10%):** Myalgia, dizziness, abdominal pain, throat irritation, vomiting, neutropenia, rhinitis, bronchospasm, urticaria.

ADVERSE REACTIONS/ TOXIC EFFECTS

Neutropenia occurs in 85%, anemia in 80%, thrombocytopenia in 72%, rash in 40%. Respiratory toxicity (16%–26%) manifested as dyspnea, cough, bronchitis, pneumonitis, pneumonia.

NURSING IMPLICATIONS

BASELINE ASSESSMENT

Pretreatment with acetaminophen and diphenhydramine before each infusion may prevent infusion-related side effects. CBC, platelet count should be obtained frequently during and after therapy to assess for neutropenia, anemia, thrombocytopenia.

INTERVENTION/EVALUATION

Monitor for an infusion-related symptoms complex consisting mainly of rigors, fever, chills, hypotension, generally occurring 30 min–2 hrs from beginning of first infusion. Slowing drip rate or slowing infusion resolves symptoms. Monitor for hematologic toxicity (fever, sore throat, signs of local infection, easy bruising, or unusual bleeding from any site), symptoms of anemia (excessive tiredness, weakness).

PATIENT/FAMILY TEACHING

Avoid crowds, those with known infection. Avoid contact with anyone who recently received live virus vaccine; do not receive vaccinations.

alendronate sodium

ah-**len**-drew-nate
(Fosamax)
Do not confuse with Flomax.

CLASSIFICATION

PHARMACOTHERAPEUTIC: Bisphosphonate. **CLINICAL:** Bone resorption inhibitor, calcium regulator.

ACTION

Inhibits normal and abnormal bone resorption, without retarding mineralization. **Therapeutic Effect:** Leads to significant increased bone mineral density, reverses the progression of osteoporosis.

PHARMACOKINETICS

Poorly absorbed after PO administration. Protein binding: 78%. After PO administration, rapidly taken into bone, with uptake greatest at sites of active bone turnover. Excreted in urine. **Terminal half-life:** >10 yrs (reflects release from skeleton as bone is resorbed).

USES

Treatment of osteoporosis, glucocorticoid-induced osteoporosis, Paget's disease; prevention of osteoporosis, vertebral compression fractures in postmenopausal women. **Unlabeled:** Treatment of breast cancer.

PRECAUTIONS

CONTRAINDICATIONS: GI disease (e.g., dysphagia, frequent heartburn, GERD, hiatal hernia, ulcers), renal function impairment, sensitivity to alendronate, inability to stand/sit upright for at least 30 min. **CAUTIONS:** Hypocalcemia, vitamin D deficiency.

LIFESPAN CONSIDERATIONS: Pregnancy/lactation: Possible incomplete fetal ossification, decreased maternal weight gain, delay in delivery. Excretion in breast milk unknown. Do not give to nursing women. **Pregnancy Category C. Children:** Safety and efficacy not established. **Elderly:** No age-related precautions noted.

INTERACTIONS

DRUG: Concurrent **dietary supplements, food, beverages** may interfere with alendronate absorption. IV **ranitidine** may double drug bioavailability. **Aspirin** may increase GI disturbances. **HERBAL:** None known. **FOOD:** None known. **LAB VALUES:** Reduces serum calcium, phosphate concentrations. Significant decrease in serum alkaline phosphatase noted in those with Paget's disease.

AVAILABILITY (Rx)

TABLETS: 5 mg, 10 mg, 35 mg, 40 mg, 70 mg.

ADMINISTRATION/HANDLING

PO

• Give first thing in morning, at least 30 min before first food, beverage, or medication of the day. • Give with 6–8 oz plain water only (mineral water, coffee, tea, juice will decrease absorption). • Instruct patient **not** to lie down for at least 30 min after administering medication and until eating first food of the day (plain water and not lying down allows medication to reach stomach quickly, minimizing esophageal irritation).

INDICATIONS/ROUTES/DOSAGE

Alert: Take with full glass plain water only, 30 min before first food, beverage, or medication.

TREATMENT OF OSTEOPOROSIS, PREVENTION OF FRACTURES

PO: ADULTS, ELDERLY: 10 mg once daily, in the morning or 70 mg once/wk.

PAGET'S DISEASE

PO: ADULTS, ELDERLY: 40 mg once daily, in the morning.

GLUCOCORTICOID INDUCED OSTEOPOROSIS

PO: ADULTS, ELDERLY: 5 mg/day (10 mg/day in postmenopausal women not receiving estrogen).

PREVENTION OF OSTEOPOROSIS

PO: ADULTS, ELDERLY: 5 mg once daily, in the morning or 35 mg once/week.

SIDE EFFECTS

FREQUENT (7%–8%): Back pain, abdominal pain. **OCCASIONAL (2%–3%):** Nausea, abdominal distention, constipation/diarrhea, flatulence. **RARE (<2%):** Skin rash.

ADVERSE REACTIONS/ TOXIC EFFECTS

Hypocalcemia, hypophosphatemia, significant GI disturbances result from overdosage. Esophageal irritation occurs if not given with 6–8 oz/ plain water or if pt lies down within 30 min of administration.

NURSING IMPLICATIONS

BASELINE ASSESSMENT

Hypocalcemia, vitamin D deficiency must be corrected before therapy. Check electrolytes (esp. calcium and alkaline phosphatase serum levels).

INTERVENTION/EVALUATION

Monitor electrolytes (esp. calcium and alkaline phosphatase serum levels).

PATIENT/FAMILY TEACHING

Instruct pt that expected benefits occur only when medication is taken with full glass (6–8 oz) of plain water, first thing in the morning and at least 30 min before first food, beverage, or medication of the day is taken. Any other beverage (mineral water, orange juice, coffee) significantly reduces absorption of medication. Do not lie down for at least 30 min after taking medication (potentiates delivery to stomach, reducing risk of esophageal irritation). Consider weight-bearing exercises, modify behavioral factors (e.g., cigarette smoking, alcohol consumption).

alfentanil

(Alfenta)

See Classification section under: Opioid analgesics

alfuzosin hydrochloride

ale-few-**zoe**-sin

(Uroxatrel)

CLASSIFICATION

PHARMACOTHERAPEUTIC: Alpha$_1$-adrenergic blocker. **CLINICAL:** Benign prostatic hyperplasia agent.

ACTION

An alpha$_1$ antagonist targets receptors around bladder neck and prostate capsule. **Therapeutic Effect:** Results in relaxation of smooth muscle, improvement in urinary flow, symptoms of prostate hyperplasia.

PHARMACOKINETICS

Rapidly absorbed following PO administration. Widely distributed. Protein binding: 90%. Extensively metabolized in liver. Primarily excreted in urine. **Half-life:** 3–9 hrs.

USES

Treatment of signs and symptoms of benign prostatic hyperplasia.

PRECAUTIONS

CONTRAINDICATIONS: None known. **CAUTIONS:** Coronary artery disease, hepatic disease, orthostatic hypotension, general anesthesia.

LIFESPAN CONSIDERATIONS: Pregnancy/lactation: Not indicated for use in women. **Children:** Not indicated in this pt population. **Elderly:** No age-related precautions noted.

INTERACTIONS

DRUG: Other alpha-blocking agents **(prazosin, terazosin, doxazosin, tamsulosin)** may have additive effect. **Cimetidine** may increase alfuzosin concentration. **HERBAL:** None known. **FOOD:** None known. **LAB VALUES:** None known.

AVAILABILITY (Rx)

TABLETS, EXTENDED-RELEASE: 10 mg.

ADMINISTRATION/HANDLING

PO

- Give after the same meal each day. Do not chew or crush extended-release tablet.

INDICATIONS/ROUTES/DOSAGE

BENIGN PROSTATIC HYPERTROPHY

PO: ADULTS: 10 mg once daily, approx. 30 min after same meal each day.

SIDE EFFECTS

FREQUENT: (6%–7%): Dizziness, headache, malaise. **OCCASIONAL (4%):** Dry mouth. **RARE (2%–3%):** Nausea, dyspepsia (heartburn, epigastric discomfort), diarrhea, orthostatic hypotension, tachycardia, drowsiness.

ADVERSE REACTIONS/ TOXIC EFFECTS

Ischemia-related chest pain may occur rarely (2%).

NURSING CONSIDERATIONS

BASELINE ASSESSMENT

Question for sensitivity to alfuzosin, use of other alpha-blocking agents (prazosin, terazosin, doxazosin, tamsulosin).

INTERVENTION/EVALUATION

Assist with ambulation if dizziness occurs. Report headache.

PATIENT/FAMILY TEACHING

Take after the same meal each day. Avoid tasks that require alertness, motor skills until response to drug is established. Do not chew or crush extended-release tablet.

alitretinoin

al-**lee**-tret-ih-nown
(Panretin)

CLASSIFICATION

PHARMACOTHERAPEUTIC: Second-generation retinoid. **CLINICAL:** Antineoplastic (see p. 69C).

ACTION

Binds to and activates all known retinoid receptors. Once activated, receptors act as transcription factors, regulating genes that control cellular differentiation and proliferation. **Therapeutic Effect:** Inhibits growth of Kaposi's sarcoma cells.

USES

Topical treatment of cutaneous lesions in those with AIDS-related Kaposi's sarcoma. **Unlabeled:** Breast, cervical, ovarian, prostatic carcinomas; myelodysplastic syndrome; psoriasis.

PRECAUTIONS

CONTRAINDICATIONS: When systemic therapy is required (>10 new Kaposi's sarcoma [KS] lesions in previous month), symptomatic pulmonary KS, symptomatic visceral involvement or symptomatic lymphedema in KS. **CAUTIONS:** None known. **Pregnancy Category D.**

INTERACTIONS

DRUG: Increased risk of toxicity to products containing **DEET** (component of insect repellent). **HERBAL:** None known. **FOOD:** None known. **LAB VALUES:** None known.

AVAILABILITY (Rx)

GEL: 0.1%.

INDICATIONS/ROUTES/DOSAGE

KAPOSI'S SARCOMA

Topical: ADULTS: Initially, apply 2 times/day to lesions. May increase to 3–4 times/day. Allow gel to dry 3–5 min before covering with clothing.

SIDE EFFECTS

FREQUENT (>5%): Rash (erythema, scaling, irritation, redness, dermatitis), itching, exfoliative dermatitis (flaking, peeling, desquamation, exfoliation), stinging, tingling, edema skin disorders (scabbing, crusting, drainage).

ADVERSE REACTIONS/ TOXIC EFFECTS

Severe local skin reaction (intense erythema, edema, vesiculation) may limit treatment.

NURSING IMPLICATIONS

PATIENT/FAMILY TEACHING

Do not apply dressings over medication gel. Do not apply gel to healthy skin surrounding lesions or apply gel on or near mucosal surfaces. If severe irritation occurs, frequency of application can be reduced or discontinued for a few days until symptoms subside.

Allegra

see fexofenadine

allopurinol

al-low-**pure**-ih-nawl
(Aloprim, Apo-Allopurinol, Purinol, Zyloprim)

CLASSIFICATION

PHARMACOTHERAPEUTIC: Xanthine oxidase inhibitor. **CLINICAL:** Antigout.

ACTION

Decreases uric acid production by inhibition of xanthine oxidase, an enzyme. **Therapeutic Effect:** Reduces uric acid concentrations in both serum and urine.

PHARMACOKINETICS

Onset	Peak	Duration
PO/IV		
2–3 days	1–3 wks	1–2 wks

Well absorbed from GI tract. Widely distributed. Metabolized in liver to active metabolite. Excreted primarily in urine. Removed by hemodialysis. **Half-life:** 1–3 hrs; metabolite: 12–30 hrs.

USES

Treatment of chronic gouty arthritis, uric acid nephropathy. Prevents or treats hyperuricemia secondary to blood dyscrasias, cancer chemotherapy. Prevents recurrence of uric acid or calcium stone formation. **Aloprim:** Management of elevated uric acid in cancer pts unable to tolerate oral therapy. **Unlabeled:** Used in mouthwash following fluorouracil therapy to prevent stomatitis.

PRECAUTIONS

CONTRAINDICATIONS: Asymptomatic hyperuricemia. **CAUTIONS:** Impaired renal, hepatic function, CHF, diabetes mellitus, hypertension.

LIFESPAN CONSIDERATIONS: Pregnancy/lactation: Unknown if drug crosses placenta or is distributed in breast milk. **Pregnancy Category C. Children/elderly:** No age-related precautions noted.

INTERACTIONS

DRUG: Thiazide diuretics may decrease effect. May increase effect of **oral anticoagulants.** May increase effect, toxicity of **azathioprine, mercaptopurine. Ampicillin, amoxicillin** may increase incidence of skin rash. **HERBAL:** None known. **FOOD:** None known. **LAB VALUES:** May increase alkaline phosphatase, SGOT (AST), SGPT (ALT), BUN, creatinine.

AVAILABILITY (Rx)

TABLETS: 100 mg, 300 mg. **POWDER FOR INJECTION:** 500 mg.

ADMINISTRATION/HANDLING

PO

• May give with or immediately after meals or milk. • Instruct pt to drink at least 10–12 eight-oz glasses of water/day. • Dosages >300 mg/day to be administered in divided doses.

IV

Storage • Store unreconstituted vials at room temperature. • May store reconstituted solution at room temperature and give within 10 hrs. Do not use if precipitate forms or solution is discolored.

Reconstitution • Reconstitute 500-mg vial with 25 ml Sterile Water for Injection, giving a clear, almost colorless solution (concentration of 20 mg/ml). • Further dilute with 0.9% NaCl or D_5W (19 ml of added diluent yields 1 mg/ml, 9 ml yields 2 mg/ml, 2.3 ml yields maximum concentration of 6 mg/ml).

Rate of administration • Infuse over 30–60 min.

IV INCOMPATIBILITIES

Amikacin (Amikin), carmustine (BiCNU), cefotaxime (Claforan), chlorpromazine (Thorazine), cimetidine (Tagamet), clindamycin (Cleocin), cytarabine (Ara-C), dacarbazine (DTIC), diphenhydramine (Benadryl), doxorubicin (Adriamycin), doxycycline (Vibramycin), droperidol (Inapsine), fludarabine (Fludara), gentamicin (Garamycin), haloperidol (Haldol), hydroxyzine (Vistaril), idarubicin (Idamycin), imipenem-cilastatin (Primaxin), meperidine (Demerol), methylprednisolone (Solu-Medrol), metoclopramide (Reglan), ondansetron (Zofran), prochlorperazine (Compazine), promethazine (Phenergan), streptozocin (Zanosar), tobramycin (Nebcin), vinorelbine (Navelbine).

IV COMPATIBILITIES

Bumetanide (Bumex), calcium gluconate, furosemide (Lasix), heparin, hydromorphone (Dilaudid), lorazepam (Ativan), morphine, potassium chloride.

INDICATIONS/ROUTES/DOSAGE

ANTIGOUT

PO: ADULTS, CHILDREN >10 YRS: Initially, 100 mg/day; may increase by 100 mg/day at weekly intervals. **Maximum:** 800 mg/day. MAINTENANCE: 100–200 mg 2–3 times/day or 300 mg/day.

NEOPLASTIC DISEASE THERAPY

PO: ADULTS: Initially, 600–800 mg/day starting 2–3 days prior to initiation of chemotherapy or radiation therapy. CHILDREN 6–10 YRS: 100 mg 3 times/day or 300 mg once daily. CHILDREN <6 YRS: 50 mg 3 times/day.

IV: ADULTS: 200–400 mg/m^2/day beginning 24–48 hrs prior to initiation of chemotherapy. CHILDREN: 200 mg/m^2/day. **Maximum:** 600 mg/day.

URIC ACID CALCULI

PO: ADULTS: 100–200 mg 1–4 times/day or 300 mg once daily.

CALCIUM OXALATE CALCULI

PO: ADULTS: 200–300 mg/day.

USUAL ELDERLY DOSAGE

PO: Initially, 100 mg/day, gradually increased to optimal uric acid level.

DOSAGE IN RENAL IMPAIRMENT

Creatinine Clearance (ml/min)	Dosage Adjustment
>50	No change
10–50	50%
<10	30%

SIDE EFFECTS

OCCASIONAL: PO: Drowsiness, unusual hair loss. **IV:** Rash, nausea, vomiting. **RARE:** Diarrhea, headache.

ADVERSE REACTIONS/ TOXIC EFFECTS

Pruritic maculopapular rash should be considered a toxic reaction. May be accompanied by malaise, fever, chills, joint pain, nausea, vomiting. Severe hypersensitivity may follow appearance of rash. Bone marrow depression, hepatotoxicity, peripheral neuritis, or acute renal failure occurs rarely.

NURSING IMPLICATIONS

BASELINE ASSESSMENT

Instruct pt to drink 10–12 glasses (8 oz) of fluid daily while taking medication.

INTERVENTION/EVALUATION

Discontinue medication immediately if rash or other evidence of allergic reaction appears. Encourage high fluid intake (3,000 ml/day). Monitor I&O (output should be at least 2,000 ml/day). Assess CBC, uric acid and liver function serum levels. Assess urine for cloudiness, unusual color, odor. Assess for therapeutic response (reduced joint tenderness, swelling, redness, limitation of motion).

PATIENT/FAMILY TEACHING

May take ≥1 wk for full therapeutic effect. Encourage drinking 10–12 glasses (8 oz) of fluid daily while taking medication. Avoid tasks that require alertness, motor skills until response to drug is established.

almotriptan malate

ale-moe-**trip**-**tan**
(Axert)

CLASSIFICATION

PHARMACOTHERAPEUTIC: Serotonin receptor agonist. **CLINICAL:** Antimigraine (see p. 54C).

ACTION

Binds selectively to vascular receptors, producing a vasoconstrictive effect on cranial blood vessels. **Therapeutic Effect:** Produces relief of migraine headache.

PHARMACOKINETICS

Well absorbed following PO administration. Metabolized by the liver, excreted in urine.

USES

Acute treatment of migraine headache with or without aura.

PRECAUTIONS

CONTRAINDICATIONS: Coronary artery disease, uncontrolled hypertension, ischemic heart disease (angina pectoris, history of MI, silent ischemia), Prinzmetal's angina, concurrent use (or within 24 hrs) of ergotamine-containing preparations, concurrent (or within 2 wks) of MAO therapy, hemiplegic or basilar migraine, within 24 hrs of another serotonin receptor agonist, Wolff-Parkinson-White syndrome, arrhythmias associated with cardiac conduction pathway disorders. **CAUTIONS:** Mild to moderate renal/hepatic impairment, pt profile suggesting cardiovascular risks, controlled hypertension, history of CVA.

LIFESPAN CONSIDERATIONS: Pregnancy/lactation: Unknown if distributed in breast milk. **Pregnancy Category C. Children:** Safety and efficacy not established in pts <12 yrs. **Elderly:** No age-related precautions noted.

INTERACTIONS

DRUG: Ergotamine-containing drugs may produce vasospastic reaction. **MAOIs** may increase concentration. Combined use of **fluoxetine, fluvoxamine, paroxetine, sertraline** may produce weakness, hyperreflexia, incoordination. Avoid taking **ketoconazole, itraconazole, ritonavir, erythromycin** in last 7 days. **HERBAL:** None known. **FOOD:** None known. **LAB VALUES:** None known.

AVAILABILITY (Rx)

TABLETS: 6.5 mg, 12.5 mg.

ADMINISTRATION/HANDLING

PO

• Swallow tablets whole. • Take with full glass of water.

INDICATIONS/ROUTES/DOSAGE

MIGRAINE HEADACHE

PO: ADULTS, ELDERLY: 6.25–12.5 mg. If headache returns, dose may be repeated after 2 hrs. **Maximum:** No more than 2 doses within 24 hrs.

DOSAGE IN RENAL IMPAIRMENT

PO: ADULTS, ELDERLY: Initially, 6.25 mg. **Maximum:** 12.5 mg daily.

SIDE EFFECTS

FREQUENT: Nausea, dry mouth, paresthesia, flushing. **OCCASIONAL:** Sensation of warm/hot, weakness, dizziness.

ADVERSE REACTIONS/TOXIC EFFECTS

Excessive dosage may produce tremor, redness of extremities, reduced respirations, cyanosis, seizures, chest pain. Serious arrhythmias occur rarely, but particularly in pts with hypertension, obesity, smokers, diabetics, and those with strong family history of coronary artery disease.

NURSING IMPLICATIONS

BASELINE ASSESSMENT

Question for history of peripheral vascular disease. Question pt regarding onset, location, and duration of migraine and possible precipitating symptoms.

INTERVENTION/EVALUATION

Evaluate for relief of migraine headache and resulting photophobia, phonophobia (sound sensitivity), nausea, and vomiting.

PATIENT/FAMILY TEACHING

Take a single dose as soon as symptoms of an actual migraine attack appear. Medication is intended to relieve migraine, not to prevent or reduce number of attacks. Lie down in quiet, dark room for additional benefit after taking medication. Avoid tasks that require alertness, motor skills until response to drug is established. If palpitations, pain/tightness in chest or throat, or pain or weakness of extremities occurs, contact physician immediately.

alosetron

al-**ohs**-eh-tron
(Lotronex)

CLASSIFICATION

PHARMACOTHERAPEUTIC: $5\text{-}HT_3$ receptor antagonist. **CLINICAL:** GI agent.

ACTION

$5\text{-}HT_3$ receptors are nonselective cation channels extensively distributed on enteric neurons in the GI tract. Mediates peristalsis, secretory reflexes, nausea, vomiting, bloating, and abdominal pain. **Therapeutic Effect:** Reduces gastric pain, alleviates exaggerated motor response (diarrhea).

PHARMACOKINETICS

Rapidly absorbed after PO administration. Extensively metabolized in liver. Primarily excreted in urine, with a lesser amount in feces. **Half-life:** 1.5 hrs.

USES

Treatment of severe diarrhea-predominant irritable bowel syndrome in women who have failed to respond to conventional therapy. **Unlabeled:** Treatment of irritable bowel syndrome in men; carcinoid diarrhea.

PRECAUTIONS

CONTRAINDICATIONS: Breast-feeding; history of colitis; constipation; GI bleeding, obstruction, or perforation; history of ischemic colitis or Crohn's disease; thrombophlebitis; ulcerative colitis; history of or active diverticulitis. **CAUTIONS:** Hepatic function impairment.

LIFESPAN CONSIDERATIONS: Pregnancy/lactation: Unknown if excreted in breast milk. **Pregnancy Category B. Children:** Safety and efficacy not established. **Elderly:** No age-related precautions noted.

INTERACTIONS

DRUG: May alter effect of **isoniazid, procainamide, hydralazine. HERBAL: St. John's wort** may increase concentration. **FOOD:** Concurrent use of food may decrease absorption, delay peak concentration. **LAB VALUES:** May increase SGOT (AST), SGPT (ALT), alkaline phosphatase, bilirubin.

AVAILABILITY (Rx)

TABLETS: 1 mg.

ADMINISTRATION/HANDLING

PO

- May give without regard to food.

INDICATIONS/DOSAGE/ROUTES

Warning: Safety and efficacy not established in men.

IRRITABLE BOWEL SYNDROME

Oral: ADULTS (WOMEN >18 YRS): 1 mg 2 times/day. **Maximum:** 2 mg/day.

SIDE EFFECTS

FREQUENT (28%): Constipation. **OCCASIONAL (2%–10%):** Nausea, GI or abdominal discomfort/pain, dyspepsia, flatulence, increased B/P, clinical depression. **RARE:** Sedation, abnormal dreams, anxiety.

ADVERSE REACTIONS/ TOXIC EFFECTS

Acute ischemic colitis, serious complications of constipation have resulted in blood transfusions, surgery.

NURSING IMPLICATIONS

BASELINE ASSESSMENT

Question for history of diarrhea, blood in stool, abdominal distress, bloating, abdominal pain/discomfort.

INTERVENTION/EVALUATION

Assess for decrease in symptoms. Monitor liver function tests.

PATIENT/FAMILY TEACHING

Therapeutic response may take 1–4 wks; urgency and diarrhea may be reduced within 1 wk of treatment. Constipation can become persistent and may require interruption of treatment and/or medication management. Inform physician/nurse if bloody diarrhea, severe constipation, or sudden worsening of stomach pain occurs.

alpha$_1$-proteinase inhibitor (human, alpha$_1$-PI)

(Aralast, Prolastin, Zemaisa)

CLASSIFICATION

PHARMACOTHERAPEUTIC: Proteinase inhibitor. **CLINICAL:** Alveolar protectant.

ACTION

Protects alveolar epithelial lining of lower respiratory tract by alleviating imbalance between elastase (enzyme capable of degrading elastin tissue in lower respiratory tract) and alpha$_1$-proteinase inhibitor (inhibits neutrophil elastase). **Therapeutic Effect:** Allows for subsequent protection from degradation of elastin tissue.

USES

Chronic replacement therapy in those with clinically demonstrable panacinar emphysema. Do not use in patients with PiMZ or PiMS phenotypes (small risk of panacinar emphysema).

PRECAUTIONS

CONTRAINDICATIONS: Pts with known antibody reaction against IgA (may experience severe reaction, including anaphylaxis). **CAUTIONS:** Those at risk for circulatory overload. **Pregnancy Category C.**

INTERACTIONS

DRUG: None known. **HERBAL:** None known. **FOOD:** None known. **LAB VALUES:** None known.

AVAILABILITY (Rx)

POWDER FOR INJECTION: 500 mg, 1,000 mg.

ADMINISTRATION/HANDLING

IV

Storage • Refrigerate vials. Do not exceed 77°F. • Do not freeze. Do not refrigerate once reconstituted. • After reconstitution, administer within 3 hrs.

Reconstitution • Reconstitute with Sterile Water for Injection (supplied by manufacturer).

Rate of administration • Rate of 0.08 ml/kg/min as IV infusion.

IV INCOMPATIBILITY

Do not mix with any other medication.

INDICATIONS/ROUTES/DOSAGE

REPLACEMENT THERAPY

IV infusion: ADULTS, ELDERLY: 60 mg/kg once weekly at rate of at least 0.08 ml/kg/min.

SIDE EFFECTS

RARE (<1%): Delayed fever, lightheadedness, dizziness.

ADVERSE REACTIONS/ TOXIC EFFECTS

Mild leukocytosis occurs rarely.

NURSING IMPLICATIONS

BASELINE ASSESSMENT

All pts should be immunized against hepatitis B before initial dose is given.

INTERVENTION/EVALUATION

Maintain blood levels of $alpha_1$-PI at 80 mg/dl. Monitor respiratory status throughout therapy.

PATIENT/FAMILY TEACHING

Explain purpose of medication, importance of hepatitis B vaccine, periodic pulmonary function tests. Avoid smoking.

alprazolam

ale-**praz**-oh-lam

(Apo-Alpraz ✤, Novo-Alprazol ✤, Xanax, Xanax XR)

Do not confuse with lorazepam, Tenex, Zantac.

◆CLASSIFICATION

PHARMACOTHERAPEUTIC: Benzodiazepine **(Schedule IV). CLINICAL:** Antianxiety (see p. 10C).

ACTION

Enhances action of inhibitory neurotransmitters in the brain. **Therapeutic Effect:** Produces anxiolytic effect due to CNS depressant action.

PHARMACOKINETICS

Well absorbed from GI tract. Protein binding: 80%. Metabolized in liver. Primarily excreted in urine. Minimal removal by hemodialysis. **Half-life:** 11–16 hrs.

USES

Management of anxiety disorders associated with depression, panic disorder. **Unlabeled:** Improves mood, relieves cramps, prevents insomnia with premenstrual syndrome. Management of irritable bowel syndrome.

PRECAUTIONS

CONTRAINDICATIONS: Acute narrow-angle glaucoma, acute alcohol intoxication with depressed vital signs, severe chronic obstructive pulmonary disease, myasthenia gravis, concurrent use of ketoconazole, itraconazole. **CAUTIONS:** Impaired renal/hepatic function.

LIFESPAN CONSIDERATIONS: Pregnancy/lactation: Crosses placenta; distributed in breast milk. Chronic ingestion during pregnancy may produce withdrawal symptoms, CNS depression in neonates. **Pregnancy Category D. Children:** Safety and efficacy not established. **Elderly:** Use small initial doses with gradual increase to avoid ataxia (muscular incoordination) or excessive sedation.

INTERACTIONS

DRUG: Potentiated effects when used with **other CNS depressants (including alcohol). Ketoconazole, nefazodone, fluvoxamine** may inhibit liver metabolism, increase serum concentrations. **HERBAL: Kava kava, valerian** may increase CNS depressant effect. **FOOD: Grapefruit juice** may inhibit metabolism. **LAB VALUES:** None known.

AVAILABILITY (Rx)

TABLETS: 0.25 mg, 0.5 mg, 1 mg, 2 mg. **TABLETS (extended-release):** 0.5 mg, 1 mg, 2 mg, 3 mg. **ORAL SOLUTION:** 1 mg/ml.

ADMINISTRATION/HANDLING

PO

- May be given without regard to meals.
- Tablets may be crushed.

INDICATIONS/ROUTES/DOSAGE

ANXIETY DISORDERS

PO: ADULTS >18 YRS: Initially, 0.25–0.5 mg 3 times daily. Titrate to maximum of 4 mg daily in divided doses. ELDERLY/DEBILITATED/LIVER DISEASE/LOW SERUM ALBUMIN: Initially, 0.25 mg 2–3 times daily. Gradually increase to optimum therapeutic response.

PANIC DISORDER

PO: ADULTS: Initially, 0.5 mg 3 times/day. May increase at 3- to 4-day intervals at no more than 1 mg/day. RANGE: 1–10 mg/day.

PANIC ATTACK (extended release):

PO: ADULTS, ELDERLY: 0.5–1 mg once daily. May increase q3–4 days up to a maximum of 10 mg/day.

USUAL ELDERLY DOSAGE

PO: Initially, 0.125–0.25 mg 2 times/day; may increase in 0.125-mg increments until desired effect attained.

PREMENSTRUAL SYNDROME

PO: ADULTS: 0.25 mg 3 times/day.

SIDE EFFECTS

FREQUENT: Muscular incoordination (ataxia), lightheadedness, transient mild drowsiness, slurred speech (particularly in elderly, debilitated). **OCCASIONAL:** Confusion, depression, blurred vision, constipation/diarrhea, dry mouth, headache, nausea. **RARE:** Behavioral problems (e.g., anger), impaired memory, paradoxical reaction (insomnia, nervousness, irritability).

ADVERSE REACTIONS/ TOXIC EFFECTS

Abrupt or too rapid withdrawal may result in pronounced restlessness, irritability, insomnia, hand tremors, abdominal/muscle cramps, sweating, vomiting, seizures. Overdosage results in somnolence, confusion, diminished reflexes, coma. Blood dyscrasias noted rarely.

NURSING IMPLICATIONS

BASELINE ASSESSMENT

Offer emotional support to anxious pt. Assess motor responses (agitation, trembling, tension), autonomic responses (cold/clammy hands, sweating).

INTERVENTION/EVALUATION

For those on long-term therapy, liver/renal function tests, perform blood counts periodically. Assess for paradoxical reaction, particularly during early therapy. Evaluate for therapeutic response: calm facial expression, decreased restlessness, and/or insomnia.

PATIENT/FAMILY TEACHING

Drowsiness usually disappears during continued therapy. If dizziness occurs, change positions slowly from recumbent to sitting position before standing. Avoid tasks that require alertness, motor skills until response to drug is established. Smoking reduces drug effectiveness. Sour hard candy, gum, sips of tepid water may relieve dry mouth. Do not abruptly withdraw medication after long-term therapy. Avoid alcohol. Do not take other medications without consulting physician.

alprostadil (prostaglandin E_1; PGE_1)

ale-**pros**-tah-dill
(Caverject, Edex, Muse, Prostin VR Pediatric)

CLASSIFICATION

PHARMACOTHERAPEUTIC: Prostaglandin. **CLINICAL:** Patent ductus arteriosus agent, anti-impotence.

ACTION

Direct effect on vascular and ductus arteriosus smooth muscle; relaxes trabecular smooth muscle. **Therapeutic Effect:** Causes vasodilation. Dilates cavernosal arteries, allowing blood flow to and entrapment in the lacunar spaces of the penis.

USES

Temporarily maintains patency of ductus arteriosus until surgery is performed in those with congenital heart defects and dependent on patent ductus for survival (e.g., pulmonary atresia or stenosis). Treatment of erectile dysfunction due to neurogenic, vasculogenic, psychogenic causes; adjunct in diagnosis of erectile dysfunction. **Unlabeled:** Treatment of atherosclerosis, gangrene, pain due to severe peripheral arterial occlusive disease.

PRECAUTIONS

CONTRAINDICATIONS: Respiratory distress syndrome (hyaline membrane disease). Conditions predisposing to priapism, anatomic deformation of penis, penile implants. **CAUTIONS:** Severe liver disease, coagulation defects, leukemia, multiple myeloma, polycythemia, sickle cell disease, thrombocythemia. **Pregnancy Category C.**

INTERACTIONS

DRUG: **Anticoagulants, heparin, thrombolytics** may increase risk of bleeding. **Sympathomimetics** may decrease effect. **Vasodilators** may increase risk of hypotension. **HERBAL:** None known. **FOOD:** None known. **LAB VALUES:** May increase bilirubin. May decrease calcium, glucose, potassium.

AVAILABILITY (Rx)

INJECTION: 500 mcg/ml. **POWDER FOR INJECTION:** 10 mcg, 20 mcg, 40 mcg. **URETHRAL PELLET (MUSE):** 125 mcg, 250 mcg, 500 mcg, 1,000 mcg.

ADMINISTRATION/HANDLING

URETHRAL PELLET

Storage • Refrigerate pellet unless used within 14 days.

IV

Storage • Store parenteral form in refrigerator. • Must dilute before use. • Prepare fresh q24h. • Discard unused portions.

Reconstitution • Dilute 500-mcg ampoule with D_5W or 0.9% NaCl to volume dependent on infusion pump capabilities.

Rate of administration • Infuse for shortest time, lowest dose possible. • If significant decrease in arterial pressure is noted via umbilical artery catheter, auscultation, or Doppler transducer, decrease infusion rate immediately. • Discontinue infusion immediately if apnea or bradycardia occurs (overdosage).

∅ **IV INCOMPATIBILITY**

No information available via Y-site administration.

INDICATIONS/ROUTES/DOSAGE

Alert: Give by continuous IV infusion or through umbilical artery catheter placed at ductal opening.

MAINTAIN PATENCY DUCTUS ARTERIOSUS

IV infusion: NEONATES: Initially, 0.05–0.1 mcg/kg/min. After therapeutic response achieved, use lowest dosage to maintain response. **Maximum:** 0.4 mcg/kg/min.

IMPOTENCE

Pellet, intracavernosal: Individualized. Doses >40 mcg (Edex) or 60 mcg (Caverjet) not recommended.

SIDE EFFECTS

FREQUENT: Intracavernosal (1%–4%): Penile pain (37%), prolonged erection, hypertension, local pain, penile fibrosis, injection site hematoma/ecchymosis, headache, respiratory infection, flulike symptoms. **Intraurethral (3%):** Penile pain (36%), urethral pain/burning, testicular pain, urethral bleeding, headache, dizziness, respiratory infection, flulike symptoms. **Systemic (>1%):** Fever, seizures, flushing, bradycardia, hypotension, tachycardia, apnea, diarrhea, sepsis. **OCCASIONAL: Intracavernosal (<1%):** Hypotension, pelvic pain, back pain, dizziness, cough, nasal congestion. **Intraurethral (<3%):** Fainting, sinusitis, back/pelvic pain. **Systemic (<1%):** Jitteriness, lethargy, stiffness, arrhythmias, respiratory depression, anemia, bleeding, thrombocytopenia, hematuria.

ADVERSE REACTIONS/ TOXIC EFFECTS

Overdosage manifested as apnea, flushing of face/arms, bradycardia. Cardiac arrest, sepsis occur rarely.

NURSING IMPLICATIONS

INTERVENTION/EVALUATION

Patent Ductus Arteriosus: Monitor arterial pressure by umbilical artery catheter, auscultation, or Doppler transducer. If significant decrease in arterial pressure occurs, decrease infusion rate immediately. Maintain continuous cardiac monitoring. Assess heart sounds, femoral pulse (circulation to lower extremities), and respiratory status frequently. Monitor for symptoms of hypotension. Assess B/P, arterial blood gases, temperature. If apnea or bradycardia occurs, discontinue infusion and notify physician.

PATIENT/FAMILY TEACHING

Patent Ductus Arteriosus: Explain purpose of this palliative therapy to parents. **Impotence:** Erection is to occur within 2–5 min. Do not use if female is pregnant (unless using condom barrier). Inform physician if erection lasts >4 hrs or becomes painful.

Altace

see ramipril

alteplase, recombinant

all-teh-place
(Activase, Cathflo Activase)

♦CLASSIFICATION

PHARMACOTHERAPEUTIC: Tissue plasminogen activator (tPA). **CLINICAL:** Thrombolytic (see p. 30C).

ACTION

An enzyme, binds to fibrin in a thrombus and converts entrapped plasminogen to plasmin, initiating fibrinolysis. **Therapeutic Effect:** Degrades fibrin clots, fibrinogen, other plasma proteins.

PHARMACOKINETICS

Rapidly metabolized in liver. Primarily excreted in urine. **Half-life:** 35 min.

USES

Treatment of acute MI, acute ischemic stroke, and acute massive pulmonary embolism. Treatment of occluded central venous catheters. **Unlabeled:** Coronary thrombolysis, decrease ischemic events in unstable angina.

PRECAUTIONS

CONTRAINDICATIONS: Active internal bleeding, recent (≤2 mos) cerebrovascular accident, intracranial or intraspinal surgery or trauma, intracranial neoplasm, AV malformation or aneurysm, bleeding diathesis, severe uncontrolled hypertension. **CAUTIONS:** Recent (≤10 days) major surgery or GI bleeding, OB delivery, organ biopsy, recent trauma (CPR, left heart thrombus, endocarditis, severe hepatic/renal disease, pregnancy, elderly, cerebrovascular disease, diabetic retinopathy, thrombophlebitis, occluded AV cannula at infected site).

LIFESPAN CONSIDERATIONS: Pregnancy/lactation: Use only when benefit outweighs potential risk to fetus. Unknown if drug crosses placenta or is distributed in breast milk. **Pregnancy Category C. Children:** Safety and efficacy not established. **Elderly:** Risk of bleeding with thrombolytic therapy increased, careful pt selection, monitoring recommended.

INTERACTIONS

DRUG: Anticoagulants, heparin, cefotetan, plicamycin, valproic acid may increase risk of hemorrhage. **Platelet aggregation inhibitors (e.g., aspirin), NSAIDs, ticlopidine** may increase risk of bleeding. **HERBAL:** None known. **FOOD:** None known. **LAB VALUES:** Decreases plasminogen and fibrinogen level during infusion, decreasing clotting time (confirms presence of lysis). Decreases Hgb, Hct.

AVAILABILITY (Rx)

POWDER FOR INJECTION: 2 mg, 50 mg, 100 mg.

ADMINISTRATION/HANDLING

IV

Storage • Store vials at room temperature. • After reconstitution, solutions appear colorless to pale yellow. • Solution is stable for 8 hrs after reconstitution. Discard unused portions.

Reconstitution • Reconstitute immediately prior to use with Sterile Water for Injection. • Reconstitute 100-mg vial with 100 ml Sterile Water for Injection (50-mg vial with 50 ml sterile water) without preservative to provide a concentration of 1 mg/ml. May be further diluted with equal volume D_5W or 0.9% NaCl to provide a concentration of 0.5 mg/ml. • Avoid excessive agitation; gently swirl or slowly invert vial to reconstitute.

Rate of administration • Give by IV infusion via infusion pump. See individual dosages. • If minor bleeding occurs at puncture sites, apply pressure for 30 sec; if unrelieved, apply pressure dressing. • If uncontrolled hemorrhage occurs, discontinue infusion immediately (slowing rate of infusion may produce worsening hemorrhage). • Avoid undue pressure when drug is injected into catheter (can rupture catheter or expel clot into circulation).

∅ IV INCOMPATIBILITIES

Do not add any other medication to the container of alteplase solution or administer other medications through the same IV line.

IV COMPATIBILITIES

Lidocaine, metoprolol (Lopressor), morphine, nitroglycerin, propranolol (Inderal).

INDICATIONS/ROUTES/DOSAGE

ACUTE MI

IV infusion: ADULTS: 100 mg over 90 min. (>67 KG): 15-mg bolus given over 1–2 min; then 50 mg over 30 min; then 35 mg over 60 min. (<67 KG): 15-mg bolus, then 0.75 mg/kg over next 30 min (**Maximum:** 50 mg), then 0.5 mg/kg over 60 min (**Maximum:** 35 mg). **Three-hour infusion** (>67 KG): 60 mg over first hr (6–10 mg as bolus over 1–2 min), 20 mg over second hr and 20 mg over third hr. (<67 KG): 1.25 mg/kg given over 3 hrs as 60% of dose over first hr (6%–10% as 1- to 2-min bolus), 20% over second hr and 20% over third hr.

ACUTE PULMONARY EMBOLI

IV infusion: ADULTS: 100 mg over 2 hrs. Institute or reinstitute heparin near end or immediately after infusion (when PTT or thrombin time returns to twice normal or less).

ACUTE ISCHEMIC STROKE

IV infusion: ADULTS: 0.9 mg/kg over 60 min (10% total dose as initial IV bolus over 1 min).

CATHETER CLEARANCE

IV: ADULTS, ELDERLY: 2 mg; may repeat in >120 min.

SIDE EFFECTS

FREQUENT: Superficial bleeding at puncture sites, decreased B/P. **OCCASIONAL:** Allergic reaction (rash, wheezing), bruising.

ADVERSE REACTIONS/ TOXIC EFFECTS

Severe internal hemorrhage may occur. Lysis of coronary thrombi may produce atrial or ventricular arrhythmias, stroke.

NURSING IMPLICATIONS

BASELINE ASSESSMENT

Obtain baseline B/P, apical pulse. Record weight. Evaluate 12-lead EKG, CPK, CPK-MB, electrolytes. Assess Hct, platelet count, thrombin (TT), activated partial thromboplastin time (aPTT), prothrombin time (PT), fibrinogen level before therapy is instituted. Type and hold blood.

INTERVENTION/EVALUATION

Perform continuous cardiac monitoring for arrhythmias. Check B/P, pulse, and respirations q15min until stable, then hourly. Check peripheral pulses, heart and lung sounds. Monitor chest pain relief and notify physician of continuation or recurrence (note location, type, and intensity). Assess for bleeding: overt blood, blood in any body substance. Monitor PTT per protocol. Maintain B/P; avoid any trauma that might increase risk of bleeding (e.g., injections, shaving). Assess neurologic status.

altretamine (hexamethyl-melamine)

(Hexalen)

See Classification section under: Antineoplastics (p. 69C)

aluminum hydroxide

(Alternagel, Alu-Cap, Alu-Tab, Amphojel, Basaljel✤)

FIXED-COMBINATION(S)

With magnesium, an antacid **(Gaviscon, Maalox)**; with magnesium and simethicone, an antiflatulent **(Gelusil, Maalox Plus, Mylanta, Silain-Gel)**

◆ CLASSIFICATION

CLINICAL: Antacid (p. 8C).

ACTION

Reduces gastric acid. Binds with phosphate in intestine, then excreted in feces. May increase absorption of calcium (due to decreased serum phosphate levels). Astringent, adsorbent properties. **Therapeutic Effect:** Neutralizes or increases gastric pH; reduces phosphates in urine, preventing formation of phosphate urinary stones; reduces serum phosphate levels; decreases fluidity of stools.

USES

Symptomatic relief of upset stomach associated with hyperacidity (heartburn, acid indigestion, sour stomach). Hyperacidity associated with gastric, duodenal ulcers. Symptomatic treatment of gastroesophageal reflux disease. Prophylactic treatment of GI bleeding secondary to gastritis and stress ulceration. In conjunction with low-phosphate diet, prevents formation of phosphate urinary stones, reduces elevated phosphate levels.

PRECAUTIONS

CONTRAINDICATIONS: Intestinal obstruction, very young. **CAUTIONS:** Impaired renal function, gastric outlet obstruction, elderly, dehydration, fluid restriction, Alzheimer's disease, symptoms of appendicitis, GI/rectal bleeding, constipation, fecal impaction, chronic diarrhea. **Pregnancy:** Considered safe unless chronic, high-dose usage. **Pregnancy Category C.**

INTERACTIONS

DRUG: May decrease excretion of **quinidine, anticholinergics.** May decrease effects of **methenamine.** May increase **salicylate** excretion. May decrease absorption of **quinolones, iron preparations, isoniazid, ketoconazole, tetracyclines.** **HERBAL:** None known. **FOOD:** None known. **LAB VALUES:** May increase gastrin, systemic/urinary pH. May decrease serum phosphate.

AVAILABILITY (OTC)

ALUMINUM HYDROXIDE: **CAPSULES:** 475 mg. **SUSPENSION:** 320 mg/5 ml, 600 mg/5 ml.

ADMINISTRATION/HANDLING

PO

• Usually administered 1–3 hrs after meals. • Individualize dose (based on neutralizing capacity of antacids). • Chewable tablets: Thoroughly chew tablets before swallowing (follow with glass of water or milk). • If administering suspension, shake well before use.

INDICATIONS/ROUTES/DOSAGE

Alert: Usual dose is 30–60 ml.

PEPTIC ULCER DISEASE

PO: ADULTS, ELDERLY: 15–45 ml q3–6h or 1 and 3 hrs after meals and at bedtime. CHILDREN: 5–15 ml as above.

ANTACID

PO: ADULTS, ELDERLY: 30 ml 1 and 3 hrs after meals and at bedtime.

GI BLEEDING PREVENTION

PO: ADULTS, ELDERLY: 30–60 ml/hr. CHILDREN: 5–15 ml q1–2h.

HYPERPHOSPHATEMIA

PO: ADULTS, ELDERLY: 500–1,800 mg 1 and 3 hrs after meals and at bedtime. CHILDREN: 50–150 mg/kg/24 hrs q4–6h.

SIDE EFFECTS

FREQUENT: Chalky taste, mild constipation, stomach cramps. **OCCASIONAL:** Nausea, vomiting, speckling/whitish discoloration of stools.

ADVERSE REACTIONS/ TOXIC EFFECTS

Prolonged constipation may result in intestinal obstruction. Excessive or chronic use may produce hypophosphatemia (anorexia, malaise, muscle weakness, bone pain) resulting in osteomalacia, osteoporosis. Prolonged use may produce urinary calculi.

NURSING IMPLICATIONS

BASELINE ASSESSMENT

Do not give other PO medication within 1–2 hrs of antacid administration.

INTERVENTION/EVALUATION

Assess pattern of daily bowel activity and stool consistency. Monitor serum phosphate, calcium, uric acid, aluminum levels. Assess for relief of gastric distress.

PATIENT/FAMILY TEACHING

Chewable Tablets: Chew tablets thoroughly before swallowing (may be followed by water or milk). Tablets may discolor stool. Maintain adequate fluid intake.

amantadine hydrochloride

ah-**man**-tih-deen
(Endantadine✤, PMS-Amantadine✤, Symmetrel)

CLASSIFICATION

PHARMACOTHERAPEUTIC: Dopaminergic agonist. **CLINICAL:** Antiviral, antiparkinson agent (see p. 58C).

ACTION

Blocks uncoating of influenza A virus, preventing penetration into the host and inhibits M2 protein in the assembly of progeny virions. Blocks reuptake of dopamine into presynaptic neurons and causes direct stimulation of postsynaptic receptors. **Therapeutic Effect:** Antiviral, antiparkinson activity.

PHARMACOKINETICS

Rapidly, completely absorbed from GI tract. Protein binding: 67%. Widely distributed. Primarily excreted in urine. Minimally removed by hemodialysis. **Half-life:** 11–15 hrs (half-life increased in elderly, decreased in impaired renal function).

USES

Prevention, treatment of respiratory tract infections due to influenza virus, Parkinson's disease, drug-induced extrapyramidal reactions. **Unlabeled:** Treatment of fatigue associated with multiple sclerosis, AHDH.

PRECAUTIONS

CONTRAINDICATIONS: None known. **CAUTIONS:** History of seizures, orthostatic hypotension, CHF, peripheral edema, liver disease, recurrent eczematoid dermatitis, cerebrovascular disease, renal dysfunction, those receiving CNS stimulants.

LIFESPAN CONSIDERATIONS: Pregnancy/lactation: Unknown if drug crosses placenta; distributed in breast milk. **Pregnancy Category C. Children:** No age-related precautions noted in those >1 yr. **Elderly:** May exhibit increased sensitivity to anticholinergic effects. Age-related decreased renal function may require dosage adjustment.

INTERACTIONS

DRUG: **Tricyclic antidepressants, antihistamines, phenothiazine, anticholinergics** may increase anticholinergic effects. **Hydrochlorothiazide, triamterene** may increase concentration, toxicity. **HERBAL:** None known. **FOOD:** None known. **LAB VALUES:** None known.

AVAILABILITY (Rx)

LIQUID: 50 mg/5 ml. **SYRUP:** 50 mg/5 ml. **TABLETS:** 100 mg.

ADMINISTRATION/HANDLING

PO

- May give without regard to food.
- Administer nighttime dose several hours before bedtime (prevents insomnia).

INDICATIONS/ROUTES/DOSAGE

PROPHYLAXIS, SYMPTOMATIC TREATMENT RESPIRATORY ILLNESS DUE TO INFLUENZA A VIRUS

Alert: Give as single or in 2 divided doses.

PO: ADULTS 10–64 YRS: 200 mg daily. ADULTS >64 YRS: 100 mg daily. CHILDREN 9–12 YRS: 100 mg 2 times/day. CHILDREN 1–9 YRS: 5 mg/kg/day (up to 150 mg/day).

PARKINSON'S DISEASE, EXTRAPYRAMIDAL SYMPTOMS

PO: ADULTS, ELDERLY: 100 mg 2 times/day. May increase up to 300 mg/day in divided doses.

DOSAGE IN RENAL IMPAIRMENT

Dose and/or frequency is modified based on creatinine clearance (Ccr).

Creatinine Clearance	Dosage
30–50 ml/min	200 mg first day; 100 mg/day thereafter
15–29 ml/min	200 mg first day; 100 mg on alternate days
<15 ml/min	200 mg every 7 days

SIDE EFFECTS

FREQUENT (5%–10%): Nausea, dizziness, poor concentration, insomnia, nervousness. **OCCASIONAL (1%–5%):** Orthostatic hypotension, anorexia, headache, livedo reticularis (reddish blue, netlike blotching of skin), blurred vision, urinary retention, dry mouth/nose. **RARE:** Vomiting, depression, irritation/swelling of eyes, rash.

ADVERSE REACTIONS/TOXIC EFFECTS

CHF, leukopenia, neutropenia occur rarely. Hyperexcitability, convulsions, ventricular arrhythmias may occur.

NURSING IMPLICATIONS

BASELINE ASSESSMENT

When treating infections caused by influenza A virus, obtain specimens for viral diagnostic tests before giving first dose (therapy may begin before results are known).

INTERVENTION/EVALUATION

Monitor I&O, renal function tests if ordered; check for peripheral edema. Evaluate food tolerance, vomiting. Assess skin for rash, blotching. Assess for dizziness. **Parkinson's Disease:** Assess for clinical reversal of symptoms (improvement of tremor of head/hands at rest, masklike facial expression, shuffling gait, muscular rigidity).

PATIENT/FAMILY TEACHING

Continue therapy for full length of treatment. Doses should be evenly spaced. Do not take any other medications without consulting physician.

Avoid alcoholic beverages. Do not drive, use machinery, or engage in other activities that require mental acuity if experiencing dizziness, blurred vision. Get up slowly from a sitting or lying position. Inform physician of new symptoms, esp. blotching, rash, dizziness, blurred vision, nausea/vomiting. Take nighttime dose several hours before bedtime to prevent insomnia.

Amaryl

see glimepiride

Ambien

see zolpidem

AmBisome

see amphotericin B

amcinonide

(Cyclocort)

See Classification section under: Corticosteroids: topical (p. 84C)

amifostine

am-ih-**fos**-teen
(Ethyol)
Do not confuse with ethanol.

◆CLASSIFICATION

PHARMACOTHERAPEUTIC: Antineoplastic adjunct. **CLINICAL:** Protective agent.

ACTION

Converted by alkaline phosphatase in tissues, allowing its ability to protect normal tissue relative to tumor tissue. **Therapeutic Effect:** Reduces the toxic effect of chemotherapeutic agent cisplatin.

USES

Reduces cumulative renal toxicity associated with repeated administration of cisplatin in those with advanced ovarian cancer. Treatment of postop radiation-induced dry mouth in pts with head or neck cancer. **Unlabeled:** Protects lung fibroblasts from damaging effects of chemotherapeutic agent paclitaxel.

PRECAUTIONS

CONTRAINDICATIONS: Sensitivity to aminothiol compounds or mannitol. **CAUTION:** Uncorrected dehydration or hypotensive pts, those receiving antihypertensive therapy that cannot be interrupted prior to 24 hrs before amifostine treatment, preexisting cardiovascular or cerebrovascular conditions (i.e., ischemic heart disease, arrhythmias, CHF, history of stroke or TIA), pts receiving chemotherapy for malignancies that are potentially curable (e.g., certain malignancies of germ cell origin). **Pregnancy Category C.**

INTERACTIONS

DRUG: Pts receiving **antihypertensive medication** or drugs that may potentiate hypotension. **HERBAL:** None known. **FOOD:** None known. **LAB VALUES:** May reduce calcium serum levels, esp. those with nephrotic syndrome.

AVAILABILITY (Rx)

POWDER FOR INJECTION: 500 mg (10-ml single-use vial).

ADMINISTRATION/HANDLING

IV

Storage • Reconstituted solution stable for 5 hrs at room temperature, 24 hrs under refrigeration. • Do not use if discolored or contains particulate matter.

Reconstitution • Reconstitute with 9.7 ml 0.9% NaCl. • Further dilute with 0.9% NaCl for a concentration of 5–40 mg/ml.

Rate of administration • Administer over 15 min (30 min prior to chemotherapy). • If hypotension requires interruption of therapy, place pt in Trendelenburg position; give an infusion of normal saline using a separate IV line. • An antiemetic, dexamethasone 20 mg IV and serotonin 5-HT_3 (receptor antagonist) should be given prior to and concurrently with amifostine.

IV INCOMPATIBILITY

Do not mix in solution other than 0.9% NaCl.

IV COMPATIBILITIES

Mannitol, potassium chloride.

INDICATIONS/ROUTES/DOSAGE

CYTOPROTECTIVE (chemotherapy)

IV infusion: ADULTS: 910 mg/m^2 once daily as 15-min infusion, beginning 30 min prior to chemotherapy (15-min infusion is better tolerated than extended infusions). If full dose cannot be administered, dose for subsequent cycles should be 740 mg/m^2.

TREATMENT OF DRY MOUTH

IV infusion: ADULTS: 200 mg/m^2 once daily as 3-min infusion, starting 15–30 min before radiation therapy.

SIDE EFFECTS

FREQUENT (62%): Transient reduction in B/P (with onset 14 min into infusion and lasts about 6 min). B/P generally returns to normal in 5–15 min; severe nausea, vomiting. **OCCASIONAL (10%–20%):** Flushing/feeling of warmth or chills/feeling of coldness, dizziness, hiccups, sneezing, somnolence. **RARE (<1%):** Clinically relevant hypocalcemia, mild skin rash.

ADVERSE REACTIONS/ TOXIC EFFECTS

A pronounced drop in B/P may require temporary cessation of amifostine.

NURSING IMPLICATIONS

BASELINE ASSESSMENT

Be sure pt is adequately hydrated prior to infusion. Pt should maintain supine position during the infusion. Monitor B/P q5min during infusion. Interrupt infusion if systolic B/P decreases significantly from baseline (for baseline of <100, B/P drop by 20 mm Hg; for baseline of 100–119, a drop by 25 mm Hg; for baseline of 120–139, a drop by 30 mm Hg; for baseline of 140–179, a drop by 40 mm Hg; for baseline of >180, a drop by 50 mm Hg). If B/P returns to normal within 5 min and pt appears asymptomatic, begin infusion again so that full dose can be administered.

INTERVENTION/EVALUATION

Carefully monitor pt for fluid balance, adequate hydration. Monitor serum calcium levels in those at risk of hypocalcemia (nephrotic syndrome). Monitor B/P q5min during infusion.

amikacin sulfate

am-ih-**kay**-sin

(Amikin)

Do not confuse with Amicar.

◆ CLASSIFICATION

PHARMACOTHERAPEUTIC: Aminoglycoside. **CLINICAL:** Antibiotic (see p. 18C).

ACTION

Irreversibly binds to protein on bacterial ribosome. **Therapeutic Effect:** Interferes in protein synthesis of susceptible microorganisms.

PHARMACOKINETICS

Rapid, complete absorption after IM administration. Protein binding: 0%–10%. Widely distributed (does not cross blood-brain barrier, low concentrations in CSF). Excreted unchanged in urine. Removed by hemodialysis. **Half-life:** 2–4 hrs (increased in reduced renal function, neonates; decreased in cystic fibrosis, burn or febrile pts).

USES

Treatment of skin/skin structure, bone, joint, respiratory tract, intra-abdominal and complicated urinary tract infections; postop, burns, septicemia, meningitis.

PRECAUTIONS

CONTRAINDICATIONS: Sensitivity to amikacin or any component. **CAUTIONS:** Myasthenia gravis, parkinsonism, decreased renal function, 8th cranial nerve impairment (vestibulocochlear nerve).

LIFESPAN CONSIDERATIONS: Pregnancy/lactation: Readily crosses placenta; small amounts distributed in breast milk. May produce fetal nephrotoxicity. **Pregnancy Category C. Children:** Neonates, premature infants may be more susceptible to toxicity due to immature renal function. **Elderly:** Higher risk of toxicity due to age-related renal impairment, increased risk of hearing loss.

INTERACTIONS

DRUG: Other aminoglycosides, nephrotoxic- and ototoxic-producing medications may increase toxicity. May increase effects of **neuromuscular blocking agents. HERBAL:** None known. **FOOD:** None known. **LAB VALUES:** May increase BUN, SGOT (AST), SGPT (ALT), bilirubin, creatinine, LDH concentrations; may decrease serum calcium, magnesium, potassium, sodium concentrations. Therapeutic blood serum level: Peak: 20–30 mcg/ml; toxic serum level: >30 mcg/ml; Trough: 1–9 mcg/ml; toxic serum level: >10 mcg/ml.

AVAILABILITY (Rx)

INJECTION: 50 mg/ml, 250 mg/ml.

ADMINISTRATION/HANDLING

IM

• To minimize discomfort, give deep IM slowly. • Less painful if injected into gluteus maximus rather than in lateral aspect of thigh.

IV

Storage • Store vials at room temperature. • Solutions appear clear but may become pale yellow (does not affect potency). • Intermittent IV infusion (piggyback) is stable for 24 hrs at room temperature. • Discard if precipitate forms or dark discoloration occurs.

Reconstitution • Dilute each 500 mg with 100 ml 0.9% NaCl or D_5W.

Rate of administration • Infuse over 30–60 min for adults, older children; over 60–120 min for infants, young children.

∅ IV INCOMPATIBILITIES

Amphotericin ampicillin, cefazolin (Ancef), heparin, propofol (Diprivan).

IV COMPATIBILITIES

Amiodarone (Cordarone), aztreonam (Azactam), calcium gluconate, cefepime (Maxipime), cimetidine (Tagamet), ciprofloxacin (Cipro), clindamycin (Cleocin), diltiazem (Cardizem), enalapril (Vasotec), esmolol (BreviBloc), fluconazole (Diflucan), furosemide (Lasix), levofloxacin (Levaquin), lorazepam (Ativan), magnesium sulfate, midazolam (Versed), morphine, ondansetron (Zofran), potassium chloride, ranitidine (Zantac), vancomycin.

INDICATIONS/ROUTES/DOSAGE

Alert: Space doses evenly around the clock. Dosage based on ideal body weight. Peak, trough serum levels are determined periodically to maintain desired serum concentrations (minimizes risk of toxicity).

UNCOMPLICATED URINARY TRACT INFECTIONS

IM/IV: ADULTS, ELDERLY: 250 mg q12h.

MODERATE TO SEVERE INFECTIONS

IM/IV: ADULTS, ELDERLY, CHILDREN: 15 mg/kg/day in divided doses q8–12h. Do not exceed 15 mg/kg or 1.5 g/day. NEONATES: LOADING DOSE: 10 mg/kg, then 7.5 mg/kg q12h.

DOSAGE IN RENAL IMPAIRMENT

Dose and/or frequency is modified based on degree of renal impairment, serum concentration of drug. After loading dose of 5–7.5 mg/kg, maintenance dose/frequency based on serum creatinine or creatinine clearance.

SIDE EFFECTS

FREQUENT: Pain, induration at IM injection site; phlebitis, thrombophlebitis with IV administration. **OCCASIONAL:** Hypersensitivity reactions (rash, fever, urticaria, pruritus). **RARE:** Neuromuscular blockade (difficulty breathing, drowsiness, weakness).

ADVERSE REACTIONS/ TOXIC EFFECTS

Nephrotoxicity (increased thirst, decreased appetite, nausea, vomiting, increased BUN and serum creatinine, decreased creatinine clearance), neurotoxicity (muscle twitching, visual disturbances, seizures, tingling), ototoxicity (tinnitus, dizziness any loss of hearing).

NURSING IMPLICATIONS

BASELINE ASSESSMENT

Dehydration must be treated before aminoglycoside therapy. Establish pt's baseline hearing acuity before beginning therapy. Question for history of allergies, esp. to aminoglycosides and sulfite. Obtain specimen for culture, sensitivity before giving the first dose (therapy may begin before results are known).

INTERVENTION/EVALUATION

Monitor I&O (maintain hydration), urinalysis (casts, RBC, WBC, decrease in specific gravity). Monitor results of peak/trough blood tests. Be alert to ototoxic, neurotoxic symptoms (see Adverse Reactions/Toxic Effects). Check IM injection site for pain, induration. Evaluate IV site for phlebitis (heat, pain, red streaking over vein). Assess for skin rash, superinfection (particularly genital/anal pruritus), changes of oral mucosa, diarrhea. When treating pts with neuromuscular disorders, assess respiratory response carefully. Therapeutic blood serum level: Peak: 20–30 mcg/ml; toxic serum level: >30 mcg/ml; trough: 1–9 mcg/ml; toxic serum level: >10 mcg/ml.

PATIENT/FAMILY TEACHING

Continue antibiotic for full length of treatment. Space doses evenly. IM injection may cause discomfort. Notify physician in event of any hearing, visual, balance, urinary problems even after therapy is completed. Do not take other medication without consulting physician. Lab tests are essential part of therapy.

amiloride hydrochloride

ah-**mill**-or-ride
(Midamor)

Do not confuse with amiodarone, amlodipine.

FIXED-COMBINATION(S)

Moduretic: amiloride/hydrochlorothiazide (a diuretic): 5 mg/50 mg.

CLASSIFICATION

PHARMACOTHERAPEUTIC: Guanidine derivative. **CLINICAL:** Potassium-sparing diuretic, antihypertensive, antihypokalemic (see p. 87C).

ACTION

Directly interferes with sodium reabsorption in distal tubule. **Therapeutic Effect:** Increases sodium and water excretion and decreases potassium excretion.

PHARMACOKINETICS

Onset	Peak	Duration
PO		
2 hrs	6–10 hrs	24 hrs

Incompletely absorbed from GI tract. Protein binding: Minimal. Primarily excreted in urine; partially eliminated in feces. **Half-life:** 6–9 hrs.

USES

Counteracts potassium loss induced by other diuretics in treatment of hypertension, CHF, hepatic cirrhosis, hypoaldosteronism. **Unlabeled:** Reduction of lithium-induced polyuria; slows pulmonary function reduction in cystic fibrosis; treatment of edema associated with CHF, hepatic cirrhosis, nephrotic syndrome; hypertension.

PRECAUTIONS

CONTRAINDICATIONS: Serum potassium >5.5 mEq/L, pts on other potassium-sparing diuretics, anuria, acute or chronic renal insufficiency, diabetic nephropathy. **CAUTIONS:** BUN >30 mg/dl or serum creatinine >1.5 mg/dl, elderly, debilitated, hepatic insufficiency, cardiopulmonary disease, or diabetes mellitus.

LIFESPAN CONSIDERATIONS: Pregnancy/lactation: Unknown if drug crosses placenta or is distributed in breast milk. **Pregnancy Category B (D if used in pregnancy-induced hypertension). Children:** No age-related precautions noted. **Elderly:** Increased risk of hyperkalemia, age-related decreased renal function may require caution.

INTERACTIONS

DRUG: May decrease effect of **anticoagulants, heparin. NSAIDs** may decrease antihypertensive effect. **ACE inhibitors (e.g., captopril), potassium-containing diuretics, potassium supplements** may increase potassium. May decrease **lithium** clearance, increase toxicity. **HERBAL:** None known. **FOOD:** None known. **LAB VALUES:** May increase BUN, calcium excretion, creatinine, glucose, magnesium, potassium, uric acid. May decrease sodium.

AVAILABILITY (Rx)

TABLETS: 5 mg.

ADMINISTRATION/HANDLING

PO

- Give with food to avoid GI distress.

INDICATIONS/ROUTES/DOSAGE

PO: ADULTS: 5–10 mg/day up to 20 mg. ELDERLY: Initially, 5 mg/day or every other day. CHILDREN 6–20 KG: 0.625 mg/kg/day. **Maximum:** 10 mg/day.

DOSAGE IN RENAL IMPAIRMENT

Creatinine Clearance	Dosage
10–50 ml/min	50% of normal
<10 ml/min	Avoid

SIDE EFFECTS

FREQUENT (3%–8%): Headache, nausea, diarrhea, vomiting, decreased appetite. **OCCASIONAL (<3%):** Dizziness, constipation, abdominal pain, weakness, fatigue, cough, impotence. **RARE (<1%):** Tremors, vertigo, confusion, nervousness, insomnia, thirst, dry mouth, heartburn, shortness of breath, increased urination, hypotension, rash.

ADVERSE REACTIONS/ TOXIC EFFECTS

Severe hyperkalemia may produce irritability, anxiety, heaviness of legs, paresthesia of hands/face/lips, hypotension, bradycardia, tented T waves, widening of QRS, ST depression.

NURSING IMPLICATIONS

BASELINE ASSESSMENT

Assess baseline electrolytes, particularly for low potassium. Assess renal/hepatic functions. Assess edema (note location, extent), skin turgor, mucous membranes for hydration status. Assess muscle strength, mental status. Note skin temperature, moisture. Obtain baseline weight. Initiate strict I&O. Obtain baseline 12-lead EKG. Note pulse rate/rhythm.

INTERVENTION/EVALUATION

Monitor B/P, vital signs, electrolytes (particularly potassium), I&O, weight. Note extent of diuresis. Watch for changes from initial assessment; hyperkalemia may result in muscle strength changes, tremor, muscle cramps, change in mental status (orientation, alertness, confusion), cardiac arrhythmias. Monitor potassium level, particularly during initial therapy. Weigh daily. Assess lung sounds for rales, wheezing.

PATIENT/FAMILY TEACHING

Expect increase in volume and frequency of urination. Therapeutic effect takes several days to begin and can last for several days when drug is discontinued. High-potassium diet/potassium supplements can be dangerous, esp. if pt has renal/hepatic problems. Avoid foods high in potassium such as whole grains (cereals), legumes, meat, bananas, apricots, orange juice, potatoes (white, sweet), raisins. Contact physician if confusion, irregular heartbeat, nervousness, numbness of hands/feet/lips, difficulty breathing, unusual tiredness, weakness in legs occur (hyperkalemia).

aminocaproic acid

ah-meen-oh-kah-**pro**-ick
(Amicar)

Do not confuse with amikacin, Amikin.

CLASSIFICATION

PHARMACOTHERAPEUTIC: Systemic hemostatic. **CLINICAL:** Antifibrinolytic, antihemorrhagic.

ACTION

Inhibits activation of plasminogen activator substances. **Therapeutic Effect:** Prevents fibrin clots from forming.

USES

Treatment of excessive bleeding from hyperfibrinolysis or urinary fibrinolysis as noted in anemia, abruptio placentae, cirrhosis, carcinoma of prostate, lung, stomach, cervix. **Unlabeled:** Prevents reoccurrence of subarachnoid hemorrhage. Prevents hemorrhage in hemophiliacs following dental surgery.

PRECAUTIONS

CONTRAINDICATIONS: Evidence of active intravascular clotting process, disseminated intravascular coagulation without concurrent heparin therapy, hematuria of upper urinary tract origin (unless benefits outweigh risk). **Parenteral:** Newborns. **CAUTION:** Impaired cardiac, hepatic, or renal disease, those with hyperfibrinolysis. **Pregnancy Category C.**

INTERACTIONS

DRUG: None known. **HERBAL:** None known. **FOOD:** None known. **LAB VALUES:** May elevate serum potassium level.

AVAILABILITY (Rx)

TABLETS: 500 mg. **SYRUP:** 250 mg/ml. **INJECTION:** 250 mg/ml.

ADMINISTRATION/HANDLING

IV

Reconstitution • Dilute each 1 g in up to 50 ml 0.9% NaCl, D_5W, Ringer's, or Sterile Water for Injection (do not use Sterile Water for Injection in pts with subarachnoid hemorrhage).

Rate of administration • Give only by IV infusion. • Infuse ≤5 g over first hr in 250 ml of solution; give each succeeding 1 g over 1 hr in 50–100 ml solution.

Administration precautions • Monitor for hypotension during infusion. Rapid infusion may produce bradycardia, arrhythmias.

IV INCOMPATIBILITY

Sodium lactate. Do not mix with other medications.

INDICATIONS/ROUTES/DOSAGE

Alert: Reduce dosage in presence of cardiac, renal, or hepatic impairment.

ACUTE BLEEDING

PO/IV infusion: ADULTS, ELDERLY: Initially, 4–5 g over 1 hr, then 1–1.25 g/hr. Continue for 8 hrs or until bleeding is controlled. **Maximum:** Up to 30 g/24 hrs. CHILDREN: 3 g/m^2 over first hr, then 1 g/m^2/hr. **Maximum:** 18 g/m^2/24 hrs.

DOSAGE IN RENAL IMPAIRMENT

Decrease dose to 25% of normal.

SIDE EFFECTS

OCCASIONAL: Nausea, diarrhea, cramps, decreased urination, decreased B/P, dizziness, headache, muscle fatigue/weakness (myopathy), bloodshot eyes.

ADVERSE REACTIONS/ TOXIC EFFECTS

Too rapid IV administration produces tinnitus, skin rash, arrhythmias, unusual tiredness, weakness. Rarely, grand mal seizure occurs, generally preceded by weakness, dizziness, headache.

NURSING IMPLICATIONS

INTERVENTION/EVALUATION

Question any change in skeletal strength as noted by pt (consider possibility of cardiac damage as a result). Skeletal myopathy characterized by increase in creatine kinase, SGOT (AST) serum levels. Monitor these lab results frequently. Monitor heart rhythm. Assess for decrease in B/P, increase in pulse rate, abdominal or back pain, severe headache (may be evidence of hemorrhage). Assess peripheral pulses, skin for bruises, petechiae. Question for increase in amount of discharge during menses. Check for excessive bleeding from minor cuts, scratches. Assess gums for erythema, gingival bleeding. Assess urine output for hematuria.

PATIENT/FAMILY TEACHING

Report any sign of red/dark urine, black/red stool, coffee-ground vomitus, red-speckled mucus from cough.

aminophylline (theophylline ethylenediamine)

am-in-**ah**-phil-lin
(Aminophylline)
Do not confuse with amitriptyline, ampicillin.

theophylline

(SloBid, Theo-Dur, Theolair, Uniphyl)
Immediate-release: **Aerolate, Theolair.** Extended-release: **Theo-24, Uniphyl.**
Do not confuse with Dolobid.

CLASSIFICATION

PHARMACOTHERAPEUTIC: Xanthine derivative. **CLINICAL:** Bronchodilator (see p. 63C).

ACTION

Directly relaxes smooth muscle of bronchial airway, pulmonary blood vessels. **Therapeutic Effect:** Relieves bronchospasm, increases vital capacity. Produces cardiac, skeletal muscle stimulation.

USES

Symptomatic relief, prevention of bronchial asthma, reversible bronchospasm due to chronic bronchitis, emphysema, or COPD. **Unlabeled:** Treatment of apnea in neonates.

PRECAUTIONS

CONTRAINDICATIONS: History of hypersensitivity to xanthine, caffeine. **CAUTIONS:** Impaired cardiac, renal, or hepatic function; hypertension; hyperthyroidism; diabetes mellitus; peptic ulcer; glaucoma; severe hypoxemia; underlying seizure disorder. **Pregnancy Category C.**

INTERACTIONS

DRUG: **Glucocorticoids** may produce hypernatremia. **Phenytoin, primidone, rifampin** may increase metabolism. **Beta-blockers** may decrease effects. **Cimetidine, ciprofloxacin, erythromycin, norfloxacin** may increase concentration, toxicity. Smoking may decrease concentration. **HERBAL:** None known. **FOOD:** None known. **LAB VALUES:** None known.

AVAILABILITY (Rx)

CAPSULES 125 mg. **CAPSULES (sustained release):** 65 mg, 125 mg, 130 mg, 200 mg, 260 mg, 300 mg. **CAPSULES (sustained release 24 hrs):** 100 mg, 200 mg, 300 mg, 400 mg. **ELIXIR:** 80 mg/15 ml. **INJECTION:** 800 mg/500 ml. **LIQUID:** 80 mg/15 ml. **TABLET:** 125 mg, 250 mg, 300 mg. **TABLET (controlled release):** 100 mg, 200 mg, 300 mg, 400 mg, 450 mg, 600 mg. **TABLETS (controlled release 12 hrs):** 100 mg, 200 mg, 300 mg. **INJECTION:** 25 mg/ml.

ADMINISTRATION/HANDLING

PO

- Give with food to avoid GI distress.
- Do not crush or break extended-release forms.

IV

Storage • Store at room temperature. • Discard if solution contains a precipitate.

Dilution • Give loading dose diluted in 100–200 ml of D_5W or 0.9% NaCl. Prepare maintenance dose in larger volume parenteral infusion.

Rate of administration • Do not exceed flow rate of 1 ml/min (25 mg/min) for either piggyback or infusion. • Administer loading dose over 20–30 min. • Use infusion pump or microdrip to regulate IV administration.

∅ IV INCOMPATIBILITIES

Amiodarone (Cordarone), ciprofloxacin (Cipro), dobutamine (Dobutrex), ondansetron (Zofran).

IV COMPATIBILITIES

Aztreonam (Azactam), ceftazidime (Fortaz), fluconazole (Diflucan), heparin, morphine, potassium chloride.

INDICATIONS/ROUTES/DOSAGE

Alert: Dosage calculated on basis of lean body weight. Dosage based on peak serum theophylline concentrations, clinical condition, presence of toxicity.

CHRONIC BRONCHOSPASM

PO: ADULTS, ELDERLY, CHILDREN: Initially, 16 mg/kg or 400 mg/day (whichever is less) in 2–4 divided doses (6- to 12-hr intervals). May increase by 25% every 2–3 days up to maximum of 24 mg/kg/day (1–9 YRS); 20 mg/kg/day (9–12 YRS); 18 mg/kg/day (12–16 YRS); 13 mg/kg/day (>16 YRS). Doses above maximum based on serum theophylline concentrations, clinical condition, presence of toxicity.

ACUTE BRONCHOSPASM IN PTS NOT CURRENTLY TAKING THEOPHYLLINE

IV loading dose: ADULTS, CHILDREN >1 YR: Initially, 6 mg/kg (aminophylline), then begin maintenance aminophylline dosage based on pt group. NEONATES: 5 mg/kg.

Pt Group	Maintenance Dosage
Neonates	5 mg/kg q12h
6 wk–6 mo	0.5 mg/kg/hr
7 mo–11 mo	0.6–0.7 mg/kg/hr
1–9 yrs	1–1.2 mg/kg/hr
10–12 yrs, young adult smokers	0.9 mg/kg/hr
13–16 yrs	0.7 mg/kg/hr
Adult, nonsmoker	0.7 mg/kg/hr
Older pt, cor pulmonale, CHF, liver impairment	0.25 mg/kg/hr

PO/loading dose: ADULTS, CHILDREN >1 YR: Initially, 5 mg/kg (theophylline), then begin maintenance theophylline dosage based on pt group.

Pt Group	Maintenance Theophylline Dosage
Children (1–9 yrs)	4 mg/kg q6h
Children (10–16 yrs), young adult smokers	3 mg/kg q6h
Healthy, nonsmoking adults	3 mg/kg q8h
Older pts, pts with cor pulmonale	2 mg/kg q8h
Pts with CHF, liver disease	1–2 mg/kg q12h

ACUTE BRONCHOSPASM IN PTS CURRENTLY TAKING THEOPHYLLINE

PO/IV: ADULTS, CHILDREN >1 YR: Obtain serum theophylline level. If not possible and pt in respiratory distress and not experiencing toxicity, may give 2.5 mg/kg dose. MAINTENANCE: Dosage based on peak serum theophylline concentrations, clinical condition, presence of toxicity.

SIDE EFFECTS

FREQUENT: Momentary change in sense of smell during IV administration; shakiness, restlessness, tachycardia, trembling. **OCCASIONAL:** Heartburn, vomiting, headache, mild diuresis, insomnia, nausea.

ADVERSE REACTIONS/ TOXIC EFFECTS

Too rapid rate of IV administration may produce marked fall in B/P with accompanying faintness and lightheadedness, palpitations, tachycardia, hyperventilation, nausea, vomiting, angina-like pain, seizures, ventricular fibrillation, cardiac standstill.

NURSING IMPLICATIONS

BASELINE ASSESSMENT

Offer emotional support (high incidence of anxiety due to difficulty in breathing and sympathomimetic response to drug). Peak serum concentration should be taken 1 hr following IV dose, 1–2 hrs after immediate-release dose, 3–8 hrs after extended-release dose. Take trough level just before next dose.

INTERVENTION/EVALUATION

Monitor rate, depth, rhythm, type of respiration; quality and rate of pulse. Assess lung sounds for rhonchi, wheezing, rales. Monitor ABGs. Observe lips, fingernails for blue or dusky color in light-skinned pts; gray in dark-skinned pts. Observe for clavicular retractions, hand tremor. Evaluate for clinical improvement (quieter, slower respirations, relaxed facial expression, cessation of clavicular retractions). Monitor theophylline blood serum levels (therapeutic serum level range: 10–20 mcg/ml).

PATIENT/FAMILY TEACHING

Increase fluid intake (decreases lung secretion viscosity). Avoid excessive use of caffeine derivatives (chocolate, coffee, tea, cola, cocoa). Smoking, charcoal-broiled food, high-protein, low-carbohydrate diet may decrease theophylline level.

amiodarone hydrochloride

ah-me-**oh**-dah-roan

(Cordarone, Pacerone)

Do not confuse with amiloride, Cardura.

CLASSIFICATION

PHARMACOTHERAPEUTIC: Cardiac agent. **CLINICAL:** Antiarrhythmic (see p. 15C).

ACTION

Prolongs myocardial cell action potential duration and refractory period by direct action on all cardiac tissue. **Therapeutic Effect:** Decreases AV conduction, sinus node function.

PHARMACOKINETICS

Onset	Peak	Duration
PO		
3 days–3 wks	1 wk–5 mos	7–50 days after discontinuation

Slowly, variably absorbed from GI tract. Protein binding: 96%. Extensively metabolized in liver to active metabolite. Excreted via bile; not removed by hemodialysis. **Half-life:** 26–107 days; metabolite: 61 days.

USES

Management of life-threatening recurrent ventricular fibrillation or hemodynamically unstable ventricular tachycardia. **Unlabeled:** Treatment/prophylaxis of supraventricular arrhythmias refractory to conventional treatment, symptomatic atrial flutter.

PRECAUTIONS

CONTRAINDICATIONS: Severe sinus-node dysfunction, second- and third-degree AV block, bradycardia-induced syncope (except in presence of pacemaker), severe hepatic disease. **CAUTIONS:** Thyroid disease.

LIFESPAN CONSIDERATIONS: Pregnancy/lactation: Crosses placenta; distributed in breast milk. May adversely affect fetal development. **Pregnancy Category D. Children:** Safety and efficacy not established. **Elderly:** May be more sensitive to effects on thyroid function. May experience increased incidence ataxia, other neurotoxic effects.

INTERACTIONS

DRUG: May increase cardiac effects with **other antiarrhythmics.** May increase effect of **beta-blockers, oral anticoagulants.** May increase concentration, toxicity of **digoxin, phenytoin.** **HERBAL:** None known. **FOOD:** None known. **LAB VALUES:** May increase SGOT (AST), SGPT (ALT), alkaline phosphatase, ANA titer. May cause changes in EKG, thyroid function tests. Therapeutic blood serum level: 0.5–2.5 mcg/ml; toxic serum level: not established.

AVAILABILITY (Rx)

TABLETS: 200 mg, 400 mg. **INJECTION:** 50 mg/ml.

ADMINISTRATION/HANDLING

PO

- Give with meals to reduce GI distress.
- Tablets may be crushed.

IV

Storage • Store at room temperature. • Use in PVC containers within 2 hrs of dilution; within 24 hrs with glass or polyolefin containers.

Reconstitution • Use glass or polyolefin containers for dilution. • Dilute loading dose (150 mg) in 100 ml D_5W (1.5 mg/ml). • Dilute maintenance dose (900 mg) in 500 ml D_5W (1.8 mg/ml). Concentrations >3 mg/ml cause peripheral vein phlebitis.

Rate of administration • Does not need protection from light during administration. • Administer through central venous catheter (CVC) if possible, using in-line filter. • Bolus over 10 min (15 mg/min) not to exceed 30 mg/min; then 1 mg/min over 6 hrs; then 0.5 mg/min over 18 hrs. • Infusions >1 hr, concentration not to exceed 2 mg/ml (unless CVC used).

∅ IV INCOMPATIBILITIES

Aminophylline (Theophylline), cefazolin (Ancef), heparin, sodium bicarbonate.

IV COMPATIBILITIES

Dobutamine (Dobutrex), dopamine (Intropin), furosemide (Lasix), insulin (regular), labetalol (Normodyne), lidocaine, midazolam (Versed), morphine, nitroglycerin, norepinephrine (Levophed), phenylephrine (Neo-Synephrine), potassium chloride, vancomycin.

INDICATIONS/ROUTES/DOSAGE

LIFE-THREATENING VENTRICULAR ARRHYTHMIAS

PO: ADULTS, ELDERLY: Initially, 800–1,600 mg/day in 2–4 divided doses for 1–3 wks. After arrhythmias controlled or side effects occur, reduce to 600–800 mg/day for about 4 wks. MAINTENANCE: 200–600 mg/day. CHILDREN: Initially, 10–15 mg/kg/day for 4–14 days, then 5 mg/kg/day for several wks. MAINTENANCE: 2.5 mg/kg minimal dose for 5 of 7 days/wk.

IV infusion: ADULTS: Initially, 1,050 mg over 24 hrs: 150 mg over 10 min, follow by 360 mg over 6 hrs, follow by 540 mg over 18 hrs. May continue at 0.5 mg/min up to 2–3 wks regardless of age, renal or left ventricular function.

SIDE EFFECTS

Corneal microdeposits are noted in almost all pts treated for >6 mos (can lead to blurry vision). **FREQUENT (>3%): Parenteral:** Hypotension, nausea, fever, bradycardia. **PO:** Constipation, headache, decreased appetite, nausea, vomiting, numbness of fingers/toes, photosensitivity, muscular incoordination. **OCCASIONAL** (<3%): **PO:** Bitter/metallic taste; decreased sexual ability/interest; dizziness; facial flushing; blue-gray coloring of skin of face, arms, neck; blurred vision; slow heartbeat; asymptomatic corneal deposits. **RARE** (<1%): **PO:** Skin rash, vision loss, blindness.

ADVERSE REACTIONS/ TOXIC EFFECTS

Serious, potentially fatal pulmonary toxicity (alveolitis, pulmonary fibrosis, pneumonitis, adult respiratory distress syndrome) may begin with progressive dyspnea and cough with rales, decreased breath sounds, pleurisy. CHF, hepatotoxicity may be noted. May worsen existing arrhythmias or produce new arrhythmias.

NURSING IMPLICATIONS

BASELINE ASSESSMENT

Obtain baseline pulmonary function tests, chest x-ray, liver enzyme tests, SGOT (AST), SGPT (ALT), alkaline phosphatase, 12-lead EKG. Assess B/P, apical pulse immediately before drug is administered (if pulse is ≤60/min or systolic B/P is <90 mm Hg, withhold medication, contact physician).

INTERVENTION/EVALUATION

Monitor for symptoms of pulmonary toxicity (progressively worsening dyspnea, cough). Dosage should be discontinued or reduced if toxicity occurs. Assess pulse for quality/weakness, irregular rhythm, bradycardia. Monitor EKG for cardiac changes, particularly widening of QRS, prolongation of PR and QT intervals. Notify physician of any significant interval changes. Assess for nausea, fatigue, paresthesia, tremor. Monitor for signs of hypothyroidism (periorbital edema, lethargy, pudgy hands/feet, cool/pale skin, vertigo, night cramps) and hyperthyroidism (hot/dry skin, bulging eyes [exophthalmos], frequent urination, eyelid edema, weight loss, breathlessness). Monitor SGOT (AST), SGPT (ALT), alkaline phosphatase for evidence of liver toxicity. Assess skin, cornea for bluish discoloration in those who have been on drug therapy >2 mos. Monitor liver function tests, thyroid test results. If elevated liver enzymes occur, dosage reduction or discontinuation is necessary. Monitor for therapeutic serum level (0.5–2.5 mcg/ml). Toxic serum level not established.

PATIENT/FAMILY TEACHING

Protect against photosensitivity reaction on skin exposed to sunlight. Bluish skin discoloration gradually disappears when drug is discontinued. Report shortness of breath, cough. Outpatients should monitor pulse before taking medication. Do not abruptly discontinue medication. Compliance with therapy regimen is essential to control arrhythmias. Restrict salt, alcohol intake. Recommend ophthalmic exams q6mo. Report any vision changes.

amitriptyline hydrochloride

a-me-**trip**-tih-leen
(Apo-Amitriptyline♣, Elavil, Levate♣, Novo-Triptyn♣)

Do not confuse with Mellaril, nortriptyline.

FIXED-COMBINATION(S)

Limbitrol: amitriptyline/chlordiazepoxide (an antianxiety): 12.5 mg/5 mg; 25 mg/10 mg. **Etrafon, Triavil:** amitriptyline/perphenazine (an antipsychotic): 10 mg/2 mg; 25 mg/2 mg; 10 mg/4 mg; 25 mg/4 mg.

CLASSIFICATION

PHARMACOTHERAPEUTIC: Tricyclic. **CLINICAL:** Antidepressant, antineuralgic, antibulimic (see p. 34C).

ACTION

Blocks reuptake of neurotransmitters (norepinephrine, serotonin) at presynaptic membranes, increasing synaptic concentration at postsynaptic receptor sites. Has strong anticholinergic activity. **Therapeutic Effect:** Results in antidepressant effect.

PHARMACOKINETICS

Rapid, well absorbed from GI tract. Protein binding: 90%. Metabolized in liver, undergoes first-pass metabolism. Primarily excreted in urine. Minimal removal by hemodialysis. **Half-life:** 10–26 hrs.

USES

Treatment of various forms of depression, exhibited as persistent, prominent dysphoria (occurring nearly every day for at least 2 wks) manifested by 4 of 8 symptoms: appetite change, sleep pattern change, increased fatigue, impaired concentration, feelings of guilt or worthlessness, loss of interest in usual activities, psychomotor agitation or retardation, suicidal tendencies. **Unlabeled:** Relieves neuropathic pain (e.g., diabetic neuropathy, postherpetic neuralgia, treatment of bulimia nervosa).

PRECAUTIONS

CONTRAINDICATIONS: Acute recovery period after MI, ≤14 days of MAOI ingestion. **CAUTIONS:** Prostatic hypertrophy, history of urinary retention or obstruction, glaucoma, diabetes mellitus, history of seizures, hyperthyroidism, cardiac/hepatic/renal disease, schizophrenia, increased intraocular pressure, hiatal hernia.

LIFESPAN CONSIDERATIONS: Pregnancy/lactation: Crosses placenta; minimally distributed in breast milk. **Pregnancy Category C. Children:** More sensitive to increased dosage, toxicity. **Elderly:** Increased risk of toxicity. Increased sensitivity to anticholinergic effects. Cautions in those with cardiovascular disease.

INTERACTIONS

DRUG: CNS depressants (including alcohol, barbiturates, phenothiazines, sedative-hypnotics, anticonvulsants) may increase sedation, respiratory depression, hypotensive effects. **Antithyroid agents** may increase risk of agranulocytosis. **Phenothiazines** may increase sedative, anticholinergic effects. **Cimetidine, valproic acid** may increase concentration, toxicity. May decrease effects of **clonidine, guanadrel.** May increase cardiac effects with **sympathomimetics.** May increase risk of hypertensive crisis, hyperpyresis, seizures with **MAOIs. HERBAL:** None known. **FOOD:** None known. **LAB VALUES:** May alter EKG readings (flattens T wave), glucose. Therapeutic blood serum level: Peak: 120–250 ng/ml; toxic serum level: >500 ng/ml.

AVAILABILITY (Rx)

TABLETS: 10 mg, 25 mg, 50 mg, 75 mg, 100 mg, 150 mg. **INJECTION:** 10 mg/ml.

ADMINISTRATION/HANDLING

PO

- Give with food or milk if GI distress occurs.

IM

- Give by IM only if PO administration is not feasible.
- Crystals may form in injection. Redissolve by immersing ampoule in hot water for 1 min.
- Give deep IM slowly.

INDICATIONS/ROUTES/DOSAGE

DEPRESSION

PO: ADULTS: 30–100 mg/day as a single

dose at bedtime or in divided doses. May gradually increase up to 300 mg/day. Titrate to lowest effective dosage. ELDERLY: Initially, 10–25 mg at bedtime. May increase by 10–25 mg/wk at weekly intervals. RANGE: 25–150 mg/day. CHILDREN 6–12 YRS: 1–5 mg/kg/day in 2 divided doses.

IM: ADULTS: 20–30 mg 4 times/day.

PAIN MANAGEMENT

PO: ADULTS, ELDERLY: 25–100 mg at bedtime.

SIDE EFFECTS

FREQUENT: Dizziness, drowsiness, dry mouth, orthostatic hypotension, headache, increased appetite/weight, nausea, unusual tiredness, unpleasant taste. **OCCASIONAL:** Blurred vision, confusion, constipation, hallucinations, delayed micturition, eye pain, arrhythmias, fine muscle tremors, parkinsonian syndrome, nervousness, diarrhea, increased sweating, heartburn, insomnia. **RARE:** Hypersensitivity, alopecia, tinnitus, breast enlargement.

ADVERSE REACTIONS/ TOXIC EFFECTS

High dosage may produce confusion, seizures, severe drowsiness, fast/slow/irregular heartbeat, fever, hallucinations, agitation, shortness of breath, vomiting, unusual tiredness/weakness. Abrupt withdrawal from prolonged therapy may produce headache, malaise, nausea, vomiting, vivid dreams. Blood dyscrasias, cholestatic jaundice occur rarely.

NURSING IMPLICATIONS

BASELINE ASSESSMENT

Observe/record behavior. Assess psychological status, thought content, sleep patterns, appearance, interest in environment. For those on long-term therapy, liver/renal function tests, blood counts should be performed periodically.

INTERVENTION/EVALUATION

Supervise suicidal-risk pt closely during early therapy (as depression lessens, energy level improves, increasing suicide potential). Assess appearance, behavior, speech pattern, level of interest, mood. Monitor B/P, pulse for hypotension, arrhythmias. Therapeutic blood serum level: Peak: 120–250 ng/ml; toxic serum level: >500 ng/ml.

PATIENT/FAMILY TEACHING

Change positions slowly to avoid hypotensive effect. Tolerance to postural hypotension, sedative and anticholinergic effects usually develop during early therapy. Maximum therapeutic effect may be noted in 2–4 wks. Sensitivity to sun may occur. Report visual disturbances. Do not abruptly discontinue medication. Avoid tasks that require alertness, motor skills until response to drug is established. Sips of tepid water may relieve dry mouth.

amlodipine

am-**low**-dih-peen
(Norvasc)

Do not confuse with Navane, Vascor.

FIXED-COMBINATION(S)

Lotrel: amlodipine/benazepril (an ACE inhibitor): 2.5 mg/10 mg; 5 mg/10 mg; 5 mg/20 mg; 10 mg/20 mg.

◆CLASSIFICATION

PHARMACOTHERAPEUTIC: Calcium channel blocker. **CLINICAL:** Antihypertensive, antianginal (see p. 67C).

ACTION

Inhibits calcium movement across cell membranes of cardiac and vascular smooth muscle. **Therapeutic Effect:** Dilates coronary arteries, peripheral arteries/arterioles. Decreases total peripheral vascular resistance by vasodilation.

PHARMACOKINETICS

Onset	Peak	Duration
PO		
0.5–1 hr	6–12 hrs	24 hrs

Slowly absorbed from GI tract. Protein binding: 93%. Undergoes first-pass metabolism in liver. Excreted primarily in urine. Not removed by hemodialysis. **Half-life:** 30–50 hrs (half-life increased in elderly, those with hepatic cirrhosis).

USES

Management of hypertension, chronic stable angina, vasospastic (Prinzmetal's or variant) angina. May be used alone or with other antihypertensives or antianginals.

PRECAUTIONS

CONTRAINDICATIONS: Severe hypotension. **CAUTIONS:** Impaired hepatic function, aortic stenosis, CHF.

LIFESPAN CONSIDERATIONS: Pregnancy/lactation: Unknown if drug crosses placenta or is distributed in breast milk. **Pregnancy Category C. Children:** Safety and efficacy not established. **Elderly:** Half-life may be increased, more sensitive to hypotensive effects.

INTERACTIONS

DRUG: None known. **HERBAL:** None known. **FOOD: Grapefruit/grapefruit juice** may increase concentration, hypotensive effects. **LAB VALUES:** None known.

AVAILABILITY (Rx)

TABLETS: 2.5 mg, 5 mg, 10 mg.

ADMINISTRATION/HANDLING

PO

- May give without regard to food.
- Grapefruit juice may increase drug concentration.

INDICATIONS/ROUTES/DOSAGE

Alert: Dosage should be titrated over 7–14 days.

HYPERTENSION

PO: ADULTS: Initially, 5 mg/day as single dose. **Maximum:** 10 mg/day.

PO: SMALL-FRAME, FRAGILE, ELDERLY: Initially, 2.5 mg/day as single dose.

ANGINA (chronic stable or vasospastic)

PO: ADULTS: 5–10 mg. ELDERLY, HEPATIC INSUFFICIENCY: 5 mg.

DOSAGE IN LIVER IMPAIRMENT

PO: ADULTS, ELDERLY: Initially, 2.5 mg/day.

SIDE EFFECTS

FREQUENT (>5%): Peripheral edema, headache, flushing. **OCCASIONAL (<5%):** Dizziness, palpitations, nausea, unusual tiredness/weakness (asthenia). **RARE (<1%):** Chest pain, bradycardia, orthostatic hypotension.

ADVERSE REACTIONS/ TOXIC EFFECTS

Overdosage may produce excessive peripheral vasodilation, marked hypotension with reflex tachycardia.

NURSING IMPLICATIONS

BASELINE ASSESSMENT

Assess baseline renal/liver function tests, B/P, and apical pulse.

INTERVENTION/EVALUATION

Assess B/P (if systolic B/P is <90 mm Hg, withhold medication, contact physician). Assess for peripheral edema behind medial malleolus (sacral area in bedridden pts). Assess skin for flushing. Question for headache, asthenia.

PATIENT/FAMILY TEACHING

Do not abruptly discontinue medication. Compliance with therapy regimen is essential to control hypertension. Avoid tasks that require alertness, motor skills until response to drug is established. Avoid concomitant ingestion of grapefruit juice.

amoxicillin

ah-**mocks**-ih-sill-in

(Amoxil, Apo-Amoxi✦, DisperMox, Novamoxin✦, Polymox, Trimox, Wymox)

Do not confuse with amoxapine, Tylox.

◆ CLASSIFICATION

PHARMACOTHERAPEUTIC: Penicillin. **CLINICAL:** Antibiotic (see p. 27C).

ACTION

Bactericidal in susceptible microorganisms. **Therapeutic Effect:** Inhibits cell wall synthesis.

PHARMACOKINETICS

Well absorbed from GI tract. Protein binding: 20%. Partially metabolized in liver. Primarily excreted in urine. Removed by hemodialysis. **Half-life:** 1–1.3 hrs (half-life increased in reduced renal function).

USES

Treatment of skin/skin structure infections; respiratory tract, GI tract, and GU tract infections; otitis media; gonorrhea. Treatment of *H. pylori* associated with peptic ulcer. **Unlabeled:** Lyme disease, typhoid fever.

PRECAUTIONS

CONTRAINDICATIONS: Infectious mononucleosis, hypersensitivity to any penicillin. **CAUTIONS:** History of allergies (esp. cephalosporins), antibiotic-associated colitis.

LIFESPAN CONSIDERATIONS: Pregnancy/lactation: Crosses placenta, appears in cord blood, amniotic fluid. Distributed in breast milk in low concentrations. May lead to allergic sensitization, diarrhea, candidiasis, skin rash in infant. **Pregnancy Category B. Children:** Immature renal function in neonate/young infant may delay renal excretion. **Elderly:** Age-related renal impairment may require dosage adjustment.

INTERACTIONS

DRUG: **Allopurinol** may increase incidence of rash. **Probenecid** may increase concentration, toxicity risk. May decrease effects of **oral contraceptives. HERBAL:** None known. **FOOD:** None known. **LAB VALUES:** May increase SGOT (AST), SGPT (ALT), LDH, bilirubin, creatinine, BUN. May cause positive Coombs' test.

AVAILABILITY (Rx)

TABLETS (chewable): 125 mg, 200 mg, 250 mg, 400 mg. **TABLETS:** 500 mg, 875 mg. **TABLETS FOR PO SUSPENSION:** 200 mg, 400 mg. **CAPSULES:** 250 mg, 500 mg. **POWDER FOR PO SUSPENSION:** 50 mg/ml, 125 mg/5 ml, 200 mg/ml, 250 mg/5 ml, 400 mg/5 ml.

ADMINISTRATION/HANDLING

PO

• Store capsules, tablets at room temperature. • After reconstitution, oral solution is stable for 14 days at either room temperature or refrigerated. • Give without regard to meals. • Instruct pt to chew or crush chewable tablets thoroughly before swallowing.

INDICATIONS/ROUTES/DOSAGE

EAR, NOSE, THROAT, GU, SKIN/SKIN STRUCTURE INFECTIONS

PO: ADULTS, ELDERLY, CHILDREN >20 KG: 250–500 mg q8h (or 500–875 mg tablets 2 times/day). CHILDREN <20 KG: 20–40 mg/kg/day in divided doses q8–12h.

LOWER RESPIRATORY TRACT INFECTIONS

PO: ADULTS, ELDERLY, CHILDREN >20 KG: 500 mg q8h (or 875 mg tablets 2 times/day). CHILDREN <20 KG: 40 mg/kg/day in divided doses q8–12h.

ACUTE, UNCOMPLICATED GONORRHEA

PO: ADULTS: 3 g one time with 1 g probenecid. Follow with tetracycline or erythromycin therapy. CHILDREN ≥2 YRS: 50 mg/kg plus probenecid 25 mg/kg as a single dose.

ACUTE OTITIS MEDIA

PO: CHILDREN: 80–90 mg/kg/day in divided doses q12h.

H. PYLORI

PO: ADULTS, ELDERLY (in combination): 1 g 2 times/day for 10 days. NEONATES, CHILDREN ≤3 MOS: 20–30 mg/kg/day in divided doses q12h.

ENDOCARDITIS PROPHYLAXIS

PO: ADULTS, ELDERLY: 2 g 1 hr prior to procedure. CHILDREN: 50 mg/kg as above.

RENAL FUNCTION IMPAIRMENT

Creatinine clearance 10–30 ml/min: Administer q12h. **Creatinine clearance <10 ml/min:** Administer q24h.

SIDE EFFECTS

FREQUENT: GI disturbances (mild diarrhea, nausea, or vomiting), headache, oral/vaginal candidiasis. **OCCASIONAL:** Generalized rash, urticaria.

ADVERSE REACTIONS/ TOXIC EFFECTS

Superinfections, potentially fatal antibiotic-associated colitis (abdominal cramps, watery severe diarrhea, fever) may result from altered bacterial balance. Severe hypersensitivity reactions, including anaphylaxis, acute interstitial nephritis, occur rarely.

NURSING IMPLICATIONS

BASELINE ASSESSMENT

Question for history of allergies, esp. penicillins, cephalosporins.

INTERVENTION/EVALUATION

Hold medication and promptly report rash or diarrhea (with fever, abdominal pain, mucus and blood in stool may indicate antibiotic-associated colitis). Be alert for superinfection: increased fever, sore throat, vomiting, diarrhea, black/hairy tongue, ulceration or changes of oral mucosa, anal/genital pruritus.

PATIENT/FAMILY TEACHING

Continue antibiotic for full length of treatment. Space doses evenly. Take with meals if GI upset occurs. Thoroughly chew the chewable tablets before swallowing. Notify physician in event of rash, diarrhea, or other new symptom.

amoxicillin/ clavulanate potassium

a-**mocks**-ih-sill-in/klah-view-**lan**-ate
(Augmentin, Augmentin ES 600, Augmentin XR, Clavulin)

CLASSIFICATION

PHARMACOTHERAPEUTIC: Penicillin. **CLINICAL:** Antibiotic (see p. 27C).

ACTION

Amoxicillin is bactericidal in susceptible microorganisms. Clavulanate inhibits bacterial beta-lactamase. **Therapeutic Effect:** Amoxicillin inhibits cell wall synthesis. Clavulanate protects amoxicillin from enzymatic degradation.

PHARMACOKINETICS

Well absorbed from GI tract. Protein binding: 20%. Partially metabolized in liver. Primarily excreted in urine. Removed by hemodialysis. **Half-life:** 1–1.3 hrs (half-life increased in reduced renal function).

USES

Treatment of skin/skin structure, lower respiratory tract and urinary infections, otitis media, sinusitis. **Unlabeled:** Treatment of bronchitis, chancroid.

PRECAUTIONS

CONTRAINDICATIONS: Infectious mononucleosis, hypersensitivity to any penicillin. **CAUTIONS:** History of allergies, esp. cephalosporins; antibiotic-associated colitis.

LIFESPAN CONSIDERATIONS: Pregnancy/lactation: Crosses placenta, appears in cord blood, amniotic fluid. Distributed in breast milk in low concentrations. May lead to allergic sensitization, diarrhea, candidiasis, skin rash in infant. **Pregnancy Category B. Children:** Immature renal function in neonate/young infant may delay renal excretion. **Elderly:** Age-related renal impairment may require dosage adjustment.

INTERACTIONS

DRUG: **Allopurinol** may increase incidence of rash. **Probenecid** may increase concentration, toxicity risk. May decrease effects of **oral contraceptives. HERBAL:** None known. **FOOD:** None known. **LAB VALUES:** May increase SGOT (AST), SGPT (ALT). May cause positive Coombs' test.

AVAILABILITY (Rx)

TABLETS (chewable): 125 mg, 200 mg, 250 mg, 400 mg. **TABLETS:** 250 mg, 500 mg, 875 mg, 1,000 mg. **POWDER FOR PO SUSPENSION:** 125 mg/5 ml, 200 mg/5 ml, 250 mg/5 ml, 400 mg/5 ml, 600 mg/5 ml.

ADMINISTRATION/HANDLING

PO

• Store tablets at room temperature. • After reconstitution, oral solution is stable for 14 days at either room temperature or refrigeration. • Give without regard to meals. • Instruct pt to chew or crush chewable tablets thoroughly before swallowing.

INDICATIONS/ROUTES/DOSAGE

Alert: Dosage expressed in terms of amoxicillin. Alternative dosing in adults: 500–875 mg 2 times/day; in children: 200–400 mg 2 times/day.

MILD TO MODERATE INFECTIONS

PO: ADULTS, ELDERLY, CHILDREN >40 KG: 250 mg q8h or 500 mg q12h. CHILDREN <40 KG: 20 mg/kg/day in divided doses q8h.

RESPIRATORY TRACT INFECTIONS, SEVERE INFECTIONS

PO: ADULTS, ELDERLY, CHILDREN >40 KG: 500 mg q8h or 875 mg q12h. CHILDREN <40 KG: 40 mg/kg/day in divided doses q8h.

OTITIS MEDIA

PO: CHILDREN: 90 mg/kg/day in divided doses q12h for 10 days.

SINUSITIS, LOWER RESPIRATORY TRACT INFECTIONS

PO: CHILDREN: 40 mg/kg/day in divided doses q8h **or** 45 mg/kg/day in divided doses q12h.

USUAL NEONATE DOSAGE

PO: NEONATES, CHILDREN ≤3 MOS: 30 mg/kg/day in divided doses q12h.

DOSAGE IN RENAL IMPAIRMENT

Creatinine clearance 10–30 ml/min: 250–500 mg q12h. **Creatinine clearance <10 ml/min:** 250–500 mg q24h.

SIDE EFFECTS

FREQUENT: GI disturbances (mild diarrhea, nausea, vomiting), headache, oral/vaginal candidiasis. **OCCASIONAL:** Generalized rash, urticaria.

ADVERSE REACTIONS/ TOXIC EFFECTS

Superinfections, potentially fatal antibiotic-associated colitis (abdominal cramps, watery severe diarrhea, fever) may result from altered bacterial balance. Severe hypersensitivity reactions, including anaphylaxis, acute interstitial nephritis, occur rarely.

NURSING IMPLICATIONS

BASELINE ASSESSMENT

Question for history of allergies, esp. penicillins, cephalosporins.

INTERVENTION/EVALUATION

Hold medication and promptly report rash or diarrhea (with fever, abdominal pain, mucus and blood in stool may indicate antibiotic-associated colitis). Be alert for superinfection: increased fever, sore throat, vomiting, diarrhea, black/hairy tongue, ulceration or changes of oral mucosa, anal/genital pruritus.

PATIENT/FAMILY TEACHING

Continue antibiotic for full length of treatment. Space doses evenly. Take with meals if GI upset occurs. Thoroughly chew the chewable tablets before swallowing. Notify physician in event of rash, diarrhea, or other new symptom.

amphotericin B

am-foe-**tear**-ih-sin

(Abelcet, AmBisome, Amphotec, Fungizone)

CLASSIFICATION

CLINICAL: Antifungal, antiprotozoal.

ACTION

Generally fungistatic but may be fungicidal with high dosage or very susceptible microorganisms. Binds to sterols in fungal cell membrane. **Therapeutic Effect:** Increases membrane permeability, allowing loss of potassium, other cellular components.

PHARMACOKINETICS

Protein binding: 90%. Widely distributed. Metabolic fate unknown. Cleared by nonrenal pathways. Minimal removal by hemodialysis. **Half-life:** 24 hrs (half-life increased in neonates, children). **Amphotec: Half-life:** 26–28 hrs. Not dialyzable. **Abelcet: Half-life:** 7.2 days. Not dialyzable. **AmBisome: Half-life:** 100–153 hrs.

USES

Abelcet: Treatment of invasive fungal infections refractory or intolerant to Fungizone. **AmBisome:** Empiric treatment for fungal infection in febrile neutropenic pts. *Aspergillus,* candida, or cryptococcus infections refractory to Fungizone or pts with renal impairment or toxicity with Fungizone. Treatment of visceral leishmaniasis. **Amphotec:** Treatment of invasive aspergillosis in pts with renal impairment or toxicity or prior treatment failure with Fungizone. **Fungizone:** Treatment of cryptococcosis, blastomycosis, systemic candidiasis, disseminated forms of moniliasis, coccidioidomycosis, and histoplasmosis, zygomycosis, sporotrichosis, aspergillosis. **Topical:** Treatment of cutaneous/mucocutaneous infections caused by *Candida albicans* (paronychia, oral thrush, perlèche, diaper rash, intertriginous candidiasis).

PRECAUTIONS

CONTRAINDICATIONS: Hypersensitivity to amphotericin B, sulfite. **CAUTIONS:** Renal impairment, in combination with antineoplastic therapy. Give only for progressive, potentially fatal fungal infection.

LIFESPAN CONSIDERATIONS: Pregnancy/lactation: Crosses placenta; unknown if distributed in breast milk. **Pregnancy Category B. Children:** Safety and efficacy not established, but use the least amount for therapeutic regimen. **Elderly:** No age-related precautions noted.

INTERACTIONS

DRUG: **Steroids** may cause severe hypokalemia. **Bone marrow depressants** may increase anemia. May increase **digoxin** toxicity (due to hypokalemia). **Nephrotoxic medications** may increase nephrotoxicity. **HERBAL:** None known. **FOOD:** None known. **LAB VALUES:** May increase SGOT (AST), SGPT (ALT), alkaline phosphatase, BUN, serum creatinine. May decrease calcium, magnesium, potassium.

AVAILABILITY (Rx)

INJECTION: 50 mg (Fungizone), 50 mg, 100 mg (Amphotec), 50 mg (AmBisone). **SUSPENSION FOR INJECTION:** 5 mg/ml (lipid complex: Abelcet). **CREAM, LOTION, OINTMENT.**

ADMINISTRATION/HANDLING

IV

Storage

ABELCET

• Refrigerate unreconstituted solution. Reconstituted solution is stable for 48 hrs if refrigerated; 6 hrs at room temperature.

AMBISOME

• Refrigerate unreconstituted solution. Reconstituted solution of 4 mg/ml is stable for 24 hrs. Concentration of 1–2 mg/ml is stable for 6 hrs.

AMPHOTEC

• Store unreconstituted solution at room temperature. Reconstituted solution stable for 24 hrs.

FUNGIZONE

• Refrigerate unreconstituted solution. Reconstituted solution is stable for 24 hrs at room temperature or 7 days if refrigerated. Diluted solution $\leq$0.1 mg/ml to be used promptly. Do not use if cloudy or contains a precipitate.

Reconstitution

ABELCET

• Shake 20-ml (100-mg) vial gently until contents are dissolved. Withdraw required dose using 5-micron filter needle (supplied by manufacturer). • Inject dose into D_5W; 4 ml D_5W required for each 1 ml (5 mg) to final concentration of 1 mg/ml. Reduce dose by half for pediatric, fluid-restricted pts (2 mg/ml).

AMBISOME

• Reconstitute each 50-mg vial with 12 ml Sterile Water for Injection to provide concentration of 4 mg/ml. • Shake vial vigorously for 30 sec. Withdraw required dose and empty syringe contents through a 5-micron filter into an infusion of D_5W to provide final concentration of 1–2 mg/ml.

AMPHOTEC

• Add 10 ml Sterile Water for Injection to each 50-mg vial to provide concentration of 5 mg/ml. Shake gently. • Further dilute **only** with D_5W using specific amount recommended by manufacturer to provide concentration of 0.16–0.83 mg/ml.

FUNGIZONE

• Rapidly inject 10 ml Sterile Water for Injection to each 50-mg vial to provide concentration of 5 mg/ml. Immediately shake vial until solution is clear. • Further dilute each 1 mg in at least 10 ml D_5W to provide a concentration of 0.1 mg/ml.

Rate of administration • Give by slow IV infusion. Infuse conventional amphotericin or Fungizone over 2–6 hrs; Abelcet over 2 hrs (shake contents if infusion >2 hrs); Amphotec over 2–4 hrs; AmBisome over 1–2 hrs.

ADMINISTRATION/PRECAUTIONS

• Monitor B/P, temperature, pulse, respirations; assess for adverse reactions q15min twice, then q30min for 4 hrs of initial infusion. • Potential for thrombophlebitis may be less with use of pediatric scalp vein needles or (with physician order) adding dilute heparin solution. • Observe strict aseptic technique because no bacteriostatic agent or preservative is present in diluent.

∅ IV INCOMPATIBILITIES

Abelcet/AmBisome/Amphotec: Do not mix with any other drug, diluent, or solution. **Fungizone:** Allopurinol (Aloprim), amifostine (Ethyol), aztreonam (Azactam), calcium gluconate, cefepime (Maxipime), cimetidine (Tagamet), ciprofloxacin (Cipro), docetaxel (Taxotere), dopamine (Intropin), doxorubicin (Adriamycin), enalapril (Vasotec), etoposide (VP-16), filgrastim (Neupogen), fluconazole (Diflucan), fludarabine (Fludara), foscarnet (Foscavir), gemcitabine (Gemzar), magnesium sulfate, meropenem (Merrem IV), ondansetron (Zofran), paclitaxel (Taxol), piperacillin/tazobactam (Zosyn), potassium chloride, propofol (Diprivan), vinorelbine (Navelbine).

IV COMPATIBILITIES

None known; do not mix with other medications or electrolytes.

INDICATIONS/ROUTES/DOSAGE

USUAL ABELCET DOSAGE

IV infusion: ADULTS, CHILDREN: 5 mg/kg at rate of 2.5 mg/kg/hr.

USUAL AMBISOME DOSAGE

IV infusion: ADULTS, CHILDREN: 3–5 mg/kg over 1 hr.

USUAL AMPHOTEC DOSAGE

IV infusion: ADULTS, CHILDREN: 3–4 mg/kg over 2–4 hrs.

CUTANEOUS INFECTIONS

Topical: ADULTS, ELDERLY, CHILDREN: Apply liberally and rub in 2–4 times/day.

USUAL FUNGIZONE DOSAGE

IV infusion: ADULTS, ELDERLY: Dosage based on pt tolerance, severity of infection. Initially, 1-mg test dose is given over 20–30 min. If test dose is tolerated, 5-mg dose may be given the same day. Subsequently, increases of 5 mg/dose are made q12–24h until desired daily dose is reached. Alternatively, if test dose is tolerated, a dose of 0.25 mg/kg is given same day; increased to 0.5 mg/kg the second day. Dose increased until desired daily dose reached. **Total daily dose:** 1 mg/kg/day up to 1.5 mg/kg every other day. Do not exceed maximum total daily dose of 1.5 mg/kg. CHILDREN: **Test dose:** 0.1 mg/kg/dose (**maximum:** 1 mg) infused over 20–60 min. If tolerated, then initial dose: 0.4 mg/kg same day. Dose may be increased in 0.25 mg/kg increments. **Maintenance dose:** 0.25–1 mg/kg/day.

SIDE EFFECTS

FREQUENT (>10%): **Abelcet:** Chills, fever, increased serum creatinine, multiple organ failure. **AmBisome:** Hypokalemia, hypomagnesemia, hyperglycemia, hypocalcemia, edema, abdominal pain, back pain, chills, chest pain, hypotension, diarrhea, nausea, vomiting, headache, fever, rigors, insomnia, dyspnea, epistaxis, increased liver/renal function tests. **Amphotec:** Chills, fever, hypotension, tachycardia, increased creatinine, hypokalemia, bilirubinemia. **Fungizone:** Fever, chills, headache, anemia, hypokalemia, hypomagnesemia, anorexia, malaise, generalized pain, nephrotoxicity. **Topical:** Local irritation, dry skin. **RARE: Topical:** Skin rash.

ADVERSE REACTIONS/ TOXIC EFFECTS

Each alternative formulation is less nephrotoxic than conventional amphotericin (Fungizone). Cardiovascular toxicity (hypotension, ventricular fibrillation), anaphylactic reaction occur rarely. Vision and hearing alterations, seizures, hepatic failure, coagulation defects, multiple organ failure, sepsis may be noted.

NURSING IMPLICATIONS

BASELINE ASSESSMENT

Question for history of allergies, esp. to amphotericin B, sulfite. Avoid, if possible, other nephrotoxic medications. Check for/obtain orders to reduce adverse reactions during IV therapy (antipyretics, antihistamines, antiemetics, or small doses of corticosteroids given before or during amphotericin administration may control reactions).

INTERVENTION/EVALUATION

Monitor B/P, temperature, pulse, respirations; assess for adverse reactions (fever, shaking, chills, anorexia, nausea, vomiting, abdominal pain) q15min twice, then q30min for 4 hrs of initial infusion. If symptoms occur, slow infusion, administer medication for symptomatic relief. For severe reaction or without symptomatic relief orders, stop infusion and notify physician. Evaluate IV site for phlebitis (heat, pain, red streaking over vein). Monitor I&O, renal function tests for nephrotoxicity. Check potassium and magnesium levels, hematologic and hepatic function test results. **Topical:** Assess for itching, irritation, burning.

PATIENT/FAMILY TEACHING

Prolonged therapy (weeks or months) is usually necessary. Fever reaction may decrease with continued therapy. Muscle weakness may be noted during therapy (due to hypokalemia). **Topical:** Application may cause staining of skin or nails; soap and water or dry cleaning will remove fabric stains. Do not use other preparations or occlusive coverings without consulting physician. Keep areas clean, dry; wear light clothing. Separate personal items with direct contact to area.

ampicillin sodium

amp-ih-**sill**-in
(Apo-Ampi ✤, Novo-Ampicillin ✤, Nu-Ampi ✤, Polycillin)

Do not confuse with aminophylline, Imipenem, Unipen.

CLASSIFICATION

PHARMACOTHERAPEUTIC: Penicillin. **CLINICAL:** Antibiotic (see p. 27C).

ACTION

Inhibits cell wall synthesis in susceptible

microorganisms. **Therapeutic Effect:** Produces bactericidal effect.

PHARMACOKINETICS

Moderately absorbed from GI tract. Protein binding: 28%. Widely distributed. Partially metabolized in liver. Primarily excreted in urine. Removed by hemodialysis. **Half-life:** 1–1.5 hrs (half-life increased in impaired renal function).

USES

Treatment of respiratory, GI, and GU tract infections; skin/skin structure, bone, and joint infections; otitis media; gonorrhea; endocarditis; meningitis; septicemia; mild to moderate typhoid fever; perioperative prophylaxis.

PRECAUTIONS

CONTRAINDICATIONS: Infectious mononucleosis, hypersensitivity to any penicillin. **CAUTIONS:** History of allergies, particularly cephalosporins, antibiotic-associated colitis.

LIFESPAN CONSIDERATIONS: Pregnancy/lactation: Readily crosses placenta; appears in cord blood, amniotic fluid. Distributed in breast milk in low concentrations. May lead to allergic sensitization, diarrhea, candidiasis, skin rash in infant. **Pregnancy Category B. Children:** Immature renal function in neonates/young infants may delay renal excretion. **Elderly:** Age-related renal impairment may require dosage adjustment.

INTERACTIONS

DRUG: Allopurinol may increase incidence of rash. **Probenecid** may increase concentration, toxicity risk. May decrease effects of **oral contraceptives. HERBAL:** None known. **FOOD:** None known. **LAB VALUES:** May increase SGOT (AST), SGPT (ALT). May cause positive Coombs' test.

AVAILABILITY (Rx)

CAPSULES: 250 mg, 500 mg. **POWDER FOR PO SUSPENSION:** 125 mg/5 ml, 250 mg/5 ml, 500 mg/5 ml. **POWDER FOR INJECTION:** 125 mg, 250 mg, 500 mg, 1 g, 2 g.

ADMINISTRATION/HANDLING

PO

• Store capsules at room temperature. • Oral suspension, after reconstituted, is stable for 7 days at room temperature, 14 days if refrigerated. • Give orally 1 hr before or 2 hrs after meals for maximum absorption.

IM

• Reconstitute each vial with Sterile Water for Injection or Bacteriostatic Water for Injection (consult individual vial for specific volume of diluent). • Stable for 1 hr. • Give deeply in large muscle mass.

IV

Storage • The IV solution, diluted with 0.9% NaCl, is stable for 2–8 hrs at room temperature or 3 days if refrigerated. • If diluted with D_5W, is stable for 2 hrs at room temperature or 3 hrs if refrigerated. • Discard if precipitate forms.

Reconstitution • For IV injection, dilute each vial with 5 ml Sterile Water for Injection (10 ml for 1- and 2-g vials). • For intermittent IV infusion (piggyback), further dilute with 50–100 ml 0.9% NaCl or D_5W.

Rate of administration • For IV injection, give over 3–5 min (10–15 min for 1- to 2-g dose). • For intermittent IV infusion (piggyback), infuse over 20–30 min. • Due to potential for hypersensitivity/anaphylaxis, start initial dose at few drops per min, increase slowly to ordered rate; stay with pt first 10–15 min, then check q10min. • Change to PO as soon as possible.

⊘ IV INCOMPATIBILITIES
Amikacin (Amikin), diltiazem (Cardizem), gentamicin, midazolam (Versed).

IV COMPATIBILITIES
Calcium gluconate, cefepime (Maxipime), dopamine (Intropin), famotidine (Pepcid), furosemide (Lasix), heparin, hydromorphone (Dilaudid), insulin (regular), levofloxacin (Levaquin), magnesium sulfate, morphine, multivitamins, potassium chloride, propofol (Diprivan).

INDICATIONS/ROUTES/DOSAGE

RESPIRATORY TRACT, SKIN/SKIN STRUCTURE INFECTIONS
PO: ADULTS, ELDERLY, CHILDREN >20 KG: 250–500 mg q6h. CHILDREN <20 KG: 50 mg/kg/day in divided doses q6h.

IM/IV: ADULTS, ELDERLY, CHILDREN >40 KG: 250–500 mg q6h. CHILDREN <40 KG: 25–50 mg/kg/day in divided doses q6–8h.

BACTERIAL MENINGITIS, SEPTICEMIA
IM/IV: ADULTS, ELDERLY: 2 g q4h or 3 g q6h. CHILDREN: 100–200 mg/kg/day in divided doses q4h.

GONOCOCCAL INFECTIONS
PO: ADULTS: 3.5 g one time with 1 g probenecid.

PERIOPERATIVE PROPHYLAXIS
IM/IV: ADULTS, ELDERLY: 2 g 30 min prior to procedure. May repeat in 8 hrs. CHILDREN: 50 mg/kg using same dosage regimen.

USUAL DOSAGE (NEONATES)

Alert: Higher dosages may be needed for neonatal meningitis.

IM/IV: NEONATES 7–28 DAYS: 75 mg/kg/day in divided doses q8h up to 200 mg/kg/day in divided doses q6h. NEONATES 0–7 DAYS: 50 mg/kg/day in divided doses q12h up to 150 mg/kg/day in divided doses q8h.

SIDE EFFECTS

FREQUENT: Pain at IM injection site, GI disturbances (mild diarrhea, nausea, or vomiting), oral/vaginal candidiasis. **OCCASIONAL:** Generalized rash, urticaria, phlebitis, thrombophlebitis with IV administration, headache. **RARE:** Dizziness, seizures, esp. with IV therapy.

ADVERSE REACTIONS/ TOXIC EFFECTS

Superinfections, potentially fatal antibiotic-associated colitis (abdominal cramps, watery severe diarrhea, fever) may result from altered bacterial balance. Severe hypersensitivity reactions, including anaphylaxis, acute interstitial nephritis, occur rarely.

NURSING IMPLICATIONS

BASELINE ASSESSMENT
Question for history of allergies, esp. penicillins, cephalosporins.

INTERVENTION/EVALUATION
Hold medication and promptly report rash (although common with ampicillin, may indicate hypersensitivity) or diarrhea (with fever, abdominal pain, mucus and blood in stool may indicate antibiotic-associated colitis). Evaluate IV site for phlebitis (heat, pain, red streaking over vein). Check IM injection site for pain, induration. Monitor I&O, urinalysis, renal function tests. Assess for signs of superinfection: increased fever, sore throat, vomiting, diarrhea, anal/genital pruritus, oral ulcerations or pain, black/hairy tongue.

PATIENT/FAMILY TEACHING
Space doses evenly. Take antibiotic for full length of treatment. More effective if taken 1 hr before or 2 hrs after food/

A

beverages. Discomfort may occur with IM injection. Notify physician of rash, diarrhea, or other new symptom.

ampicillin/ sulbactam sodium

amp-ih-**sill**-in/sull-**bak**-tam (Unasyn)

◆ CLASSIFICATION

PHARMACOTHERAPEUTIC: Penicillin. **CLINICAL:** Antibiotic (see p. 27C).

ACTION

Ampicillin is bactericidal in susceptible microorganisms. Sulbactam inhibits bacterial beta-lactamase. **Therapeutic Effect:** Ampicillin inhibits cell wall synthesis. Sulbactam protects ampicillin from enzymatic degradation.

PHARMACOKINETICS

Protein binding: 28%–38%. Widely distributed. Partially metabolized in liver. Primarily excreted in urine. Removed by hemodialysis. **Half-life:** 1 hr (half-life increased in impaired renal function).

USES

Treatment of intra-abdominal, skin/skin structure, gynecologic infections.

PRECAUTIONS

CONTRAINDICATIONS: Infectious mononucleosis, hypersensitivity to any penicillin. **CAUTIONS:** History of allergies, particularly to cephalosporins, antibiotic-associated colitis.

LIFESPAN CONSIDERATIONS: Pregnancy/lactation: Readily crosses placenta; appears in cord blood, amniotic fluid. Distributed in breast milk in low concentrations. May lead to allergic sensitization, diarrhea, candidiasis, skin rash in infant. **Pregnancy Category B. Children:** Safety and efficacy not established in children <1 yr. **Elderly:** Age-related renal impairment may require dosage adjustment.

INTERACTIONS

DRUG: Allopurinol may increase incidence of rash. **Probenecid** may increase concentration, toxicity risk. May decrease effects of **oral contraceptives. HERBAL:** None known. **FOOD:** None known. **LAB VALUES:** May increase SGOT (AST), SGPT (ALT), alkaline phosphatase, LDH, creatinine. May cause positive Coombs' test.

AVAILABILITY (Rx)

POWDER FOR INJECTION: 1.5 g, 3 g.

ADMINISTRATION/HANDLING

IM

• Reconstitute each 1.5-g vial with 3.2 ml Sterile Water for Injection to provide concentration of 250 mg ampicillin/125 mg sulbactam/ml. • Give deeply into large muscle mass within 1 hr after preparation.

IV

Storage • When reconstituted with 0.9% NaCl, IV solution is stable for 8 hrs at room temperature, 48 hrs if refrigerated. Stability may be different with other diluents. • Discard if precipitate forms.

Reconstitution • For IV injection, dilute with 10–20 ml Sterile Water for Injection. • For intermittent IV infusion (piggyback), further dilute with 50–100 ml D_5W or 0.9% NaCl.

Rate of administration • For IV injection, give slowly over minimum of 10–15 min. • For intermittent IV infusion (piggyback), infuse over 15–30 min. • Due to potential for hypersensitivity/anaphylaxis, start initial dose at few drops per min, increase slowly to ordered rate; stay with pt first 10–15 min, then check q10min. • Change to PO antibiotic as soon as possible.

⊘ IV INCOMPATIBILITIES
Diltiazem (Cardizem), idarubicin (Idamycin), ondansetron (Zofran), sargramostim (Leukine).

IV COMPATIBILITIES
Famotidine (Pepcid), heparin, insulin (regular), morphine.

INDICATIONS/ROUTES/DOSAGE

SKIN/SKIN STRUCTURE, INTRA-ABDOMINAL, GYNECOLOGIC INFECTIONS
IM/IV: ADULTS, ELDERLY: 1.5 g (1 g ampicillin/500 mg sulbactam) to 3 g (2 g ampicillin/1 g sulbactam) q6h.

SKIN/SKIN STRUCTURE INFECTIONS
IV: CHILDREN 1–12 YRS: 150–300 mg/kg/day in divided doses q6h.

DOSAGE IN RENAL IMPAIRMENT
Modification of dose and/or frequency based on creatinine clearance and/or severity of infection.

Creatinine Clearance	Dosage
>30 ml/min	0.5–3 g q6–8h
15–29 ml/min	1.5–3 g q12h
5–14 ml/min	1.5–3 g q24h
<5 ml/min	Not recommended

SIDE EFFECTS

FREQUENT: Diarrhea and rash (most common), urticaria, pain at IM injection site; thrombophlebitis with IV administration; oral/vaginal candidiasis. **OCCASIONAL:** Nausea, vomiting, headache, malaise, urinary retention.

ADVERSE REACTIONS/ TOXIC EFFECTS

Severe hypersensitivity reactions, including anaphylaxis, acute interstitial nephritis, blood dyscrasias, may be noted. Superinfections, potentially fatal antibiotic-associated colitis (abdominal cramps, watery severe diarrhea, fever) may result from altered bacterial balance. Overdose may produce seizures.

NURSING IMPLICATIONS

BASELINE ASSESSMENT
Question for history of allergies, esp. penicillins, cephalosporins.

INTERVENTION/EVALUATION
Hold medication and promptly report rash (although common with ampicillin, may indicate hypersensitivity) or diarrhea (with fever, mucus and blood in stool, abdominal pain may indicate antibiotic-associated colitis). Evaluate IV site for phlebitis (heat, pain, red streaking over vein). Check IM injection site for pain, induration. Monitor I&O, urinalysis, renal function tests. Assess for initial signs of superinfection: increased fever, sore throat onset, vomiting, diarrhea, anal/genital pruritus, ulceration or changes of oral mucosa.

PATIENT/FAMILY TEACHING
Space doses evenly. Take antibiotic for full length of treatment. Discomfort may occur with IM injection. Notify physician of rash, diarrhea, or other new symptom.

amprenavir

am-**prenn**-ah-veer
(Agenerase)

CLASSIFICATION

PHARMACOTHERAPEUTIC: Antiviral. **CLINICAL:** Protease inhibitor (see pp. 58C, 99C).

ACTION

Inhibits HIV-1 protease by binding to active site of HIV-1 protease, preventing processing of viral precursors and forming immature noninfectious viral particles. **Therapeutic Effect:** Produces impairment of HIV viral replication and proliferation.

PHARMACOKINETICS

Rapidly absorbed after PO administration. Protein binding: 90%. Metabolized in the liver. Primarily excreted in feces. **Half-life:** 7.1–10.6 hrs.

USES

Treatment of HIV-1 infection in combination with other antiretroviral agents.

PRECAUTIONS

CONTRAINDICATIONS: None known. **CAUTIONS:** Liver function impairment, diabetes mellitus, hemophilia, hypersensitivity to sulfas, vitamin K deficiency due to anticoagulant/malabsorption.

LIFESPAN CONSIDERATIONS: Pregnancy/lactation: Unknown if drug crosses placenta or is distributed in breast milk. **Pregnancy Category C. Children:** Safety and efficacy not established in those <4 yrs. **Elderly:** Age-related liver impairment may require decreased dosage.

INTERACTIONS

DRUG: May interfere with metabolism of **amiodarone, lidocaine, oral contraceptives, midazolam, triazolam, tricyclic antidepressants, quinidine, bepridil, ergotamine. Antacids, didanosine** may decrease absorption. **Carbamazepine, phenobarbital, phenytoin, rifampin** may decrease concentration. **Amprenavir** may increase concentration of **clozapine, HMG-CoA reductase inhibitors (statins), warfarin. HERBAL: St. John's wort** may decrease concentration. **FOOD: High-fat meal** may decrease absorption. **LAB VALUES:** May increase glucose, cholesterol, triglycerides.

AVAILABILITY (Rx)

CAPSULES: 50 mg, 150 mg. **ORAL SOLUTION:** 15 mg/ml.

ADMINISTRATION/HANDLING

PO

- May give without regard to food.

INDICATIONS/ROUTES/DOSAGE

HIV-1 INFECTION

PO: ADULTS, CHILDREN 13–16 YRS (CAPSULES): 1,200 mg 2 times/day. CHILDREN 4–12 YRS, 13–16 YRS <50 KG: 20 mg/kg 2 times/day or 15 mg/kg 3 times/day. **Maximum:** 2,400 mg/day.

Oral solution: CHILDREN 4–12, 13–16 YRS <50 KG: 22.5 mg/kg/day (1.5 ml/kg) 2 times/day or 17 mg/kg/day (1.1 ml/kg) 3 times/day. **Maximum:** 2,800 mg/day.

DOSAGE IN LIVER IMPAIRMENT

Child-Pugh Score	Capsules	Oral Solution
5–8	450 mg bid	513 mg bid
9–12	300 mg bid	342 mg bid

SIDE EFFECTS

FREQUENT: Diarrhea/loose stools (56%), nausea (38%), oral paresthesia (30%), rash (25%), vomiting (20%). **OCCASIONAL:** Rash (18%), peripheral paresthesia (12%), depression (4%).

ADVERSE REACTIONS/ TOXIC EFFECTS

Severe hypersensitivity reactions, Stevens-Johnson syndrome (blisters, peeling of skin, loosening skin/mucous membranes, fever).

NURSING IMPLICATIONS

BASELINE ASSESSMENT

Obtain baseline laboratory testing before beginning therapy and at periodic intervals during therapy. Offer emotional support.

INTERVENTION/EVALUATION

Assess for nausea, vomiting. Determine pattern of bowel activity and stool consistency. Assess eating pattern; monitor for weight loss. Assess tingling/numbness of peripheral extremities. Assess skin for rash.

PATIENT/FAMILY TEACHING

Avoid high-fat meals (decreases drug absorption). Small, frequent meals may offset anorexia, nausea. Amprenavir is not a cure for HIV infection, nor does it reduce risk of transmission to others.

anagrelide

an-ah-**gree**-lide
(Agrylin)

CLASSIFICATION

PHARMACOTHERAPEUTIC: Hematologic agent. **CLINICAL:** Antiplatelet (see p. 29C).

ACTION

Reduces platelet production and prevents platelet shape changes caused by platelet aggregating agents. **Therapeutic Effect:** Inhibits platelet aggregation.

PHARMACOKINETICS

After PO administration, peak plasma concentration occurs within 1 hr. Extensively metabolized. Primarily excreted in urine. **Half-life:** About 3 days.

USES

Treatment of essential thrombocythemia, reducing elevated platelet count and risk of thrombosis. Treatment of thrombocythemia due to myeloproliferative disorders.

PRECAUTIONS

CONTRAINDICATIONS: None known. **CAUTIONS:** Cardiac disease; renal, liver impairment.

LIFESPAN CONSIDERATIONS: Pregnancy/lactation: Unknown if crosses placenta or is distributed in breast milk. May cause fetal harm. **Pregnancy Category C. Children:** Safety and efficacy in those <16 yrs not established. **Elderly:** Age-related decreased renal/liver function, cardiac disease requires caution.

INTERACTIONS

DRUG: None known. **HERBAL:** None known. **FOOD:** None known. **LAB VALUES:** May increase liver enzymes (rare).

AVAILABILITY (Rx)

CAPSULES: 0.5 mg, 1 mg.

ADMINISTRATION/HANDLING

PO

- May give without regard to food.

INDICATIONS/ROUTES/DOSAGE

THROMBOCYTHEMIA

PO: ADULTS, ELDERLY: Initially, 0.5 mg 4 times/day or 1 mg 2 times/day. Adjust to lowest effective dosage, increasing by ≤0.5 mg/day in any 1 wk. **Maximum:** 10 mg/day or 2.5 mg/dose.

SIDE EFFECTS

FREQUENT (≥5%): Headache, palpitations, diarrhea, abdominal pain, nausea, flatulence, bloating, asthenia (loss of strength and energy), pain, dizziness. **OCCASIONAL (<5%):** Tachycardia, chest pain, vomiting, paresthesia, peripheral edema, anorexia, dyspepsia, rash. **RARE:** Confusion, insomnia.

ADVERSE REACTIONS/ TOXIC EFFECTS

Angina, heart failure, arrhythmias occur rarely.

NURSING IMPLICATIONS

BASELINE ASSESSMENT

Assess platelet count, Hgb, Hct, WBC prior to treatment and q2days during first week of treatment and weekly thereafter until therapeutic range is achieved. Ask if pt is breast-feeding, pregnant, or planning to become pregnant (may cause fetal harm).

INTERVENTION/EVALUATION

Monitor liver function test results, BUN, creatinine, and pts with suspected heart disease. Assess skin for bruises, petechiae, also catheter insertion site, needle site, GI sites.

PATIENT/FAMILY TEACHING

Platelet count responds within 7–14 days. Not recommended in pregnancy. Use contraceptives while taking anagrelide.

anakinra

ana-**kin**-rah
(Kineret)

CLASSIFICATION

PHARMACOTHERAPEUTIC: Interleukin-1 receptor antagonist. **CLINICAL:** Anti-inflammatory.

ACTION

Blocks the binding of interleukin-1 (IL-1), a protein that is a major mediator of joint pathology that is present in excess in pts with rheumatoid arthritis. **Therapeutic Effect:** Inhibits inflammatory response.

PHARMACOKINETICS

No accumulation of anakinra in tissues or organs was observed following daily subcutaneous doses. Excreted in the urine. **Half-life:** 4–6 hrs.

USES

Treatment of signs and symptoms or slowing the progression of structural damage of moderate to severely active rheumatoid arthritis in pts who have failed treatment with one or more disease modifying antirheumatic drug.

PRECAUTIONS

CONTRAINDICATIONS: Known hypersensitivity to *E. coli*–derived proteins, serious infection. **CAUTIONS:** Renal function impairment (risk of toxic reaction is increased), asthma (higher incidence of serious infection).

LIFESPAN CONSIDERATIONS: Pregnancy/lactation: Unknown if distributed in breast milk. **Pregnancy Category B. Children:** Safety and efficacy not established. **Elderly:** Age-related decreased renal function may require caution.

INTERACTIONS

DRUG: Live virus vaccines may be ineffective. **HERBAL:** None known. **FOOD:** None known. **LAB VALUES:** May decrease WBC count, platelet count, absolute neutrophil count (ANC). May increase eosinophil count.

AVAILABILITY (Rx)

SOLUTION: 100-mg syringe.

ADMINISTRATION/HANDLING

SUBCUTANEOUS

• Store in refrigerator. Do not freeze or shake. • Do not use if particulate or discoloration is noted. • Give by subcutaneous injection.

INDICATIONS/ROUTES/DOSAGE

RHEUMATOID ARTHRITIS

Subcutaneous: ADULTS >18 YRS, EL-

DERLY: 100 mg/day, given at same time each day.

SIDE EFFECTS

OCCASIONAL: Injection site reactions (erythema, inflammation, ecchymosis). **RARE:** Headache, nausea, diarrhea, abdominal pain.

ADVERSE REACTIONS/ TOXIC EFFECTS

Infection (upper respiratory tract infection, sinusitis, influenza-like symptoms, cellulitis) has been noted. Neutropenia may occur, particularly when used in combination with tumor necrosis factor (TNF)-blocking agents.

NURSING IMPLICATIONS

BASELINE ASSESSMENT

Do not give live vaccine concurrently (vaccination may not be effective in those receiving anakinra).

INTERVENTION/EVALUATION

Monitor neutrophil count before therapy begins, monthly for 3 mos while receiving therapy and then quarterly for up to 1 yr. Assess for inflammatory reaction, esp. during first 4 wks of therapy (uncommon after the first month of therapy).

PATIENT/FAMILY TEACHING

Instruct pt on proper dosage and administration, correct procedure to administer subcutaneous dosage. Advise pt on importance of proper disposal of syringes and needles.

anastrozole

ah-**nas**-trow-zole

(Arimidex)

Do not confuse with Imitrex.

CLASSIFICATION

PHARMACOTHERAPEUTIC: Aromatase inhibitor. **CLINICAL:** Antineoplastic, hormone (see p. 69C).

ACTION

Decreases circulating estrogen by inhibiting aromatase, an enzyme that catalyzes the final step in estrogen production. **Therapeutic Effect:** Because growth of many breast cancers are stimulated by estrogens, drug significantly lowers serum estradiol (estrogen) concentration.

PHARMACOKINETICS

Well absorbed into systemic circulation. Protein binding: 40%. Food does not affect extent of absorption. Extensively metabolized. Eliminated by hepatic metabolism and, to a lesser extent, renal excretion. **Mean half-life:** 50 hrs in postmenopausal women. Plasma concentrations reach steady-state levels at about 7 days.

USES

Treatment of advanced breast cancer in postmenopausal women who have developed progressive disease while receiving tamoxifen therapy. First-line therapy in advanced/metastatic breast cancer. Adjuvant treatment in early breast cancer.

PRECAUTIONS

CONTRAINDICATIONS: None known. **CAUTIONS:** None known.

LIFESPAN CONSIDERATIONS: Pregnancy/lactation: Crosses placenta; may cause fetal harm. Unknown if excreted in breast milk. **Pregnancy Category D. Children:** Safety and efficacy not established. **Elderly:** No age-related precautions noted.

INTERACTIONS

DRUG: None known. **HERBAL:** None known. **FOOD:** None known. **LAB VALUES:** May elevate serum GGT level in those with liver metastases. May increase SGOT (AST), SGPT (ALT), alkaline phosphate, total cholesterol, LDL cholesterol.

AVAILABILITY (Rx)

TABLETS: 1 mg.

ADMINISTRATION/HANDLING

PO

- May give without regard to food.

INDICATIONS/ROUTES/DOSAGE

BREAST CANCER

PO: ADULTS, ELDERLY: 1 mg once daily.

SIDE EFFECTS

FREQUENT (8%–16%): Asthenia (loss of strength/energy), nausea, headache, hot flashes, back pain, vomiting, cough, diarrhea. **OCCASIONAL (4%–6%):** Constipation, abdominal pain, anorexia, bone pain, pharyngitis, dizziness, rash, dry mouth, peripheral edema, pelvic pain, depression, chest pain, paresthesia. **RARE (1%–2%):** Weight gain, sweating.

ADVERSE REACTIONS/ TOXIC EFFECTS

Thrombophlebitis, anemia, leukopenia occur rarely. Vaginal hemorrhage occurs rarely (2%).

NURSING IMPLICATIONS

INTERVENTION/EVALUATION

Monitor for/assist with ambulation if asthenia/dizziness occurs. Assess for headache. Offer antiemetic for nausea/vomiting. Monitor for onset of diarrhea; offer antidiarrheal medication.

PATIENT/FAMILY TEACHING

Notify physician if nausea, asthenia, hot flashes become unmanageable.

Ancef

see cefazolin

antihemophilic factor (factor viii, AHF)

(Advate, Alphanate, Bioclate, Helixate, Hyate C, Koate-HP, Kogenate, Monoclate-P)

CLASSIFICATION

PHARMACOTHERAPEUTIC: Antihemophilic agent. **CLINICAL:** Hemostatic.

ACTION

Assists in conversion of prothrombin to thrombin (essential for blood coagulation). **Therapeutic Effect:** Produces hemostasis. Replaces missing clotting factor, correcting or preventing bleeding episodes.

PHARMACOKINETICS

Rapidly cleared from plasma. Peak effect in 1–2 hrs. **Half-life:** 10–18 hrs.

USES

Treatment, prevention of bleeding in pts with hemophilia A factor XIII deficiency, hypofibrinogenemia. **Unlabeled:** Treatment of disseminated intravascular coagulation (DIC).

PRECAUTIONS

CONTRAINDICATIONS: Hypersensitivity to bovine, hamster, or mouse protein or to porcine or murine factor. **CAUTIONS:** Hepatic disease, those with blood types A, B, AB.

LIFESPAN CONSIDERATIONS: Pregnancy/lactation: Unknown if drug crosses placenta or is distributed in breast milk. **Pregnancy Category C. Children/Elderly:** No age-related precautions noted.

INTERACTIONS

DRUG: None known. **HERBAL:** None known. **FOOD:** None known. **LAB VALUES:** None known.

ADMINISTRATION/HANDLING

IV

Storage • Refrigerate.

Reconstitution • Warm concentrate and diluent to room temperature. Using needle supplied by the manufacturer, add diluent to powder to dissolve, gently agitate or rotate. Do not shake vigorously. Complete dissolution may take 5–10 min. Use second filtered needle supplied by the manufacturer, and add to infusion bag.

Rate of administration • Administer IV at rate of approx. 2 ml/min. May give up to 10 ml/min.

Administration precautions

• Check pulse rate prior to and following administration. If pulse rate increases, reduce or stop administration. • After administration, apply prolonged pressure on venipuncture site. Monitor IV site for oozing q5–15min for 1–2 hrs following administration.

IV INCOMPATIBILITIES

Do not mix antihemophilic factor with other IV solutions or medications.

AVAILABILITY (Rx)

INJECTION: Actual number of AHF units listed on each vial.

INDICATIONS/ROUTES/DOSAGE

Note: Dosage is highly individualized, based on pt weight, severity of bleeding, coagulation studies.

PROPHYLAXIS OF SPONTANEOUS HEMORRHAGE

IV: ADULTS, ELDERLY, CHILDREN: 10 AHF/international units/kg as a single infusion.

MODERATE HEMORRHAGE, MINOR SURGERY

IV: ADULTS, ELDERLY, CHILDREN: Initially, 15–25 AHF/international units/kg. MAINTENANCE: 10–15 international units/kg q8–12h.

SEVERE HEMORRHAGE (near vital organ)

IV: ADULTS, ELDERLY, CHILDREN: Initially, 40–50 AHF/international units/kg. MAINTENANCE: 20–25 international units/kg q8–12h.

MAJOR SURGERY

IV: ADULTS, ELDERLY, CHILDREN: 40–50 AHF/international units/kg 1 hr prior to surgery, 20–25 international units/kg 5 hrs later, then 10–15 international units/kg/day for 10–14 days.

SIDE EFFECTS

OCCASIONAL: Allergic reaction (fever, chills, urticaria [hives], wheezing, slight hypotension, nausea, feeling of chest tightness), stinging at injection site, dizziness, dry mouth, headache, unpleasant taste.

ADVERSE REACTIONS/ TOXIC EFFECTS

There is a risk of transmitting viral hepatitis and a slight risk of transmitting AIDS. Possibility of intravascular hemolysis is present if large or frequent doses used in those with blood types A, B, AB.

NURSING IMPLICATIONS

BASELINE ASSESSMENT

When monitoring B/P, avoid overinflation of cuff. Remove adhesive tape from any pressure dressing very carefully and slowly.

INTERVENTION/EVALUATION

Following IV administration, apply prolonged pressure on venipuncture site.

Monitor IV site for oozing q5–15min for 1–2 hrs following administration. Assess for allergic reaction. Report any evidence of hematuria or change in vital signs immediately. Assess for decrease in B/P, increased pulse rate, complaint of abdominal or back pain, severe headache (may be evidence of hemorrhage). Question for increased discharge during menses. Assess skin for bruises, petechiae. Check for excessive bleeding from minor cuts, scratches. Assess gums for erythema, gingival bleeding. Assess urine for hematuria. Evaluate for therapeutic relief of pain, reduction of swelling, and restricted joint movement.

PATIENT/FAMILY TEACHING

Use electric razor, soft toothbrush to prevent bleeding. Report any sign of red or dark urine, black/red stool, coffee-ground vomitus, red-speckled mucus from cough.

Anzemet

see dolasetron

apraclonidine

(Iopidine)

See Classification section under: Antiglaucoma agents (p. 45C)

aprepitant

ah-**prep**-ih-tant

(Emend)

◆ CLASSIFICATION

PHARMACOTHERAPEUTIC: Selective receptor antagonist. **CLINICAL:** Antinausea, antiemetic.

ACTION

Inhibits chemotherapy-induced nausea/vomiting centrally in the chemoreceptor trigger zone. **Therapeutic Effect:** Prevents the acute and delayed phases of chemotherapy-induced emesis, including high-dose cisplatin.

PHARMACOKINETICS

Crosses the blood-brain barrier. Extensively metabolized in liver. Eliminated primarily by metabolism (not excreted renally). **Half-life:** 9–13 hrs.

USES

Prevention of acute and delayed nausea/vomiting associated with initial and repeat courses with a high potential for emetogenic cancer chemotherapy, including high-dose cisplatin.

PRECAUTIONS

CONTRAINDICATIONS: Concurrent use with pimozide (Orap), breast-feeding. **CAUTIONS:** None known.

LIFESPAN CONSIDERATIONS: Pregnancy/lactation: Unknown if drug crosses placenta or is distributed in breast milk. **Pregnancy Category B. Children:** Safety and efficacy not established. **Elderly:** No age-related precautions noted.

INTERACTIONS

DRUG: Carbamazepine, phenytoin, rifampin reduce aprepitant plasma concentration. **Antifungals, nefazodone, clarithromycin, ritonavir, nelfinavir, diltiazem** increase aprepitant plasma concentration. **Docetaxel, paclitaxol, etoposide, irinotecan, ifosfamide, imatinib, vinorelbine, vinblastine, vincristine, midazolam, alprazolam, triazolam,** plasma concentrations may be elevated. May decrease effectiveness of **contraceptives**. Increases exposure to **steroids** (IV steroid dose should be reduced by 25%, oral dose by 50%). **Paroxetine** may decrease effectiveness of either drug. May decrease effectiveness of **warfarin**. **HERBAL:** None known. **FOOD:** None known. **LAB VALUES:** May increase SGOT (AST), SGPT (ALT), BUN, serum creatine. May produce proteinuria.

AVAILABILITY: (Rx)

CAPSULES: 80 mg, 125 mg.

ADMINISTRATION/HANDLING

PO

- Give without regard to food.

INDICATIONS/ROUTE/DOSAGE

Alert: Give medication concurrently with 12 mg dexamethasone PO and 32 mg ondansetron IV on day 1, and 8 mg dexamethasone PO on days 2 to 4.

NAUSEA, VOMITING: CHEMOTHERAPY

PO: ADULTS, ELDERLY: 125 mg 1 hr prior to chemotherapy on day 1 and 80 mg once daily in the morning on days 2 and 3.

SIDE EFFECTS

FREQUENT (10%–17%): Fatigue, nausea, hiccups, diarrhea, constipation, anorexia. **OCCASIONAL (4%–8%):** Headache, vomiting, dizziness, dehydration, heartburn. **RARE (<2%–3%):** Abdominal pain, epigastric discomfort, gastritis, tinnitus, insomnia.

ADVERSE REACTIONS/ TOXIC EFFECTS

Neutropenia, mucous membrane disorder occur rarely.

NURSING IMPLICATIONS

BASELINE ASSESSMENT

Assess for dehydration if excessive vomiting occurs (poor skin turgor, dry mucous membranes, longitudinal furrows in tongue). Provide emotional support.

INTERVENTION/EVALUATION

Monitor pt in environment. Assess bowel sounds for peristalsis. Assist with ambulation if dizziness occurs. Provide supportive measures. Monitor daily bowel activity, stool consistency (watery, loose, soft, semisolid, solid) and record time of evacuation.

PATIENT/FAMILY TEACHING

Relief from nausea/vomiting generally occurs shortly after drug administration. Report persistent vomiting, headache.

Aranesp

see darbepoetin alfa

Arava

see leflunomide

argatroban

our-ga-**trow**-ban

CLASSIFICATION

PHARMACOTHERAPEUTIC: Thrombin inhibitor. **CLINICAL:** Anticoagulant.

ACTION

A direct thrombin inhibitor that reversibly binds to thrombin active site. Exerts its effect by inhibiting thrombin catalyzed or induced reactions. **Therapeutic Effect:** Produces anticoagulation.

PHARMACOKINETICS

Following IV administration, distributed primarily in extracellular fluid. Protein binding: 54%. Metabolized in the liver. Primarily excreted in the feces, presumably through biliary secretion. **Half-life:** 39–51 min.

USES

Prophylaxis or treatment of thrombosis in heparin-induced thrombocytopenia (HIT). Prevention of HIT during percutaneous coronary procedures.

PRECAUTIONS

CONTRAINDICATIONS: Overt major bleeding. **CAUTIONS:** Severe hypertension, immediately following lumbar puncture, spinal anesthesia, major surgery, patients with congenital or acquired bleeding disorders, ulcerations, liver function impairment.

LIFESPAN CONSIDERATIONS: Pregnancy/lactation: Unknown if excreted in breast milk. **Pregnancy Category B. Children:** Safety and efficacy not established in those <18 yrs. **Elderly:** No age-related precautions noted.

INTERACTIONS

DRUG: Antiplatelet agents, thrombolytics, other anticoagulants may increase risk of bleeding. **HERBAL:** None known. **FOOD:** None known. **LAB VALUES:** Increased aPTT, prothrombin time, INR.

AVAILABILITY (Rx)

INJECTION: 100 mg/ml.

ADMINISTRATION/HANDLING

IV

Storage • Discard if solution appears cloudy or an insoluble precipitate is noted. • Following reconstitution, stable for 24 hrs at room temperature, 48 hrs if refrigerated. • Avoid direct sunlight.

Reconstitution • Must be diluted 100-fold prior to infusion in 0.9% NaCl, D_5W, or lactated Ringer's to provide a final concentration of 1 mg/ml. • The solution must be mixed by repeated inversion of the diluent bag for 1 min. • After reconstitution, solution may show a brief haziness due to formation of microprecipitates that rapidly dissolve upon mixing.

Rate of administration • Rate of administration is based on body weight at 2 mcg/kg/min (e.g., 50-kg pt infuse at 6 ml/hr).

IV INCOMPATIBILITY

Do not mix with any other medications or solutions.

INDICATIONS/ROUTES/DOSAGE

HEPARIN-INDUCED THROMBOCYTOPENIA

IV infusion: ADULTS, ELDERLY: Initially, 2 mcg/kg/min administered as a continuous infusion. After initial infusion, dose may be adjusted until steady state aPTT is 1.5–3 times initial baseline value not to exceed 100 sec. LIVER IMPAIRMENT: Initially, 0.5 mcg/kg/min.

SIDE EFFECTS

FREQUENT (3%–8%): Dyspnea, hypotension, fever, diarrhea, nausea, pain, vomiting, infection, cough.

ADVERSE REACTIONS/ TOXIC EFFECTS

Ventricular tachycardia, atrial fibrillation occur occasionally. Major bleeding, sepsis occur rarely.

NURSING IMPLICATIONS

BASELINE ASSESSMENT

Assess CBC, including platelet count. Check PT, PTT. Determine initial B/P. Minimize need for numerous injection sites, blood draws, catheters.

INTERVENTION/EVALUATION

Assess for any sign of bleeding: bleeding at surgical site, hematuria, blood in stool, bleeding from gums, petechiae, bruising, bleeding from injection sites. Handle pt carefully and as infrequently as possible to prevent bleeding. Do not obtain B/P in lower extremities (possible deep vein thrombi). Assess for decrease in B/P, increase in pulse rate, complaint of abdominal/back pain, severe headache (indicates evidence of hemorrhage). Monitor ACT, PT, aPTT, platelet count. Question for increase in discharge during menses. Assess urine output for hematuria. Monitor for any occurring hematoma. Use care in removing any dressing, tape.

PATIENT/FAMILY TEACHING

Use electric razor, soft toothbrush to prevent bleeding. Report any sign of red/dark urine, black/red stool, coffee-ground vomitus, red-speckled mucus from cough.

Aricept

see donepezil

Arimidex

see anastrozole

aripiprazole

air-ee-**pip**-rah-zole
(Abilify)

CLASSIFICATION

PHARMACOTHERAPEUTIC: Dopamine agonist. **CLINICAL:** Antipsychotic agent.

PHARMACOKINETICS

Well absorbed through the GI tract. Reaches steady levels in 2 wks. Metabolized in liver. Protein binding: 99%, primarily albumin. Eliminated primarily in the feces with a lesser extent excreted in the urine. **Half-life:** 75 hrs. Not removed by hemodialysis.

ACTION

Provides partial agonist activity at dopamine and serotonin ($5\text{-}HT_{1A}$) receptors and antagonist activity at serotonin ($5\text{-}HT_{2A}$) receptors. **Therapeutic Effect:** Improves and achieves target goals in schizophrenia.

USES

Treatment of schizophrenia. Maintains stability in pts with schizophrenia. **Unlabeled:** Schizoaffective disorder.

PRECAUTIONS

CONTRAINDICATIONS: None known. **CAUTIONS:** Concurrent use of CNS depressants (including alcohol), cardiovascular or cerebrovascular diseases (may induce hypotension), Parkinson's disease (potential for exacerbation), history of seizures or conditions that may lower seizure threshold (Alzheimer disease), renal or liver impairment.

LIFESPAN CONSIDERATIONS: Pregnancy/lactation: Unknown if drug crosses placenta. May be distributed in breast milk; avoid breast-feeding. **Pregnancy Category C. Children:** Safety and efficacy not established. **Elderly:** No age-related precautions noted.

INTERACTIONS

DRUG: Carbamazepine may decrease concentration. **Ketoconazole, quinidine, fluoxetine, paroxetine** may increase concentrations. **HERBAL:** None known. **FOOD:** None known. **LAB VAL-**

UES: None known.

AVAILABILITY (Rx)

TABLETS: 10 mg, 15 mg, 20 mg, 30 mg.

ADMINISTRATION/HANDLING

PO

- May give without regard to meals.

INDICATIONS/ROUTES/DOSAGE

Alert: Dosage adjustment should not be made at intervals of less then 2 wks.

SCHIZOPHRENIA

PO: ADULTS, ELDERLY: Initially, 10–15 mg once daily. May increase up to 30 mg/day.

SIDE EFFECTS

FREQUENT (5%–11%): Weight gain, headache, insomnia, vomiting. **OCCASIONAL (3%–4%):** Lightheadedness, nausea, akathisia (motor restlessness), somnolence. **RARE (≤2%):** Blurred vision, constipation, asthenia (loss of energy, strength), anxiety, fever, rash, cough, rhinitis, orthostatic hypotension.

ADVERSE REACTONS/TOXIC EFFECT

Extrapyramidal symptoms, neuroleptic malignant syndrome occur rarely.

NURSING IMPLICATIONS

BASELINE ASSESSMENT

Assess behavior, appearance, emotional status, response to environment, speech pattern, thought content. Correct dehydration, hypovolemia.

INTERVENTION/EVALUATION

Periodically monitor weight. Monitor for extrapyramidal symptoms (abnormal movement), tardive dyskinesia (protrusion of tongue, puffing of cheeks, chewing/puckering of the mouth). Periodically monitor B/P, pulse (particularly in those with preexisting cardiovascular disease). Assess for therapeutic response (greater interest in surroundings, improved self-care, increased ability to concentrate, relaxed facial expression).

PATIENT/FAMILY TEACHING

Avoid alcohol. Avoid tasks that require alertness, motor skills until response to drug is established.

Arixtra

see fondaparinux

Aromasin

see exemestane

arsenic trioxide

are-sih-nic try-**ox**-ide
(Trisenox)

CLASSIFICATION

CLINICAL: Antineoplastic (see p. 69C).

ACTION

Produces morphologic changes and DNA fragmentation in promyelocytic leukemia cells. **Therapeutic Effect:** Produces cell death.

USES

Induction of remission and consolidations in pts with acute promyelocytic leukemia (APL) who are refractory to or have relapsed from retinoid and anthracycline chemotherapy.

PRECAUTIONS

CONTRAINDICATIONS: None known. **CAUTIONS:** Renal impairment, cardiac abnormalities. **Pregnancy Category D.**

INTERACTIONS

DRUG: May prolong QT interval in those taking **antiarrhythmics, thioridazine. Diuretics, amphotericin B** may produce electrolyte abnormalities. **HERBAL:** None known. **FOOD:** None known. **LAB VALUES:** May decrease WBC count, Hgb, platelet count, magnesium, calcium. May increase SGOT (AST), SGPT (ALT). Higher risk of hypokalemia than hyperkalemia, hyperglycemia than hypoglycemia.

AVAILABILITY (Rx)

INJECTION: 1 mg/ml.

ADMINISTRATION/HANDLING

IV

Alert: A central venous line is not required for drug administration.

Storage • Store at room temperature. • Diluted solution is stable for 24 hrs at room temperature, 48 hrs if refrigerated.

Reconstitution • After withdrawing drug from ampoule, dilute with 100–250 ml D_5W or 0.9% NaCl.

Rate of administration • Infuse over 1–2 hrs. Duration of infusion may be extended up to 4 hrs.

IV INCOMPATIBILITY

Do not mix with any other medications.

INDICATIONS/ROUTES/DOSAGE

ACUTE PROMYELOCYTIC LEUKEMIA (APL), INDUCTION TREATMENT

IV: ADULTS, ELDERLY: 0.15 mg/kg/day until bone marrow suppression occurs. Total induction dose should not exceed 60 doses.

ACUTE PROMYELOCYTIC LEUKEMIA (APL), CONSOLIDATION TREATMENT

IV: ADULTS, ELDERLY: Consolidation treatment should begin 3–6 wks after completion of induction therapy. Give dose of 0.15 mg/kg/day for 25 doses up to 5 wks.

SIDE EFFECTS

COMMON (50%–75%): Nausea, cough, fatigue, fever, headache, vomiting, abdominal pain, tachycardia, diarrhea, dyspnea. **FREQUENT (30%–43%):** Dermatitis, insomnia, edema, rigors, prolonged QT interval, sore throat, pruritus, arthralgia, paresthesia, anxiety. **OCCASIONAL (20%–28%):** Constipation, myalgia, hypotension, epistaxis, anorexia, dizziness, sinusitis. **OCCASIONAL (8%–15%):** Ecchymosis, nonspecific pain, weight gain, herpes simplex, wheezing, flushing, increased sweating, tremor, hypertension, palpitations, dyspepsia, eye irritation, blurred vision, weakness, decreased breath sounds, rales. **RARE:** Confusion, petechiae, dry mouth oral candidiasis, incontinence, rhonchi.

ADVERSE REACTIONS/ TOXIC EFFECTS

Seizures, GI hemorrhage, renal impairment or failure, pleural or pericardial effusion, hemoptysis, sepsis occur rarely. Prolonged QT interval, complete AV block, unexplained fever, dyspnea, weight gain, effusion are evidence of arsenic toxicity. Treatment should be halted, steroid treatment instituted.

NURSING IMPLICATIONS

BASELINE ASSESSMENT

Assess platelet count, Hgb, Hct, WBC prior to and frequently during treatment. Ask if pt is breast-feeding, pregnant, or planning to become pregnant (may cause fetal harm).

INTERVENTION/EVALUATION

Monitor liver function test results, CBC, serum values. Monitor for arsenic toxicity syndrome (fever, dyspnea, weight gain, confusion, muscle weakness, seizures).

PATIENT/FAMILY TEACHING

Avoid crowds, those with known infection. Avoid contact with anyone who recently received live virus vaccine; do not receive vaccinations.

artificial tears

(Eye Tears, Hypotears, Isopto Tears, Refresh Aquasite, Tears Naturale, Tears Plus, Ultra Fresh Eyes, Visine Tears, Viva Drops)

◆CLASSIFICATION

PHARMACOTHERAPEUTIC: Ophthalmic lubricant.

ACTION

Stabilizes/thickens precorneal tear film, lengthening tear film breakup time. **Therapeutic Effect:** Protects and lubricates the eyes.

USES

Relief of dryness and irritation due to deficient tear production; ocular lubricant for artificial eyes; some products may be used with hard contact lenses. **Unlabeled:** Treatment of recurrent corneal erosions, decreased corneal sensitivity.

PRECAUTIONS

CONTRAINDICATIONS: Hypersensitivity to any component of preparation. **CAUTIONS:** None known.

INTERACTIONS

DRUG: None known. **HERBAL:** None known. **FOOD:** None known. **LAB VALUES:** None known.

INDICATIONS/ROUTES/DOSAGE

OPHTHALMIC LUBRICANT

ADULTS, ELDERLY: 1–2 drops 3–4 times/day as needed.

SIDE EFFECTS

OCCASIONAL: Eye irritation, blurred vision, stickiness of eyelashes.

ADVERSE REACTIONS/TOXIC EFFECTS

None known.

NURSING IMPLICATIONS

BASELINE ASSESSMENT

Determine extent of dryness, irritation.

INTERVENTION/EVALUATION

Monitor for increased irritation or discomfort. Assess therapeutic response.

PATIENT/FAMILY TEACHING

Wash hands thoroughly before use. Do not touch the tip of the dropper or container to any surface.

ascorbic acid (vitamin C)

(Apo-C✱, Cecon, Cenolate, Redoxon✱)

◆CLASSIFICATION

CLINICAL: Vitamin (see p. 137C).

ACTION

Assists in collagen formation, tissue repair; involved in oxidation reduction reactions, other metabolic reactions. **Therapeutic Effect:** Involved in metabolism; carbohydrate utilization; synthesis of lipids, proteins, carnitine. Preserves blood vessel integrity.

PHARMACOKINETICS

Readily absorbed from GI tract. Protein binding: 25%. Metabolized in liver. Excreted in urine. Removed by hemodialysis.

USES

Prevention and treatment of scurvy, acidification of urine, dietary supplement, prevention of and reduction in the severity of colds. **Unlabeled:** Prevention of common cold, urinary acidifier, control of idiopathic methemoglobinemia.

PRECAUTIONS

CONTRAINDICATIONS: None known. **CAUTIONS:** Those on sodium restriction, daily salicylate treatment, warfarin therapy; diabetes mellitus; history of renal stones.

LIFESPAN CONSIDERATIONS: Pregnancy/lactation: Crosses placenta, excreted in breast milk. Large doses during pregnancy may produce scurvy in neonates. **Pregnancy Category A** (**C** if used in doses above RDA). **Children/elderly:** No age-related precautions noted.

INTERACTIONS

DRUG: May increase iron toxicity with **deferoxamine. HERBAL:** None known. **FOOD:** None known. **LAB VALUES:** May decrease bilirubin, urinary pH. May increase uric acid, urine oxalate.

AVAILABILITY (OTC)

CAPSULES (controlled release): 500 mg. **INJECTION:** 250 mg/ml, 500 mg/ml. **LIQUID:** 500 mg/5 ml. **SYRUP:** 500 mg/5 ml. **TABLET:** 100 mg, 250 mg, 500 mg, 1 g. **TABLET (chewable):** 60 mg, 100 mg, 250 mg, 500 mg. **TABLET (controlled release):** 500 mg, 1 g, 1,500 mg.

ADMINISTRATION/HANDLING

PO

- May give without regard to food.

IV

Storage • Refrigerate. • Protect from freezing/light.

Rate of administration • May give undiluted or dilute in D_5W, 0.9% NaCl, lactated Ringer's. • For IV push, dilute with equal volume D_5W or 0.9% NaCl and infuse over 10 min. For IV solution, infuse over 4–12 hrs.

IV INCOMPATIBILITY

No information available via Y-site administration.

IV COMPATIBILITIES

Calcium gluconate, heparin

INDICATIONS/ROUTES/DOSAGE

DIETARY SUPPLEMENT

PO: ADULTS, ELDERLY: 45–60 mg/day. CHILDREN >4 YRS: 30–40 mg/day.

DEFICIENCY

PO/IM/IV: ADULTS, ELDERLY: 75–150 mg/day.

SCURVY

PO: ADULTS, ELDERLY: 300 mg–1 g/day.

BURNS

PO: ADULTS, ELDERLY: Up to 2 g/day.

ENHANCE WOUND HEALING

PO: ADULTS, ELDERLY: 300–500 mg/day for 7–10 days.

SIDE EFFECTS

RARE: Abdominal cramps, nausea, vomiting, diarrhea, increased urination with doses exceeding 1 g. **Parenteral:** Flushing, headache, dizziness, sleepiness or insomnia, soreness at injection site.

ADVERSE REACTIONS/ TOXIC EFFECTS

May produce urine acidification, leading to crystalluria. Large doses given IV may lead to deep vein thrombosis. Prolonged use of large doses may result in scurvy when dosage is reduced to normal.

NURSING IMPLICATIONS

INTERVENTION/EVALUATION

Assess for clinical improvement (improved sense of well-being and sleep patterns). Observe for reversal of deficiency symptoms (gingivitis, bleeding gums, poor wound healing, digestive difficulties, joint pain).

PATIENT/FAMILY TEACHING

Abrupt vitamin C withdrawal may produce rebound deficiency. Reduce dosage gradually. Foods rich in vitamin C include rose hips, guava, black currant jelly, brussels sprouts, green peppers, spinach, watercress, strawberries, citrus fruits.

asparaginase

ah-spa-**raj**-in-ace
(Elspar, Kidrolase❋)

CLASSIFICATION

PHARMACOTHERAPEUTIC: Enzyme. **CLINICAL:** Antineoplastic (see p. 69C).

ACTION

Inhibits protein synthesis by deaminating asparagine and depriving tumor cells of this essential amino acid. **Therapeutic Effect:** Interferes with DNA, RNA, protein synthesis in leukemic cells. Cell cycle–specific for G_1 phase of cell division.

PHARMACOKINETICS

Metabolized via slow sequestration by reticuloendothelial system. **Half-life:** 39–49 hrs IM; 8–30 hrs IV.

USES

Treatment of acute lymphocytic leukemia (ALL), lymphoma in combination with other therapy. **Unlabeled:** Treatment of acute myelocytic leukemia, acute myelomonocytic leukemia, chronic lymphocytic leukemia, Hodgkin's disease, lymphosarcoma, reticulum cell sarcoma, melanosarcoma.

PRECAUTIONS

CONTRAINDICATIONS: Hypersensitivity to *E. coli,* pancreatitis. **CAUTIONS:** Existing or recent chickenpox, herpes zoster, diabetes mellitus, gout, infection, liver/renal function impairment, recent cytotoxic/radiation therapy.

LIFESPAN CONSIDERATIONS: Pregnancy/lactation: If possible, avoid use during pregnancy, esp. first trimester. Breast-feeding not recommended. **Pregnancy Category C. Children/elderly:** No age-related precautions noted.

INTERACTIONS

DRUG: Steroids, vincristine may increase hyperglycemia, risk of neuropathy, disturbances of erythropoiesis. May decrease effect of **antigout medications.** May block effects of **methotrexate. Live virus vaccines** may potentiate virus replication, increase vaccine side effects, decrease pt's antibody response to vaccine. **HERBAL:** None known. **FOOD:** None known. **LAB VALUES:** May increase blood ammonia, BUN, uric acid, glucose, partial thromboplastin time (PTT), platelet count, prothrombin time (PT), thrombin time (TT), SGOT (AST), SGPT (ALT), alkaline phosphatase, bilirubin. May decrease blood clotting factors (plasma fibrinogen, antithrombin, plasminogen), albumin, calcium, cholesterol.

AVAILABILITY (Rx)

POWDER FOR INJECTION: 10,000 international units.

ADMINISTRATION/HANDLING

Alert: May be carcinogenic, mutagenic, or teratogenic. Handle with extreme care during preparation/administration. Handle voided urine as infectious waste. Powder, solution may irritate skin on contact. Wash area for 15 min if contact occurs.

IM

• Add 2 ml 0.9% NaCl injection to 10,000 international units vial to provide a concentration of 5,000 international units/ml. • Administer no more than 2 ml at any one site.

IV

Storage • Refrigerate powder for injection. • Reconstituted solutions stable for 8 hrs if refrigerated. • Gelatinous fiberlike particles may develop (remove via 5-micron filter during administration).

Reconstitution

Alert: Administer intradermal test dose (2 international units) prior to initiating therapy or when >1 wk has elapsed between doses. Observe pt for 1 hr for appearance of wheal or erythema.

Test Solution: Reconstitute 10,000 international units vial with 5 ml Sterile Water for Injection or 0.9% NaCl. Shake to dissolve. Withdraw 0.1 ml, inject into vial containing 9.9 ml same diluent for concentration of 20 international units/ml.

• Reconstitute 10,000 international units vial with 5 ml Sterile Water for Injection or 0.9% NaCl to provide a concentration of 2,000 international units/ml. • Shake gently to ensure complete dissolution (vigorous shaking produces foam, some loss of potency).

Rate of administration • For IV injection, administer into tubing of freely running IV solution of D_5W or 0.9% NaCl over at least 30 min. • For IV infusion, further dilute with up to 1,000 ml D_5W or 0.9% NaCl.

IV INCOMPATIBILITY

None known. Consult pharmacy.

INDICATIONS/ROUTES/DOSAGE

Alert: Dosage individualized based on clinical response, tolerance to adverse effects. When used in combination therapy, consult specific protocols for optimum dosage, sequence of drug administration.

ACUTE LYMPHOCYTIC LEUKEMIA

IV: ADULTS, ELDERLY, CHILDREN (combination therapy): 1,000 units/kg/day for 10 days. (Single drug therapy): 200 units/kg/day for 28 days.

IM: ADULTS, ELDERLY, CHILDREN (combination therapy): 6–10,000 units/m^2/dose 3 times/wk for 3 wks.

SIDE EFFECTS

FREQUENT: Allergic reaction (rash, urticaria, arthralgia, facial edema, hypotension, respiratory distress), pancreatitis (severe stomach pain with nausea/vomiting). **OCCASIONAL:** CNS effects (confusion, drowsiness, depression, nervousness, tiredness), stomatitis (sores in mouth/lips), hypoalbuminemia/uric acid nephropathy (swelling of feet or lower legs), hyperglycemia. **RARE:** Hyperthermia (fever or chills), thrombosis, seizures.

ADVERSE REACTIONS/ TOXIC EFFECTS

Hepatotoxicity usually occurs within 2 wks of initial treatment. Increased risk of allergic reaction, including anaphylaxis, after repeated therapy, severe bone marrow depression.

NURSING IMPLICATIONS

BASELINE ASSESSMENT

Before giving medication, agents for adequate airway and allergic reaction (antihistamine, epinephrine, O_2, IV corticosteroid) should be readily available. Assess baseline CNS functions.

Hepatic, renal, pancreatic, CBC, blood chemistry should be performed before therapy begins and when ≥1 wk has elapsed between doses.

INTERVENTION/EVALUATION

Assess serum amylase concentration frequently during therapy. Discontinue medication at first sign of renal failure (oliguria, anuria), pancreatitis (abdominal pain, nausea, vomiting). Monitor for hematologic toxicity (fever, sore throat, signs of local infection, easy bruising, unusual bleeding), symptoms of anemia (excessive tiredness, weakness).

PATIENT/FAMILY TEACHING

Increase fluid intake (protects against renal impairment). Nausea may decrease during therapy. Do not have immunizations without physician's approval (drug lowers body's resistance). Avoid contact with those who have recently taken live virus vaccine.

aspirin (acetylsalicylic acid, ASA)

ass-purr-in

(Ascriptin, Bayer, Bufferin, Ecotrin, Entrophen✤, Halfprin, Novasen✤)

FIXED-COMBINATION(S)

Aggrenox: aspirin/dipyridamole (an antiplatelet agent): 25 mg/200 mg. **Fiorinal:** aspirin/butalbital/caffeine (a barbiturate): 325 mg/50 mg/40 mg. **Lortab/ASA:** aspirin/hydrocodone (an analgesic): 325 mg/5 mg. **Percodan:** aspirin/oxycodone (an analgesic): 325 mg/4.5 mg; 325 mg/2.25 mg. **Pravigard:** aspirin/pravastatin (a cholesterol lowering agent): 81 mg/20 mg, 81 mg/40 mg, 81 mg/80 mg, 325 mg/20 mg, 325 mg/40 mg, 325 mg/80 mg.

◆CLASSIFICATION

PHARMACOTHERAPEUTIC: Nonsteroidal salicylate. **CLINICAL:** Anti-inflammatory, antipyretic, anticoagulant (see pp. 29C, 109C).

ACTION

Inhibits prostaglandin synthesis, acts on the hypothalamus heat-regulating center, blocks prostaglandin synthetase action. **Therapeutic Effect:** Reduces inflammatory response and intensity of pain stimulus reaching sensory nerve endings. Decreases elevated body temperature. Inhibits platelet aggregation.

PHARMACOKINETICS

Onset	Peak	Duration
PO		
1 hr	2–4 hrs	24 hrs

Rapidly, completely absorbed from GI tract; enteric-coated absorption delayed; rectal absorption delayed, incomplete. Protein binding: High. Widely distributed. Rapidly hydrolyzed to salicylate. **Half-life:** 15–20 min (aspirin); salicylate: 2–3 hrs at low dose; >20 hrs at high dose.

USES

Treatment of mild to moderate pain, fever, inflammatory conditions. Treatment of transient ischemic attack, ischemic stroke, angina, acute MI, recurrent MI, specific revascularization procedures, rheumatologic diseases. **Unlabeled:** Prophylaxis against thromboembolism, treatment of Kawasaki disease.

PRECAUTIONS

CONTRAINDICATIONS: Chickenpox or flu in children/teenagers, GI bleeding/ulceration, bleeding disorders, history of hypersensitivity to aspirin or NSAIDs, allergy to tartrazine dye, impaired hepatic function. **CAUTIONS:** Vitamin K deficiency, chronic renal insufficiency, those with "aspirin triad" (rhinitis, nasal polyps, asthma).

LIFESPAN CONSIDERATIONS: Pregnancy/lactation: Readily crosses placenta; distributed in breast milk. May prolong gestation and labor; decrease fetal birth weight; increase incidence of stillbirths, neonatal mortality, hemorrhage. Avoid use during last trimester (may adversely affect fetal cardiovascular system: premature closure of ductus arteriosus). **Pregnancy Category C** (**D** if full dose used in third trimester). **Children:** Caution in children with acute febrile illness (Reye's syndrome). **Elderly:** May be more susceptible to toxicity; lower dosages recommended.

INTERACTIONS

DRUG: Alcohol, NSAIDs may increase risk of GI effects (e.g., ulceration). **Urinary alkalinizers, antacids** increase excretion. **Anticoagulants, heparin, thrombolytics** increase risk of bleeding. Large dose may increase effect of **insulin, oral hypoglycemics. Valproic acid, platelet aggregation inhibitors** may increase risk of bleeding. May increase toxicity of **methotrexate, zidovudine. Ototoxic medications, vancomycin** may increase ototoxicity. May decrease effect of **probenecid, sulfinpyrazone. HERBAL:** None known. **FOOD:** None known. **LAB VALUES:** May alter SGOT (AST), SGPT (ALT), alkaline phosphatase, uric acid; prolongs prothrombin time, bleeding time. May decrease cholesterol, potassium, T_3, T_4.

AVAILABILITY (OTC)

SUPPOSITORY: 60 mg, 120 mg, 200 mg, 300 mg, 600 mg. **TABLET:** 81 mg, 325 mg, 500 mg, 650 mg. **TABLET (chewable):** 81 mg. **TABLET (controlled release):** 650 mg, 800 mg, 975 mg. **TABLET (enteric-coated):** 81 mg, 162 mg, 325 mg, 500 mg, 650 mg, 975 mg.

ADMINISTRATION/HANDLING

PO

• Do not crush or break enteric-coated/sustained-release form. • May give with water, milk, meals if GI distress occurs.

RECTAL

• Refrigerate suppositories. • If suppository is too soft, chill for 30 min in refrigerator or run cold water over foil wrapper. • Moisten suppository with cold water before inserting well into rectum.

INDICATIONS/ROUTES/DOSAGE

ANALGESIC/ANTIPYRETIC

PO/rectal: ADULTS, ELDERLY: 325–1,000 mg q4–6h. CHILDREN: 10–15 mg/kg/dose q4–6h. **Maximum:** 4 g/day.

ANTI-INFLAMMATORY

PO: ADULTS, ELDERLY: Initially, 2.4–3.6 g/day in divided doses, then 3.6–5.4 g/day. CHILDREN: 60–90 mg/kg/day in divided doses, then 80–100 mg/kg/day.

SUSPECT MI

PO: ADULTS, ELDERLY: Initially, 162 mg as soon as MI suspected, then daily for 30 days post-MI.

MI PROPHYLAXIS

PO: ADULTS, ELDERLY: 75–325 mg/day.

STROKE PREVENTION FOLLOWING TIA

PO: ADULTS, ELDERLY: 50–325 mg/day.

KAWASAKI DISEASE

PO: CHILDREN: 80–100 mg/kg/day in divided doses.

SIDE EFFECTS

OCCASIONAL: GI distress (cramping, heartburn, abdominal distention, mild nausea), allergic reaction (pruritus, urticaria, bronchospasm).

ADVERSE REACTIONS/ TOXIC EFFECTS

High dosages may produce GI bleeding and/or gastric mucosal lesions. Low-grade toxicity characterized by ringing in ears, generalized pruritus (may be severe), headache, dizziness, flushing, tachycardia, hyperventilation, sweating, thirst. Febrile, dehydrated children can reach toxic levels quickly. Marked toxicity manifested by hyperthermia, restlessness, abnormal breathing pattern, convulsions, respiratory failure, coma.

NURSING IMPLICATIONS

BASELINE ASSESSMENT

Do not give to children/teenagers who have flu or chickenpox (increases risk of Reye's syndrome). Do not use if vinegar-like odor is noted (indicates chemical breakdown). Assess type, location, duration of pain, inflammation. Inspect appearance of affected joints for immobility, deformities, skin condition. Therapeutic serum level for antiarthritic effect: 20–30 mg/dl (toxicity occurs if levels are >30 mg/dl).

INTERVENTION/EVALUATION

Monitor urinary pH (sudden acidification, pH from 6.5 to 5.5), may result in toxicity. Assess skin for evidence of bruising. If given as antipyretic, assess temperature directly before and 1 hr after giving medication. Evaluate for therapeutic response: relief of pain, stiffness, swelling; increase in joint mobility; reduced joint tenderness; improved grip strength.

PATIENT/FAMILY TEACHING

Do not crush or chew sustained-release or enteric-coated form. Report ringing in ears or persistent GI pain. Therapeutic anti-inflammatory effect noted in 1–3 wks.

Atacand

see candesartan

atazanavir sulfate

ah-tah-**zan**-ah-veer
(Reyataz)

◆ CLASSIFICATION

PHARMACOTHERAPEUTIC: Antiretroviral. **CLINICAL:** Protease inhibitor.

ACTION

An HIV-1 protease inhibitor, selectively prevents the processing of viral polyproteins found in HIV-1 infected cells. **Therapeutic Effect:** Prevents formation of the mature HIV viral cell.

PHARMACOKINETICS

Rapidly absorbed following oral administration. Protein binding: 86%. Extensively metabolized in the liver. Primarily excreted in urine with a lesser extent in the feces. **Half-life:** 5–8 hrs.

USES

Treatment of HIV-1 infection in combination with other antiretroviral agents.

PRECAUTIONS

CONTRAINDICATIONS: Concurrent use with midazolam, triazolam, ergot derivatives, pimozide, severe hepatic insufficiency. **EXTREME CAUTION:** Hepatic impairment. **CAUTIONS:** Preexisting conduction system disease (first-degree AV block or second- or third-degree AV block), diabetes mellitus, elderly, impaired renal function.

LIFESPAN CONSIDERATIONS: Pregnancy/lactation: Unknown if drug crosses placenta or distributed in breast milk. Lactic acidosis syndrome, hyperbilirubinemia, kernicterus has been reported. **Pregnancy Category B. Children:** Safety and efficacy not established in those <3 mos of age. **Elderly:** Age-related hepatic impairment may require dose reduction.

INTERACTIONS

DRUG: Calcium channel blockers, lovastatin, simvastatin, atorvastatin, immunosuppressants, sildenafil, irinotecan, tricyclic antidepressants may result in increased plasma concentrations. **Rifampin, antacids, H_2 receptor antagonists, proton pump inhibitors** decreases plasma concentrations. **HERBAL: St. Johns wort** may decrease concentration. **FOOD:** High-fat meal may decrease absorption. **LAB VALUES:** May increase bilirubin, SGOT (AST), SGPT (ALT), amylase, lipase. May decrease, Hgb, neutrophil count, platelets. May alter LDL cholesterol, triglycerides.

AVAILABILITY (Rx)

CAPSULES: 100 mg, 150 mg, 200 mg.

ADMINISTRATION/HANDLING

PO

- Give with food.

INDICATIONS/ROUTES/DOSAGE

HIV-1 INFECTION

PO: ADULTS, ELDERLY: 400 mg (2 capsules) once daily given with food.

CONCURRENT THERAPY WITH EFAVIRENZ

PO: ADULTS, ELDERLY: 300 mg atazanavir and 100 mg ritonavir and 600 mg efavirenz given as a single daily dose with food.

CONCURRENT THERAPY WITH DIDANOSINE

PO: ADULTS, ELDERLY: Give atazanavir with food 2 hrs prior to or 1 hr following didanosine.

MILD TO MODERATE HEPATIC FUNCTION IMPAIRMENT

PO: ADULTS, ELDERLY: 300 mg once daily given with food.

SIDE EFFECTS

FREQUENT (14%–16%): Nausea, headache. **OCCASIONAL (4%–9%):** Rash, vomiting, depression, diarrhea, abdominal pain, fever. **RARE: (≤3%):** Dizziness, insomnia, cough, fatigue, back pain.

ADVERSE REACTIONS/ TOXIC EFFECTS

Severe hypersensitivity reaction (angioedema, chest pain), jaundice may occur.

NURSING IMPLICATIONS

BASELINE ASSESSMENT

Obtain baseline laboratory testing, CBC, hepatic function tests, before beginning therapy and at periodic intervals during therapy. Offer emotional support.

INTERVENTION/EVALUATION

Assess for nausea, vomiting; assess eating pattern. Determine pattern of bowel activity, stool consistency. Assess skin for rash. Question for evidence of headache. Monitor for onset of depression.

PATIENT/FAMILY TEACHING

Take with food. Small, frequent meals may offset nausea, vomiting. Atazanavir is not a cure for HIV infection, nor does it reduce risk of transmission to others.

atenolol

ay-**ten**-oh-lol

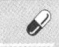

(Apo-Atenol ✤, Tenolin ✤, Tenormin)

Do not confuse with albuterol.

FIXED-COMBINATION(S)

Tenoretic: atenolol/chlorthalidone (a diuretic): 50 mg/25 mg; 100 mg/25 mg.

CLASSIFICATION

PHARMACOTHERAPEUTIC: $Beta_1$-adrenergic blocker. **CLINICAL:** Antihypertensive, antianginal, antiarrhythmic (see p. 61C).

ACTION

Blocks $beta_1$-adrenergic receptors in cardiac tissue. **Therapeutic Effect:** Slows sinus heart rate, decreasing cardiac output, decreasing B/P. Decreases myocardial O_2 demand.

PHARMACOKINETICS

Onset	Peak	Duration
PO		
1 hr	2–4 hrs	24 hrs

Incompletely absorbed from GI tract. Protein binding: 6%–16%. Minimal liver metabolism. Primarily excreted unchanged in urine. Removed by hemodialysis. **Half-life:** 6–7 hrs (half-life increased in impaired renal function).

USES

Treatment of hypertension, alone or in combination with other agents; management of angina pectoris; reduces cardiovascular mortality in those with definite or suspected acute MI. **Unlabeled:** Hypertrophic cardiomyopathy, pheochromocytoma, prophylaxis of migraine, tremors, thyrotoxicosis, syndrome of mitral valve prolapse. Improves survival in diabetics with heart disease.

PRECAUTIONS

CONTRAINDICATIONS: Overt cardiac failure, cardiogenic shock, heart block greater than first degree, severe bradycardia. **CAUTIONS:** Impaired renal or hepatic function, peripheral vascular disease, hyperthyroidism, diabetes, inadequate cardiac function, bronchospastic disease.

LIFESPAN CONSIDERATIONS: Pregnancy/lactation: Readily crosses placenta; distributed in breast milk. Avoid use during first trimester. May produce bradycardia, apnea, hypoglycemia, hypothermia during delivery, low-birth-weight infants. **Pregnancy Category D.** **Children:** No age-related precautions noted. **Elderly:** Age-related peripheral vascular disease, renal function requires caution.

INTERACTIONS

DRUG: **Diuretics, other hypotensives** may increase hypotensive effect; **sympathomimetics, xanthines** may mutually inhibit effects; may mask symptoms of hypoglycemia, prolong hypoglycemic effect of **insulin, oral hypoglycemics; NSAIDs** may decrease antihypertensive effect; **cimetidine** may increase concentration. **HERBAL:** None known. **FOOD:** None known. **LAB VALUES:** May increase ANA titer, BUN, creatinine, potassium, uric acid, lipoproteins, triglycerides.

AVAILABILITY (Rx)

TABLETS: 25 mg, 50 mg, 100 mg. **INJECTION:** 5 mg/10 ml.

ADMINISTRATION/HANDLING

PO

- May give without regard to meals.
- Tablets may be crushed.

IV

Storage • Store at room temperature. • After reconstitution, parenteral form is stable for 48 hrs at room temperature.

Reconstitution • May give undiluted or dilute in 10–50 ml 0.9% NaCl or D_5W.

Rate of administration • Give IV push over 5 min. • Give IV infusion over 15 min.

IV INCOMPATIBILITIES
Amphotericin complex (Abelcet, AmBisome, Amphotec).

INDICATIONS/ROUTES/DOSAGE

HYPERTENSION

PO: ADULTS: Initially, 25–50 mg once/day. May increase up to 100 mg once/day.

ANGINA PECTORIS

PO: ADULTS: Initially, 50 mg once daily. May increase up to 200 mg once daily.

USUAL ELDERLY DOSAGE

PO: Initially, 25 mg/day for angina/hypertension.

USUAL PEDIATRIC DOSE

PO: Initially, 0.8–1 mg/kg/dose.

ACUTE MYOCARDIAL INFARCTION

IV: Give 5 mg over 5 min, may repeat in 10 min. In those who tolerate full 10-mg IV dose, begin 50-mg tablets 10 min after last IV dose followed by another 50-mg oral dose 12 hrs later. Thereafter, give 100 mg once/day or 50 mg twice/day for 6–9 days. (Alternatively, for those who do not tolerate full IV dose, give 50 mg orally 2 times/day or 100 mg once/day for at least 7 days.)

DOSAGE IN RENAL IMPAIRMENT

Creatinine Clearance	Dosage
15–35 ml/min	50 mg daily
<15 ml/min	50 mg every other day

SIDE EFFECTS

Generally well tolerated with mild and transient side effects. **FREQUENT:** Hypotension manifested as dizziness, nausea, diaphoresis, headache, cold extremities, fatigue, constipation/diarrhea. **OCCASIONAL:** Insomnia, flatulence, urinary frequency, impotence or decreased libido. **RARE:** Rash, arthralgia, myalgia, confusion (esp. in elderly), change in taste.

ADVERSE REACTIONS/ TOXIC EFFECTS

Overdosage may produce profound bradycardia, hypotension. Abrupt withdrawal may result in sweating, palpitations, headache, tremulousness. May precipitate CHF, MI in those with cardiac disease; thyroid storm in those with thyrotoxicosis; peripheral ischemia in those with existing peripheral vascular disease. Hypoglycemia may occur in previously controlled diabetics. Thrombocytopenia (unusual bruising, bleeding) occurs rarely.

NURSING IMPLICATIONS

BASELINE ASSESSMENT

Assess B/P, apical pulse immediately before drug is administered (if pulse is ≤60/min, or systolic B/P is <90 mm Hg, withhold medication, contact physician). **Antianginal:** Record onset, type (sharp, dull, squeezing), radiation, location, intensity, and duration of anginal pain, precipitating factors (exertion, emotional stress). Assess baseline renal/liver function tests.

INTERVENTION/EVALUATION

Monitor B/P for hypotension, pulse for bradycardia, respiration for difficulty in breathing. Assess pattern of daily bowel activity and stool consistency. Assess for evidence of CHF: dyspnea (particularly on exertion or lying down), night cough, peripheral edema, distended neck veins. Monitor I&O (increase in weight, decrease in urine output may indicate CHF). Assess extremities for coldness. Assist with ambulation if dizziness occurs.

PATIENT/FAMILY TEACHING

Do not abruptly discontinue medication. Compliance with therapy essential to control hypertension, angina. To reduce hypotensive effect, rise slowly from lying to sitting position and permit legs to dangle from bed momentarily before standing. Avoid tasks that require alertness, motor skills until drug reaction is established. Report dizziness, depression, confusion, rash, unusual bruising/bleeding. Outpatients should monitor B/P, pulse before taking medication (teach correct technique). Restrict salt, alcohol intake. Therapeutic antihypertensive effect noted in 1–2 wks.

Ativan

see lorazepam

atomoxetine

ah-toe-**mocks**-eh-teen
(Strattera)

CLASSIFICATION

PHARMACOTHERAPEUTIC: Norepinephrine re-uptake inhibitor. **CLINICAL:** Psychotherapeutic agent.

ACTION

Enhances noradrenergic function by selective inhibition of the presynaptic norepinephrine transporter. **Therapeutic Effect:** Improves symptoms of attention deficit hyperactivity disorder (ADHD).

PHARMACOKINETICS

Rapidly absorbed after oral administration. 98% bound to protein, primarily albumin. Eliminated primarily in the urine, with less excreted in the feces. Not removed by hemodialysis. **Half-life:** 4–5 hrs found in the major population, 22 hrs in 7% Caucasians, and 2% in African-Americans. Half-life increased in moderate to severe hepatic insufficiency.

USES

Treatment of ADHD.

PRECAUTIONS

CONTRAINDICATIONS: Concurrent use of MAOIs or within 2 wks of discontinuing an MAOI; narrow-angle glaucoma. **CAUTIONS:** Hypertension; tachycardia; cardiovascular disease; pts at risk of urinary retention, moderate or severe hepatic impairment.

LIFESPAN CONSIDERATIONS: Pregnancy/lactation: Unknown if excreted in breast milk. **Pregnancy Category C. Children:** Safety and efficacy in pts <6 yrs have not been established. **Elderly:** Age-related decreased hepatic impairment, renal impairment, cardiovascular or cerebrovascular disease may increase risk of effects.

INTERACTIONS

DRUG: MAOIs may increase toxic effects. **Paroxetine, fluoxetine, quinidine** may increase concentrations. Avoid concurrent use of medications that can increase heart rate or blood pressure. **HERBAL:** None known. **FOOD:** None known. **LAB VALUES:** None known.

AVAILABILITY (Rx)

CAPSULES: 10 mg, 18 mg, 25 mg, 40 mg, 60 mg.

ADMINISTRATION/HANDLING

PO

- Give without regard to meals.

INDICATIONS/ROUTES/DOSAGE

Alert: Reduce dosage to 50% in those with moderate liver impairment and to 25% in those with severe liver impairment.

ADHD

PO: ADULTS, CHILDREN >70 KG: 40 mg once daily. May increase after a minimum of 3 days to 80 mg as a single daily dose or in divided doses. **Maximum:** 100 mg. CHILDREN <70 KG: Initially, 0.5 mg/kg/day. May increase to 1.2 mg/kg/day after minimum of 3 days. **Maximum:** 1.4 mg/kg/day.

SIDE EFFECTS

FREQUENT: Headache, dyspepsia (epigastric distress, heartburn), nausea, vomiting, fatigue, reduced appetite, dizziness, changes in mood. **OCCASIONAL:** Increase in heart rate, B/P, weight loss, slowing of growth. **RARE:** Insomnia, sexual dysfunction in adults (desire, performance, satisfaction).

ADVERSE REACTIONS/TOXIC EFFECT

Urinary retention or urinary hesitance may occur. In overdose, gastric emptying, repeated activated charcoal may prevent systemic absorption.

NURSING IMPLICATIONS

BASELINE ASSESSMENT

Assess pulse, B/P prior to therapy, following dose increases, and periodically while on therapy.

INTERVENTION/EVALUATION

Monitor urinary output; a complaint of urinary retention or hesitancy may be a related adverse reaction. Assist with ambulation if dizziness occurs. Be alert to mood changes. Monitor fluid and electrolyte status in those with significant vomiting.

PATIENT/FAMILY TEACHING

Avoid tasks that require alertness, motor skills until response to drug is established. Take last dose early in evening to avoid insomnia. Report nervousness, palpitations, fever, vomiting, skin rash.

atorvastatin

ah-tore-**vah**-stah-tin

(Lipitor)

Do not confuse with Levatol.

CLASSIFICATION

PHARMACOTHERAPEUTIC: HMG-CoA reductase inhibitor. **CLINICAL:** Antihyperlipidemic (see p. 50C).

ACTION

Inhibits HMG-CoA reductase, the enzyme that catalyzes the early step in cholesterol synthesis. **Therapeutic Effect:** Decreases LDL cholesterol, VLDL cholesterol, and plasma triglycerides; increases HDL cholesterol.

PHARMACOKINETICS

Poorly absorbed from GI tract. Protein binding: >98%. Metabolized in liver. Minimally eliminated in urine. Plasma levels markedly increased with chronic alcoholic liver disease, unaffected by renal disease. **Half-life:** 14 hrs.

USES

Adjunct to diet therapy to decrease elevated total and LDL cholesterol concentrations in pts with primary hypercholesterolemia (types IIa and IIb) and in those with combined hypercholesterolemia and hypertriglyceridemia. Treatment of familial hypercholesterolemia in children 10–17 yrs.

PRECAUTIONS

CONTRAINDICATIONS: Active liver disease, unexplained elevated liver function tests, pregnancy, lactation. **CAUTIONS:** Anticoagulant therapy, history of liver disease, substantial alcohol consumption, major surgery, severe acute infection, trauma, hypotension, severe metabolic, endocrine, or electrolyte disorders, uncontrolled seizures.

LIFESPAN CONSIDERATIONS: Pregnancy/lactation: Distributed in breast milk. Contraindicated during pregnancy. May produce skeletal malformation. **Pregnancy Category X. Children:** Safety and efficacy not established. **Elderly:** No age-related precautions noted.

INTERACTIONS

DRUG: **Antacids, colestipol, propranolol** decreases atorvastatin activity. **Warfarin, digoxin, oral contraceptives, itraconazole** levels may increase concentration, producing severe muscle pain, inflammation, weakness. Increased risk of rhabdomyolysis, acute renal failure with **cyclosporine, erythromycin, gemfibrozil, nicotinic acid.** **HERBAL:** None known. **FOOD:** May be given without regard to meals. **LAB VALUES:** May increase creatinine kinase, serum transaminase concentrations.

AVAILABILITY (Rx)

TABLETS: 10 mg, 20 mg, 40 mg, 80 mg.

ADMINISTRATION/HANDLING

PO

- May be given without regard to food.
- Do not break film-coated tablets.

INDICATIONS/ROUTES/DOSAGE

HYPERLIPIDEMIA

PO: ADULTS, ELDERLY: Initially, 10–40 mg/day given as a single daily dose. DOSE RANGE: Increase at 2- to 4-wk intervals up to maximum of 80 mg/day.

SIDE EFFECTS

Generally well tolerated. Side effects usually mild and transient. **FREQUENT (16%):** Headache. **OCCASIONAL (2%–5%):** Myalgia, rash/pruritus, allergy. **RARE:** Flatulence, dyspepsia.

ADVERSE REACTIONS/ TOXIC EFFECTS

Potential for cataracts, photosensitivity.

NURSING IMPLICATIONS

BASELINE ASSESSMENT

Question for possibility of pregnancy before initiating therapy (Pregnancy Category X). Assess baseline lab results: cholesterol, triglycerides, liver function tests.

INTERVENTION/EVALUATION

Monitor for headache. Assess for rash, pruritus, malaise. Monitor cholesterol and triglyceride lab values for therapeutic response.

PATIENT/FAMILY TEACHING

Follow special diet (important part of treatment). Periodic lab tests are essential part of therapy. Do not take other medications without physician's knowledge.

atovaquone

ah-**tow**-vah-quon
(Mepron)

CLASSIFICATION

PHARMACOTHERAPEUTIC: Systemic anti-infective. **CLINICAL:** Antiprotozoal.

ACTION

Inhibits mitochondrial electron-transport system at the cytochrome bc_1 complex (Complex III). **Therapeutic Effect:** Interrupts nucleic acid and ATP synthesis.

USES

Treatment or prevention of mild to moderate *Pneumocystis carinii* pneumonia

(PCP) in those intolerant to trimethoprim-sulfamethoxazole (TMP-SMZ).

PRECAUTIONS

CONTRAINDICATIONS: Development or history of potentially life-threatening allergic reaction to drug. **CAUTIONS:** Elderly, pts with severe PCP, chronic diarrhea, malabsorption syndromes. **Pregnancy Category C.**

INTERACTIONS

DRUG: **Rifampin** may decrease concentration, **atovaquone** may increase rifampin concentration. **HERBAL:** None known. **FOOD:** None known. **LAB VALUES:** May elevate SGOT (AST), SGPT (ALT), alkaline phosphatase, amylase. May decrease sodium.

AVAILABILITY (Rx)

SUSPENSION: 750 mg/5 ml.

INDICATIONS/ROUTES/DOSAGE

PNEUMOCYSTIS CARINII PNEUMONIA (PCP)

PO: ADULTS: 750 mg with food 2 times/day for 21 days.

PREVENTION OF PCP

PO: ADULTS: 1,500 mg once daily with food.

USUAL PEDIATRIC DOSAGE

PO: 40 mg/kg/day.

SIDE EFFECTS

FREQUENT (>10%): Rash, nausea, diarrhea, headache, vomiting, fever, insomnia, cough. **OCCASIONAL (<10%):** Abdominal discomfort, thrush, asthenia (loss of strength, energy), anemia, neutropenia.

ADVERSE REACTIONS/ TOXIC EFFECTS

None known.

NURSING IMPLICATIONS

INTERVENTION/EVALUATION

Assess for GI discomfort, nausea, vomiting. Check consistency and frequency of stools. Assess skin for rash. Monitor I&O, renal function tests, Hgb. Monitor elderly closely because of decreased hepatic, renal, and cardiac function.

PATIENT/FAMILY TEACHING

Continue therapy for full length of treatment. Do not take any other medication unless approved by physician. Notify physician in event of rash, diarrhea, or other new symptom.

atracurium

(Tracrium)

See Classification section under: Neuromuscular blockers **(p. 106C)**

atropine sulfate

ah-trow-peen
(Atropine Sulfate, Atropisol✤)

FIXED-COMBINATION(S)

Lomotil: atropine/diphenoxylate: 0.025 mg/2.5 mg.

◆ CLASSIFICATION

PHARMACOTHERAPEUTIC: Acetylcholine antagonist. **CLINICAL:** Antiarrhythmic, antispasmodic, antidote, cycloplegic, antisecretory, anticholinergic.

ACTION

Competes with acetylcholine for common binding sites on muscarinic receptor, blocking all muscarinic effects (exocrine glands, cardiac/smooth muscle ganglia and intramural neurons). **Therapeutic Effect:** Inhibits action of acetylcholine; decreases GI motility and secretory activity, GU muscle tone (ureter, bladder); produces ophthalmic cycloplegia, mydriasis.

USES

Treatment in cardiopulmonary (ACLS) resuscitation for treatment of sinus bradycardia accompanied by hemodynamic compromise (hypotension, altered mental status, frequent ventricular ectopy or ventricular asystole. Treatment of functional disturbances of GI motility (hypermotility, diarrhea, irritable bowel syndrome), hypermotility disorders of lower urinary tract (urinary incontinence). Preop medication to prevent or reduce salivation, excessive secretions of respiratory tract. Prevention of cholinergic effects during surgery: cardiac arrhythmias, hypotension, reflex bradycardia. Blocks adverse muscarinic effects of anticholinesterase agents (e.g., neostigmine). Used for cycloplegic refraction to dilate pupil in inflammatory conditions of iris and uveal tract of the eye.

PRECAUTIONS

CONTRAINDICATIONS: Narrow-angle glaucoma, severe ulcerative colitis, toxic megacolon, obstructive disease of GI tract, paralytic ileus, intestinal atony, bladder neck obstruction due to prostatic hypertrophy, myasthenia gravis in those not treated with neostigmine, tachycardia secondary to cardiac insufficiency or thyrotoxicosis, cardiospasm, unstable cardiovascular status in acute hemorrhage. **EXTREME CAUTION:** Autonomic neuropathy, known or suspected GI infections, diarrhea, mild to moderate ulcerative colitis. **CAUTIONS:** Hyperthyroidism, hepatic or renal disease, hypertension, tachyarrhythmias, CHF, coronary artery disease, gastric ulcer, esophageal reflux or hiatal hernia associated with reflux esophagitis, infants, elderly, systemic administration in those with COPD. **Pregnancy Category C.**

INTERACTIONS

DRUG: Antacids, antidiarrheals may decrease absorption. **Anticholinergics** may increase effects. May decrease absorption of **ketoconazole.** May increase severity of GI lesions with **KCl (wax matrix). HERBAL:** None known. **FOOD:** None known. **LAB VALUES:** None known.

AVAILABILITY (Rx)

INJECTION: 0.05 mg/ml, 0.1 mg/ml, 0.4 mg/0.5 ml, 0.4 mg/ml, 0.5 mg/ml, 1 mg/ml.

ADMINISTRATION/HANDLING

IM

- May be given subcutaneous or IM.

IV

- Must be given rapidly (prevents paradoxical slowing of heart rate).

IV INCOMPATIBILITY

Pentothal (Thiopental).

IV COMPATIBILITIES

Diphenhydramine (Benadryl), droperidol (Inapsine), fentanyl (Sublimaze), glycopyrrolate (Robinul), heparin, hydromorphone (Dilaudid), midazolam (Versed), morphine, potassium chloride, propofol (Diprivan).

INDICATIONS/ROUTES/DOSAGE

ASYSTOLE, SLOW PULSELESS ELECTRICAL ACTIVITY

IV: ADULTS, ELDERLY: 1 mg may repeat q3–5min up to total dose of 0.04 mg/kg.

PREANESTHETIC

IV/IM/subcutaneous: ADULTS, ELDERLY: 0.4–0.6 mg 30–60 min preop. CHILDREN >5 KG: 0.01–0.02 mg/kg/dose to maximum of 0.4 mg/dose. <5 KG: 0.02 mg/kg/dose 30–60 min preop.

BRADYCARDIA

IV: ADULTS, ELDERLY: 0.5–1 mg q5min

not to exceed 2 mg or 0.04 mg/kg. CHILDREN: 0.02 mg/kg (minimum 0.1 mg; maximum 0.5 mg in children, 1 mg in adolescents) may repeat in 5 min. **Maximum total dose:** 1 mg children, 2 mg adolescents.

SIDE EFFECTS

Alert: Discontinue medication immediately if dizziness, increased pulse, or blurring of vision occurs.

FREQUENT: Dry mouth/nose/throat (may be severe), decreased sweating, constipation, irritation at subcutaneous/IM injection site. **OCCASIONAL:** Swallowing difficulty, blurred vision, bloated feeling, impotence, urinary hesitancy. **RARE:** Allergic reaction (rash, urticaria), mental confusion/excitement (particularly children), fatigue.

ADVERSE REACTIONS/ TOXIC EFFECTS

Overdosage may produce tachycardia, palpitations, hot/dry/flushed skin, absence of bowel sounds, increased respiratory rate, nausea, vomiting, confusion, drowsiness, slurred speech, CNS stimulation, psychosis (agitation, restlessness, rambling speech, visual hallucinations, paranoid behavior, delusions), followed by depression.

NURSING IMPLICATIONS

BASELINE ASSESSMENT

Before giving medication, instruct pt to void (reduces risk of urinary retention).

INTERVENTION/EVALUATION

Monitor changes in B/P, pulse, temperature. Observe for tachycardia if pt has cardiac abnormalities. Assess skin turgor, mucous membranes to evaluate hydration status (encourage adequate fluid intake unless NPO for surgery), bowel sounds for peristalsis. Be alert for fever (increased risk of hyperthermia). Monitor I&O, palpate bladder for urinary retention. Assess stool frequency, consistency.

PATIENT/FAMILY TEACHING

For preop use, explain that warm, dry, flushing feeling may occur. Remind pt to remain in bed and not eat or drink anything.

auranofin

aur-an-**oh**-fin
(Ridaura)
Do not confuse with Cardura.

aurothioglucose

ah-row-thigh-oh-**glue**-cose
(Solganal)

CLASSIFICATION

PHARMACOTHERAPEUTIC: Gold compound. **CLINICAL:** Antirheumatic.

ACTION

Alters cellular mechanisms, enzyme systems, immune responses, collagen biosynthesis. **Therapeutic Effect:** Suppresses synovitis of the active stage of rheumatoid arthritis.

PHARMACOKINETICS

Auranofin (29% gold): Moderately absorbed from GI tract. Protein binding: 60%. Rapidly metabolized. Primarily excreted in urine. **Half-life:** 21–31 days. **Aurothioglucose (≈50% gold):** Slow, erratic absorption after IM administration. Protein binding: 95%–99%. Primarily excreted in urine. **Half-life:** 3–27 days (half-life increased with increased number of doses).

USES

Management of rheumatoid arthritis in

those with insufficient therapeutic response to NSAIDs. **Unlabeled:** Treatment of pemphigus, psoriatic arthritis.

PRECAUTIONS

CONTRAINDICATIONS: History of gold-induced pathologies (necrotizing enterocolitis, exfoliative dermatitis, pulmonary fibrosis, blood dyscrasias), bone marrow aplasia, severe blood dyscrasias, serious adverse effects with previous gold therapy. **CAUTIONS:** Renal/hepatic disease, marked hypertension, compromised cerebral/cardiovascular circulation. Blood dyscrasias, severe debilitation, history of sensitivity to gold compounds, Sjögren's syndrome in rheumatoid arthritis, systemic lupus erythematosus, eczema.

LIFESPAN CONSIDERATIONS: Pregnancy/lactation: Crosses placenta; distributed in breast milk. Use only when benefits outweigh hazard to fetus. **Pregnancy Category C. Children:** No age-related precautions noted. **Elderly:** Age-related decreased renal function may require caution.

INTERACTIONS

DRUG: Bone marrow depressants; hepatotoxic, nephrotoxic medications may increase toxicity. **Penicillamine** may increase risk of hematologic or renal adverse effects. **HERBAL:** None known. **FOOD:** None known. **LAB VALUES:** May decrease Hgb, Hct, platelets, WBC count. May alter liver function tests. May increase urine protein.

AVAILABILITY (Rx)

CAPSULES: 3 mg. **INJECTION:** 50 mg/ml suspension.

ADMINISTRATION/HANDLING

PO

- Give without regard to food.

IM

- Give in upper outer quadrant of gluteus.

INDICATIONS/ROUTES/DOSAGE

RHEUMATOID ARTHRITIS

Alert: Give as weekly injections.

IM: ADULTS, ELDERLY: Initially, 10 mg, then 25 mg for 2 doses, then 50 mg weekly thereafter until total dose of 0.8–1 g given. If pt is improved and there are no signs of toxicity, may give 50 mg at 3- to 4-wk intervals for many months. CHILDREN: 0.25 mg/kg, may increase by 0.25 mg/kg each week. **Maintenance:** 0.75–1 mg/kg/dose. **Maximum:** 25 mg dose for total of 20 doses, then q2–4wks.

PO: ADULTS, ELDERLY: 6 mg/day in 1 or 2 divided doses. If there is no response in 6 mos, may increase to 9 mg/day (in 3 divided doses). If response is still inadequate, discontinue. CHILDREN: 0.1 mg/kg/day in 1–2 divided doses. **Maintenance:** 0.15 mg/kg/day. **Maximum:** 0.2 mg/kg/day.

SIDE EFFECTS

FREQUENT: Auranofin: Diarrhea (50%), pruritic rash (26%), abdominal pain (14%), stomatitis (13%), nausea (10%). **Aurothioglucose:** Rash (39%), stomatitis (19%), diarrhea (13%). **OCCASIONAL:** Nausea, vomiting, anorexia, abdominal cramps.

ADVERSE REACTIONS/ TOXIC EFFECTS

Signs of gold toxicity: decreased hemoglobin, leukopenia (WBC count <4,000/mm^3), reduced granulocyte counts (<150,000/mm^3), proteinuria, hematuria, stomatitis (ulcers, sores, white spots in mouth, throat), blood dyscrasias (anemia, leukopenia, thrombocytopenia, eosinophilia), glomerulonephritis, nephrotic syndrome, cholestatic jaundice.

NURSING IMPLICATIONS

BASELINE ASSESSMENT

Rule out pregnancy before beginning treatment. CBC, urinalysis, platelet count, renal/liver function tests should be performed before therapy begins.

INTERVENTION/EVALUATION

Monitor daily bowel activity and stool consistency. Assess urine tests for proteinuria, hematuria. Monitor CBC, blood chemistries, renal/hepatic function studies. Question for pruritus (may be first sign of impending rash). Assess skin daily for rash, purpura, or ecchymoses. Assess oral mucous membranes, borders of tongue, palate, pharynx for ulceration, complaint of metallic taste sensation (sign of stomatitis). Evaluate for therapeutic response: relief of pain, stiffness, swelling, increase in joint mobility, reduced joint tenderness, improved grip strength.

PATIENT/FAMILY TEACHING

Therapeutic response may be expected in 3–6 mos. Avoid exposure to sunlight (gray to blue pigment may appear). Contact physician if pruritus, rash, sore mouth, indigestion, or metallic taste occurs. Maintain diligent oral hygiene.

Avandia

see rosiglitazone

Avapro

see irbesartan

Avelox

see moxifloxacin

Avodart

see dutasteride

Axid

see nizatidine

azathioprine

asia-**thigh**-oh-preen
(Alti-Azathioprine ✱, Azasan, Imuran)

Do not confuse with Azulfidine, Elmiron, Imferon.

◆CLASSIFICATION

PHARMACOTHERAPEUTIC: Immunologic agent. **CLINICAL:** Immunosuppressant.

ACTION

Antagonizes metabolism, inhibits RNA, DNA, and protein synthesis. **Therapeutic Effect:** Suppresses cell-mediated hypersensitivities; alters antibody production, immune response in transplant recipients. Reduces arthritis severity.

USES

Adjunct in prevention of rejection in kidney transplantation; treatment of rheumatoid arthritis in those unresponsive to conventional therapy. **Unlabeled:** Treatment of inflammatory bowel disease, chronic active hepatitis, biliary cirrhosis, systemic lupus erythematosus, glomerulonephritis, nephrotic syndrome, inflammatory myopathy, myasthenia gravis, polymyositis, pemphigus, pemphigoid, multiple sclerosis.

PRECAUTIONS

CONTRAINDICATIONS: Pregnant rheumatoid arthritis pts. **CAUTIONS:** Immunosuppressed pts, those previously treated for rheumatoid arthritis with alkylating agents (cyclophosphamide, chlorambucil, melphalan), chickenpox (current or recent), herpes zoster, gout, decreased liver/renal function, infection. **Pregnancy Category D.**

INTERACTIONS

DRUG: **Allopurinol** may increase activity, toxicity. **Bone marrow depressants** may increase bone marrow depression. **Other immunosuppressants** may increase risk of infection or development of neoplasms. **Live virus vaccines** may potentiate virus replication, increase vaccine side effects, decrease pt's antibody response to vaccine. **HERBAL:** None known. **FOOD:** None known. **LAB VALUES:** May decrease Hgb, albumin, uric acid. May increase SGOT (AST), SGPT (ALT), alkaline phosphatase, amylase, bilirubin.

AVAILABILITY (Rx)

TABLETS: 50 mg, 75 mg, 100 mg. **INJECTION:** 100-mg vial.

ADMINISTRATION/HANDLING

PO

• Give during or after meal to reduce potential for GI disturbances. • Store oral form at room temperature.

IV

Storage • Store parenteral form at room temperature. • After reconstitution, IV solution stable for 24 hrs.

Reconstitution • Reconstitute 100-mg vial with 10 ml Sterile Water for Injection to provide concentration of 10 mg/ml. • Swirl vial gently to mix and dissolve solution. • May further dilute in 50 ml D_5W or 0.9% NaCl.

Rate of administration • Infuse over 30–60 min. Range: 5 min–8 hrs.

IV INCOMPATIBILITIES

Methyl and propyl parabens, phenol.

INDICATIONS/ROUTES/DOSAGE

KIDNEY TRANSPLANTATION

IV/PO: ADULTS, ELDERLY, CHILDREN: Initially, 2–5 mg/kg/day on day of transplant, then 1–3 mg/kg/day as maintenance dose.

RHEUMATOID ARTHRITIS

PO: ADULTS: Initially, 1 mg/kg/day as single or in 2 divided doses. May increase by 0.5 mg/kg/day after 6–8 wks at 4-wk intervals up to maximum dose of 2.5 mg/kg/day. MAINTENANCE: Lowest effective dosage. May decrease dose by 0.5 mg/kg or 25 mg/day q4wks (other therapy maintained). ELDERLY: Initially, 1 mg/kg/day (50–100 mg); may increase by 25 mg/day until response or toxicity.

RENAL IMPAIRMENT

Creatinine Clearance	Dose
10–50 ml/min	75%
<10 ml/min	50%

SIDE EFFECTS

FREQUENT: Nausea, vomiting, anorexia, particularly during early treatment and with large doses. **OCCASIONAL:** Rash. **RARE:** Severe nausea, vomiting with diarrhea, stomach pain, hypersensitivity reaction.

ADVERSE REACTIONS/ TOXIC EFFECTS

Increased risk of neoplasia (new, abnormal growth tumors). Significant leukopenia, thrombocytopenia may occur, particularly in those undergoing kidney rejection. Hepatotoxicity occurs rarely.

NURSING IMPLICATIONS

BASELINE ASSESSMENT

Arthritis: Assess onset, type, location, and duration of pain, fever, inflammation. Inspect appearance of affected joints for immobility, deformities, skin condition.

INTERVENTION/EVALUATION

CBC, platelet count, liver function studies should be performed weekly during first month of therapy, twice monthly during second and third months of treatment, then monthly thereafter. If rapid fall in WBC occurs, dosage should be reduced or discontinued. Assess particularly for delayed bone marrow suppression. Routinely watch for any change from normal. **Arthritis:** Evaluate for therapeutic response: relief of pain, stiffness, swelling, increase in joint mobility, reduced joint tenderness, improved grip strength.

PATIENT/FAMILY TEACHING

Contact physician if unusual bleeding/bruising, sore throat, mouth sores, abdominal pain, fever occurs. Therapeutic response in rheumatoid arthritis may take up to 12 wks. Women of childbearing age must avoid pregnancy.

azelastine

aye-zeh-**las**-teen
(Astelin, Optivar)

CLASSIFICATION

PHARMACOTHERAPEUTIC: Antihistamine. **CLINICAL:** Antiallergy.

ACTION

Competes with histamine for histamine receptor sites on cells in the GI tract, blood vessels, respiratory tract. **Therapeutic Effect:** Inhibits symptoms associated with seasonal allergic rhinitis (e.g., sneezing, increased mucus production).

PHARMACOKINETICS

Onset	Peak	Duration
Nasal spray		
0.5–1 hr	2–3 hrs	12 hrs
Ophthalmic		
—	3 min	8 hrs

Well absorbed through nasal mucosa. Primarily excreted in feces. **Half-life:** 22 hrs.

USES

Treatment of symptoms of seasonal allergic rhinitis and conjunctivitis.

PRECAUTIONS

CONTRAINDICATIONS: History of hypersensitivity to antihistamines, newborn/premature infants, nursing mothers, third trimester of pregnancy. **CAUTIONS:** Renal function impairment.

LIFESPAN CONSIDERATIONS: Pregnancy/lactation: Unknown if drug crosses placenta or is distributed in breast milk. Do not use during third trimester. **Pregnancy Category C. Children:** Safety and efficacy not established in those <12 yrs. **Elderly:** No age-related precautions noted.

INTERACTIONS

DRUG: Alcohol, CNS depressants may increase CNS depression. **Cimetidine** may increase plasma concentration. **HERBAL:** None known. **FOOD:** None known. **LAB VALUES:** May suppress wheal and flare reaction to antigen skin testing unless drug is discontinued 4 days before testing. May increase SGPT (ALT).

AVAILABILITY (Rx)

NASAL SPRAY: 137 mcg. **OPHTHALMIC SOLUTION:** 0.05%.

ADMINISTRATION/HANDLING

NASAL

• Clear nasal passages as much as possible before use. • Tilt head slightly forward. • Insert spray tip into nostril, pointing toward nasal passage, away from nasal septum. • Spray into nostril while holding the other nostril closed and concurrently inhale through nose to permit medication as high into nasal passages as possible.

OPHTHALMIC

• Tilt pt's head back; place solution in conjunctival sac. • Have pt close eyes; press gently on lacrimal sac for 1 min.

INDICATIONS/ROUTES/DOSAGE

ALLERGIC RHINITIS

Nasal: ADULTS, CHILDREN, CHILDREN ≥12 YRS: 2 sprays 2 times/day. CHILDREN, 5–11 YRS: 1 spray 2 times/day.

VASOMOTOR RHINITIS

Nasal: ADULTS, ELDERLY, CHILDREN ≥12 YRS: 2 sprays twice daily.

ALLERGIC CONJUNCTIVITIS

Ophthalmic: ADULTS, ELDERLY, CHILDREN ≥3 YRS: 1 drop twice daily.

SIDE EFFECTS

FREQUENT (15%–20%): Headache, bitter taste. **RARE:** Nasal burning, paroxysmal sneezing. **Ophthalmic:** Transient eye burning/stinging, bitter taste, headache.

ADVERSE REACTIONS/ TOXIC EFFECTS

Epistaxis (nosebleed) occurs rarely.

NURSING IMPLICATIONS

BASELINE ASSESSMENT

Question for hypersensitivity to antihistamines.

INTERVENTION/EVALUATION

Assess therapeutic response to medication.

azithromycin

aye-**zith**-row-my-sin
(Zithromax)
Do not confuse with erythromycin.

◆CLASSIFICATION

PHARMACOTHERAPEUTIC: Macrolide. **CLINICAL:** Antibiotic (see p. 24C).

ACTION

Binds to ribosomal receptor sites of susceptible organisms. **Therapeutic Effect:** Inhibits protein synthesis.

PHARMACOKINETICS

Rapidly absorbed from GI tract. Protein binding: 7%–50%. Widely distributed. Eliminated primarily unchanged via biliary excretion. **Half-life:** 68 hrs.

USES

Treatment of mild to moderate infections of upper respiratory tract (pharyngitis, tonsillitis), lower respiratory tract (acute bacterial exacerbations, COPD, pneumonia), uncomplicated skin/skin structure infections, and sexually transmitted diseases (nongonococcal urethritis, cervicitis due to *Chlamydia trachomatis*), gonorrhea, chancroid. Prevents disseminated *Mycobacterium avium* complex (MAC). Treatment of mycoplasma pneumonia. **Injection:** Community-acquired pneumonia, PID, acne. **Unlabeled:** Uncomplicated gonococcal infections of cervix, urethra, rectum; gonococcal pharyngitis, chlamydial infections.

PRECAUTIONS

CONTRAINDICATIONS: Hypersensitivity to azithromycin, erythromycins, any macrolide antibiotic. **CAUTIONS:** Hepatic/renal dysfunction.

LIFESPAN CONSIDERATIONS: Pregnancy/lactation: Unknown if distributed in breast milk. **Pregnancy Category B. Children:** Safety and efficacy not established in those <16 yrs for IV use and <6 mos for oral use. **Elderly:** No age-related precautions in those with normal renal function.

INTERACTIONS

DRUG: May increase serum concentrations of **carbamazepine, cyclosporine, theophylline, warfarin. Aluminum/magnesium-containing antacids** may decrease concentration (give 1 hr before or 2 hrs after antacid). **HERBAL:** None known. **FOOD:** None known. **LAB VALUES:** May increase serum CPK, SGOT (AST), SGPT (ALT).

AVAILABILITY (Rx)

TABLETS: 250 mg, 500 mg, 600 mg. **INJECTION:** 500 mg. **ORAL SUSPENSION:** 100 mg/5 ml, 200 mg/5 ml.

ADMINISTRATION/HANDLING

PO

• May give tablets without regard to food. • May store suspension at room temperature. Stable for 10 days after reconstitution. • Do not administer oral suspension with food. Give at least 1 hr before or 2 hrs after meals.

IV

Storage • Store vials at room temperature. • Following reconstitution, is stable for 24 hrs at room temperature or 7 days if refrigerated.

Reconstitution • Reconstitute each 500-mg vial with 4.8 ml Sterile Water for Injection to provide concentration of 100 mg/ml. • Shake well to ensure dissolution. • Further dilute with 250 or 500 ml 0.9% NaCl or D_5W to provide final concentration of 2 mg with 250 ml diluent or 1 mg/ml with 500 ml diluent.

Rate of administration • Infuse over 60 min.

IV INCOMPATIBILITY

Information not available.

IV COMPATIBILITIES

None known; do not mix with other medication.

INDICATIONS/ROUTES/DOSAGE

RESPIRATORY TRACT INFECTIONS

PO: ADULTS, ELDERLY: 500 mg once, then 250 mg daily for 4 days. CHILDREN >6 MONTHS: 10 mg/kg once (maximum 500 mg) then 5 mg/kg/day for 4 days (maximum 250 mg).

ACUTE BACTERIAL EXACERBATIONS OF COPD

PO: ADULTS: 500 mg/day for 3 days.

SKIN, SKIN STRUCTURE INFECTIONS

PO: ADULTS, ELDERLY: 500 mg once, then 250 mg daily for 4 days.

OTITIS MEDIA

CHILDREN >6 MONTHS: 10 mg/kg once (maximum 500 mg) then 5 mg/kg/day for 4 days (maximum 250 mg).

PHARYNGITIS, TONSILLITIS

PO: CHILDREN >2 YRS: 12 mg/kg/day (maximum: 500 mg) for 5 days.

TREATMENT OF MAC

PO: ADULTS, ELDERLY: 500 mg/day in combination. CHILDREN: 5 mg/kg/day (maximum 250 mg) in combination.

MAC PREVENTION

PO: ADULTS, ELDERLY: 1,200 mg/wk alone or with rifabutin. CHILDREN: 5 mg/kg/day (maximum 250 mg) **or** 20 mg/kg/wk (maximum 1,200 mg) alone or with rifabutin.

NONGONOCOCCAL URETHRITIS, CERVICITIS DUE TO *C. TRACHOMATIS*
PO: ADULTS: 1 g as a single dose.

USUAL PARENTERAL DOSAGE
IV: ADULTS: 500 mg/day followed by oral therapy.

SIDE EFFECTS

OCCASIONAL: Nausea, vomiting, diarrhea, abdominal pain. **RARE:** Headache, dizziness, allergic reaction.

ADVERSE REACTIONS/ TOXIC EFFECTS

Superinfections, esp. antibiotic-associated colitis (abdominal cramps, watery severe diarrhea, fever), may result from altered bacterial balance. Acute interstitial nephritis occurs rarely.

NURSING IMPLICATIONS

BASELINE ASSESSMENT

Question for history of hepatitis, allergies to azithromycin, erythromycins.

INTERVENTION/EVALUATION

Check for GI discomfort, nausea, vomiting. Determine pattern of bowel activity and stool consistency. Monitor hepatic function tests, assess for hepatotoxicity: malaise, fever, abdominal pain, GI disturbances. Evaluate for superinfection: genital/anal pruritus, sore mouth or tongue, moderate to severe diarrhea.

PATIENT/FAMILY TEACHING

Continue therapy for full length of treatment. Doses should be evenly spaced. Take oral medication with 8 oz water at least 1 hr before or 2 hrs after food/beverage.

aztreonam

az-**tree**-oh-nam
(Azactam)

CLASSIFICATION

PHARMACOTHERAPEUTIC: Monobactam. **CLINICAL:** Antibiotic.

ACTION

Bactericidal effects due to inhibition of cell wall synthesis. **Therapeutic Effect:** Produces cell lysis, death.

PHARMACOKINETICS

Completely absorbed after IM administration. Protein binding: 56%–60%. Partially metabolized by hydrolysis. Primarily excreted unchanged in urine. Removed by hemodialysis. **Half-life:** 1.4–2.2 hrs (half-life increased in reduced renal, liver function).

USES

Lower respiratory tract, skin/skin structure, intra-abdominal, gynecologic, complicated/uncomplicated urinary tract infections; septicemia, cystic fibrosis. **Unlabeled:** Treatment of bone/joint infections.

PRECAUTIONS

CONTRAINDICATIONS: None known. **CAUTIONS:** History of allergy, esp. antibiotics, hepatic or renal impairment.

LIFESPAN CONSIDERATIONS: Pregnancy/lactation: Crosses placenta, distributed in amniotic fluid; low concentration in breast milk. **Pregnancy Category B. Children:** Safety and efficacy not established in children <9 mos. **Elderly:** Age-related renal impairment may require dosage adjustment.

INTERACTIONS

DRUG: None known. **HERBAL:** None known. **FOOD:** None known. **LAB VAL-**

UES: Positive Coombs' test. May increase SGOT (AST), SGPT (ALT), LDH, alkaline phosphatase, creatinine.

AVAILABILITY (Rx)

INJECTION: 500 mg, 1 g, 2 g.

ADMINISTRATION/HANDLING

IM

• Shake immediately, vigorously after adding diluent. • Inject deeply into large muscle mass. • Following reconstitution for IM injection, solution is stable for 48 hrs at room temperature, or 7 days if refrigerated.

IV

Storage • Store vials at room temperature. • Solution appears colorless to light yellow. • Following reconstitution, solution is stable for 48 hrs at room temperature, or 7 days if refrigerated. • Discard if precipitate forms. Discard unused portions.

Reconstitution • For IV push, dilute each gram with 6–10 ml Sterile Water for Injection. • For intermittent IV infusion, further dilute with 50–100 ml D_5W or 0.9% NaCl.

Rate of administration • For IV push, give over 3–5 min. • For IV infusion, administer over 20–60 min.

IV INCOMPATIBILITIES

Acyclovir (Zovirax), amphotericin (Fungizone), daunorubicin (Cerubidine), ganciclovir (Cytovene), lorazepam (Ativan), metronidazole (Flagyl), vancomycin (Vancocin).

IV COMPATIBILITIES

Aminophylline, bumetanide (Bumex), calcium gluconate, cimetidine (Tagamet), diltiazem (Cardizem), dobutamine (Dobutrex), dopamine (Intropin), famotidine (Pepcid), furosemide (Lasix), heparin, hydromorphone (Dilaudid), insulin (Regular), magnesium sulfate, morphine, potassium chloride, propofol (Diprivan).

INDICATIONS/ROUTES/DOSAGE

URINARY TRACT INFECTIONS

IM/IV: ADULTS, ELDERLY: 500 mg–1 g q8–12h.

MODERATE TO SEVERE SYSTEMIC INFECTIONS

IM/IV: ADULTS, ELDERLY: 1–2 g q8–12h.

SEVERE OR LIFE-THREATENING INFECTIONS

IV: ADULTS, ELDERLY: 2 g q6–8h.

USUAL PEDIATRIC DOSAGE

IV: 30 mg/kg q6–8h. **Maximum:** 120 mg/kg/day.

DOSAGE IN RENAL IMPAIRMENT

Dose and/or frequency is modified based on creatinine clearance, severity of infection:

Creatinine Clearance	Dosage
10–30 ml/min	1–2 g initially; then ½ the usual dose at usual intervals
<10 ml/min	1–2 g initially; then ¼ the usual dose at usual intervals

SIDE EFFECTS

OCCASIONAL (<3%): Discomfort/swelling at IM injection site, nausea, vomiting, diarrhea, rash. **RARE (<1%):** Phlebitis/thrombophlebitis at IV injection site, abdominal cramps, headache, hypotension.

ADVERSE REACTIONS/ TOXIC EFFECTS

Superinfection, antibiotic-associated colitis (abdominal cramps, watery severe diarrhea, fever) may result from altered bacterial balance. Severe hypersensitivity

B

reactions, including anaphylaxis, occur rarely.

NURSING IMPLICATIONS

BASELINE ASSESSMENT:

Question for history of allergies, esp. to aztreonam, other antibiotics.

INTERVENTION/EVALUATION

Evaluate for phlebitis (heat, pain, red streaking over vein), pain at IM injection site. Assess for GI discomfort, nausea, vomiting. Monitor stool frequency and consistency. Assess skin for rash. Be alert for superinfection: increased temperature, sore throat, vomiting, diarrhea, black/hairy tongue, ulceration or changes of oral mucosa, anal/genital pruritus.

PATIENT/FAMILY TEACHING

Report nausea, vomiting, diarrhea, rash.

bacitracin

bah-cih-**tray**-sin

(Bacitracin, Baci-IM)

Do not confuse with Bactrim, Bactroban.

FIXED-COMBINATION(S)

With polymyxin B, an antibiotic **(Polysporin);** with polymyxin B and neomycin, antibiotics **(Mycitracin, Neosporin).**

◆CLASSIFICATION

PHARMACOTHERAPEUTIC: Anti-infective. **CLINICAL:** Antibiotic.

ACTION

Interferes with plasma membrane permeability in susceptible microorganisms. **Therapeutic Effect:** Inhibits cell wall synthesis. Bacteriostatic.

USES

Ophthalmic: Superficial ocular infections (conjunctivitis, keratitis, corneal ulcers, blepharitis). **Topical:** Minor skin abrasions, superficial infections. **Irrigation:** Treatment, prophylaxis of surgical procedures.

PRECAUTIONS

CONTRAINDICATIONS: None known. **CAUTIONS:** None known. **Pregnancy Category C.**

INTERACTIONS

DRUG: None known. **HERBAL:** None known. **FOOD:** None known. **LAB VALUES:** None known.

AVAILABILITY (Rx)

POWDER FOR IRRIGATION: 50,000 units. **OPHTHALMIC OINTMENT. (OTC) TOPICAL OINTMENT.**

ADMINISTRATION/HANDLING

OPHTHALMIC

• Place finger on lower eyelid. Pull out until a pocket is formed between eye and lower lid. Place ¼–½ inch ointment in pocket. • Close eye gently for 1–2 min, rolling eyeball (increases contact area of drug to eye). Remove excess ointment around eye with tissue.

INDICATIONS/ROUTES/DOSAGE

USUAL OPHTHALMIC DOSAGE

ADULTS: ½-inch ribbon in conjunctival sac q3–4h.

USUAL TOPICAL DOSAGE

ADULTS, CHILDREN: Apply 1–5 times/day to affected area.

IRRIGATION

ADULTS, ELDERLY: 50,000–150,000 units, as needed.

SIDE EFFECTS

Alert: It is important to know side effects of components when bacitracin is used in fixed-combination.

RARE: Topical: Hypersensitivity reaction (itching, burning, inflammation), allergic contact dermatitis. **Ophthalmic:** Burning, itching, redness, swelling, pain.

ADVERSE REACTIONS/ TOXIC EFFECTS

Severe hypersensitivity reaction (hypotension, apnea) occurs rarely.

NURSING IMPLICATIONS

INTERVENTION/EVALUATION

Topical: Evaluate for hypersensitivity: itching, burning, inflammation. With preparations containing corticosteroids, consider masking effect on clinical signs. **Ophthalmic:** Assess eye for therapeutic response or increased redness, swelling, burning, itching (hypersensitivity reaction).

PATIENT/FAMILY TEACHING

Continue therapy for full length of treatment. Doses should be evenly spaced. Report burning, itching, rash, increased irritation.

baclofen

back-low-fin

(Apo-Baclofen♣, Kemstro, Liotec♣)

Do not confuse with Bactroban, Beclovent, lisinopril.

CLASSIFICATION

PHARMACOTHERAPEUTIC: Skeletal muscle relaxant. **CLINICAL:** Antispastic, analgesic in trigeminal neuralgia (see p. 131C).

ACTION

Inhibits transmission of reflexes at the spinal cord level. **Therapeutic Effect:** Relieves muscle spasticity.

PHARMACOKINETICS

Well absorbed from GI tract. Protein binding: 30%. Partially metabolized in liver. Primarily excreted in urine. **Half-life:** 2.5–4 hrs. Intrathecal: 1.5 hrs.

USES

Treatment of reversible spasticity associated with multiple sclerosis or spinal cord lesions. **Unlabeled:** Treatment of trigeminal neuralgia.

PRECAUTIONS

CONTRAINDICATIONS: Skeletal muscle spasm due to rheumatic disorders, stroke, cerebral palsy, Parkinson's disease. **CAUTIONS:** Impaired renal function, CVA, diabetes mellitus, epilepsy, preexisting psychiatric disorders.

LIFESPAN CONSIDERATIONS: Pregnancy/lactation: Unknown if drug crosses placenta or is distributed in breast milk. **Pregnancy Category C. Children:** Safety and efficacy not established in those <12 yrs. **Elderly:** Increased risk of CNS toxicity (hallucinations, sedation, confusion, mental depression); age-related renal impairment may require decreased dosage.

INTERACTIONS

DRUG: Potentiated effects when used with other **CNS depressants (including alcohol). HERBAL:** None known. **FOOD:** None known. **LAB VALUES:** May increase SGOT (AST), SGPT (ALT), alkaline phosphatase, blood sugar.

AVAILABILITY (Rx)

TABLETS: 10 mg, 20 mg. **AMPS:** 500 mcg/ml. **ORAL DISINTEGRATING TABLET:** 10 mg.

ADMINISTRATION/HANDLING

PO

• Give without regard to meals. • Tablets may be crushed.

B

INDICATIONS/ROUTES/DOSAGE

MUSCULOSKELETAL SPASM

PO: ADULTS: Initially, 5 mg 3 times/day. May increase by 15 mg/day at 3-day intervals. RANGE: 40–80 mg/day. Total dose not to exceed 80 mg/day. ELDERLY: Initially, 5 mg 2–3 times/day. May gradually increase dosage. CHILDREN 2–7 YRS: Initially, 10–15 mg/day in divided doses q8hr. May increase at 3-day intervals by 5–15 mg/day. **Maximum:** 40 mg/day. **Children ≥8 yrs:** Maximum: 60 mg/day.

USUAL INTRATHECAL DOSAGE

ADULTS, ELDERLY, CHILDREN >12 YRS: 300–800 mcg/day. CHILDREN ≤12 YRS: 100–300 mcg/day.

SIDE EFFECTS

FREQUENT (>10%): Transient drowsiness, weakness, dizziness, lightheadedness, nausea, vomiting. **OCCASIONAL (2%–10%):** Headache, paresthesia of hands/feet, constipation, anorexia, hypotension, confusion, nasal congestion. **RARE (<1%):** Paradoxical CNS excitement/restlessness, slurred speech, tremor, dry mouth, diarrhea, nocturia, impotence.

ADVERSE REACTIONS/ TOXIC EFFECTS

Abrupt withdrawal may produce hallucinations, seizures. Overdosage results in blurred vision, convulsions, myosis, mydriasis, severe muscle weakness, strabismus, respiratory depression, vomiting.

NURSING IMPLICATIONS

BASELINE ASSESSMENT

Record onset, type, location, duration of muscular spasm. Check for immobility, stiffness, swelling.

INTERVENTION/EVALUATION

Assess for paradoxical reaction. Assist with ambulation at all times. For those on long-term therapy, liver/renal function tests, blood counts should be performed periodically. Evaluate for therapeutic response: decreased intensity of skeletal muscle pain. Be alert to signs of infection.

PATIENT/FAMILY TEACHING

Drowsiness usually diminishes with continued therapy. Avoid tasks that require alertness, motor skills until response to drug is established. Do not abruptly withdraw medication after long-term therapy. Avoid alcohol, CNS depressants.

Bactrim

see co-trimoxazole

basiliximab

bay-zul-**ix**-ah-mab
(Simulect)

◆CLASSIFICATION

PHARMACOTHERAPEUTIC: Monoclonal antibody. **CLINICAL:** Immunosuppressive (see p. 102C).

ACTION

Binds to interleukin-2 (IL-2) receptor complex and inhibits IL-2 binding. **Therapeutic Effect:** Prevents lymphocytic activity, and response of the immune system to antigens is impaired.

PHARMACOKINETICS

Half-life: adults: 4–10 days; children: 5–17 days.

USES

Adjunct with cyclosporine, corticosteroids in the prevention of acute organ rejection in pts receiving renal transplant.

PRECAUTIONS

CONTRAINDICATIONS: None known. **CAUTIONS:** Infection, history of malignancy.

LIFESPAN CONSIDERATIONS: Pregnancy/lactation: Unknown if crosses placenta or is distributed in breast milk. **Pregnancy Category B. Children/elderly:** No age-related precautions noted.

INTERACTONS

DRUG: None known. **HERBAL:** None known. **FOOD:** None known. **LAB VALUES:** Alters calcium, glucose, potassium, Hgb, Hct. Increases cholesterol, BUN, serum creatinine, uric acid. Decreases magnesium, phosphate, platelet count.

AVAILABILITY (Rx)

POWDER FOR INJECTION: 10 mg, 20 mg.

ADMINISTRATION/HANDLING

IV

Storage • Refrigerate. • After reconstitution, use within 4 hrs (24 hrs if refrigerated) • Discard if precipitate forms.

Reconstitution • Reconstitute with 5 ml Sterile Water for Injection. • Shake gently to dissolve. • Further dilute with 50 ml 0.9% NaCl or D_5W. Gently invert to avoid foaming.

Rate of administration • Infuse over 20–30 min.

IV INCOMPATIBILITY

Specific information not available. Other medications should not be added simultaneously through same IV line.

INDICATIONS/ROUTES/DOSAGE

PROPHYLAXIS OF ORGAN REJECTION

IV: ADULTS, ELDERLY, CHILDREN ≥35 KG: Two doses of 20 mg each in reconstituted volume of 50 ml given as IV infusion over 20–30 min. Give first dose of 20 mg within 2 hrs before transplant surgery and the second dose of 20 mg 4 days after transplant. CHILDREN: 12 mg/m^2 as above. CHILDREN <35 KG: 10-mg dose as above.

SIDE EFFECTS

FREQUENT (>10%): GI disturbances (constipation, diarrhea, dyspepsia), CNS effects (headache, tremor, dizziness, insomnia), respiratory infection, dysuria, acne, leg/back pain, peripheral edema, hypertension. **OCCASIONAL (3%–10%):** Angina, neuropathy, abdominal distention, tachycardia, rash, hypotension, urinary disturbances (hematuria, frequent micturition, genital edema), joint pain, increased hair growth, muscle pain.

ADVERSE REACTIONS/ TOXIC EFFECTS

None known.

NURSING IMPLICATIONS

BASELINE ASSESSMENT

Obtain baseline BUN, creatinine, potassium, uric acid, glucose, calcium, phosphatase blood serum levels and vital signs, particularly B/P, pulse rate. Breast-feeding not recommended.

INTERVENTION/EVALUATION

Diligently monitor CBC, all blood serum levels. Assess B/P for hypertension/hypotension; pulse for evidence of tachycardia. Question for GI disturbances, CNS effects, urinary changes. Monitor for presence of wound infection, signs of infection (fever, sore throat, unusual bleeding/bruising).

PATIENT/FAMILY TEACHING

Report difficulty in breathing/swallowing, rapid heartbeat, rash, itching, swelling of lower extremities and weakness. Avoid pregnancy.

B

BCG, intravesical

(Immu Cyst, Pacis, TheraCys, Tice BCG)

See Classification section under: Cancer Chemotherapeutic Agents (p. 69C)

becaplermin

beh-**cap**-lear-min
(Regranex)

Do not confuse with Repronex.

CLASSIFICATION

PHARMACOTHERAPEUTIC: Biologic response modifier. **CLINICAL:** Growth factor.

ACTION

Platelet-derived growth factor. **Therapeutic Effect:** Stimulates body to grow new tissue to heal open wounds.

USES

Treatment of lower extremity diabetic neuropathic ulcers extending into subcutaneous tissue or beyond.

PRECAUTIONS

CONTRAINDICATIONS: Skin neoplasms at site of application. **CAUTIONS:** Wounds showing exposed joints, tendons, ligaments, bones.

LIFESPAN CONSIDERATIONS: Pregnancy/lactation: Unknown if distributed in breast milk. **Pregnancy Category C. Children:** Safety and efficacy not established in those <16 yrs. **Elderly:** No age-related precautions noted.

INTERACTIONS

DRUG: None known. **HERBAL:** None known. **FOOD:** None known. **LAB VALUES:** None known.

AVAILABILITY (Rx)

GEL: 0.01%.

ADMINISTRATION/HANDLING

• Refrigerate gel. • Measure gel on a clean, nonabsorbable surface. • Transfer to ulcer and spread as a thin, continuous layer onto the ulcer. • With a gauze pad moistened with 0.9% NaCl, cover ulcer for 12 hrs; remove and wash any residual gel from ulcer and replace with new gauze pad moistened with 0.9% NaCl until time of next application.

INDICATIONS/ROUTES/DOSAGE

ULCERS

Topical: ADULTS, ELDERLY: Apply once daily (spread evenly; cover with saline-moistened gauze dressing). After 12 hrs, rinse ulcer, recover with saline gauze.

SIDE EFFECTS

OCCASIONAL (2%): Local rash near ulcer.

ADVERSE REACTIONS/ TOXIC EFFECTS

None known.

NURSING IMPLICATIONS

INTERVENTION/EVALUATION

Do not allow tip of tube to come in contact with the ulcer.

PATIENT/FAMILY TEACHING

Dosage requires recalculation weekly or biweekly, depending on rate of change in the width and length of ulcer.

B

beclomethasone dipropionate

beck-low-**meth**-ah-sewn
(Beclodisk♣, Becloforte inhaler♣, Beconase AQ, Qvar)

Do not confuse with baclofen.

CLASSIFICATION

PHARMACOTHERAPEUTIC: Adrenocorticosteroid. **CLINICAL:** Anti-inflammatory, immunosuppressant (see pp. 65C, 81C).

ACTION

Controls rate of protein synthesis; depresses migration of polymorphonuclear leukocytes, fibroblasts; reverses capillary permeability; prevents or controls inflammation. **Therapeutic Effect: Inhalation:** Inhibits bronchoconstriction, produces smooth muscle relaxation, decreases mucus secretion. **Intranasal:** Decreases response to seasonal and perennial rhinitis.

PHARMACOKINETICS

Rapidly absorbed from pulmonary, nasal, GI tissue. Protein binding: 87%. Metabolized in liver, undergoes extensive first-pass effect. Primarily eliminated in feces. **Half-life:** 15 hrs.

USES

Inhalation: Control of bronchial asthma in pts requiring chronic steroid therapy. **Intranasal:** Relief of seasonal/perennial rhinitis; prevention of nasal polyps from recurring after surgical removal; treatment of nonallergic rhinitis. **Unlabeled: Nasal:** Prophylaxis of seasonal rhinitis.

PRECAUTIONS

CONTRAINDICATIONS: Status asthmaticus, hypersensitivity to beclomethasone. **CAUTIONS:** Cirrhosis, glaucoma, hypothyroidism, untreated systemic infections, osteoporosis, tuberculosis.

LIFESPAN CONSIDERATIONS: Pregnancy/lactation: Unknown if drug crosses placenta or is distributed in breast milk. **Pregnancy Category C. Children:** Prolonged treatment/high dosages may decrease short-term growth rate, cortisol secretion. **Elderly:** No age-related precautions noted.

INTERACTIONS

DRUG: None known. **HERBAL:** None known. **FOOD:** None known. **LAB VALUES:** None known.

AVAILABILITY (Rx)

AEROSOL FOR INHALATION. INTRANASAL: 42 mcg, 84 mcg per spray.

ADMINISTRATION/HANDLING

INHALATION

• Shake container well, exhale completely, place mouthpiece between lips, inhale, hold breath as long as possible before exhaling. • Allow at least 1 min between inhalations. • Rinse mouth after each use to decrease dry mouth, hoarseness.

INTRANASAL

• Clear nasal passages as much as possible. • Insert spray tip into nostril, pointing toward nasal passages, away from nasal septum. • Spray into nostril while holding other nostril closed, concurrently inspire through nose to permit medication as high into nasal passages as possible.

INDICATIONS/ROUTES/DOSAGE

Oral inhalation: ADULTS, ELDERLY CHILDREN ≥12 YRS: 2 puffs 3–4 times/day. **Maximum:** 20 puffs/day. CHILDREN 6–12 YRS: 1–2 puffs 3–4 times/day. **Maximum:** 10 puffs/day.

Nasal inhalation: ADULTS, ELDERLY, CHILDREN >12 YRS: 1–2 sprays in each nostril 2 times/day. CHILDREN 6–12 YRS:

B

1 spray each nostril 2 times/day. May increase up to 2 sprays 2 times/day each nostril.

SIDE EFFECTS

FREQUENT: Inhalation (4%–14%): Throat irritation, dry mouth, hoarseness, cough. **Intranasal:** Burning, dryness inside nose. **OCCASIONAL: Inhalation (2%–3%):** Localized fungal infection (thrush). **Intranasal:** Nasal-crusting nosebleed, sore throat, ulceration of nasal mucosa. **RARE: Inhalation:** Transient bronchospasm, esophageal candidiasis. **Intranasal:** Nasal/pharyngeal candidiasis, eye pain.

ADVERSE REACTIONS/ TOXIC EFFECTS

Acute hypersensitivity reaction (urticaria, angioedema, severe bronchospasm) occurs rarely. Transfer from systemic to local steroid therapy may unmask previously suppressed bronchial asthma condition.

NURSING IMPLICATIONS

BASELINE ASSESSMENT

Question for hypersensitivity to any corticosteroids.

INTERVENTION/EVALUATION

In those receiving bronchodilators by inhalation concomitantly with inhalation of steroid therapy, advise to use bronchodilator several minutes before corticosteroid aerosol (enhances penetration of steroid into bronchial tree).

PATIENT/FAMILY TEACHING

Do not change dose schedule or stop taking drug; must taper off gradually under medical supervision. **Inhalation:** Maintain careful mouth hygiene. Rinse mouth with water immediately after inhalation (prevents mouth/throat dryness, fungal infection of mouth). Contact physician/nurse if sore throat or mouth occurs. **Intranasal:** Contact physician if no improvement in symptoms, sneezing, or nasal irritation occurs. Clear nasal passages prior to use. Improvement noted in several days.

Benadryl

see diphenydramine

benazepril

ben-**ayz**-ah-prill

(Lotensin)

Do not confuse with Benadryl, Loniten, lovastatin.

FIXED-COMBINATION(S)

Lotensin HCT: benazepril/hydrochlorothiazide (a diuretic): 5 mg/625 mg; 10 mg/12.5 mg; 20 mg/12.5 mg; 20 mg/25 mg. **Lotrel:** benazepril/amlodipine (a calcium blocker): 2.5 mg/10 mg; 5 mg/10 mg; 5 mg/20 mg; 10 mg/20 mg.

CLASSIFICATION

PHARMACOTHERAPEUTIC: Angiotensin-converting enzyme (ACE) inhibitor. **CLINICAL:** Antihypertensive (see p. 6C).

ACTION

Decreases rate of conversion of angiotensin I to angiotensin II, a potent vasoconstrictor. Reduces peripheral arterial resistance. **Therapeutic Effect:** Lowers B/P.

PHARMACOKINETICS

Onset	Peak	Duration
PO		
1 hr	2–4 hrs	24 hrs

Partially absorbed from GI tract. Protein

binding: 97%. Metabolized in liver to active metabolite. Primarily excreted in urine. Minimal removal by hemodialysis. **Half-life:** 35 min; metabolite: 10–11 hrs.

USES

Treatment of hypertension. Used alone or in combination with other antihypertensives. **Unlabeled:** Treatment of CHF.

PRECAUTIONS

CONTRAINDICATIONS: History of angioedema with previous treatment with ACE inhibitors. **CAUTIONS:** Renal impairment, sodium depletion, diuretic therapy, dialysis, hypovolemia, coronary or cerebrovascular insufficiency, liver impairment, diabetes mellitus.

LIFESPAN CONSIDERATIONS: Pregnancy/lactation: Crosses placenta. Unknown if distributed in breast milk. May cause fetal-neonatal mortality/morbidity. **Pregnancy Category C** (**D** if used in second or third trimester). **Children:** Safety and efficacy not established. **Elderly:** May be more sensitive to hypotensive effects.

INTERACTIONS

DRUG: **Alcohol, diuretics, hypotensive agents** may increase effects. **NSAIDs** may decrease effect. **Potassium-sparing diuretics, potassium supplements** may cause hyperkalemia. May increase **lithium** concentration, toxicity. **HERBAL:** None known. **FOOD:** None known. **LAB VALUES:** May increase potassium, SGOT (AST), SGPT (ALT), alkaline phosphatase, bilirubin, BUN, creatinine. May decrease sodium. May cause positive ANA titer.

AVAILABILITY (Rx)

TABLETS: 5 mg, 10 mg, 20 mg, 40 mg.

ADMINISTRATION/HANDLING

- May give without regard to food.

INDICATIONS/ROUTES/DOSAGE

HYPERTENSION (used alone)

PO: ADULTS: Initially, 10 mg/day. MAINTENANCE: 20–40 mg/day as single dose. **Maximum:** 80 mg/day.

USUAL ELDERLY DOSAGE

PO: Initially, 5–10 mg/day. RANGE: 20–40 mg/day.

HYPERTENSION (combination therapy)

Alert: Discontinue diuretic 2–3 days prior to initiating benazepril therapy.

PO: ADULTS: Initially, 5 mg/day titrated to pt's needs.

DOSAGE IN RENAL IMPAIRMENT (creatinine clearance <30 ml/min)
Initially, 5 mg/day titrated up to maximum of 40 mg/day.

SIDE EFFECTS

FREQUENT (3%–6%): Cough, headache, dizziness. **OCCASIONAL (2%):** Fatigue, somnolence/drowsiness, nausea. **RARE (<1%):** Skin rash, fever, joint pain, diarrhea, loss of taste.

ADVERSE REACTIONS/ TOXIC EFFECTS

Excessive hypotension ("first-dose syncope") may occur in those with CHF, severe salt/volume depletion. Angioedema (swelling of face/lips), hyperkalemia occur rarely. Agranulocytosis, neutropenia may be noted in those with impaired renal function or collagen vascular disease (systemic lupus erythematosus, scleroderma). Nephrotic syndrome may be noted in pts with history of renal disease.

NURSING IMPLICATIONS

BASELINE ASSESSMENT

Obtain B/P immediately prior to each dose, in addition to regular monitoring (be alert to fluctuations). If excessive reduction in B/P occurs, place pt in supine position with legs elevated. In pts with renal impairment, autoimmune

B

disease, or taking drugs that affect leukocytes or immune response, CBC should be performed before therapy begins and q2wks for 3 mos, then periodically thereafter.

INTERVENTION/EVALUATION

Assist with ambulation if dizziness occurs. Monitor B/P, renal function, urinary protein, leukocyte count.

PATIENT/FAMILY TEACHING

To reduce hypotensive effect, rise slowly from lying to sitting position, permit legs to dangle from bed momentarily before standing. Full therapeutic effect may take 2–4 wks. Skipping doses or noncompliance with drug therapy may produce severe, rebound hypertension.

Benicar

see olmesartan

benzocaine

(Americaine, Anbesol, Cetacaine, Chloraseptic Lozenges, Dermoplast, Hurricane, Orajel)

See Classification section under: Anesthetics: local

benzonatate

ben-**zow**-nah-tate
(Tessalon Perles)

◆ CLASSIFICATION

PHARMACOTHERAPEUTIC: Non-narcotic antitussive. **CLINICAL:** Anticough.

ACTION

Anesthetizes stretch receptors in respiratory passages, lungs, pleura. **Therapeutic Effect:** Reduces cough production.

USES

Relief of nonproductive cough, including acute cough of minor throat/bronchial irritation.

PRECAUTIONS

CONTRAINDICATIONS: None known. **CAUTIONS:** Productive cough. **Pregnancy Category C.**

INTERACTIONS

DRUG: **CNS depressants** may increase effect. **HERBAL:** None known. **FOOD:** None known. **LAB VALUES:** None known.

AVAILABILITY (Rx)

CAPSULES: 100 mg, 200 mg.

ADMINISTRATION/HANDLING

PO

• Give without regard to meals. • Swallow whole, do not chew/dissolve in mouth (may produce temporary local anesthesia/choking).

INDICATIONS/ROUTES/DOSAGE

ANTITUSSIVE

PO: ADULTS, ELDERLY, CHILDREN >10 YRS: 100 mg 3 times/day, up to 600 mg/day.

SIDE EFFECTS

OCCASIONAL: Mild drowsiness, mild dizziness, constipation, GI upset, skin eruptions, nasal congestion.

ADVERSE REACTIONS/ TOXIC EFFECTS

Paradoxical reaction (restlessness, insomnia, euphoria, nervousness, tremors) has been noted.

NURSING IMPLICATIONS

BASELINE ASSESSMENT

Assess type, severity, frequency of cough; monitor amount, color, consistency of sputum.

INTERVENTION/EVALUATION

Initiate deep breathing/coughing exercises, particularly in pts with impaired pulmonary function. Monitor for paradoxical reaction. Increase fluid intake, environmental humidity to lower viscosity of lung secretions. Assess for clinical improvement and record onset of relief of cough.

PATIENT/FAMILY TEACHING

Avoid tasks that require alertness, motor skills until response to drug is established. Dry mouth, drowsiness, dizziness may be an expected response of drug.

benztropine mesylate ℮

benz-**trow**-peen
(Apo-Benztropine♣, Cogentin)

Do not confuse with bromocriptine.

CLASSIFICATION

PHARMACOTHERAPEUTIC: Anticholinergic. **CLINICAL:** Antiparkinson agent.

ACTION

Selectively blocks central cholinergic receptors, assists in balancing cholinergic/dopaminergic activity. **Therapeutic Effect:** Reduces incidence, severity of akinesia, rigidity, tremor.

USES

Treatment of Parkinson's disease, drug-induced extrapyramidal reactions, except tardive dyskinesia.

PRECAUTIONS

CONTRAINDICATIONS: Angle-closure glaucoma, GI obstruction, paralytic ileus, intestinal atony, severe ulcerative colitis, prostatic hypertrophy, myasthenia gravis, megacolon, children <3 yrs. **CAUTIONS:** Treated open-angle glaucoma, heart disease, hypertension; pts with tachycardia, arrhythmias, prostatic hypertrophy, liver/renal impairment, obstructive diseases of the GI/GU tract, urinary retention. **Pregnancy Category C.**

INTERACTIONS

DRUG: **Alcohol, CNS depressants** may increase sedation. **Amantadine, anticholinergics, MAOIs** may increase effects. **Antacids, antidiarrheals** may decrease absorption, effects. **HERBAL:** None known. **FOOD:** None known. **LAB VALUES:** None known.

AVAILABILITY (Rx)

TABLETS: 0.5 mg, 1 mg, 2 mg. **INJECTION:** 1 mg/ml.

INDICATIONS/ROUTES/DOSAGE

PARKINSONISM

PO: ADULTS: 0.5–6 mg/day in 1–2 divided doses. Titrate by 0.5 mg at 5- to 6-day intervals. ELDERLY: Initially, 0.5 mg 1–2 times/day. Titrate by 0.5 mg at 5- to 6-day intervals. **Maximum:** 4 mg/day.

DRUG-INDUCED EXTRAPYRAMIDAL SYMPTOMS

PO/IM: ADULTS: 1–4 mg 1–2 times/day.

ACUTE DYSTONIC REACTIONS

IM/IV: ADULTS: 1–2 mg, then 1–2 mg PO 2 times/day to prevent recurrence.

B

SIDE EFFECTS

Alert: Elderly (>60 yrs) tend to develop mental confusion, disorientation, agitation, psychotic-like symptoms.

FREQUENT: Drowsiness, dry mouth, blurred vision, constipation, decreased sweating/urination, GI upset, photosensitivity. **OCCASIONAL:** Headache, memory loss, muscle cramping, nervousness, peripheral paresthesia, orthostatic hypotension, abdominal cramping. **RARE:** Rash, confusion, eye pain.

ADVERSE REACTIONS/ TOXIC EFFECTS

Overdosage may vary from severe anticholinergic effects (unsteadiness, severe drowsiness, severe dryness of mouth/nose/throat, tachycardia, shortness of breath, skin flushing). Also produces severe paradoxical reaction (hallucinations, tremor, seizures, toxic psychosis).

NURSING IMPLICATIONS

BASELINE ASSESSMENT

Assess mental status for confusion, disorientation, agitation, psychotic-like symptoms (medication frequently produces such side effects in those >60 yrs).

INTERVENTION/EVALUATION

Be alert to neurologic effects: headache, lethargy, mental confusion, agitation. Assess for clinical reversal of symptoms (improvement of tremor of head/hands at rest, masklike facial expression, shuffling gait, muscular rigidity).

PATIENT/FAMILY TEACHING

Avoid tasks that require alertness, motor skills until response to drug is established. Dry mouth, drowsiness, dizziness may be an expected response of drug. Avoid alcoholic beverages during therapy. Drowsiness tends to diminish/disappear with continued therapy.

beractant

burr-**act**-ant
(Survanta)
Do not confuse with Sufenta.

CLASSIFICATION

PHARMACOTHERAPEUTIC: Natural bovine lung extract. **CLINICAL:** Pulmonary surfactant.

ACTION

Lowers surface tension on alveolar surfaces during respiration, stabilizes alveoli vs. collapse that may occur at resting transpulmonary pressures. **Therapeutic Effect:** Replenishes surfactant, restores surface activity to lungs.

PHARMACOKINETICS

Not absorbed systemically.

USES

Prevention/treatment (rescue) of respiratory distress syndrome (RDS—hyaline membrane disease) in premature infants. Oxygenation improves within minutes of administration.

PRECAUTIONS

CONTRAINDICATIONS: None known. **CAUTIONS:** Those at risk for circulatory overload.

LIFESPAN CONSIDERATIONS: Neonate: No age-related precautions noted.

INTERACTIONS

DRUG: None known. **HERBAL:** None known. **FOOD:** None known. **LAB VALUES:** None known.

AVAILABILITY (Rx)

SUSPENSION: 25 mg/ml vial.

ADMINISTRATION/HANDLING

INTRATRACHEAL

Storage • Refrigerate vials. • Warm by standing vial at room temperature for 20 min or warm in hand 8 min. • If settling occurs, gently swirl vial (do not shake) to redisperse. • After warming, may return to refrigerator within 8 hrs one time only. • Each vial should be injected with a needle only one time; discard unused portions. • Color appears off-white to light brown.

Administration • Instill through catheter inserted into infant's endotracheal tube. Do not instill into main stem bronchus. • Monitor for bradycardia, decreased O_2 saturation during administration. Stop dosing procedure if these effects occur; begin appropriate measures before reinstituting therapy.

INDICATIONS/ROUTES/DOSAGE

USUAL DOSAGE

Intratracheal: INFANTS: 100 mg of phospholipids/kg birth weight (4 ml/kg). Give within 15 min of birth if infant <1,250 g with evidence of surfactant deficiency; give within 8 hrs when RDS confirmed by x-ray and requiring mechanical ventilation. May repeat ≥6 hrs after preceding dose. As many as 4 doses may be given during the first 48 hrs of life.

SIDE EFFECTS

FREQUENT: Transient bradycardia, O_2 desaturation; increased CO_2 retention. **OCCASIONAL:** Endotracheal tube reflux. **RARE:** Apnea, endotracheal tube blockage, hypotension/hypertension, pallor, vasoconstriction.

ADVERSE REACTIONS/ TOXIC EFFECTS

Nosocomial sepsis may occur (associated with increased mortality).

NURSING IMPLICATIONS

BASELINE ASSESSMENT

Drug must be administered in highly supervised setting. Clinicians in care of neonate must be experienced with intubation, ventilator management. Offer emotional support to parents.

INTERVENTION/EVALUATION

Monitor infant with arterial or transcutaneous measurement of systemic O_2, CO_2. Assess lung sounds for rales, moist breath sounds.

betamethasone

bay-tah-**meth**-a-sone

(Betaderm✤, Beta-Val, Betnesol✤, Celestone, Diprolene, Diprosone, Luxiq Foam)

FIXED-COMBINATION(S)

Lotrisone: betamethasone/clotrimazole (an antifungal): 0.05%/1%.

◆ CLASSIFICATION

PHARMACOTHERAPEUTIC: Adrenocorticosteroid. **CLINICAL:** Anti-inflammatory, immunosuppressant (see pp. 81C, 84C).

ACTION

Controls rate of protein synthesis; depresses migration of polymorphonuclear leukocytes, fibroblasts; reverses capillary permeability; prevents or controls inflammation. **Therapeutic Effect:** Decreases tissue response to inflammatory process.

USES

Systemic: Anti-inflammatory, immunosuppressant, corticosteroid replacement therapy. **Topical:** Relief of inflammatory and pruritic dermatoses. **Foam:**

Relief of inflammation, itching associated with dermatosis.

PRECAUTIONS

CONTRAINDICATIONS: Hypersensitivity to betamethasone, systemic fungal infections. **CAUTIONS:** Hypothyroidism, cirrhosis, nonspecific ulcerative colitis, pts at increased risk of peptic ulcer. **Pregnancy Category C (D if used in first trimester).**

INTERACTIONS

DRUG: **Amphotericin** may increase hypokalemia. May decrease effect of **oral hypoglycemics, insulin, diuretics, potassium supplements.** May increase **digoxin** toxicity (due to hypokalemia). **Hepatic enzyme inducers** may decrease effect. **Live virus vaccines** may potentiate virus replication, increase vaccine side effects, decrease pt's antibody response to vaccine. **HERBAL:** None known. **FOOD:** None known. **LAB VALUES:** May decrease calcium, potassium, thyroxine. May increase cholesterol, lipids, glucose, sodium, amylase.

AVAILABILITY (Rx)

AEROSOL: 0.1%. **CREAM:** 0.1%, 0.05%. **FOAM:** 0.12% **LOTION:** 0.1%, 0.05%. **OINTMENT:** 0.05%. **SYRUP:** 0.6 mg/5 ml.

ADMINISTRATION/HANDLING

PO

• Give with milk or food (decreases GI upset). • Give single doses prior to 9 AM; multiple doses should be given at evenly spaced intervals.

TOPICAL

• Gently cleanse area prior to application. • Use occlusive dressings only as ordered. • Apply sparingly and rub into area thoroughly. • When using aerosol, spray area 3 sec from 15-cm distance; avoid inhalation.

INDICATIONS/ROUTES/DOSAGE

USUAL DOSAGE

PO: ADULTS, ELDERLY: 0.6–7.2 mg/day. CHILDREN: 0.063–0.25 mg/kg/day in 3–4 divided doses.

Topical: ADULTS, ELDERLY: 2–4 times/day. FOAM: Apply twice daily.

SIDE EFFECTS

FREQUENT: Systemic: Increased appetite, abdominal distention, nervousness, insomnia, false sense of well-being. **Foam:** Burning, stinging, pruritus. **OCCASIONAL: Systemic:** Dizziness, facial flushing, diaphoresis, decreased/blurred vision, mood swings. **Topical:** Allergic contact dermatitis, purpura (blood-containing blisters, thinning of skin with easy bruising), telangiectasis (raised dark red spots on skin).

ADVERSE REACTIONS/TOXIC EFFECTS

When taken in excessive quantities, systemic hypercorticism and adrenal suppression may occur.

NURSING IMPLICATIONS

BASELINE ASSESSMENT

Question for hypersensitivity to any of the corticosteroids, sulfite. Obtain baselines for height, weight, B/P, glucose, electrolytes. Check results of initial tests (TB skin test, x-rays, EKG).

INTERVENTION/EVALUATION

Monitor B/P, blood glucose, electrolytes. Apply topical preparation sparingly. Not for use on broken skin or in areas of infection. Do not apply to wet skin, face, inguinal areas.

PATIENT/FAMILY TEACHING

Take with food, milk. Take single daily dose in the morning. Do not stop abruptly. Apply topical preparations in a thin layer.

betaxolol

beh-**tax**-oh-lol
(Betoptic-S, Kerlone)
Do not confuse with bethanechol.

CLASSIFICATION

PHARMACOTHERAPEUTIC: Beta-adrenergic blocker. **CLINICAL:** Antihypertensive; antiglaucoma (see pp. 45C, 61C).

ACTION

Blocks $beta_1$-adrenergic receptors in cardiac tissue. Reduces aqueous humor production. **Therapeutic Effect:** Slows sinus heart rate, decreases B/P. Reduces intraocular pressure (IOP).

USES

Ophthalmic: Treatment of chronic open-angle glaucoma, ocular hypertension. **Systemic:** Management of hypertension. **Unlabeled:** With miotics, decreases IOP in acute/chronic angle-closure glaucoma, treatment of secondary glaucoma, malignant glaucoma, angle-closure glaucoma during/after iridectomy.

PRECAUTIONS

CONTRAINDICATIONS: Sinus bradycardia, overt cardiac failure, cardiogenic shock, heart block greater than first degree. **CAUTIONS:** Impaired renal or hepatic function, peripheral vascular disease, hyperthyroidism, diabetes, inadequate cardiac function. **Pregnancy Category C (D** if used in second or third trimester).

INTERACTIONS

DRUG: Diuretics, other hypotensives may increase hypotensive effect; **sympathomimetics, xanthines** may mutually inhibit effect; may mask symptoms of hypoglycemia, prolong hypoglycemic effect of **insulin, oral hypoglycemics; NSAIDs** may decrease antihypertensive effect; **cimetidine** may increase concentration. **HERBAL:** None known. **FOOD:** None known. **LAB VALUES:** May increase ANA titer, BUN, creatinine, potassium, uric acid, lipoproteins, triglycerides.

AVAILABILITY (Rx)

TABLETS: 10 mg, 20 mg. **OPHTHALMIC SOLUTION:** 0.5%. **OPHTHALMIC SUSPENSION:** 0.25%.

INDICATIONS/ROUTES/DOSAGE

HYPERTENSION

PO: ADULTS: Initially, 10 mg/day alone or added to diuretic therapy. Dose may be doubled if no response in 7–14 days. If used alone, addition of another antihypertensive to be considered.

USUAL ELDERLY DOSAGE

PO: Initially, 5 mg/day.

DOSAGE IN RENAL IMPAIRMENT (dialysis)

Initially, 5 mg/day, increase by 5 mg/day q2wks. **Maximum:** 20 mg/day.

GLAUCOMA

Eyedrops: ADULTS, ELDERLY: 1 drop 2 times/day.

SIDE EFFECTS

Generally well tolerated, with mild and transient side effects. **FREQUENT: Systemic:** Hypotension manifested as dizziness, nausea, diaphoresis, headache, fatigue, constipation/diarrhea; shortness of breath. **Ophthalmic:** Eye irritation, visual disturbances. **OCCASIONAL: Systemic:** Insomnia, flatulence, urinary frequency, impotence/decreased libido. **Ophthalmic:** Increased light sensitivity, watering of eye. **RARE: Systemic:** Rash, arrhythmias, arthralgia, myalgia, confusion, change in taste, increased urina-

B

tion. **Ophthalmic:** Dry eye, conjunctivitis, eye pain.

ADVERSE REACTIONS/ TOXIC EFFECTS

Oral form may produce profound bradycardia, hypotension, bronchospasm. Abrupt withdrawal may result in sweating, palpitations, headache, tremulousness. May precipitate CHF, MI in those with cardiac disease; thyroid storm in those with thyrotoxicosis; peripheral ischemia in those with existing peripheral vascular disease. Hypoglycemia may occur in previously controlled diabetics. Ophthalmic overdosage may produce bradycardia, hypotension, bronchospasm, acute cardiac failure.

NURSING IMPLICATIONS

BASELINE ASSESSMENT

PO: Assess baseline renal/liver function tests. Assess B/P, apical pulse immediately before drug is administered (if pulse is ≤60/min or systolic B/P is <90 mm Hg, withhold medication, contact physician).

INTERVENTION/EVALUATION

Monitor B/P for hypotension. Assess pulse for quality, irregular rate, bradycardia. Monitor daily bowel/stool activity. Assist with ambulation if dizziness occurs. Assess for evidence of CHF: dyspnea (particularly on exertion or lying down), night cough, peripheral edema, distended neck veins, increase in weight, decrease in urine output. Assess for nausea, diaphoresis, headache, fatigue.

PATIENT/FAMILY TEACHING

Do not abruptly discontinue medication. Compliance with therapy regimen is essential to control glaucoma, hypertension. To avoid hypotensive effect, rise slowly from lying to sitting position, wait momentarily before standing. Avoid tasks that require alertness, motor skills until response to drug is established. Report shortness of breath, excessive fatigue, prolonged dizziness, headache. Do not use nasal decongestants, OTC cold preparations (stimulants) without physician approval. Restrict salt, alcohol intake.

bethanechol chloride

be-**than**-eh-coal
(Duvoid✱, Myotonachol✱, Urecholine)

Do not confuse with betaxolol.

◆ CLASSIFICATION

PHARMACOTHERAPEUTIC: Cholinergic (see p. 79C).

ACTION

Acts directly at cholinergic receptors of smooth muscle of urinary bladder, GI tract. Increases tone of detrusor muscle. **Therapeutic Effect:** May initiate micturition, bladder emptying. Stimulates gastric, intestinal motility.

USES

Treatment of nonobstructive urinary retention, retention due to neurogenic bladder. **Unlabeled:** Treatment of postop gastric atony, congenital megacolon, gastroesophageal reflux.

PRECAUTIONS

CONTRAINDICATIONS: Hyperthyroidism, peptic ulcer, latent or active bronchial asthma, mechanical GI/urinary obstruction, recent GI resection, acute inflammatory GI tract conditions, anastomosis, bladder wall instability, pronounced bradycardia, hypotension, hypertension, cardiac disease, coronary artery disease, vasomotor instability, epilepsy, parkinsonism. **CAUTIONS:** None known. **Pregnancy Category C.**

INTERACTIONS

DRUG: Cholinesterase inhibitors may increase effects/toxicity. **Procainamide, quinidine** may decrease effect. **HERBAL:** None known. **FOOD:** None known. **LAB VALUES:** May increase amylase, lipase, SGOT (AST).

AVAILABILITY (Rx)

TABLETS: 5 mg, 10 mg, 25 mg, 50 mg. **INJECTION:** 5 mg/ml.

INDICATIONS/ROUTES/DOSAGE

POSTOP/POSTPARTUM URINARY RETENTION, ATONY OF BLADDER

PO: ADULTS, ELDERLY: 10–50 mg 3–4 times/day. Minimum effective dose determined by initially giving 5–10 mg, and repeating same amount at 1-hr intervals until desired response achieved, or maximum of 50 mg reached. CHILDREN: 0.6 mg/kg/day in 3–4 divided doses.

Subcutaneous: ADULTS, ELDERLY: Initially, 2.5–5 mg. Minimum effective dose determined by giving 2.5 mg (0.5 ml), repeating same amount at 15- to 30-min intervals up to a maximum of 4 doses. Minimum dose repeated 3–4 times/day. CHILDREN: 0.2 mg/kg/day in 3–4 divided doses.

SIDE EFFECTS

Alert: Effects more noticeable with subcutaneous administration.

OCCASIONAL: Belching, change in vision, blurred vision, diarrhea, frequent urinary urgency. **RARE: Subcutaneous:** Shortness of breath, chest tightness, bronchospasm.

ADVERSE REACTIONS/ TOXIC EFFECTS

Overdosage produces CNS stimulation (insomnia, nervousness, orthostatic hypotension), cholinergic stimulation (headache, increased salivation/sweating, nausea, vomiting, flushed skin, stomach pain, seizures).

NURSING IMPLICATIONS

BASELINE ASSESSMENT

Violent cholinergic reaction if given IM or IV (circulatory collapse, severe hypotension, bloody diarrhea, shock, cardiac arrest). **Antidote:** 0.6–1.2 mg atropine sulfate.

INTERVENTION/EVALUATION

Assess for cholinergic reaction: GI discomfort/cramping, feeling of facial warmth, excessive salivation and sweating, lacrimation, pallor, urinary urgency, blurred vision. Question for complaints of difficulty chewing, swallowing, progressive muscle weakness (see Adverse Reactions/Toxic Effects).

PATIENT/FAMILY TEACHING

Report nausea, vomiting, diarrhea, sweating, increased salivary secretions, irregular heartbeat, muscle weakness, severe abdominal pain, difficulty in breathing.

bexarotene

becks-**aye**-row-teen
(Targretin)

CLASSIFICATION

PHARMACOTHERAPEUTIC: Retinoid. **CLINICAL:** Antineoplastic (see p. 69C).

ACTION

Binds to and activates retinoid X receptor subtypes that regulate the genes that control cellular differentiation and proliferation. **Therapeutic Effect:** Inhib-

B

its growth of tumor cell lines of hematopoietic and squamous cell and induces tumor regression.

PHARMACOKINETICS

Metabolized in liver. Moderately absorbed from GI tract. Protein binding: >99%. Primarily eliminated through hepatobiliary system. **Half-life:** 7 hrs.

USES

Treatment of cutaneous T-cell lymphoma (CTCL) in those refractory to at least one prior systemic therapy. **Unlabeled:** Treatment of diabetes mellitus; head, neck, lung, renal cell carcinomas; Kaposi's sarcoma.

PRECAUTONS

CONTRAINDICATIONS: None known. **CAUTIONS:** Liver impairment, diabetes mellitus, lipid abnormalities.

LIFESPAN CONSIDERATIONS: Pregnancy/lactation: May cause fetal harm. Unknown if distributed in breast milk. **Pregnancy Category X. Children:** Safety and efficacy not established. **Elderly:** No age-related precautions noted.

INTERACTIONS

DRUG: **Phenytoin, rifampin** may decrease concentrations. **Erythromycin, ketoconazole, itraconazole** may increase concentrations; bexarotene may enhance effect of **antidiabetic agents.** **HERBAL:** None known. **FOOD: Grapefruit juice** may increase concentration/toxicity. **LAB VALUES:** CA-125 in ovarian cancer may be increased. May produce abnormal liver function tests; increase cholesterol, triglycerides, total and LDL cholesterol; decrease HDL cholesterol.

AVAILABILITY (Rx)

CAPSULES (soft gelatin): 75 mg.

ADMINISTRATION/HANDLING

PO

- Give with food.

INDICATIONS/ROUTES/DOSAGE

CTCL

PO: ADULTS: 300 mg/m^2/day. If no response and initial dose well tolerated, may be increased to 400 mg/m^2/day. If not tolerated, may decrease to 200 mg/m^2/day or 100 mg/m^2/day.

SIDE EFFECTS

FREQUENT: Hyperlipemia (79%), headache (30%), hypothyroidism (29%), asthenia (loss of strength and energy) (20%). **OCCASIONAL:** Rash (17%); nausea (15%); peripheral edema (13%); dry skin, abdominal pain (11%); chills, exfoliative dermatitis (10%); diarrhea (7%).

ADVERSE REACTIONS/ TOXIC EFFECTS

Pancreatitis, liver failure, pneumonia occur rarely.

NURSING IMPLICATIONS

BASELINE ASSESSMENT

Assess baseline lipid profile, WBC, liver function, thyroid function. Question about possibility of pregnancy (Pregnancy Category X). Warn women of childbearing age about potential fetal risk if pregnancy occurs. Instruct in need for use of 2 reliable forms of contraceptives concurrently during therapy and for 1 mo after discontinuation of therapy, even in infertile, premenopausal woman.

INTERVENTION/EVALUATION

Monitor cholesterol, triglycerides, liver and thyroid function tests, CBC.

PATIENT/FAMILY TEACHING

Do not use medicated, drying, abrasive soaps; wash with bland soap. Inform physician if you are pregnant or are planning to become pregnant (Pregnancy Category X).

Bextra

see valdecoxib

Biaxin

see clarithromycin

bicalutamide

by-kale-**yew**-tah-myd
(Casodex)

CLASSIFICATION

PHARMACOTHERAPEUTIC: Antiandrogen hormone. **CLINICAL:** Antineoplastic (see p. 69C).

ACTION

Competitively inhibits androgen action by binding to androgen receptors in target tissue. **Therapeutic Effect:** Decreases growth of prostatic carcinoma.

PHARMACOKINETICS

Well absorbed from GI tract. Protein binding: 96%. Metabolized in liver to inactive metabolite. Excreted in urine, feces. Not removed by hemodialysis. **Half-life:** 5.8 days.

USES

Treatment of advanced metastatic prostatic carcinoma (in combination with luteinizing hormone-releasing hormone [LHRH] agonistic analogues—i.e., leuprolide). Treatment with both drugs must be started at same time.

PRECAUTIONS

CONTRAINDICATIONS: None known. **CAUTIONS:** Moderate to severe liver impairment.

LIFESPAN CONSIDERATIONS: Pregnancy/lactation: May inhibit spermatogenesis, not used in women. **Pregnancy Category X. Children:** Safety and efficacy not established. **Elderly:** No age-related precautions noted.

INTERACTIONS

DRUG: May displace **warfarin** from protein-binding sites, increase warfarin effect. **HERBAL:** None known. **FOOD:** None known. **LAB VALUES:** May increase SGOT (AST), SGPT (ALT), alkaline phosphatase, serum creatinine, bilirubin, BUN. May increase WBC, Hgb.

AVAILABILITY (Rx)

TABLETS: 50 mg.

ADMINISTRATION/HANDLING

PO

- May be given without regard to food.
- Take at same time each day.

INDICATIONS/ROUTES/DOSAGE

PROSTATIC CARCINOMA

PO: ADULTS, ELDERLY: 50 mg once daily (morning or evening). Use concurrently with an LHRH analogue or after surgical castration.

SIDE EFFECTS

FREQUENT: Hot flashes (49%), breast pain (38%), muscle pain (27%), constipation (17%), diarrhea (10%), asthenia (15%), nausea (11%). **OCCASIONAL (8%–9%):** Nocturia, abdominal pain, peripheral edema. **RARE (3%–7%):** Vomiting, weight loss, dizziness, insomnia, rash, impotence, gynecomastia.

ADVERSE REACTIONS/ TOXIC EFFECTS

Sepsis, CHF, hypertension, iron deficiency anemia may be noted.

B

NURSING IMPLICATIONS

INTERVENTION/EVALUATION

Check for diarrhea, nausea, vomiting.

PATIENT/FAMILY TEACHING

Do not stop taking medication (both drugs must be continued). Take medications at same time each day. Explain possible expectancy of frequent side effects. Contact physician for persistent nausea/vomiting.

bimatoprost

(Lumigan)

See Classification section under: Antiglaucoma agents (p. 45C)

bisacodyl

bise-ah-**co**-dahl

(Apo-Bisacodyl✱, Dulcolax)

◆CLASSIFICATION

PHARMACOTHERAPEUTIC: GI stimulant. **CLINICAL:** Laxative (see p. 105C).

ACTION

Direct effect on colonic smooth musculature (stimulates intramural nerve plexi). **Therapeutic Effect:** Promotes fluid and ion accumulation in colon to increase peristalsis, laxative effect.

PHARMACOKINETICS

Onset	Peak	Duration
PO		
6–12 hrs	—	—
Rectal		
15–60 min	—	—

Minimal absorption following PO, rectal administration. Absorbed drug excreted in urine; remainder eliminated in feces.

USES

Treatment of constipation, colonic evacuation before examinations/procedures.

PRECAUTIONS

CONTRAINDICATIONS: Abdominal pain, nausea, vomiting, appendicitis, intestinal obstruction, undiagnosed rectal bleeding. **CAUTIONS:** Excessive use may lead to fluid, electrolyte imbalance.

LIFESPAN CONSIDERATIONS: Pregnancy/lactation: Unknown if drug crosses placenta or is distributed in breast milk. **Pregnancy Category C. Children:** Avoid in children <6 yrs (usually unable to describe symptoms or more severe side effects). **Elderly:** Repeated use may cause weakness, orthostatic hypotension due to electrolyte loss.

INTERACTIONS

DRUG: Antacids, cimetidine, ranitidine, famotidine; milk may cause rapid dissolution of bisacodyl (produces abdominal cramping, vomiting). May decrease transit time of concurrently administered PO medication, decreasing absorption. **HERBAL:** None known. **FOOD:** None known. **LAB VALUES:** None known.

AVAILABILITY (OTC)

TABLETS (enteric-coated): 5 mg. **SUPPOSITORY:** 10 mg.

ADMINISTRATION/HANDLING

PO

• Give on empty stomach (faster action). • Offer 6–8 glasses of water/day (aids stool softening). • Administer tablets whole; do not chew or crush. • Avoid giving within 1 hr of antacids, milk, other oral medication.

RECTAL

• If suppository is too soft, chill for 30

min in refrigerator or run cold water over foil wrapper. • Moisten suppository with cold water before inserting well into rectum.

INDICATIONS/ROUTES/DOSAGE

LAXATIVE

PO: ADULTS: 5–15 mg as needed. CHILDREN 3–12 YRS: 5–10 mg (0.3 mg/kg) at bedtime or after breakfast.

Rectal: ADULTS, CHILDREN ≥12 YRS: 10 mg to induce bowel movement. CHILDREN 2–11 YRS: 5–10 mg as a single dose. CHILDREN <2 YRS: 5 mg.

USUAL ELDERLY DOSAGE

PO: Initially, 5 mg/day.

Rectal: 5–10 mg/day.

SIDE EFFECTS

FREQUENT: Some degree of abdominal discomfort, nausea, mild cramps, faintness. **OCCASIONAL:** Rectal administration may produce burning of rectal mucosa, mild proctitis.

ADVERSE REACTIONS/ TOXIC EFFECTS

Long-term use may result in laxative dependence, chronic constipation, loss of normal bowel function. Chronic use or overdosage may result in electrolyte disturbances (hypokalemia, hypocalcemia, metabolic acidosis, alkalosis), persistent diarrhea, malabsorption, weight loss. Electrolyte disturbance may produce vomiting, muscle weakness.

NURSING IMPLICATIONS

INTERVENTION/EVALUATION

Encourage adequate fluid intake. Assess bowel sounds for peristalsis. Monitor daily bowel activity, stool consistency (watery, loose, soft, semisolid, solid); record time of evacuation. Assess for abdominal disturbances. Monitor serum electrolytes in those exposed to prolonged, frequent, or excessive use of medication.

PATIENT/FAMILY TEACHING

Institute measures to promote defecation: increase fluid intake, exercise, high-fiber diet. Do not take antacids, milk, or other medication within 1 hr of taking medication (decreased effectiveness). Report unrelieved constipation, rectal bleeding, muscle pain/cramps, dizziness, weakness.

bismuth subsalicylate

bis-muth sub-sal-**ih**-sah-late (Bismed ✤, Pepto-Bismol)

FIXED-COMBINATION(S)

Helidac: bismuth/metronidazole/tetracycline: 262 mg/250 mg/500 mg.

CLASSIFICATION

PHARMACOTHERAPEUTIC: Antisecretory, antimicrobial. **CLINICAL:** Antidiarrheal, antinauseant, antiulcer (see p. 41C).

ACTION

Absorbs water, toxins in large intestine, forms a protective coat in intestinal mucosa. Also possesses antisecretory and antimicrobial effects. **Therapeutic Effect:** Prevents diarrhea.

USES

Treatment of diarrhea, indigestion, nausea, traveler's diarrhea. Adjunct in treatment of *H. pylori*–associated peptic ulcer disease. **Unlabeled:** Prevents traveler's diarrhea.

B

PRECAUTIONS

CONTRAINDICATIONS: Bleeding ulcers, hemorrhagic states, gout, hemophilia, renal function impairment. **CAUTIONS:** Elderly, diabetic pts. **Pregnancy Category C.**

INTERACTIONS

DRUG: **Anticoagulants, heparin, thrombolytics** may increase risk of bleeding. Large dose may increase **oral hypoglycemic, insulin** effects. **Other salicylates** may increase toxicity. May decrease absorption of **tetracyclines.** **HERBAL:** None known. **FOOD:** None known. **LAB VALUES:** May alter SGOT (AST), SGPT (ALT), alkaline phosphatase, uric acid. May decrease potassium. May prolong prothrombin time.

AVAILABILITY (OTC)

TABLETS: 262 mg. **TABLETS (chewable):** 262 mg, 300 mg. **SUSPENSION:** 262 mg/5 ml, 525 mg/5 ml.

INDICATIONS/ROUTES/DOSAGE

DIARRHEA, GASTRIC DISTRESS

PO: ADULTS, ELDERLY: 2 tablets (30 ml) q30–60min up to 8 doses/24 hrs. CHILDREN 9–12 YRS: 1 tablet or 15 ml q30–60min up to 8 doses/24 hrs. CHILDREN 6–9 YRS: ⅔ tablet or 10 ml q30–60min up to 8 doses/24 hrs. CHILDREN 3–6 YRS: ⅓ tablet or 5 ml q30–60min up to 8 doses/24 hrs.

H. PYLORI–ASSOCIATED DUODENAL ULCER, GASTRITIS

PO: ADULTS, ELDERLY: 525 mg 4 times/day (with 500 mg amoxicillin and 500 mg metronidazole 3 times/day after meals) for 7–14 days.

SIDE EFFECTS

FREQUENT: Grayish black stools. **RARE:** Constipation.

ADVERSE REACTIONS/ TOXIC EFFECTS

Debilitated pts and infants may develop impaction.

NURSING IMPLICATIONS

INTERVENTION/EVALUATION

Encourage adequate fluid intake. Assess bowel sounds for peristaltic activity. Monitor stool frequency, consistency (watery, loose, soft, semisolid, solid).

PATIENT/FAMILY TEACHING

Stool may appear gray/black. Chew tablets thoroughly before swallowing.

bisoprolol fumarate

bye-**sew**-prow-lol
(Zebeta)
Do not confuse with DiaBeta.

FIXED-COMBINATION(S)

Ziac: bisoprolol/hydrochlorothiazide (a diuretic): 2.5 mg/6.25 mg; 5 mg/6.25 mg; 10 mg/6.25 mg.

◆CLASSIFICATION

PHARMACOTHERAPEUTIC: Beta-adrenergic blocker. **CLINICAL:** Antihypertensive (see p. 62C).

ACTION

Blocks $beta_1$-adrenergic receptors in cardiac tissue. **Therapeutic Effect:** Slows sinus heart rate, decreases B/P.

PHARMACOKINETICS

Well absorbed from GI tract. Protein binding: 26%–33%. Metabolized in liver. Primarily excreted in urine. Not removed by hemodialysis. **Half-life:** 9–12 hrs (half-life increased in impaired renal function).

B

USES

Management of hypertension, alone or in combination with diuretics, other medications. **Unlabeled:** Angina pectoris, supraventricular arrhythmias, premature ventricular contractions (PVCs).

PRECAUTIONS

CONTRAINDICATIONS: Overt cardiac failure, cardiogenic shock, heart block greater than first degree. **CAUTIONS:** Impaired renal or hepatic function, peripheral vascular disease, hyperthyroidism, diabetes, inadequate cardiac function, bronchospastic disease.

LIFESPAN CONSIDERATIONS: Pregnancy/lactation: Readily crosses placenta; distributed in breast milk. Avoid use during first trimester. May produce bradycardia, apnea, hypoglycemia, hypothermia during delivery, low birth-weight infants. **Pregnancy Category C.** (**D** if used in second or third trimester). **Children:** Safety and efficacy not established. **Elderly:** Age-related peripheral vascular disease may increase risk of decreased peripheral circulation.

INTERACTIONS

DRUG: **Diuretics, other hypotensives** may increase hypotensive effect; **sympathomimetics, xanthines** may mutually inhibit effects; may mask symptoms of hypoglycemia, prolong hypoglycemic effect of **insulin, oral hypoglycemics; NSAIDs** may decrease antihypertensive effect; **cimetidine** may increase concentration. **HERBAL:** None known. **FOOD:** None known. **LAB VALUES:** May increase ANA titer, BUN, creatinine, potassium, uric acid, lipoproteins, triglycerides.

AVAILABILITY (Rx)

TABLETS: 5 mg, 10 mg.

ADMINISTRATION/HANDLING

PO

- May give without regard to food.
- Scored tablet may be crushed.

INDICATIONS/ROUTES/DOSAGE

HYPERTENSION

PO: ADULTS: Initially, 5 mg/day. May increase up to 20 mg/day. ELDERLY: Initially, 2.5–5 mg/day. May increase by 2.5–5 mg/day. **Maximum:** 20 mg/day.

DOSAGE IN RENAL/HEPATIC IMPAIRMENT

Creatinine Clearance	Dosage
<40 ml/min	Initially, 2.5 mg/day Increase cautiously

SIDE EFFECTS

FREQUENT: Hypotension manifested as dizziness, nausea, diaphoresis, headache, cold extremities, fatigue, constipation/diarrhea. **OCCASIONAL:** Insomnia, flatulence, urinary frequency, impotence/decreased libido. **RARE:** Rash, arthralgia, myalgia, confusion (esp. elderly), change in taste.

ADVERSE REACTIONS/ TOXIC EFFECTS

Overdosage may produce profound bradycardia, hypotension. Abrupt withdrawal may result in sweating, palpitations, headache, tremulousness. May precipitate CHF, MI in those with cardiac disease; thyroid storm in those with thyrotoxicosis; peripheral ischemia in those with existing peripheral vascular disease. Hypoglycemia may occur in previously controlled diabetics. Thrombocytopenia (unusual bruising, bleeding) occurs rarely.

NURSING IMPLICATIONS

BASELINE ASSESSMENT

Assess baseline renal/liver function tests. Assess B/P, apical pulse immediately before drug is administered (if

B

pulse is ≤60/min or systolic B/P is <90 mm Hg, withhold medications, contact physician).

INTERVENTION/EVALUATION

Assess pulse for quality, irregular rate, bradycardia. Assist with ambulation if dizziness occurs. Assess for peripheral edema of hands, feet (usually, first area of lower extremity swelling is behind medial malleolus in ambulatory, sacral area in bedridden). Monitor stool frequency, consistency.

PATIENT/FAMILY TEACHING

Do not abruptly discontinue medication. Compliance with therapy regimen is essential to control hypertension. If dizziness occurs, sit or lie down immediately. Avoid tasks that require alertness, motor skills until response to drug is established. Teach pts how to take pulse properly before each dose and to report excessively slow pulse rate (<60 beats/min), peripheral numbness, dizziness. Do not use nasal decongestants, OTC cold preparations (stimulants) without physician approval. Restrict salt, alcohol intake.

bivalirudin

bye-**vail**-ih-rhu-din
(Angiomax)

CLASSIFICATION

PHARMACOTHERAPEUTIC: Thrombin inhibitor. **CLINICAL:** Anticoagulant.

ACTION

Specifically and reversibly inhibits thrombin by binding to its receptor sites. **Therapeutic Effect:** Decreases acute ischemic complications in pts with unstable angina pectoris.

PHARMACOKINETICS

Onset	Peak	Duration
IV		
Immediate	—	1 hr

Primarily eliminated by kidneys. **Half-life:** 25 min (half-life increased with moderate to severe renal function); 25% is removed by hemodialysis.

USES

Anticoagulant in pts with unstable angina undergoing percutaneous transluminal coronary angioplasty (PTCA).

PRECAUTIONS

CONTRAINDICATIONS: Active major bleeding. **CAUTIONS:** Conditions associated with increased risk of bleeding (e.g., bacterial endocarditis, recent major bleeding, cerebrovascular accident [CVA], stroke, intracerebral surgery, hemorrhagic diathesis, severe hypertension, severe renal/liver function impairment, recent major surgery).

LIFESPAN CONSIDERATIONS: Pregnancy/lactation: Unknown if distributed in breast milk or crosses placenta. **Pregnancy Category B. Children:** Safety and efficacy not established. **Elderly:** Age-related renal function impairment may require dosage adjustment.

INTERACTIONS

DRUG: Warfarin, platelet aggregation inhibitors other than aspirin, **thrombolytics** may increase risk of bleeding complications. **HERBAL: Ginkgo biloba** may increase risk of bleeding. **FOOD:** None known. **LAB VALUES:** Prolongs aPTT, PT time.

AVAILABILITY (Rx)

INJECTION, LYOPHILIZED: 250 mg.

ADMINISTRATION/HANDLING

IV

Storage • Store unreconstituted vials at room temperature. • Reconstituted solution may be refrigerated for ≤24 hrs. • Diluted drug with a concentration of 0.5–5 mg/ml is stable at room temperature for ≤24 hrs.

Reconstitution • To each 250-mg vial add 5 ml Sterile Water for Injection. • Gently swirl until all material is dissolved. • Further dilute each vial in 50 ml D_5W or 0.9% NaCl to yield final concentration of 5 mg/ml (1 vial in 50 ml, 2 vials in 100 ml, 5 vials in 250 ml). • If low-rate infusion is used after the initial infusion, reconstitute the 250-mg vial with added 5 ml Sterile Water for Injection. • Gently swirl until all material is dissolved. • Further dilute each vial in 500 ml D_5W or 0.9% NaCl to yield final concentration of 0.5 mg/ml. • Produces a clear, colorless solution (do not use if cloudy or contains a precipitate).

Rate of administration • Adjust IV infusion based on APTT or pt's body weight.

IV INCOMPATIBILITY

Do not mix with any other medication.

INDICATIONS/ROUTES/DOSAGE

Alert: Intended for use with aspirin (300–325 mg daily).

ANTICOAGULANT

Alert: Treatment should be initiated just prior to angioplasty.

IV: ADULTS, ELDERLY: 1 mg/kg given as IV bolus followed by a 4-hr IV infusion at rate of 2.5 mg/kg/hr. After initial 4-hr infusion is completed, give additional IV infusion at rate of 0.2 mg/kg/hr for ≤20 hrs, if necessary.

DOSAGE IN RENAL IMPAIRMENT

GFR (ml/min)	Dosage Reduced by
30–59	20%
10–29	60%
Dialysis	90%

SIDE EFFECTS

FREQUENT (42%): Back pain. **OCCASIONAL (12%–15%):** Nausea, headache, hypotension, generalized pain. **RARE (4%–8%):** Injection site pain, insomnia, hypertension, anxiety, vomiting, pelvic/abdominal pain, bradycardia, nervousness, dyspepsia, fever, urinary retention.

ADVERSE REACTIONS/ TOXIC EFFECTS

Hemorrhagic event occurs rarely and is characterized by fall in B/P or Hct.

NURSING IMPLICATIONS

BASELINE ASSESSMENT

Assess CBC, bleeding time, renal function. Determine initial B/P.

INTERVENTION/EVALUATION

Monitor aPTT, Hct, urine/stool culture for occult blood, renal function studies. Assess for decrease in B/P, increase in pulse rate. Question for increase in amount of discharge during menses. Assess urine for hematuria.

black cohosh

Also known as baneberry, bugbane, bugwort, fairy candles (Black Cohosh Softgel, Remifemin)

CLASSIFICATION

HERBAL.

ACTION

Mechanism of action unknown. A phytoestrogen that may have estrogen-like

B

effects. **Effect:** Reduces symptoms of menopause (e.g., hot flashes).

USES

Treatment of symptoms of menopause, inducing labor in pregnant women. May reduce lipids and/or blood pressure (esp. when combined with prescription medications). Mild sedative action.

PRECAUTIONS

CONTRAINDICATIONS: Pregnancy (has menstrual and uterine stimulant effects that may increase risk of miscarriage). Not to be taken for >6 mos. **CAUTIONS:** Pts with breast, uterine, ovarian cancer; endometriosis; uterine fibroids.

LIFESPAN CONSIDERATIONS: Pregnancy/lactation: Contraindicated. **Children:** Safety and efficacy not established. **Elderly:** No age-related precautions noted.

INTERACTIONS

DRUG: May have additive antiproliferative effect with **tamoxifen.** May increase action of **antihypertensives. HERBAL:** None known. **FOOD:** None known. **LAB VALUES:** May decrease serum LH concentration.

AVAILABILITY

CAPSULES (soft gelatin): 40 mg. **TABLETS:** 20 mg.

INDICATIONS/ROUTES/DOSAGE

MENOPAUSE, INDUCING LABOR, LIPIDS AND/OR B/P, SEDATIVE

PO: ADULTS, ELDERLY: 20–80 mg 2 times/day.

SIDE EFFECTS

Nausea, headache, dizziness, increase in weight, visual changes, migraines.

ADVERSE REACTIONS/ TOXIC EFFECTS

Overdosage may cause nausea/vomiting, decreased heart rate, diaphoresis.

NURSING IMPLICATIONS

BASELINE ASSESSMENT

Assess if pt is pregnant/breast-feeding (contraindicated).

INTERVENTION/EVALUATION

Monitor B/P, lipid levels.

PATIENT/FAMILY TEACHING

Inform physician if pregnancy occurs or planning to become pregnant, breast-feeding. Do not take for >6 mos.

bleomycin sulfate

blee-oh-**my**-sin
(Blenoxane)

CLASSIFICATION

PHARMACOTHERAPEUTIC: Glycopeptide antibiotic. **CLINICAL:** Antineoplastic, sclerosing agent (see p. 70C).

ACTION

Mechanism of action unknown. Most effective in G_2 phase of cell division. **Therapeutic Effect:** Appears to inhibit DNA synthesis and, to a lesser extent, RNA, protein synthesis.

USES

Treatment of lymphomas: Hodgkin's disease, reticulum cell sarcoma, lymphosarcoma and squamous cell carcinomas: head and neck, including mouth, tongue, tonsil, nasopharynx, oropharynx, sinus, palate, lip, buccal mucosa, gingiva, epiglottis, larynx. Treatment of testicular carcinoma, choriocarcinoma. Treatment of malignant pleural effusions, prevention of recurrent pleural effusions. **Unlabeled:** Treatment of renal carcinoma, soft tissue sarcoma, osteosarcoma, ovarian tumors, mycosis fungoides.

PRECAUTIONS

CONTRAINDICATIONS: Previous allergic reaction. **CAUTION:** Severe renal/pulmonary impairment. **Pregnancy Category D.**

INTERACTIONS

DRUG: **Other antineoplastics** may increase toxicity. **Cisplatin**-induced renal impairment may decrease clearance, increase toxicity. **HERBAL:** None known. **FOOD:** None known. **LAB VALUES:** None known.

AVAILABILITY (Rx)

POWDER FOR INJECTION: 15 units, 30 units.

ADMINISTRATION/HANDLING

Alert: May be carcinogenic, mutagenic, or teratogenic. Handle with extreme care during preparation/administration.

Storage • Refrigerate powder. • After reconstitution with 0.9% NaCl, solution is stable for 24 hrs at room temperature.

SUBCUTANEOUS/IM

Reconstitution • Reconstitute 15-unit vial with 1–5 ml (30-unit vial with 2–10 ml) Sterile Water for Injection, 0.9% NaCl injection, or Bacteriostatic Water for Injection to provide concentration of 3–15 units/ml. Do not use D_5W.

IV

Reconstitution • Reconstitute 15-unit vial with at least 5 ml (30-unit vial with at least 10 ml) 0.9% NaCl to provide a concentration not greater than 3 unit/ml.

Rate of administration • Administer over at least 10 min for IV injection.

∅ IV INCOMPATIBILITY

None known via Y-site administration.

IV COMPATIBILITIES

Cefepime (Maxipime), dacarbazine (DTIC), dexamethasone (Decadron), diphenhydramine (Benadryl), fludarabine (Fludara), gemcitabine (Gemzar), ondansetron (Zofran), paclitaxel (Taxol), piperacillin/tazobactam (Zosyn), vinblastine (Velban), vinorelbine (Navelbine).

INDICATIONS/ROUTES/DOSAGE

Alert: Dosage individualized based on clinical response, tolerance to adverse effects. When used in combination therapy, consult specific protocols for optimum dosage, sequence of drug administration. Cumulative doses >400 units increase risk of pulmonary toxicity. Test doses of ≤2 units for first 2 doses recommended due to increased possibility of anaphylactoid reaction in lymphoma pts.

SINGLE AGENT THERAPY

IV/IM/subcutaneous: ADULTS, ELDERLY: 10–20 units/m^2 (0.25–0.5 units/kg) 1–2 times/wk. **Continuous IV:** 15 units/m^2 over 24 hrs for 4 days.

COMBINATION THERAPY

IV/IM: 3–4 units/m^2.

PLEURAL SCLEROSING

IV infusion: 60–240 units as a single infusion.

SIDE EFFECTS

FREQUENT: Anorexia, weight loss, erythematous skin swelling, urticaria, rash, striae (streaking), vesiculation (small blisters), hyperpigmentation (particularly at areas of pressure, skin folds, nail cuticles, IM injection sites, scars), mucosal lesions of lips, tongue (stomatitis). Usually evident 1–3 wks after initial therapy. May be accompanied by decreased skin sensitivity followed by hypersensitivity of skin, nausea, vomiting, alopecia, fever/chills with parenteral form (particularly noted few hours after large single dose, lasts 4–12 hrs).

B

ADVERSE REACTIONS/ TOXIC EFFECTS

Interstitial pneumonitis occurs in 10% of pts, occasionally progressing to pulmonary fibrosis. Appears to be dose/age related (>70 yrs, those receiving total dose >400 units). Renal, hepatic toxicity occur infrequently.

NURSING IMPLICATIONS

BASELINE ASSESSMENT

Obtain chest x-rays q1–2wks.

INTERVENTION/EVALUATION

Monitor lung sounds for pulmonary toxicity (dyspnea, fine lung rales). Monitor hematologic, pulmonary function, hepatic, renal function tests. Assess skin daily for cutaneous toxicity. Monitor for stomatitis (burning/erythema of oral mucosa at inner margin of lips), hematologic toxicity (fever, sore throat, signs of local infection, easy bruising, unusual bleeding), symptoms of anemia (excessive tiredness, weakness).

PATIENT/FAMILY TEACHING

Fever/chills reaction occurs less frequently with continued therapy. Improvement of Hodgkin's disease, testicular tumors noted within 2 wks, squamous cell carcinoma within 3 wks. Do not have immunizations without doctor's approval (drug lowers body's resistance). Avoid contact with those who have recently taken live virus vaccine.

bortezomib

bor-**teh**-zoe-mib
(Velcade)

CLASSIFICATION

PHARMACOTHERAPEUTIC: Proteasome inhibitor. **CLINICAL:** Antineoplastic.

ACTION

Degrades conjugated proteins, required for cell-cycle progression/mitosis; disrupts cell proliferation. **Therapeutic Effect:** Produces antitumor/chemosensitizing activity, cell death.

PHARMACOKINETICS

Distributed to tissues/organs, with highest level in GI tract, liver. Protein binding: 83%. Primarily metabolized by enzymatic action. Rapidly cleared from the circulation. Significant biliary excretion, with lesser amount excreted in the urine. **Half-life:** 9–15 hrs.

USES

Treatment of refractory/relapsed multiple myeloma in those who have received at least 2 prior therapies and have demonstrated disease progression on the last therapy.

PRECAUTIONS

CONTRAINDICATIONS: Hypersensitivity to boron, mannitol. **CAUTIONS:** History of syncope, pts receiving medication known to be associated with hypotension, dehydrated pts, renal/hepatic function impairment.

LIFESPAN CONSIDERATIONS: Pregnancy/lactation: May induce degenerative effects in the ovary, degenerative changes in the testes. May affect male/female fertility. Breast-feeding not recommended. **Pregnancy Category D. Children:** Safety and efficacy not established. **Elderly:** Increased incidence of grades 3 and 4 thrombocytopenia.

INTERACTIONS

DRUG: May alter **oral hypoglycemic** response. **HERBAL:** None known. **FOOD:**

None known. **LAB VALUES:** May significantly decrease WBC, Hgb, Hct, platelet count, neutrophils.

AVAILABILITY (Rx)

POWDER FOR INJECTION: 3.5 mg.

ADMINISTRATION/HANDLING

IV

Storage • Store unopened vials at room temperature. Once reconstituted, solution may be stored at room temperature up to 8 hrs after preparation.

Reconstitution • Reconstitute vial with 3.5 ml 0.9% NaCl.

Rate of administration Give as a bolus IV injection.

INDICATIONS/ROUTES/DOSAGE

MULTIPLE MYELOMA

IV injection: ADULTS, ELDERLY: 1.3 mg/m^2/dose twice weekly for 2 weeks (days 1, 4, 8, 11) followed by a 10-day rest period (days 12–21). This is considered a treatment cycle. Separate consecutive doses by at least 72 hrs.

Dose modification: Withhold therapy at onset of any grade 3 nonhematologic or grade 4 hematologic toxicities, excluding neuropathy. Once symptoms have resolved, reinitiate therapy at a 25% reduction in dosage.

NEUROPATHIC PAIN/PERIPHERAL SENSORY NEUROPATHY

Grade 1 with pain or grade 2 (interfering with function but not activities of daily living): Reduce dose to 1 mg/m^2. **Grade 2 with pain or grade 3 (interfering with activities of daily living):** Withhold until toxicity resolved then reinitiate with 0.7 mg/m^2. **Grade 4 (permanent sensory loss that interferes with function):** Discontinue bortezomib.

SIDE EFFECTS

COMMON (36%–65%): Fatigue, malaise, weakness, nausea, diarrhea, anorexia, constipation, fever, vomiting. **FREQUENT (21%–28%):** Headache, insomnia, arthralgia, limb pain, edema, paresthesia, dizziness, rash. **OCCASIONAL (11%–18%):** Dehydration, cough, anxiety, bone pain, muscle cramps, myalgia, back pain, abdominal pain, taste alteration, dyspepsia (heartburn, epigastric distress), pruritus, hypotension, rigors, blurred vision.

ADVERSE REACTIONS/ TOXIC EFFECTS

Thrombocytopenia occurs in 40% of pts, is maximal at day 11, returns to baseline by day 21. GI, intracerebral hemorrhage are associated with drug-induced thrombocytopenia. Anemia occurs in 32% of pts. New onset/worsening of existing neuropathy occurs in 37% of pts. Symptoms may improve/return to baseline in some pts upon drug discontinuation. Pneumonia occurs occasionally.

NURSING IMPLICATIONS

BASELINE ASSESSMENT

Obtain baseline CBC; monitor CBC, especially platelet count, throughout treatment. Antiemetics, antidiarrheals may be effective in preventing, treating nausea, vomiting, diarrhea.

INTERVENTION/EVALUATION

Routinely assess B/P; monitor pt for orthostatic hypotension. Maintain strict I&O. Encourage fluid intake to prevent dehydration. Monitor temperature and be alert to high potential for fever. Monitor for peripheral neuropathy (burning sensation, neuropathic pain, paresthesia, hyperesthesia). Avoid IM injections, rectal temperatures, other traumas that may induce bleeding.

B

PATIENT/FAMILY TEACHING

Discuss importance of pregnancy testing, avoidance of pregnancy, measures to prevent pregnancy. Increase fluid intake. Avoid tasks requiring mental alertness, motor skills until response to drug is established.

bosentan

baws-en-tan
(Tracleer)

CLASSIFICATION

PHARMACOTHERAPEUTIC: Endothelin receptor antagonist. **CLINICAL:** Vasodilator, neurohormonal blocker.

ACTION

Blocks the neurohormone that constricts pulmonary arteries. **Therapeutic Effect:** Improves exercise ability. Decreases rate of clinical worsening of pulmonary arterial hypertension.

PHARMACOKINETICS

Highly bound to plasma proteins, mainly albumin. Metabolized in the liver. Eliminated by biliary excretion. **Half-life:** Approx. 5 hrs.

USES

Treatment of pulmonary arterial hypertension (PAH) in those with class III or IV symptoms (World Health Organization).

PRECAUTIONS

CONTRAINDICATIONS: Pregnancy, coadministration with cyclosporine, glyburide. **EXTREME CAUTION:** Moderate to severe hepatic function impairment. **CAUTIONS:** Mildly impaired hepatic impairment.

LIFESPAN CONSIDERATIONS: Pregnancy/lactation: May induce male infertility, atrophy of seminiferous tubules of the testes; reduce sperm count. Expected to cause fetal harm, teratogenic effects, including malformations of head, mouth, face, large vessels. Breast-feeding is not recommended. **Pregnancy Category X. Children:** Safety and efficacy not established. **Elderly:** Use caution in dosage due to higher frequency of decreased hepatic, renal, cardiac function.

INTERACTIONS

DRUG: Cyclosporine, ketoconazole may increase plasma concentration of bosentan. May decrease plasma concentrations of **warfarin, glyburide, hormonal contraceptives,** including oral, injectable, and implantable; **simvastatin, lovastatin, atorvastatin. HERBAL:** None known. **FOOD:** None known. **LAB VALUES:** May increase SGOT (AST), SGPT (ALT), bilirubin. May decrease Hgb, Hct.

AVAILABILITY (Rx)

TABLETS: 62.5 mg, 125 mg.

ADMINISTRATION/HANDLING

• Give in the morning and evening, with or without food. • Do not crush or chew film-coated tablets.

INDICATIONS/ROUTES/DOSAGE

PULMONARY ARTERIAL HYPERTENSION (PAH)

PO: ADULTS, ELDERLY: 62.5 mg twice daily for 4 wks, then increase to maintenance dose of 125 mg twice daily. BODY WEIGHT <40 KG BUT >12 YRS: 62.5 mg twice daily.

SIDE EFFECTS

OCCASIONAL: Headache, nasopharyngitis, flushing. **RARE:** Dyspepsia (heartburn, epigastric distress), fatigue, pruritus, hypotension.

ADVERSE REACTIONS/ TOXIC EFFECTS

Abnormal hepatic function, edema of lower extremities, palpitations occur rarely.

NURSING IMPLICATIONS

BASELINE ASSESSMENT

Pregnancy must be excluded before the start of treatment and prevented thereafter. A negative result from a urine or serum pregnancy test performed during the first 5 days of a normal menstrual period and at least 11 days after the last act of sexual intercourse must be obtained. Monthly follow-up pregnancy tests must be maintained.

INTERVENTION/EVALUATION

Assess liver enzyme levels (aminotransferase) before initiating therapy and then monthly thereafter. If elevation in liver enzymes is noted, changes in monitoring and treatment must be initiated. If clinical symptoms of liver injury (nausea, vomiting, fever, abdominal pain, fatigue, jaundice) occur or if bilirubin level increases, stop treatment. Monitor Hgb levels at 1 and 3 mos of treatment, then every 3 mos. Monitor Hgb, Hct levels for decrease.

PATIENT/FAMILY TEACHING

Discuss importance of pregnancy testing, avoidance of pregnancy, measures to prevent pregnancy.

botulinum toxin type A

botch-you-lin-em toxin
(Botox)

◆CLASSIFICATION

PHARMACOTHERAPEUTIC: Neurotoxin. **CLINICAL:** Neuromuscular conduction blocker.

ACTION

Blocks neuromuscular conduction by binding to receptor sites on motor nerve endings, entering the nerve terminals, inhibiting release of acetylcholine, producing denervation of the muscle. **Therapeutic Effect:** Results in reduction of muscle activity.

USE

Treatment of strabismus, blepharospasm associated with dystonia; cervical dystonia. Temporary improvement of brow furrow lines in those ≤65 yrs. **Unlabeled:** Treatment of hemifacial spasms, oromandibular dystonia, spasmoditic torticollis, laryngeal dystonia, writer's cramp, focal task-specific dystonia, head and neck tremor unresponsive to drug therapy, dynamic muscle contracture in pediatric cerebral palsy pts.

PRECAUTIONS

CONTRAINDICATIONS: Presence of infection at proposed injection site(s). **CAUTIONS:** Pts with neuromuscular junctional disorders (amyotrophic lateral sclerosis, motor neuropathy, myasthenia gravis, Lambert-Eaton syndrome) may experience significant systemic effects (severe dysphagia, respiratory compromise). **Pregnancy Category C.**

INTERACTIONS

DRUG: **Aminoglycoside antibiotics,** other drugs that interfere with neuromuscular transmission **(curare-like compounds)** may potentiate effect of botulinum toxin. **HERBAL:** None known.

B

FOOD: None known. **LAB VALUES:** None known.

AVAILABILITY (Rx)

INJECTION: 100 units.

ADMINISTRATION/HANDLING

IM

Storage • Store in freezer. • Administer within 4 hrs after removal from freezer and reconstituted. • May store reconstituted solution in refrigerator for up to 4 hrs. • Appears as a clear, colorless solution (discard if particulate matter is present).

Reconstitution • 0.9% NaCl is recommended diluent. • For resulting dose of units/0.1 ml, draw up 1 ml diluent to provide 10 units, 2 ml to provide 5 units, 4 ml to provide 2.5 units, or 8 ml to provide 1.25 units. • Slowly, gently inject diluent into the vial, avoid bubbles, rotate vial gently to mix.

Rate of administration • Administer within 4 hrs after reconstitution. • To be injected into affected muscle using 25-, 27-, or 30-gauge needle for superficial muscles and a 22-gauge needle for deeper musculature.

INDICATIONS/ROUTES/DOSAGE

Alert: To be administered into affected muscle by physician.

CERVICAL DYSTONIA, PTS WITH KNOWN HISTORY OF TOLERATING TOXIN

IM: ADULTS, ELDERLY: Mean dose is 236 units with range of 198–300 units divided among the affected muscles, based on pt's head/neck position, localization of pain, muscle hypertrophy, pt response, adverse event history.

CERVICAL DYSTONIA, PTS WITHOUT PRIOR USE

IM: ADULTS, ELDERLY: Administer at lower dosage than for pts with known history of tolerance.

SIDE EFFECTS

Alert: Side effects usually occur within first week following injection.

FREQUENT (11%–15%): Localized pain, tenderness, bruising at injection site, localized weakness of injected muscle, upper respiratory tract infection, neck pain, headache. **OCCASIONAL (2%–10%):** Increased cough, flu syndrome, back pain, rhinitis, dizziness, hypertonia, soreness at injection site, asthenia, dry mouth, nausea, drowsiness. **RARE:** Stiffness, numbness, double vision, ptosis (drooping of upper eyelid).

ADVERSE REACTIONS/ TOXIC EFFECTS

Dysphagia, mild to moderate in severity, occurs in approx. 20% of pts. Cardiac arrhythmias, severe dysphagia manifested as aspiration, dyspnea, pneumonia occur rarely. Overdosage produces systemic weakness, muscle paralysis.

NURSING IMPLICATIONS

BASELINE ASSESSMENT

Assess onset, type, location, duration of dystonia.

INTERVENTION/EVALUATION

Clinical improvement begins within first 2 wks after injection. Maximum benefit appears at approx. 6 wks after injection.

PATIENT/FAMILY TEACHING

Resume activity slowly and carefully. Seek medical attention immediately if swallowing, speech, respiratory difficulties appear.

botulinum toxin type B

botch-you-lin-em toxin
(Myobloc)

♦CLASSIFICATION

PHARMACOTHERAPEUTIC: Neurotoxin. **CLINICAL:** Neuromuscular conduction blocker.

ACTION

Inhibits acetylcholine release at the neuromuscular junction by binding, internalization, translocation of the toxin where it acts as an endoprotease, an enzyme. **Therapeutic Effect:** Splits polypeptides essential for neurotransmitter release.

USES

Treatment of cervical dystonia (CD) to reduce severity of abnormal head position, neck pain associated with CD.

PRECAUTIONS

CONTRAINDICATIONS: None known. **CAUTIONS:** Pts with neuromuscular junctional disorders (amyotrophic lateral sclerosis, motor neuropathy, myasthenia gravis, Lambert-Eaton syndrome) may experience significant systemic effects (severe dysphagia, respiratory compromise). **Pregnancy Category C.**

INTERACTIONS

DRUG: **Aminoglycoside antibiotics,** other drugs that interfere with neuromuscular transmission **(curare-like compounds)** may potentiate effect of botulinum toxin. **HERBAL:** None known. **FOOD:** None known. **LAB VALUES:** None known.

AVAILABILITY (Rx)

INJECTION: 2,500 units, 5,000 units, 10,000 units.

ADMINISTRATION/HANDLING

IM

Storage • May be refrigerated for up to 21 mos. Do not freeze. • Administer within 4 hrs after removal from refrigerator and reconstituted. • May store reconstituted solution in refrigerator for up to 4 hrs. • Appears as a clear, colorless solution (discard if particulate matter is present).

Reconstitution • 0.9% NaCl is recommended diluent. • Slowly, gently inject diluent into the vial; avoid bubbles, rotate vial gently to mix.

Rate of administration • Administer within 4 hrs after reconstitution. • To be injected into affected muscle using 25-, 27-, or 30-gauge needle for superficial muscles and a 22-gauge needle for deeper musculature.

INDICATIONS/ROUTES/DOSAGE

Alert: To be administered into affected muscle by physician.

CERVICAL DYSTONIA IN PTS WITH HISTORY OF TOLERATING TOXIN

IM: ADULTS, ELDERLY: 2,500–5,000 units divided among the affected muscles.

CERVICAL DYSTONIA, PTS WITHOUT PRIOR USE

IM: ADULTS, ELDERLY: Administer at lower dosage than for pts with known history of tolerance.

SIDE EFFECTS

Alert: Side effects usually occur within first week after injection.

FREQUENT (12%–19%): Infection, neck pain, headache, injection site pain, dry mouth. **OCCASIONAL (4%–10%):** Flu syndrome, generalized pain, increased cough, back pain, myasthenia. **RARE:**

B

Dizziness, nausea, rhinitis, headache, vomiting, edema, allergic reaction.

ADVERSE REACTIONS/ TOXIC EFFECTS

Dysphagia, mild to moderate in severity, occurs in approx. 10% of pts. Cardiac arrhythmias, severe dysphagia manifested as aspiration, dyspnea, pneumonia occur rarely. Overdosage produces systemic weakness, muscle paralysis.

NURSING IMPLICATIONS

BASELINE ASSESSMENT

Assess onset, type, location, duration of dystonia.

INTERVENTION/EVALUATION

Duration of effect lasts between 12–16 wks at doses of 5,000 units or 10,000 units.

PATIENT/FAMILY TEACHING

Resume activity slowly and carefully. Seek medical attention immediately if swallowing, speech, respiratory difficulties appear.

bretylium tosylate

bre-**till**-ee-um

(Bretylate ✱, Bretylol)

See Classification section under: Antiarrhythmics

brimonidine

(Alphagan)

See Classification section under: Antiglaucoma agents (p. 45C)

brinzolamide

(Azopt)

See Classification section under: Antiglaucoma agents (p. 46C)

bromocriptine mesylate

brom-oh-**crip**-teen

(Apo-Bromocriptine ✱, Parlodel)

Do not confuse with benztropine, pindolol.

♦CLASSIFICATION

PHARMACOTHERAPEUTIC: Dopamine agonist. **CLINICAL:** Infertility therapy adjunct, antihyperprolactinemic, lactation inhibitor, antidyskinetic, growth hormone suppressant.

ACTION

Inhibits prolactin secretion, directly stimulates dopamine receptors in the corpus striatum. **Therapeutic Effect:** Suppresses galactorrhea, improves symptoms of parkinsonism.

PHARMACOKINETICS

Onset	Peak	Duration
Prolactin lowering		
2 hrs	8 hrs	24 hrs
Antiparkinson		
0.5–1.5 hrs	2 hrs	—
Growth hormone		
1–2 hrs	4–8 wks	4–8 hrs

Minimal absorption from GI tract. Protein binding: 90%–96%. Metabolized in liver. Excreted in feces via biliary secretion. **Half-life:** 15 hrs.

USES

Treatment of parkinsonism in pts unresponsive or allergic to levodopa. Used in conditions associated with hyperprolactinemia, acromegaly. **Unlabeled:** Treatment of neuroleptic malignant syndrome, cocaine addiction, hyperprolactinemia associated with pituitary adenomas.

PRECAUTIONS

CONTRAINDICATIONS: Pregnancy, peripheral vascular disease, severe ischemic heart disease, uncontrolled hypertension, hypersensitivity to ergot alkaloids. **CAUTIONS:** Impaired hepatic/cardiac function, hypertension, psychiatric disorders.

LIFESPAN CONSIDERATIONS: Pregnancy/lactation: Not recommended during pregnancy or while breast-feeding. **Pregnancy Category C. Children:** Safety and efficacy not established. **Elderly:** CNS effects may occur more frequently.

INTERACTIONS

DRUG: Disulfiram reaction (chest pain, confusion, flushed face, nausea, vomiting) may occur with **alcohol. Estrogens, progestins** may decrease effects. **Phenothiazines, haloperidol, MAOIs** may decrease prolactin effect. **Hypotensive agents** may increase hypotension. **Levodopa** may increase effects. **Erythromycin, ritonavir** may increase concentration, toxicity. **Risperidone** may increase serum prolactin concentrations, interfere with bromocriptine effects. **HERBAL:** None known. **FOOD:** None known. **LAB VALUES:** May increase plasma concentration of growth hormone.

AVAILABILITY (Rx)

TABLETS: 2.5 mg. **CAPSULES:** 5 mg.

ADMINISTRATION/HANDLING

PO

• Pt should be lying down before administering first dose. • Give after food intake (decreases incidence of nausea).

INDICATIONS/ROUTES/DOSAGE

HYPERPROLACTINEMIA

PO: ADULTS, ELDERLY: Initially, 1.25–2.5 mg/day. May increase by 2.5 mg/day at 3- to 7-day intervals. RANGE: 2.5 mg 2–3 times/day.

PARKINSON'S DISEASE

PO: ADULTS, ELDERLY: Initially, 1.25 mg 2 times/day. Increase by 2.5 mg/day q14–28days. RANGE: 30–90 mg/day.

ACROMEGALY

PO: ADULTS, ELDERLY: Initially, 1.25–2.5 mg/day at bedtime for 3 days. May increase by 1.25–2.5 mg/day q3–7days. RANGE: 20–30 mg/day. **Maximum:** 100 mg/day.

SIDE EFFECTS

Alert: Incidence of side effects is high, esp. at beginning of therapy or with high dosage.

FREQUENT: Nausea (49%), headache (19%), dizziness (17%). **OCCASIONAL (3%–7%):** Fatigue, lightheadedness, vomiting, abdominal cramps, diarrhea, constipation, nasal congestion, drowsiness, dry mouth. **RARE:** Muscle cramping, urinary hesitancy.

ADVERSE REACTIONS/ TOXIC EFFECTS

Visual/auditory hallucinations noted in parkinsonism syndrome. Long-term, high-dose therapy may produce continuing rhinorrhea, fainting, GI hemorrhage, peptic ulcer, severe abdominal/stomach pain.

NURSING IMPLICATIONS

BASELINE ASSESSMENT

Evaluation of pituitary (rule out tumor) should be done prior to treatment for hyperprolactinemia with amenorrhea/galactorrhea, infertility. Obtain pregnancy test.

B

INTERVENTION/EVALUATION

Assist with ambulation if dizziness is noted after administration. Assess for therapeutic response (decrease in engorgement, parkinsonism symptoms). Monitor for constipation.

PATIENT/FAMILY TEACHING

To reduce lightheadedness, rise slowly from lying to sitting position, permit legs to dangle momentarily before standing. Avoid sudden posture changes. Avoid tasks that require alertness, motor skills until response to drug is established. Must use contraceptive measures (other than oral) during treatment. Report any watery nasal discharge to physician.

brompheniramine

(Brovex, Brovex CT)

See Classification section under: Antihistamines (p. 47C)

budesonide

byew-**des**-oh-nyd

(Entocort, Pulmicort, Rhinocort, Rhinocort Aqua)

CLASSIFICATION

PHARMACOTHERAPEUTIC: Glucocorticosteroid. **CLINICAL:** Anti-inflammatory, antiallergy (see pp. 65C, 81C).

ACTION

Decreases/prevents tissue response to inflammatory process. **Therapeutic Effect:** Inhibits accumulation of inflammatory cells.

PHARMACOKINETICS

Minimally absorbed from nasal tissue, moderately absorbed from inhalation. Protein binding: 88%. Primarily metabolized in liver. **Half-life:** 2–3 hrs.

USES

Oral Inhalation, Nasal: Management of symptoms of seasonal or perennial allergic rhinitis in adults and children and nonallergic perennial rhinitis in adults. Maintenance treatment of asthma. **Capsule:** Treatment of Crohn's disease. **Unlabeled:** Treatment of vasomotor rhinitis.

PRECAUTIONS

CONTRAINDICATIONS: Hypersensitivity to any corticosteroid or components, primary treatment of status asthmaticus, systemic fungal infections, persistently positive sputum cultures for *Candida albicans,* untreated localized infection involving nasal mucosa. **CAUTIONS:** Adrenal insufficiency, cirrhosis, glaucoma, hypothyroidism, untreated infection, osteoporosis, tuberculosis.

LIFESPAN CONSIDERATIONS: Pregnancy/lactation: Unknown if drug crosses placenta or is distributed in breast milk. **Pregnancy Category B. Children:** Prolonged treatment/high dosages may decrease short-term growth rate, cortisol secretion. **Elderly:** No age-related precautions noted.

INTERACTIONS

DRUG: None known. **HERBAL:** None known. **FOOD:** None known. **LAB VALUES:** None known.

AVAILABILITY (Rx)

CAPSULES: 3 mg (Entocort EC). **POWDER FOR ORAL INHALATION:** 200 mcg (Pulmicort Turbuhaler). **SUSPENSION FOR NASAL INHALATION:** 50 mcg/inhalation (Pulmicort). **SUSPENSION FOR ORAL INHALATION:** 0.25 mg/2 ml, 0.5 mg/2 mg (Pulmicort Respules). **NASAL**

SPRAY SUSPENSION: 32 mcg/spray (Rhinocort Aqua).

ADMINISTRATION/HANDLING

INHALATION

• Shake container well, exhale completely, place mouthpiece between lips, inhale, hold breath as long as possible before exhaling. • Allow at least 1 min between inhalations. • Rinse mouth after each use to decrease dry mouth, hoarseness.

INTRANASAL

• Clear nasal passages before use. • Tilt head slightly forward. • Insert spray tip into nostril, pointing toward nasal passages, away from nasal septum. • Spray into 1 nostril while holding other nostril closed, concurrently inspire through nostril to allow medication as high into nasal passages as possible.

INDICATIONS/ROUTES/DOSAGE

Intranasal: ADULTS, ELDERLY, CHILDREN ≥6 YRS: RHINOCORT: 2 sprays to each nostril 2 times/day or 4 sprays to each nostril in morning. RHINOCORT AQUA: 1 spray to each nostril once daily. **Maximum:** ADULTS, CHILDREN ≥12 YRS: 8 sprays/day. CHILDREN <12 YRS: 4 sprays/day.

Nebulization: CHILDREN 6 MOS–8 YRS: 0.25–1 mg/day titrated to lowest effective dosage.

Inhalation: ADULTS, ELDERLY, CHILDREN ≥6 YRS: Initially, 200–400 mcg 2 times/day. **Maximum:** ADULTS: 800 mcg 2 times/day. CHILDREN: 400 mcg 2 times/day.

CROHN'S DISEASE

PO: ADULTS, ELDERLY: 9 mg once daily for up to 8 wks.

SIDE EFFECTS

FREQUENT (>3%): Nasal: Mild nasopharyngeal irritation, burning, stinging, dryness, headache, cough. **Inhalation:** Flulike syndrome, headache, pharyngitis. **OCCASIONAL (1%–3%): Nasal:** Dry mouth, dyspepsia, rebound congestion, rhinorrhea, loss of sense of taste. **Inhalation:** Back pain, vomiting, altered taste/voice, abdominal pain, nausea, dyspepsia.

ADVERSE REACTIONS/ TOXIC EFFECTS

Acute hypersensitivity reaction (urticaria, angioedema, severe bronchospasm) occurs rarely.

NURSING IMPLICATIONS

BASELINE ASSESSMENT

Question for hypersensitivity to any corticosteroids, components.

INTERVENTION/EVALUATION

Monitor for relief of symptoms.

PATIENT/FAMILY TEACHING

Improvement noted in 24 hrs, but full effect may take 3–7 days. Contact physician if no improvement in symptoms, sneezing, nasal irritation occurs.

bumetanide

byew-**met**-ah-nide
(Bumex, Burinex ✤)

CLASSIFICATION

PHARMACOTHERAPEUTIC: Loop. **CLINICAL:** Diuretic (see p. 87C).

ACTION

Enhances excretion of sodium, chloride, and, to lesser degree, potassium by direct action at ascending limb of loop of Henle and in the proximal tubule. **Therapeutic Effect:** Produces diuresis.

B

PHARMACOKINETICS

Onset	Peak	Duration
PO		
30–60 min	60–120 min	4–6 hrs
IM		
40 min	60–120 min	4–6 hrs
IV		
Rapid	15–30 min	2–3 hrs

Completely absorbed from GI tract (absorption decreased in CHF, nephrotic syndrome). Protein binding: 94%–96%. Partially metabolized in liver. Primarily excreted in urine. Not removed by hemodialysis. **Half-life:** 1–1.5 hrs.

USES

Treatment of edema associated with CHF, chronic renal failure (including nephrotic syndrome), hepatic cirrhosis with ascites; treatment of acute pulmonary edema. **Unlabeled:** Treatment of hypertension, hypercalcemia.

PRECAUTIONS

CONTRAINDICATIONS: Anuria, hepatic coma, severe electrolyte depletion. **CAUTIONS:** Hypersensitivity to sulfonamides, impaired renal/hepatic function, diabetes mellitus, elderly/debilitated.

LIFESPAN CONSIDERATIONS: Pregnancy/lactation: Unknown if drug is distributed in breast milk. **Pregnancy Category C** (**D** if used in pregnancy-induced hypertension). **Children:** Safety and efficacy not established. **Elderly:** May be more sensitive to hypotension/electrolyte effects. Increased risk for circulatory collapse or thrombolytic episode. Age-related renal impairment may require reduced or extended dosage interval.

INTERACTIONS

DRUG: Amphotericin, ototoxic, nephrotoxic agents may increase toxicity. May decrease effect of **anticoagulants, heparin. Hypokalemia-causing agents** may increase risk of hypokalemia. May increase risk of **lithium** toxicity. **HERBAL:** None known. **FOOD:** None known. **LAB VALUES:** May increase glucose, BUN, uric acid, urinary phosphate. May decrease calcium, chloride, magnesium, potassium, sodium.

AVAILABILITY (Rx)

TABLETS: 0.5 mg, 1 mg, 2 mg. **INJECTION:** 0.25 mg/ml.

ADMINISTRATION/HANDLING

PO

• Give with food to avoid GI upset, preferably with breakfast (may prevent nocturia).

IV

Storage • Store at room temperature. • Stable for 24 hrs if diluted.

Rate of administration • May give undiluted but is compatible with D_5W, 0.9% NaCl, or lactated Ringer's. • Administer IV push >1–2 min. • May give through Y tube or 3-way stopcock. • May give as continuous infusion.

IV INCOMPATIBILITIES

Midazolam (Versed).

IV COMPATIBILITIES

Aztreonam, (Azactam), cefepime (Maxipime), diltiazem (Cardizem), dobutamine (Dobutrex), furosemide (Lasix), lorazepam (Ativan), milrinone (Primacor), morphine, piperacillin tazobactam (Zosyn), propofol (Diprivan).

INDICATIONS/ROUTES/DOSAGE

EDEMA

PO: ADULTS >18 YRS: 0.5–2 mg given as single dose in AM. May repeat at 4- to 5-hr intervals. ELDERLY: 0.5 mg/day, increase as needed.

IM/IV: ADULTS, ELDERLY: 0.5–2 mg/dose. May repeat in 2–3 hrs. **Continuous IV:** 0.5–1 mg/hr.

HYPERTENSION

PO: ADULTS, ELDERLY: Initially, 0.5 mg/

day. Range: 1–4 mg/day. **Maximum:** 5 mg/day. For larger doses may divide in 2–3 doses/day.

USUAL PEDIATRIC DOSE
IV/IM/PO: 0.015–0.1 mg/kg/dose q6–24h.

SIDE EFFECTS

EXPECTED: Increase in urine frequency/volume. **FREQUENT:** Orthostatic hypotension, dizziness. **OCCASIONAL:** Blurred vision, diarrhea, headache, anorexia, premature ejaculation, impotence, GI upset. **RARE:** Rash, urticaria, pruritus, weakness, muscle cramps, nipple tenderness.

ADVERSE REACTIONS/ TOXIC EFFECTS

Vigorous diuresis may lead to profound water/electrolyte depletion, resulting in hypokalemia, hyponatremia, dehydration, coma, circulatory collapse. Acute hypotensive episodes may occur. Ototoxicity manifested as deafness, vertigo, tinnitus (ringing/roaring in ears) may occur, esp. in pts with severe renal impairment or who are on other ototoxic drugs. Blood dyscrasias have been reported.

NURSING IMPLICATIONS

BASELINE ASSESSMENT

Check vital signs, esp. B/P for hypotension, prior to administration. Assess baseline electrolytes; particularly check for low potassium. Assess edema, skin turgor, mucous membranes for hydration status. Initiate I&O.

INTERVENTION/EVALUATION

Continue to monitor B/P, vital signs, electrolytes, I&O, weight. Note extent of diuresis. Watch for changes from initial assessment (hypokalemia may result in muscle strength changes, tremor, muscle cramps, change in mental status, cardiac arrhythmias; hyponatremia may result in confusion, thirst, cold/clammy skin).

PATIENT/FAMILY TEACHING

Expect increased frequency and volume of urination, hearing abnormalities (e.g., sense of fullness in ears, ringing/roaring in ears). Eat foods high in potassium such as whole grains (cereals), legumes, meat, bananas, apricots, orange juice, potatoes (white, sweet), raisins. Get up slowly from sitting/lying position.

Bumex

see bumetanide

bupivacaine

(Marcaine, Sensorcaine)
See Classification section under: Anesthetics: local (p. 4C)

buprenorphine

(Buprenex)
See Classification section under: Opioid analgesics

bupropion

byew-**pro**-peon
(Wellbutrin, Wellbutrin SR, Wellbutrin XL, Zyban)
Do not confuse with buspirone, Wellcovorin, Wellferon, Zagam.

◆CLASSIFICATION

PHARMACOTHERAPEUTIC: Aminoketone. **CLINICAL:** Antidepressant, smoking cessation aid (see p. 36C).

B

ACTION

Blocks reuptake of neurotransmitters (serotonin, norepinephrine) at CNS presynaptic membranes, increasing availability at postsynaptic receptor sites. Reduces firing rate of noradrenergic neurons, eliminating nicotine withdrawal symptoms. **Therapeutic Effect:** Resulting enhancement of synaptic activity produces antidepressant effect.

PHARMACOKINETICS

Rapidly absorbed from GI tract. Crosses blood-brain barrier. Protein binding: 84%. Extensive first-pass metabolism in liver to active metabolite. Primarily excreted in urine. **Half-life:** 14 hrs.

USES

Treatment of depression, particularly endogenous depression, exhibited as persistent and prominent dysphoria (occurring nearly every day for at least 2 wks) manifested by 4 of 8 symptoms: change in appetite, change in sleep pattern, increased fatigue, impaired concentration, feelings of guilt/worthlessness, loss of interest in usual activities, psychomotor agitation/retardation, or suicidal tendencies. Also used to assist in smoking cessation. **Unlabeled:** Attention deficit hyperactivity disorder in adults, children.

PRECAUTIONS

CONTRAINDICATIONS: Pts with seizure disorder, current or prior diagnosis of bulimia or anorexia nervosa, concurrent use of MAOI. **CAUTIONS:** History of seizure, cranial trauma; those currently taking antipsychotics, antidepressants; impaired renal, hepatic function.

LIFESPAN CONSIDERATIONS: Pregnancy/lactation: Unknown if drug crosses placenta or is distributed in breast milk. **Pregnancy Category B. Children:** Safety and efficacy not established in those <18 yrs. **Elderly:** More sensitive to anticholinergic, sedative, cardiovascular effects. Age-related impaired renal function may require dosage adjustment.

INTERACTIONS

DRUG: Alcohol, tricyclic antidepressants, lithium, ritonavir, trazodone may increase risk of seizures. May increase risk of acute toxicity with **MAOIs. HERBAL:** None known. **FOOD:** None known. **LAB VALUES:** May decrease WBCs.

AVAILABILITY (Rx)

TABLETS: 75 mg, 100 mg. **TABLETS (sustained-release):** 100 mg, 150 mg, 200 mg. **TABLETS (extended-release):** 150 mg, 300 mg.

ADMINISTRATION/HANDLING

PO

• May take with/without food (take with food to reduce GI irritation). • Give at least 4-hr interval for immediate onset and 8-hr interval for sustained-release tablet to avoid seizures. • Avoid bedtime dosage (decreases risk of insomnia). • Do not crush sustained-release preparations.

INDICATIONS/ROUTES/DOSAGE

DEPRESSION

Alert: Gradually increase dosage to minimize agitation, motor restlessness, insomnia.

PO: ADULTS: **Immediate-release:** Initially, 100 mg 2 times/day, may increase to 100 mg 3 times/day no sooner than 3 days after beginning therapy. **Maximum:** 450 mg/day. ELDERLY: 37.5 mg 2 times/day. May increase by 37.5 mg q3–4days. MAINTENANCE: Lowest effective dosage. **Sustained-release:** Initially, 150 mg/day as single dose in the morning. May increase to 300 mg/day at 150 mg 2 times/day as early as day 4 of dosing. **Extended-release:** 150 mg once daily. May increase to 300 mg once daily. **Max-**

imum: 400 mg/day. ELDERLY: 50–100 mg/day. May increase by 50–100 mg q3–4days. MAINTENANCE: Lowest effective dosage.

SMOKING CESSATION

PO: ADULTS: Initially, 150 mg daily for 3 days; then 150 mg 2 times/day. Continue for 7–12 wks.

SIDE EFFECTS

Alert: Fewer side effects noted with sustained-release form.

FREQUENT (18%–32%): Constipation, weight gain/loss, nausea, vomiting, anorexia, dry mouth, headache, increased sweating, tremor, sedation, insomnia, dizziness, agitation. **OCCASIONAL (5%–10%):** Diarrhea, akinesia, blurred vision, tachycardia, confusion, hostility, fatigue.

ADVERSE REACTIONS/ TOXIC EFFECTS

Increased risk of seizures with increase in dosage >150 mg/dose, in pts with history of bulimia or seizure disorders, or discontinuing agents that may lower seizure threshold.

NURSING IMPLICATIONS

BASELINE ASSESSMENT

For those on long-term therapy, liver/renal function tests should be performed periodically.

INTERVENTION/EVALUATION

Closely supervise suicidal-risk pt during early therapy (as depression lessens, energy level improves, increasing suicide potential). Assess appearance, behavior, speech pattern, level of interest, mood.

PATIENT/FAMILY TEACHING

Full therapeutic effect may be noted in 4 wks. Avoid tasks that require alertness, motor skills until response to drug is established.

buspirone hydrochloride

byew-spear-own
(BuSpar, Buspirex ✤, Bustab ✤)
Do not confuse with bupropion.

CLASSIFICATION

PHARMACOTHERAPEUTIC: Nonbarbiturate. **CLINICAL:** Antianxiety (see p. 11C).

ACTION

Binds to serotonin, dopamine at presynaptic neurotransmitter receptors in the CNS. **Therapeutic Effect:** Produces antianxiety effect.

PHARMACOKINETICS

Rapidly completely absorbed from GI tract. Protein binding: 95%. Undergoes extensive first-pass metabolism. Metabolized in liver to active metabolite. Primarily excreted in urine. Not removed by hemodialysis. **Half-life:** 2–3 hrs.

USES

Short-term management (up to 4 wks) of anxiety disorders. **Unlabeled:** Management of symptoms of premenstrual syndrome (PMS) (e.g., aches, pain, fatigue, irritability), panic attack.

PRECAUTIONS

CONTRAINDICATIONS: Severe renal/hepatic impairment, MAOI therapy. **CAUTIONS:** Renal/hepatic impairment.

LIFESPAN CONSIDERATIONS: Pregnancy/lactation: Unknown if drug crosses placenta or is distributed in breast milk. **Pregnancy Category B. Children:** Safety and efficacy not established. **Elderly:** No age-related precautions noted.

INTERACTIONS

DRUG: **Alcohol, CNS depressants** may increase sedation. **Erythromycin, itraconazole** may increase concentration, risk of toxicity. **MAOIs** may increase B/P. **HERBAL:** **Kava kava** may increase sedation. **FOOD:** **Grapefruit/grapefruit juice** may increase concentration, toxicity. **LAB VALUES:** None known.

AVAILABILITY (Rx)

TABLETS: 5 mg, 7.5 mg, 10 mg, 15 mg, 30 mg.

ADMINISTRATION/HANDLING

PO

• Give without regard to meals. • Tablets may be crushed.

INDICATIONS/ROUTES/DOSAGE

PO: ADULTS: 5 mg 2–3 times daily or 7.5 mg 2 times/day. May increase in 5-mg increments/day at intervals of 2–4 days. MAINTENANCE: 15–30 mg/day in 2–3 divided doses. Do not exceed 60 mg/day. ELDERLY: Initially, 5 mg 2 times/day. May increase by 5 mg q2–3days. **Maximum:** 60 mg. CHILDREN: Initially, 5 mg/day. May increase by 5 mg/day at weekly intervals. **Maximum:** 60 mg/day.

SIDE EFFECTS

FREQUENT (6%–12%): Dizziness, drowsiness, nausea, headache. **OCCASIONAL (2%–5%):** Nervousness, fatigue, insomnia, dry mouth, lightheadedness, mood swings, blurred vision, poor concentration, diarrhea, numbness in hands/feet. **RARE:** Muscle pain/stiffness, nightmares, chest pain, involuntary movements.

ADVERSE REACTIONS/ TOXIC EFFECTS

No evidence of tolerance or psychological and/or physical dependence, no withdrawal syndrome. Overdosage may produce severe nausea, vomiting, dizziness, drowsiness, abdominal distention, excessive pupil contraction.

NURSING IMPLICATIONS

BASELINE ASSESSMENT

Offer emotional support to anxious pt. Assess motor responses (agitation, trembling, tension), autonomic responses (cold, clammy hands; sweating).

INTERVENTION/EVALUATION

For those on long-term therapy, liver/renal function tests, blood counts should be performed periodically. Assist with ambulation if drowsiness, lightheadedness occur. Evaluate for therapeutic response: calm, facial expression, decreased restlessness, insomnia.

PATIENT/FAMILY TEACHING

Improvement may be noted in 7–10 days, but optimum therapeutic effect generally takes 3–4 wks. Drowsiness usually disappears during continued therapy. If dizziness occurs, change position slowly from recumbent to sitting position before standing. Avoid tasks that require alertness, motor skills until response to drug is established.

busulfan

bew-**sull**-fan
(Busulfex, Myleran)
Do not confuse with Alkeran, Leukeran.

◆ CLASSIFICATION

PHARMACOTHERAPEUTIC: Alkylating agent. **CLINICAL:** Antineoplastic (see p. 70C).

ACTION

Cell cycle–phase nonspecific. Interferes with DNA replication, RNA synthesis. **Therapeutic Effect:** Disrupts nucleic acid function. Myelosuppressant.

PHARMACOKINETICS

Completely absorbed from GI tract. Protein binding: 33%. Metabolized in liver. Primarily excreted in urine. Minimal removal by hemodialysis. **Half-life:** 2.5 hrs.

USES

Treatment of chronic myelogenous leukemia (CML). **Injection:** Combined with cyclophosphamide as conditioning regimen before allogeneic hematopoietic cell transplantation in pts with CML. **Unlabeled:** Treatment of acute myelocytic leukemia (AML).

PRECAUTIONS

CONTRAINDICATIONS: Disease resistance to previous therapy with drug. **EXTREME CAUTION:** Compromised bone marrow reserve. **CAUTIONS:** Chickenpox, herpes zoster, infection, history of gout.

LIFESPAN CONSIDERATIONS: Pregnancy/lactation: If possible, avoid use during pregnancy, esp. first trimester. May cause fetal harm. Unknown if distributed in breast milk. Breast-feeding not recommended. **Pregnancy Category D. Children/elderly:** No age-related precautions noted.

INTERACTIONS

DRUG: May decrease effect of **antigout medications. Bone marrow depressant** may increase risk of bone marrow depression. **Live virus vaccines** may potentiate virus replication, increase vaccine side effects, decrease antibody response to vaccine. **HERBAL:** None known. **FOOD:** None known. **LAB VALUES:** May decrease magnesium, potassium, phosphates, sodium. May increase glucose, calcium, bilirubin, SGPT (ALT), creatinine, alkaline phosphatase, BUN.

AVAILABILITY (Rx)

TABLETS: 2 mg. **INJECTION:** 60-mg ampoule.

ADMINISTRATION/HANDLING

Alert: May be carcinogenic, mutagenic, or teratogenic. Handle with extreme care during administration. Use of gloves recommended. If contact occurs with skin/mucosa, wash thoroughly with water.

PO

• Give at same time each day. • Give on empty stomach if nausea/vomiting occur.

IV

Storage • Refrigerate ampoules. • Following dilution, stable for 8 hrs at room temperature, 12 hrs if refrigerated when diluted with 0.9% NaCl.

Reconstitution • Dilute with 0.9% NaCl or D_5W only. The diluent quantity must be 10 times the volume of busulfan (e.g., 9.3 ml busulfan must be diluted with 93 ml diluent). • Use filter to withdraw busulfan from ampoule. • Add busulfan to calculated diluent. • Use infusion pump to administer busulfan.

Rate of administration • Infuse over 2 hrs. • Prior to and after infusion, flush catheter line with 5 ml 0.9% NaCl or D_5W.

IV INCOMPATIBILITY

Do not mix with any other medications.

INDICATIONS/ROUTES/DOSAGE

Alert: Dosage individualized based on clinical response, tolerance to adverse effects. When used in combination therapy, consult specific protocols for optimum dosage, sequence of drug administration.

REMISSION INDUCTION

PO: ADULTS: 4–8 mg/day. Withdraw

B

drug when WBC falls below 15,000/mm^3. CHILDREN: 0.06–0.12 mg/kg once daily.

MAINTENANCE THERAPY

PO: ADULTS: Induction dose (4–8 mg/day) when total leukocyte count reaches 50,000/mm^3. If remission occurs in <3 mos, 1–3 mg/day may produce satisfactory response.

USUAL ELDERLY DOSAGE

PO: Initially, lowest dosage for adults.

USUAL PARENTERAL DOSAGE

Alert: Premedicate with phenytoin to decrease risk of seizures.

IV infusion: ADULTS: 0.8 mg/kg q6h (as 2-hr infusion) for total of 16 doses. CHILDREN: 60–120 mcg/kg/day or 1.8–4.6 mg/m^2/day.

SIDE EFFECTS

VERY FREQUENT (72%–98%): Nausea, stomatitis, vomiting, anorexia, insomnia, diarrhea, fever, abdominal pain, anxiety. **FREQUENT (44%–69%):** Headache, rash, asthenia (loss of strength, energy), infection, chills, tachycardia, dyspepsia. **OCCASIONAL (16%–38%):** Constipation, dizziness, edema, pruritus, cough, dry mouth, depression, abdominal enlargement, pharyngitis, hiccups, back pain, alopecia, myalgia. **RARE (5%–13%):** Injection site pain, arthralgia, confusion, hypotension, lethargy.

ADVERSE REACTIONS/ TOXIC EFFECTS

Major adverse reaction is bone marrow depression resulting in hematologic toxicity (severe leukopenia, anemia, severe thrombocytopenia). Very high dosages may produce blurred vision, muscle twitching, tonic-clonic seizures. Long-term therapy (>4 yrs) may produce pulmonary syndrome ("busulfan lung") characterized by persistent cough, congestion, rales, dyspnea. Hyperuricemia may produce uric acid nephropathy, renal stones, acute renal failure.

NURSING IMPLICATIONS

BASELINE ASSESSMENT

CBC with differential, hepatic/renal function studies should be performed weekly (dosage based on hematologic values). Institute pt/family teaching regarding expected effects of treatment.

INTERVENTION/EVALUATION

Monitor lab values diligently for evidence of bone marrow depression. Assess mouth for onset of stomatitis (redness/ulceration of oral mucous membranes, gum inflammation, difficulty swallowing). Initiate antiemetics to prevent nausea/vomiting. Monitor daily bowel activity, stool consistency.

PATIENT/FAMILY TEACHING

Maintain adequate daily fluid intake (may protect against renal impairment). Report consistent cough, congestion, difficulty breathing. Promptly report fever, sore throat, signs of local infection, easy bruising, unusual bleeding from any site. Do not have immunizations without physician's approval (drug lowers body's resistance). Avoid contact with those who have recently taken live virus vaccine. Take at same time each day. Contraception is recommended during therapy.

butenafine

(Mentax)

See Classification section under: Antifungals: topical (p. 42C)

butorphanol tartrate

byew-**tore**-phen-awl
(Stadol, Stadol NS)
Do not confuse with Haldol.

CLASSIFICATION

PHARMACOTHERAPEUTIC: Opioid **(Schedule IV). CLINICAL:** Analgesic, anesthesia adjunct (see p. 120C).

ACTION

Binds at opiate receptor sites in CNS. Reduces intensity of pain stimuli incoming from sensory nerve endings. **Therapeutic Effect:** Alters pain perception, emotional response to pain.

PHARMACOKINETICS

Onset	Peak	Duration
IM		
10–30 min	30–60 min	3–4 hrs
IV		
<1 min	30 min	2–4 hrs
Nasal		
15 min	1–2 hrs	4–5 hrs

Rapidly absorbed from IM injection. Protein binding: 80%. Extensively metabolized in liver. Primarily excreted in urine. **Half-life:** 2.5–4 hrs.

USES

Management of pain (including postop pain). **Nasal:** Migraine headache pain. **Parenteral:** Preop, preanesthetic medication, supplement balanced anesthesia, relief of pain during labor.

PRECAUTIONS

CONTRAINDICATIONS: CNS disease that affects respirations, pulmonary disease, preexisting respiratory depression, physical dependence on other opioid analgesics. **CAUTIONS:** Impaired hepatic/renal function, elderly, debilitated, head injury, hypertension, prior to biliary tract surgery (produces spasm of sphincter of Oddi), MI.

LIFESPAN CONSIDERATIONS: Pregnancy/lactation: Readily crosses placenta. Distributed in breast milk. Breastfeeding not recommended. **Pregnancy Category C** (**D** if used for prolonged time, high dose at term). **Children:** Safety and efficacy not known in those <18 yrs. **Elderly:** May be more sensitive to effects; adjust dose and interval.

INTERACTIONS

DRUG: Alcohol, CNS depressants may increase CNS or respiratory depression, hypotension. **MAOIs** may produce severe, fatal reaction (reduce dose to one-fourth usual dose). Effects may be decreased with **buprenorphine. HERBAL:** None known. **FOOD:** None known. **LAB VALUES:** None known.

AVAILABILITY (Rx)

INJECTION: 1 mg/ml, 2 mg/ml. **NASAL SPRAY:** 10 mg/ml.

ADMINISTRATION/HANDLING

INTRANASAL

• Instruct pt to blow nose to clear nasal passages as much as possible. • Tilt head slightly forward, insert spray tip into nostril, pointing toward nasal passages, away from nasal septum. • Spray into nostril while holding other nostril closed, concurrently inspire through nose to permit medication as high into nasal passages as possible.

IV

Storage • Store at room temperature.

Rate of administration • May give undiluted. • Administer over 3–5 min.

IV INCOMPATIBILITIES

Amphotericin B complex (Abelcet, AmBisome, Amphotec).

IV COMPATIBILITIES

Atropine, diphenhydramine (Benadryl),

droperidol (Inapsine), hydroxyzine (Vistaril), morphine, promethazine (Phenergan), propofol (Diprivan).

INDICATIONS/ROUTES/DOSAGE

Alert: May be given by IM or IV push.

ANALGESIA

IM: ADULTS: 1–4 mg q3–4h as needed.

IV: ADULTS: 0.5–2 mg q3–4h as needed.

USUAL ELDERLY DOSAGE

IM/IV: 1 mg q4–6h as needed.

Nasal: ADULTS: 1 mg (1 spray in one nostril). May repeat in 60–90 min. May repeat 2-dose sequence q3–4h as needed. Alternatively, 2 mg (1 spray each nostril if pt remains recumbent), may repeat in 3–4 hrs.

SIDE EFFECTS

FREQUENT: Parenteral: Drowsiness (43%), dizziness (19%). **Nasal:** Nasal congestion (13%), insomnia (11%). **OCCASIONAL: Parenteral (3%–9%):** Confusion, sweating/clammy skin, lethargy, headache, nausea, vomiting, dry mouth. **Nasal (3%–9%):** Vasodilation, constipation, unpleasant taste, dyspnea, epistaxis, nasal irritation, upper respiratory infection, tinnitus. **RARE: Parenteral:** Hypotension, pruritus, blurred vision, sensation of heat, CNS stimulation, insomnia. **Nasal:** Hypertension, tremor, ear pain, paresthesia, depression, sinusitis.

ADVERSE REACTIONS/ TOXIC EFFECTS

Abrupt withdrawal after prolonged use may produce symptoms of narcotic withdrawal (abdominal cramping, rhinorrhea, lacrimation, anxiety, increased temperature, piloerection [goose bumps]). Overdosage results in severe respiratory depression, skeletal muscle flaccidity, cyanosis, extreme somnolence progressing to convulsions, stupor, coma. Tolerance to analgesic effect, physical dependence may occur with chronic use.

NURSING IMPLICATIONS

BASELINE ASSESSMENT

Obtain vital signs before giving medication. If respirations are ≤12/min (≤20/min in children), withhold medication, contact physician. Assess onset, type, location, duration of pain. Effect of medication is reduced if full pain recurs before next dose. Protect from falls. During labor, assess fetal heart tones, uterine contractions.

INTERVENTION/EVALUATION

Monitor for change in respirations, B/P, rate/quality of pulse. Initiate deep breathing, coughing exercises, particularly in those with impaired pulmonary function. Change pt's position q2–4h. Assess for clinical improvement, record onset of relief of pain.

PATIENT/FAMILY TEACHING

Change positions slowly to avoid dizziness. Avoid tasks that require alertness, motor skills until response to drug is established. Instruct pt on proper use of nasal spray. Avoid use of alcohol, CNS depressants.

cabergoline

cab-**err**-go-leen
(Dostinex)

◆CLASSIFICATION

CLINICAL: Antihyperprolactinemic.

ACTION

Agonist at dopamine D_2 receptors suppressing prolactin secretion. **Therapeutic Effect:** Shrinks prolactinomas, restores gonadal function.

USES

Treatment of hyperprolactinemic disorders, either idiopathic or due to pituitary adenomas.

PRECAUTIONS

CONTRAINDICATIONS: Uncontrolled hypertension, hypersensitivity to ergot alkaloids. **CAUTIONS:** Hepatic function impairment. **Pregnancy Category B.**

INTERACTIONS

DRUG: May increase hypotensive effect if given with other **antihypertensives.** **HERBAL:** None known. **FOOD:** None known. **LAB VALUES:** None known.

INDICATIONS/ROUTES/DOSAGE

HYPERPROLACTINEMIA

PO: ADULTS, ELDERLY: Initially, 0.25 mg 2 times/wk. May increase by 0.25 mg/wk at 4-wk intervals up to a maximum of 1 mg 2 times/wk.

SIDE EFFECTS

FREQUENT (29%): Nausea. **OCCASIONAL (5%–20%):** Headache, vertigo, dizziness, dyspepsia, postural hypotension, constipation. **RARE (2%–4%):** Vomiting, dry mouth, diarrhea, flatulence.

ADVERSE REACTIONS/ TOXIC EFFECTS

Overdosage may produce nasal congestion, syncope, hallucinations.

NURSING IMPLICATIONS

BASELINE ASSESSMENT

Obtain baseline liver function tests.

INTERVENTION/EVALUATION

Monitor prolactin levels monthly until prolactin levels equalize.

PATIENT/FAMILY TEACHING

To reduce hypotensive effect, rise slowly from lying to sitting position, permit legs to dangle momentarily before rising.

caffeine citrate

(Cafcit)

C

ACTION

Stimulates medullary respiratory center. Appears to increase sensitivity of respiratory center to stimulatory effects of CO_2. **Therapeutic Effect:** Increases alveolar ventilation, reducing severity, frequency of apneic episodes.

USES

Short-term treatment of apnea in premature infants from 28 to <33 wks' gestational age.

PRECAUTIONS

CAUTION: Pregnancy Category B.

AVAILABILITY (Rx)

INJECTION: 20 mg/ml. **ORAL SOLUTION:** 20 mg/ml.

INDICATIONS/ROUTES/DOSAGE

APNEA

PO/IV: LOADING DOSE: 10–20 mg/kg as caffeine citrate (5–10 mg/kg as caffeine base). If theophylline given within previous 72 hrs a modified dose (50%–75%) may be given. MAINTENANCE: 5 mg/kg/day as caffeine citrate (2.5 mg/kg/day as caffeine base). Dosage adjusted based on patient response.

SIDE EFFECTS

FREQUENT (5%–10%): Feeding intolerance, rash.

ADVERSE REACTIONS/ TOXIC EFFECTS

Sepsis, necrotizing enterocolitis may be noted.

C

NURSING IMPLICATIONS

INTERVENTION/EVALUATION

Monitor respirations diligently. Assess skin for rash.

calcipotriene

kal-sih-**poe**-tree-in
(Dovonex)

CLASSIFICATION

CLINICAL: Antipsoriatic.

ACTION

Synthetic vitamin D_3 analogue. Regulates skin cell (keratinocyte) production and development. **Therapeutic Effect:** Prevents abnormal growth, production of psoriasis (abnormal keratinocyte growth).

USES

Treatment of mild to moderate plaque psoriasis. **Solution:** Treatment of chronic, moderately severe scalp psoriasis.

PRECAUTIONS

CONTRAINDICATIONS: Hypercalcemia, evidence of vitamin D toxicity, use on face. **CAUTIONS:** History of nephrolithiasis. **Pregnancy Category C.**

INTERACTIONS

DRUG: None known. **HERBAL:** None known. **FOOD:** None known. **LAB VALUES:** Excessive use may increase serum calcium level.

AVAILABILITY (Rx)

CREAM: 0.005%. **OINTMENT:** 0.005%. **SOLUTION:** 0.005%.

INDICATIONS/ROUTES/DOSAGE

PSORIASIS

Topical: ADULTS, ELDERLY: Apply thin layer to affected skin twice daily (morning and evening); rub in gently, completely. **Solution:** Apply to lesions after combing hair.

SIDE EFFECTS

FREQUENT (10%–15%): Burning, itching, skin irritation. **OCCASIONAL (2%–10%):** Erythema, dry skin, peeling, rash, worsening of psoriasis, dermatitis. **RARE (≤1%):** Skin atrophy, hyperpigmentation, folliculitis.

ADVERSE REACTIONS/ TOXIC EFFECTS

Potential for hypercalcemia (abdominal pain, depression, easy fatigability, high B/P, anorexia, nausea, thirst) may occur.

NURSING IMPLICATIONS

BASELINE ASSESSMENT

Establish baseline electrolytes, particularly serum, urine calcium.

INTERVENTION/EVALUATION

Monitor healing of lesions, serum calcium concentrations. Assess skin for irritation, erythema, worsening of psoriasis (children, those >65 yrs are at greater risk of reactions). If irritation of lesions or surrounding uninvolved skin develops or serum calcium level increases outside normal range, medication should be discontinued.

PATIENT/FAMILY TEACHING

Avoid contact with face/eyes. Wash hands after application. Report any sign of local reaction. Improvement noted usually beginning after 2 wks of therapy, with marked improvement after 8 wks.

calcitonin

kal-sih-**toe**-nin
(Caltine, Miacalcin)

◆ CLASSIFICATION

PHARMACOTHERAPEUTIC: Synthetic hormone. **CLINICAL:** Calcium regulator, bone resorption inhibitor, osteoporosis therapy.

ACTION

Acts on bone to decrease osteoclast activity; decreases tubular reabsorption of sodium, calcium in kidneys; increases absorption of calcium in the GI tract. **Therapeutic Effect:** Regulates serum calcium concentrations.

PHARMACOKINETICS

Injection: Rapidly metabolized (primarily in kidney). Primarily excreted in urine. **Half-life:** 70–90 min. **Nasal:** Rapid absorption. **Half-life:** 43 min.

USES

Treatment of Paget's disease of bone, adjunctive therapy for hypercalcemia, treatment of osteoporosis in postmenopausal women. **Unlabeled:** Treatment of secondary osteoporosis due to hormone disturbance, drug therapy.

PRECAUTIONS

CONTRAINDICATIONS: Hypersensitivity to salmon protein, gelatin desserts. **CAUTIONS:** History of allergy, renal dysfunction.

LIFESPAN CONSIDERATIONS: Pregnancy/lactation: Drug does not cross placenta; unknown if distributed in breast milk. Safe usage during lactation not established (inhibits lactation in animals). **Pregnancy Category C. Children:** Safety and efficacy not established. **Elderly:** No age-related precautions noted.

INTERACTIONS

DRUG: None known. **HERBAL:** None known. **FOOD:** None known. **LAB VALUES:** None known.

AVAILABILITY (Rx)

INJECTION: 200 international units/ml. **NASAL SPRAY:** 200 international units/activation.

ADMINISTRATION/HANDLING

INTRANASAL

• Refrigerate. Nasal preparation can be stored at room temperature once pump is activated. • Clear nasal passages as much as possible. • Tilt head slightly forward, insert spray tip into nostril, pointing toward nasal passages, away from nasal septum. • Spray into nostril while holding other nostril closed and concurrently inspire through nose to permit medication as high into nasal passage as possible.

IM/SUBCUTANEOUS

• May be administered subcutaneously or IM. No more than 2-ml dose should be given IM. • Skin test should be performed before therapy in pts suspected of sensitivity to calcitonin. • Bedtime administration may reduce nausea, flushing.

INDICATIONS/ROUTES/DOSAGE

SKIN TESTING

Prepare a 10 unit/ml dilution; withdraw 0.05 ml from 200 international unit/ml vial solution in tuberculin syringe; fill up to 1 ml with 0.9% NaCl. Take 0.1 ml, inject intracutaneously on inner aspect of forearm. Observe after 15 min (positive response: appearance of more than mild erythema or wheal).

PAGET'S DISEASE

Subcutaneous/IM: ADULTS, ELDERLY: Initially, 100 international units/day (improvement in biochemical abnormalities, bone pain seen in first few months; in neurologic lesion, often longer than 1 yr). MAINTENANCE: 50 international units/day or 50–100 units every other day.

Intranasal: 200–400 units/day.

C

OSTEOPOROSIS IMPERFECTA

Subcutaneous/IM: ADULTS: 2 units/kg 3 times/wk.

POSTMENOPAUSAL OSTEOPOROSIS

Subcutaneous/IM: ADULTS, ELDERLY: 100 international units/day (with adequate calcium and vitamin D intake).

Intranasal: 200 international units as single daily spray, alternating nostrils daily.

HYPERCALCEMIA

Subcutaneous/IM: ADULTS, ELDERLY: Initially, 4 international units/kg q12h; may increase to 8 international units/kg q12h if no response in 2 days; may further increase to 8 international units/kg q6h if no response in 2 days.

SIDE EFFECTS

FREQUENT: Subcutaneous/IM (10%): Nausea (may occur 30 min after injection, usually diminishes with continued therapy), inflammation at injection site. **Nasal (10%–12%):** Rhinitis, nasal irritation, redness, sores. **OCCASIONAL: Subcutaneous/IM (2%–5%):** Flushing of face or hands. **Nasal (3%–5%):** Back pain, arthralgia, epistaxis (nosebleed), headache. **RARE: Subcutaneous/IM:** Epigastric discomfort, dry mouth, diarrhea, flatulence. **Nasal:** Itching of earlobes, edema of feet, rash, increased sweating.

ADVERSE REACTIONS/ TOXIC EFFECTS

Potential hypersensitivity reaction with protein allergy.

NURSING IMPLICATIONS

BASELINE ASSESSMENT

Establish baseline electrolytes.

INTERVENTION/EVALUATION

Ensure rotation of injection sites; check for inflammation. Assess vertebral bone mass (document stabilization/improvement). Assess for allergic response: rash, urticaria, swelling, shortness of breath, tachycardia, hypotension.

PATIENT/FAMILY TEACHING

Instruct pt/family on aseptic technique, proper injection of medication, including rotation of sites. Nausea is transient and usually decreases with continued therapy. Notify physician immediately if rash, itching, shortness of breath, significant nasal irritation occur.

calcium acetate

(PhosLo)

calcium carbonate

(Apo-Cal✤, Calsan✤, Caltrate✤, Dicarbosil, OsCal, Titralac, Tums)

calcium chloride

(Calcijex✤)

calcium citrate

(Citracal, Calcitrate)

calcium glubionate

(Calcione, Calciquid)

calcium gluconate

Do not confuse with Asacol, Citrucel, PhosChol.

◆ CLASSIFICATION

PHARMACOTHERAPEUTIC: Electrolyte replenisher. **CLINICAL:** Antacid, antihypocalcemic, antihyperkalemic, antihypermagnesemic, antihyperphosphatemic (see p. 9C).

ACTION

Calcium is essential for function, integrity of nervous, muscular, skeletal systems. Important role in normal cardiac/renal function, respiration, blood coagulation, cell membrane and capillary permeability. Assists in regulating release/storage of neurotransmitter/hormones. Neutralizes/reduces gastric acid (increase pH). **Calcium Acetate:** Combines with dietary phosphate, forming insoluble calcium phosphate. **Therapeutic Effect:** Replaces calcium in deficiency states, controls hyperphosphatemia in end-stage renal disease.

PHARMACOKINETICS

Moderately absorbed from small intestine (dependent on presence of vitamin D metabolites, pH). Primarily eliminated in feces.

USES

Parenteral: Acute hypocalcemia (e.g., neonatal hypocalcemic tetany, alkalosis), electrolyte depletion, cardiac arrest (strengthens myocardial contractions), hyperkalemia (reverses cardiac depression), hypermagnesemia (aids in reversing CNS depression). **PO:** Chronic hypocalcemia, calcium deficiency, antacid. **Calcium Acetate:** Controls hyperphosphatemia in end-stage renal disease. **Unlabeled: Calcium Carbonate:** Treatment of hyperphosphatemia.

PRECAUTIONS

CONTRAINDICATIONS: Ventricular fibrillation, hypercalcemia, hypercalciuria, calcium renal calculi, sarcoidosis, digoxin toxicity. **Calcium acetate:** Hypoparathyroidism, decreased renal function. **CAUTIONS:** Dehydration, history of renal calculi, chronic renal impairment, decreased cardiac function, ventricular fibrillation during cardiac resuscitation.

LIFESPAN CONSIDERATIONS: Pregnancy/lactation: Distributed in breast milk. Unknown whether calcium chloride or gluconate is distributed in breast milk. **Pregnancy Category C. Children:** Extreme irritation, possible tissue necrosis/sloughing with IV. Restrict IV use due to small vasculature. **Elderly:** Oral absorption may be decreased.

INTERACTIONS

DRUG: May antagonize **etidronate, gallium** effects. May decrease absorption of **ketoconazole, phenytoin, tetracyclines.** May decrease effects of **methenamine, parenteral magnesium.** May increase risk of arrhythmias with **digoxin. HERBAL:** None known. **FOOD:** None known. **LAB VALUES:** May increase calcium gastrin, pH. May decrease phosphate, potassium.

AVAILABILITY (OTC)

CALCIUM ACETATE: **TABLETS:** 667 mg. **CAPSULES:** 667 mg.

CALCIUM CARBONATE: **TABLETS:** 500 mg, 650 mg, 1,250 mg, 1,500 mg. **TABLETS (chewable):** 350 mg, 500 mg, 750 mg, 1,250 mg. **CAPSULES:** 1,250 mg.

CALCIUM CHLORIDE (Rx): **INJECTION:** 10%.

CALCIUM CITRATE: **TABLETS:** 950 mg.

CALCIUM GLUBIONATE: **SYRUP.**

CALCIUM GLUCONATE: **TABLETS:** 500 mg, 650 mg, 975 mg, 1,000 mg. **INJECTION: (Rx):** 10%.

ADMINISTRATION/HANDLING

PO

• Take tablets with full glass of water 0.5–1 hr after meals. Give syrup before meals (increases absorption), diluted in juice, water. • Chew chewable tablets well before swallowing.

IV

Storage • Store at room temperature.

Dilution

CALCIUM CHLORIDE

• May give undiluted or may dilute with

equal amount 0.9% NaCl or Sterile Water for Injection.

C

CALCIUM GLUCONATE
• May give undiluted or may dilute in up to 1,000 ml NaCl.

Rate of administration

CALCIUM CHLORIDE
• Give by slow IV push: 0.5–1 ml/min (rapid administration may produce bradycardia, metallic/chalky taste, drop in B/P, sensation of heat, peripheral vasodilation).

CALCIUM GLUCONATE
• Give by IV push: 0.5–1 ml/min (rapid administration may produce vasodilation, drop in B/P, arrhythmias, syncope, cardiac arrest). • Maximum rate for intermittent IV infusion is 200 mg/min (e.g., 10 ml/min when 1 g diluted with 50 ml diluent).

∅ IV INCOMPATIBILITIES

Calcium chloride: Amphotericin B complex (AmBisome, Abelcet), propofol (Diprivan), sodium bicarbonate. **Calcium gluconate:** Amphotericin C complex (AmBisome, Abelcet), fluconazole (Diflucan).

IV COMPATIBILITIES

Calcium chloride: amikacin (Amikin), dobutamine (Dobutrex), lidocaine, milrinone (Primacor), morphine, norepinephrine (Levophed). **Calcium gluconate:** Ampicillin, aztreonam (Azactam), cefazolin (Ancef), cefepime (Maxipime), ciprofloxacin (Cipro), dobutamine (Dobutrex), enalapril (Vasotec), famotidire (Pepcid), furosemide (Lasix), heparin, lidocaine, magnesium sulfate, meropenem (Merrem IV), midazolam (Versed), milrinone (Primacor), norepinephrine (Levophed), piperacillin tazobactam (Zosyn), potassium chloride, propofol (Diprivan).

INDICATIONS/ROUTES/DOSAGE

CALCIUM ACETATE

HYPOPHOSPHATEMIA

PO: ADULTS, ELDERLY: 2 tablets 3 times/day with meals.

CALCIUM CARBONATE

HYPOCALCEMIA

PO: ADULTS, ELDERLY: 1–2 g/day in 3–4 divided doses. CHILDREN: 45–65 mg/kg/day in 3–4 divided doses.

ANTACID

PO: ADULTS, ELDERLY: 1–2 tabs (5–10 ml) q2h as needed.

OSTEOPOROSIS

PO: ADULTS, ELDERLY: 1,200 mg/day.

CALCIUM GLUBIONATE

ANTIHYPOCALCEMIC

PO: ADULTS, ELDERLY: 15 ml 3–4 times/day. CHILDREN 1–4 YRS: 10 ml 3 times/day. CHILDREN <1 YR: 5 ml 5 times/day.

CALCIUM CHLORIDE

CARDIAC ARREST

IV: ADULTS, ELDERLY: 2–4 mg/kg. May repeat q10min. CHILDREN: 20 mg/kg. May repeat in 10 min.

HYPOCALCEMIA

IV: ADULTS, ELDERLY: 0.5–1 g repeated q4–6h as needed. CHILDREN: 2.5–5 mg/kg/dose q4–6h.

HYPOCALCEMIC TETANY

IV: ADULTS, ELDERLY: 1 g may repeat in 6 hrs. CHILDREN: 10 mg/kg over 5–10 min. May repeat in 6–8 hrs.

CALCIUM GLUCONATE

HYPOCALCEMIA

IV: ADULTS, ELDERLY: 2–15 g/24 hrs. CHILDREN: 200–500 mg/kg/day.

HYPOCALCEMIC TETANY

IV: ADULTS, ELDERLY: 1–3 g until therapeutic response. CHILDREN: 100–200 mg/kg/dose q6–8h.

SIDE EFFECTS

FREQUENT: Parenteral: Hypotension, flushing, feeling of warmth, nausea, vomiting; pain, rash, redness, burning at injection site; sweating, decreased B/P. **PO:** Chalky taste. **OCCASIONAL: PO:** Mild constipation, fecal impaction, swelling of hands/feet, metabolic alkalosis (muscle pain, restlessness, slow breathing, poor taste). **Calcium carbonate:** Milk-alkali syndrome (headache, decreased appetite, nausea, vomiting, unusual tiredness). **RARE: PO:** Difficult/painful urination.

ADVERSE REACTIONS/ TOXIC EFFECTS

HYPERCALCEMIA: Early signs: Constipation, headache, dry mouth, increased thirst, irritability, decreased appetite, metallic taste, fatigue, weakness, depression. **Later signs:** Confusion, drowsiness/increased B/P, light sensitivity, urination; irregular heartbeat; nausea, vomiting.

NURSING IMPLICATIONS

BASELINE ASSESSMENT

Assess B/P, EKG readings, renal function, magnesium, phosphate, potassium concentrations.

INTERVENTION/EVALUATION

Monitor B/P; EKG; renal function; magnesium, phosphate, potassium, serum, urine calcium concentrations. Monitor for signs of hypercalcemia.

PATIENT/FAMILY TEACHING

Stress importance of diet. Take tablets with full glass of water, ½–1 hr after meals. Give liquid before meals. Do not take within 1–2 hrs of other oral medications, fiber-containing foods. Avoid excessive alcohol, tobacco, caffeine.

calfactant

cal-**fak**-tant
(Infasurf)

◆ CLASSIFICATION

PHARMACOTHERAPEUTIC: Natural lung extract. **CLINICAL:** Pulmonary surfactant.

ACTION

Modifies alveolar surface tension, stabilizing the alveoli. **Therapeutic Effect:** Restores surface activity to infant lungs; improves lung compliance, respiratory gas exchange.

PHARMACOKINETICS

No studies performed.

USES

Prevention of respiratory distress syndrome (RDS) in premature infants <29 wks of gestational age; treatment of premature infants <72 hrs of age who develop RDS and require endotracheal intubation.

PRECAUTIONS

CONTRAINDICATIONS: None known. **CAUTIONS:** Hypersensitivity to calfactant.

LIFESPAN CONSIDERATIONS: Used only in neonates. No age-related precautions noted.

INTERACTIONS

DRUG: None known. **HERBAL:** None known. **FOOD:** None known. **LAB VALUES:** None known.

AVAILABILITY (Rx)

INTRATRACHEAL SUSPENSION: 35 mg/ml vials.

ADMINISTRATION/HANDLING

INTRATRACHEAL

• Refrigerate. • Unopened, unused vi-

C

als may be returned to refrigerator only once after having been warmed to room temperature. • Do not shake. • Enter only once, discard unused suspension.

INDICATIONS/ROUTES/DOSAGE

RDS

Intratracheal: INFANTS: Instill 3 ml/kg of birth weight as soon as possible after birth, administered as 2 doses of 1.5 ml/kg. Repeat doses of 3 ml/kg of birth weight, up to a total of 3 doses, 12 hrs apart.

SIDE EFFECTS

FREQUENT: Cyanosis (65%), airway obstruction (39%), bradycardia (34%), reflux of surfactant into endotracheal tube (21%), requirement of manual ventilation (16%). **OCCASIONAL (3%):** Reintubation.

ADVERSE REACTIONS/ TOXIC EFFECTS

Complications may occur as apnea, patent ductus arteriosus, intracranial hemorrhage, sepsis, pulmonary air leaks, pulmonary hemorrhage, necrotizing enterocolitis.

NURSING IMPLICATIONS

BASELINE ASSESSMENT

Drug must be administered in highly supervised setting. Clinicians in care of neonate must be experienced with intubation, ventilator management. Offer emotional support to parents.

INTERVENTION/EVALUATION

Monitor infant with arterial or transcutaneous measurement of systemic O_2, CO_2. Assess lung sounds for rales, moist breath sounds.

Cancidas

see caspofungin

candesartan cilexetil

can-deh-**sar-tan sill-ex**-eh-til
(Atacand)

FIXED-COMBINATION(S)

Atacand HCT: candesartan/hydrochlorothiazide (a diuretic): 16 mg/12.5 mg; 32 mg/12.5 mg.

◆CLASSIFICATION

PHARMACOTHERAPEUTIC: Angiotensin II receptor antagonist. **CLINICAL:** Antihypertensive (see p. 7C).

ACTION

Potent vasodilator. Angiotensin II receptor (type AT_1) antagonist; blocks vasoconstrictor, aldosterone-secreting effects of angiotensin II, inhibiting the binding of angiotensin II to the AT_1 receptors. **Therapeutic Effect:** Produces vasodilation; decreases peripheral resistance, B/P.

PHARMACOKINETICS

Onset	Peak	Duration
PO		
2–3 hrs	6–8 hrs	>24 hrs

Rapidly, completely absorbed. Protein binding: >99%. Undergoes minor hepatic metabolism to inactive metabolite. Excreted unchanged in urine and feces via biliary system. Not removed by hemodialysis. **Half-life:** 9 hrs.

USES

Treatment of hypertension alone or in combination with other antihypertensives. **Unlabeled:** Treatment of heart failure.

PRECAUTIONS

CONTRAINDICATIONS: Hypersensitivity to candesartan. **CAUTIONS:** Severe CHF, dehydration (increased risk for hypotension), renal/liver impairment, renal artery stenosis.

LIFESPAN CONSIDERATIONS: Pregnancy/lactation: Unknown if distributed in breast milk. May cause fetal/neonatal morbidity/mortality. **Pregnancy Category C** (**D** if used in second or third trimester). **Children:** Safety and efficacy not established. **Elderly:** No age-related precautions noted.

INTERACTIONS

DRUG: None known. **HERBAL:** None known. **FOOD:** None known. **LAB VALUES:** May increase BUN, serum creatinine, SGOT (AST), SGPT (ALT), alkaline phosphatase, bilirubin. May decrease Hgb, Hct.

AVAILABILITY (Rx)

TABLETS: 4 mg, 8 mg, 16 mg, 32 mg.

ADMINISTRATION/HANDLING

PO

- Give without regard to food.

INDICATIONS/ROUTES/DOSAGE

HYPERTENSION

PO: ADULTS, ELDERLY, MILDLY IMPAIRED RENAL/HEPATIC FUNCTION: Initially, 16 mg once daily in those who are not volume depleted. Can be given once or twice daily with total daily doses 8–32 mg. Give lower dosage in those treated with diuretics, severely impaired renal function.

SIDE EFFECTS

OCCASIONAL (3%–6%): Upper respiratory tract infection, dizziness, back/leg pain. **RARE (1%–2%):** Pharyngitis, rhinitis, headache, fatigue, diarrhea, nausea, dry cough, peripheral edema.

ADVERSE REACTIONS/ TOXIC EFFECTS

Overdosage may manifest as hypotension, tachycardia; bradycardia occurs less often. Institute supportive measures.

NURSING IMPLICATIONS

BASELINE ASSESSMENT

Obtain B/P, apical pulse immediately before each dose, in addition to regular monitoring (be alert to fluctuations). If excessive reduction in B/P occurs, place pt in supine position, feet slightly elevated. Question possibility of pregnancy (see Pregnancy Category). Assess medication history (esp. diuretic). Question for history of hepatic/renal impairment, renal artery stenosis. Obtain BUN, serum creatinine, SGOT (AST), SGPT (ALT), alkaline phosphatase, bilirubin, Hgb, Hct.

INTERVENTION/EVALUATION

Maintain hydration (offer fluids frequently). Assess for evidence of upper respiratory infection. Assist with ambulation if dizziness occurs. Monitor all blood serum levels. Assess B/P for hypertension/hypotension.

PATIENT/FAMILY TEACHING

Inform female pt regarding consequences of second- and third-trimester exposure to candesartan. Report pregnancy to physician as soon as possible. Avoid tasks that require alertness, motor skills until response to drug is established. Report any sign of infection (sore throat, fever). Do not stop taking medication. Need for lifelong control. Caution against exercising during hot weather (risk of dehydration, hypotension).

C

capecitabine

cap-eh-**site**-ah-bean
(Xeloda)
Do not confuse with Xenical.

◆ CLASSIFICATION

PHARMACOTHERAPEUTIC: Antimetabolite. **CLINICAL:** Antineoplastic (see p. 70C).

ACTION

Enzymatically converted to 5-fluorouracil. Inhibits enzymes necessary for synthesis of essential cellular components. **Therapeutic Effect:** Interferes with DNA synthesis, RNA processing, protein synthesis.

PHARMACOKINETICS

Readily absorbed from GI tract. Protein binding: <60%. Metabolized in the liver. Primarily excreted in urine. **Half-life:** 45 min.

USES

Treatment of metastatic breast cancer resistant to other therapy, colon cancer.

PRECAUTIONS

CONTRAINDICATIONS: Severe renal function impairment. **CAUTIONS:** Existing bone marrow depression, chickenpox, herpes zoster, liver function impairment, moderate renal function impairment, previous cytotoxic therapy/radiation therapy.

LIFESPAN CONSIDERATIONS: Pregnancy/lactation: May be harmful to fetus. Unknown if distributed in breast milk. **Pregnancy Category D. Children:** Safety and efficacy in those <18 yrs not established. **Elderly:** May be more sensitive to GI side effects.

INTERACTIONS

DRUG: May alter effects of **warfarin. HERBAL:** None known. **FOOD:** None known. **LAB VALUES:** May increase alkaline phosphatase, SGPT (ALT), SGOT (AST), bilirubin. May decrease WBC, Hgb, Hct.

AVAILABILITY (Rx)

TABLETS: 150 mg, 500 mg.

ADMINISTRATION/HANDLING

- Give within 30 min of a meal.

INDICATIONS/ROUTES/DOSAGE

METASTATIC BREAST CANCER, COLON CANCER

PO: ADULTS, ELDERLY: Initially, 2,500 mg/m^2/day in 2 equally divided doses approximately 12 hrs apart for 2 wks. Follow with a 1-wk rest period; given in 3-wk cycles.

SIDE EFFECTS

FREQUENT (>5%): Diarrhea (sometimes severe), nausea, vomiting, stomatitis (painful erythema, ulcers of mouth or tongue), hand-and-foot syndrome (painful palmar-plantar erythema and swelling with paresthesia, tingling, blistering), fatigue, anorexia, dermatitis. **OCCASIONAL (<5%):** Constipation, dyspepsia, nail disorder, headache, dizziness, insomnia, edema, myalgia.

ADVERSE REACTIONS/ TOXIC EFFECTS

Bone marrow depression (neutropenia, thrombocytopenia, anemia), cardiovascular toxicity noted as angina, cardiomyopathy, deep venous thrombosis (DVT), lymphedema. Respiratory toxicity noted as dyspnea, epistaxis, pneumonia.

NURSING IMPLICATIONS

BASELINE ASSESSMENT

Assess sensitivity to capecitabine or 5-fluorouracil. Obtain baseline Hgb, Hct, blood chemistries.

INTERVENTION/EVALUATION

Monitor for severe diarrhea; if dehydration occurs, fluid/electrolyte replacement therapy should be ordered. Assess hands/feet for erythema (chemotherapy induced). Monitor CBC for evidence of bone marrow depression. Monitor for blood dyscrasias (fever, sore throat, signs of local infection, easy bruising, unusual bleeding from any site), symptoms of anemia (excessive tiredness, weakness).

PATIENT/FAMILY TEACHING

Inform pt of potential for and notify physician if nausea, vomiting, possibly severe diarrhea, hand-and-foot syndrome, stomatitis occur. Do not have immunizations without physician's approval (drug lowers body's resistance). Avoid contact with those who have recently received live virus vaccine. Promptly report fever >100.5°F, sore throat, signs of local infection, easy bruising, unusual bleeding from any site.

Capoten

see captopril

capsaicin

cap-**say**-sin

(Arthritis Formula Capsaicin, Arthritis Pain Relief, Capsin, MediGen, Zostrix-HP)

Do not confuse with Zestril, Zovirax.

CLASSIFICATION

PHARMACOTHERAPEUTIC: Counterirritant. **CLINICAL:** Topical analgesic.

ACTION

Depletes/prevents reaccumulation of the chemomediator of pain impulses (substance P) from peripheral sensory neurons to CNS. **Therapeutic Effect:** Relieves pain.

USES

Treatment of neuralgia (e.g., pain with shingles, painful diabetic neuropathy), osteoarthritis, rheumatoid arthritis. **Unlabeled:** Treatment of neurogenic pain.

PRECAUTIONS

CONTRAINDICATIONS: None known. **CAUTIONS:** For external use only.

LIFESPAN CONSIDERATIONS: Pregnancy/lactation: Unknown if distributed in breast milk. **Pregnancy Category C:** Problems in humans not detected. **Children:** Not recommended in those <2 yrs. **Elderly:** No age-related precautions noted.

INTERACTIONS

DRUG: None known. **HERBAL:** None known. **FOOD:** None known. **LAB VALUES:** None known.

AVAILABILITY (Rx)

CREAM: 0.025%, 0.075%. **LOTION:** 0.025%. **SOLUTION:** 0.04%. **STICK:** 0.075%.

INDICATIONS/ROUTES/DOSAGE

USUAL TOPICAL DOSAGE

Topical: ADULTS, ELDERLY, CHILDREN >2 YRS: Apply directly to affected area 3–4 times/day. Continue for 14–28 days for optimal clinical response.

SIDE EFFECTS

FREQUENT (>30%): Burning, stinging, erythema at application site.

ADVERSE REACTIONS/ TOXIC EFFECTS

None known.

C

NURSING IMPLICATIONS

PATIENT/FAMILY TEACHING

Avoid contact with eyes, broken/irritated skin. Transient burning may occur on application; usually disappears after 72 hrs. Wash hands immediately after application. If there is no improvement or condition deteriorates after 28 days, discontinue use and consult physician.

captopril

cap-toe-prill
(Capoten, Novo-Captoril ✤)

Do not confuse with Capitrol.

FIXED-COMBINATION(S)

Capozide: captopril/hydrachlorothiazide (a diuretic): 25 mg/15 mg; 25 mg/25 mg; 50 mg/15 mg; 50 mg/25 mg.

◆CLASSIFICATION

PHARMACOTHERAPEUTIC: Angiotensin-converting enzyme (ACE) inhibitor. **CLINICAL:** Antihypertensive, vasodilator (see p. 6C).

ACTION

Suppresses renin-angiotensin-aldosterone system (prevents conversion of angiotensin I to angiotensin II, a potent vasoconstrictor; may inhibit angiotensin II at local vascular and renal sites). Decreases plasma angiotensin II, increases plasma renin activity, decreases aldosterone secretion. **Therapeutic Effect:** Reduces peripheral arterial resistance, pulmonary capillary wedge pressure; improves cardiac output, exercise tolerance.

PHARMACOKINETICS

Onset	Peak	Duration
PO		
0.25 hrs	0.5–1.5 hrs	Dose related

Rapidly, well absorbed from GI tract (decreased in presence of food). Protein binding: 25%–30%. Metabolized in liver. Primarily excreted in urine. Removed by hemodialysis. **Half-life:** <3 hrs (half-life increased with impaired renal function).

USES

Treatment of hypertension, CHF, Raynaud's phenomenon, diabetic nephropathy, post-MI for prevention of ventricular failure. **Unlabeled:** Hypertensive crisis, rheumatoid arthritis, diagnosis of anatomic renal artery stenosis.

PRECAUTIONS

CONTRAINDICATIONS: History of angioedema with previous treatment with ACE inhibitors. **CAUTIONS:** Renal impairment, those with sodium depletion or on diuretic therapy, dialysis, hypovolemia, coronary/cerebrovascular insufficiency.

LIFESPAN CONSIDERATIONS: Pregnancy/lactation: Crosses placenta; distributed in breast milk. May cause fetal/neonatal mortality/morbidity. **Pregnancy Category C (D** if used in second or third trimester). **Children:** Safety and efficacy not established. **Elderly:** May be more sensitive to hypotensive effects; caution recommended.

INTERACTIONS

DRUG: Alcohol, diuretics, hypotensive agents may increase effect. **NSAIDs** may decrease effect. **Potassium-sparing diuretics, potassium supplements** may cause hyperkalemia. May increase **lithium** concentration, toxicity. **HERBAL:** None known. **FOOD:** None known. **LAB VALUES:** May increase potassium, SGOT (AST), SGPT (ALT), alkaline phosphatase, bilirubin, BUN, creatinine. May decrease sodium. May cause positive ANA titer.

AVAILABILITY (Rx)

TABLETS: 12.5 mg, 25 mg, 50 mg, 100 mg.

ADMINISTRATION/HANDLING

PO

• Best taken 1 hr before meals for maximum absorption (food significantly decreases drug absorption). • Tablets may be crushed.

INDICATIONS/ROUTES/DOSAGE

HYPERTENSION

PO: ADULTS, ELDERLY: Initially, 12.5–25 mg 2–3 times/day. After 1–2 wks, may increase to 50 mg 2–3 times/day. Diuretic may be added if no response in additional 1–2 wks. If taken in combination with diuretic, may increase to 100–150 mg 2–3 times/day after 1–2 wks. MAINTENANCE: 25–150 mg 2–3 times/day. **Maximum:** 450 mg/day.

CHF

PO: ADULTS, ELDERLY: Initially, 6.25–25 mg 3 times/day. Increase to 50 mg 3 times/day. After at least 2 wks, may increase to 50–100 mg 3 times/day. **Maximum:** 450 mg/day.

POST-MI, IMPAIRED LIVER FUNCTION

PO: ADULTS, ELDERLY: 6.25 mg once, then 12.5 mg 3 times/day. Increase to 25 mg 3 times/day over several days up to 50 mg 3 times/day over several weeks.

NEPHROPATHY/PREVENTION OF KIDNEY FAILURE

PO: ADULTS, ELDERLY: 25 mg 3 times/day.

USUAL PEDIATRIC DOSE

PO: CHILDREN: Initially, 0.3–0.5 mg/kg/dose titrated up to maximum of 6 mg/kg/day in 2–4 divided doses. NEONATES: Initially, 0.05–0.1 mg/kg/dose q8–24h titrated up to 0.5 mg/kg/dose given q6–24h.

SIDE EFFECTS

FREQUENT (4%–7%): Rash. **OCCASIONAL (2%–4%):** Pruritus, dysgeusia (change in sense of taste). **RARE (0.5% – <2%):** Headache, cough, insomnia, dizziness, fatigue, paresthesia, malaise, nausea, diarrhea/constipation, dry mouth, tachycardia.

ADVERSE REACTIONS/ TOXIC EFFECTS

Excessive hypotension ("first-dose syncope") may occur in those with CHF, severely salt/volume depleted. Angioedema (swelling of face/lips), hyperkalemia occur rarely. Agranulocytosis, neutropenia may be noted in those with impaired renal function or collagen vascular disease (systemic lupus erythematosus, scleroderma). Nephrotic syndrome may be noted in those with history of renal disease.

NURSING IMPLICATIONS

BASELINE ASSESSMENT

Obtain B/P immediately before each dose, in addition to regular monitoring (be alert to fluctuations). If excessive reduction in B/P occurs, place pt in supine position with legs elevated. In pts with prior renal disease or receiving dosages >150 mg/day, urine test for protein by dipstick method should be made with first urine of day before therapy begins and periodically thereafter. In pts with renal impairment, autoimmune disease, or taking drugs that affect leukocytes or immune response, CBC should be performed prior to beginning therapy, q2wks for 3 mos, then periodically thereafter.

INTERVENTION/EVALUATION

Assess skin for rash, pruritus. Assist with ambulation if dizziness occurs. Monitor urinalysis for proteinuria. Assess for anorexia secondary to decreased taste perception. Monitor serum potassium levels in those on concurrent diuretic therapy.

PATIENT/FAMILY TEACHING

Several weeks may be needed for full therapeutic effect of B/P reduction.

Skipping doses or voluntarily discontinuing drug may produce severe, rebound hypertension. Avoid alcohol.

C

carbachol

(Isopto-Carbachol)

See Classification section under: Antiglaucoma agents (p. 44C)

carbamazepine

car-bah-**may**-zeh-peen

(Apo-Carbamazepine❋, Carbatrol, Epitol, Tegretol, Tegretol XR, Teril)

Do not confuse with Toradol, Trental.

◆ CLASSIFICATION

PHARMACOTHERAPEUTIC: Iminostilbene derivative. **CLINICAL:** Anticonvulsant, antineuralgic, antimanic, antipsychotic (see p. 32C).

ACTION

Decreases sodium, calcium ion influx into neuronal membranes, reducing posttetanic potentiation at synapse. **Therapeutic Effect:** Produces anticonvulsant effect.

PHARMACOKINETICS

Slowly, completely absorbed from GI tract. Protein binding: 75%. Metabolized in liver to active metabolite. Primarily excreted in urine. Not removed by hemodialysis. **Half-life:** 25–65 hrs (half-life decreased with chronic use).

USES

Partial seizures with complex symptomatology, generalized tonic-clonic seizures, mixed seizure patterns, pain relief of trigeminal neuralgia, diabetic neuropathy. **Unlabeled:** Treatment of neurogenic pain, bipolar disorder, diabetes insipidus, alcohol withdrawal, psychotic disorders.

PRECAUTIONS

CONTRAINDICATIONS: History of bone marrow depression, history of hypersensitivity to tricyclic antidepressants, concomitant use of MAOIs. **CAUTIONS:** Impaired cardiac, hepatic, renal function.

LIFESPAN CONSIDERATIONS: Pregnancy/lactation: Crosses placenta; distributed in breast milk. Accumulates in fetal tissue. **Pregnancy Category D. Children:** Behavioral changes more likely to occur. **Elderly:** More susceptible to confusion, agitation, AV block, bradycardia, syndrome of inappropriate antidiuretic hormone (SIADH).

INTERACTIONS

DRUG: May decrease effect of **steroids, anticoagulants.** May increase metabolism of **anticonvulsants, barbiturates, benzodiazepines, valproic acid. Tricyclic antidepressants, haloperidol, antipsychotics** may increase CNS depressant effects. **Cimetidine** may increase concentration, toxicity. May decrease effects of **estrogens, quinidine, clarithromycin, diltiazem, erythromycin, propoxyphene. Verapamil** may increase toxicity. May increase metabolism of **isoniazid** (hepatotoxicity). **Isoniazid** may increase concentration, toxicity. **MAOIs** may cause hypertensive crises, convulsions. **HERBAL:** None known. **FOOD: Grapefruit** can increase absorption, concentration. **LAB VALUES:** May increase BUN, glucose, protein, SGOT (AST), SGPT (ALT), alkaline phosphatase, bilirubin, cholesterol, HDL, triglycerides. May decrease calcium, T_3, T_4,

T_4 index. Therapeutic blood serum level: 4–12 mcg/ml; toxic serum level: >12 mcg/ml.

AVAILABILITY (Rx)

CAPSULES (controlled-release) Cabatrol: 200 mg, 300 mg. **SUSPENSION:** 100 mg/5 ml. **TABLETS:** 200 mg. **TABLETS (chewable):** 100 mg, 200 mg. **TABLETS (controlled release):** 100 mg, 400 mg.

ADMINISTRATION/HANDLING

PO

• Store oral suspension, tablets at room temperature. • Give with meals to reduce risk of GI distress. • Shake oral suspension well. Do not administer simultaneously with other liquid medicine. • Do not crush extended-release tablets.

INDICATIONS/ROUTES/DOSAGE

Alert: When replacement by another anticonvulsant is necessary, decrease carbamazepine gradually as therapy begins with low replacement dose. When transferring from tablets to suspension, divide total tablet daily dose into smaller, more frequent doses of suspension. Administer extended-release tablets in 2 divided doses.

SEIZURE CONTROL

PO: ADULTS, CHILDREN >12 YRS: Initially, 200 mg 2 times/day. Increase dosage up to 200 mg/day at weekly intervals until response is attained. MAINTENANCE: 800–1,200 mg/day. Do not exceed 1,000 mg/day in children 12–15 yrs, 1,200 mg/day in pts >15 yrs. ELDERLY: Initially, 100 mg 1–2 time/day. May increase by 100 mg at weekly intervals. RANGE: 400–1,000 mg/day. CHILDREN 6–12 YRS: Initially, 100 mg 2 times/day. Increase by 100 mg/day until response is attained. MAINTENANCE: 400–800 mg/day. Give dosage ≥200 mg/day in 3–4 equally divided doses. **Suspension:** ELDERLY: Initially, 100 mg 1–2 times/day. May increase by 100 mg at weekly intervals. RANGE: 400–1,000 mg/day. CHILDREN 6–12 YRS: Initially, 50 mg 4 times/day. Increase dosage slowly (reduces sedation risk). CHILDREN <6 YRS: 10–20 mg/kg/day in 2–4 divided doses. **Maximum:** 35 mg/kg/day.

TRIGEMINAL NEURALGIA

PO: ADULTS, ELDERLY: 100 mg 2 times/day on day 1. Increase by 100 mg q12h until pain is relieved. MAINTENANCE: 200–1,200 mg/day. Do not exceed 1,200 mg/day.

SIDE EFFECTS

FREQUENT: Drowsiness, dizziness, nausea, vomiting. **OCCASIONAL:** Visual abnormalities (spots before eyes, difficulty focusing, blurred vision), dry mouth/pharynx, tongue irritation, headache, water retention, increased sweating, constipation/diarrhea.

ADVERSE REACTIONS/ TOXIC EFFECTS

Toxic reactions appear as blood dyscrasias (aplastic anemia, agranulocytosis, thrombocytopenia, leukopenia, leukocytosis, eosinophilia), cardiovascular disturbances (CHF, hypotension/hypertension, thrombophlebitis, arrhythmias), dermatologic effects (rash, urticaria, pruritus, photosensitivity). Abrupt withdrawal may precipitate status epilepticus.

NURSING IMPLICATIONS

BASELINE ASSESSMENT

Seizures: Review history of seizure disorder (intensity, frequency, duration, loss of consciousness [LOC]). Provide safety precautions, quiet, dark environment. CBC, serum iron determination, urinalysis, BUN should be performed before therapy begins and periodically during therapy.

C

INTERVENTION/EVALUATION

Seizures: Observe frequently for recurrence of seizure activity. Monitor for therapeutic serum levels. Assess for clinical improvement (decrease in intensity/frequency of seizures). Assess for clinical evidence of early toxic signs (fever, sore throat, mouth ulcerations, easy bruising, unusual bleeding, joint pain). **Neuralgia:** Avoid triggering tic douloureux (draft, talking, washing face, jarring bed, hot/warm/cold food or liquids). Therapeutic blood serum level: 4–12 mcg/ml; toxic serum level: >12 mcg/ml.

PATIENT/FAMILY TEACHING

Do not abruptly withdraw medication after long-term use (may precipitate seizures). Strict maintenance of drug therapy is essential for seizure control. Drowsiness usually disappears during continued therapy. Avoid tasks that require alertness, motor skills until response to drug is established. Report visual abnormalities. Blood tests should be repeated frequently during first 3 mos of therapy and at monthly intervals thereafter for 2–3 yrs. Do not take oral suspension simultaneously with other liquid medicine. Do not take with grapefruit juice.

carbenicillin

(Geocillin)

See Classification section under: Antibiotic: penicillins (p. 27C)

carbidopa/levodopa

car-bih-dope-ah/**lev**-oh-dope-ah (Apo-Levocarb♣, Sinemet, Sinemet CR)

FIXED-COMBINATION(S)

Stavelo: carbidopa/levodopa/entacapone (antiparkinson agent): 12.5 mg/50 mg/200 mg, 25 mg/100 mg/200 mg, 37.5 mg/150 mg/200 mg

◆ CLASSIFICATION

PHARMACOTHERAPEUTIC: Dopamine precursor. **CLINICAL:** Antiparkinson agent.

ACTION

Converted to dopamine in basal ganglia. Increases dopamine concentration in brain, inhibiting hyperactive cholinergic activity. Carbidopa prevents peripheral breakdown of levodopa, allowing more levodopa to be available for transport into brain. **Therapeutic Effect:** Reduces tremor.

PHARMACOKINETICS

Carbidopa: Rapidly, completely absorbed from GI tract. Widely distributed. Excreted primarily in urine. **Half-life:** 1–2 hrs. **Levodopa:** Converted to dopamine. Excreted primarily in urine. **Half-life:** 1–3 hrs.

USES

Treatment of idiopathic Parkinson's disease (paralysis agitans), postencephalitic parkinsonism, symptomatic parkinsonism following injury to nervous system by CO_2 poisoning, manganese intoxication.

PRECAUTIONS

CONTRAINDICATIONS: Narrow-angle glaucoma, those on MAOI therapy. **CAUTIONS:** History of MI, bronchial asthma (tartrazine sensitivity), emphysema; severe cardiac, pulmonary, renal, hepatic, endocrine disease; active peptic ulcer; treated open-angle glaucoma.

LIFESPAN CONSIDERATIONS: Pregnancy/lactation: Unknown if drug crosses placenta or is distributed in breast milk. May inhibit lactation. Do not nurse. **Pregnancy Category C. Children:** Safety and efficacy not established in those <18 yrs. **Elderly:** More sensitive to effects of levodopa. Anxiety, confusion, nervousness more common when receiving anticholinergics.

INTERACTIONS

DRUG: Anticonvulsants, benzodiazepines, haloperidol, phenothiazines may decrease effect. **MAOIs** may increase risk of hypertensive crises. **Selegiline** may increase dyskinesias, nausea, orthostatic hypotension, confusion, hallucinations. **HERBAL:** None known. **FOOD:** None known. **LAB VALUES:** May increase alkaline phosphatase, SGOT (AST), SGPT (ALT), LDH, bilirubin, BUN.

AVAILABILITY (Rx)

TABLETS (expressed as carbidopa/levodopa): 10 mg/100 mg, 25 mg/100 mg, 25 mg/250 mg. **TABLETS (extended-release):** 25 mg/100 mg, 50 mg/200 mg.

ADMINISTRATION/HANDLING

PO

- Scored tablets may be crushed.
- May be given without regard to meals.
- Do not crush sustained-release tablet; may cut in half.

INDICATIONS/ROUTES/DOSAGE

PARKINSONISM

PO: ADULTS: Initially, 25/100 mg 2–4 times/day. May increase up to a maximum of 200/2,000 mg. ELDERLY: Initially, 25/100 mg 2 times/day. May increase as necessary. Conversion from Sinemet (based on total daily dose of levodopa) to Sinemet CR (50/200 mg):

Sinemet	Sinemet CR
300–400 mg	1 tab 2×/day
500–600 mg	1.5 tab 2×/day or 1 tab 3×/day
700–800 mg	4 tabs in 3 or more divided doses
900–1,000 mg	5 tabs in 3 or more divided doses

Intervals between Sinemet CR should be 4–8 hrs while awake.

RECEIVING ONLY LEVODOPA

Alert: Discontinue levodopa at least 8 hrs prior to carbidopa/levodopa. Initiate with dose providing at least 25% of previous levodopa dosage.

PO: ADULTS, ≤1,500 MG LEVODOPA/DAY: 1 tablet (25/100 mg) 3–4 times/day. ADULTS, >1,500 MG LEVODOPA/DAY: 1 tablet (25/250 mg) 3–4 times/day. **Sustained-release:** ADULTS: 1 tablet 2 times/day.

RECEIVING CARBIDOPA/LEVODOPA

ADULTS: Provide about 10% more levodopa; may increase up to 30% more at 4- to 8-hr dosing intervals.

SIDE EFFECTS

FREQUENT (10%–90%): Uncontrolled body movements (including face, tongue, arms, upper body), nausea/vomiting (80%), anorexia (50%). **OCCASIONAL:** Depression, anxiety, confusion, nervousness, difficulty urinating, irregular heartbeats, dizziness, lightheadedness, decreased appetite, blurred vision, constipation, dry mouth, flushed skin, headache, insomnia, diarrhea, unusual tiredness, darkening of urine. **RARE:** Hypertension, ulcer, hemolytic anemia (tiredness/weakness).

ADVERSE REACTIONS/ TOXIC EFFECTS

High incidence of involuntary choreiform, dystonic, dyskinetic movements may be noted in pts on long-term therapy. Mental changes (paranoid ideation, psychotic episodes, depression) may be noted. Numerous mild to severe CNS, psychiatric disturbances may include reduced attention span, anxiety, nightmares, daytime somnolence, euphoria, fatigue, paranoia, hallucinations.

C

NURSING IMPLICATIONS

BASELINE ASSESSMENT

Instruct pt to void before giving medication (reduces risk of urinary retention).

INTERVENTION/EVALUATION

Be alert to neurologic effects: headache, lethargy, mental confusion, agitation. Monitor for evidence of dyskinesia (difficulty with movement). Assess for clinical reversal of symptoms (improvement of tremor of head/hands at rest, masklike facial expression, shuffling gait, muscular rigidity).

PATIENT/FAMILY TEACHING

Avoid tasks that require alertness, motor skills until response to drug is established. Avoid alcoholic beverages during therapy. Sugarless gum, sips of tepid water may relieve dry mouth. Take with food to minimize GI upset. Effects may be delayed from several weeks to months. May cause darkening in urine/sweat (not harmful). Report any uncontrolled movement of face, eyelids, mouth, tongue, arms, hands, legs; mental changes; palpitations; irregular heartbeats; severe/persistent nausea/vomiting; difficulty urinating.

carboplatin

car-bow-**play-tin**
(Paraplatin)

Do not confuse with Cisplatin, Platinol.

CLASSIFICATION

PHARMACOTHERAPEUTIC: Platinum coordination complex. **CLINICAL:** Antineoplastic (see p. 70C).

ACTION

Inhibits DNA synthesis by cross-linking with DNA strands. Cell cycle–phase nonspecific. **Therapeutic Effect:** Prevents cellular division, interferes with DNA function.

PHARMACOKINETICS

Protein binding: Low. Hydrolyzed in solution to active form. Primarily excreted in urine. **Half-life:** 2.6–5.9 hrs.

USES

Treatment of ovarian carcinomoa. **Unlabeled:** Treatment of small cell lung cancer; squamous cell carcinoma of the esophagus; solid tumors of the bladder, cervix, testes; pediatric brain tumor; neuroblastoma; bony/soft tissue sarcomas; germ cell tumors.

PRECAUTIONS

CONTRAINDICATIONS: History of severe allergic reaction to cisplatin, platinum compounds, mannitol; severe myelosuppression, severe bleeding. **CAUTIONS:** Infection, chickenpox, herpes zoster, renal function impairment.

LIFESPAN CONSIDERATIONS: Pregnancy/lactation: If possible, avoid use during pregnancy, esp. first trimester. May cause fetal harm. Unknown if distributed in breast milk. Breast-feeding not recommended. **Pregnancy Category D. Children:** Safety and efficacy not established. **Elderly:** Peripheral neurotoxicity increased, myelotoxicity may be more severe. Age-related decreased renal function may require decreased dosage, more careful monitoring of blood counts.

INTERACTIONS

DRUG: Bone marrow depressants may increase bone marrow depression. **Nephrotoxic-, ototoxic-producing agents** may increase toxicity. **Live virus vaccines** may potentiate virus replication, increase vaccine side effects, decrease antibody response to vaccine. **HERBAL:** None known. **FOOD:** None known. **LAB VALUES:** May decrease electrolytes (sodium, magnesium, calcium, potassium). High dosages (>4 times recommended dosage) may elevate alkaline phosphatase, SGOT (AST), total bilirubin, BUN, serum creatinine concentrations.

AVAILABILITY (Rx)

POWDER FOR INJECTION: 50 mg, 150 mg, 450 mg.

ADMINISTRATION/HANDLING

Alert: May be carcinogenic, mutagenic, or teratogenic. Handle with extreme care during preparation/administration.

IV

Storage • Store vials at room temperature. • After reconstitution, solution is stable for 8 hrs. Discard unused portion after 8 hrs.

Reconstitution • Reconstitute immediately before use. • Do not use aluminum needles or administration sets that come in contact with drug (may produce black precipitate, loss of potency). • Reconstitute each 50 mg with 5 ml Sterile Water for Injection, D_5W, or 0.9% NaCl to provide concentration of 10 mg/ml. • May be further diluted with D_5W or 0.9% NaCl to provide concentration as low as 0.5 mg/ml.

Rate of administration • Infuse over 15–60 min. • Rarely, anaphylactic reaction occurs minutes after administration. Use of epinephrine, corticosteroids alleviates symptoms.

IV INCOMPATIBILITIES
Amphotericin B complex (AmBisome, Amphotec, Abelcet).

IV COMPATIBILITIES
Cisplatin (Platinol), etoposide (VePesid), filgrastim (Neupogen), granisetron (Kytril), ondansetron (Zofran), paclitaxel (Taxol), propofol (Diprivan).

INDICATIONS/ROUTES/DOSAGE

Alert: Dosage individualized based on clinical response, tolerance to adverse effects. Platelets must be >100,000 mm^3, neutrophils >2,000 mm^3 before giving any dosage.

OVARIAN CARCINOMA (single agent)
IV: ADULTS: 360 mg/m^2 on day 1, q4wks. Do not repeat dose until neutrophil, platelet counts are within acceptable levels. Adjust dosage in pts previously treated based on lowest posttreatment platelet or neutrophil value.

Alert: Make only one escalation, not >125% of starting dose.

OVARIAN CARCINOMA (combination therapy)
IV: ADULTS: 300 mg/m^2 (with cyclophosphamide) on day 1, q4wks. Do not repeat dose until neutrophil, platelet counts are within acceptable levels.

DOSAGE IN RENAL IMPAIRMENT
Initial dosage based on creatinine clearance; subsequent dosages based on pt's tolerance, degree of myelosuppression.

Creatinine Clearance	Dosage Day 1
>60 ml/min	360 mg/m^2
41–59 ml/min	250 mg/m^2
16–40 ml/min	200 mg/m^2

USUAL PEDIATRIC DOSAGE
IV: SOLID TUMOR: 300–600 mg/m^2 q4wks. BRAIN TUMOR: 175 mg/m^2 q4wks.

SIDE EFFECTS

FREQUENT: Nausea (75%–80%), vomiting (65%). **OCCASIONAL:** Generalized pain (17%), diarrhea/constipation (6%), peripheral neuropathy (4%). **RARE (2%–**

C

3%): Alopecia, asthenia (loss of energy, strength), hypersensitivity reaction (rash, urticaria, pruritus, erythema).

ADVERSE REACTIONS/ TOXIC EFFECTS

Bone marrow suppression may be severe, resulting in anemia, infection, bleeding (GI bleeding, sepsis, pneumonia). Prolonged treatment may result in peripheral neurotoxicity.

NURSING IMPLICATIONS

BASELINE ASSESSMENT

Offer emotional support. Do not repeat treatment until WBC recovers from previous therapy. Transfusions may be needed in those receiving prolonged therapy (myelosuppression increased in those with previous therapy, impaired kidney function).

INTERVENTION/EVALUATION

Monitor hematologic status, pulmonary function studies, hepatic and renal function tests. Monitor for fever, sore throat, signs of local infection, easy bruising, unusual bleeding from any site, symptoms of anemia (excessive tiredness, weakness).

PATIENT/FAMILY TEACHING

Nausea, vomiting generally abates in <24 hrs. Do not have immunizations without physician's approval (drug lowers body's resistance). Avoid contact with those who have recently received live virus vaccine.

Cardizem

see diltiazem

carisoprodol

(Soma)

See Classification section under: Skeletal muscle relaxants

carmustine

car-**muss**-teen

(BiCNU, Gliadel)

CLASSIFICATION

PHARMACOTHERAPEUTIC: Alkylating agent, nitrosourea. **CLINICAL:** Antineoplastic (see p. 70C).

ACTION

Inhibits DNA, RNA synthesis by cross-linking with DNA, RNA strands, preventing cellular division. Cell cycle–phase nonspecific. **Therapeutic Effect:** Interferes with DNA/RNA function.

USES

Treatment of primary and metastatic brain tumors, multiple myeloma, disseminated Hodgkin's disease, non-Hodgkin's lymphoma. **Gliadel Wafer:** Adjunct to surgery to prolong survival in recurrent glioblastoma multiforme. **Unlabeled:** Treatment of hepatic, GI carcinoma; malignant melanoma; mycosis fungoides.

PRECAUTIONS

CONTRAINDICATIONS: None known. **CAUTIONS:** Pts with decreased platelet, leukocyte, erythrocyte counts. **Pregnancy Category D.**

INTERACTIONS

DRUG: Bone marrow depressants, cimetidine may enhance myelosuppressive effect. **Hepatotoxic, nephrotoxic drugs** may enhance respective toxicities. **Live virus vaccines** may potentiate virus replication, increase vaccine side effects, decrease antibody response to vaccine. **HERBAL:** None known. **FOOD:** None known. **LAB VALUES:** May increase BUN, SGOT (AST), SGPT (ALT), alkaline phosphatase, bilirubin.

AVAILABILITY (Rx)

POWDER FOR INJECTION: 100 mg. **WAFER:** 7.7 mg.

ADMINISTRATION/HANDLING

Alert: May be carcinogenic, mutagenic, or teratogenic. Wear protective gloves during preparation of drug; may cause transient burning, brown staining of skin.

IV

Storage • Refrigerate unopened vials of dry powder. • Reconstituted vials are stable for 8 hrs at room temperature or 24 hrs if refrigerated. • Solutions further diluted to 0.2 mg/ml with D_5W or 0.9% NaCl are stable for 48 hrs if refrigerated or an additional 8 hrs at room temperature. • Solutions appear clear, colorless to yellow. • Discard if precipitate forms, color change occurs, or oily film develops on bottom of vial.

Reconstitution • Reconstitute 100-mg vial with 3 ml sterile dehydrated (absolute) alcohol, followed by 27 ml Sterile Water for Injection to provide concentration of 3.3 mg/ml. • Further dilute with 50–250 ml D_5W or 0.9% NaCl.

Rate of administration • Infuse over 1–2 hrs (shorter duration may produce intense burning pain at injection site, intense flushing of skin, conjunctiva). • Flush IV line with 5–10 ml 0.9% NaCl or D_5W before and after administration to prevent irritation at injection site.

IV INCOMPATIBILITY
Allopurinol (Aloprim).

IV COMPATIBILITIES
Etoposide (VePesid), filgrastim (Neupogen), gemcitabine (Gemzar), granisetron (Kytril), ondansetron (Zofran), sargramostim (Leukine), vinorelbine (Navelbine).

INDICATIONS/ROUTES/DOSAGE

Alert: Dosage individualized based on clinical response, tolerance to adverse effects. When used in combination therapy, consult specific protocols for optimum dosage, sequence of drug administration.

SINGLE AGENT IN PREVIOUSLY UNTREATED PT

IV infusion: ADULTS, ELDERLY: 150–200 mg/m² as single dose or 75–100 mg/m² on 2 successive days. CHILDREN: 200–250 mg/m² q4–6wks as a single dose.

SIDE EFFECTS

FREQUENT: Nausea and vomiting within minutes to 2 hrs after administration (may last up to 6 hrs). **OCCASIONAL:** Diarrhea, esophagitis, anorexia, dysphagia. **RARE:** Thrombophlebitis.

ADVERSE REACTIONS/TOXIC EFFECTS

Hematologic toxicity, due to bone marrow depression, occurs frequently. Thrombocytopenia occurs at about 4 wks, lasts 1–2 wks; leukopenia evident at about 5–6 wks, lasts 1–2 wks. Anemia occurs less frequently, is less severe. Mild, reversible hepatotoxicity also occurs frequently. Prolonged therapy with high dosage may produce impaired renal function, pulmonary toxicity (pulmonary infiltrate and/or fibrosis).

NURSING IMPLICATIONS

BASELINE ASSESSMENT

Perform CBC, renal/liver function studies prior to beginning therapy and periodically thereafter. Perform blood counts weekly during and for at least 6 wks after therapy ends.

C

INTERVENTION/EVALUATION

Monitor CBC, BUN, serum transaminase, alkaline phosphatase, bilirubin; pulmonary, renal/liver function tests. Monitor for hematologic toxicity (fever, sore throat, signs of local infection, easy bruising, unusual bleeding from any site) or symptoms of anemia (excessive tiredness, weakness). Monitor lung sounds for pulmonary toxicity (dyspnea, fine lung rales).

PATIENT/FAMILY TEACHING

Maintain adequate daily fluid intake (may protect against renal impairment). Do not have immunizations without doctor's approval (drug lowers body's resistance). Avoid contact with those who have recently received live virus vaccine. Contact physician if nausea/vomiting continues at home.

carteolol

(Cartrol, Ocupress)

See Classification section under: Beta-adrenergic blockers (pp. 45C, 62C)

carvedilol

car-**veh**-dih-lol

(Coreg)

Do not confuse with carteolol.

CLASSIFICATION

PHARMACOTHERAPEUTIC: Beta-adrenergic blocker. **CLINICAL:** Antihypertensive (see p. 62C).

ACTION

Possesses nonselective beta-blocking and alpha-adrenergic blocking activity. Causes vasodilation. **Therapeutic Effect:** Reduces cardiac output, exercise-induced tachycardia, reflex orthostatic tachycardia, peripheral vascular resistance.

PHARMACOKINETICS

Onset	Peak	Duration
PO		
30 min	1–2 hrs	24 hrs

Rapidly and extensively absorbed from GI tract. Protein binding: 98%. Metabolized in liver. Excreted primarily via bile into feces. Minimally removed by hemodialysis. **Half-life:** 7–10 hrs. Food delays rate of absorption.

USES

Management of essential hypertension. Used alone or in combination with diuretics, esp. thiazide type. Treatment of CHF. Reduces cardiovascular mortality. **Unlabeled:** Treatment of angina pectoris, idiopathic cardiomyopathy.

PRECAUTIONS

CONTRAINDICATIONS: Pulmonary edema, bronchial asthma or related bronchospastic conditions, second- or third-degree AV block, cardiogenic shock, severe bradycardia. **CAUTIONS:** CHF controlled with digitalis, diuretics, angiotensin-converting enzyme inhibitor; peripheral vascular disease; anesthesia; diabetes mellitus; hypoglycemia; thyrotoxicosis; impaired hepatic function.

LIFESPAN CONSIDERATIONS: Pregnancy/lactation: Unknown if drug crosses placenta or is distributed in breast milk. May produce bradycardia, apnea, hypoglycemia, hypothermia during delivery, low birth-weight infants. **Pregnancy Category C.** (**D** if used in second or third trimester). **Children:** Safety and efficacy not established. **El-**

derly: Incidence of dizziness may be increased.

INTERACTIONS

DRUG: Diuretics, other hypotensives may increase hypotensive effect; may mask symptoms of hypoglycemia, prolong hypoglycemic effect of **insulin, oral hypoglycemics. Catapres** may potentiate B/P effects. **Calcium blockers** increase risk of conduction disturbances, increase **digoxin** concentrations. **Cimetidine** may increase concentration. **Rifampin** decreases concentration. **HERBAL:** None known. **FOOD:** None known. **LAB VALUES:** None known.

AVAILABILITY (Rx)

TABLETS: 3.125 mg, 6.25 mg, 12.5 mg, 25 mg.

ADMINISTRATION/HANDLING

PO

- Give with food (slows rate of absorption, reduces risk of orthostatic effects).
- Take standing systolic B/P 1 hr after dosing as guide for tolerance.

INDICATIONS/ROUTES/DOSAGE

HYPERTENSION/REDUCING CARDIOVASCULAR MORTALITY

PO: ADULTS, ELDERLY: Initially, 6.25 mg twice daily. May double at 7- to 14-day intervals to highest tolerated dosage. **Maximum:** 50 mg/day.

CHF

PO: ADULTS, ELDERLY: Initially, 3.125 mg twice daily. May double at 2-wk intervals to highest tolerated dosage. **Maximum: <85 kg:** 25 mg twice daily; **>85 kg:** 50 mg twice daily.

SIDE EFFECTS

Generally well tolerated, with mild and transient side effects. **FREQUENT (4%–6%):** Fatigue, dizziness. **OCCASIONAL (2%):** Diarrhea, bradycardia, rhinitis, back pain. **RARE (<2%):** Postural hypotension, somnolence, urinary tract infection, viral infection.

ADVERSE REACTIONS/ TOXIC EFFECTS

Overdosage may produce profound bradycardia, hypotension, bronchospasm, cardiac insufficiency, cardiogenic shock, cardiac arrest. Abrupt withdrawal may result in sweating, palpitations, headache, tremulousness. May precipitate CHF, MI in those with cardiac disease, thyroid storm in those with thyrotoxicosis, peripheral ischemia in pts with existing peripheral vascular disease. Hypoglycemia may occur in pts with previously controlled diabetes.

NURSING IMPLICATIONS

BASELINE ASSESSMENT

Assess B/P, apical pulse immediately before drug is administered (if pulse is ≤60/min or systolic B/P is <90 mm Hg, withhold medication, contact physician).

INTERVENTION/EVALUATION

Monitor B/P for hypotension, respiration for breathlessness. Assess pulse for quality, irregular rate, bradycardia. Monitor EKG for cardiac arrhythmias. Assist with ambulation if dizziness occurs. Assess for evidence of CHF: dyspnea (particularly on exertion or lying down), night cough, peripheral edema, distended neck veins. Monitor I&O (increase in weight, decrease in urine output may indicate CHF).

PATIENT/FAMILY TEACHING

Full antihypertensive effect noted in 1–2 wks. Contact lens wearers may experience decreased lacrimation. Take with food. Do not abruptly discontinue medication. Compliance with therapy regimen is essential to control hypertension. Avoid tasks that require alertness, motor skills until response to

C

drug is established. Report excessive fatigue, prolonged dizziness. Do not use nasal decongestants, OTC cold preparations (stimulants) without physician approval. Monitor B/P, pulse before taking medication. Restrict salt, alcohol intake.

cascara sagrada

cass-**care**-ah sah-**graud**-ah
(Cascara Sagrada)

FIXED-COMBINATION(S)

With milk of magnesia, a saline laxative **(SAMe).**

◆CLASSIFICATION

PHARMACOTHERAPEUTIC: GI stimulant. **CLINICAL:** Laxative (see p. 105C).

ACTION

Increases peristalsis by direct effect on colonic smooth musculature (stimulates intramural nerve plexi). **Therapeutic Effect:** Promotes fluid, ion accumulation in colon to increase laxative effect.

USES

Temporary relief of constipation, sometimes used with milk of magnesia.

PRECAUTIONS

CONTRAINDICATIONS: Abdominal pain, nausea, vomiting, appendicitis, intestinal obstruction. **CAUTIONS:** None known. **Pregnancy Category C.**

INTERACTIONS

DRUG: May decrease transit time of concurrently administered oral medication, decreasing absorption. **HERBAL:** None known. **FOOD:** None known. **LAB VALUES:** May increase blood glucose. May decrease potassium, calcium.

AVAILABILITY (Rx)

TABLETS: 325 mg. **LIQUID:** (18% alcohol).

INDICATIONS/ROUTES/DOSAGE

LAXATIVE

PO: ADULTS, ELDERLY: 1 tablet (or 5 ml) at bedtime. CHILDREN 2–11 YRS: 2.5 ml (1–3 ml) as a single dose. INFANTS: 1.25 ml (0.5–2 ml) as a single dose.

SIDE EFFECTS

FREQUENT: Pink-red, red-violet, red-brown, yellow-brown discoloration of urine. **OCCASIONAL:** Some degree of abdominal discomfort, nausea, mild cramps, faintness.

ADVERSE REACTIONS/ TOXIC EFFECTS

Long-term use may result in laxative dependence, chronic constipation, loss of normal bowel function. Chronic use or overdosage may result in electrolyte disturbances (hypokalemia, hypocalcemia, metabolic acidosis or alkalosis), persistent diarrhea, malabsorption, weight loss. Electrolyte disturbance may produce vomiting, muscle weakness.

NURSING IMPLICATIONS

INTERVENTION/EVALUATION

Encourage adequate fluid intake. Assess bowel sounds for peristalsis. Monitor daily bowel activity/stool consistency (watery, loose, soft, semisolid, solid); record time of evacuation. Assess for abdominal disturbances. Monitor serum electrolytes in those exposed to prolonged/frequent/excessive use of medication.

PATIENT/FAMILY TEACHING

Urine may turn pink-red, red-violet, red-brown, yellow-brown (only temporary, not harmful). Institute measures to promote defecation: increase fluid intake, exercise, high-fiber diet. Laxative effect generally occurs in 6–12 hrs but may take 24 hrs. Do not use in presence of nausea, vomiting, abdominal pain >1 wk. Do not take other oral medication within 1 hr of taking this medicine (decreased effectiveness due to increased peristalsis).

caspofungin acetate

cas-poe-**fun**-gin
(Cancidas)

CLASSIFICATION

CLINICAL: Antifungal.

ACTION

Inhibits synthesis of glucan (vital component of fungal cell formation), damaging fungal cell membrane. **Therapeutic Effect:** Fungistatic.

PHARMACOKINETICS

Distributed in tissue. Extensively bound to albumin. Protein binding: 97%. Slowly metabolized in liver to active metabolite. Primarily excreted in urine and to a lesser extent in feces. Not removed by hemodialysis. **Half-life:** 40–50 hrs.

USES

Treatment of invasive aspergillosis in pts refractory to or intolerant of other fungal therapies.

PRECAUTIONS

CONTRAINDICATIONS: None known. **CAUTIONS:** Hepatic function impairment.

LIFESPAN CONSIDERATIONS: Pregnancy/lactation: May be embryotoxic. Crosses placental barrier. Distributed in breast milk. **Pregnancy Category C. Children:** Safety and efficacy not established. **Elderly:** Age-related moderate renal impairment may require dosage adjustment.

INTERACTIONS

DRUG: May decrease effect of **tacrolimus. Cyclosporine, efavirenz, nelfinavir, nevirapine, phenytoin, rifampin, dexamethasone, carbamazepine** may increase concentration of caspofungin. **HERBAL:** None known. **FOOD:** None known. **LAB VALUES:** May increase SGOT (AST), SGPT (ALT), alkaline phosphatase, LDH, bilirubin, creatinine, serum uric acid, urine pH, urine protein, urine RBCs, urine WBCs, prothrombin time. May decrease serum albumin, serum bicarbonate, serum protein, potassium, Hgb, Hct, WBCs, platelet count.

AVAILABILITY (Rx)

POWDER FOR INJECTION: 50-mg, 70-mg vials.

ADMINISTRATION/HANDLING

IV

Storage • Refrigerate but warm to room temperature before preparing with diluent. • Reconstituted solution, prior to preparation of pt infusion solution, may be stored at room temperature for 1 hr before infusion. • Final infusion solution can be stored at room temperature for 24 hrs. • Discard if solution contains particulate or is discolored.

Reconstitution • For 50- to 70-mg loading dose, add 10.5 ml 0.9% NaCl to the vial. • Transfer 10 ml of reconstituted solution to 250 ml 0.9% NaCl. • For 35-mg dose in pts with moderate hepatic insufficiency, add 10.5 ml 0.9% NaCl to the vial. • Transfer 10 ml of reconstituted solution to 100 or 250 ml 0.9% NaCl for 50- to 70-mg daily dose. For moderate hepatic insufficiency, transfer 7 ml to 100 or 250 ml 0.9% NaCl.

Rate of administration • Infuse over 60 min.

C

∅ **IV INCOMPATIBILITY**

Do not mix with any other medication or use dextrose as a diluent.

INDICATIONS/ROUTES/DOSAGE

ASPERGILLOSIS

IV: ADULTS, ELDERLY: Give single 70-mg loading dose on day 1, followed by 50 mg daily thereafter. Pts with moderate liver insufficiency, daily dose reduced to 35 mg.

SIDE EFFECTS

FREQUENT (26%): Fever. **OCCASIONAL (4%–11%):** Headache, nausea, phlebitis. **RARE (≤3%):** Paresthesia, vomiting, diarrhea, abdominal pain, myalgia, chills, tremor, insomnia.

ADVERSE REACTIONS/ TOXIC EFFECTS

Hypersensitivity reaction characterized by rash, facial swelling, pruritus, sensation of warmth.

NURSING IMPLICATIONS

BASELINE ASSESSMENT

Determine baseline temperature, liver function tests. Assess allergies.

INTERVENTION/EVALUATION

Assess for signs/symptoms of liver dysfunction. Monitor hepatic enzyme test results in pts with preexisting liver dysfunction.

Catapres

see clonidine

cefaclor

sef-ah-klor

(Apo-Cefaclor✱, Ceclor, Ceclor CD)

◆ CLASSIFICATION

PHARMACOTHERAPEUTIC: Second-generation cephalosporin. **CLINICAL:** Antibiotic (see p. 20C).

ACTION

Binds to bacterial membranes. **Therapeutic Effect:** Inhibits synthesis of bacterial cell wall. Bactericidal.

PHARMACOKINETICS

Well absorbed from GI tract. Protein binding: 25%. Widely distributed. Primarily excreted unchanged in urine. Moderately removed by hemodialysis. **Half-life:** 0.6–0.9 hrs (half-life increased with impaired renal function).

USES

Treatment of respiratory, skin/skin structure infections, otitis media, urinary tract infection (UTI). **Extended-Release:** Bacterial infections of acute or chronic bronchitis, skin/skin structure infection, pharyngitis, tonsillitis.

PRECAUTIONS

CONTRAINDICATIONS: History of hypersensitivity to cephalosporins, anaphylactic reaction to penicillins. **CAUTIONS:** Renal impairment, history of GI disease (esp. ulcerative colitis, antibiotic-associated colitis), concurrent use of nephrotoxic medications.

LIFESPAN CONSIDERATIONS: Pregnancy/lactation: Readily crosses placenta. Distributed in breast milk. **Pregnancy Category B. Children:** No age-related precautions noted in those >1 mo. **Elderly:** Age-related decreased renal function may require dosage adjustment.

INTERACTIONS

DRUG: Probenecid may increase serum concentrations of cefaclor. **HERBAL:** None known. **FOOD:** None known. **LAB VALUES:** Positive direct/indirect Coombs' test. May increase BUN, serum creatinine, SGPT (ALT), SGOT (AST), alkaline phosphatase, bilirubin, LDH concentrations.

AVAILABILITY (Rx)

CAPSULES: 250 mg, 500 mg. **TABLETS (extended-release):** 375 mg, 500 mg. **ORAL SUSPENSION:** 125 mg/5 ml, 187 mg/5 ml, 250 mg/5 ml, 375 mg/5 ml.

ADMINISTRATION/HANDLING

PO

• After reconstitution, oral solution is stable for 14 days if refrigerated. • Shake oral suspension well before using. • Give without regard to meals; if GI upset occurs, give with food or milk. • Do not cut, crush, or chew extended-release tablets.

INDICATIONS/ROUTES/DOSAGE

MILD TO MODERATE INFECTIONS

PO: ADULTS, ELDERLY: 250 mg q8h. CHILDREN >1 MO: 20 mg/kg/day in divided doses q8h.

SEVERE INFECTIONS

PO: ADULTS, ELDERLY: 500 mg q8h. **Maximum:** 4 g/day. CHILDREN >1 MO: 40 mg/kg/day in divided doses q8h. **Maximum:** 2 g/day.

USUAL DOSAGE FOR EXTENDED-RELEASE TABLETS

PO: ADULTS, CHILDREN >16 YRS: 375–500 mg q12h.

OTITIS MEDIA

PO: CHILDREN >1 MO: 40 mg/kg/day in divided doses q8h. **Maximum:** 1 g/day.

DOSAGE IN RENAL IMPAIRMENT

Reduced dosage may be necessary in those with creatinine clearance <40 ml/min.

SIDE EFFECTS

FREQUENT: Oral candidiasis (sore mouth/tongue), mild diarrhea, mild abdominal cramping, vaginal candidiasis (itching, discharge). **OCCASIONAL:** Nausea, serum sickness reaction (joint pain, fever); usually occurs after second course of therapy, resolves after drug discontinuation. **RARE:** Allergic reaction (rash, pruritus, urticaria).

ADVERSE REACTIONS/ TOXIC EFFECTS

Antibiotic-associated colitis (severe abdominal pain, tenderness; fever; watery, severe diarrhea), other superinfections may result from altered bacterial balance. Nephrotoxicity may occur, esp. with preexisting renal disease. Severe hypersensitivity reaction (severe pruritus, angioedema, bronchospasm, anaphylaxis), particularly in pts with history of allergies, esp. penicillin.

NURSING IMPLICATIONS

BASELINE ASSESSMENT

Question for history of allergies, particularly cephalosporins, penicillins.

INTERVENTION/EVALUATION

Assess mouth for white patches on mucous membranes, tongue. Monitor bowel activity/stool consistency carefully; mild GI effects may be tolerable, but increasing severity may indicate onset of antibiotic-associated colitis. Monitor I&O, renal function reports for nephrotoxicity. Be alert for superinfection: severe genital/anal pruritus, abdominal pain, severe mouth soreness, moderate to severe diarrhea.

PATIENT/FAMILY TEACHING

Continue therapy for full length of treatment. Doses should be evenly spaced. May cause GI upset (may take with food or milk). Refrigerate oral suspension.

C

cefadroxil

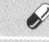

sef-ah-**drocks**-ill
(Duricef)

CLASSIFICATION

PHARMACOTHERAPEUTIC: First-generation cephalosporin. **CLINICAL:** Antibiotic (see p. 20C).

ACTION

Binds to bacterial membranes. **Therapeutic Effect:** Inhibits synthesis of bacterial cell wall. Bactericidal.

PHARMACOKINETICS

Well absorbed from GI tract. Protein binding: 15%–20%. Widely distributed. Primarily excreted unchanged in urine. Removed by hemodialysis. **Half-life:** 1.2–1.5 hrs (half-life increased with impaired renal function).

USES

Treatment of respiratory, GU tract, skin, soft tissue infections; pharyngitis; tonsillitis; follow-up to parenteral therapy.

PRECAUTIONS

CONTRAINDICATIONS: History of hypersensitivity to cephalosporins, anaphylactic reaction to penicillins. **CAUTIONS:** Renal impairment, history of GI disease (esp. ulcerative colitis, antibiotic-associated colitis), concurrent use of nephrotoxic medications.

LIFESPAN CONSIDERATIONS: Pregnancy/lactation: Readily crosses placenta. Distributed in breast milk. **Pregnancy Category B. Children:** No age-related precautions noted. **Elderly:** Age-related decreased renal function may require dosage adjustment.

INTERACTIONS

DRUG: Probenecid increases serum concentrations of cefadroxil. **HERBAL:** None known. **FOOD:** None known. **LAB VALUES:** Positive direct/indirect Coombs' test. May increase BUN, serum creatinine, SGPT (ALT), SGOT (AST), alkaline phosphatase, bilirubin, LDH concentrations.

AVAILABILITY (Rx)

CAPSULES: 500 mg. **TABLETS:** 1,000 mg. **ORAL SUSPENSION:** 250 mg/5 ml, 500 mg/5 ml.

ADMINISTRATION/HANDLING

PO

- After reconstitution, oral solution is stable for 14 days if refrigerated.
- Shake oral suspension well before using.
- Give without regard to meals; if GI upset occurs, give with food or milk.

INDICATIONS/ROUTES/DOSAGE

URINARY TRACT INFECTIONS

PO: ADULTS, ELDERLY: 1–2 g/day in 1–2 divided doses.

SKIN/SKIN STRUCTURE INFECTIONS, GROUP A BETA-HEMOLYTIC STREPTOCOCCAL PHARYNGITIS, TONSILLITIS

PO: ADULTS, ELDERLY: 1–2 g in 2 divided doses.

USUAL DOSAGE FOR CHILDREN

PO: CHILDREN: 30 mg/kg/day in 2 divided doses. **Maximum:** 2 g/day.

DOSAGE IN RENAL IMPAIRMENT

Dose and/or frequency is based on degree of renal impairment and/or severity of infection. After initial 1-g dose:

Creatinine Clearance	Dosage Interval
26–50 ml/min	500 mg q12h
10–25 ml/min	500 mg q24h
<10 ml/min	500 mg q36h

SIDE EFFECTS

FREQUENT: Oral candidiasis (sore mouth/tongue), mild diarrhea, mild abdominal cramping, vaginal candidiasis (itching, discharge). **OCCASIONAL:** Nausea, unusual bruising/bleeding, serum sickness reaction (joint pain, fever) (usually occurs following second course of therapy, resolves after drug discontinuation). **RARE:** Allergic reaction (rash, pruritus, urticaria), thrombophlebitis (pain, redness, swelling at injection site).

ADVERSE REACTIONS/ TOXIC EFFECTS

Antibiotic-associated colitis (severe abdominal pain, tenderness; fever; watery, severe diarrhea), other superinfections may result from altered bacterial balance. Nephrotoxicity may occur, esp. with preexisting renal disease. Severe hypersensitivity reaction (severe pruritus, angioedema, bronchospasm, anaphylaxis), particularly in pts with history of allergies, esp. penicillin.

NURSING IMPLICATIONS

BASELINE ASSESSMENT

Question for history of allergies, particularly cephalosporins, penicillins.

INTERVENTION/EVALUATION

Assess mouth for white patches on mucous membranes, tongue. Monitor bowel activity/stool consistency carefully; mild GI effects may be tolerable, but increasing severity may indicate onset of antibiotic-associated colitis. Monitor I&O, renal function reports for nephrotoxicity. Be alert for superinfection: genital/anal pruritus, moniliasis, abdominal pain, sore mouth/tongue, moderate to severe diarrhea.

PATIENT/FAMILY TEACHING

Continue therapy for full length of treatment. Doses should be evenly spaced. May cause GI upset (may take with food or milk). Refrigerate oral suspension.

cefazolin sodium

cef-ah-**zoe**-lin

(Ancef, Kefzol)

Do not confuse with cefprozil, Cefzil.

CLASSIFICATION

PHARMACOTHERAPEUTIC: First-generation cephalosporin. **CLINICAL:** Antibiotic (see p. 20C).

ACTION

Binds to bacterial membranes. **Therapeutic Effect:** Inhibits synthesis of bacterial cell wall. Bactericidal.

PHARMACOKINETICS

Widely distributed. Protein binding: 85%. Primarily excreted unchanged in urine. Moderately removed by hemodialysis. **Half-life:** 1.4–1.8 hrs (half-life increased with impaired renal function).

USES

Treatment of respiratory tract, skin, soft tissue, bone, joint, GU tract, serious intra-abdominal, biliary infections; septicemia. Preferred first-generation cephalosporin for perioperative prophylaxis.

PRECAUTIONS

CONTRAINDICATIONS: History of hypersensitivity to cephalosporins, anaphylactic reaction to penicillins. **CAUTIONS:** Renal impairment, history of GI disease (esp. ulcerative colitis, antibiotic-associated colitis), concurrent use of nephrotoxic medications.

LIFESPAN CONSIDERATIONS: Pregnancy/lactation: Readily crosses placenta; distributed in breast milk. **Pregnancy Category B. Children:** No age-related precautions noted. **Elderly:** Age-related renal impairment may require reduced dosage.

C

INTERACTIONS

DRUG: **Probenecid** increases serum concentrations of cefazolin. **HERBAL:** None known. **FOOD:** None known. **LAB VALUES:** Positive direct/indirect Coombs' test. May increase BUN, serum creatinine, SGPT (ALT), SGOT (AST), alkaline phosphatase, bilirubin, LDH concentrations.

AVAILABILITY (Rx)

INJECTION: 500 mg, 1 g. **READY-TO-HANG INFUSION:** 1 g/50 ml, 2 g/100 ml.

ADMINISTRATION/HANDLING

IM

• To minimize discomfort, inject deep IM slowly. • Less painful if injected into gluteus maximus than lateral aspect of thigh.

IV

Storage • Solution appears light yellow to yellow. • IV infusion (piggyback) stable for 24 hrs at room temperature, 96 hrs if refrigerated. • Discard if precipitate forms.

Reconstitution • Reconstitute each 1 g with at least 10 ml Sterile Water for Injection. • May further dilute in 50–100 ml D_5W or 0.9% NaCl (decreases incidence of thrombophlebitis).

Rate of administration • For IV push, administer over 3–5 min. • For intermittent IV infusion (piggyback), infuse over 20–30 min.

∅ IV INCOMPATIBILITIES

Amikacin (Amikin), amiodarone (Cordarone), hydromorphone (Dilaudid).

IV COMPATIBILITIES

Calcium gluconate, diltiazem (Cardizem), famotidine (Pepcid), heparin, insulin (Regular), lidocaine, magnesium sulfate, midazolam (Versed), morphine, multivitamins, potassium chloride, propofol (Diprivan).

INDICATIONS/ROUTES/DOSAGE

UNCOMPLICATED UTI

IM/IV: ADULTS, ELDERLY: 1 g q12h.

MILD TO MODERATE INFECTIONS

IM/IV: ADULTS, ELDERLY: 250–500 mg q8–12h.

SEVERE INFECTIONS

IM/IV: ADULTS, ELDERLY: 0.5–1 g q6–8h.

LIFE-THREATENING INFECTIONS

IM/IV: ADULTS, ELDERLY: 1–1.5 g q6h. **Maximum:** 12 g/day.

PERIOPERATIVE PROPHYLAXIS

IM/IV: ADULTS, ELDERLY: 1 g 30–60 min before surgery, 0.5–1 g during surgery, and q6–8h for up to 24 hrs postop.

USUAL PEDIATRIC DOSAGE

IM/IV: NEONATES ≤7 DAYS: 40 mg/kg/day in divided doses q12h. >7 DAYS: 40–60 mg/kg/day in divided doses q8–12h. CHILDREN: 50–100 mg/kg/day in divided doses q8h.

DOSAGE IN RENAL IMPAIRMENT

Creatinine Clearance	Dosing Interval
10–30 ml/min	q12h
<10 ml/min	q24h

SIDE EFFECTS

FREQUENT: Discomfort with IM administration, oral candidiasis (sore mouth/tongue), mild diarrhea, mild abdominal cramping, vaginal candidiasis (itching, discharge). **OCCASIONAL:** Nausea, serum sickness reaction (joint pain, fever); usually occurs after second course of therapy, resolves after drug discontinuation. **RARE:** Allergic reaction (rash, pruritus, urticaria), thrombophlebitis (pain, redness, swelling at injection site).

ADVERSE REACTIONS/ TOXIC EFFECTS

Antibiotic-associated colitis (severe abdominal pain, tenderness; fever; watery, severe diarrhea), other superinfections may result from altered bacterial balance. Nephrotoxicity may occur, esp. with preexisting renal disease. Severe hypersensitivity reaction (severe pruritus, angioedema, bronchospasm, anaphylaxis), particularly in pts with history of allergies, esp. penicillin.

NURSING IMPLICATIONS

BASELINE ASSESSMENT

Question for history of allergies, particularly cephalosporins, penicillins.

INTERVENTION/EVALUATION

Evaluate IM site for induration and tenderness. Assess mouth for white patches on mucous membranes, tongue. Monitor bowel activity/stool consistency carefully; mild GI effects may be tolerable, but increasing severity may indicate onset of antibiotic-associated colitis. Monitor I&O, renal function reports for nephrotoxicity. Be alert for superinfection: severe genital/anal pruritus, abdominal pain, severe mouth soreness, moderate to severe diarrhea.

PATIENT/FAMILY TEACHING

Discomfort may occur with IM injection. Doses should be evenly spaced. Continue antibiotic therapy for full length of treatment.

cefdinir

cef-din-ur
(Omnicef)

CLASSIFICATION

PHARMACOTHERAPEUTIC: Third-generation cephalosporin. **CLINICAL:** Antibiotic (see p. 21C).

ACTION

Binds to bacterial membranes. **Therapeutic Effect:** Inhibits synthesis of bacterial cell wall. Bactericidal.

PHARMACOKINETICS

Moderately absorbed from GI tract. Protein binding: 60%–70%. Widely distributed. Not appreciably metabolized. Primarily excreted unchanged in urine. Minimally removed by hemodialysis. **Half-life:** 1–2 hrs (half-life increased in those with impaired renal function).

USES

Treatment of community-acquired pneumonia, acute exacerbation of chronic bronchitis, acute maxillary sinusitis, pharyngitis, tonsillitis, uncomplicated skin/skin structure infections, otitis media.

PRECAUTIONS

CONTRAINDICATIONS: Hypersensitivity to cephalosporins. **CAUTIONS:** Hypersensitivity to penicillins or other drugs; history of GI disease (e.g., colitis); renal impairment, impaired hepatic function.

LIFESPAN CONSIDERATIONS: Pregnancy/lactation: Crosses placenta. Not detected in breast milk. **Pregnancy Category B. Children:** Newborn, infants may have lower renal clearance. **Elderly:** Age-related decrease in renal function may require decreased dosage or increased dosing interval.

INTERACTIONS

DRUG: Probenecid increases serum concentration of cefdinir. **Antacids** decrease cefdinir plasma concentration. **HERBAL:** None known. **FOOD:** None known. **LAB VALUES:** May produce a false-positive reaction for ketones in urine. May increase SGPT (AST), SGOT (ALT), alkaline phosphatase, bilirubin, LDH concentrations.

C

AVAILABILITY (Rx)

CAPSULES: 300 mg. **ORAL SUSPENSION:** 125 mg/5 ml.

ADMINISTRATION/HANDLING

PO

• Give without regard to meals. • To reconstitute oral suspension, for the 60-ml bottle, add 39 ml water; for the 120-ml bottle, add 65 ml water. • Shake oral suspension well before administering. • Store mixed suspension at room temperature. Discard unused portion after 10 days.

INDICATIONS/ROUTES/DOSAGE

COMMUNITY-ACQUIRED PNEUMONIA

PO: ADULTS, ELDERLY, CHILDREN ≥13 YRS: 300 mg q12h for 10 days.

ACUTE EXACERBATION OF CHRONIC BRONCHITIS

PO: ADULTS, ELDERLY: 300 mg q12h for 5 days.

ACUTE MAXILLARY SINUSITIS

PO: ADULTS, ELDERLY, CHILDREN ≥13 YRS: 300 mg q12h or 600 mg q24h for 10 days. CHILDREN 6 MOS–12 YRS: 7 mg/kg q12h or 14 mg/kg q24h for 10 days.

PHARYNGITIS/TONSILLITIS

PO: ADULTS, ELDERLY, CHILDREN ≥13 YRS: 300 mg q12h for 5–10 days or 600 mg q24h for 10 days. CHILDREN 6 MOS–12 YRS: 7 mg/kg q12h for 5–10 days or 14 mg/kg q24h for 10 days.

UNCOMPLICATED SKIN AND SKIN STRUCTURE INFECTIONS

PO: ADULTS, ELDERLY, CHILDREN ≥13 YRS: 300 mg q12h for 10 days. CHILDREN 6 MOS–12 YRS: 7 mg/kg q12h for 10 days.

ACUTE BACTERIAL OTITIS MEDIA

PO: CHILDREN 6 MOS–12 YRS: 7 mg/kg q12h or 14 mg/kg q24h for 10 days.

Oral suspension: PEDIATRIC <20 LBS: 2.5 ml (½ tsp) q12h or 5 ml (1 tsp) q24h. PEDIATRIC 20–40 LBS: 5 ml (1 tsp) q12h or 10 ml (2 tsp) q24h. PEDIATRIC 41–60 LBS: 7.5 ml (1½ tsp) q12h or 15 ml (3 tsp) q24h. PEDIATRIC 61–80 LBS: 10 ml (2 tsp) q12h or 20 ml (4 tsp) q24h. PEDIATRIC 81–95 LBS: 12.5 ml (2½ tsp) q12h or 25 ml (5 tsp) q24h.

DOSAGE IN RENAL IMPAIRMENT

Creatinine clearance <30 ml/min: 300 mg/day as single daily dose. **Hemodialysis pts:** 300 mg or 7 mg/kg dose every other day.

SIDE EFFECTS

FREQUENT: Oral candidiasis (sore mouth/tongue), mild diarrhea, mild abdominal cramping, vaginal candidiasis (itching, discharge). **OCCASIONAL:** Nausea, serum sickness reaction (joint pain, fever) usually occurs after second course of therapy, resolves after drug discontinuation. **RARE:** Allergic reaction (rash, pruritus, urticaria).

ADVERSE REACTIONS/ TOXIC EFFECTS

Antibiotic-associated colitis (severe abdominal pain, tenderness; fever; watery, severe diarrhea) may result from altered bacterial balance. Nephrotoxicity may occur, esp. with preexisting renal disease. Severe hypersensitivity reaction (severe pruritus, angioedema, bronchospasm, anaphylaxis), particularly in pts with history of allergies, esp. penicillin.

NURSING IMPLICATIONS

BASELINE ASSESSMENT

Question for hypersensitivity to cefdinir or other cephalosporins, penicillins.

INTERVENTION/EVALUATION

Monitor bowel activity/stool consistency carefully; mild GI effects may be tolerable, but increasing severity may indicate onset of antibiotic-associated colitis. Be alert for superinfection (e.g., genital/anal pruritus, ulceration/changes in oral mucosa, moderate to severe diarrhea, new/increased fever). Monitor hematology reports.

PATIENT/FAMILY TEACHING

Take antacids 2 hrs prior to or following medication. Continue medication for full length of treatment; do not skip doses. Doses should be evenly spaced. Report persistent diarrhea to nurse/physician.

cefditoren

sef-dih-**tore**-inn
(Spectracef)
See Classification section under: Antibiotic: cephalosporins (p. 21C)

cefepime

sef-eh-**peem**
(Maxipime)

◆CLASSIFICATION

PHARMACOTHERAPEUTIC: Fourth-generation cephalosporin. **CLINICAL:** Antibiotic (see p. 22C).

ACTION

Binds to bacterial membranes. **Therapeutic Effect:** Inhibits synthesis of bacterial cell wall. Bactericidal.

PHARMACOKINETICS

Well absorbed after IM administration. Protein binding: 20%. Widely distributed. Primarily excreted unchanged in urine. Removed by hemodialysis. **Half-life:** 2–2.3 hrs (half-life increased with impaired renal function, in elderly).

USES

Treatment of pneumonia; bronchitis; urinary tract, skin/skin structure, intra-abdominal infections; bacteremia; septicemia, fever, neutropenia in cancer pts; complicated intra-abdominal infections (with metronidazole).

PRECAUTIONS

CONTRAINDICATIONS: History of hypersensitivity to cephalosporins, anaphylactic reaction to penicillins. **CAUTIONS:** Renal impairment.

LIFESPAN CONSIDERATIONS: Pregnancy/lactation: Unknown whether distributed in breast milk. **Pregnancy Category B. Children:** No age-related precautions noted in those >2 mos. **Elderly:** Age-related decreased renal function may require reduced dosage or increased dosing interval.

INTERACTIONS

DRUG: Probenecid may increase concentration of cefepime. **HERBAL:** None known. **FOOD:** None known. **LAB VALUES:** Positive direct/indirect Coombs' test may occur. May increase SGOT (AST), SGPT (ALT), alkaline phosphatase, LDH, bilirubin.

AVAILABILITY (Rx)

POWDER FOR INJECTION: 500 mg, 1 g, 2 g.

ADMINISTRATION/HANDLING

IM

• Add 1.3 ml Sterile Water for Injection, 0.9% NaCl, or D_5W to 500-mg vial. (2.4 ml for 1-g and 2-g vials) • Inject into a large muscle mass (e.g., upper gluteus maximus).

IV

Storage • Solution is stable for 24 hrs at room temperature or 7 days if refrigerated.

C

Reconstitution • Add 5 ml to 500-mg vial (10 ml for 1-g and 2-g vials). • Further dilute with 50–100 ml 0.9% NaCl, or D_5W.

Rate of administration • For IV push, administer over 3–5 min. • For intermittent IV infusion (piggyback), infuse over 30 min.

IV INCOMPATIBILITIES

Acyclovir (Zovirax), amphotericin (Fungizone), cimetidine (Tagamet), ciprofloxacin (Cipro), cisplatin (Platinol), dacarbazine (DTIC), daunorubicin (Cerubidine), diazepam (Valium), diphenhydramine (Benadryl), dobutamine (Dobutrex), dopamine (Intropin), doxorubicin (Adriamycin), etoposide (VePesid), droperidol (Inapsine), famotidine (Pepcid), ganciclovir (Cytovene), haloperidol (Haldol), magnesium sulfate, mannitol, meperidine (Demerol), metoclopramide (Reglan), morphine, ofloxacin (Floxin), ondansetron (Zofran), vancomycin (Vancocin).

IV COMPATIBILITIES

Bumetanide (Bumex), calcium gluconate, furosemide (Lasix), hydromorphone (Dilaudid), lorazepam (Ativan), propofol (Diprivan).

INDICATIONS/ROUTES/DOSAGE

USUAL ADULT DOSAGE

IM/IV: 1–2 g q12h.

URINARY TRACT INFECTIONS

IM/IV: ADULTS, ELDERLY: 500 mg q12h.

EMPIRIC THERAPY FOR FEBRILE NEUTROPENIA

IV: ADULTS: 2 g q8h.

USUAL PEDIATRIC DOSAGE

IM/IV: CHILDREN 2 MOS–16 YRS: 50 mg/kg q8–12h. Do not exceed maximum adult dose.

DOSAGE IN RENAL IMPAIRMENT

Dose and/or frequency is based on degree of renal impairment (creatinine clearance) and/or severity of infection.

Creatinine Clearance	Dose
30–60 ml/min	0.5–2 g q24h
11–29 ml/min	0.5–1 g q24h
≤10 ml/min	0.25–0.5 g q24h

SIDE EFFECTS

FREQUENT: Discomfort with IM administration, oral candidiasis (sore mouth/tongue), mild diarrhea, mild abdominal cramping, vaginal candidiasis (itching, discharge). **OCCASIONAL:** Nausea, serum sickness reaction (joint pain, fever); usually occurs after second course of therapy, resolves after drug discontinuation. **RARE:** Allergic reaction (rash, pruritus, urticaria), thrombophlebitis (pain, redness, swelling at injection site).

ADVERSE REACTIONS/ TOXIC EFFECTS

Antibiotic-associated colitis (severe abdominal pain, tenderness; fever; watery, severe diarrhea), other superinfections may result from altered bacterial balance. Nephrotoxicity may occur, esp. with preexisting renal disease. Severe hypersensitivity reaction (severe pruritus, angioedema, bronchospasm, anaphylaxis), particularly in pts with history of allergies, esp. penicillin.

NURSING IMPLICATIONS

BASELINE ASSESSMENT

Question for history of allergies, particularly cephalosporins, penicillins.

INTERVENTION/EVALUATION

Evaluate IM site for induration and tenderness. Assess mouth for white patches on mucous membranes, tongue. Monitor bowel activity/stool consistency carefully; mild GI effects may be tolerable, but increasing severity may indicate onset of antibiotic-associated colitis. Monitor I&O, renal function reports for nephrotoxicity. Be alert for superinfection: severe genital/anal pruritus, abdominal pain, severe mouth soreness, moderate to severe diarrhea.

PATIENT/FAMILY TEACHING

Discomfort may occur with IM injection. Continue therapy for full length of treatment. Doses should be evenly spaced.

cefotaxime sodium

seh-fo-**tax**-eem

(Claforan)

Do not confuse with cefoxitin, ceftizoxime, cefuroxime.

CLASSIFICATION

PHARMACOTHERAPEUTIC: Third-generation cephalosporin. **CLINICAL:** Antibiotic (see p. 21C).

ACTION

Binds to bacterial membranes. **Therapeutic Effect:** Inhibits synthesis of bacterial cell wall. Bactericidal.

PHARMACOKINETICS

Widely distributed (including CSF). Protein binding: 30%–50%. Partially metabolized in liver to active metabolite. Primarily excreted in urine. Moderately removed by hemodialysis. **Half-life:** 1 hr (half-life increased with impaired renal function).

USES

Treatment of respiratory tract, GU tract, skin, bone infections; septicemia; gonorrhea; gynecologic, intra-abdominal, biliary infections; meningitis; perioperative prophylaxis. **Unlabeled:** Treatment of Lyme disease.

PRECAUTIONS

CONTRAINDICATIONS: History of hypersensitivity to cephalosporins, anaphylactic reaction to penicillins. **CAUTIONS:** Concurrent use of nephrotoxic medications, history of GI disease (esp. ulcerative colitis, antibiotic-associated colitis), renal impairment with creatinine clearance <20 ml/min.

LIFESPAN CONSIDERATIONS: Pregnancy/lactation: Readily crosses placenta. Distributed in breast milk. **Pregnancy Category B. Children:** No age-related precautions noted. **Elderly:** Age-related renal impairment may require dosage adjustment.

INTERACTIONS

DRUG: Probenecid increases serum concentration of cefotaxime. **HERBAL:** None known. **FOOD:** None known. **LAB VALUES:** Positive direct/indirect Coombs' test may occur. May increase liver function tests.

AVAILABILITY (Rx)

POWDER FOR INJECTION: 500 mg, 1 g, 2 g.

ADMINISTRATION/HANDLING

IM

• Reconstitute with Sterile Water for Injection or Bacteriostatic Water for Injection. • Add 2, 3, or 5 ml to 500-mg, 1-g, or 2-g vial, respectively, providing a concentration of 230 mg, 300 mg, or 330 mg/ml, respectively. • To minimize discomfort, inject deep IM slowly. Less painful if injected into gluteus maximus than lateral aspect of thigh. For 2-g IM dose, give at 2 separate sites.

IV

Storage • Solution appears light yellow to amber. IV infusion (piggyback) may darken in color (does not indicate loss of potency). • IV infusion (piggy-

C

back) is stable for 24 hrs at room temperature, 5 days if refrigerated. • Discard if precipitate forms.

Reconstitution • Reconstitute with 10 ml Sterile Water for Injection to provide a concentration of 50 mg, 95 mg, or 180 mg/ml for 500-mg, 1-g, or 2-g vials, respectively. • May further dilute with 50–100 ml 0.9% NaCl or D_5W.

Rate of administration • For IV push, administer over 3–5 min. • For intermittent IV infusion (piggyback), infuse over 20–30 min.

∅ IV INCOMPATIBILITIES
Allopurinol (Aloprim), filgrastim (Neupogen), fluconazole (Diflucan), hetastarch (Hespan), pentamidine (Pentam IV), vancomycin (Vancocin).

IV COMPATIBILITIES
Diltiazem (Cardizem), famotidine (Pepcid), hydromorphone (Dilaudid), lorazepam (Ativan), magnesium sulfate, midazolam (Versed), morphine, propofol (Diprivan).

INDICATIONS/ROUTES/DOSAGE

Alert: Space doses evenly around the clock.

UNCOMPLICATED INFECTIONS
IM/IV: ADULTS, ELDERLY: 1 g q12h.

MILD TO MODERATE INFECTIONS
IM/IV: ADULTS, ELDERLY: 1–2 g q8h.

SEVERE INFECTIONS
IM/IV: ADULTS, ELDERLY: 2 g q6–8h.

LIFE-THREATENING INFECTIONS
IM/IV: ADULTS, ELDERLY: 2 g q4h.

UNCOMPLICATED GONORRHEA
IM: ADULTS: 1 g one time.

PERIOPERATIVE PROPHYLAXIS
IM/IV: ADULTS, ELDERLY: 1 g 30–90 min before surgery.

CESAREAN SECTION
IV: ADULTS: 1 g as soon as umbilical cord is clamped, then 1 g 6 hrs and 12 hrs after first dose.

USUAL DOSAGE FOR CHILDREN
IM/IV: 1 MO–12 YRS (<50 KG): 100–200 mg/kg/day in divided doses q6–8h; (≥50 KG): 1–2 g q6–8h; **life-threatening infection:** 2 g q4h. **Maximum:** 12 g/day.

DOSAGE IN RENAL IMPAIRMENT
Creatinine clearance <20 ml/min: Give ½ dose at usual dosing intervals.

SIDE EFFECTS

FREQUENT: Discomfort with IM administration, oral candidiasis (sore mouth/tongue), mild diarrhea, mild abdominal cramping, vaginal candidiasis (itching, discharge). **OCCASIONAL:** Nausea, serum sickness reaction (joint pain, fever) usually occurs after second course of therapy, resolves after drug discontinuation. **RARE:** Allergic reaction (rash, pruritus, urticaria), thrombophlebitis (pain, redness, swelling at injection site).

ADVERSE REACTIONS/ TOXIC EFFECTS

Antibiotic-associated colitis (severe abdominal pain, tenderness; fever; watery, severe diarrhea), other superinfections may result from altered bacterial balance. Nephrotoxicity may occur, esp. with preexisting renal disease. Severe hypersensitivity reaction (severe pruritus, angioedema, bronchospasm, anaphylaxis), particularly in pts with history of allergies, esp. penicillin.

NURSING IMPLICATIONS

BASELINE ASSESSMENT

Question for history of allergies, particularly cephalosporins, penicillins.

INTERVENTION/EVALUATION

Check IM injection sites for induration, tenderness. Assess mouth for white patches on mucous membranes, tongue. Monitor bowel activity/stool consistency carefully; mild GI effects may be tolerable, but increasing severity may indicate onset of antibiotic-associated colitis. Monitor I&O, renal function reports for nephrotoxicity. Be alert for superinfection: severe genital/anal pruritus, abdominal pain, severe mouth soreness, moderate to severe diarrhea.

PATIENT/FAMILY TEACHING

Discomfort may occur with IM injection. Doses should be evenly spaced. Continue antibiotic therapy for full length of treatment.

cefotetan disodium

seh-fo-**teh**-tan

(Cefotan)

Do not confuse with cefoxitin, Ceftin.

CLASSIFICATION

PHARMACOTHERAPEUTIC: Second-generation cephalosporin. **CLINICAL:** Antibiotic (see p. 20C).

ACTION

Binds to bacterial membranes. **Therapeutic Effect:** Inhibits synthesis of bacterial cell wall. Bactericidal.

PHARMACOKINETICS

Widely distributed. Protein binding: 78%–91%. Primarily excreted unchanged in urine. Minimally removed by hemodialysis. **Half-life:** 3–4.6 hrs (half-life increased with impaired renal function).

USES

Treatment of respiratory tract, GU tract, skin, bone, gynecologic, intra-abdominal infections; perioperative prophylaxis.

PRECAUTIONS

CONTRAINDICATIONS: History of hypersensitivity to cephalosporins, anaphylactic reaction to penicillins. **CAUTIONS:** Renal impairment, history of GI disease (esp. ulcerative colitis, antibiotic-associated colitis), concurrent use of nephrotoxic medications.

LIFESPAN CONSIDERATIONS: Pregnancy/lactation: Readily crosses placenta. Distributed in breast milk. **Pregnancy Category B. Children:** Safety and efficacy not established. **Elderly:** Age-related renal impairment may require dosage adjustment.

INTERACTIONS

DRUG: Disulfiram reaction (facial flushing, nausea, sweating, headache, tachycardia) may occur when **alcohol** is ingested. May increase bleeding risk with **anticoagulants, heparin, thrombolytics. HERBAL:** None known. **FOOD:** None known. **LAB VALUES:** Positive direct/indirect Coombs' test may occur (interferes with hematologic tests, cross-matching procedures). Prothrombin times may be increased. May increase BUN, serum creatinine, SGOT (AST), SGPT (ALT), alkaline phosphatase concentrations.

AVAILABILITY (Rx)

POWDER FOR INJECTION: 1 g, 2 g.

ADMINISTRATION/HANDLING

Alert: Give by IM injection, IV push, intermittent IV infusion (piggyback).

IM

• Add 2, 3 ml Sterile Water for Injection or other appropriate diluent to 1 g, 2 g providing a concentration of 400 mg/ml or 500 mg/ml, respectively. • Less painful if injected deep IM slowly into gluteus maximus than lateral aspect of thigh.

IV

Storage • Solution appears colorless

C

to light yellow. • Color change to deep yellow does not indicate loss of potency. • IV infusion (piggyback) is stable for 24 hrs at room temperature, 96 hrs if refrigerated. • Discard if precipitate forms.

Reconstitution • Reconstitute each 1 g with 10 ml Sterile Water for Injection to provide a concentration of 95 mg/ml. • May further dilute with 50–100 ml 0.9% NaCl or D_5W.

Rate of administration • For IV push, administer over 3–5 min. • For intermittent IV infusion (piggyback), infuse over 20–30 min.

IV INCOMPATIBILITY
Vancomycin (Vancocin).

IV COMPATIBILITIES
Diltiazem (Cardizem), famotidine (Pepcid), heparin, insulin (Regular), morphine, propofol (Diprivan).

INDICATIONS/ROUTES/DOSAGE

URINARY TRACT INFECTIONS
IM/IV: ADULTS, ELDERLY: 1–2 g in divided doses q12–24h.

MILD TO MODERATE INFECTIONS
IM/IV: ADULTS, ELDERLY: 1–2 g q12h.

SEVERE INFECTIONS
IM/IV: ADULTS, ELDERLY: 2 g q12h.

LIFE-THREATENING INFECTIONS
IM/IV: ADULTS, ELDERLY: 3 g q12h.

PERIOPERATIVE PROPHYLAXIS
IV: ADULTS, ELDERLY: 1–2 g 30–60 min before surgery.

CESAREAN SECTION
IV: ADULTS: 1–2 g as soon as umbilical cord is clamped.

USUAL PEDIATRIC DOSAGE
IM/IV: 40–80 mg/kg/day in divided doses q12h. **Maximum:** 6 g/day.

DOSAGE IN RENAL IMPAIRMENT
Dose and/or frequency modified on basis of creatinine clearance and/or severity of infection.

Creatinine Clearance	Dosage Interval
10–30 ml/min	Usual dose q24h
<10 ml/min	Usual dose q48h

SIDE EFFECTS

FREQUENT: Discomfort with IM administration, oral candidiasis (sore mouth/tongue), mild diarrhea, mild abdominal cramping, vaginal candidiasis (itching, discharge). **OCCASIONAL:** Nausea, unusual bruising/bleeding, serum sickness reaction (joint pain, fever) usually occurs after second course of therapy, resolves after drug discontinuation. **RARE:** Allergic reaction (rash, pruritus, urticaria), thrombophlebitis (pain, redness, swelling at injection site).

ADVERSE REACTIONS/ TOXIC EFFECTS

Antibiotic-associated colitis (severe abdominal pain/tenderness; fever; watery, severe diarrhea), other superinfections may result from altered bacterial balance. Nephrotoxicity may occur, esp. with preexisting renal disease. Severe hypersensitivity reaction (severe pruritus, angioedema, bronchospasm, anaphylaxis), particularly in pts with history of allergies, esp. penicillin.

NURSING IMPLICATIONS

BASELINE ASSESSMENT
Question for history of allergies, particularly cephalosporins, penicillins.

INTERVENTION/EVALUATION
Evaluate IV site for phlebitis (heat, pain, red streaking over vein). Check IM injection sites for induration, tenderness. Assess mouth for white patches on mucous membranes, tongue. Monitor

bowel activity/stool consistency carefully; mild GI effects may be tolerable, but increasing severity may indicate onset of antibiotic-associated colitis. Monitor I&O, renal function reports for nephrotoxicity. Be alert for superinfection: severe genital/anal pruritus, abdominal pain, severe mouth soreness, moderate to severe diarrhea.

PATIENT/FAMILY TEACHING

Discomfort may occur with IM injection. Doses should be evenly spaced. Continue antibiotic therapy for full length of treatment. Avoid alcohol/alcohol-containing preparations (salad dressings, sauces, cough syrups) during and for 72 hrs after last dose of cefotetan.

cefoxitin sodium

seh-**fox**-ih-tin
(Mefoxin)
Do not confuse with cefotaxime, cefotetan, Cytoxan.

CLASSIFICATION

PHARMACOTHERAPEUTIC: Second-generation cephalosporin. **CLINICAL:** Antibiotic (see p. 20C).

ACTION

Binds to bacterial membranes. **Therapeutic Effect:** Inhibits synthesis of bacterial cell wall. Bactericidal.

USES

Treatment of respiratory tract, GU tract, skin, bone, intra-abdominal, gynecologic infections; gonorrhea, septicemia, perioperative prophylaxis.

PRECAUTIONS

CONTRAINDICATIONS: History of hypersensitivity to cephalosporins, anaphylactic reaction to penicillins. **CAUTIONS:** Renal impairment, history of GI disease (esp. ulcerative colitis, antibiotic-associated colitis), concurrent use of nephrotoxic medications. **Pregnancy Category B.**

INTERACTIONS

DRUG: **Probenecid** increases serum concentrations of cefoxitin. **HERBAL:** None known. **FOOD:** None known. **LAB VALUES:** Positive direct/indirect Coombs' test may occur (interferes with hematologic tests, cross-matching procedures). May increase BUN, serum creatinine, SGOT (AST), SGPT (ALT), alkaline phosphatase concentrations.

AVAILABILITY (Rx)

POWDER FOR INJECTION: 1 g, 2 g.

ADMINISTRATION/HANDLING

Alert: Give IM, IV push, intermittent IV infusion (piggyback).

IM

• Reconstitute each 1 g with 2 ml Sterile Water for Injection or lidocaine to provide concentration of 400 mg/ml. • To minimize discomfort, inject deep IM slowly. Less painful if injected into gluteus maximus than lateral aspect of thigh.

IV

Storage • Solution appears colorless to light amber but may darken (does not indicate loss of potency). • IV infusion (piggyback) is stable for 24 hrs at room temperature, 48 hrs if refrigerated. • Discard if precipitate forms.

Reconstitution • Reconstitute each 1 g with 10 ml Sterile Water for Injection to provide concentration of 95 mg/ml.

• May further dilute with 50–100 ml 0.9% Sterile Water for Injection, NaCl, or D_5W.

C

Rate of administration • For IV push, administer over 3–5 min. • For intermittent IV infusion (piggyback), infuse over 15–30 min.

IV INCOMPATIBILITIES
Filgrastim (Neupogen), pentamidine (Pentam IV), vancomycin (Vancocin).

IV COMPATIBILITIES
Diltiazem (Cardizem), famotidine (Pepcid), heparin, hydromorphone (Dilaudid), magnesium sulfate, morphine, multivitamins, propofol (Diprivan).

INDICATIONS/ROUTES/DOSAGE

Alert: Space doses evenly around the clock.

MILD TO MODERATE INFECTIONS
IM/IV: ADULTS, ELDERLY: 1–2 g q6–8h.

SEVERE INFECTIONS
IM/IV: ADULTS, ELDERLY: 1 g q4h or 2 g q6–8h up to 2 g q4h.

UNCOMPLICATED GONORRHEA
IM: ADULTS: 2 g one time with 1 g probenecid.

PERIOPERATIVE PROPHYLAXIS
IM/IV: ADULTS, ELDERLY: 2 g 30–60 min before surgery and q6h up to 24 hrs postop. CHILDREN >3 MOS: 30–40 mg/kg 30–60 min before surgery and q6h postop for no more than 24 hrs.

CESAREAN SECTION
IV: ADULTS: 2 g as soon as umbilical cord is clamped, then 2 g 4 hrs and 8 hrs after first dose, then q6h for no more than 24 hrs.

USUAL DOSAGE FOR CHILDREN
IM/IV: CHILDREN >3 MOS: 80–160 mg/kg/day in 4–6 divided doses. **Maximum:** 12 g/day. NEONATES: 90–100 mg/kg/day in divided doses q6–8h.

DOSAGE IN RENAL IMPAIRMENT
After loading dose of 1–2 g, dose and/or frequency is modified based on creatinine clearance and/or severity of infection.

Creatinine Clearance	Dosage
30–50 ml/min	1–2 g q8–12h
10–29 ml/min	1–2 g q12–24h
5–9 ml/min	500 mg–1 g q12–24h
<5 ml/min	500 mg–1 g q24–48h

SIDE EFFECTS

FREQUENT: Discomfort with IM administration, oral candidiasis (sore mouth/tongue), mild diarrhea, mild abdominal cramping, vaginal candidiasis (itching, discharge). **OCCASIONAL:** Nausea, serum sickness reaction (joint pain, fever) (usually occurs after second course of therapy, resolves after drug discontinuation). **RARE:** Allergic reaction (rash, pruritus, urticaria), thrombophlebitis (pain, redness, swelling at injection site).

ADVERSE REACTIONS/ TOXIC EFFECTS

Antibiotic-associated colitis (severe abdominal pain and tenderness, fever, watery and severe diarrhea), other superinfections may result from altered bacterial balance. Nephrotoxicity may occur, esp. with preexisting renal disease. Severe hypersensitivity reaction (severe pruritus, angioedema, bronchospasm, anaphylaxis), particularly in pts with history of allergies, esp. penicillin.

NURSING IMPLICATIONS

BASELINE ASSESSMENT
Question for history of allergies, particularly cephalosporins, penicillins.

INTERVENTION/EVALUATION
Evaluate IV site for phlebitis (heat, pain, red streaking over vein). Assess IM injection sites for induration, tenderness. Assess mouth for white patches on mucous membranes, tongue. Monitor bowel activity/stool consistency care-

fully; mild GI effects may be tolerable, but increasing severity may indicate onset of antibiotic-associated colitis. Monitor I&O, renal function reports for nephrotoxicity. Be alert for superinfection: severe genital/anal pruritus, abdominal pain, severe mouth soreness, moderate to severe diarrhea.

PATIENT/FAMILY TEACHING

Discomfort may occur with IM injection. Doses should be evenly spaced. Continue antibiotic therapy for full length of treatment.

cefpodoxime proxetil

sef-poe-**docks**-em
(Vantin)
Do not confuse with Ventolin.

CLASSIFICATION

PHARMACOTHERAPEUTIC: Third-generation cephalosporin. **CLINICAL:** Antibiotic (see p. 21C).

ACTION

Binds to bacterial membranes. **Therapeutic Effect:** Inhibits synthesis of bacterial cell wall. Bactericidal.

PHARMACOKINETICS

Well absorbed from GI tract (food increases absorption). Protein binding: 21%–40%. Widely distributed. Primarily excreted unchanged in urine. Partially removed by hemodialysis. **Half-life:** 2.3 hrs (half-life increased with impaired renal function, elderly).

USES

Treatment of lower respiratory tract infections (pneumonia, chronic bronchitis), upper respiratory tract infections (otitis media, pharyngitis/tonsillitis), acute maxillary sinusitis, sexually transmitted diseases (urethral and cervical gonorrhea, anorectal infection), skin and skin structure infections, urinary tract infections.

PRECAUTIONS

CONTRAINDICATIONS: History of hypersensitivity to cephalosporins, anaphylactic reaction to penicillins. **CAUTIONS:** Renal impairment, history of allergies or GI disease (esp. ulcerative colitis, antibiotic-associated colitis), concurrent use of nephrotoxic medications.

LIFESPAN CONSIDERATIONS: Pregnancy/lactation: Readily crosses placenta. Distributed in breast milk. **Pregnancy Category B. Children:** Safety and efficacy not established in those <6 mos. **Elderly:** Age-related renal impairment may require dosage adjustment.

INTERACTIONS

DRUG: Antacids, H_2 antagonists may decrease absorption. **Probenecid** may increase concentration. **HERBAL:** None known. **FOOD:** None known. **LAB VALUES:** Positive direct/indirect Coombs' test may occur. May increase SGOT (AST), SGPT (ALT), alkaline phosphatase, LDH, bilirubin, BUN, serum creatinine.

AVAILABILITY (Rx)

TABLETS: 100 mg, 200 mg. **ORAL SUSPENSION:** 50 mg/5 ml, 100 mg/5 ml.

ADMINISTRATION/HANDLING

PO

• Administer with food to enhance absorption. • After reconstitution, oral suspension is stable for 14 days if refrigerated.

INDICATIONS/ROUTES/DOSAGE

PNEUMONIA, CHRONIC BRONCHITIS

PO: ADULTS, ELDERLY, CHILDREN >13 YRS: 200 mg q12h for 10–14 days.

C

GONORRHEA, RECTAL GONOCOCCAL INFECTIONS (women only)
PO: ADULTS, CHILDREN >13 YRS: 200 mg as single dose.

SKIN/SKIN STRUCTURE INFECTIONS
PO: ADULTS, ELDERLY, CHILDREN >13 YRS: 400 mg q12h for 7–14 days.

PHARYNGITIS/TONSILLITIS
PO: ADULTS, ELDERLY, CHILDREN >13 YRS: 100 mg q12h for 5–10 days. CHILDREN 6 MOS–12 YRS: 5 mg/kg q12h for 5–10 days. **Maximum:** 100 mg/dose.

ACUTE MAXILLARY SINUSITIS
PO: ADULTS, CHILDREN >13 YRS: 200 mg twice daily for 10 days. CHILDREN 2 MOS–12 YRS: 5 mg/kg q12h for 10 days. **Maximum:** 400 mg/day.

URINARY TRACT INFECTIONS
PO: ADULTS, ELDERLY, CHILDREN >13 YRS: 100 mg q12h for 7 days.

ACUTE OTITIS MEDIA
PO: CHILDREN 6 MOS–12 YRS: 5 mg/kg q12h for 5 days. **Maximum:** 400 mg/dose.

DOSAGE IN RENAL IMPAIRMENT
Dose and/or frequency is based on degree of renal impairment (creatinine clearance). Creatinine clearance <30 ml/min: dose q24h; on hemodialysis: 3 times/wk after dialysis.

SIDE EFFECTS

FREQUENT: Oral candidiasis (sore mouth/tongue), mild diarrhea, mild abdominal cramping, vaginal candidiasis (itching, discharge). **OCCASIONAL:** Nausea, serum sickness reaction (joint pain, fever) usually occurs after second course of therapy, resolves after drug discontinuation. **RARE:** Allergic reaction (rash, pruritus, urticaria).

ADVERSE REACTIONS/ TOXIC EFFECTS

Antibiotic-associated colitis (severe abdominal pain, tenderness; fever; watery, severe diarrhea), other superinfections may result from altered bacterial balance. Nephrotoxicity may occur, esp. with preexisting renal disease. Severe hypersensitivity reaction (severe pruritus, angioedema, bronchospasm, anaphylaxis), particularly in pts with history of allergies, esp. penicillin.

NURSING IMPLICATIONS

BASELINE ASSESSMENT

Question for history of allergies, particularly cephalosporins, penicillins.

INTERVENTION/EVALUATION

Assess mouth for white patches on mucous membranes, tongue. Monitor bowel activity/stool consistency carefully; mild GI effects may be tolerable, but increasing severity may indicate onset of antibiotic-associated colitis. Monitor I&O, renal function reports for nephrotoxicity. Be alert for superinfection: severe genital/anal pruritus, abdominal pain, severe mouth soreness, moderate to severe diarrhea.

PATIENT/FAMILY TEACHING

Doses should be evenly spaced. Shake oral suspension well before using. Continue antibiotic therapy for full length of treatment. Take with food. Refrigerate oral suspension.

cefprozil

sef-**proz**-ill
(Cefzil)
Do not confuse with Cefazolin, Ceftin.

CLASSIFICATION

PHARMACOTHERAPEUTIC: Second-generation cephalosporin. **CLINICAL:** Antibiotic (see p. 21C).

ACTION

Binds to bacterial membranes. **Therapeutic Effect:** Inhibits synthesis of bacterial cell wall. Bactericidal.

PHARMACOKINETICS

Well absorbed from GI tract. Protein binding: 36%–45%. Widely distributed. Primarily excreted unchanged in urine. Moderately removed by hemodialysis. **Half-life:** 1.3 hrs (half-life increased with impaired renal function).

USES

Treatment of pharyngitis/tonsillitis, otitis media, secondary bacterial infection of acute bronchitis, acute bacterial exacerbation of chronic bronchitis, uncomplicated skin/skin structure infections, acute sinusitis.

PRECAUTIONS

CONTRAINDICATIONS: History of hypersensitivity to cephalosporins, anaphylactic reaction to penicillins. **CAUTIONS:** Renal impairment, history of GI disease (esp. ulcerative colitis, antibiotic-associated colitis), concurrent use of nephrotoxic medications.

LIFESPAN CONSIDERATIONS: Pregnancy/lactation: Readily crosses placenta. Distributed in breast milk. **Pregnancy Category B. Children:** Safety and efficacy not established in those <6 mos. **Elderly:** Age-related renal impairment may require dosage adjustment.

INTERACTIONS

DRUG: Probenecid increases serum concentrations of cefprozil. **HERBAL:** None known. **FOOD:** None known. **LAB VALUES:** Positive direct/indirect Coombs' test may occur (interferes with hematologic tests, cross-matching procedures). May increase liver function tests.

AVAILABILITY (Rx)

TABLETS: 250 mg, 500 mg. **ORAL SUSPENSION:** 125 mg/5 ml, 250 mg/5 ml.

ADMINISTRATION/HANDLING

PO

• After reconstitution, oral suspension is stable for 14 days if refrigerated. • Shake oral suspension well before using. • Give without regard to meals; if GI upset occurs, give with food or milk.

INDICATIONS/ROUTES/DOSAGE

PHARYNGITIS, TONSILLITIS

PO: ADULTS, ELDERLY: 500 mg q24h for 10 days. CHILDREN 2–12 YRS: 7.5 mg/kg q12h for 10 days.

SECONDARY BACTERIAL INFECTION OF ACUTE BRONCHITIS; ACUTE BACTERIAL EXACERBATION OF CHRONIC BRONCHITIS

PO: ADULTS, ELDERLY: 500 mg q12h for 10 days.

SKIN/SKIN STRUCTURE INFECTIONS

PO: ADULTS, ELDERLY: 250–500 mg q12h for 10 days. CHILDREN: 20 mg/kg q24h.

ACUTE SINUSITIS

PO: ADULTS, ELDERLY: 250–500 mg q12h. CHILDREN 6 MOS–12 YRS: 7.5–15 mg/kg q12h.

OTITIS MEDIA

PO: CHILDREN 6 MOS–12 YRS: 15 mg/kg q12h for 10 days. **Maximum:** 1 g/day.

DOSAGE IN RENAL IMPAIRMENT

Dose and/or frequency is based on degree of renal impairment (creatinine clearance). Creatinine clearance <30 ml/min: 50% dosage at usual interval.

SIDE EFFECTS

FREQUENT: Oral candidiasis (sore mouth/tongue), mild diarrhea, mild abdominal cramping, vaginal candidiasis (itching, discharge). **OCCASIONAL:** Nausea, serum sickness reaction (joint pain, fever) usually occurs after second course of therapy, resolves after drug discontinuation.

RARE: Allergic reaction (rash, pruritus, urticaria).

ADVERSE REACTIONS/ TOXIC EFFECTS

Antibiotic-associated colitis (severe abdominal pain, tenderness; fever; watery, severe diarrhea), other superinfections may result from altered bacterial balance. Nephrotoxicity may occur, esp. with preexisting renal disease. Severe hypersensitivity reaction (severe pruritus, angioedema, bronchospasm, anaphylaxis), particularly in pts with history of allergies, esp. penicillin.

NURSING IMPLICATIONS

BASELINE ASSESSMENT

Question for history of allergies, particularly cephalosporins, penicillins.

INTERVENTION/EVALUATION

Assess mouth for white patches on mucous membranes, tongue. Monitor bowel activity/stool consistency carefully; mild GI effects may be tolerable, but increasing severity may indicate onset of antibiotic-associated colitis. Monitor I&O, renal function reports for nephrotoxicity. Be alert for superinfection: severe genital/anal pruritus, abdominal pain, severe mouth soreness, moderate to severe diarrhea.

PATIENT/FAMILY TEACHING

Doses should be evenly spaced. Continue antibiotic therapy for full length of treatment. May cause GI upset (may take with food or milk).

ceftazidime

sef-**taz**-ih-deem

(Ceptaz, Fortaz, Tazicef, Tazidime)

Do not confuse with ceftizoxime.

CLASSIFICATION

PHARMACOTHERAPEUTIC: Third-generation cephalosporin. **CLINICAL:** Antibiotic (see p. 21C).

ACTION

Binds to bacterial membranes. **Therapeutic Effect:** Inhibits synthesis of bacterial cell wall. Bactericidal.

PHARMACOKINETICS

Widely distributed (including CSF). Protein binding: 5%–17%. Primarily excreted unchanged in urine. Removed by hemodialysis. **Half-life:** 2 hrs (half-life increased with impaired renal function).

USES

Treatment of intra-abdominal, biliary tract, respiratory tract, GU tract, skin, bone infections; meningitis; septicemia.

PRECAUTIONS

CONTRAINDICATIONS: History of hypersensitivity to cephalosporins, anaphylactic reactions to penicillins. **CAUTIONS:** Renal impairment, history of GI disease (esp. ulcerative colitis, antibiotic-associated colitis) concurrent use of nephrotoxic medications.

LIFESPAN CONSIDERATIONS: Pregnancy/lactation: Readily crosses placenta. Distributed in breast milk. **Pregnancy Category B. Children:** No age-related precautions noted. **Elderly:** Age-related renal impairment may require dosage adjustment.

INTERACTIONS

DRUG: None known. **HERBAL:** None known. **FOOD:** None known. **LAB VALUES:** Positive direct/indirect Coombs' test may occur (interferes with hematologic tests, cross-matching procedures). May increase BUN, serum creatinine, SGOT (AST), SGPT (ALT), alkaline phosphatase, LDH concentrations.

AVAILABILITY (Rx)

POWDER FOR INJECTION: 500 mg, 1 g, 2 g.

ADMINISTRATION/HANDLING

Alert: Give by IM injection, direct IV injection, intermittent IV infusion (piggyback).

IM

• For reconstitution, add 1.5 ml Sterile Water for Injection or lidocaine 1% to 500 mg or 3 ml to 1-g vial to provide a concentration of 280 mg/ml. • To minimize discomfort, inject deep IM slowly. Less painful if injected into gluteus maximus than lateral aspect of thigh.

IV

Storage • Solution appears light yellow to amber, tends to darken (color change does not indicate loss of potency). • IV infusion (piggyback) stable for 18 hrs at room temperature, 7 days if refrigerated. • Discard if precipitate forms.

Reconstitution • Add 10 ml Sterile Water for Injection to each 1 g to provide concentration of 90 mg/ml. • May further dilute with 50–100 ml 0.9% NaCl, D_5W, or other compatible diluent.

Rate of administration • For IV push, administer over 3–5 min. • For intermittent IV infusion (piggyback), infuse over 15–30 min.

IV INCOMPATIBILITIES

Amphotericin B complex (AmBisome, Amphotec, Abelcet), doxorubicin liposome (Doxil), fluconazole (Diflucan), idarubicin (Idamycin), midazolam (Versed), pentamidine (Pentam IV), vancomycin (Vancocin).

IV COMPATIBILITIES

Diltiazem (Cardizem), famotidine (Pepcid), heparin, hydromorphone (Dilaudid), morphine, propofol (Diprivan).

INDICATIONS/ROUTES/DOSAGE

URINARY TRACT INFECTIONS
IM/IV: ADULTS: 250–500 mg q8–12h.

MILD TO MODERATE INFECTIONS
IM/IV: ADULTS: 1 g q8–12h.

UNCOMPLICATED PNEUMONIA, SKIN/SKIN STRUCTURE INFECTION
IM/IV: ADULTS: 0.5–1 g q8h.

BONE, JOINT INFECTION
IM/IV: ADULTS: 2 g q12h.

MENINGITIS, SERIOUS GYNECOLOGIC, INTRA-ABDOMINAL INFECTIONS
IM/IV: ADULTS: 2 g q8h.

PSEUDOMONAL PULMONARY INFECTIONS IN PTS WITH CYSTIC FIBROSIS
IV: ADULTS: 30–50 mg/kg q8h. **Maximum:** 6 g/day.

USUAL ELDERLY DOSAGE
IM/IV: Normal renal function: 500 mg–1 g q12h.

USUAL DOSAGE FOR CHILDREN
IM/IV: CHILDREN 1 MO–12 YRS: 100–150 mg/kg/day in divided doses q8h. **Maximum:** 6 g/day. NEONATES 0–4 WKS: 100–150 mg/kg/day in divided doses q8–12h.

DOSAGE IN RENAL IMPAIRMENT
After initial 1-g dose, dose and/or frequency is modified based on creatinine clearance and/or severity of infection.

Creatinine Clearance (ml/min)	Dosage Interval
30–50	q12h
10–29	q24h
<10	q24–48h

SIDE EFFECTS

FREQUENT: Discomfort with IM administration, oral candidiasis (sore mouth/tongue), mild diarrhea, mild abdominal

C

cramping, vaginal candidiasis (itching, discharge). **OCCASIONAL:** Nausea, serum sickness reaction (joint pain, fever) (usually occurs after second course of therapy, resolves after drug discontinuation). **RARE:** Allergic reaction (rash, pruritus, urticaria), thrombophlebitis (pain, redness, swelling at injection site).

ADVERSE REACTIONS/ TOXIC EFFECTS

Antibiotic-associated colitis (severe abdominal pain, tenderness; fever; watery, severe diarrhea), other superinfections may result from altered bacterial balance. Nephrotoxicity may occur, esp. with preexisting renal disease. Severe hypersensitivity reaction (severe pruritus, angioedema, bronchospasm, anaphylaxis), particularly in pts with history of allergies, esp. penicillin.

NURSING IMPLICATIONS

BASELINE ASSESSMENT

Question for history of allergies, particularly cephalosporins, penicillins.

INTERVENTION/EVALUATION

Evaluate IV site for phlebitis (heat, pain, red streaking over vein). Assess IM injection sites for induration, tenderness. Check mouth for white patches on mucous membranes, tongue. Monitor bowel activity/stool consistency carefully; mild GI effects may be tolerable, but increasing severity may indicate onset of antibiotic-associated colitis. Monitor I&O, renal function reports for nephrotoxicity. Be alert for superinfection: severe genital/anal pruritus, abdominal pain, severe mouth soreness, moderate to severe diarrhea.

PATIENT/FAMILY TEACHING

Discomfort may occur with IM injection. Doses should be evenly spaced. Continue antibiotic therapy for full length of treatment.

ceftibuten

sef-tih-**byew**-ten
(Cedax)

CLASSIFICATION

PHARMACOTHERAPEUTIC: Third-generation cephalosporin. **CLINICAL:** Antibiotic (see p. 21C).

ACTION

Binds to bacterial cell membranes. **Therapeutic Effect:** Inhibits bacterial cell wall synthesis. Bactericidal.

USES

Treatment of chronic bronchitis, acute bacterial otitis media, pharyngitis, tonsillitis.

PRECAUTIONS

CONTRAINDICATIONS: Hypersensitivity to cephalosporins. **CAUTIONS:** Hypersensitivity to penicillins or other drugs; allergies; history of GI disease (e.g., colitis); renal impairment. **Pregnancy Category B.**

INTERACTIONS

DRUG: **Probenecid** increases cephalosporin serum levels. Increased risk of nephrotoxicity with concurrent use of **aminoglycosides.** **HERBAL:** None known. **FOOD:** None known. **LAB VALUES:** Positive direct/indirect Coombs' test. May increase BUN, serum creatinine, SGOT (AST), SGPT (ALT), alkaline phosphatase, bilirubin, LDH concentrations.

AVAILABILITY (Rx)

CAPSULES: 400 mg. **ORAL SUSPENSION:** 90 mg/5 ml.

INDICATIONS/ROUTES/DOSAGE

Alert: Use oral suspension to treat otitis media (achieves higher peak blood level).

USUAL PO DOSAGE

PO: ADULTS, ELDERLY, CHILDREN ≥12 YRS: 400 mg/day as single daily dose for 10 days. CHILDREN <12 YRS: 9 mg/kg/day as single dose for 10 days. **Maximum:** 400 mg/day.

DOSAGE IN RENAL IMPAIRMENT

Based on creatinine clearance.

Creatinine Clearance	Dosage
≥50 ml/min	400 mg or 9 mg/kg q24h
30–49 ml/min	200 mg or 4.5 mg/kg q24h
<30 ml/min	100 mg or 2.25 mg/kg q24h

SIDE EFFECTS

FREQUENT: Oral candidiasis (sore mouth/tongue), mild diarrhea, mild abdominal cramping, vaginal candidiasis (itching, discharge). **OCCASIONAL:** Nausea, serum sickness reaction (joint pain, fever) usually occurs after second course of therapy, resolves after drug discontinuation. **RARE:** Allergic reaction (rash, pruritus, urticaria).

ADVERSE REACTIONS/ TOXIC EFFECTS

Antibiotic-associated colitis (severe abdominal pain, tenderness; fever; watery, severe diarrhea), other superinfections may result from altered bacterial balance. Nephrotoxicity may occur, esp. with preexisting renal disease. Severe hypersensitivity reaction (severe pruritus, angioedema, bronchospasm, anaphylaxis), particularly in pts with history of allergies, esp. penicillin.

NURSING IMPLICATIONS

BASELINE ASSESSMENT

Question for history of allergies, particularly cephalosporins, penicillins.

INTERVENTION/EVALUATION

Assess mouth for white patches on mucous membranes, tongue. Monitor bowel activity/stool consistency carefully; mild GI effects may be tolerable, but increasing severity may indicate onset of antibiotic-associated colitis. Monitor I&O, renal function reports for nephrotoxicity. Be alert for superinfection: severe genital/anal pruritus, abdominal pain, severe mouth soreness, moderate to severe diarrhea.

PATIENT/FAMILY TEACHING

Continue medication for full length of treatment; do not skip doses. Doses should be evenly spaced. May cause GI upset (may take with food or milk).

Ceftin

see cefuroxime

ceftizoxime sodium

cef-tih-**zox**-eem
(Cefizox)

Do not confuse with cefotaxime, ceftazidime.

✦CLASSIFICATION

PHARMACOTHERAPEUTIC: Third-generation cephalosporin. **CLINICAL:** Antibiotic (see p. 22C).

ACTION

Binds to bacterial membranes. **Therapeutic Effect:** Inhibits synthesis of bacterial cell wall. Bactericidal.

PHARMACOKINETICS

Widely distributed (including CSF). Protein binding: 30%. Primarily excreted unchanged in urine. Moderately removed by hemodialysis. **Half-life:** 1.7 hrs (half-life increased with impaired renal function).

C

USES

Treatment of intra-abdominal, biliary tract, respiratory tract, GU tract, skin, bone infections; gonorrhea; meningitis; septicemia; pelvic inflammatory disease (PID).

PRECAUTIONS

CONTRAINDICATIONS: History of hypersensitivity to cephalosporins, anaphylactic reaction to penicillins. **CAUTIONS:** History of GI disease (esp. ulcerative colitis, antibiotic-associated colitis), hepatic/renal impairment.

LIFESPAN CONSIDERATIONS: Pregnancy/lactation: Readily crosses placenta. Distributed in breast milk. **Pregnancy Category B. Children:** Associated with transient elevations of eosinophils, SGOT (AST), SGPT (ALT), or creatine kinase. **Elderly:** Age-related renal impairment may require dosage adjustment.

INTERACTIONS

DRUG: Probenecid increases serum concentration of ceftizoxime. **HERBAL:** None known. **FOOD:** None known. **LAB VALUES:** Positive direct/indirect Coombs' test may occur. May increase BUN, serum creatinine, SGOT (AST), SGPT (ALT), alkaline phosphatase concentrations.

AVAILABILITY (Rx)

POWDER FOR INJECTION: 1 g, 2 g.

ADMINISTRATION/HANDLING

IM

• Add 1.5 ml Sterile Water for Injection to each 0.5 g to provide concentration of 270 mg/ml. • Inject deep IM slowly to minimize discomfort. • When giving 2-g dose, divide dose and give in different large muscle masses.

IV

Storage • Solutions appears clear to pale yellow. Color change from yellow to amber does not indicate loss of potency. • IV infusion (piggyback) is stable for 24 hrs at room temperature, 96 hrs if refrigerated. • Discard if precipitate forms.

Reconstitution • Add 5 ml Sterile Water for Injection to each 0.5 g to provide concentration of 95 mg/ml. • May further dilute with 50–100 ml 0.9% NaCl, D_5W, or other compatible fluid.

Rate of administration • For IV push, administer over 3–5 min. • For intermittent IV infusion (piggyback), infuse over 15–30 min.

IV INCOMPATIBILITY

Filgrastim (Neupogen).

IV COMPATIBILITIES

Hydromorphone (Dilaudid), morphine, propofol (Diprivan).

INDICATIONS/ROUTES/DOSAGE

UNCOMPLICATED UTI

IM/IV: ADULTS, ELDERLY: 500 mg q12h.

MILD TO MODERATE TO SEVERE INFECTION

IM/IV: ADULTS, ELDERLY: 1–2 g q8–12h.

PID

IV: ADULTS: 2 g q4–8h.

LIFE-THREATENING INFECTIONS

IV: ADULTS, ELDERLY: 3–4 g q8h, up to 2 g q4h.

UNCOMPLICATED GONORRHEA

IM: ADULTS: 1 g one time.

USUAL DOSAGE FOR CHILDREN

IM/IV: CHILDREN >6 MOS: 50 mg/kg q6–8h. **Maximum:** 12 g/day.

DOSAGE IN RENAL IMPAIRMENT

After loading dose of 0.5–1 g, dose and/or frequency is modified on basis of creatinine clearance and/or severity of infection.

Creatinine Clearance	Dosage Interval
≥50 ml/min	q8–12h
10–49 ml/min	q36–48h
<10 ml/min	q48–72h

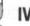

SIDE EFFECTS

FREQUENT: Discomfort with IM administration, oral candidiasis (sore mouth/tongue), mild diarrhea, mild abdominal cramping, vaginal candidiasis (itching, discharge). **OCCASIONAL:** Nausea, serum sickness reaction (joint pain, fever) usually occurs after second course of therapy, resolves after drug discontinuation. **RARE:** Allergic reaction (rash, pruritus, urticaria), thrombophlebitis (pain, redness, swelling at injection site).

ADVERSE REACTIONS/ TOXIC EFFECTS

Antibiotic-associated colitis (severe abdominal pain, tenderness; fever; watery, severe diarrhea), other superinfections may result from altered bacterial balance. Nephrotoxicity may occur, esp. with preexisting renal disease. Severe hypersensitivity reaction (severe pruritus, angioedema, bronchospasm, anaphylaxis) particularly in pts with history of allergies, esp. penicillin.

NURSING IMPLICATIONS

BASELINE ASSESSMENT

Question for history of allergies, particularly cephalosporins, penicillins.

INTERVENTION/EVALUATION

Assess mouth for white patches on mucous membranes, tongue. Monitor bowel activity and stool consistency carefully; mild GI effects may be tolerable, but increasing severity may indicate onset of antibiotic-associated colitis. Monitor I&O, renal function reports for nephrotoxicity. Be alert for superinfection: severe genital/anal pruritus, abdominal pain, severe mouth soreness, moderate to severe diarrhea.

PATIENT/FAMILY TEACHING

Doses should be evenly spaced. Continue therapy for full length of treatment. Discomfort may occur with IM injection.

ceftriaxone sodium

cef-try-**ax**-zone
(Rocephin)

◆ CLASSIFICATION

PHARMACOTHERAPEUTIC: Third-generation cephalosporin. **CLINICAL:** Antibiotic (see p. 22C).

ACTION

Binds to bacterial membranes. **Therapeutic Effect:** Inhibits synthesis of bacterial cell wall. Bactericidal.

PHARMACOKINETICS

Widely distributed (including CSF). Protein binding: 83%–96%. Primarily excreted unchanged in urine. Not removed by hemodialysis. **Half-life:** 4.3–4.6 hrs IV; 5.8–8.7 hrs IM (half-life increased with impaired renal function).

USES

Treatment of respiratory tract, GU tracts, skin, bone, intra-abdominal, biliary tract infections; septicemia; meningitis; gonorrhea; Lyme disease; acute bacterial otitis media.

PRECAUTIONS

CONTRAINDICATIONS: History of hypersensitivity to cephalosporins, anaphylactic reactions to penicillins. **CAUTIONS:** Renal/hepatic impairment, history of GI disease (esp. ulcerative colitis, antibiotic-associated colitis), concurrent administration of nephrotoxic medications.

LIFESPAN CONSIDERATIONS: Pregnancy/lactation: Readily crosses placenta. Distributed in breast milk. **Pregnancy Category B. Children:** May displace bilirubin from serum albumin. Caution in hyperbilirubinemic neonates.

C

Elderly: Age-related renal impairment may require dosage adjustment.

INTERACTIONS

DRUG: None known. **HERBAL:** None known. **FOOD:** None known. **LAB VALUES:** Positive direct/indirect Coombs' test may occur (interferes with hematologic tests, cross-matching procedures). May increase BUN, serum creatinine, SGOT (AST), SGPT (ALT), alkaline phosphatase, bilirubin concentrations.

AVAILABILITY (Rx)

POWDER FOR INJECTION: 250 mg, 500 mg, 1 g, 2 g.

ADMINISTRATION/HANDLING

IM

• Add 0.9 ml Sterile Water for Injection, 0.9% NaCl, D_5W, Bacteriostatic Water and 0.9% Benzyl Alcohol or lidocaine to each 250 mg to provide concentration of 250 mg/ml. • To minimize discomfort, inject deep IM slowly. Less painful if injected into gluteus maximus than lateral aspect of thigh.

IV

Storage • Solution appears light yellow to amber. • IV infusion (piggyback) is stable for 3 days at room temperature, 10 days if refrigerated. • Discard if precipitate forms.

Reconstitution • Add 2.4 ml Sterile Water for Injection to each 250 mg to provide concentration of 100 mg/ml. • May further dilute with 50–100 ml 0.9% NaCl, D_5W.

Rate of administration • For intermittent IV infusion (piggyback), infuse over 15–30 min for adults, 10–30 min in children, neonates. • Alternating IV sites, use large veins to reduce potential for phlebitis.

IV INCOMPATIBILITIES

Aminophylline, amphotericin B complex (AmBisome, Amphotec, Abelcet), filgrastim (Neupogen), fluconazole (Diflucan), labetalol (Normodyne), pentamidine (Pentam IV), vancomycin (Vancocin).

IV COMPATIBILITIES

Diltiazem (Cardizem), heparin, lidocaine, morphine, propofol (Diprivan).

INDICATIONS/ROUTES/DOSAGE

MILD TO MODERATE INFECTIONS

IM/IV: ADULTS, ELDERLY: 1–2 g given as single dose or 2 divided doses.

SERIOUS INFECTIONS

IM/IV: ADULTS, ELDERLY: Up to 4 g/day in 2 divided doses. CHILDREN: 50–75 mg/kg/day in divided doses q12h. **Maximum:** 2 g/day.

SKIN/SKIN STRUCTURE INFECTIONS

IM/IV: CHILDREN: 50–75 mg/kg/day as single or 2 divided doses. **Maximum:** 2 g/day.

MENINGITIS

IV: CHILDREN: Initially, 75 mg/kg, then 100 mg/kg/day as single or in divided doses q12h. **Maximum:** 4 g/day.

LYME DISEASE

IV: ADULTS, ELDERLY: 2–4 g daily for 10–14 days.

ACUTE BACTERIAL OTITIS MEDIA

IM: CHILDREN: 50 mg/kg daily for 3 days as single dose. **Maximum:** 1 g/day.

PERIOPERATIVE PROPHYLAXIS

IM/IV: ADULTS, ELDERLY: 1 g 0.5–2 hrs before surgery.

UNCOMPLICATED GONORRHEA

IM: ADULTS: 250 mg one time plus doxycycline.

DOSAGE IN RENAL IMPAIRMENT

Dosage modification usually unnecessary

but should be monitored in pts with both renal and hepatic impairment or severe renal impairment.

SIDE EFFECTS

FREQUENT: Discomfort with IM administration, oral candidiasis (sore mouth/tongue), mild diarrhea, mild abdominal cramping, vaginal candidiasis (itching, discharge). **OCCASIONAL:** Nausea, serum sickness reaction (joint pain, fever) usually occurs after second course of therapy, resolves after drug discontinuation. **RARE:** Allergic reaction (rash, pruritus, urticaria), thrombophlebitis (pain, redness, swelling at injection site).

ADVERSE REACTIONS/ TOXIC EFFECTS

Antibiotic-associated colitis (severe abdominal pain, tenderness; fever; watery, severe diarrhea), other superinfections may result from altered bacterial balance. Nephrotoxicity may occur, esp. with preexisting renal disease. Severe hypersensitivity reaction (severe pruritus, angioedema, bronchospasm, anaphylaxis), particularly in pts with history of allergies, esp. penicillin.

NURSING IMPLICATIONS

BASELINE ASSESSMENT

Question for history of allergies, particularly cephalosporins, penicillins.

INTERVENTION/EVALUATION

Assess mouth for white patches on mucous membranes, tongue. Monitor bowel activity/stool consistency carefully; mild GI effects may be tolerable, but increasing severity may indicate onset of antibiotic-associated colitis. Monitor I&O, renal function reports for nephrotoxicity. Be alert for superinfection: severe genital/anal pruritus, abdominal pain, severe mouth soreness, moderate to severe diarrhea.

PATIENT/FAMILY TEACHING

Discomfort may occur with IM injection. Doses should be evenly spaced. Continue antibiotic therapy for full length of treatment.

cefuroxime axetil

sef-yur-**ox**-ime
(Ceftin)
Do not confuse with cefotaxime, Cefzil.

cefuroxime sodium

(Kefurox, Zinacef)

CLASSIFICATION

PHARMACOTHERAPEUTIC: Second-generation cephalosporin. **CLINICAL:** Antibiotic (see p. 21C).

ACTION

Binds to bacterial membranes. **Therapeutic Effect:** Inhibits synthesis of bacterial cell wall. Bactericidal.

PHARMACOKINETICS

Rapidly absorbed from GI tract. Protein binding: 33%–50%. Widely distributed (including CSF). Primarily excreted unchanged in urine. Moderately removed by hemodialysis. **Half-life:** 1.3 hrs (half-life increased with impaired renal function).

USES

Treatment of otitis media, respiratory tract, GU tract, gynecologic, skin, bone infections; septicemia; bacterial meningitis; gonorrhea and other gonococcal infections; ampicillin-resistant influenza; perioperative prophylaxis; impetigo; acute bacterial maxillary sinusitis; early Lyme disease.

C

PRECAUTIONS

CONTRAINDICATIONS: History of hypersensitivity to cephalosporins, anaphylactic reaction to penicillins. **CAUTIONS:** Renal impairment, history of GI disease (esp. ulcerative colitis, antibiotic-associated colitis), concurrent use of nephrotoxic medications.

LIFESPAN CONSIDERATIONS: Pregnancy/lactation: Readily crosses placenta. Distributed in breast milk. **Pregnancy Category B. Children:** No age-related precautions noted. **Elderly:** Age-related renal impairment may require dosage adjustment.

INTERACTIONS

DRUG: Probenecid increases serum concentration of cefuroxime. **HERBAL:** None known. **FOOD:** None known. **LAB VALUES:** Positive direct/indirect Coombs' test may occur (interferes with hematologic tests, cross-matching procedures). May increase SGOT (AST), SGPT (ALT), alkaline phosphatase, bilirubin, LDH concentrations.

AVAILABILITY (Rx)

TABLETS: 250 mg, 500 mg. **ORAL SUSPENSION:** 125 mg/5 ml, 250 mg/5 ml. **POWDER FOR INJECTION:** 750 mg, 1.5 g.

ADMINISTRATION/HANDLING

PO

• Give without regard to meals. If GI upset occurs, give with food or milk. • Avoid crushing tablets due to bitter taste. • Suspension must be given with food.

IM

• To minimize discomfort, inject deep IM slowly. Less painful if injected into gluteus maximus than lateral aspect of thigh.

IV

Storage • Solution appears light yellow to amber; may darken, but color change does not indicate loss of potency. • IV infusion (piggyback) is stable for 24 hrs at room temperature, 7 days if refrigerated. • Discard if precipitate forms.

Reconstitution • Reconstitute 750 mg in 8 ml (1.5 g in 14 ml) Sterile Water for Injection to provide a concentration of 100 mg/ml. • For intermittent IV infusion (piggyback), further dilute with 50–100 ml 0.9% NaCl or D_5W.

Rate of administration • For IV push, administer over 3–5 min. • For intermittent IV infusion (piggyback), infuse over 15–60 min.

IV INCOMPATIBILITIES

Filgrastim (Neupogen), fluconazole (Diflucan), midazolam (Versed), vancomycin (Vancocin).

IV COMPATIBILITIES

Diltiazem (Cardizem), hydromorphone (Dilaudid), morphine, propofol (Diprivan).

INDICATIONS/ROUTES/DOSAGE

IM/IV: ADULTS, ELDERLY: 750 mg to 1.5 g q8h. CHILDREN: 75–100 mg/kg/day divided q8h. **Maximum:** 8 g/day. NEONATES: 50–100 mg/kg/day divided q12h.

PO: ADULTS, ELDERLY: 125–500 mg 2 times/day depending on the infection.

PHARYNGITIS, TONSILLITIS

PO: CHILDREN 3 MOS–12 YRS: **Tablet:** 125 mg q12h. **Suspension:** 20 mg/kg/day in 2 divided doses.

ACUTE OTITIS MEDIA, ACUTE BACTERIAL MAXILLARY SINUSITIS, IMPETIGO

PO: CHILDREN 3 MOS–12 YRS: **Tablet:** 250 mg q12h. **Suspension:** 30 mg/kg/day in 2 divided doses.

BACTERIAL MENINGITIS

IV: CHILDREN 3 MOS–12 YRS: 200–240 mg/kg/day in divided doses q6–8h.

PERIOPERATIVE PROPHYLAXIS

IV: ADULTS, ELDERLY: 1.5 g 30–60 min before surgery and 750 mg q8h postop.

IM/IV: NEONATES: 20–100 mg/kg/day in divided doses q12h.

DOSAGE IN RENAL IMPAIRMENT

Adult dosage is modified based on creatinine clearance and/or severity of infection.

Creatinine Clearance	Dosage Interval
10–20 ml/min	q12h
<10 ml/min	q24h

SIDE EFFECTS

FREQUENT: Discomfort with IM administration, oral candidiasis (sore mouth/tongue), mild diarrhea, mild abdominal cramping, vaginal candidiasis (itching, discharge). **OCCASIONAL:** Nausea, serum sickness reaction (joint pain, fever) usually occurs after second course of therapy, resolves after drug discontinuation. **RARE:** Allergic reaction (rash, pruritus, urticaria), thrombophlebitis (pain, redness, swelling at injection site).

ADVERSE REACTIONS/ TOXIC EFFECTS

Antibiotic-associated colitis (severe abdominal pain, tenderness; fever; watery, severe diarrhea), other superinfections may result from altered bacterial balance. Nephrotoxicity may occur, esp. with preexisting renal disease. Severe hypersensitivity reaction (severe pruritus, angioedema, bronchospasm, anaphylaxis), particularly in pts with history of allergies, esp. penicillin.

NURSING IMPLICATIONS

BASELINE ASSESSMENT

Question for history of allergies, particularly cephalosporins, penicillins.

INTERVENTION/EVALUATION

Assess mouth for white patches on mucous membranes, tongue. Monitor bowel activity/stool consistency carefully; mild GI effects may be tolerable, but increasing severity may indicate onset of antibiotic-associated colitis. Monitor I&O, renal function reports for nephrotoxicity. Be alert for superinfection: severe genital/anal pruritus, abdominal pain, severe mouth soreness, moderate to severe diarrhea.

PATIENT/FAMILY TEACHING

Discomfort may occur with IM injection. Doses should be evenly spaced. Continue antibiotic therapy for full length of treatment. May cause GI upset (may take with food or milk).

Celebrex

see celecoxib

celecoxib

sell-eh-**cox**-ib

(Celebrex, Panixine DisperDose)

Do not confuse with Celexa, Cerebyx.

CLASSIFICATION

PHARMACOTHERAPEUTIC: Nonsteroidal anti-inflammatory. **CLINICAL:** Anti-inflammatory (see p. 110C).

ACTION

Inhibits cyclo-oxygenase-2, the enzyme responsible for producing prostaglandins that cause pain and inflammation. **Therapeutic Effect:** Produces anti-inflammatory effects.

PHARMACOKINETICS

Widely distributed. Protein binding: 97%. Metabolized in the liver. Primarily eliminated in feces. **Half-life:** 11.2 hrs.

USES

Relief of signs/symptoms of osteoarthri-

C

tis, rheumatoid arthritis in adults. Treatment of acute pain, menstrual pain. Used to reduce number of adenomatous colorectal polyps in familial adenomatous polyposis (FAP).

PRECAUTIONS

CONTRAINDICATIONS: Hypersensitivity to sulfonamides, NSAIDs, aspirin. **CAUTIONS:** Past history of peptic ulcer, >60 yrs, those receiving anticoagulant therapy, steroids, alcohol consumption, smoking.

LIFESPAN CONSIDERATIONS: Pregnancy/lactation: Unknown if drug crosses placenta or is distributed in breast milk. Avoid use during third trimester (may adversely affect fetal cardiovascular system: premature closure of ductus arteriosus). **Pregnancy Category C (D** if used in third trimester or near delivery). **Children:** Safety and efficacy not established in those <18 yrs. **Elderly:** No age-related precautions noted.

INTERACTIONS

DRUG: May increase risk of bleeding with **warfarin.** Significant interactions may occur with **lithium, fluconazole. HERBAL:** None known. **FOOD:** None known. **LAB VALUES:** May increase liver function test results.

AVAILABILITY (Rx)

CAPSULES: 100 mg, 200 mg, 400 mg.

ADMINISTRATION/HANDLING

PO

• May give without regard to food. • Do not crush or break capsules.

INDICATIONS/ROUTES/DOSAGE

OSTEOARTHRITIS

PO: ADULTS, ELDERLY: 200 mg/day as single dose or 100 mg twice daily.

RHEUMATOID ARTHRITIS

PO: ADULTS, ELDERLY: 100–200 mg twice daily.

FAMILIAL ADENOMATOUS POLYPOSIS (FAP)

PO: ADULTS, ELDERLY: 400 mg twice daily (give with food).

SIDE EFFECTS

FREQUENT (>5%): Diarrhea, dyspepsia, headache, upper respiratory tract infection. **OCCASIONAL (1%–5%):** Abdominal pain, flatulence, nausea, back pain, peripheral edema, dizziness, rash.

ADVERSE REACTIONS/ TOXIC EFFECTS

None known.

NURSING IMPLICATIONS

BASELINE ASSESSMENT

Assess onset, type, location, duration of pain/inflammation. Inspect appearance of affected joints for immobility, deformity, skin condition.

INTERVENTION/EVALUATION

Evaluate for therapeutic response: pain relief, decreased stiffness, swelling, increased joint mobility, decreased tenderness, improved grip strength.

PATIENT/FAMILY TEACHING

If GI upset occurs, take with food. Avoid aspirin, alcohol (increases risk of GI bleeding).

cephalexin

cef-ah-**lex**-in

(Apo-Cephalex, Keflex, Keftab, Novolexin)

CLASSIFICATION

PHARMACOTHERAPEUTIC: First-generation cephalosporin. **CLINICAL:** Antibiotic (see p. 20C).

C

ACTION

Binds to bacterial membranes. **Therapeutic Effect:** Inhibits synthesis of bacterial cell wall. Bactericidal.

PHARMACOKINETICS

Rapidly absorbed from GI tract. Protein binding: 10%–15%. Widely distributed. Primarily excreted unchanged in urine. Moderately removed by hemodialysis. **Half-life:** 0.9–1.2 hrs (half-life increased with impaired renal function).

USES

Treatment of respiratory tract, GU tract, skin, soft tissue, bone infections; otitis media, rheumatic fever prophylaxis; follow-up to parenteral therapy.

PRECAUTIONS

CONTRAINDICATIONS: History of hypersensitivity to cephalosporins, anaphylactic reaction to penicillins. **CAUTIONS:** Renal impairment, history of GI disease (esp. ulcerative colitis, antibiotic-associated colitis), concurrent use of nephrotoxic medications.

LIFESPAN CONSIDERATIONS: Pregnancy/lactation: Readily crosses placenta. Distributed in breast milk. **Pregnancy Category B. Children:** No age-related precautions noted. **Elderly:** Age-related renal impairment may require dosage adjustment.

INTERACTIONS

DRUG: Probenecid increases serum concentration of cephalexin. **HERBAL:** None known. **FOOD:** None known. **LAB VALUES:** Positive direct/indirect Coombs' test may occur (interferes with hematologic test, cross-matching procedures). May increase SGOT (AST), SGPT (ALT), alkaline phosphatase concentrations.

AVAILABILITY (Rx)

CAPSULES: 250 mg, 500 mg. **TABLETS:** 250 mg, 500 mg, 1 g. **ORAL SUSPENSION:** 125 mg/5 ml, 250 mg/5 ml. **TABLETS FOR ORAL SUSPENSION:** 125 mg, 250 mg.

ADMINISTRATION/HANDLING

PO

• After reconstitution, oral suspension is stable for 14 days if refrigerated. • Shake oral suspension well before using. • Give without regard to meals. If GI upset occurs, give with food or milk.

INDICATIONS/ROUTES/DOSAGE

Alert: Space doses evenly around the clock.

USUAL DOSAGE FOR ADULTS

PO: ADULTS, ELDERLY: 250–500 mg q6h up to 4 g/day.

STREPTOCOCCAL PHARYNGITIS, SKIN/SKIN STRUCTURE INFECTIONS, UNCOMPLICATED CYSTITIS

PO: ADULTS, ELDERLY: 500 mg q12h.

USUAL DOSAGE FOR CHILDREN

PO: CHILDREN: 25–100 mg/kg/day in 2–4 divided doses.

OTITIS MEDIA

PO: CHILDREN: 75–100 mg/kg/day in 4 divided doses.

DOSAGE IN RENAL IMPAIRMENT

After usual initial dose, dose and/or frequency is modified based on creatinine clearance and/or severity of infection.

Creatinine Clearance	Dosage Interval
10–40 ml/min	q8–12h
<10 ml/min	q12–24h

SIDE EFFECTS

FREQUENT: Oral candidiasis (sore mouth/tongue), mild diarrhea, mild abdominal cramping, vaginal candidiasis (itching, discharge). **OCCASIONAL:** Nausea, serum sickness reaction (joint pain, fever) usually occurs after second course of therapy, resolves after drug discontinuation. **RARE:** Allergic reaction (rash, pruritus, urticaria).

C

ADVERSE REACTIONS/ TOXIC EFFECTS

Antibiotic-associated colitis (severe abdominal pain, tenderness; fever; watery, severe diarrhea), other superinfections may result from altered bacterial balance. Nephrotoxicity may occur, esp. with preexisting renal disease. Severe hypersensitivity reaction (severe pruritus, angioedema, bronchospasm, anaphylaxis), particularly in pts with history of allergies, esp. penicillin.

NURSING IMPLICATIONS

BASELINE ASSESSMENT

Question for history of allergies, particularly cephalosporins, penicillins.

INTERVENTION/EVALUATION

Assess mouth for white patches on mucous membranes, tongue. Monitor bowel activity/stool consistency carefully; mild GI effects may be tolerable, but increasing severity may indicate onset of antibiotic-associated colitis. Monitor I&O, renal function reports for nephrotoxicity. Be alert for superinfection: severe genital/anal pruritus, abdominal pain, severe mouth soreness, moderate to severe diarrhea.

PATIENT/FAMILY TEACHING

Doses should be evenly spaced. Continue therapy for full length of treatment. May cause GI upset (may take with food or milk). Refrigerate oral suspension.

cetirizine

sih-**tier**-eh-zeen

(Reactine, Zyrtec)

Do not confuse with Zyprexa.

FIXED-COMBINATION(S)

Zyrtec D 12 hour Tablets: cetirizine/pseudoephedrine: 5 mg/120 mg.

CLASSIFICATION

PHARMACOTHERAPEUTIC: Second-generation piperazine. **CLINICAL:** Antihistamine (see p. 47C).

ACTION

Competes with histamine for H_1-receptor sites on effector cells in the GI tract, blood vessels, respiratory tract. **Therapeutic Effect:** Prevents allergic response, produces mild bronchodilation, blocks histamine-induced bronchitis.

PHARMACOKINETICS

Onset	Peak	Duration
PO		
<1 hr	4–8 hrs	<24 hrs

Rapidly, almost completely absorbed from GI tract. Protein binding: 93%. Food has no effect on absorption. Undergoes low first-pass metabolism; not extensively metabolized. Primarily excreted in urine (>80% as unchanged drug). **Half-life:** 6.5–10 hrs.

USES

Relief of symptoms (sneezing, rhinorrhea, postnasal discharge, nasal pruritus, ocular pruritus, tearing) of seasonal and perennial allergic rhinitis (hay fever). Treatment of chronic urticaria (hives). **Unlabeled:** Treatment of bronchial asthma.

PRECAUTIONS

CONTRAINDICATIONS: Hypersensitivity to cetirizine, hydroxyzine. **CAUTIONS:** Impaired liver/renal function. May cause drowsiness at dosage >10 mg/day.

LIFESPAN CONSIDERATIONS: Pregnancy/lactation: Not recommended during early months of pregnancy. Unknown if excreted in breast milk (breast-feeding not recommended). **Pregnancy Category B.** **Children:** Less likely to cause anticholinergic effects. **Elderly:** More sensitive to anticholinergic effects (e.g., dry mouth, urinary retention). Dizziness, sedation, confusion more likely to occur.

INTERACTIONS

DRUG: **Alcohol, CNS depressants** may increase CNS depression. **HERBAL:** None known. **FOOD:** None known. **LAB VALUES:** May suppress wheal and flare reactions to antigen skin testing, unless antihistamines are discontinued 4 days before testing.

AVAILABILITY (Rx)

TABLETS: 5 mg, 10 mg. **SYRUP:** 5 mg/5 ml.

ADMINISTRATION/HANDLING

PO

- Give without regard to meals.

INDICATIONS/ROUTES/DOSAGE

ALLERGIC RHINITIS, HIVES

PO: ADULTS: 5–10 mg/day. May increase up to 20 mg/day. ELDERLY: Initially, 5 mg/day. May increase to 10 mg/day. CHILDREN 2–5 YRS: Initially, 2.5 mg once daily. **Maximum:** 5 mg once daily or 2.5 mg q12h. CHILDREN 6–11 YRS: 5–10 mg once daily.

RENAL IMPAIRMENT (creatinine clearance 11–31 ml/min), HEMODIALYSIS (creatinine clearance <7 ml/min), HEPATIC IMPAIRMENT

PO: ADULTS, ELDERLY: 5 mg once daily.

SIDE EFFECTS

Minimal anticholinergic effects. **OCCASIONAL (2%–10%):** Pharyngitis, dry mouth, nose, throat, nausea, vomiting, abdominal pain, headache, dizziness, fatigue, thickening mucus, drowsiness, increased sensitivity of skin to sun.

ADVERSE REACTIONS/TOXIC EFFECTS

Children may experience dominant paradoxical reaction (restlessness, insomnia, euphoria, nervousness, tremors). Dizziness, sedation, confusion more likely to occur in elderly pts.

NURSING IMPLICATIONS

BASELINE ASSESSMENT

Assess lung sounds. Assess severity of rhinitis, urticaria, other symptoms. Obtain baseline liver function tests.

INTERVENTION/EVALUATION

For upper respiratory allergies, increase fluids to maintain thin secretions and offset thirst. Monitor symptoms for therapeutic response.

PATIENT/FAMILY TEACHING

If drowsiness occurs, do not drive or perform tasks requiring fine motor skills. Avoid alcohol during antihistamine therapy. Avoid prolonged exposure to sunlight.

cetrorelix

(Cetrotide)

See Classification section under: Fertility agents (p. 88C)

cevimeline

sev-ee-**me**-line

(Evoxac)

Do not confuse with Eurax.

CLASSIFICATION

PHARMACOTHERAPEUTIC: Cholinergic agonist. **CLINICAL:** Mouth, throat agent.

C

ACTION

Binds to muscarinic receptors. **Therapeutic Effect:** Increases secretion of exocrine glands (e.g., salivary glands), relieving dry mouth symptoms.

USES

Treatment of dry mouth symptoms in pts with Sjögren's syndrome.

PRECAUTIONS

CONTRAINDICATIONS: Uncontrolled asthma, acute iritis, narrow-angle glaucoma. **CAUTIONS:** Cholelithiasis, history of nephrolithiasis, cardiovascular disease, chronic bronchitis, chronic obstructive pulmonary disease (COPD). **Pregnancy Category C.**

INTERACTIONS

DRUG: Amiodarone, diltiazem, erythromycin, fluoxetine, itraconazole, ketoconazole, paroxetine, quinidine, ritonavir, verapamil may increase effect. **Atropine, tricyclic antidepressants, phenothiazines** may decrease effect. **Beta-blockers** may increase potential for conduction disturbances. **HERBAL:** None known. **FOOD:** Food decreases absorption rate. **LAB VALUES:** None known.

AVAILABILITY (Rx)

CAPSULES: 30 mg.

INDICATIONS/ROUTES/DOSAGE

DRY MOUTH

PO: ADULTS: 30 mg 3 times/day.

SIDE EFFECTS

FREQUENT (11%–19%): Excessive sweating, headache, nausea, sinusitis, rhinitis, upper respiratory tract infections, diarrhea. **OCCASIONAL (3%–10%):** Dyspepsia, abdominal pain, coughing, urinary tract infection, vomiting, back pain, rash, dizziness, fatigue. **RARE (1%–2%):** Skeletal pain, insomnia, hot flashes, excessive salivation, rigors, anxiety.

ADVERSE REACTIONS/TOXIC EFFECTS

May produce decreased visual acuity, esp. at night, and impairment of depth perception.

NURSING IMPLICATIONS

PATIENT/FAMILY TEACHING

Advise caution while driving at night or performing hazardous duties in reduced lighting. Drink extra fluids to prevent possibility of dehydration. May be taken without regard to food. May cause decreased visual acuity (especially at night) and impaired depth perception.

chamomile

ka-mow-meal

Also known as German chamomile, pinheads

(Blossom 120/jar, 45/jar, 30/jar)

CLASSIFICATION

HERBAL.

ACTION

Antiallergic, anti-inflammatory action due to inhibiting release of histamine. Possesses antiallergic, antiflatulent, antispasmodic, mild sedative, anti-inflammatory action.

USES

Treatment of symptoms of flatulence, travel sickness, diarrhea, insomnia, GI spasms. Topically used for hemorrhoids.

PRECAUTIONS

CONTRAINDICATIONS: Pregnancy. **CAUTIONS:** Pts with asthma (may exacerbate condition) and those allergic to ragweed, aster, daisies, chrysanthemums.

LIFESPAN CONSIDERATIONS: Pregnancy/lactation: Contraindicated. A teratogen, affects menstrual cycle, has uterine stimulant effects. **Children:** Safety and efficacy not established. **Elderly:** No age-related precautions noted.

INTERACTIONS

DRUG: May increase anticoagulation, risk of bleeding with **aspirin, clopidogrel, dalteparin, enoxaparin, heparin, warfarin.** May have additive effects with **benzodiazepines. HERBAL:** Sedative effects may increase with **ginseng, kava, St. John's wort, valerian.** May increase risk of bleeding with **feverfew, garlic, ginger, ginkgo, licorice. FOOD:** None known. **LAB VALUES:** None known.

AVAILABILITY

WHOLE FLOWERS: 120/jar, 45/jar, 30/jar (chamomile whole flowers); 120 g, 45 g, 30 g.

INDICATIONS/ROUTES/DOSAGE

FLATULENCE, TRAVEL SICKNESS, DIARRHEA, INSOMNIA, GI SPASMS

PO: ADULTS, ELDERLY: 2–8 g of dried flower heads 3 times/day or 1 cup of tea 3–4 times/day.

SIDE EFFECTS

Allergic reaction (e.g., contact dermatitis, severe hypersensitivity reaction, anaphylactic reaction), eye irritation.

ADVERSE REACTIONS/ TOXIC EFFECTS

Anaphylactic reaction (bronchospasm, severe pruritus, angioedema).

NURSING IMPLICATIONS

BASELINE ASSESSMENT

Assess if pt is pregnant/breast-feeding/asthmatic. Assess if pt is taking other medications, esp. those that increase risk of bleeding or have sedative properties. Assess for allergies to ragweed, aster, daisies, chrysanthemums.

INTERVENTION/EVALUATION

Monitor for signs of allergic reaction.

PATIENT/FAMILY TEACHING

Inform physician if pregnancy occurs or if planning to become pregnant or breast-feed. May cause mild sedation; do not drive, operate machinery until effect of herbal is known. Avoid use with other sedatives, alcohol, anticoagulants.

charcoal, activated

(Actidose, Aqueous Charcodote ✽)

CLASSIFICATION

CLINICAL: Antidote.

ACTION

Adsorbs toxic substances, irritants. **Therapeutic Effect:** Inhibits GI absorption.

USES

Emergency antidote in treatment of poisoning.

PRECAUTIONS

CONTRAINDICATIONS: Unprotected airway; those at increased risk of aspiration; those at risk of GI perforation, hemorrhage. **CAUTIONS:** When using ipecac, induce vomiting with ipecac before giving charcoal. Induce vomiting in those taking petroleum distillate and caustic substances. May cause decreased

C

absorption of maintenance medications, placing the patient at risk. **Pregnancy Category:** Problems in humans have not been encountered.

INTERACTIONS

DRUG: May decrease absorption, effects of orally administered medications. **HERBAL:** None known. **FOOD:** None known. **LAB VALUES:** None known.

AVAILABILITY

CAPSULES, TABLETS: 250 mg. **GRANULES:** 15 g. **LIQUID (aqueous base):** 15 g, 25 g, 30 g, 50 g. **LIQUID (sorbitol):** 25 g, 50 g.

INDICATIONS/ROUTES/DOSAGE

ACUTE POISONING: SINGLE DOSE

PO: ADULTS, ELDERLY: 30–100 g or 1–2 g/kg. CHILDREN: 25–50 g or 1–2 g/kg.

MULTIPLE DOSES

PO: ADULTS, ELDERLY: 25–60 g or 1–2 g/kg. CHILDREN: 15–30 g or 1–2 g/kg.

SIDE EFFECTS

OCCASIONAL: Diarrhea, GI discomfort, intestinal gas.

ADVERSE REACTIONS/ TOXIC EFFECTS

None known.

NURSING IMPLICATIONS

INTERVENTION/EVALUATION

Monitor vital signs, level of consciousness, other clinical signs related to specific drug ingested.

chloral hydrate

klor-al **high**-drate
(Aquachloral Supprettes, PMS-Chloral Hydrate, Somnote)

CLASSIFICATION

PHARMACOTHERAPEUTIC: Nonbarbiturate chloral derivative. **CLINICAL:** Sedative, hypnotic.

ACTION

Produces CNS depression. **Therapeutic Effect:** Induces quiet, deep sleep, with only slight decrease in respiration, B/P.

USES

Sedative/hypnotic for dental/diagnostic procedures, sedative before EEG evaluations.

PRECAUTIONS

CONTRAINDICATIONS: Marked hepatic/renal impairment; severe cardiac disease; presence of gastritis. **CAUTIONS:** History of drug abuse, clinical depression. **Pregnancy Category C.**

INTERACTIONS

DRUG: **Alcohol, CNS depressants** may increase effects. May increase effect of **warfarin.** IV **furosemide** given within 24 hrs following chloral hydrate may alter B/P, cause diaphoresis. **HERBAL:** None known. **FOOD:** None known. **LAB VALUES:** None known.

AVAILABILITY (Rx)

CAPSULES: 500 mg. **SYRUP:** 500 mg/5 ml. **SUPPOSITORY:** 324 mg, 500 mg, 648 mg.

INDICATIONS/ROUTES/DOSAGE

PREMEDICATION FOR DENTAL/MEDICAL PROCEDURES

PO/rectal: ADULTS: 0.5–1 g. CHILDREN: 75 mg/kg up to 1 g total.

PREMEDICATION FOR EEG

PO/rectal: ADULTS: 0.5–1.5 g. CHILDREN: 25–50 mg/kg/dose.

SIDE EFFECTS

OCCASIONAL: Gastric irritation (nausea, vomiting, flatulence, diarrhea), rash, sleepwalking. **RARE:** Headache, paradoxical CNS hyperactivity/nervousness in children, excitement/restlessness in elderly (esp. when given in presence of pain).

ADVERSE REACTIONS/ TOXIC EFFECTS

Overdosage may produce somnolence, confusion, slurred speech, severe incoordination, respiratory depression, coma. Tolerance, psychological dependence may occur by second week of therapy.

NURSING IMPLICATIONS

BASELINE ASSESSMENT

Assess B/P, pulse, respirations immediately prior to administration. Raise bed rails. Provide environment conducive to sleep (back rub, quiet environment, low lighting).

INTERVENTION/EVALUATION

Monitor mental status, vital signs. Gastric irritation decreased by diluting dose in water. Assess sleep pattern. Assess elderly/children for paradoxical reaction. Evaluate for therapeutic response to insomnia: decrease in number of nocturnal awakenings, increase in length of sleep.

PATIENT/FAMILY TEACHING

Take capsule with a full glass of water or fruit juice. Swallow capsules whole; do not chew. If taking at home before procedure, do not drive. Do not abruptly withdraw medication after long-term use. Tolerance, dependence may occur with prolonged use.

chlorambucil

klor-**am**-bew-sill

(Leukeran)

Do not confuse with Alkeran, Chloromycetin, Myleran.

CLASSIFICATION

PHARMACOTHERAPEUTIC: Alkylating agent, nitrogen mustard. **CLINICAL:** Antineoplastic (see p. 70C).

ACTION

Inhibits DNA, RNA synthesis by cross-linking with DNA and RNA strands. Cell cycle–phase nonspecific. **Therapeutic Effect:** Interferes with nucleic acid function.

PHARMACOKINETICS

Rapidly, completely absorbed from GI tract. Protein binding: 99%. Rapidly metabolized in liver to active metabolite. Not removed by hemodialysis. **Half-life:** 1.5 hrs; metabolite: 2.5 hrs.

USES

Palliative treatment of chronic lymphocytic leukemia, advanced malignant (non-Hodgkin's) lymphomas, lymphosarcoma, giant follicular lymphomas, advanced Hodgkin's disease. **Unlabeled:** Treatment of ovarian, testicular carcinoma; hairy cell leukemia; polycythemia vera; nephrotic syndrome.

PRECAUTIONS

CONTRAINDICATIONS: Previous allergic reaction, disease resistance to previous therapy with drug. **EXTREME CAUTION:** Within 4 wks after full-course radiation therapy or myelosuppressive drug regimen.

LIFESPAN CONSIDERATIONS: Pregnancy/lactation: If possible, avoid use during pregnancy, esp. first trimester. Breast-feeding not recommended. **Pregnancy Category D. Children:** No age-related precautions. When taken for nephritic syndrome, may increase seizures. **Elderly:** No age-related precautions noted.

C

INTERACTIONS

DRUG: May decrease effect of **antigout medications. Bone marrow depressants** may increase bone marrow depression. **Other immunosuppressants (e.g., steroids)** may increase risk of infection or development of neoplasms. **Live virus vaccines** may potentiate virus replication, increase vaccine side effects, decrease antibody response to vaccine. **HERBAL:** None known. **FOOD:** None known. **LAB VALUES:** May increase SGOT (AST), alkaline phosphatase, uric acid.

AVAILABILITY (Rx)

TABLETS: 2 mg.

ADMINISTRATION/HANDLING

PO

- Give without regard to food.

INDICATIONS/ROUTES/DOSAGE

Alert: May be carcinogenic, mutagenic, or teratogenic. Handle with extreme care during administration. Dosage individualized based on clinical response, tolerance to adverse effects. When used in combination therapy, consult specific protocols for optimum dosage, sequence of drug administration.

USUAL DOSAGE (initial or short-course therapy)

PO: ADULTS, ELDERLY, CHILDREN: 0.1–0.2 mg/kg/day as single or divided dose for 3–6 wks. AVERAGE DOSE: 4–10 mg/day. SINGLE DAILY DOSE Q2WKS: 0.4 mg/kg initially. Increase by 0.1 mg/kg q2wks until response and/or myelosuppression.

USUAL DOSAGE (maintenance)

PO: ADULTS, ELDERLY, CHILDREN: 0.03–0.1 mg/kg/day. AVERAGE DOSE: 2–4 mg/day.

SIDE EFFECTS

GI effects (nausea, vomiting, anorexia, diarrhea, abdominal distress) are generally mild, last <24 hrs, and occur only if single dose exceeds 20 mg. **OCCASIONAL:** Rash, dermatitis, pruritus, cold sores. **RARE:** Alopecia, urticaria (hives), erythema, hyperuricemia.

ADVERSE REACTIONS/ TOXIC EFFECTS

Bone marrow depression manifested as hematologic toxicity (neutropenia, leukopenia, progressive lymphopenia, anemia, thrombocytopenia). After discontinuation of therapy, thrombocytopenia, leukopenia usually occur at 1–3 wks and lasts 1–4 wks. Neutrophil count decreases up to 10 days following last dose. Toxicity appears to be less severe with intermittent rather than continuous drug administration. Overdosage may produce seizures in children. Excessive uric acid level, hepatotoxicity occurs rarely.

NURSING IMPLICATIONS

BASELINE ASSESSMENT

CBC should be performed prior to and each week during therapy, WBC count performed 3–4 days following each weekly CBC during first 3–6 wks of therapy (4–6 wks if pt on intermittent dosing schedule).

INTERVENTION/EVALUATION

Monitor for hematologic toxicity (fever, sore throat, signs of local infection, easy bruising, unusual bleeding from any site), symptoms of anemia (excessive tiredness, weakness). Assess skin for rash, pruritus, urticaria.

PATIENT/FAMILY TEACHING

Increase fluid intake (may protect against hyperuricemia). Do not have immunizations without doctor's approval (drug lowers body's resistance). Avoid contact with those who have recently received live virus vaccine. Promptly report fever, sore throat, signs of local infection, easy bruising, unusual bleeding from any site.

chloramphenicol

klor-am-**fen**-ih-call
(Chloromycetin, Chloroptic)
Do not confuse with chlorambucil.

CLASSIFICATION

PHARMACOTHERAPEUTIC: Dichloroacetic acid derivative. **CLINICAL:** Antibiotic.

ACTION

Bacteriostatic (may be bactericidal in high concentrations). Binds to ribosomal receptor sites. **Therapeutic Effect:** Inhibits protein synthesis.

USES

Treatment of serious infection due to organisms resistant to other less toxic antibiotics.

PRECAUTIONS

CONTRAINDICATIONS: Hypersensitivity to chloramphenicol. **CAUTIONS:** Bone marrow depression, previous cytotoxic drug therapy, radiation therapy, hepatic or renal impairment, infants/children <2 yrs. **Pregnancy Category C.**

INTERACTIONS

DRUG: **Anticonvulsants, bone marrow depressants** may increase bone marrow depression. May increase effect of **oral hypoglycemics.** May antagonize effects of **clindamycin, erythromycin.** May increase concentration of **phenobarbital, phenytoin, warfarin.** **HERBAL:** None known. **FOOD:** None known. **LAB VALUES:** None known. Therapeutic blood serum level: 10–20 mcg/ml; toxic serum level: >25 mcg/ml.

AVAILABILITY (Rx)

CAPSULES: 250 mg. **ORAL SUSPENSION:** 150 mg/5 ml. **POWDER FOR INJECTION:** 100 mg/ml. **OPHTHALMIC SOLUTION:** 5 mg/ml. **OPHTHALMIC OINTMENT:** 10 mg/g.

INDICATIONS/ROUTES/DOSAGE

MILD TO MODERATE INFECTIONS

PO/IV: ADULTS, ELDERLY, CHILDREN: 50 mg/kg/day in divided doses q6h.

SEVERE INFECTIONS, INFECTIONS DUE TO MODERATELY RESISTANT ORGANISMS

PO/IV: ADULTS, ELDERLY, CHILDREN: 50–100 mg/kg/day in divided doses q6h.

DOSAGE IN RENAL OR HEPATIC IMPAIRMENT

Dosage is reduced based on degree of renal impairment, plasma concentration of drug. Initially, 1 g, then 500 mg q6h.

USUAL DOSAGE FOR NEONATES

PO/IV: NEWBORN INFANTS: 25 mg/kg/day in 4 doses q6h. INFANTS >2 WKS: 50 mg/kg/day in 4 doses q6h. NEONATES <2 KG: 25 mg/kg once daily. NEONATES <7 DAYS, >2 KG: 25 mg/kg once daily. NEONATES >7 DAYS, >2 KG: 50 mg/kg/day in divided doses q12h.

USUAL OPHTHALMIC DOSAGE

Ointment: ADULTS, ELDERLY, CHILDREN: Apply thin strip to conjunctiva q3–4h.

Drops: ADULTS, ELDERLY, CHILDREN: 1–2 drops 4–6 times/day.

USUAL OTIC DOSAGE

Otic: ADULTS, ELDERLY, CHILDREN: 2–3 drops into ear 3 times/day.

SIDE EFFECTS

OCCASIONAL: **Systemic:** Nausea, vomiting, diarrhea. **Ophthalmic:** Blurred vision, burning, stinging, hypersensitivity reaction. **Otic:** Hypersensitivity reaction. **RARE:** "Gray baby" syndrome (abdominal distention, blue-gray skin color, cardiovascular collapse, unresponsiveness) (in neonates), rash, shortness of breath, confusion, headache, optic neuritis (eye pain, blurred vision), peripheral neuritis (numbness/weakness in hands/feet).

ADVERSE REACTIONS/ TOXIC EFFECTS

Superinfection due to bacterial or fungal overgrowth. Narrow margin between effective therapy and toxic levels producing blood dyscrasias. Bone marrow depression with resulting aplastic anemia, hypoplastic anemia, pancytopenia (may occur weeks, months later).

NURSING IMPLICATIONS

BASELINE ASSESSMENT

Avoid, if possible, other drugs that cause bone marrow depression. Establish baseline blood studies before therapy.

INTERVENTION/EVALUATION

Assess for nausea/vomiting. Evaluate mental status. Check for visual disturbances. Assess skin for rash. Determine pattern of bowel activity/stool consistency. Watch for superinfection: diarrhea, anal/genital pruritus, change in oral mucosa, increased fever. Therapeutic blood serum level: 10–20 mcg/ml; toxic serum level: >25 mcg/ml.

PATIENT/FAMILY TEACHING

Continue therapy for full length of treatment; ophthalmic treatment should continue at least 48 hrs after eye returns to normal appearance. Doses should be evenly spaced. Take oral doses on empty stomach, 1 hr before or 2 hrs after meals (may take with food if GI upset occurs, but not with iron or vitamins).

chlordiazepoxide

klor-dye-az-eh-**pox**-eyd (Apo-Chlordiazepoxide, Librium, Lipoxide, Libritabs, Novopoxide)

FIXED-COMBINATION(S)

Limbitrol: amitriptyline/chlordiazepoxide: 5 mg/12.5 mg; 10 mg/25 mg. **Librax:** chlordiazepoxide-clidinium: 5 mg/2.5 mg.

CLASSIFICATION

PHARMACOTHERAPEUTIC: Benzodiazepine. **CLINICAL:** Antianxiety (see p. 10C).

ACTION

Enhances action of gamma-aminobutyric acid (GABA) neurotransmission at CNS. **Therapeutic Effect:** Produces anxiolytic effect.

USES

Management of anxiety disorders, acute alcohol withdrawal symptoms; short-term relief of symptoms of anxiety, preop anxiety, tension. **Unlabeled:** Treatment of panic disorder, tension headache, tremors.

PRECAUTIONS

CONTRAINDICATIONS: Acute narrow-angle glaucoma, acute alcohol intoxication. **CAUTIONS:** Impaired kidney/liver function. **Pregnancy Category D.**

INTERACTIONS

DRUG: **Alcohol, CNS depressants** may increase CNS depressant effect. **HERBAL:** **Kava kava, valerian** may increase CNS depression. **FOOD:** None known. **LAB VALUES:** None known. Therapeutic blood serum level: 1–3 mcg/ml; toxic serum level: >5 mcg/ml.

AVAILABILITY (Rx)

CAPSULES: 5 mg, 10 mg, 25 mg. **TABLETS:** 25 mg.

INDICATIONS/ROUTES/DOSAGE

Alert: Use smallest effective dosage in elderly or debilitated; those with liver disease, low serum albumin.

ALCOHOL WITHDRAWAL SYMPTOMS

PO: ADULTS, ELDERLY: 50–100 mg. May repeat q2–4h. **Maximum:** 300 mg/24 hrs.

ANXIETY

PO: ADULTS: 15–100 mg/day in 3–4 divided doses. ELDERLY: 5 mg 2–4 times/day.

SIDE EFFECTS

FREQUENT: Pain with IM injection; drowsiness, ataxia, dizziness, confusion with oral dose, particularly in elderly, debilitated. **OCCASIONAL:** Rash, peripheral edema, GI disturbances. **RARE:** Paradoxical CNS hyperactivity/nervousness in children, excitement/restlessness in elderly (generally noted during first 2 wks of therapy, esp. in presence of uncontrolled pain).

ADVERSE REACTIONS/ TOXIC EFFECTS

IV route may produce pain, swelling, thrombophlebitis, carpal tunnel syndrome. Abrupt or too rapid withdrawal may result in pronounced restlessness, irritability, insomnia, hand tremors, abdominal/muscle cramps, sweating, vomiting, seizures. Overdosage results in somnolence, confusion, diminished reflexes, coma.

NURSING IMPLICATIONS

BASELINE ASSESSMENT

Assess B/P, pulse, respirations immediately prior to administration. Pt must remain recumbent for up to 3 hrs (individualized) after parenteral administration to reduce hypotensive effect.

INTERVENTION/EVALUATION

Assess motor responses (agitation, trembling, tension), autonomic responses (cold/clammy hands, sweating). Assess children, elderly for paradoxical reaction, particularly during early therapy. Assist with ambulation if drowsiness, ataxia occur. Therapeutic blood serum level: 1–3 mcg/ml; toxic serum level: >5 mcg/ml.

PATIENT/FAMILY TEACHING

Discomfort may occur with IM injection. Drowsiness usually disappears during continued therapy. If dizziness occurs, change positions slowly from recumbent to sitting before standing. Smoking reduces drug effectiveness. Do not abruptly withdraw medication after long-term therapy.

chloroprocaine

(Nesacaine)

See Classification section under: Anesthetics: local (p. 4C)

chloroquine

klor-oh-kwin
(Aralen)

CLASSIFICATION

PHARMACOTHERAPEUTIC: Amebacide. **CLINICAL:** Antimalarial.

ACTION

Concentrates in parasite acid vesicles. May interfere with parasite protein synthesis. **Therapeutic Effect:** Increases pH (inhibits parasite growth).

C

USES

Suppression/chemoprophylaxis of malaria in chloroquine-sensitive areas. Treatment of uncomplicated or mild to moderate malaria, extraintestinal amebiasis. **Unlabeled:** Treatment of sarcoid-associated hypercalcemia, juvenile arthritis, rheumatoid arthritis, systemic lupus erythematosus, solar urticaria, chronic cutaneous vasculitis.

PRECAUTIONS

CONTRAINDICATIONS: Hypersensitivity to 4-aminoquinolones, retinal/visual field changes, psoriasis, porphyria. **CAUTIONS:** Alcoholism, severe blood disorders, liver disease, neurologic disorders, G6PD deficiency. Children are esp. susceptible to chloroquine fatalities. **Pregnancy Category C.**

INTERACTIONS

DRUG: May increase concentration of **penicillamine,** increase risk of hematologic/renal or severe skin reaction. **HERBAL:** None known. **FOOD:** None known. **LAB VALUES:** Acute decrease in Hct, Hgb, RBC count may occur.

AVAILABILITY (Rx)

TABLETS: 250 mg, 500 mg. **INJECTION:** 50 mg/ml.

INDICATIONS/ROUTES/DOSAGE

Alert: Chloroquine PO_4 500 mg = 300 mg base; chloroquine HCl 50 mg = 40 mg base.

CHLOROQUINE PHOSPHATE

TREATMENT OF MALARIA (acute attack): Dose (mg base)

Dose	Time	Adults	Children
Initial	Day 1	600 mg	10 mg/kg
Second	6 hrs later	300 mg	5 mg/kg
Third	Day 2	300 mg	5 mg/kg
Fourth	Day 3	300 mg	5 mg/kg

SUPPRESSION OF MALARIA

PO: ADULTS: 300 mg (base)/wk on same day each week beginning 2 wks before exposure; continue for 6–8 wks after leaving endemic area. CHILDREN: 5 mg base/kg/wk. If therapy is not begun prior to exposure, then: **PO:** ADULTS: 600 mg base initially given in 2 divided doses 6 hrs apart. CHILDREN: 10 mg base/kg.

AMEBIASIS

PO: ADULTS: 1 g (600 mg base) daily for 2 days; then, 500 mg (300 mg base)/day for at least 2–3 wks. CHILDREN: 10 mg base/kg once daily for 2–3 wks.

CHLOROQUINE HCL

TREATMENT OF MALARIA

IM: ADULTS: Initially, 160–200 mg base (4–5 ml), repeat in 6 hrs. **Maximum:** 800 mg base in first 24 hrs. Begin oral therapy as soon as possible and continue for 3 days until approximately 1.5 g base given. CHILDREN: Initially, 5 mg base/kg, repeat in 6 hrs. Do not exceed 10 mg base/kg/24 hrs.

AMEBIASIS

IM: ADULTS: 160–200 mg base (4–5 ml) daily for 10–12 days. Change to oral therapy as soon as possible.

SIDE EFFECTS

FREQUENT: Discomfort with IM administration, mild transient headache, anorexia, nausea/vomiting. **OCCASIONAL:** Visual disturbances (blurring, difficulty focusing); nervousness; fatigue; pruritus, esp. of palms, soles, scalp; bleaching of hair; irritability; personality changes; diarrhea; skin eruptions. **RARE:** Stomatitis (redness/burning of oral mucosa, gingivitis, glossitis), exfoliative dermatitis.

ADVERSE REACTIONS/ TOXIC EFFECTS

Ocular toxicity (tinnitus), ototoxicity (reduced hearing). Prolonged therapy: peripheral neuritis and neuromyopathy, hypotension, EKG changes, agranulocytosis, aplastic anemia, thrombocytopenia, convulsions, psychosis. Overdosage: headache, vomiting, visual disturbance, drowsiness, convulsions, hypokalemia followed by cardiovascular collapse, death.

NURSING IMPLICATIONS

INTERVENTION/EVALUATION

Check for, promptly report any visual disturbances. Evaluate for GI distress. Monitor hepatic function tests, assess for fatigue, jaundice, other signs of hepatic effects. Assess skin/buccal mucosa, inquire about pruritus. Check vital signs, be alert to signs/symptoms of overdosage (esp. with parenteral administration, children). Notify physician of tinnitus, reduced hearing. With prolonged therapy, test for muscle weakness.

PATIENT/FAMILY TEACHING

IM administration may cause local discomfort. Continue drug for full length of treatment. Notify physician of **any** new symptom, visual difficulties, decreased hearing, tinnitus immediately. Periodic lab, visual tests are important part of therapy.

chlorothiazide

(Diuril)

See Classification section under: Diuretics (p. 86C)

chlorpheniramine

(Chlor-Trimeton, Teldrin)

See Classification section under: Antihistamines (p. 48C)

chlorpromazine

klor-**pro**-mah-zeen

(Chlorpromanyl♣, Largactil♣, Thorazine)

Do not confuse with chlorpropamide, thiamide, thioridazine.

CLASSIFICATION

PHARMACOTHERAPEUTIC: Phenothiazine. **CLINICAL:** Antipsychotic, antiemetic, antianxiety, antineuralgia adjunct (see p. 56C).

ACTION

Blocks dopamine neurotransmission at postsynaptic dopamine receptor sites. Possesses strong anticholinergic, sedative, antiemetic effects; moderate extrapyramidal effects; slight antihistamine action. **Therapeutic Effect:** Reduces psychosis; relieves nausea/vomiting; controls intractable hiccups, porphyria.

USES

Management of psychotic disorders, manic phase of manic-depressive illness, severe nausea/vomiting, preop sedation, severe behavioral disturbances in children. Relief of intractable hiccups, acute intermittent porphyria. **Unlabeled:** Treatment of choreiform movement of Huntington's disease.

PRECAUTIONS

CONTRAINDICATIONS: Severe CNS depression, comatose states, severe cardiovascular disease, bone marrow depression, subcortical brain damage. **CAUTIONS:** Impaired respiratory/hepatic/renal/cardiac function, alcohol withdrawal, history of seizures, urinary retention, glaucoma, prostatic hypertrophy, hypocalcemia (increases susceptibility to dystonias). **Pregnancy Category C.**

C

INTERACTIONS

DRUG: **Alcohol, CNS depressants** may increase respiratory depression; hypotensive effects. **Tricyclic antidepressants, MAOIs** may increase sedative, anticholinergic effects. **Antithyroid agents** may increase risk of agranulocytosis. Increased risk of extrapyramidal symptoms (EPS) with **EPS-producing medications. Hypotensives** may increase hypotension. May decrease **levodopa** effects. **Lithium** may decrease absorption, produce adverse neurologic effects. **HERBAL:** None known. **FOOD:** None known. **LAB VALUES:** May produce false-positive pregnancy test, phenylketonuria (PKU). EKG changes may occur, including Q- and T-wave disturbances. Therapeutic blood serum level: 50–300 mcg/ml; toxic serum level: >750 mcg/ml.

AVAILABILITY (Rx)

INJECTION: 25 mg/ml. **LIQUID:** 30 mg/ml, 100 mg/ml. **SUPPOSITORY:** 100 mg. **SYRUP:** 10 mg/5 ml. **TABLET:** 10 mg, 25 mg, 50 mg, 100 mg.

INDICATIONS/ROUTES/DOSAGE

PSYCHOSIS

IM/IV: ADULTS, ELDERLY: Initially, 25 mg; may repeat in 1–4 hrs. May gradually increase to 400 mg q4–6h. **Maximum:** 300–800 mg/day. CHILDREN >6 MOS: 0.5–1 mg/kg q6–8h. **Maximum:** <5 YRS: 40 mg/day. 5–12 YRS: 75 mg/day.

PO: ADULTS, ELDERLY: 30–800 mg/day in 1–4 divided doses. CHILDREN >6 MOS: 0.5–1 mg/kg q4–6h.

NAUSEA/VOMITING

IM/IV: ADULTS, ELDERLY: 25–50 mg q4–6h. CHILDREN: 0.5–1 mg/kg q6–8h.

PO: ADULTS, ELDERLY: 10–25 mg q4–6h. CHILDREN: 0.5–1 mg/kg q4–6h.

Rectal: ADULTS, ELDERLY: 50–100 mg q6–8h. CHILDREN: 1 mg/kg q6–8h.

HICCUPS

PO: ADULTS: 25–50 mg 3 times/day. May give IM/IV.

SIDE EFFECTS

FREQUENT: Drowsiness, blurred vision, hypotension, abnormal color vision, difficulty in night vision, dizziness, decreased sweating, constipation, dry mouth, nasal congestion. **OCCASIONAL:** Difficulty urinating, increased skin sensitivity to sun, skin rash, decreased sexual function, swelling/pain in breasts, weight gain, nausea, vomiting, stomach pain, tremors.

ADVERSE REACTIONS/ TOXIC EFFECTS

Extrapyramidal symptoms appear to be dose related (particularly high dosage) and are divided into 3 categories: akathisia (inability to sit still, tapping of feet, urge to move around), parkinsonian symptoms (masklike face, tremors, shuffling gait, hypersalivation), and acute dystonias (torticollis [neck muscle spasm], opisthotonos [rigidity of back muscles], oculogyric crisis [rolling back of eyes]). Dystonic reaction may produce profuse sweating, pallor. Tardive dyskinesia (protrusion of tongue, puffing of cheeks, chewing/puckering of the mouth) occurs rarely (may be irreversible). Abrupt withdrawal after long-term therapy may precipitate nausea, vomiting, gastritis, dizziness, tremors. Blood dyscrasias, particularly agranulocytosis, mild leukopenia, may occur. May lower seizure threshold.

NURSING IMPLICATIONS

BASELINE ASSESSMENT

Avoid skin contact with solution (contact dermatitis). **Antiemetic:** Assess for dehydration (poor skin turgor, dry mucous membranes, longitudinal furrows in tongue). **Antipsychotic:** Assess behavior, appearance, emotional status, response to environment, speech pattern, thought content.

INTERVENTION/EVALUATION

Monitor B/P for hypotension. Assess for EPS. Monitor WBC, differential count for blood dyscrasias, fine tongue movement (may be early sign of tardive dyskinesia). Supervise suicidal-risk pt closely during early therapy (as depression lessens, energy level improves, increasing suicide potential). Assess for therapeutic response (interest in surroundings, improvement in self-care, increased ability to concentrate, relaxed facial expression). Therapeutic blood serum level: 50–300 mcg/ml; toxic serum level: >750 mcg/ml.

PATIENT/FAMILY TEACHING

Full therapeutic response may take up to 6 wks. Urine may darken. Do not abruptly withdraw from long-term drug therapy. Report visual disturbances. Drowsiness generally subsides during continued therapy. Avoid tasks that require alertness, motor skills until response to drug is established. Avoid alcohol, exposure to sunlight.

chlorpropamide

(Diabinese)

See Classification section under: Antidiabetics (p. 39C)

chlorthalidone

klor-**thal**-ih-doan

(Apo-Chlorthalidone✤, Thalitone)

FIXED-COMBINATION(S)

Combipres: chlorthalidone/clonidine (an antihypertensive): 15 mg/0.1 mg; 15 mg/0.2 mg; 15 mg/0.3 mg. **Tenoretic:** chlorthalidone/atenolol (a beta-blocker): 25 mg/50 mg, 25 mg/100 mg.

CLASSIFICATION

PHARMACOTHERAPEUTIC: Thiazide. **CLINICAL:** Diuretic (see p. 86C).

ACTION

Diuretic: Blocks reabsorption of sodium, potassium, chloride at distal convoluted tubule. **Antihypertensive:** Reduces plasma, extracellular fluid volume, peripheral vascular resistance. **Therapeutic Effect:** As diuretic, promotes renal excretion. As antihypertensive, lowers B/P.

PHARMACOKINETICS

Onset	Peak	Duration
PO (diuretic)		
2 hrs	2–6 hrs	Up to 36 hrs

Rapidly absorbed from GI tract. Excreted unchanged in urine. **Half-life:** 35–50 hrs; onset antihypertensive effect: 3–4 days; optimal therapeutic effect: 3–4 wks.

USES

Adjunctive therapy in edema associated with CHF, hepatic cirrhosis, corticoid/estrogen therapy, renal impairment. In treatment of hypertension, may be used alone or with other antihypertensive agents.

PRECAUTIONS

CONTRAINDICATIONS: History of hypersensitivity to sulfonamides or thiazide diuretics, renal decompensation, anuria. **CAUTIONS:** Severe renal disease, impaired hepatic function, diabetes mellitus, elderly/debilitated, gout, hypercholesterolemia.

C

LIFESPAN CONSIDERATIONS: Pregnancy/lactation: Crosses placenta: small amount distributed in breast milk: nursing not advised. **Pregnancy Category B** (**D** if used in pregnancy-induced hypertension). **Children:** No age-related precautions noted. **Elderly:** May be more sensitive to hypotensive and electrolyte effects.

INTERACTIONS

DRUG: **Cholestyramine, colestipol** may decrease absorption, effects. May increase **digoxin** toxicity (due to hypokalemia). May increase **lithium** toxicity. **HERBAL:** None known. **FOOD:** None known. **LAB VALUES:** May increase bilirubin, serum calcium, LDL, cholesterol, triglycerides, creatinine, glucose, uric acid. May decrease urinary calcium, magnesium, potassium, sodium.

AVAILABILITY (Rx)

TABLETS: 15 mg, 25 mg, 50 mg, 100 mg.

ADMINISTRATION/HANDLING

PO

• Give with food or milk if GI upset occurs, preferably with breakfast (may prevent nocturia). • Scored tablets may be crushed.

INDICATIONS/ROUTES/DOSAGE

HYPERTENSION/EDEMA

PO: ADULTS: 25–100 mg/day or 100 mg 3 times/wk. ELDERLY: Initially, 12.5–25 mg/day or every other day.

SIDE EFFECTS

EXPECTED: Increased urine frequency/volume. **FREQUENT:** Potassium depletion (rarely produces symptoms). **OCCASIONAL:** Anorexia, impotence, diarrhea, orthostatic hypotension, GI upset, photosensitivity. **RARE:** Rash.

ADVERSE REACTIONS/ TOXIC EFFECTS

Vigorous diuresis may lead to profound water loss and electrolyte depletion, resulting in hypokalemia, hyponatremia, dehydration. Acute hypotensive episodes may occur. Hyperglycemia may be noted during prolonged therapy. Overdosage can lead to lethargy, coma without changes in electrolytes or hydration.

NURSING IMPLICATIONS

BASELINE ASSESSMENT

Check vital signs, esp. B/P, for hypotension before administration. Assess baseline electrolytes, particularly potassium. Assess edema, skin turgor, mucous membranes for hydration status. Evaluate muscle strength, mental status.

INTERVENTION/EVALUATION

Watch for electrolyte disturbances (hypokalemia may result in weakness, tremor, muscle cramps, nausea, vomiting, change in mental status, tachycardia; hyponatremia may result in confusion, thirst, cold/clammy skin). Periodically check blood sugar for hyperglycemia in prolonged therapy.

PATIENT/FAMILY TEACHING

To reduce hypotensive effect, rise slowly from lying to sitting position, permit legs to dangle momentarily before standing. Eat foods high in potassium, such as whole grains (cereals), legumes, meat, bananas, apricots, orange juice, potatoes (white, sweet), raisins. Avoid prolonged exposure to sunlight.

chlorzoxazone

(Paraflex, Parafon Forte DSC)

See Classification section under: Skeletal muscle relaxants

cholestyramine resin

coal-es-**tie**-rah-mean
(Novo-Cholamine✱, Prevalite, Questran✱, Questran Lite)

Do not confuse with Quarzan.

CLASSIFICATION

PHARMACOTHERAPEUTIC: Bile acid sequestrant. **CLINICAL:** Antihyperlipoproteinemic (see p. 50C).

ACTION

Binds with bile acids in intestine, forming insoluble complex. Binding results in partial removal of bile acid from enterohepatic circulation. **Therapeutic Effect:** Removes LDL and cholesterol from plasma.

PHARMACOKINETICS

Not absorbed from GI tract. Decreases in LDL apparent in 5–7 days, serum cholesterol in 1 mo. Serum cholesterol returns to baseline levels about 1 mo after discontinuing drug.

USES

Adjunct to dietary therapy to decrease elevated serum cholesterol levels in pts with primary hypercholesterolemia. Relief of pruritus associated with partial biliary obstruction. **Unlabeled:** Treatment of diarrhea (due to bile acids); hyperoxaluria.

PRECAUTIONS

CONTRAINDICATIONS: Hypersensitivity to cholestyramine or tartrazine (frequently seen in aspirin hypersensitivity), complete biliary obstruction. **CAUTIONS:** GI dysfunction (esp. constipation), hemorrhoids, bleeding disorders, osteoporosis.

LIFESPAN CONSIDERATIONS: Pregnancy/lactation: Not systemically absorbed. May interfere with maternal absorption of fat-soluble vitamins. **Pregnancy Category B. Children:** No age-related precautions noted. Limited experience in those <10 yrs. **Elderly:** Increased risk of GI side effects, adverse nutritional effects.

INTERACTIONS

DRUG: May increase effects of **anticoagulants** by decreasing vitamin K. May decrease **warfarin** absorption. May bind, decrease absorption of **digoxin, thiazides, penicillins, propranolol, tetracyclines, folic acid, thyroid hormones, other medications.** Binds, decreases effect of **oral vancomycin. HERBAL:** None known. **FOOD:** None known. **LAB VALUES:** May increase SGOT (AST), SGPT (ALT), alkaline phosphatase, magnesium. May decrease calcium, potassium, sodium. May prolong prothrombin time.

AVAILABILITY (Rx)

POWDER: 4 g.

ADMINISTRATION/HANDLING

PO

• Give other drugs at least 1 hr prior to or 4–6 hrs following cholestyramine (capable of binding drugs in GI tract). • Do not give in dry form (highly irritating). Mix with 3–6 oz water, milk, fruit juice, soup. • Place powder on surface for 1–2 min (prevents lumping), then mix thoroughly. • Excessive foaming with carbonated beverages; use extra large glass and stir slowly. • Administer before meals.

INDICATIONS/ROUTES/DOSAGE

PRIMARY HYPERCHOLESTEROLEMIA

PO: ADULTS, ELDERLY: 3–4 g 3–4 times/day. **Maximum:** 16–32 g/day in 2–4 divided doses. CHILDREN >10 YRS: 2 g/day up to 8 g/day. CHILDREN ≤10 YRS: Initially, 2 g/day. RANGE: 1–4 g/day.

C

SIDE EFFECTS

FREQUENT: Constipation (may lead to fecal impaction), nausea, vomiting, stomach pain, indigestion. **OCCASIONAL:** Diarrhea, belching, bloating, headache, dizziness. **RARE:** Gallstones, peptic ulcer, malabsorption syndrome.

ADVERSE REACTIONS/ TOXIC EFFECT

GI tract obstruction, hyperchloremic acidosis, osteoporosis secondary to calcium excretion. High dosage may interfere with fat absorption, resulting in steatorrhea.

NURSING IMPLICATIONS

BASELINE ASSESSMENT

Question for history of hypersensitivity to cholestyramine, tartrazine, aspirin. Obtain baseline serum cholesterol, triglycerides, electrolytes.

INTERVENTION/EVALUATION

Determine pattern of bowel activity. Evaluate food tolerance, abdominal discomfort, flatulence. Monitor blood chemistries. Encourage several glasses of water between meals.

PATIENT/FAMILY TEACHING

Complete full course; do not omit or change doses. Take other drugs at least 1 hr before or 4–6 hrs after cholestyramine. Never take in dry form; mix with 3–6 oz water, milk, fruit juice, soup (place powder on surface for 1–2 min to prevent lumping, then mix well). Use extra large glass, stir slowly when mixing with carbonated beverages due to foaming. Take before meals, drink several glasses of water between meals. Eat high-fiber foods (whole grain cereals, fruits, vegetables) to reduce potential for constipation.

chorionic gonadotropin, hCG

kore-ee-**on**-ik goe-**nad**-oh-troe-pin (APL, Chorex-10, Novarel, Pregnyl, Profasi)

◆ CLASSIFICATION

PHARMACOTHERAPEUTIC: Sex hormone. **CLINICAL:** Androgen, progesterone stimulant (see p. 89C).

ACTION

Stimulates production of gonadal steroid hormones by stimulating interstitial cells (Leydig cells) of the testes to produce androgen and the corpus luteum of the ovary to produce progesterone. **Therapeutic Effect:** Androgen stimulation in the male causes production of secondary sex characteristics and may stimulate descent of testes when no anatomic impediment exists. In women of childbearing age with normally functioning ovaries, causes maturation of corpus luteum and triggers ovulation.

USES

Treatment of hypogonadotropic hypogonadism, prepubertal cryptorchidism. Induces ovulation. **Unlabeled:** Diagnosis of male hypogonadism, treatment of corpus luteum dysfunction.

PRECAUTIONS

CONTRAINDICATIONS: Precocious puberty, carcinoma of the prostate or other androgen-dependent neoplasia. **CAUTIONS:** Prepubertal males, conditions aggravated by fluid retention (cardiac/renal disease, epilepsy, migraine, asthma). **Pregnancy Category C.**

INTERACTIONS

DRUG: None known. **HERBAL:** None known. **FOOD:** None known. **LAB VALUES:** None known.

AVAILABILITY (Rx)

POWDER FOR INJECTION: 500 units/ml, 1,000 units/ml, 10,000-unit vial.

INDICATIONS/ROUTES/DOSAGE

PREPUBERTAL CRYPTORCHIDISM, HYPOGONADOTROPIC HYPOGONADISM

IM: CHILDREN: Dosage is individualized based on indication, age, weight of pt, and physician preference.

INDUCTION OF OVULATION AND PREGNANCY

IM: ADULTS (after pretreatment with menotropins): 5,000–10,000 international units 1 day after last dose of menotropins.

SIDE EFFECTS

FREQUENT: Pain at injection site. **Induction of ovulation:** Ovarian cysts, uncomplicated ovarian enlargement. **OCCASIONAL:** Enlarged breasts, headache, irritability, fatigue, depression. **Induction of ovulation:** Severe ovarian hyperstimulation, peripheral edema. **Cryptorchidism:** Precocious puberty (acne, deepening voice, penile growth, pubic/axillary hair).

ADVERSE REACTIONS/ TOXIC EFFECTS

When used with menotropins: increased risk of arterial thromboembolism, ovarian hyperstimulation with high incidence (20%) of multiple births (premature deliveries and neonatal prematurity), ruptured ovarian cysts.

NURSING IMPLICATIONS

BASELINE ASSESSMENT

Obtain baseline weight, B/P.

INTERVENTION/EVALUATION

Assess for edema: weigh every 2–3 days, report gain >5 lbs/wk; monitor B/P periodically during treatment; check for decreased urinary output, peripheral edema.

PATIENT/FAMILY TEACHING

Promptly report abdominal pain, vaginal bleeding, signs of precocious puberty in males (deepening of voice; axillary, facial, pubic hair; acne; penile growth), signs of edema. In anovulation treatment, begin recording daily basal temperature; initiate intercourse daily beginning the day preceding human chorionic gonadotropin (hCG) treatment. Possibility of multiple births.

ciclopirox

(Loprox, Penlac)

See Classification section under: Antifungals: topical (p. 42C)

cidofovir

sid-**dough**-foe-vir

(Vistide)

CLASSIFICATION

PHARMACOTHERAPEUTIC: Anti-infective. **CLINICAL:** Antiviral (see p. 58C).

ACTION

Suppresses cytomegalovirus (CMV) replication. **Therapeutic Effect:** Inhibits viral DNA synthesis. Incorporation of cidofovir in growing viral DNA chain results in reduced rate of viral DNA synthesis.

PHARMACOKINETICS

Protein binding: <6%. Excreted primarily unchanged in urine. Effect of hemodialysis unknown. **Half-life:** 1.4–3.8 hrs.

USES

Treatment of CMV retinitis in those with acquired immunodeficiency syndrome (AIDS). **Unlabeled:** Antiviral with activity against ganciclovir-resistant CMV, foscarnet-resistant CMV, acyclovir-resistant herpes simplex virus or varicella zoster virus, and adenovirus.

PRECAUTIONS

CONTRAINDICATIONS: Hypersensitivity to cidofovir, history of clinically severe hypersensitivity to probenecid or other sulfa-containing medication, direct intraocular injection, renal function impairment (serum creatinine >1.5 mg/dl, creatinine clearance ≤55 ml/min, urine protein >100 mg/dl). **CAUTIONS:** Preexisting diabetes.

LIFESPAN CONSIDERATIONS: Pregnancy/lactation: Embryotoxic (reduced fetal body weight) in animals. Unknown if excreted in breast milk. Do not administer to nursing women. HIV-infected women should not breast-feed. **Pregnancy Category C. Children:** Safety and efficacy not established. **Elderly:** Age-related renal impairment may require dosage adjustment.

INTERACTIONS

DRUG: Avoid concurrent administration of cidofovir and medication with nephrotoxic risk **(amphotericin B, aminoglycosides, foscarnet, IV pentamidine). HERBAL:** None known. **FOOD:** None known. **LAB VALUES:** May decrease neutrophil count, serum phosphate, uric acid, bicarbonate; elevate serum creatinine.

AVAILABILITY (Rx)

INJECTION: 75 mg/ml (5-ml amp).

ADMINISTRATION/HANDLING

Alert: Do not exceed recommended dosage, frequency, infusion rate.

IV

Storage • Store at controlled room temperature (68°–77°F). • Admixtures may be refrigerated for no more than 24 hrs. • Allow refrigerated admixtures to warm to room temperature before use.

Dilution • Dilute in 100 ml 0.9% NaCl.

Rate of administration • Infuse over 1 hr. • IV hydration with 0.9% NaCl and probenecid therapy **must** be used with each cidofovir infusion (minimizes risk of nephrotoxicity). • Ingestion of food before each dose of probenecid may reduce nausea/vomiting. An antiemetic may also reduce potential for nausea.

IV INCOMPATIBILITY

No information available via Y-site administration.

INDICATIONS/ROUTES/DOSAGE

PROBENECID

PO: ADULTS: Give 2 g 3 hrs prior to cidofovir dose, and 1 g given 2 hrs and again 8 hrs after completion of the 1-hr cidofovir infusion (total of 4 g).

HYDRATION

IV: ADULTS: 1 liter 0.9% NaCl given over 1–2 hrs immediately before cidofovir infusion. If tolerated, a second liter may be given at start or immediately after cidofovir infusion and infused over 1–3 hrs.

USUAL DOSAGE

IV Infusion: ADULTS: INDUCTION: 5 mg/kg at constant rate over 1 hr once weekly for 2 consecutive wks. MAINTENANCE: 5 mg/kg at constant rate over 1 hr once every 2 wks.

RENAL FUNCTION IMPAIRMENT

Dose based on creatinine clearance.

Creatinine Clearance	Induction Dose	Maintenance Dose
41–55 ml/min	2 mg/kg	2 mg/kg
30–40 ml/min	1.5 mg/kg	1.5 mg/kg
20–29 ml/min	1 mg/kg	1 mg/kg
≤19 ml/min	0.5 mg/kg	0.5 mg/kg

SIDE EFFECTS

FREQUENT: Nausea, vomiting (65%), fever (57%), asthenia (46%), rash (30%), diarrhea (27%), headache (27%), alopecia (25%), chills (24%), anorexia (22%), dyspnea (22%), abdominal pain (17%).

ADVERSE REACTIONS/ TOXIC EFFECTS

Proteinuria (80%), nephrotoxicity (53%), neutropenia (31%), serum creatinine elevations (29%), infection (24%), anemia (20%), ocular hypotony (12%) (decrease in intraocular pressure), pneumonia (9%). Probenecid may produce hypersensitivity reaction (rash, fever, chills, anaphylaxis). Acute renal failure occurs rarely.

NURSING IMPLICATIONS

BASELINE ASSESSMENT

For those taking zidovudine, temporarily discontinue zidovudine administration or decrease zidovudine dose by 50% on days of infusion (probenecid reduces metabolic clearance of zidovudine). Closely monitor renal function (urinalysis, serum creatinine) during therapy.

INTERVENTION/EVALUATION

Monitor serum creatinine, urine protein, WBC count prior to each dose. Monitor for proteinuria (may be early indicator of dose-dependent nephrotoxicity). Periodically monitor visual acuity, ocular symptoms.

PATIENT/FAMILY TEACHING

Obtain regular follow-up ophthalmologic exams. Those of childbearing age should use effective contraception during and for 1 mo after treatment. Men should practice barrier contraceptive methods during and for 3 mos after treatment. Do not breast-feed. Must complete full course of probenecid with each cidofovir dose.

cilostazol

sill-oh-**stay**-zole
(Pletal)
Do not confuse with Plendil.

CLASSIFICATION

PHARMACOTHERAPEUTIC: Phosphodiesterase III inhibitor. **CLINICAL:** Antiplatelet.

ACTION

Inhibits platelet aggregation. Dilation of vascular beds with greatest dilation in femoral beds. **Therapeutic Effect:** Improves walking distance in those with intermittent claudication.

PHARMACOKINETICS

Moderately absorbed from GI tract. Protein binding: 95%–98%. Extensively metabolized in the liver. Excreted primarily in the urine and, to a lesser extent, in the feces. Not removed by hemodialysis. **Half-life:** 11–13 hrs. Therapeutic effect noted in 2–4 wks but may take as long as 12 wks before beneficial effect is experienced.

USES

Reduction of symptoms of intermittent claudication indicated by increased walking distance without leg pain.

PRECAUTIONS

CONTRAINDICATIONS: CHF of any severity. **CAUTIONS:** None known.

LIFESPAN CONSIDERATIONS: Preg-

C

nancy/lactation: Unknown if drug crosses placenta or is distributed in breast milk. **Pregnancy Category C. Children:** Safety and efficacy not established. **Elderly:** No age-related precautions noted.

INTERACTIONS

DRUG: None known. **HERBAL:** None known. **FOOD:** **Grapefruit juice** may increase concentration, toxicity. **LAB VALUES:** May decrease Hgb, Hct. May increase creatinine, BUN.

AVAILABILITY (Rx)

TABLETS: 50 mg, 100 mg.

ADMINISTRATION/HANDLING

PO

• Give at least 30 min before or 2 hrs after meals. • Do not take with grapefruit juice.

INDICATIONS/ROUTES/DOSAGE

INTERMITTENT CLAUDICATION

PO: ADULTS, ELDERLY: 100 mg 2 times/day at least 30 min before or 2 hrs after meals.

SIDE EFFECTS

FREQUENT (10%–34%): Headache, diarrhea, palpitations, dizziness, pharyngitis. **OCCASIONAL (3%–7%):** Nausea, rhinitis, back pain, peripheral edema, dyspepsia, abdominal pain, tachycardia, cough, flatulence, myalgia. **RARE (1%–2%):** Leg cramps, paresthesia, rash, vomiting.

ADVERSE REACTIONS/ TOXIC EFFECTS

Overdosage noted by severe headache, diarrhea, hypotension, cardiac arrhythmias.

NURSING IMPLICATIONS

BASELINE ASSESSMENT

Assess platelet count, Hgb, Hct prior to treatment and periodically during treatment.

PATIENT/FAMILY TEACHING

Take on an empty stomach (at least 30 min before or 2 hrs after meals). Do not take with grapefruit juice.

cimetidine

sih-**met**-ih-deen
(Apo-Cimetidine ✦, Novocimetine ✦, Peptol ✦, Tagamet, Tagamet HB)

Do not confuse with simethicone.

◆CLASSIFICATION

PHARMACOTHERAPEUTIC: H_2 receptor antagonist. **CLINICAL:** Antiulcer, gastric acid secretion inhibitor (see p. 91C).

ACTION

Inhibits histamine action at H_2 receptor sites of parietal cells. **Therapeutic Effect:** Inhibits gastric acid secretion (fasting, nocturnal, or when stimulated by food, caffeine, insulin).

PHARMACOKINETICS

Well absorbed from GI tract. Protein binding: 15%–20%. Widely distributed. Metabolized in liver. Primarily excreted in urine. Not removed by hemodialysis. **Half-life:** 2 hrs (half-life increased with impaired renal function).

USES

Short-term treatment of active duodenal ulcer. Prevention of duodenal ulcer recurrence, upper GI bleeding in critically ill pts. Treatment of active benign gastric ulcer, pathologic GI hypersecretory conditions, gastroesophageal reflux disease (GERD). **Unlabeled:** Treatment of upper GI bleeding; prophylaxis of aspiration pneumonia, acute urticaria, chronic warts.

PRECAUTIONS

CONTRAINDICATIONS: None known. **CAUTIONS:** Impaired renal/hepatic function, elderly.

LIFESPAN CONSIDERATIONS: Pregnancy/lactation: Crosses placenta. Distributed in breast milk. In infants, may suppress gastric acidity, inhibit drug metabolism, produce CNS stimulation. **Pregnancy Category B. Children:** Long-term use may induce cerebral toxicity, affect hormonal system. **Elderly:** More likely to experience confusion, esp. in pts with impaired renal function.

INTERACTIONS

DRUG: Antacids may decrease absorption (do not give within ½–1 hr). May decrease absorption of **ketoconazole** (give at least 2 hrs after). May decrease metabolism, increase concentration of **oral anticoagulants, tricyclic antidepressants, oral hypoglycemics, metoprolol, metronidazole, phenytoin, propranolol, theophylline, calcium channel blockers, cyclosporine, lidocaine. HERBAL:** None known. **FOOD:** None known. **LAB VALUES:** Interferes with skin tests using allergen extracts. May increase creatinine, prolactin, transaminase. May decrease parathyroid hormone concentration.

AVAILABILITY (Rx)

TABLETS: 100 mg (OTC), 200 mg, 300 mg, 400 mg, 800 mg. **ORAL LIQUID:** 300 mg/5 ml. **INJECTION:** 300 mg/2 ml. **SUSPENSION:** 200 mg/5 ml.

ADMINISTRATION/HANDLING

PO

• Give without regard to meals. Best given with meals and at bedtime. • Do not administer within 1 hr of antacids.

IM

• Administer undiluted. • Inject deep into large muscle mass.

IV

Storage • Store at room temperature. • Reconstituted IV is stable for 48 hrs at room temperature.

Dilution • Dilute each 300 mg (2 ml) with 18 ml 0.9% NaCl, 0.45% NaCl, 0.2% NaCl, D_5W, $D_{10}W$, Ringer's solution, or lactated Ringer's to a total volume of 20 ml.

Rate of administration • For IV push, administer over not less than 2 min (prevents arrhythmias, hypotension). • For intermittent IV (piggyback) administration, infuse over 15–20 min. • For IV infusion, dilute with 100–1,000 ml 0.9% NaCl, D_5W, or other compatible solution (see Dilution) and infuse over 24 hrs.

IV INCOMPATIBILITIES

Allopurinol (Aloprim), amphotericin B complex (AmBisome, Amphotec, Abelcet), cefepime (Maxipime).

IV COMPATIBILITIES

Aminophylline, diltiazem (Cardizem), furosemide (Lasix), heparin, hydromorphone (Dilaudid), insulin (Regular), lidocaine, lorazepam (Ativan), midazolam (Versed), morphine, potassium chloride, propofol (Diprivan).

INDICATIONS/ROUTES/DOSAGE

ACTIVE ULCER

IM/IV: ADULTS, ELDERLY: 300 mg q6h or 150 mg as single dose followed by 37.5 mg/hr continuous infusion.

PO: 300 mg 4 times/day or 400 mg 2 times/day or 800 mg at bedtime.

PROPHYLAXIS DUODENAL ULCER

PO: ADULTS, ELDERLY: 400–800 mg at bedtime.

GASTRIC HYPERSECRETORY CONDITIONS

IM/IV/PO: ADULTS, ELDERLY: 300–600 mg q6h. **Maximum:** 2,400 mg/day.

C

GERD

PO: ADULTS, ELDERLY: 800 mg 2 times/day or 400 mg 4 times/day for 12 wks.

OTC USE

PO: ADULTS, ELDERLY: 100 mg up to 30 min before meals. **Maximum:** 2 doses/day.

PREVENTION OF UPPER GI BLEEDING

IV infusion: ADULTS, ELDERLY: 50 mg/hr.

USUAL DOSAGE FOR CHILDREN

IM/IV/PO: CHILDREN: 20–40 mg/kg/day in divided doses q6h. INFANTS: 10–20 mg/kg/day in divided doses q6–12h. NEONATES: 5–10 mg/kg/day in divided doses q8–12h.

DOSAGE IN RENAL IMPAIRMENT

Based on 300-mg dose in adults.

Creatinine Clearance	Dosage Interval
>40 ml/min	q6h
20–40 ml/min	q8h or decrease dose by 25%
<20 ml/min	q12h or decrease dose by 50%
Give after hemodialysis and q12h between dialysis periods	

SIDE EFFECTS

OCCASIONAL (2%–4%): Headache. **Elderly, severely ill, impaired renal function:** Confusion, agitation, psychosis, depression, anxiety, disorientation, hallucinations (effects reverse 3–4 days after discontinuance). **RARE (<2%):** Diarrhea, dizziness, drowsiness, headache, nausea, vomiting, gynecomastia, rash, impotence.

ADVERSE REACTIONS/ TOXIC EFFECTS

Rapid IV may produce cardiac arrhythmias, hypotension.

NURSING IMPLICATIONS

BASELINE ASSESSMENT

Do not administer antacids concurrently (separate by 1 hr).

INTERVENTION/EVALUATION

Monitor B/P for hypotension during IV infusion. Assess for GI bleeding: hematemesis, blood in stool. Check mental status in elderly, severely ill, those with impaired renal function.

PATIENT/FAMILY TEACHING

May produce transient discomfort at IM injection site. Do not take antacids within 1 hr of cimetidine administration. Avoid tasks that require alertness, motor skills until drug response is established. Avoid smoking. Report any blood in vomitus/stool, or dark, tarry stool.

ciprofloxacin hydrochloride

sip-row-**flocks**-ah-sin

(Ciloxan, Cipro)

Do not confuse with cinoxacin, Cytoxan.

FIXED-COMBINATION(S)

Cipro HC Otic: ciprofloxacin/hydrocortisone (a steroid): 0.2%/1%. **CiproDex Otic** ciprofloxacin/dexamethasone (a corticosteroid): 0.3%/0.1%.

CLASSIFICATION

PHARMACOTHERAPEUTIC: Fluoroquinolone. **CLINICAL:** Anti-infective (see p. 23C).

ACTION

Inhibits DNA enzyme in susceptible microorganisms. **Therapeutic Effect:**

Interferes with bacterial DNA replication. Bactericidal.

PHARMACOKINETICS

Well absorbed from GI tract (delayed by food). Protein binding: 20%–40%. Widely distributed (including CSF). Metabolized in liver to active metabolite. Primarily excreted in urine. Minimal removal by hemodialysis. **Half-life:** 4–6 hrs (half-life increased with impaired renal function, in elderly).

USES

Treatment of chronic bacterial prostatitis; skin/skin structure, GI tract, bone/joint, lower respiratory tract, urinary tract infections; infectious diarrhea; uncomplicated gonorrhea; empiric treatment of febrile neutropenia, acute sinusitis. **Ophthalmic:** Conjunctival keratitis, keratoconjunctivitis, corneal ulcers, blepharitis, dacryocystitis, blepharoconjunctivitis, acute meibomianitis. **Unlabeled:** Treatment of chancroid.

PRECAUTIONS

CONTRAINDICATIONS: Hypersensitivity to ciprofloxacin, quinolones. **Ophthalmic:** Vaccinia, varicella, epithelial herpes simplex, keratitis, mycobacterial infection, fungal disease of ocular structure. Not for use after uncomplicated removal of foreign body. **CAUTIONS:** Renal impairment, CNS disorders, seizures, those taking theophylline, caffeine. Suspension not for use in an NG tube.

LIFESPAN CONSIDERATIONS: Pregnancy/lactation: Unknown if distributed in breast milk. If possible, do not use during pregnancy/lactation (risk of arthropathy to fetus/infant). **Pregnancy Category C. Children:** Safety and efficacy not established in those <18 yrs. **Elderly:** Age-related renal impairment may require dosage adjustment.

INTERACTIONS

DRUG: Antacids, iron preparations, sucralfate may decrease absorption. Decreases clearance, may increase concentration, toxicity of **theophylline.** May increase effects of **oral anticoagulants. HERBAL:** None known. **FOOD:** None known. **LAB VALUES:** May increase SGOT (AST), SGPT (ALT), alkaline phosphatase, LDH, bilirubin, BUN, creatinine.

AVAILABILITY (Rx)

TABLETS: 100 mg, 250 mg, 500 mg, 750 mg. **TABLETS (extended-release):** 500 mg. **ORAL SUSPENSION.** 50 mg/ml, 100 mg/ml. **INJECTION:** 200 mg, 400 mg. **OPHTHALMIC SOLUTION:** 0.03%. **OPHTHALMIC OINTMENT:** 0.3%.

ADMINISTRATION/HANDLING

PO

• May be given without regard to meals (preferred dosing time: 2 hrs after meals). • Do not administer antacids (aluminum, magnesium) within 2 hrs of ciprofloxacin. • Encourage cranberry juice, citrus fruits (acidifies urine). • Suspension may be stored for 14 days at room temperature.

IV

Storage • Store at room temperature. • Solution appears clear, colorless to slightly yellow.

Reconstitution • Available prediluted in infusion container ready for use.

Rate of administration • Infuse over 60 min.

OPHTHALMIC

• Tilt pt's head back; place solution in conjunctival sac. • Have pt close eyes; press gently on lacrimal sac for 1 min. • Do not use ophthalmic solutions for injection. • Unless infection is very superficial, systemic administration generally accompanies ophthalmic use.

IV INCOMPATIBILITIES

Aminophylline, ampicillin/sulbactam (Unasyn), cefepime (Maxipime), dexamethasone (Decadron), furosemide (Lasix), heparin, hydrocortisone (Solu-Cortef), methylprednisolone (Solu-Medrol), phenytoin (Dilantin), sodium bicarbonate.

C

IV COMPATIBILITIES

Calcium gluconate, diltiazem (Cardizem), dobutamine (Dobutrex), dopamine (Intropin), lidocaine, lorazepam (Ativan), magnesium, midazolam (Versed), potassium chloride.

INDICATIONS/ROUTES/DOSAGE

MILD TO MODERATE URINARY TRACT INFECTIONS

PO: ADULTS, ELDERLY: 250 mg q12h.

IV: ADULTS, ELDERLY: 200 mg q12h.

COMPLICATED URINARY TRACT, MILD TO MODERATE RESPIRATORY TRACT, SKIN/SKIN STRUCTURE, BONES, JOINT INFECTIONS, INFECTIOUS DIARRHEA

PO: ADULTS, ELDERLY: 500 mg q12h.

IV: ADULTS, ELDERLY: 400 mg q12h.

SEVERE, COMPLICATED INFECTIONS

PO: ADULTS, ELDERLY: 750 mg q12h.

IV: ADULTS, ELDERLY: 400 mg q12h.

PROSTATITIS

PO: ADULTS, ELDERLY: 500 mg q12h for 28 days.

UNCOMPLICATED BLADDER INFECTIONS

PO: ADULTS: 100 mg 2 times/day for 3 days.

ACUTE SINUSITIS

PO: ADULTS: 500 mg q12h.

UNCOMPLICATED GONORRHEA

PO: ADULTS: 250 mg as single dose.

USUAL DOSAGE FOR CHILDREN

PO: 20–30 mg/kg/day in 2 divided doses. **Maximum:** 1.5 g/day.

IV: 20–30 mg/kg/day in 2 divided doses q12h. **Maximum:** 800 mg/day.

DOSAGE IN RENAL IMPAIRMENT

Dose and/or frequency is modified in pts based on severity of infection, degree of renal impairment.

Creatinine Clearance	Dosage Interval
<30 ml/min	q18–24h

Hemodialysis, peritoneal dialysis 250–500 mg q24h (after dialysis).

USUAL OPHTHALMIC DOSAGE

Corneal ulcer: ADULTS, ELDERLY: 2 drops q15min for 6 hrs, then 2 drops q30min for remainder of first day; 2 drops q1h for second day; then 2 drops q4h days 3–14.

Conjunctivitis: ADULTS, ELDERLY: 1–2 drops q2h for 2 days, then 2 drops q4h next 5 days.

SIDE EFFECTS

FREQUENT (2%–5%): Nausea, diarrhea, dyspepsia, vomiting, constipation, flatulence, confusion, crystalluria. **Ophthalmic:** Burning, crusting in corner of eye. **OCCASIONAL (<2%):** Abdominal pain/discomfort, headache, rash. **Ophthalmic:** Bad taste, sense of something in eye, redness of eyelids, eyelid itching. **RARE (<1%):** Dizziness, confusion, tremors, hallucinations, hypersensitivity reaction, insomnia, dry mouth, paresthesia.

ADVERSE REACTIONS/ TOXIC EFFECTS

Superinfection (esp. enterococcal, fungal), nephropathy, cardiopulmonary arrest, cerebral thrombosis may occur. Arthropathy may occur if given to children <18 yrs. **Ophthalmic:** Sensitization may contraindicate later systemic use of ciprofloxacin.

NURSING IMPLICATIONS

BASELINE ASSESSMENT

Question for history of hypersensitivity to ciprofloxacin, quinolones.

INTERVENTION/EVALUATION

Evaluate food tolerance. Determine pattern of bowel activity. Check for dizziness, headache, visual difficulties, tremors. Assess for chest, joint pain. **Ophthalmic:** Observe therapeutic response.

PATIENT/FAMILY TEACHING

Do not skip doses; take full course of therapy. Take with 8 oz water; drink several glasses of water between meals. Eat/drink high sources of ascorbic acid (cranberry juice, citrus fruits) to prevent crystalluria. Do not take antacids (reduces/destroys effectiveness). Shake suspension well before using; do not chew microcapsules in suspension. Sugarless gum/hard candy may relieve bad taste. **Ophthalmic:** Explain possibility of crystal precipitate forming, usual resolution in 1–7 days.

cisatracurium

(Nimbex)

See Classification section under: Neuromuscular blockers (p. 106C)

cisplatin

sis-**plah**-tin

(Platinol-AQ)

Do not confuse with carboplatin, Paraplatin, Patanol.

◆CLASSIFICATION

PHARMACOTHERAPEUTIC: Platinum coordination complex. **CLINICAL:** Antineoplastic (see p. 70C).

ACTION

Inhibits DNA and, to lesser extent, RNA, protein synthesis by cross-linking with DNA strands. Cell cycle–phase nonspecific. **Therapeutic Effect:** Prevents cellular division.

PHARMACOKINETICS

Widely distributed. Protein binding: >90%. Undergoes rapid nonenzymatic conversion to inactive metabolite. Excreted in urine. Removed by hemodialysis. **Half-life:** 58–73 hrs (half-life increased with impaired renal function).

USES

Treatment of metastatic testicular tumors, metastatic ovarian tumors, advanced bladder carcinoma. **Unlabeled:** Treatment of carcinoma of breast, cervical, endometrial, gastric, lung, prostate, head/neck, neuroblastoma, germ cell tumors, osteosarcoma.

PRECAUTIONS

CONTRAINDICATIONS: Myelosuppression, hearing impairment, pregnancy. **CAUTIONS:** Previous therapy with other antineoplastic agents, radiation.

LIFESPAN CONSIDERATIONS: Pregnancy/lactation: If possible, avoid use during pregnancy, esp. first trimester. Breast-feeding not recommended. **Pregnancy Category D. Children:** Ototoxic effects may be more severe. **Elderly:** Age-related renal impairment may require dosage adjustment.

INTERACTIONS

DRUG: May decrease effect of **antigout medications. Bone marrow depressants** may increase bone marrow depression. **Nephrotoxic, ototoxic agents** may increase toxicity. **Live virus vaccines** may potentiate virus replication, increase vaccine side effects, decrease pt's antibody response to vaccine. **HERBAL:** None known. **FOOD:** None known. **LAB VALUES:** May cause posi-

C

tive Coombs' test. May increase BUN, creatinine, uric acid, SGOT (AST). May decrease creatinine clearance, calcium, magnesium, phosphate, potassium, sodium.

AVAILABILITY (Rx)

INJECTION: 50-mg, 100-mg vials.

ADMINISTRATION/HANDLING

Alert: Wear protective gloves during handling of cisplatin. May be carcinogenic, mutagenic, or teratogenic. Handle with extreme care during preparation/administration.

IV

Storage • Following reconstitution, solution should appear clear, colorless. • Protect from direct sunlight; do not refrigerate (may precipitate). • Discard if precipitate forms. • Stable for 20 hrs at room temperature.

Reconstitution • Reconstitute 10-mg vial with 10 ml Sterile Water for Injection (50 ml for 50-mg vial) to provide concentration of 1 mg/ml. • For IV infusion, dilute desired dose in up to 1,000 ml D_5W, 0.33% or 0.45% NaCl containing 12.5–50 g mannitol/L.

Rate of administration • Infuse over 2–24 hrs. • Avoid rapid infusion (increases risk of nephrotoxicity, ototoxicity). • Monitor for anaphylactic reaction during first few minutes of IV infusion.

IV INCOMPATIBILITIES

Amifostine (Ethyol), amphotericin B complex (AmBisome, Amphotec, Abelcet), cefepime (Maxipime), piperacillin/tazobactam (Zosyn), thiotepa.

IV COMPATIBILITIES

Etoposide (VePesid), granisetron (Kytril), heparin, hydromorphone (Dilaudid), lorazepam (Ativan), magnesium sulfate, mannitol, morphine, ondansetron (Zofran).

INDICATIONS/ROUTES/DOSAGE

Alert: Verify any cisplatin dose exceeding 120 mg/m^2 per course. Dosage individualized based on clinical response, tolerance to adverse effects. When used in combination therapy, consult specific protocols for optimum dosage, sequence of drug administration. Repeat courses should not be given more frequently than q3–4wks. Do not repeat unless auditory acuity within normal limits, serum creatinine <1.5 mg/dl, BUN <25 mg/dl, circulating blood elements (platelets, WBC) are within acceptable levels.

INTERMITTENT DOSAGE SCHEDULE

IV: ADULTS, ELDERLY, CHILDREN: 37–75 mg/m^2 once every 2–3 wks or 50–100 mg/m^2 over 4–8 hrs once every 21–28 days.

DAILY DOSAGE SCHEDULE

IV: ADULTS, ELDERLY, CHILDREN: 15–20 mg/m^2/day for 5 days every 3–4 wks.

DOSAGE IN RENAL IMPAIRMENT

Creatinine Clearance	% of Dose
10–50 ml/min	75%
<10 ml/min	50%

SIDE EFFECTS

FREQUENT: Nausea, vomiting (begins 1–4 hrs after administration, generally last up to 24 hrs). Myelosuppression occurs in 25%–30% of pts. Recovery can generally be expected in 18–23 days. **OCCASIONAL:** Peripheral neuropathy (numbness, tingling of fingers, toes, face) may occur with prolonged therapy (4–7 mos), pain/redness at injection site, loss of taste/appetite. **RARE:** Hemolytic anemia, blurred vision, stomatitis.

ADVERSE REACTIONS/ TOXIC EFFECTS

Anaphylactic reaction (facial edema, wheezing, tachycardia, hypotension) may occur in first few minutes of IV administration in those previously exposed to cisplatin. Nephrotoxicity in 28%–36% of pts treated with single dose of cisplatin, usually during second week of therapy. Ototoxicity (tinnitus, hearing loss) in 31% of pts treated with single dose of cisplatin (more severe in children). May become more frequent, severe with repeated doses.

NURSING IMPLICATIONS

BASELINE ASSESSMENT

Pts should be well hydrated prior to and 24 hrs after medication to ensure good urinary output, decrease risk of nephrotoxicity.

INTERVENTION/EVALUATION

Measure all vomitus (general guideline requiring immediate notification of physician: 750 ml/8 hrs, urinary output <100 ml/hr). Monitor I&O q1–2h beginning with pretreatment hydration, continue for 48 hrs after cisplatin therapy. Assess vital signs q1–2h during infusion. Monitor urinalysis, renal function reports for nephrotoxicity.

PATIENT/FAMILY TEACHING

Report signs of ototoxicity (ringing/roaring in ears, hearing loss). Do not have immunizations without physician's approval (lowers body's resistance). Avoid contact with those who have recently taken oral polio vaccine. Contact physician if nausea/vomiting continues at home. Teach signs of peripheral neuropathy.

citalopram hydrobromide

sigh-**tail**-oh-pram high-dro-**broh**-mide

(Celexa)

Do not confuse with Celebrex, Cerebyx, Zyprexa.

CLASSIFICATION

PHARMACOTHERAPEUTIC: Serotonin reuptake inhibitor. **CLINICAL:** Antidepressant (see p. 35C).

ACTION

Blocks uptake of the neurotransmitter serotonin at CNS neuronal presynaptic membranes, increasing availability at postsynaptic receptor sites. **Therapeutic Effect:** Enhances postsynaptic activity, producing antidepressant effect.

PHARMACOKINETICS

Well absorbed after PO administration. Protein binding: 80%. Primarily metabolized in the liver. Primarily excreted in the feces with a lesser amount eliminated in the urine. **Half-life:** 35 hrs.

USES

Treatment of depression. **Unlabeled:** Treatment of dementia, smoking cessation, alcohol abuse, obsessive-compulsive disorder, diabetic neuropathy.

PRECAUTIONS

CONTRAINDICATIONS: Sensitivity to citalopram, concurrent use of MAOIs. **CAUTIONS:** Liver/renal impairment, history of seizures, mania, hypomania.

LIFESPAN CONSIDERATIONS: Pregnancy/lactation: Distributed in breast milk. **Pregnancy Category C. Children:** May cause increased anticholinergic effects, hyperexcitability. **Elderly:** More sensitive to anticholinergic effects (e.g., dry mouth), more likely to experience dizziness, sedation, confusion, hypotension, hyperexcitability.

INTERACTIONS

DRUG: MAOIs may cause serotonergic syndrome (excitement, diaphoresis, rigidity, hyperthermia, autonomic hyperactivity, coma). **Antifungals, macrolide antibiotics, cimetidine** may increase plasma levels; **carbamazepine** may decrease plasma levels. Increases **metoprolol** plasma levels. **HERBAL:** None known. **FOOD:** None known. **LAB VALUES:** May reduce serum sodium.

C

AVAILABILITY (Rx)

TABLETS: 10 mg, 20 mg, 40 mg. **ORAL SOLUTION:** 10 mg/5 ml.

ADMINISTRATION/HANDLING

PO

• Give without regard to food. • Scored tablets may be crushed.

INDICATIONS/ROUTES/DOSAGE

ANTIDEPRESSANT

PO: ADULTS: Initially, 20 mg once daily in the morning or evening. Dosage may be increased in 20-mg increments at intervals of no less than 1 wk. **Maximum:** 60 mg/day. ELDERLY, IMPAIRED HEPATIC FUNCTION: 20 mg/day. May titrate to 40 mg/day only for nonresponding pts.

SIDE EFFECTS

FREQUENT (11%–21%): Nausea, dry mouth, somnolence, insomnia, excessive sweating. **OCCASIONAL (4%–8%):** Tremor, diarrhea/loose stools, abnormal ejaculation, dyspepsia, fatigue, anxiety, vomiting, anorexia. **RARE (2%–3%):** Sinusitis, sexual dysfunction, menstrual disorder, abdominal pain, agitation, decreased libido.

ADVERSE REACTIONS/ TOXIC EFFECTS

Overdosage manifested as dizziness, drowsiness, tachycardia, severe somnolence, confusion, seizures.

NURSING IMPLICATIONS

BASELINE ASSESSMENT

Liver/renal function tests, blood counts should be performed periodically for pts on long-term therapy. Observe/record behavior. Assess psychological status, thought content, sleep pattern, appearance, interest in environment.

INTERVENTION/EVALUATION

Closely supervise suicidal-risk pt during early therapy (as energy level improves, suicide potential increases). Assess appearance, behavior, speech pattern, level of interest, mood.

PATIENT/FAMILY TEACHING

Do not stop taking medication or increase dosage. Avoid alcohol. Avoid tasks that require alertness, motor skills until response to drug is established.

citrates

(Bicitra, Oracit, Polycitra, Urocit-K)

◆CLASSIFICATION

CLINICAL: Alkalinizer.

ACTION

Increases urinary pH, increasing solubility of cystine in urine and ionization of uric acid to urate ion. Increasing urinary pH and urinary citrate decrease calcium ion activity, saturation of calcium oxalate. Increases plasma bicarbonate, buffers excess hydrogen ion concentration. **Therapeutic Effect:** Increases blood pH, reverses acidosis.

USES

Treatment of metabolic acidosis.

CONTRAINDICATIONS: Hypersensitivity to citrate, those with sodium-restricted diet, severe renal impairment, azotemia, anuria, untreated Addison's disease, acute dehydration, heat cramps, severe myocardial damage. **Urocit-K:** Those with delayed gastric emptying, intestinal obstruction/stricture, anticholinergics, severe peptic ulcer disease. **CAU-**

TIONS: Those with CHF, hypertension, pulmonary edema. May increase risk of urolithiasis. **Pregnancy Category:** Not expected to cause fetal harm.

INTERACTIONS

DRUG: May increase **quinidine** excretion. **Antacids** may increase risk of systemic alkalosis. **NSAIDs, angiotensin-converting enzyme inhibitors, potassium-sparing diuretics, potassium-containing medication** may increase risk of hyperkalemia. May decrease effect of **methenamine.** **HERBAL:** None known. **FOOD:** None known. **LAB VALUES:** None known.

AVAILABILITY (Rx)

TABLETS: 5 mEq, 10 mEq. **SYRUP. ORAL SOLUTION.**

INDICATIONS/ROUTES/DOSAGE

USUAL DOSAGE

PO: ADULTS, ELDERLY: 15–30 ml after meals and at bedtime. Urocit-K: 30–60 mEq/day in 3–4 divided doses. CHILDREN: 5–15 ml after meals and at bedtime or 2–3 mEq/kg/day in 3–4 divided doses.

SIDE EFFECTS

OCCASIONAL: Diarrhea, mild abdominal pain, nausea, vomiting.

ADVERSE REACTIONS/ TOXIC EFFECTS

Metabolic alkalosis, bowel obstruction/perforation, hyperkalemia, hypernatremia occur rarely.

NURSING IMPLICATIONS

INTERVENTION/EVALUATION

Assess urinary pH, EKG in pts with cardiac disease, serum acid–base balance, CBC, Hgb, Hct, serum creatinine.

PATIENT/FAMILY TEACHING

Take after meals. Mix in water or juice; follow with additional liquid if desired.

cladribine

clad-rih-bean
(Leustatin)
Do not confuse with lovastatin.

◆CLASSIFICATION

PHARMACOTHERAPEUTIC: Antimetabolite. **CLINICAL:** Antineoplastic (see p. 70C).

ACTION

Disrupts cellular metabolism by incorporating into DNA of dividing cells. Cytotoxic to both actively dividing and quiescent lymphocytes, monocytes. **Therapeutic Effect:** Prevents DNA synthesis.

PHARMACOKINETICS

Primarily excreted in urine. **Half-life:** 5.4 hrs.

USES

Treatment for active hairy cell leukemia defined by clinically significant anemia, neutropenia, thrombocytopenia. **Unlabeled:** Chronic lymphocytic leukemia, non-Hodgkin's lymphoma, acute myeloid leukemia, autoimmune hemolytic anemia.

PRECAUTIONS

CONTRAINDICATIONS: None known. **CAUTIONS:** Renal/hepatic impairment, bone marrow suppression. **Pregnancy Category D.**

LIFESPAN CONSIDERATIONS: Pregnancy/lactation: May produce fetal harm; may be embryotoxic and fetotoxic; potential for serious reactions in nursing infants. **Pregnancy Category D.** **Children:** Safety and efficacy not established. **Elderly:** No age-related precautions noted.

C

INTERACTIONS

DRUG: Bone marrow depressants may increase bone marrow depression. High dosages with **cyclophosphamide** and total body irradiation may cause severe, irreversible neurologic toxicity, acute renal dysfunction. **Nephrotoxic, neurotoxic medications** may increase toxicity. **Live virus vaccines** may potentiate virus replication, increase vaccine side effects, decrease pt's antibody response to vaccine. **HERBAL:** None known. **FOOD:** None known. **LAB VALUES:** None known.

AVAILABILITY (Rx)

INJECTION: 1 mg/ml.

ADMINISTRATION/HANDLING

IV

Storage • Refrigerate unopened vials. • May refrigerate dilution solution for no more than 8 hrs before administration. • Solution is stable for at least 24 hrs at room temperature. • Discard unused portion.

Reconstitution • Must dilute before administration. • Wear gloves, protective clothing during handling; if contact with skin, rinse with copious amounts of water. • Add calculated dose (0.09 mg/kg) to 500 ml 0.9% NaCl. Avoid D_5W (increases degradation of medication).

Rate of administration • Monitor vital signs during infusion, esp. during first hour. Observe for hypotension, bradycardia (usually both do not occur during same course). • Immediately discontinue administration if severe hypersensitivity reaction occurs.

IV INCOMPATIBILITIES

Do not mix with other IV drugs/additives or infuse concurrently via a common IV line.

INDICATIONS/ROUTES/DOSAGE

HAIRY CELL LEUKEMIA

IV infusion: ADULTS, CHILDREN: 0.09 mg/kg/day as continuous infusion for 7 days.

CHRONIC LYMPHOCYTIC LEUKEMIA

IV infusion: ADULTS, ELDERLY: 0.1 mg/kg/day days 1–7.

CHRONIC MYELOGENOUS LEUKEMIA

IV infusion: ADULTS, ELDERLY: 15 mg/m^2/day days 1–5. Give as a 1 hr infusion.

SIDE EFFECTS

FREQUENT: Fever (69%), fatigue (45%), nausea (28%), rash (27%), headache (22%), injection site reactions (19%), anorexia (17%), vomiting (13%). **OCCASIONAL (5%–10%):** Diarrhea, cough, purpura, chills, diaphoresis, constipation, dizziness, petechiae, myalgia, shortness of breath, malaise, pruritus, erythema, insomnia, edema, tachycardia, abdominal/trunk pain, epistaxis, arthralgia.

ADVERSE REACTIONS/ TOXIC EFFECTS

Myelosuppression characterized as severe neutropenia (<500 cells/mm^3); severe anemia (Hgb <8.5 g/dl), thrombocytopenia occur commonly. High-dose treatment may produce acute nephrotoxicity (increased serum BUN, creatinine levels) and/or neurotoxicity (irreversible motor weakness of upper or lower extremities).

NURSING IMPLICATIONS

BASELINE ASSESSMENT

Offer emotional support to pt, family. Perform neurologic function tests before chemotherapy. Use strict asepsis; protect pt from infection.

INTERVENTION/EVALUATION

Monitor temperature, report fever promptly. Assess for signs of infection.

Assess skin for evidence of rash, purpura, petechiae. Monitor Hgb, Hct, BUN, creatinine, platelet count, WBC, potassium, sodium.

PATIENT/FAMILY TEACHING

Narrow margin between therapeutic and toxic response. Avoid crowds, persons with known infections; report signs of infection at once (fever, flulike symptoms). Do not have immunizations without physician's approval (drug lowers body's resistance). Avoid contact with those who have recently received live virus vaccine. Women of childbearing potential should not become pregnant during treatment.

Clarinex

see desloratidine

clarithromycin

clair-**rith**-row-my-sin
(Biaxin, Biaxin XL)

CLASSIFICATION

PHARMACOTHERAPEUTIC: Macrolide. **CLINICAL:** Antibiotic (see p. 24C).

ACTION

Bacteriostatic. Binds to ribosomal receptor sites. May be bactericidal with high dosage or very susceptible microorganisms. **Therapeutic Effect:** Inhibits protein synthesis of bacterial cell wall.

PHARMACOKINETICS

Well absorbed from GI tract. Protein binding: 65%–75%. Widely distributed. Metabolized in liver to active metabolite. Primarily excreted in urine. Not removed by hemodialysis. **Half-life:** 3–7 hrs; metabolite: 5–7 hrs (half-life increased with impaired renal function).

USES

Treatment of bacterial exacerbation of bronchitis, otitis media, acute maxillary sinusitis, *Mycobacterium avium* complex (MAC), pharyngitis, tonsillitis, *H. pylori* duodenal ulcer, bacterial pneumonia, skin/soft tissue infections. Prevention of MAC disease. **Biaxin XL:** Treatment of community-acquired pneumonia.

PRECAUTIONS

CONTRAINDICATIONS: Hypersensitivity to clarithromycin, erythromycins, any macrolide antibiotic. **CAUTIONS:** Hepatic/renal dysfunction, elderly with severe renal impairment.

LIFESPAN CONSIDERATIONS: Pregnancy/lactation: Unknown if distributed in breast milk. **Pregnancy Category C. Children:** Safety and efficacy not established in those <6 mos. **Elderly:** Age-related renal impairment may require dosage adjustment.

INTERACTIONS

DRUG: May increase concentration, toxicity of **carbamazepine, digoxin, theophylline.** May decrease concentration of **zidovudine.** May increase **warfarin** effects. **Rifampin** may decrease clarithromycin concentrations. **HERBAL:** None known. **FOOD:** None known. **LAB VALUES:** May rarely increase SGOT (AST), SGPT (ALT), BUN.

AVAILABILITY (Rx)

TABLETS: 250 mg, 500 mg. **TABLETS (extended-release):** 500 mg. **ORAL SUSPENSION:** 125 mg/5 ml.

ADMINISTRATION/HANDLING

PO

- Give without regard to food.
- Do not crush/break tablets.

INDICATIONS/ROUTES/DOSAGE

USUAL ADULT, ELDERLY DOSAGE

PO: Immediate-release: 250–500 mg q12h for 7–14 days. **Extended-release:** Two 500-mg tablets daily for 7–14 days.

ACUTE OTITIS MEDIA

PO: CHILDREN: 15 mg/kg/day in 2 divided doses for 10 days.

RESPIRATORY, SKIN/SKIN STRUCTURE INFECTIONS

PO: CHILDREN: 15 mg/kg/day in 2 divided doses for 7–14 days.

DOSAGE IN RENAL IMPAIRMENT

Creatinine clearance <30 ml/min: Reduce dose by 50% and administer once or twice daily.

SIDE EFFECTS

OCCASIONAL (3%–6%): Diarrhea, nausea, altered taste, abdominal pain. **RARE (1%–2%):** Headache, dyspepsia.

ADVERSE REACTIONS/ TOXIC EFFECTS

Antibiotic-associated colitis (severe abdominal pain, tenderness; fever; watery, severe diarrhea), other superinfections may result from altered bacterial balance. Hepatotoxicity, thrombocytopenia occur rarely.

NURSING IMPLICATIONS

BASELINE ASSESSMENT

Question pt for history of hepatitis, allergies to clarithromycin, erythromycins.

INTERVENTION/EVALUATION

Monitor bowel activity/stool consistency carefully; mild GI effects may be tolerable, but increasing severity may indicate onset of antibiotic-associated colitis. Be alert for superinfection: genital/anal pruritus, abdominal pain, mouth soreness, moderate to severe diarrhea.

PATIENT/FAMILY TEACHING

Continue therapy for full length of treatment. Doses should be evenly spaced. Take medication with 8 oz water without regard to food.

Claritin

see loratidine

clemastine fumarate

kleh-**mass**-teen

(Dayhist-1, Tavist, Tavist-1)

◆ CLASSIFICATION

PHARMACOTHERAPEUTIC: Ethanolamine. **CLINICAL:** Antihistamine (see p. 48C).

ACTION

Competes with histamine on effector cells in the GI tract, blood vessels, respiratory tract. **Therapeutic Effect:** Relieves allergic conditions (urticaria, pruritus). Anticholinergic effects cause drying of nasal mucosa.

PHARMACOKINETICS

Onset	Peak	Duration
PO		
15–60 min	5–7 hrs	10–12 hrs

Well absorbed from GI tract. Metabolized in liver. Excreted primarily in urine.

USES

Relief of allergic conditions (nasal allergies, allergic dermatitis), cold symptoms, hypersensitivity reaction.

PRECAUTIONS

CONTRAINDICATIONS: Hypersensitivity to clemastine, narrow-angle glaucoma, those receiving MAOIs. **CAUTIONS:** Peptic ulcer, GI/GU obstruction, asthma, prostatic hypertrophy.

LIFESPAN CONSIDERATIONS: Pregnancy/lactation: Excreted in breast milk. **Pregnancy Category B. Children:** Safety and efficacy not established in those <6 yrs. **Elderly:** Age-related renal impairment may require dosage adjustment.

INTERACTIONS

DRUG: Alcohol, CNS depressants may increase CNS depressant effects. **MAOIs** may increase anticholinergic, CNS depressant effects. **HERBAL:** None known. **FOOD:** None known. **LAB VALUES:** May suppress wheal, flare reactions to antigen skin testing, unless antihistamines discontinued 4 days prior to testing.

AVAILABILITY (Rx)

TABLETS: 1.34 mg, 2.68 mg. **ELIXIR:** 0.5 mg/5 ml. **SYRUP:** 0.5 mg/5 ml, 0.67 mg/5 ml.

ADMINISTRATION/HANDLING

PO

- Give without regard to meals.
- Scored tablets may be crushed. Do not crush extended-release or film-coated forms.

INDICATIONS/ROUTES/DOSAGE

ALLERGIC RHINITIS

PO: ADULTS, CHILDREN >12 YRS: 1.34–2.68 mg 3 times/day. **Maximum:** 8.04 mg/day. CHILDREN 6–12 YRS: 0.67–1.34 mg 2 times/day. **Maximum.** 4.02 mg/day. CHILDREN <6 YRS: 0.335–0.67 mg/day in 2–3 divided doses. **Maximum:** 1.34 mg.

ALLERGIC URTICARIA, ANGIOEDEMA

PO: ADULTS, CHILDREN >12 YRS: 2.68 mg 1–3 times/day. Do not exceed 8.04 mg/day. CHILDREN 6–11 YRS: 1.34 mg 2 times/day. Do not exceed 4.02 mg/day.

USUAL ELDERLY DOSAGE

PO: 1.34 mg 1–2 times/day.

SIDE EFFECTS

Alert: Fixed-combination form (Tavist-D) may produce mild CNS stimulation.

FREQUENT: Drowsiness, dizziness, dry mouth/nose/throat, urinary retention, thickening of bronchial secretions. **Elderly:** Sedation, dizziness, hypotension. **OCCASIONAL:** Epigastric distress, flushing, blurred vision, tinnitus, paresthesia, sweating, chills.

ADVERSE REACTIONS/ TOXIC EFFECTS

Children may experience dominant paradoxical reaction (restlessness, insomnia, euphoria, nervousness, tremors). Overdosage in children may result in hallucinations, convulsions, death. Hypersensitivity reaction (eczema, pruritus, rash, cardiac disturbances, angioedema, photosensitivity) may occur. Overdosage may vary from CNS depression (sedation, apnea, cardiovascular collapse, death) to severe paradoxical reaction (hallucinations, tremor, seizures).

NURSING IMPLICATIONS

BASELINE ASSESSMENT

If pt is experiencing allergic reaction, obtain history of recently ingested foods, drugs, environmental exposure, recent emotional stress. Monitor rate, depth, rhythm, type of respiration; quality/rate of pulse. Assess lung sounds for rhonchi, wheezing, rales.

INTERVENTION/EVALUATION

Monitor B/P, esp. in elderly (increased risk of hypotension). Monitor children closely for paradoxical reaction.

C

PATIENT/FAMILY TEACHING

Tolerance to antihistaminic effect generally does not occur; tolerance to sedative effect may occur. Avoid tasks that require alertness, motor skills until response to drug is established. Dry mouth, drowsiness, dizziness may be an expected response of drug. Avoid alcoholic beverages during antihistamine therapy. Coffee, tea may help reduce drowsiness.

Climara

see estradiol

clindamycin

klin-da-**my**-sin
(Cleocin, Dalacin)

CLASSIFICATION

PHARMACOTHERAPEUTIC: Lincosamide. **CLINICAL:** Antibiotic.

ACTION

Bacteriostatic. Binds to bacterial ribosomal receptor sites. Topically, decreases fatty acid concentration on skin. **Therapeutic Effect:** Inhibits protein synthesis of bacterial cell wall. Prevents outbreak of acne vulgaris.

PHARMACOKINETICS

Rapidly absorbed from GI tract. Protein binding: 92%–94%. Widely distributed. Metabolized in liver to some active metabolites. Primarily excreted in urine. Not removed by hemodialysis. **Half-life:** 2.4–3 hrs (half-life increased with impaired renal function, in premature infants).

USES

Treatment of respiratory tract, skin/soft tissue, chronic bone/joint infections; septicemia; intra-abdominal, female GU infections; bacterial vaginosis; endocarditis. **Topical:** Acne vulgaris. **Unlabeled:** Treatment of malaria, otitis media, *Pneumocystis carinii* pneumonia (PCP), toxoplasmosis.

PRECAUTIONS

CONTRAINDICATIONS: Hypersensitivity to clindamycin, lincomycin; known allergy to tartrazine dye; history of ulcerative colitis, regional enteritis, antibiotic-associated colitis. **CAUTIONS:** Severe renal/hepatic dysfunction, concomitant use of neuromuscular blocking agents, neonates. Topical preparations should not be applied to abraded areas or near eyes.

LIFESPAN CONSIDERATIONS: Pregnancy/lactation: Readily crosses placenta. Distributed in breast milk. **Pregnancy Category B. Topical/vaginal:** Unknown if distributed in breast milk. **Children:** Caution in those <1 mo. **Elderly:** No age-related precautions noted.

INTERACTIONS

DRUG: Adsorbent antidiarrheals may delay absorption. **Chloramphenicol, erythromycin** may antagonize effects. May increase effect of **neuromuscular blockers. HERBAL:** None known. **FOOD:** None known. **LAB VALUES:** May increase SGOT (AST), SGPT (ALT), alkaline phosphatase.

AVAILABILITY (Rx)

CAPSULES: 75 mg, 150 mg, 300 mg. **ORAL SOLUTION:** 75 mg/5 ml. **INJECTION:** 150 mg/ml. **VAGINAL CREAM:** 2%. **VAGINAL SUPPOSITORY. LOTION. TOPICAL SOLUTION.**

ADMINISTRATION/HANDLING

PO

• Store capsules at room temperature. • After reconstitution, oral solution is stable for 2 wks at room temperature. • Do not refrigerate oral solution (avoids thickening). • Give with 8 oz water. May give without regard to food.

IM

• Do not exceed 600 mg/dose. • Administer deep IM.

IV

Storage • IV infusion (piggyback) is stable for 16 days at room temperature.

Reconstitution • Dilute 300–600 mg with 50 ml D_5W or 0.9% NaCl (900–1,200 mg with 100 ml). • Never exceed concentration of 18 mg/ml.

Rate of administration • 50 ml (300–600 mg) piggyback is infused >10–20 min; 100 ml (900 mg–1.2 g) piggyback is infused >30–40 min. Severe hypotension/cardiac arrest can occur with too rapid administration. • No more than 1.2 g should be given in a single infusion.

IV INCOMPATIBILITIES

Allopurinol (Aloprim), filgrastim (Neupogen), fluconazole (Diflucan), idarubicin (Idamycin).

IV COMPATIBILITIES

Amiodarone (Cordarone), diltiazem (Cardizem), heparin, hydromorphone (Dilaudid), magnesium sulfate, midazolam (Versed), morphine, multivitamins, propofol (Diprivan).

INDICATIONS/ROUTES/DOSAGE

IV/IM: ADULTS, ELDERLY: 1.2–1.8 g/day in 2–4 divided doses. CHILDREN: 25–40 mg/kg/day in 3–4 divided doses. **Maximum:** 4.8 g/day.

PO: ADULTS, ELDERLY: 150–450 mg/dose q6–8h. CHILDREN: 10–30 mg/kg/day in 3–4 divided doses. **Maximum:** 1.8 g/day.

BACTERIAL VAGINOSIS

Intravaginal: ADULTS: One applicatorful at bedtime for 3–7 days or 1 suppository at bedtime for 3 days.

PO: ADULTS, ELDERLY: 300 mg 2 times/day for 7 days.

ACNE VULGARIS

Topical: ADULTS: Apply thin layer 2 times/day to affected area.

SIDE EFFECTS

FREQUENT: Abdominal pain, nausea, vomiting, diarrhea. **Vaginal:** Vaginitis, itching. **Topical:** Dry scaly skin. **OCCASIONAL:** Phlebitis, thrombophlebitis with IV administration; pain, induration at IM injection site; allergic reaction, urticaria, pruritus. **Vaginal:** Headache, dizziness, nausea, vomiting, abdominal pain. **Topical:** Contact dermatitis, abdominal pain, mild diarrhea, stinging/burning. **RARE: Vaginal:** Hypersensitivity reaction.

ADVERSE REACTIONS/ TOXIC EFFECTS

Antibiotic-associated colitis (severe abdominal pain, tenderness; fever; watery, severe diarrhea), during and several weeks after therapy (including topical), may occur. Blood dyscrasias (leukopenia, thrombocytopenia), nephrotoxicity (proteinuria, azotemia, oliguria) occur rarely.

NURSING IMPLICATIONS

BASELINE ASSESSMENT

Question pt for history of allergies, particularly to clindamycin, lincomycin, aspirin. Avoid, if possible, concurrent use of neuromuscular blocking agents.

INTERVENTION/EVALUATION

Monitor bowel activity, stool consistency; report diarrhea promptly due to potential for serious colitis (even with topical or vaginal). Assess skin for rash (dryness, irritation) with topical application. With all routes of administration, assess for superinfection: severe

C

diarrhea, genital/anal pruritus, increased fever, change of oral mucosa.

PATIENT/FAMILY TEACHING

Continue therapy for full length of treatment. Doses should be evenly spaced. Take oral doses with 8 oz water. Caution should be used when applying topical clindamycin concurrently with peeling/abrasive acne agents, soaps, alcohol-containing cosmetics to avoid cumulative effect. Do not apply topical preparations near eyes, abraded areas. **Vaginal:** In event of accidental contact with eyes, rinse with copious amounts of cool tap water. Do not engage in sexual intercourse during treatment.

clobetasol

(Temovate)

See Classification section under: Corticosteroids: topical (p. 84C)

clomipramine hydrochloride

klow-**mih**-prah-meen

(Anafranil, Apo-Clomipramine🍁, Novo-Clopamine🍁)

Do not confuse with alfentanil, chlorpromazine, clomiphene, enalapril, nafarelin.

◆ CLASSIFICATION

PHARMACOTHERAPEUTIC: Tricyclic. **CLINICAL:** Antidepressant (see p. 34C).

ACTION

Blocks reuptake of neurotransmitters (norepinephrine, serotonin) at CNS presynaptic membranes, increasing availability at postsynaptic receptor sites. **Therapeutic Effect:** Reduces obsessive-compulsive behavior. Possesses strong anticholinergic activity.

USES

Treatment of obsessive-compulsive disorder manifested as repetitive tasks producing marked distress, time-consuming, or significant interference with social or occupational behavior. **Unlabeled:** Treatment of mental depression, panic disorder, neurogenic pain, cataplexy associated with narcolepsy, bulimia.

PRECAUTIONS

CONTRAINDICATIONS: Acute recovery period following MI, within 14 days of MAOI ingestion. **CAUTIONS:** Prostatic hypertrophy, history of urinary retention/obstruction, glaucoma, diabetes mellitus, seizures, hyperthyroidism, cardiac/hepatic/renal disease, schizophrenia, increased intraocular pressure, hiatal hernia. **Pregnancy Category C.**

INTERACTIONS

DRUG: **Alcohol, CNS depressants** may increase CNS, respiratory depression, hypotensive effects. **Antithyroid agents** may increase risk of agranulocytosis. **Phenothiazines** may increase sedative, anticholinergic effects. **Cimetidine** may increase concentration, toxicity. May decrease effects of **clonidine, guanadrel.** May increase cardiac effects with **sympathomimetics.** May increase risk of hypertensive crisis, hyperpyretic, convulsions with **MAOIs.** **HERBAL:** None known. **FOOD:** None known. **LAB VALUES:** May alter EKG readings, glucose.

AVAILABILITY (Rx)

CAPSULES: 25 mg, 50 mg, 75 mg.

INDICATIONS/ROUTES/DOSAGE

OBSESSIVE-COMPULSIVE DISORDER

PO: ADULTS, ELDERLY: Initially, 25 mg/

day. May gradually increase to 100 mg/day in the first 2 wks. **Maximum:** 250 mg/day. CHILDREN ≥10 YRS: Initially, 25 mg/day. May gradually increase up to maximum of 200 mg/day.

SIDE EFFECTS

FREQUENT: Drowsiness, fatigue, dry mouth, blurred vision, constipation, sexual dysfunction (42%), ejaculatory failure (20%), impotence; weight gain (18%), delayed micturition, postural hypotension, excessive sweating, disturbed concentration, increased appetite, urinary retention. **OCCASIONAL:** GI disturbances (nausea, GI distress, metallic taste), asthenia, aggressiveness, muscle weakness. **RARE:** Paradoxical reactions (agitation, restlessness, nightmares, insomnia, extrapyramidal symptoms, particularly fine hand tremor), laryngitis, seizures.

ADVERSE REACTIONS/ TOXIC EFFECTS

High dosage may produce cardiovascular effects (severe postural hypotension, dizziness, tachycardia, palpitations, arrhythmias), seizures. May result in altered temperature regulation (hyperpyrexia, hypothermia). Abrupt withdrawal from prolonged therapy may produce headache, malaise, nausea, vomiting, vivid dreams. Anemia has been noted.

NURSING IMPLICATIONS

INTERVENTION/EVALUATION

Closely supervise suicidal-risk pt during early therapy (as depression lessens, energy level improves, increasing suicide potential). Assess appearance, behavior, speech pattern, level of interest, mood.

PATIENT/FAMILY TEACHING

May cause dry mouth, constipation, blurred vision. Tolerance to postural hypotension, sedative, anticholinergic effects usually develop during early therapy. Maximum therapeutic effect may be noted in 2–4 wks. Do not abruptly discontinue medication. Avoid tasks that require alertness, motor skills until response to drug is established. Avoid alcohol.

C

clonazepam

klon-**nah**-zih-pam

(Apo-Clonazepam♣, Clonapam♣, Klonopin, Rivotril♣)

Do not confuse with clonidine, lorazepam.

CLASSIFICATION

PHARMACOTHERAPEUTIC: Benzodiazepine. **CLINICAL:** Anticonvulsant, antianxiety. (see p. 32C).

ACTION

Depresses all levels of the CNS. Depresses nerve transmission in the motor cortex. **Therapeutic Effect:** Suppresses abnormal discharge in petite mal seizures. Produces anxiolytic effect.

PHARMACOKINETICS

Well absorbed from GI tract. Protein binding: 85%. Metabolized in liver. Excreted in urine. Not removed by hemodialysis. **Half-life:** 18–50 hrs.

USES

Adjunct in treatment of Lennox-Gastaut syndrome (petit mal variant epilepsy); akinetic, myoclonic seizures; absence seizures (petit mal). Treatment of panic disorder. **Unlabeled:** Adjunct treatment of seizures; treatment of simple/complex partial seizures, tonic-clonic seizures.

PRECAUTIONS

CONTRAINDICATIONS: Significant liver disease, narrow-angle glaucoma. **CAU-**

TIONS: Impaired kidney/liver function, chronic respiratory disease.

LIFESPAN CONSIDERATIONS: Pregnancy/lactation: Crosses placenta. May be distributed in breast milk. Chronic ingestion during pregnancy may produce withdrawal symptoms, CNS depression in neonates. **Pregnancy Category D. Children:** Long-term use may adversely affect physical/mental development. **Elderly:** Usually more sensitive to CNS effects (e.g., ataxia, dizziness, oversedation). Use low dosage, increase gradually.

INTERACTIONS

DRUG: Alcohol, CNS depressants may increase CNS depressant effect. **HERBAL: Kava kava** may increase CNS sedation. **FOOD:** None known. **LAB VALUES:** None known.

AVAILABILITY (Rx)

TABLETS: 0.5 mg, 1 mg, 2 mg. **ORALLY DISINTEGRATING TABLETS:** 0.125 mg, 0.25 mg, 0.5 mg, 1 mg, 2 mg.

ADMINISTRATION/HANDLING

PO

• Give without regard to meals. • Tablets may be crushed.

INDICATIONS/ROUTES/DOSAGE

ANTICONVULSANT

Alert: When replacement by another anticonvulsant is necessary, decrease clonazepam gradually as therapy begins with low replacement dosage.

PO: ADULTS, ELDERLY: 1.5 mg daily. Dosage may be increased in 0.5- to 1-mg increments at 3-day intervals until seizures are controlled. Do not exceed maintenance dosage of 20 mg daily. INFANTS, CHILDREN <10 YRS, OR <30 KG: 0.01–0.03 mg/kg daily in 2–3 divided doses. Dosage may be increased in up to 0.5-mg increments at 3-day intervals until seizures are controlled. Do not exceed maintenance dosage of 0.2 mg/kg daily.

PANIC DISORDER

PO: ADULTS, ELDERLY: Initially, 0.25 mg 2 times/day. Increase in increments of 0.125–0.25 mg 2 times/day at 3-day intervals. **Maximum:** 4 mg/day.

SIDE EFFECTS

FREQUENT: Mild, transient drowsiness; ataxia; behavioral disturbances (esp. in children) manifested as aggression, irritability, agitation. **OCCASIONAL:** Rash, ankle/facial edema, nocturia, dysuria, change in appetite/weight, dry mouth, sore gums, nausea, blurred vision. **RARE:** Paradoxical reaction (hyperactivity/nervousness in children, excitement/restlessness in elderly—particularly noted in presence of uncontrolled pain).

ADVERSE REACTIONS/ TOXIC EFFECTS

Abrupt withdrawal may result in pronounced restlessness, irritability, insomnia, hand tremors, abdominal/muscle cramps, sweating, vomiting, status epilepticus. Overdosage results in somnolence, confusion, diminished reflexes, coma.

NURSING IMPLICATIONS

BASELINE ASSESSMENT

Review history of seizure disorder (frequency, duration, intensity, level of consciousness). For panic attack, assess motor responses (agitation, trembling, tension), autonomic responses (cold/clammy hands, diaphoresis).

INTERVENTION/EVALUATION

Assess children, elderly for paradoxical reaction, particularly during early therapy. Implement safety measures and observe frequently for recurrence of seizure activity. Assist with ambulation if drowsiness, ataxia occur. For those on long-term therapy, liver/renal function tests, blood counts should be performed periodically. Evaluate for therapeutic response: decrease in intensity/frequency of seizures or, if used in panic attack, calm facial expression, decreased restlessness.

PATIENT/FAMILY TEACHING

Drowsiness usually diminishes with continued therapy. Avoid tasks that require alertness, motor skills until response to drug is established. Smoking reduces drug effectiveness. Do not abruptly withdraw medication after long-term therapy. Strict maintenance of drug therapy is essential for seizure control. Avoid alcohol.

clonidine

klon-ih-deen

(Catapres, Catapres TTS, Dixarit✱, Duraclon)

Do not confuse with Cetapred, clomiphene, Klonopin, quinidine.

FIXED-COMBINATION(S)

Combipres: clonidine/chlorthalidone (a diuretic): 0.1 mg/15 mg, 0.2 mg/15 mg, 0.3 mg/15 mg.

CLASSIFICATION

PHARMACOTHERAPEUTIC: Antiadrenergic, sympatholytic. **CLINICAL:** Antihypertensive (see p. 52C).

ACTION

EPIDURAL: Prevents pain signal transmission to the brain and produces analgesia at pre– and post–alpha-adrenergic receptors in the spinal cord. **Therapeutic Effect:** Reduces peripheral resistance; decreases B/P, heart rate.

PHARMACOKINETICS

Onset	Peak	Duration
PO		
0.5–1 hr	2–4 hrs	Up to 8 hrs

Well absorbed from GI tract. Transdermal best absorbed from chest, upper arm; least absorbed from thigh. Protein binding: 20%–40%. Metabolized in liver. Primarily excreted in urine. Minimal removal by hemodialysis. **Half-life:** 12–16 hrs (half-life increased with impaired renal function).

USES

Treatment of hypertension alone or in combination with other antihypertensive agents. Treatment of severe pain in cancer pts. **Epidural:** Combined with opiates for relief of severe pain. **Unlabeled:** Diagnosis of pheochromocytoma, prevention of migraine headaches, treatment of dysmenorrhea/menopausal flushing, opioid withdrawal. Attention deficit hyperactivity disorder (ADHD).

PRECAUTIONS

CONTRAINDICATIONS: Epidural contraindicated in those receiving anticoagulation therapy, those with bleeding diathesis or infection at the injection site. **CAUTIONS:** Severe coronary insufficiency, recent MI, cerebrovascular disease, chronic renal failure, Raynaud's disease, thromboangiitis obliterans.

LIFESPAN CONSIDERATIONS: Pregnancy/lactation: Crosses placenta. Distributed in breast milk. **Pregnancy Category C. Children:** More sensitive to effects, use caution. **Elderly:** May be more sensitive to hypotensive effect. Age-related renal impairment may require dosage adjustment.

INTERACTIONS

DRUG: Tricyclic antidepressants may decrease effect. Discontinuing concurrent **beta-blockers** may increase risk of clonidine-withdrawal hypertensive crisis. **HERBAL:** None known. **FOOD:** None known. **LAB VALUES:** None known.

C

AVAILABILITY (Rx)

TABLETS: 0.1 mg, 0.2 mg, 0.3 mg. **TRANSDERMAL PATCH:** 2.5 mg (release at 0.1 mg/24 hrs), 5 mg (release at 0.2 mg/24 hrs), 7.5 mg (release at 0.3 mg/24 hrs). **INJECTION:** 100 mcg/ml, 500 mcg/ml.

ADMINISTRATION/HANDLING

PO

• Give without regard to food. • Tablets may be crushed. • Give last oral dose just before retiring.

TRANSDERMAL

• Apply transdermal system to dry, hairless area of intact skin on upper arm or chest. • Rotate sites (prevents skin irritation). • Do not trim patch to adjust dose.

∅ IV INCOMPATIBILITIES

No known drug incompatibilities noted.

IV COMPATIBILITIES

Bupivacaine (Marcaine, Sensorcaine), fentanyl (Sublimaze), heparin, ketamine (Ketalar), lidocaine, lorazepam (Ativan).

INDICATIONS/ROUTES/DOSAGE

HYPERTENSION

PO: ADULTS: Initially, 0.1 mg 2 times/day. Increase by 0.1–0.2 mg q2–4days. MAINTENANCE: 0.2–1.2 mg/day in 2–4 divided doses up to maximum of 2.4 mg/day. CHILDREN: 5–25 mcg/kg/day in divided doses q6h; increase at 5- to 7-day intervals. **Maximum:** 0.9 mg/day.

Transdermal: ADULTS, ELDERLY: System delivering 0.1 mg/24 hrs up to 0.6 mg/24 hrs q7days.

USUAL ELDERLY DOSAGE

PO: Initially, 0.1 mg at bedtime. May increase gradually.

ADHD

PO: CHILDREN: Initially, 0.05 mg/day. may increase by 0.05 mg/day q3–7days. **Maximum:** 0.3–0.4 mg/day.

SEVERE PAIN

Epidural: ADULTS, ELDERLY: 30–40 mcg/hr. CHILDREN: Initially, 0.5 mcg/kg/hr, not to exceed adult dose.

SIDE EFFECTS

FREQUENT: Dry mouth (40%), drowsiness (33%), dizziness (16%), sedation, constipation (10%). **OCCASIONAL (1%–5%):** Depression, swelling of feet, loss of appetite, decreased sexual ability, itching eyes, dizziness, nausea, vomiting, nervousness. **Transdermal:** Itching, red skin, darkening of skin. **RARE (<1%):** Nightmares, vivid dreams, cold feeling in fingers/toes.

ADVERSE REACTIONS/ TOXIC EFFECTS

Overdosage produces profound hypotension, irritability, bradycardia, respiratory depression, hypothermia, miosis (pupillary constriction), arrhythmias, apnea. Abrupt withdrawal may result in rebound hypertension associated with nervousness, agitation, anxiety, insomnia, hand tingling, tremor, flushing, sweating.

NURSING IMPLICATIONS

BASELINE ASSESSMENT

Obtain B/P immediately before each dose is administered, in addition to regular monitoring (be alert to B/P fluctuations).

INTERVENTION/EVALUATION

Monitor pattern of daily bowel activity/stool consistency. If clonidine is to be withdrawn, discontinue concurrent beta-blocker therapy several days before discontinuing clonidine (prevents clonidine withdrawal hypertensive crisis). Slowly reduce clonidine dosage over 2–4 days.

PATIENT/FAMILY TEACHING

Sugarless gum, sips of tepid water may relieve dry mouth. To reduce hypotensive effect, rise slowly from lying to sitting position, permit legs to dangle momentarily before standing. Skipping doses or voluntarily discontinuing drug may produce severe, rebound hypertension. Side effects tend to diminish during therapy.

clopidogrel

klow-**pih**-duh-grel
(Plavix)

CLASSIFICATION

PHARMACOTHERAPEUTIC: Thienopyridine derivative. **CLINICAL:** Antiplatelet (see p. 29C).

ACTION

Inhibits binding of the enzyme adenosine diphosphate (ADP) to its platelet receptor and subsequent ADP-mediated activation of a glycoprotein complex. **Therapeutic Effect:** Inhibits platelet aggregation.

PHARMACOKINETICS

Onset	Peak	Duration
PO		
1 hr	2 hrs	—

Rapidly absorbed. Protein binding: 98%. Extensively metabolized by the liver. Eliminated equally in the urine and feces. **Half-life:** 8 hrs.

USES

Reduction of MI, stroke, vascular death in pts with documented atherosclerosis. Treatment of acute coronary syndrome.

PRECAUTIONS

CONTRAINDICATIONS: Active bleeding, coagulation disorders, severe liver disease. **CAUTIONS:** Hypertension, liver/renal impairment, history of bleeding, hematologic disorders, scheduled for surgery.

LIFESPAN CONSIDERATIONS: Pregnancy/lactation: Unknown if drug crosses placenta or is distributed in breast milk. **Pregnancy Category B. Children:** Safety and efficacy not established. **Elderly:** No age-related precautions noted.

INTERACTIONS

DRUG: May interfere with metabolism of **phenytoin, tamoxifen, tolbutamide, warfarin, torsemide, fluvastatin, other NSAIDs. HERBAL: Ginger, ginkgo** may increase bleeding. **FOOD:** None known. **LAB VALUES:** Prolongs bleeding time.

AVAILABILITY (Rx)

TABLETS: 75 mg.

ADMINISTRATION/HANDLING

PO

Give without regard to food. • Do not crush coated tablets.

INDICATIONS/ROUTES/DOSAGE

INHIBITION OF PLATELET AGGREGATION

PO: ADULTS, ELDERLY: 75 mg once daily.

SIDE EFFECTS

FREQUENT (15%): Skin disorders. **OCCASIONAL (6%–8%):** Upper respiratory tract infection, chest pain, flulike symptoms, headache, dizziness, arthralgia. **RARE (3%–5%):** Fatigue, edema, hypertension, abdominal pain, dyspepsia, diarrhea, nausea, epistaxis, dyspnea, rhinitis.

ADVERSE REACTIONS/ TOXIC EFFECTS

None known.

C

NURSING IMPLICATIONS

BASELINE ASSESSMENT

Perform platelet counts prior to drug therapy, q2days during the first week of treatment and weekly thereafter until therapeutic maintenance dose is reached. Abrupt discontinuation of drug therapy produces an elevation of platelet count within 5 days.

INTERVENTION/EVALUATION

Monitor platelet count for evidence of thrombocytopenia. Assess BUN, creatinine, bilirubin, SGOT (AST), SGPT (ALT), WBC, Hgb, signs/symptoms of hepatic insufficiency during therapy.

PATIENT/FAMILY TEACHING

Inform pt it may take longer to stop bleeding during drug therapy. Report any unusual bleeding. All physicians and dentists must be informed if clopidogrel is being taken, esp. before surgery is scheduled or before taking any new drug.

clorazepate dipotassium

klor-**az**-eh-payt
(Novoclopate, Tranxene)
Do not confuse with clofibrate.

CLASSIFICATION

PHARMACOTHERAPEUTIC: Benzodiazepine. **CLINICAL:** Antianxiety, anticonvulsant (see p. 10C).

ACTION

Depresses all levels of the CNS, including limbic and reticular formation, by binding to benzodiazepine site on the GABA receptor complex. Modulates GABA, which is a major inhibitory neurotransmitter in the brain. **Therapeutic Effect:** Produces anxiolytic effect, suppresses seizure activity.

USES

Management of anxiety disorders, short-term relief of anxiety symptoms, partial seizures, acute alcohol withdrawal symptoms.

PRECAUTIONS

CONTRAINDICATIONS: Acute narrow-angle glaucoma. **CAUTIONS:** Impaired renal/hepatic function, acute alcohol intoxication. **Pregnancy Category D.**

INTERACTIONS

DRUG: **Alcohol, CNS depressants** may increase CNS depressant effect. **HERBAL:** **Kava kava, valerian** may increase CNS depression. **FOOD:** None known. **LAB VALUES:** None known. Therapeutic blood serum level: Peak: 0.12–1.5 mcg/ml; toxic serum level: >5 mcg/ml.

AVAILABILITY (Rx)

CAPSULES: 3.75 mg, 7.5 mg, 15 mg. **TABLETS:** 3.75 mg, 7.5 mg, 15 mg. **TABLETS (single dose):** 11.5 mg, 22.5 mg.

INDICATIONS/ROUTES/DOSAGE

Alert: When replacement by another anticonvulsant is necessary, decrease clorazepate gradually as therapy begins with low-replacement dosage.

ANXIETY

PO: ADULTS: 30 mg daily in divided doses or single bedtime dose. ELDERLY, DEBILITATED: 7.5–15 mg in divided doses or single bedtime dose. DAILY DOSE RANGE: 15–60 mg.

PARTIAL SEIZURES

PO: ADULTS, CHILDREN >12 YRS: Initially, up to 7.5 mg 3 times daily. Do not increase dosage more than 7.5 mg/wk or exceed 90 mg/day. CHILDREN 9–12 YRS: 3.75–7.5 mg/dose 2 times/day. **Maximum:** 60 mg/day in 2–3 divided doses.

ALCOHOL WITHDRAWAL

PO: ADULTS, ELDERLY: Initially, 30 mg, then 15 mg 2–4 times/day on first day. **Maximum:** 90 mg/day. Gradually decrease dosage over subsequent days.

SIDE EFFECTS

FREQUENT: Drowsiness. **OCCASIONAL:** Dizziness, GI disturbances, nervousness, blurred vision, dry mouth, headache, confusion, ataxia, rash, irritability, slurred speech. **RARE:** Paradoxical CNS hyperactivity/nervousness in children, excitement/restlessness in elderly/debilitated (generally noted during first 2 wks of therapy, particularly noted in presence of uncontrolled pain).

ADVERSE REACTIONS/ TOXIC EFFECTS

Abrupt or too rapid withdrawal may result in pronounced restlessness, irritability, insomnia, hand tremors, abdominal/muscle cramps, sweating, vomiting, seizures. Overdosage results in somnolence, confusion, diminished reflexes, coma.

NURSING IMPLICATIONS

BASELINE ASSESSMENT

Anxiety: Assess autonomic response (cold/clammy hands, sweating), motor response (agitation, trembling, tension). Offer emotional support to anxious pt. **Seizures:** Review history of seizure disorder (intensity, frequency, duration, LOC). Observe frequently for recurrence of seizure activity. Initiate seizure precautions.

INTERVENTION/EVALUATION

Assess for paradoxical reaction, particularly during early therapy. Assist with ambulation if drowsiness, dizziness occur. Evaluate for therapeutic response: **Anxiety:** Calm facial expression; decreased restlessness. **Seizures:** Decrease in intensity/frequency of seizures. Therapeutic blood serum level: Peak: 0.12–1.5 mcg/ml; toxic serum level: >5 mcg/ml.

PATIENT/FAMILY TEACHING

Do not abruptly withdraw medication after long-term use (may precipitate seizures). Strict maintenance of drug therapy is essential for seizure control. Drowsiness usually disappears during continued therapy. Avoid tasks that require alertness, motor skills until response to drug is established. If dizziness occurs, change positions slowly from recumbent to sitting position before standing. Smoking reduces drug effectiveness. Avoid alcohol.

clotrimazole

kloe-**try**-mah-zole
(Canesten ✤, Clotrimaderm ✤, Gyne-Lotrimin, Lotrimin, Mycelex, Mycelex-G)

Do not confuse with co-trimoxazole, Myoflex.

FIXED-COMBINATION(S)

Lotrisone: clotrimazole/betamethasone (a corticosteroid): 1%/0.05%.

CLASSIFICATION

PHARMACOTHERAPEUTIC: Anti-infective. **CLINICAL:** Antifungal (see p. 42C).

ACTION

Binds with phospholipids in fungal cell membrane. **Therapeutic Effect:** Altered cell membrane permeability inhibits yeast growth.

USES

Oral Lozenges: Treatment/prophylaxis of oropharyngeal candidiasis due to *Candida* sp. **Topical:** Treatment of tinea pedis, tinea cruris, tinea corporis, tinea versicolor, cutaneous candidiasis (moniliasis) due to *Candida albicans.* **Intravaginal:** Treatment of vulvovaginal candidiasis (moniliasis) due to *Candida* sp. **Unlabeled: Topical:** Treatment of paronychia, tinea barbae, tinea capitis.

PRECAUTIONS

CONTRAINDICATIONS: Hypersensitivity to clotrimazole or any ingredient in preparation, children <3 yrs. **CAUTIONS:** Hepatic disorder with oral therapy. **Pregnancy Category B.**

INTERACTIONS

DRUG: None known. **HERBAL:** None known. **FOOD:** None known. **LAB VALUES:** May increase SGOT (AST).

AVAILABILITY (Rx)

LOTION: 1%. **LOZENGES:** 10 mg. **SOLUTION:** 1%. **VAGINAL CREAM:** 1%, 2%. **VAGINAL SUPPOSITORY:** 100 mg, 200 mg. **VAGINAL TABLETS:** 100 mg, 200 mg.

ADMINISTRATION/HANDLING

PO

- Lozenges must be dissolved in mouth >15–30 min for oropharyngeal therapy.
- Swallow saliva.

TOPICAL

- Rub well into affected, surrounding areas. • Do not apply occlusive covering or other preparations to affected area.

VAGINAL

- Use vaginal applicator; insert high into vagina.

INDICATIONS/ROUTES/DOSAGE

ORAL-LOCAL/OROPHARYNGEAL

PO: ADULTS, ELDERLY, CHILDREN ≥3 YRS: 10 mg 5 times/day for 14 days.

PROPHYLAXIS VS. OROPHARYNGEAL CANDIDIASIS

PO: ADULTS, ELDERLY: 10 mg 3 times/day.

USUAL TOPICAL DOSAGE

Topical: ADULTS, ELDERLY, CHILDREN ≥3 YRS: 2 times/day. Therapeutic effect may take up to 8 wks.

VULVOVAGINAL CANDIDIASIS

Vaginal: (tablets): ADULTS, ELDERLY, CHILDREN ≥12 YRS: 1 tablet (100 mg) at bedtime for 7 days; 2 tablets (200 mg) at bedtime for 3 days; or 500-mg tablet one time.

Vaginal: (cream): ADULTS, ELDERLY, CHILDREN ≥12 YRS: 1 applicatorful at bedtime for 7–14 days.

SIDE EFFECTS

FREQUENT: PO: Nausea, vomiting, diarrhea, abdominal pain. **OCCASIONAL: Topical:** Itching, burning, stinging, erythema, urticaria. **Vaginal:** Mild burning (tablets/cream); irritation, cystitis (cream). **RARE: Vaginal:** Itching, rash, lower abdominal cramping, headache.

ADVERSE REACTIONS/ TOXIC EFFECTS

None known.

NURSING IMPLICATIONS

BASELINE ASSESSMENT

Assess pt's ability to understand/follow directions regarding use of oral lozenges.

INTERVENTION/EVALUATION

With oral therapy, assess for nausea, vomiting. With topical therapy, check skin for erythema, urticaria, blistering; inquire about itching, burning, stinging. With vaginal therapy, evaluate for vulvovaginal irritation, abdominal cramping, urinary frequency, discomfort.

PATIENT/FAMILY TEACHING

Continue for full length of therapy. Inform physician of increased irritation. Avoid contact with eyes. **Topical:** Keep areas clean, dry; wear light clothing to promote ventilation. Separate personal items, linens. **Vaginal:** Continue use during menses. Refrain from sexual intercourse or advise partner to use condom during therapy.

cloxacillin

(Tegopen)

See Classification section under: Antibiotic: penicillins (p. 26C)

clozapine

klow-zah-peen

(Clozaril)

Do not confuse with Clinoril, Cloxapen, Colazal.

CLASSIFICATION

PHARMACOTHERAPEUTIC: Dibenzodiazepine derivative. **CLINICAL:** Antipsychotic (see p. 56C).

ACTION

Interferes with binding of dopamine at dopamine receptor sites (binds primarily at nondopamine receptor sites). **Therapeutic Effect:** Diminishes schizophrenic behavior.

USES

Management of severely ill schizophrenic pts who fail to respond to other antipsychotic therapy. Recurrent suicidal behavior.

PRECAUTIONS

CONTRAINDICATIONS: Myeloproliferative disorders, history of clozapine-induced agranulocytosis or severe granulocytopenia, concurrent administration with other drugs having potential to suppress bone marrow function, severe CNS depression, comatose state. **CAUTIONS:** History of seizures, cardiovascular disease, myocarditis; impaired respiratory, hepatic, renal function; alcohol withdrawal; urinary retention; glaucoma; prostatic hypertrophy. **Pregnancy Category B.**

INTERACTIONS

DRUG: **Alcohol, CNS depressants** may increase CNS depressant effects. **Bone marrow depressants** may increase myelosuppression. **Lithium** may increase risk of seizures, confusion, dyskinesias. **Phenobarbital** decreases concentration. **HERBAL:** None known. **FOOD:** None known. **LAB VALUES:** None known.

AVAILABILITY (Rx)

TABLETS: 25 mg, 100 mg.

ADMINISTRATION/HANDLING

PO

- Give without regard to meals.

INDICATIONS/ROUTES/DOSAGE

SCHIZOPHRENIC DISORDERS

PO: ADULTS: Initially, 25 mg 1–2 times/day. May increase by 25–50 mg/day over 2 wks until dosage of 300–450 mg/day achieved. May further increase dosage by 50–100 mg/day no more frequently than 1–2 times/wk. RANGE: 200–600 mg/day. **Maximum:** 900 mg/day.

USUAL ELDERLY DOSAGE

PO: Initially, 25 mg/day. May increase by 25 mg/day. **Maximum:** 450 mg/day.

SIDE EFFECTS

FREQUENT: Drowsiness (39%), salivation (31%), tachycardia (25%), dizziness (19%), constipation (14%). **OCCASIONAL:** Hypotension (9%); headache (7%); tremor, syncope, sweating, dry mouth (6%); nausea, visual disturbances (5%); nightmares, restlessness, akinesia, agitation, hypertension, abdominal discomfort/heartburn, weight gain (4%).

RARE: Rigidity, confusion, fatigue, insomnia, diarrhea, rash.

C

ADVERSE REACTIONS/ TOXIC EFFECTS

Seizures occur occasionally (3%). Overdosage produces CNS depression (sedation, coma, delirium), respiratory depression, hypersalivation. Blood dyscrasias, particularly agranulocytosis, mild leukopenia may occur.

NURSING IMPLICATIONS

BASELINE ASSESSMENT

Obtain baseline WBC before initiating treatment and monitor WBC count every week for first 6 mos of continuous therapy, then biweekly for those with acceptable WBC counts. Assess behavior, appearance, emotional status, response to environment, speech pattern, thought content.

INTERVENTION/EVALUATION

Monitor B/P for hypertension/hypotension. Assess pulse for tachycardia (common side effect). Monitor CBC for blood dyscrasias. Supervise suicidal-risk pt closely during early therapy (as depression lessens, energy level improves, increasing suicide potential). Assess for therapeutic response (interest in surroundings, improvement in self-care, increased ability to concentrate, relaxed facial expression).

PATIENT/FAMILY TEACHING

Do not abruptly withdraw from long-term drug therapy. Drowsiness generally subsides during continued therapy. Avoid tasks that require alertness, motor skills until response to drug is established. Avoid alcohol.

cocaine

koe-**kane**

FIXED-COMBINATION(S)

AC Gel: cocaine/epinephrine (a sympathomimetic): 11.8%/1:1,000. **TAC:** tetracaine/epinephrine/cocaine: 0.5%/1:2,000/11.8%.

CLASSIFICATION

PHARMACOTHERAPEUTIC: Amide. **CLINICAL:** Topical anesthetic.

ACTION

Decreases membrane permeability; increases norepinephrine at postsynaptic receptor sites, producing intense vasoconstriction. **Therapeutic Effect:** Blocks conduction of nerve impulses.

USES

Topical anesthesia for mucous membranes of orolaryngeal, nasal areas; minor, uncomplicated facial lacerations.

PRECAUTIONS

CONTRAINDICATIONS: Hypersensitivity to cocaine, local anesthetics; systemic or ophthalmic use. **CAUTIONS:** Hypertension, severe cardiovascular disease, thyrotoxicosis, infants, those with severely traumatized mucosa in area of intended application. **Pregnancy Category C (X** if nonmedical use).

INTERACTIONS

DRUG: Tricyclic antidepressants, digoxin, methyldopa may increase arrhythmias. May decrease effects of **beta-blockers. Cholinesterase inhibitors** may increase effects, risk of toxicity. CNS stimulation-producing agents may increase effects. **Sympathomimetics** increase CNS stimulation, risk of cardiovascular effects. **HERBAL:** None known. **FOOD:** None known. **LAB VALUES:** None known.

AVAILABILITY (Rx)

TOPICAL SOLUTION: 4%, 10%.

INDICATIONS/ROUTES/DOSAGE

USUAL TOPICAL DOSAGE

Topical: ADULTS, ELDERLY: 1%–10% solution. **Maximum single dose:** 1 mg/kg.

SIDE EFFECTS

FREQUENT: Loss of sense of smell/taste.

ADVERSE REACTIONS/ TOXIC EFFECTS

Repeated nasal application may produce stuffy nose, chronic rhinitis. Early signs of overdosage produces increased B/P, increased pulse, irregular heartbeat, chills/fever, agitation, nervousness, confusion, inability to remain still, nausea, vomiting, abdominal pain, increased sweating, rapid breathing, large pupils. Advanced signs of overdosage produces arrhythmias, CNS hemorrhage, CHF, convulsions, delirium, hyperreflexia, loss of bladder/bowel control, respiratory weakness. Late signs of overdosage produces loss of reflexes, muscle paralysis, dilated pupils, LOC, cyanosis, pulmonary edema, cardiac/respiratory failure.

NURSING IMPLICATIONS

INTERVENTION/EVALUATION

Monitor for anesthetic response. Be alert to CNS stimulation. Assess for euphoria; restlessness; increased B/P, pulse, respirations. Be prepared to provide ventilatory support and emergency medications in event of progression of CNS response.

PATIENT/FAMILY TEACHING

NPO until sensation returns when used for throat anesthesia. One time or infrequent use for procedures will not cause dependence. Report feelings of euphoria, restlessness, rapid heartbeat if these develop during procedure.

codeine phosphate

koe-deen
(Codeine)

codeine sulfate

(Contin ♣)

Do not confuse with Lodine.

FIXED-COMBINATION(S)

Capital with Codeine, Tylenol with Codeine: acetaminophen/codeine: 120 mg/12 mg per 5 ml. **Tylenol with Codeine:** acetaminophen/codeine: 300 mg/15 mg, 300 mg/30 mg, 300 mg/60 mg.

◆ CLASSIFICATION

PHARMACOTHERAPEUTIC: Opioid agonist. **CLINICAL:** Analgesic: **Schedule II;** fixed-combination form: **Schedule III** (see p. 120C).

ACTION

Binds at opiate receptor sites in CNS. Has direct action in the medulla. **Therapeutic Effect:** Inhibits ascending pain pathways, altering perception of/response to pain, causes cough suppression.

USES

Relief of mild to moderate pain and/or nonproductive cough. **Unlabeled:** Treatment of diarrhea.

PRECAUTIONS

CONTRAINDICATIONS: None known. **EXTREME CAUTION:** CNS depression, anoxia, hypercapnia, respiratory depression, seizures, acute alcoholism, shock, untreated myxedema, respiratory dysfunction. **CAUTIONS:** Increased intracranial pressure, impaired hepatic function, acute abdominal conditions, hypothyroidism, prostatic hypertrophy, Addison's disease, urethral stricture, COPD. **Preg-**

nancy Category C (**D** if used for prolonged periods, high dosages at term).

INTERACTIONS

DRUG: Alcohol, CNS depressants may increase CNS or respiratory depression, hypotension. **MAOIs** may produce severe, fatal reaction (reduce dosage to ¼ usual dose). **HERBAL:** None known. **FOOD:** None known. **LAB VALUES:** May increase amylase, lipase.

AVAILABILITY (Rx)

TABLETS: 15 mg, 30 mg, 60 mg. **SOLUBLE TABLETS:** 15 mg, 30 mg, 60 mg. **INJECTION:** 30 mg, 60 mg.

INDICATIONS/ROUTES/DOSAGE

Alert: Reduce initial dosage in those with hypothyroidism, concurrent CNS depressants, Addison's disease, renal insufficiency, elderly/debilitated.

ANALGESIA

PO/subcutaneous/IM: ADULTS, ELDERLY: 30 mg q4–6h. **RANGE:** 15–60 mg. CHILDREN: 0.5–1 mg/kg q4–6h. **Maximum:** 60 mg/dose.

ANTITUSSIVE

PO: ADULTS, ELDERLY, CHILDREN >12 YRS: 10–20 mg q4–6h. CHILDREN 6–11 YRS: 5–10 mg q4–6h. CHILDREN 2–5 YRS: 2.5–5 mg q4–6h.

DOSAGE IN RENAL IMPAIRMENT

Creatinine Clearance	Dosage
10–50 ml/min	75% dose
<10 ml/min	50% dose

SIDE EFFECTS

Alert: Ambulatory pts, those not in severe pain may experience dizziness, nausea, vomiting, hypotension more frequently than those in supine position or with severe pain.

FREQUENT: Constipation, drowsiness, nausea, vomiting. **OCCASIONAL:** Paradoxical excitement, confusion, pounding heartbeat, facial flushing, decreased urination, blurred vision, dizziness, dry mouth, headache, hypotension, decreased appetite, redness/burning/pain at injection site. **RARE:** Hallucinations, depression, stomach pain, insomnia.

ADVERSE REACTIONS/ TOXIC EFFECTS

Too frequent use may result in paralytic ileus. Overdosage results in cold/clammy skin, confusion, convulsions, decreased B/P, restlessness, pinpoint pupils, bradycardia, respiratory depression, LOC, severe weakness. Tolerance to analgesic effect, physical dependence may occur with repeated use.

NURSING IMPLICATIONS

BASELINE ASSESSMENT

Analgesic: Assess onset, type, location, duration of pain. Effect of medication is reduced if full pain response recurs before next dose. **Antitussive:** Assess type, severity, frequency of cough, sputum production.

INTERVENTION/EVALUATION

Monitor daily bowel activity/stool consistency. Increase fluid intake, environmental humidity to improve viscosity of lung secretions. Initiate deep breathing, coughing exercises. Assess for clinical improvement; record onset of relief of pain, cough.

PATIENT/FAMILY TEACHING

Change positions slowly to avoid orthostatic hypotension. Avoid tasks that require alertness, motor skills until response to drug is established. Tolerance/dependence may occur with prolonged use of high dosages. Avoid alcohol.

colchicine

coal-cheh-seen
(Colchicine)

◆CLASSIFICATION

PHARMACOTHERAPEUTIC: Alkaloid.
CLINICAL: Antigout.

ACTION

Decreases leukocyte motility, phagocytosis, lactic acid production. **Therapeutic Effect:** Results in decreased urate crystal deposits, inflammatory process.

PHARMACOKINETICS

Rapidly absorbed from GI tract. Highest concentration in liver, spleen, kidney. Protein binding: 30%–50%. Reenters intestinal tract (biliary secretion), reabsorbed from intestines. Partially metabolized in liver. Eliminated primarily in feces.

USES

Treatment of acute gouty arthritis, prophylaxis of recurrent gouty arthritis. **Unlabeled:** Reduce frequency of familial Mediterranean fever; treatment of acute calcium pyrophosphate deposition, sarcoid arthritis, amyloidosis, biliary cirrhosis, recurrent pericarditis.

PRECAUTIONS

CONTRAINDICATIONS: Severe GI, renal, hepatic, cardiac disorders; blood dyscrasias. **CAUTIONS:** Impaired hepatic function, elderly, debilitated.

LIFESPAN CONSIDERATIONS: Pregnancy/lactation: Unknown if drug crosses placenta or is distributed in breast milk. **Pregnancy Category D. Children:** Safety and efficacy not established. **Elderly:** May be more susceptible to cumulative toxicity. Age-related renal impairment may increase risk of myopathy.

INTERACTIONS

DRUG: NSAIDs may increase risk of neutropenia, thrombocytopenia, bone marrow depression. **Bone marrow depressants** may increase risk of blood dyscrasias. **HERBAL:** None known. **FOOD:** None known. **LAB VALUES:** May decrease platelet count. May increase SGOT (AST), alkaline phosphatase.

AVAILABILITY (Rx)

TABLETS: 0.5 mg, 0.6 mg. **INJECTION:** 1 mg.

ADMINISTRATION/HANDLING

PO

- Give without regard to meals.

IV

Alert: Subcutaneous or IM administration produce severe local reaction. Use via IV route only.

Storage • Store at room temperature.

Reconstitution • May dilute with 0.9% NaCl or Sterile Water for Injection. • Do not dilute with D_5W.

Rate of administration • Administer over 2–5 min.

IV INCOMPATIBILITY

No information available via Y-site administration.

INDICATIONS/ROUTES/DOSAGE

ACUTE GOUTY ARTHRITIS

PO: ADULTS, ELDERLY: 0.5–1.2 mg, then 0.5–0.6 mg q1–2h or 1–1.2 mg q2h until pain relieved or nausea, vomiting, diarrhea occurs. Total dose: 4–8 mg.

IV: ADULTS, ELDERLY: Initially, 2 mg, then 0.5 mg q6h until satisfactory response. **Maximum:** 4 mg/24 hrs or 4 mg/one course of treatment.

Alert: If pain recurs, may give 1–2 mg/day for several days but no sooner than

7 days after a full course of IV therapy (4 mg).

CHRONIC GOUTY ARTHRITIS

PO: ADULTS, ELDERLY: 0.5–0.6 mg once weekly up to once daily (dependent on number of attacks per year).

SIDE EFFECTS

Alert: Those with impaired renal function may exhibit myopathy, neuropathy manifested as generalized weakness.

FREQUENT: PO: Nausea, vomiting, abdominal discomfort. **OCCASIONAL: PO:** Anorexia. **RARE:** Hypersensitivity reaction, including angioedema. **Parenteral only:** Nausea, vomiting, diarrhea, abdominal discomfort, pain/redness at injection site, neuritis in injected arm.

ADVERSE REACTIONS/ TOXIC EFFECTS

Bone marrow depression (aplastic anemia, agranulocytosis, thrombocytopenia) may occur with long-term therapy. Overdose: **INITIALLY:** Burning feeling in throat/skin, severe diarrhea, abdominal pain. **SECOND STAGE:** Fever, seizures, delirium, renal impairment (hematuria, oliguria). **THIRD STAGE:** Hair loss, leukocytosis, stomatitis.

NURSING IMPLICATIONS

BASELINE ASSESSMENT

Instruct pt to drink 8–10 glasses (8 oz) of fluid daily while taking medication. Medication should be discontinued if any GI symptoms occur.

INTERVENTION/EVALUATION

Discontinue medication immediately if GI symptoms occur. Encourage high fluid intake (3,000 ml/day). Monitor I&O (output should be at least 2,000 ml/day). Assess serum uric acid levels. Assess for therapeutic response (reduced joint tenderness, swelling, redness, limitation of motion).

PATIENT/FAMILY TEACHING

Encourage low-purine food intake, drink 8–10 glasses (8 oz) of fluid daily while taking medication. Report skin rash, sore throat, fever, unusual bruising/bleeding, weakness, tiredness, numbness. Stop medication as soon as gout pain is relieved or at first sign of nausea, vomiting, diarrhea.

colesevelam

ko-leh-**sev**-eh-lam
(Welchol)

CLASSIFICATION

PHARMACOTHERAPEUTIC: Bile acid sequestrant. **CLINICAL:** Antihyperlipidemic agent (see p. 50C).

ACTION

Nonsystemic polymer that binds with bile acids in the intestine, preventing their reabsorption and removing them from the body. **Therapeutic Effect:** Decreases LDL cholesterol.

USES

Adjunctive therapy to diet, exercise used either alone or in combination with an HMG-CoA reductase inhibitor (e.g., simvastatin) to decrease elevated LDL cholesterol in pts with primary hypercholesterolemia (Fredrickson type IIa).

PRECAUTIONS

CONTRAINDICATIONS: Hypersensitivity to colesevelam, complete biliary obstruction. **CAUTIONS:** Dysphagia, swallowing disorders, severe GI motility disorders, major GI tract surgery, those susceptible to fat-soluble vitamin deficiency.

LIFESPAN CONSIDERATIONS: Pregnancy/lactation: Not absorbed systemically. May decrease proper vitamin absorption and have effect on nursing infants. **Pregnancy Category B. Children:** Safety and efficacy not established. **Elderly:** No age-related precautions noted.

INTERACTIONS

DRUG: May decrease absorption of **vitamins A, D, E, K; NSAIDs, aspirin, clindamycin, digoxin, furosemide, glipizide, hydrocortisone, imipramine, phenytoin, propranolol, tetracyclines, thiazide diuretics. HERBAL:** None known. **FOOD:** None known. **LAB VALUES:** None known.

AVAILABILITY (Rx)

TABLETS: 625 mg.

INDICATIONS/ROUTES/DOSAGE

CHOLESTEROL LOWERING

PO: ADULTS, ELDERLY: 3 tablets with meals 2 times/day or 6 tablets once daily with meal. May increase daily dose to 7 tablets/day.

SIDE EFFECTS

FREQUENT (8%–12%): Flatulence, constipation, infection, dyspepsia.

ADVERSE REACTIONS/ TOXIC EFFECTS

GI tract obstruction may be noted.

NURSING IMPLICATIONS

BASELINE ASSESSMENT

Assess baseline lab results: cholesterol, triglycerides, liver function tests.

INTERVENTION/EVALUATION

Monitor cholesterol, triglyceride lab results for therapeutic response. Assess bowel activity.

PATIENT/FAMILY TEACHING

Follow special diet (important part of treatment). Periodic lab tests are essential part of therapy. Do not take other medications without physician's knowledge.

colestipol

(Cholestid)

See Classification section under: Antihyperlipidemics

Combivent

see albuterol or ipratropium

Combivir

see lamivudine

Concerta

see methylphenidate

conjugated estrogens

ess-troe-jenz

(Cenestin, C.E.S. ✤, Congest ✤, Premarin)

FIXED-COMBINATION(S)

Premphase, Prempro: estrogen/methyltestosterone (an androgen): 0.3 mg/1.5 mg; 0.45 mg/1.5 mg; 0.625 mg/2.5 mg; 0.625 mg/5 mg.

C

CLASSIFICATION

PHARMACOTHERAPEUTIC: Estrogen. **CLINICAL:** Hormone.

ACTION

Increases synthesis of DNA, RNA/various proteins in responsive tissues. Reduces release of gonadotropin-releasing hormone, reducing follicle-stimulating hormone (FSH), leuteinizing hormone (LH). **Therapeutic Effect:** Promotes vasomotor stability, maintains GU function, normal growth, development of female sex organs. Prevents accelerated bone loss by inhibiting bone resorption, restoring balance of bone resorption/formation. Inhibits LH, decreases serum concentration of testosterone.

PHARMACOKINETICS

Well absorbed from GI tract. Widely distributed. Protein binding: 50%–80%. Metabolized in liver. Primarily excreted in urine.

USES

Management of moderate to severe vasomotor symptoms associated with menopause. Treatment of atrophic vaginitis, kraurosis vulvae, female hypogonadism and castration, primary ovarian failure. Retardation of osteoporosis in postmenopausal women. Palliative treatment of inoperable, progressive cancer of the prostate in men and of the breast in postmenopausal women. **Unlabeled:** Prevents estrogen deficiency–induced premenopausal osteoporosis. **Cream:** Prevention of nosebleeds.

PRECAUTIONS

CONTRAINDICATIONS: Undiagnosed vaginal bleeding, thrombophlebitis, liver disease, breast cancer (some exceptions). **CAUTIONS:** Asthma, epilepsy, migraine headaches, diabetes, cardiac/renal dysfunction.

LIFESPAN CONSIDERATIONS: Pregnancy/lactation: Distributed in breast milk. May be harmful to fetus. Not for use during lactation. **Pregnancy Category X. Children:** Safety and efficacy not established. **Elderly:** No age-related precautions noted.

INTERACTIONS

DRUG: May interfere with effects of **bromocriptine.** May increase concentration of **cyclosporine,** increase hepatic, nephrotoxicity. **Hepatotoxic medications** may increase hepatotoxicity. **HERBAL:** None known. **FOOD:** None known. **LAB VALUES:** May affect metapyrone, thyroid function tests. May decrease cholesterol, LDH. May increase calcium, glucose, HDL, triglycerides.

AVAILABILITY (Rx)

TABLETS: 0.3 mg, 0.45 mg, 0.625 mg, 0.9 mg, 1.25 mg, 2.5 mg. **INJECTION:** 25 mg. **VAGINAL CREAM.**

ADMINISTRATION/HANDLING

PO

- Administer at the same time each day.
- Give with milk or food if nausea occurs.

IV

Storage • Refrigerate vials for IV use. • Reconstituted solution stable for 60 days if refrigerated. • Do not use if solution darkens or precipitate forms.

Reconstitution • Reconstitute with 5 ml Sterile Water for Injection containing benzyl alcohol (diluent provided). • Slowly add diluent, shaking gently. Avoid vigorous shaking.

Rate of administration • Give slowly to prevent flushing reaction.

IV INCOMPATIBILITY

No information available via Y-site administration.

INDICATIONS/ROUTES/DOSAGE

VASOMOTOR SYMPTOMS ASSOCIATED WITH MENOPAUSE, ATROPHIC VAGINITIS, KRAUROSIS VULVAE

PO: ADULTS, ELDERLY: 0.3–0.625 mg/day cyclically (21 days on; 7 days off or continuously).

Intravaginal: ADULTS, ELDERLY: ½–2 g/day cyclically.

FEMALE HYPOGONADISM

PO: ADULTS: 0.3–0.625 mg/day in divided doses for 20 days; rest 10 days.

FEMALE CASTRATION, PRIMARY OVARIAN FAILURE

PO: ADULTS: Initially, 1.25 mg/day cyclically.

OSTEOPOROSIS

PO: ADULTS, ELDERLY: 0.3–0.625 mg/day, cyclically.

BREAST CANCER

PO: ADULTS, ELDERLY: 10 mg 3 times/day for at least 3 mos.

PROSTATE CANCER

PO: ADULTS, ELDERLY: 1.25–2.5 mg 3 times/day.

ABNORMAL UTERINE BLEEDING

IM/IV: ADULTS: 25 mg, may repeat once in 6–12 hrs.

PO: 1.25 mg q4h for 24 hrs, then 1.25 mg/day for 7–10 days.

SIDE EFFECTS

FREQUENT: Change in vaginal bleeding (spotting, breakthrough), breast pain/tenderness, gynecomastia. **OCCASIONAL:** Headache, increased B/P, intolerance to contact lenses. **High-dose therapy:** Anorexia, nausea. **RARE:** Loss of scalp hair, clinical depression.

ADVERSE REACTIONS/ TOXIC EFFECTS

Prolonged administration may increase risk of gallbladder, thromboembolic disease; breast, cervical, vaginal, endometrial, liver carcinoma.

NURSING IMPLICATIONS

BASELINE ASSESSMENT

Question for hypersensitivity to estrogen, previous jaundice, thromboembolic disorders associated with pregnancy, estrogen therapy.

INTERVENTION/EVALUATION

Assess B/P periodically. Check for edema; weigh daily. Promptly report signs/symptoms of thromboembolic, thrombotic disorders: sudden severe headache, shortness of breath, vision/speech disturbance, weakness/numbness of an extremity, loss of coordination, pain in chest/groin/leg.

PATIENT/FAMILY TEACHING

Avoid smoking due to increased risk of heart attack/blood clots. Explain importance of diet/exercise when taken to retard osteoporosis. Teach how to perform Homans' test, signs/symptoms of blood clots (report these to physician immediately). Notify physician of abnormal vaginal bleeding, depression. Teach female pts to perform breast self-exam. Report weight gain of >5 lbs/wk. Stop taking medication and contact physician if pregnancy is suspected.

Coreg

see carvedilol

Corlopam

see fenoldopam

C

corticotropin injection

kore-tih-koe-**troe**-pin
(Acthar HP)

◆ **CLASSIFICATION**

PHARMACOTHERAPEUTIC: Adrenocortical steroid. **CLINICAL:** Corticotropin.

ACTION

Stimulates adrenal cortex to secrete cortisol, corticosterone, aldosterone, androgenic substances. Acts to stimulate synthesis of adrenocortical hormones. **Therapeutic Effect:** Suppresses immune response, inflammation.

USES

Diagnostic testing of adrenocortical function. Limited therapeutic value in conditions responsive to corticosteroid therapy. May be used for hypercalcemia associated with cancer, acute exacerbations of multiple sclerosis, nonsuppurative thyroiditis.

PRECAUTIONS

CONTRAINDICATIONS: Hypersensitivity to any corticosteroid or porcine proteins, systemic fungal infection, peptic ulcers (except life-threatening situations), scleroderma, primary adrenocortical insufficiency. Avoid live virus vaccine; long-term therapy in children. **CAUTIONS:** Thromboembolic disorders, history of tuberculosis (may reactivate disease), hypothyroidism, cirrhosis, nonspecific ulcerative colitis, CHF, hypertension, psychosis, renal insufficiency, seizures. Prolonged therapy should be discontinued slowly. **Pregnancy Category C.**

INTERACTIONS

DRUG: **Amphotericin** may increase hypokalemia. May decrease effect of **oral hypoglycemics, insulin, diuretics, potassium supplements.** May increase **digoxin** toxicity (due to hypokalemia). **Hepatic enzyme inducers** may decrease effect. **Live virus vaccines** may potentiate virus replication, increase vaccine side effects, decrease pt's antibody response to vaccine. **HERBAL:** None known. **FOOD:** None known. **LAB VALUES:** May decrease calcium, potassium, thyroxine. May increase cholesterol, lipids, glucose, sodium, amylase.

AVAILABILITY (Rx)

REPOSITORY FOR INJECTION: 40 units/ml, 80 units/ml.

INDICATIONS/ROUTES/DOSAGE

DIAGNOSTIC TESTING

IM/subcutaneous: ADULTS: 25 units.

ACUTE EXACERBATION OF MULTIPLE SCLEROSIS

IM: ADULTS: 80–120 units/day for 2–3 wks.

INFANTILE SPASMS

IM: INFANTS: 20–40 units/day or 80 units every other day for 3 mos (or 1 mo after cessation of seizures).

SIDE EFFECTS

FREQUENT: Insomnia, heartburn, nervousness, abdominal distention, increased sweating, acne, mood swings, increased appetite, facial flushing, delayed wound healing, increased susceptibility to infection, diarrhea/constipation. **OCCASIONAL:** Headache, edema, change in skin color, frequent urination. **RARE:** Tachycardia, allergic reaction (rash, hives), pain, redness, swelling at injection site, psychological changes, hallucinations, depression.

ADVERSE REACTIONS/ TOXIC EFFECTS

LONG-TERM THERAPY: Hypocalcemia, hypokalemia, muscle wasting (esp. arms, legs), osteoporosis, spontaneous fractures, amenorrhea, cataracts, glaucoma, peptic ulcer, CHF. **ABRUPT WITHDRAWAL FOLLOWING LONG-TERM THERAPY:** Anorexia, nausea, fever, headache, joint pain, rebound inflammation, fatigue, weakness, lethargy, dizziness, orthostatic hypertension.

NURSING IMPLICATIONS

BASELINE ASSESSMENT

Question for hypersensitivity to any of the corticosteroids. Obtain baseline values for weight, B/P, glucose, cholesterol, electrolytes.

INTERVENTION/EVALUATION

Be alert to infection (reduced immune response): sore throat, fever, vague symptoms. For those on long-term therapy, watch for hypocalcemia (muscle twitching, cramps, positive Trousseau's or Chvostek's signs), hypokalemia (weakness/muscle cramps, numbness/tingling [esp. lower extremities], nausea/vomiting, irritability, EKG changes). Assess emotional status, ability to sleep.

PATIENT/FAMILY TEACHING

Do not change dose/schedule or stop taking drug; **must** taper off under medical supervision. Notify physician of fever, sore throat, muscle aches, sudden weight gain/swelling. Inform dentist or other physicians of cortisone therapy now or within past 12 mos.

cortisone acetate

kore-tih-zone

(Cortone ✤)

Do not confuse with Cort-Dome.

✦CLASSIFICATION

PHARMACOTHERAPEUTIC: Adrenocortical steroid. **CLINICAL:** Glucocorticoid (see p. 81C).

ACTION

Inhibits accumulation of inflammatory cells at inflammation sites, phagocytosis, lysosomal enzyme release and synthesis and/or release of mediators of inflammation. **Therapeutic Effect:** Prevents/suppresses cell-mediated immune reactions. Decreases/prevents tissue response to inflammatory process.

USES

Management of adrenocortical insufficiency.

PRECAUTIONS

CONTRAINDICATIONS: Hypersensitivity to any corticosteroid, systemic fungal infection, peptic ulcers (except life-threatening situations). Avoid live virus vaccine. **CAUTIONS:** Thromboembolic disorders, history of tuberculosis (may reactivate disease), hypothyroidism, cirrhosis, nonspecific ulcerative colitis, CHF, hypertension, psychosis, renal insufficiency, seizure disorders. Prolonged therapy should be discontinued slowly. **Pregnancy Category C** (**D** if used in first trimester).

INTERACTIONS

DRUG: **Amphotericin** may increase hypokalemia. May decrease effect of **oral hypoglycemics, insulin, diuretics, potassium supplements.** May increase **digoxin** toxicity (due to hypokalemia). **Hepatic enzyme inducers** may decrease effect. **Live virus vaccines** may potentiate virus replication, increase vaccine side effects, decrease pt's antibody response to vaccine. **HERBAL:** None known. **FOOD:** None known. **LAB VALUES:** May decrease calcium, potassium, thyroxine. May increase cholesterol, lipids, glucose, sodium, amylase.

AVAILABILITY (Rx)

TABLETS: 25 mg.

C

INDICATIONS/ROUTES/DOSAGE

Dosage dependent on condition being treated and patient response.

ANTI-INFLAMMATORY, IMMUNOSUPPRESSIVE:
PO: ADULTS, ELDERLY: 25–300 mg/day divided doses q12–24h. CHILDREN: 2.5–10 mg/kg/day in divided doses q6–8h.

PHYSIOLOGIC REPLACEMENT:
PO: ADULTS, ELDERLY: 25–35 mg/day. CHILDREN: 0.5–0.75 mg/kg/day in divided doses q8h.

SIDE EFFECTS

FREQUENT: Insomnia, heartburn, nervousness, abdominal distention, increased sweating, acne, mood swings, increased appetite, facial flushing, delayed wound healing, increased susceptibility to infection, diarrhea/constipation. **OCCASIONAL:** Headache, edema, change in skin color, frequent urination. **RARE:** Tachycardia, allergic reaction (rash, hives), physiological changes, hallucinations, depression.

ADVERSE REACTIONS/ TOXIC EFFECTS

LONG-TERM THERAPY: Hypocalcemia, hypokalemia, muscle wasting (esp. arms, legs), osteoporosis, spontaneous fractures, amenorrhea, cataracts, glaucoma, peptic ulcer, CHF. **ABRUPT WITHDRAWAL FOLLOWING LONG-TERM THERAPY:** Anorexia, nausea, fever, headache, joint pain, rebound inflammation, fatigue, weakness, lethargy, dizziness, orthostatic hypertension.

NURSING IMPLICATIONS

BASELINE ASSESSMENT

Question for hypersensitivity to any of the corticosteroids. Obtain baseline values for weight, B/P, glucose, cholesterol, electrolytes.

INTERVENTION/EVALUATION

Be alert to infection (reduced immune response): sore throat, fever, vague symptoms. For pts on long-term therapy, monitor for hypocalcemia (muscle twitching, cramps, positive Trousseau's or Chvostek's signs), hypokalemia (weakness/muscle cramps, numbness/tingling [esp. lower extremities], nausea/vomiting, irritability, EKG changes). Assess emotional status, ability to sleep.

PATIENT/FAMILY TEACHING

Do not change dose/schedule or stop taking drug; **must** taper off under medical supervision. Notify physician of fever, sore throat, muscle aches, sudden weight gain/swelling. Inform dentist or other physicians of cortisone therapy now or within past 12 mos.

cosyntropin

koe-syn-**troe**-pin
(Cortrosyn)
Do not confuse with Cotazym.

◆CLASSIFICATION

PHARMACOTHERAPEUTIC: Adrenocortical steroid. **CLINICAL:** Glucocorticoid.

ACTION

Stimulates initial reaction in synthesis of adrenal steroids from cholesterol. **Therapeutic Effect:** Increases endogenous corticoid synthesis.

USES

Diagnostic testing of adrenocortical function.

PRECAUTIONS

CONTRAINDICATIONS: Hypersensitivity to cosyntropin or corticotropin. **CAU-**

TIONS: None known. **Pregnancy Category C.**

INTERACTIONS

DRUG: None known. **HERBAL:** None known. **FOOD:** None known. **LAB VALUES:** None known.

AVAILABILITY (Rx)

POWDER FOR INJECTION: 0.25 mg.

INDICATIONS/ROUTES/DOSAGE

SCREENING TEST FOR ADRENAL FUNCTION

IM: ADULTS: 0.25–0.75 mg one time. CHILDREN <2 YRS: 0.125 mg one time. NEONATES: 0.015 mg/kg/dose.

IV infusion: ADULTS: 0.25 mg in D_5W or 0.9% NaCl. Infuse at 0.04 mg/hr over 6 hrs.

SIDE EFFECTS

OCCASIONAL: Nausea, vomiting. **RARE:** Hypersensitivity reaction (fever, pruritus).

ADVERSE REACTIONS/ TOXIC EFFECTS

None known.

NURSING IMPLICATIONS

BASELINE ASSESSMENT

Hold cortisone, hydrocortisone, spironolactone on the test day. Ensure that baseline plasma cortisol concentration has been drawn prior to start of test or 24-hr urine for 17-KS or 17-OHCS is initiated.

INTERVENTION/EVALUATION

Adhere to time frame for blood draws; monitor collection of urine if indicated.

PATIENT/FAMILY TEACHING

Explain procedure, purpose of the test.

co-trimoxazole (sulfamethoxazole-trimethoprim)

koe-try-**mox**-oh-zole

(Apo-Sulfatrim ✱, Bactrim, Novotrimel ✱, Septra)

Do not confuse with bacitracin, clotrimazole, Sectral, Septa.

FIXED-COMBINATION(S)

Zotrim: co-trimethoxazole/phenazopyridine. **Bactrim, Septra** (sulfamethoxazole/trimethoprim): 5 : 1 ratio remains constant in all dosage forms (e.g., 400 mg/80 mg).

CLASSIFICATION

PHARMACOTHERAPEUTIC: Sulfonamide/folate antagonist. **CLINICAL:** Antibiotic.

ACTION

Blocks bacterial synthesis of essential nucleic acids. **Therapeutic Effect:** Produces bactericidal action in susceptible microorganisms.

PHARMACOKINETICS

Rapidly, well absorbed from GI tract. Widely distributed. Protein binding: 45%–60%. Metabolized in liver. Excreted in urine. Minimally removed by hemodialysis. **Half-life:** 6–12 hrs; trimethoprim 8–10 hrs (half-life increased with impaired renal function).

USES

Acute/complicated and recurrent/chronic urinary tract infection, *Pneumocystis carinii* pneumonia (PCP), shigellosis, enteritis, otitis media, chronic bronchitis, traveler's diarrhea. Prophylaxis of PCP. **Unlabeled:** Treatment of biliary tract, bone/joint, chancroid infections; bacterial endocarditis; chlamydial infection,

C

gonorrhea, intra-abdominal infection, meningitis, sinusitis, septicemia, skin/soft tissue infection.

PRECAUTIONS

CONTRAINDICATIONS: Hypersensitivity to trimethoprim or any sulfonamides, megaloblastic anemia due to folate deficiency, infants <2 mos. **CAUTIONS:** Those with G6PD deficiency, impaired renal/liver function.

LIFESPAN CONSIDERATIONS: Pregnancy/lactation: Contraindicated during pregnancy at term and during lactation. Readily crosses placenta. Distributed in breast milk. May produce kernicterus in newborns. **Pregnancy Category C. Children:** Contraindicated in those <2 mos, may increase risk of kernicterus in newborn. **Elderly:** Increased risk for severe skin reaction, bone marrow depression, or decreased platelet count.

INTERACTIONS

DRUG: May increase/prolong effects, increase toxicity with **warfarin, hydantoin anticonvulsants, oral hypoglycemics.** May increase risk of toxicity with other **hemolytics. Hepatotoxic medications** may increase risk of hepatotoxicity. **Methenamine** may form precipitate. May increase effect of **methotrexate. HERBAL:** None known. **FOOD:** None known. **LAB VALUES:** May increase SGOT (AST), SGPT (ALT), alkaline phosphatase, BUN, creatinine, potassium.

AVAILABILITY (Rx)

TABLETS: 80 mg trimethoprim/400 mg sulfamethoxazole; 160 mg/800 mg. **ORAL SUSPENSION:** 40 mg/200 mg per 5 ml. **INJECTION:** 80 mg/400 mg per 5 ml.

ADMINISTRATION/HANDLING

PO

• Store tablets, suspension at room temperature. • Administer on empty stomach with 8 oz water. • Give several extra glasses of water/day.

IV

Storage • IV infusion (piggyback) stable for 2–6 hrs (use immediately). • Discard if cloudy or precipitate forms.

Reconstitution • For IV infusion (piggyback), dilute each 5 ml with 75–125 ml D_5W. • Do not mix with other drugs or solutions.

Rate of administration • Infuse over 60–90 min. Must avoid bolus or rapid infusion. • Do not give IM. • Ensure adequate hydration.

IV INCOMPATIBILITIES

Fluconazole (Diflucan), foscarnet (Foscavir), midazolam (Versed), vinorelbine (Navelbine).

IV COMPATIBILITIES

Diltiazem (Cardizem), heparin, hydromorphone (Dilaudid), lorazepam (Ativan), magnesium sulfate, morphine.

INDICATIONS/ROUTES/DOSAGE

Alert: Potency expressed in terms of trimethoprim content.

MILD TO MODERATE INFECTIONS

PO/IV: ADULTS, ELDERLY, CHILDREN >2 MOS: 6–12 mg/kg/day in divided doses q12h.

SERIOUS INFECTIONS, PCP

PO/IV: ADULTS, ELDERLY, CHILDREN >2 MOS: 15–20 mg/kg/day in divided doses q6–8h.

PREVENTION OF *PNEUMOCYSTIS CARINII* PNEUMONIA

PO: ADULTS: One double-strength tablet/day. CHILDREN: 150 mg/m^2/day on 3 consecutive days/wk.

TRAVELER'S DIARRHEA

PO: ADULTS, ELDERLY: One double-strength tablet q12h for 5 days.

C

ACUTE EXACERBATION OF CHRONIC BRONCHITIS

PO: ADULTS, ELDERLY: One double-strength tablet q12h for 14 days.

UTI PROPHYLAXIS

PO: ADULTS, ELDERLY, CHILDREN >2 MOS: 2 mg/kg/dose once daily.

DOSAGE IN RENAL IMPAIRMENT

Dose and/or frequency is modified based on severity of infection, degree of renal impairment, serum concentration of drug. For those with creatinine clearance of 15–30 ml/min, a reduction in dose of 50% is recommended.

SIDE EFFECTS

FREQUENT: Anorexia, nausea, vomiting, rash (generally 7–14 days after therapy begins), urticaria. **OCCASIONAL:** Diarrhea, abdominal pain, local pain/irritation at IV site. **RARE:** Headache, vertigo, insomnia, seizures, hallucinations, depression.

ADVERSE REACTIONS/ TOXIC EFFECTS

Rash, fever, sore throat, pallor, purpura, cough, shortness of breath may be early signs of serious adverse reactions. Fatalities are rare but have occurred in sulfonamide therapy following Stevens-Johnson syndrome, toxic epidermal necrolysis, fulminant hepatic necrosis, agranulocytosis, aplastic anemia, other blood dyscrasias. Elderly are at increased risk of adverse reactions: bone marrow suppression, decreased platelets, severe dermatologic reactions.

NURSING IMPLICATIONS

BASELINE ASSESSMENT

Obtain history for hypersensitivity to trimethoprim or any sulfonamide, sulfite sensitivity, bronchial asthma. Determine renal, hepatic, hematologic baselines.

INTERVENTION/EVALUATION

Determine pattern of bowel activity. Assess skin for rash, pallor, purpura. Check IV site, flow rate. Monitor renal, hepatic, hematology reports. Assess I&O. Check for CNS symptoms: headache, vertigo, insomnia, hallucinations. Monitor vital signs at least twice a day. Monitor for cough, shortness of breath. Assess for overt bleeding, bruising, swelling.

PATIENT/FAMILY TEACHING

Continue medication for full length of therapy. Space doses evenly around the clock. Take oral doses with 8 oz water and drink several extra glasses of water daily. Notify physician of new symptoms immediately, esp. rash, other skin changes, bleeding/bruising, fever, sore throat.

Cozaar

see losartan

Crestor

see rosuvastatin

Crixivan

see indinavir

C

cromolyn sodium

krom-oh-lin

(Apo-Cromolyn✤, Crolom, Gastrocom, Intal, Nasalcrom, Opticrom

◆CLASSIFICATION

PHARMACOTHERAPEUTIC: Mast cell stabilizer. **CLINICAL:** Antiasthmatic, antiallergic (see p. 65C).

ACTION

Prevents mast cell release of histamine, leukotrienes, slow-reacting substances of anaphylaxis by inhibiting degranulation after contact with antigens. **Therapeutic Effect:** Prevents release of mast cells (e.g., histamine) after exposure to allergens that produce allergic reaction.

PHARMACOKINETICS

Minimal absorption after PO, inhalation, nasal administration. Absorbed portion excreted in urine or via biliary elimination. **Half-life:** 80–90 min.

USES

Oral Inhalation, Nebulization: Prophylactic management of severe bronchial asthma, exercise-induced bronchospasm. **Intranasal:** Perennial or seasonal allergic rhinitis. **Systemic:** Symptomatic treatment of systemic mastocytosis, food allergy, treatment of inflammatory bowel disease (IBD). **Ophthalmic:** Conjunctivitis.

PRECAUTIONS

CONTRAINDICATIONS: Status asthmaticus. **CAUTIONS:** Coronary artery disease, arrhythmias, tapering dose or discontinuing (symptoms may recur).

LIFESPAN CONSIDERATIONS: Pregnancy/lactation: Unknown if drug crosses placenta or is distributed in breast milk. **Pregnancy Category B. Children:** No age-related precautions noted. **Elderly:** Age-related renal/liver impairment may require dosage adjustment.

INTERACTIONS

DRUG: None known. **HERBAL:** None known. **FOOD:** None known. **LAB VALUES:** None known.

AVAILABILITY (Rx)

AEROSOL: 800 mcg. **LIQUID:** 100 mg/5 ml. **NASAL SPRAY:** 4%. **NEBULIZATION:** 20 mg/2 ml. **OPHTHALMIC DROPS:** 4%.

ADMINISTRATION/HANDLING

INHALATION

• Shake container well; exhale completely; place mouthpiece fully into mouth, inhale deeply/slowly while depressing the canister; hold breath as long as possible before exhaling. • Wait 1–10 min before inhaling second dose (allows for deeper bronchial penetration). • Rinse mouth with water immediately after inhalation (prevents mouth/throat dryness). **Nebulization, inhalation capsules:** Inhalation capsules are not to be swallowed; instruct patient on use of Spinhaler.

OPHTHALMIC

• Place finger on lower eyelid; pull down until pocket is formed between eye and lower lid. Hold dropper above pocket; place prescribed number of drops in pocket. Instruct pt to close eyes gently so that medication will not be squeezed out of sac. • Apply gentle finger pressure to the lacrimal sac at inner canthus for 1 min after installation (lessens risk of systemic absorption).

PO

• Give at least 30 min before meals. • Pour contents of capsule in hot water, stirring until completely dissolved; add equal amount cold water while stirring. • Do not mix with fruit juice, milk, food.

NASAL

• Nasal passages should be clear (may require nasal decongestant). • Inhale through nose.

INDICATIONS/ROUTES/DOSAGE

ASTHMA

Inhalation (nebulization): ADULTS, ELDERLY, CHILDREN >2 YRS: 20 mg 3–4 times/day.

Aerosol spray: ADULTS, ELDERLY, CHILDREN ≥12 YRS: Initially, 2 sprays 4 times/day. MAINTENANCE: 2–4 sprays 3–4 times/day. CHILDREN 5–12 YRS: Initially, 2 sprays 4 times/day, then 1–2 sprays 3–4 times/day.

PREVENTION OF BRONCHOSPASM

Inhalation (nebulization): ADULTS, ELDERLY, CHILDREN >2 YRS: 20 mg not longer than 1 hr prior to exercise, allergic exposure.

Aerosol spray: ADULTS, ELDERLY, CHILDREN >5 YRS: 2 sprays not longer than 1 hr prior to exercise, allergic exposure.

FOOD ALLERGY, IBD

PO: ADULTS, ELDERLY, CHILDREN >12 YRS: 200–400 mg 4 times/day. CHILDREN 2–12 YRS: 100–200 mg 4 times/day. **Maximum:** 40 mg/kg/day.

ALLERGIC RHINITIS

Intranasal: ADULTS, ELDERLY, CHILDREN >6 YRS: 1 spray each nostril 3–4 times/day. May increase up to 6 times/day.

SYSTEMIC MASTOCYTOSIS

PO: ADULTS, ELDERLY, CHILDREN >12 YRS: 200 mg 4 times/day. CHILDREN 2–12 YRS: 100 mg 4 times/day. **Maximum:** 40 mg/kg/day. CHILDREN <2 YRS: 20 mg/kg/day in 4 divided doses. **Maximum** (children 6 mos–2 yrs): 30 mg/kg/day.

USUAL OPHTHALMIC DOSE

Ophthalmic: ADULTS, ELDERLY, CHILDREN >4 YRS: 1–2 drops in both eyes 4–6 times/day.

SIDE EFFECTS

FREQUENT: Inhalation: Cough, dry mouth/throat, stuffy nose, throat irritation, unpleasant taste. **Nasal:** Burning, stinging, irritation of nose, increased sneezing. **Ophthalmic:** Burning/stinging of eye. **PO:** Headache, diarrhea. **OCCASIONAL: Inhalation:** Bronchospasm, hoarseness, watering eyes. **Nasal:** Cough, headache, unpleasant taste, postnasal drip. **Ophthalmic:** Increased watering/itching of eye. **PO:** Skin rash, abdominal pain, joint pain, nausea, insomnia. **RARE: Inhalation:** Dizziness, painful urination, muscle/joint pain, skin rash. **Nasal:** Nosebleeds, skin rash. **Ophthalmic:** Chemosis (edema of conjunctiva), eye irritation.

ADVERSE REACTIONS/ TOXIC EFFECTS

Nasal, PO, inhalation: Anaphylaxis occurs rarely.

NURSING IMPLICATIONS

INTERVENTION/EVALUATION

Monitor rate, depth, rhythm, type of respiration; quality/rate of pulse. Assess lung sounds for rhonchi, wheezing, rales. Observe lips, fingernails for blue/dusky color in light-skinned patients; gray in dark-skinned patients.

PATIENT/FAMILY TEACHING

Increase fluid intake (decreases lung secretion viscosity). Rinsing mouth with water immediately after inhalation may prevent mouth/throat dryness. Effect of therapy dependent on administration at regular intervals.

C

cyanocobalamin (vitamin B_{12})

sye-ah-no-koe-**bal**-a-min
(Bedoz, Rubion)

CLASSIFICATION

PHARMACOTHERAPEUTIC: Coenzyme. **CLINICAL:** Vitamin, antianemic (see p. 137C).

ACTION

Coenzyme for metabolic functions (fat, carbohydrate metabolism, protein synthesis). **Therapeutic Effect:** Necessary for growth, cell replication, hematopoiesis, myelin synthesis.

PHARMACOKINETICS

Absorbed in lower half of ileum in presence of calcium. Initially, bound to intrinsic factor; this complex passes down intestine, binding to receptor sites on ileal mucosa. In presence of calcium, absorbed systemically. Protein binding: High. Metabolized in liver. Primarily eliminated in urine unchanged. **Half-life:** 6 days.

USES

Prophylaxis, treatment of pernicious anemia, vitamin B_{12} deficiency. Deficiency generally occurs concurrently with other B-vitamin deficiencies.

PRECAUTIONS

CONTRAINDICATIONS: History of allergy to cobalamin, folate deficient anemia, hereditary optic nerve atrophy. **CAUTIONS:** None known.

LIFESPAN CONSIDERATIONS: Pregnancy/lactation: Crosses placenta. Excreted in breast milk. **Pregnancy Category A (C** if used at dosages greater than RDA). **Children/elderly:** No age-related precautions noted.

INTERACTIONS

DRUG: Alcohol, colchicine may decrease absorption. **Ascorbic acid** may destroy vitamin B_{12}. **Folic acid** (large doses) may decrease concentration. **HERBAL:** None known. **FOOD:** None known. **LAB VALUES:** None known.

AVAILABILITY (Rx)

TABLETS: 50 mcg, 100 mcg, 250 mcg, 500 mcg, 660 mcg, 1 mg, 2 mg, 2.5 mg. **TABLET (CONTROLLED-RELEASE):** 1,000 mcg, 1,500 mcg. **INJECTION:** 1,000 mcg/ml.

ADMINISTRATION/HANDLING

PO

- Give with meals (increases absorption).

INDICATIONS/ROUTES/DOSAGE

DEFICIENCY (SEVERE)/PERNICIOUS ANEMIA

IM/subcutaneous: ADULTS, ELDERLY: 1,000 mcg with folic acid 15 mg (IV or IM) once, then 1,000 mcg and 5 mg folic acid (oral) daily for 1 wk.

DEFICIENCY (UNCOMPLICATED)

IM/subcutaneous: ADULTS, ELDERLY: 100 mcg/day for 5–10 days then 100–200 mcg monthly.

PO: 1,000–2,000 mcg/day.

USUAL NASAL DOSAGE

ADULTS, ELDERLY: 500 mcg (1 spray) every week (after deficiency corrected).

SUPPLEMENT

PO: ADULTS, ELDERLY: 2–6 mcg/day. CHILDREN: 0.3–2 mcg/day.

SIDE EFFECTS

OCCASIONAL: Diarrhea, itching.

ADVERSE REACTIONS/ TOXIC EFFECTS

Rare allergic reaction generally due to impurities in preparation. May produce peripheral vascular thrombosis, pulmonary edema, hypokalemia, CHF.

NURSING IMPLICATIONS

INTERVENTION/EVALUATION

Assess for CHF, pulmonary edema, hypokalemia in cardiac pts receiving subcutaneous/IM therapy. Monitor potassium levels (3.5–5 mEq/L), serum B_{12} (200–800 mcg/ml), rise in reticulocyte count (peaks in 5–8 days). Assess for reversal of deficiency symptoms: hyporeflexia, loss of positional sense, ataxia, fatigue, irritability, insomnia, anorexia, pallor, palpitation on exertion. Therapeutic response to treatment usually dramatic within 48 hrs.

PATIENT/FAMILY TEACHING

Lifetime treatment may be necessary with pernicious anemia. Report symptoms of infection. Foods rich in vitamin B_{12} include organ meats, clams, oysters, herring, red snapper, muscle meats, fermented cheese, dairy products, egg yolks.

cyclobenzaprine hydrochloride

cy-klow-**benz**-ah-preen

(Flexeril, Flexitec ♣, Novo-Cycloprine ♣)

Do not confuse with cycloserine, cyproheptadine, Floxin.

CLASSIFICATION

CLINICAL: Skeletal muscle relaxant.

ACTION

Centrally acting skeletal muscle relaxant. Reduces tonic somatic motor activity influencing motor neurons. **Therapeutic Effect:** Relieves local skeletal muscle spasm.

PHARMACOKINETICS

Onset	Peak	Duration
PO		
1 hr	3–4 hrs	12–24 hrs

Well (but slowly) absorbed from GI tract. Protein binding: 93%. Metabolized in GI tract, liver. Primarily excreted in urine. **Half-life:** 1–3 days.

USES

Treatment of muscle spasm associated with acute painful musculoskeletal conditions; supportive therapy in tetanus. **Unlabeled:** Treatment of fibromyalgia.

PRECAUTIONS

CONTRAINDICATIONS: Concurrent use of MAOIs or within 14 days after their discontinuation; acute recovery phase of MI; those with arrhythmias, heart blocks, conduction disturbances, CHF, hyperthyroidism. **CAUTIONS:** Impaired renal/hepatic function, history of urinary retention, angle-closure glaucoma, increased intraocular pressure.

LIFESPAN CONSIDERATIONS: Pregnancy/lactation: Unknown if drug crosses placenta or is distributed in breast milk. **Pregnancy Category B. Children:** Safety and efficacy not established. **Elderly:** Increased sensitivity to anticholinergic effects (e.g., confusion, urinary retention).

INTERACTIONS

DRUG: Tricyclic antidepressants, CNS depression-producing medications may increase CNS depression. **MAOIs** may increase risk of hypertensive crisis, severe seizures. **HERBAL:** None

see also www.elsevierhealth.com/EVOLVE/SaundersNDH

known. **FOOD:** None known. **LAB VALUES:** None known.

C

AVAILABILITY (Rx)

TABLETS: 5 mg, 10 mg.

ADMINISTRATION/HANDLING

PO

- Give without regard to food.

INDICATIONS/ROUTES/DOSAGE

Alert: Do not use longer than 2–3 wks.

ACUTE, PAINFUL MUSCULOSKELETAL CONDITIONS

PO: ADULTS, ELDERLY: 10 mg 3 times/day. RANGE: 20–40 mg/day in 2–4 divided doses. **Maximum:** 60 mg/day.

SIDE EFFECTS

FREQUENT: Drowsiness (39%), dry mouth (27%), dizziness (11%). **RARE (1%–3%):** Fatigue, tiredness, asthenia, blurred vision, headache, nervousness, confusion, nausea, constipation, dyspepsia, unpleasant taste.

ADVERSE REACTIONS/ TOXIC EFFECTS

Overdosage may result in visual hallucinations, hyperactive reflexes, muscle rigidity, vomiting, hyperpyrexia.

NURSING IMPLICATIONS

BASELINE ASSESSMENT

Record onset, type, location, duration of muscular spasm. Check for immobility, stiffness, swelling.

INTERVENTION/EVALUATION

Assist with ambulation at all times. Evaluate for therapeutic response: decreased intensity of skeletal muscle pain/tenderness, improved mobility, decrease in stiffness.

PATIENT/FAMILY TEACHING

Drowsiness usually diminishes with continued therapy. Avoid tasks that require alertness, motor skills until response to drug is established. Avoid alcohol, other depressants while taking medication. Avoid sudden changes in posture. Sugarless gum, sips of water may relieve dry mouth.

cyclophosphamide

sigh-klo-**phos**-fah-mide
(Cytoxan, Neosar, Procytox✤)

Do not confuse with cefoxitin, Ciloxan, Cytotec.

CLASSIFICATION

PHARMACOTHERAPEUTIC: Alkylating agent. **CLINICAL:** Antineoplastic (see p. 70C).

ACTION

Inhibits DNA, RNA protein synthesis by cross-linking with DNA, RNA strands. **Therapeutic Effect:** Inhibits protein synthesis, prevents cell growth. Potent immunosuppressant.

PHARMACOKINETICS

Well absorbed from GI tract. Crosses blood-brain barrier. Protein binding: Low. Metabolized in liver to active metabolites. Primarily excreted in urine. Removed by hemodialysis. **Half-life:** 3–12 hrs.

USES

Treatment of Hodgkin's disease, non-Hodgkin's lymphoma, multiple myeloma, leukemia (acute lymphoblastic, acute myelogenous, acute monocytic, chronic granulocytic, chronic lymphocytic), mycosis fungoides, disseminated neuroblastoma, adenocarcinoma of ovary, retinoblastoma, carcinoma of breast. Biopsy-proven "minimal change" nephrotic syndrome in children. **Unlabeled:** Treatment of carcinoma of lung, cervix, endometrium, bladder, prostate, testicles; osteosarcoma; germ cell ovarian tumors; rheumatoid arthritis; systemic lupus erythematosus.

PRECAUTIONS

CONTRAINDICATIONS: None known. **CAUTIONS:** Severe leukopenia, thrombocytopenia, tumor infiltration of bone marrow, previous therapy with other antineoplastic agents, radiation.

LIFESPAN CONSIDERATIONS: Pregnancy/lactation: If possible, avoid use during pregnancy. May cause malformations (limb abnormalities, cardiac anomalies, hernias). Distributed in breast milk. Breast-feeding not recommended. **Pregnancy Category D. Children:** No age-related precautions noted. **Elderly:** Age-related renal impairment may require caution.

INTERACTIONS

DRUG: May decrease effect of **antigout medications. Allopurinol, bone marrow depressants** may increase bone marrow depression. **Cytarabine** may increase cardiomyopathy. **Immunosuppressants** may increase risk of infection, development of neoplasms. **Live virus vaccines** may potentiate virus replication, increase vaccine side effects, decrease pt's antibody response to vaccine. **HERBAL:** None known. **FOOD:** None known. **LAB VALUES:** May increase uric acid.

AVAILABILITY (Rx)

TABLETS: 25 mg, 50 mg. **POWDER FOR INJECTION:** 100 mg, 200 mg, 500 mg, 1 g, 2 g.

ADMINISTRATION/HANDLING

Alert: May be carcinogenic, mutagenic, or teratogenic. Handle with extreme care during preparation/administration.

PO

- Give on an empty stomach. If GI upset occurs, give with food.

IV

Storage • Reconstituted solution is stable for 24 hrs at room temperature or up to 6 days if refrigerated.

Reconstitution • For IV push, reconstitute each 100 mg with 5 ml Sterile Water for Injection or Bacteriostatic Water for Injection to provide concentration of 20 mg/ml. • Shake to dissolve. Allow to stand until clear.

Rate of administration • May give by IV push or further dilute with 250 ml D_5W, 0.9% NaCl, 0.45% NaCl, lactated Ringer's (LR) solution or D_5W/LR. • Infuse each 100 mg or fraction thereof over ≥15 min. • IV route may produce faintness, facial flushing, diaphoresis, oropharyngeal sensation.

IV INCOMPATIBILITIES

Amphotericin B complex (Abelcet, AmBisome, Amphotec).

IV COMPATIBILITIES

Granisetron (Kytril), heparin, hydromorphone (Dilaudid), lorazepam (Ativan), morphine, ondansetron (Zofran), propofol (Diprivan).

INDICATIONS/ROUTES/DOSAGE

Alert: Dosage individualized based on clinical response, tolerance to adverse effects. When used in combination therapy, consult specific protocols for optimum dosage, sequence of drug administration.

MALIGNANT DISEASES

PO: ADULTS: 1–5 mg/kg/day. CHILDREN: Initially, 2–8 mg/kg/day. MAINTENANCE: 2–5 mg/kg 2 times/wk.

IV: ADULTS: 40–50 mg/kg in divided doses over 2–5 days; or 10–15 mg/kg q7–10 days or 3–5 mg/kg 2 times/wk. CHILDREN: Initially, 40–50 mg/kg in divided doses over 2–5 days. MAINTENANCE: 10–15 mg/kg q7–10days or 3–5 mg/kg 2 times/wk.

see also www.elsevierhealth.com/EVOLVE/SaundersNDH

C

BIOPSY-PROVEN "MINIMAL CHANGE" NEPHROTIC SYNDROME

PO: ADULTS, CHILDREN: 2.5–3 mg/kg/day for 60–90 days.

SIDE EFFECTS

EXPECTED: Marked leukopenia 8–15 days after initial therapy. **FREQUENT:** Nausea, vomiting begins about 6 hrs after administration and lasts about 4 hrs; alopecia (33%). **OCCASIONAL:** Diarrhea, darkening of skin/fingernails, stomatitis (may include oral ulceration), headache, diaphoresis. **RARE:** Pain/redness at injection site.

ADVERSE REACTIONS/ TOXIC EFFECTS

Major toxic effect is bone marrow depression resulting in blood dyscrasias (leukopenia, anemia, thrombocytopenia, hypoprothrombinemia). Thrombocytopenia may occur 10–15 days after drug initiation. Anemia generally occurs after large doses or prolonged therapy. Hemorrhagic cystitis occurs commonly in long-term therapy (esp. in children). Pulmonary fibrosis, cardiotoxicity noted with high doses. Amenorrhea, azoospermia, hyperkalemia may occur.

NURSING IMPLICATIONS

BASELINE ASSESSMENT

Obtain WBC count weekly during therapy or until maintenance dose is established, then at 2- to 3-wk intervals.

INTERVENTION/EVALUATION

Monitor CBC, serum uric acid concentration, blood chemistries. Monitor WBC closely during initial therapy. Monitor for hematologic toxicity (fever, sore throat, signs of local infection, easy bruising, unusual bleeding from any site), symptoms of anemia (excessive tiredness, weakness). Recovery from marked leukopenia due to bone marrow depression can be expected in 17–28 days.

PATIENT/FAMILY TEACHING

Encourage copious fluid intake, frequent voiding (assists in preventing cystitis) at least 24 hrs before, during, after therapy. Do not have immunizations without physician's approval (drug lowers body's resistance). Avoid contact with those who have recently received live virus vaccine. Promptly report fever, sore throat, signs of local infection, easy bruising/unusual bleeding from any site. Alopecia is reversible, but new hair growth may have different color or texture.

cyclosporine

sigh-klo-**spore**-in

(Neoral, Restasis, Sandimmune)

Do not confuse with cycloserine, Cyklokapron.

◆ CLASSIFICATION

PHARMACOTHERAPEUTIC: Cyclic polypeptide. **CLINICAL:** Immunosuppressant (see p. 102C).

ACTION

Inhibits interleukin-2, a proliferative factor needed for T-cell activity. **Therapeutic Effect:** Inhibits both cellular and humoral immune responses.

PHARMACOKINETICS

Variably absorbed from GI tract. Widely distributed. Protein binding: 90%. Metabolized in liver. Eliminated primarily by biliary/fecal excretion. Not removed by hemodialysis. **Half-life:** adults 10–27 hrs, children 7–19 hrs.

C

USES

Prevents organ rejection of kidney, liver, heart in combination with steroid therapy. Treatment of chronic allograft rejection in those previously treated with other immunosuppressives. **Capsules/ Solution:** Treatment of severe, active rheumatoid arthritis, psoriasis. **Ophthalmic:** Chronic dry eyes. **Unlabeled:** Treatment of alopecia areata, aplastic anemia, atopic dermatitis, Behçet's disease, biliary cirrhosis, corneal transplantation.

PRECAUTIONS

CONTRAINDICATIONS: History of hypersensitivity to cyclosporine, polyoxyethylated castor oil. **CAUTIONS:** Impaired hepatic, renal, cardiac function; malabsorption syndrome; pregnancy; chickenpox; herpes zoster infection; hypokalemia. **Ophthalmic:** Active eye infection.

LIFESPAN CONSIDERATIONS: Pregnancy/lactation: Readily crosses placenta. Distributed in breast milk. Avoid nursing. **Pregnancy Category C. Children:** No age-related precautions noted in transplant patients. **Elderly:** Increased risk of hypertension, increased serum creatinine.

INTERACTIONS

DRUG: Cimetidine, danazol, diltiazem, erythromycin, ketoconazole may increase concentration, risk of hepatotoxicity, nephrotoxicity; **ACE inhibitors, potassium-sparing diuretics, potassium supplements** may cause hyperkalemia. **Immunosuppressants** may increase risk of infection, lymphoproliferative disorders. **Lovastatin** may increase risk of rhabdomyolysis, acute renal failure. **Live virus vaccines** may potentiate virus replication, increase vaccine side effects, decrease pt's antibody response to vaccine. **HERBAL: St. John's wort** may alter absorption. **FOOD: Grapefruit/grapefruit juice** may increase absorption, risk of toxicity.

LAB VALUES: May increase BUN, creatinine, SGOT (AST), SGPT (ALT), alkaline phosphatase, amylase, bilirubin, uric acid, potassium. May decrease magnesium. Therapeutic blood serum level: Peak: 50–300 ng/ml; toxic blood serum level: >400 ng/ml.

AVAILABILITY (Rx)

CAPSULES: 25 mg, 100 mg. **ORAL SOLUTION:** 100 mg/ml (in 50-ml calibrated liquid measuring device). **IV SOLUTION:** 50 mg/ml (5-ml amps). **OPHTHALMIC EMULSION:** 0.05%.

ADMINISTRATION/HANDLING

Alert: Oral solution available in bottle form with calibrated liquid measuring device. Oral form should replace IV administration as soon as possible.

PO

• Oral solution may be mixed in glass container with milk, chocolate milk, orange juice (preferably at room temperature). Stir well. Drink immediately. • Add more diluent to glass container. Mix with remaining solution to ensure total amount is given. • Dry outside of calibrated liquid measuring device before replacing in cover. Do not rinse with water. • Avoid refrigeration of oral solution (separation of solution may occur). Discard oral solution after 2 mos once bottle is opened.

IV

Storage • Store parenteral form at room temperature. • Protect IV solution from light. • After diluted, stable for 24 hrs.

Reconstitution • Dilute each ml concentrate with 20–100 ml 0.9% NaCl or D_5W.

Rate of administration • Infuse over 2–6 hrs. • Monitor pt continuously for first 30 min after instituting infusion and frequently thereafter for hypersensitivity reaction (facial flushing, dyspnea).

⊘ IV INCOMPATIBILITIES
Amphotericin B complex (AmBisome, Amphotec, Abelcet), magnesium.

IV COMPATIBILITY
Propofol (Diprivan).

INDICATIONS/ROUTES/DOSAGE

Alert: May be given with adrenal corticosteroids, but not with other immunosuppressive agents (increases susceptibility to infection, development of lymphoma).

PREVENTION OF ALLOGRAFT REJECTION
PO: ADULTS, ELDERLY, CHILDREN: Initially, 15 mg/kg as single dose 4–12 hrs prior to transplantation, continue daily dose of 10–14 mg/kg/day for 1–2 wks. Taper dose by 5%/wk over 6–8 wks. MAINTENANCE: 5–10 mg/kg/day.

IV: ADULTS, ELDERLY, CHILDREN: Give one third of oral dose: 5–6 mg/kg as single dose 4–12 hrs prior to transplantation, continue this daily single dose until pt is able to take oral medication.

PSORIASIS, RHEUMATOID ARTHRITIS
PO: ADULTS: 2.5 mg/kg daily in 2 divided doses.

DRY EYE
Ophthalmic: ADULTS, ELDERLY: Apply 2 times/day.

SIDE EFFECTS

FREQUENT: Mild to moderate hypertension (26%), increased hair growth (hirsutism) (21%), tremor (12%). **OCCASIONAL (2%–4%):** Acne, cramping, gingival hyperplasia (bleeding, tender gums), paresthesia, diarrhea, nausea, vomiting, headache. **RARE (<1%):** Hypersensitivity reaction, abdominal discomfort, gynecomastia, sinusitis.

ADVERSE REACTIONS/ TOXIC EFFECTS

Mild nephrotoxicity occurs in 25% of renal transplants after transplantation, 38% in cardiac transplants, and 37% of liver transplants. Hepatotoxicity occurs in 4% of renal, 7% of cardiac, and 4% of liver transplants. Both toxicities usually responsive to dosage reduction. Severe hyperkalemia, hyperuricemia occur occasionally.

NURSING IMPLICATIONS

BASELINE ASSESSMENT
If nephrotoxicity occurs, mild toxicity is generally noted 2–3 mos after transplantation; more severe toxicity noted early after transplantation; hepatotoxicity may be noted during first month after transplantation.

INTERVENTION/EVALUATION
Diligently monitor BUN, creatinine, bilirubin, SGOT (AST), SGPT (ALT), LDH blood serum levels for evidence of hepatotoxicity, nephrotoxicity (mild toxicity noted by slow rise in serum levels; more overt toxicity noted by rapid rise in levels; hematuria also noted in nephrotoxicity). Monitor potassium level for evidence of hyperkalemia. Encourage diligent oral hygiene (gum hyperplasia). Monitor B/P for evidence of hypertension. Therapeutic blood serum level: Peak: 50–300 ng/ml; toxic blood serum level: >400 ng/ml.

PATIENT/FAMILY TEACHING
Essential to repeat blood testing on a routine basis while receiving medication. Headache, tremor may occur as a response to medication. Avoid grapefruit, grapefruit juice (increases concentration, side effects).

cyproheptadine hydrochloride

sigh-pro-**hep**-tah-deen
(Pyrohep)

Do not confuse with cyclobenzaprine, Persantine.

CLASSIFICATION

PHARMACOTHERAPEUTIC: Phenothiazine. **CLINICAL:** Antihistamine (see p. 48C).

ACTION

Competes with histamine for H_1-receptor sites on effector cells in the GI tract, blood vessels, and respiratory tract. **Therapeutic Effect:** Relieves allergic conditions (urticaria, pruritus).

USES

Relief of nasal allergies, allergic dermatitis, urticaria, hypersensitivity reactions. **Unlabeled:** Stimulates appetite in underweight pts, those with anorexia nervosa. Treatment of vascular cluster headaches.

PRECAUTIONS

CONTRAINDICATIONS: Exacerbation of asthma, pts receiving MAOIs. **CAUTIONS:** Narrow-angle glaucoma, peptic ulcer, prostatic hypertrophy, pyloroduodenal or bladder neck obstruction, asthma, COPD, increased intraocular pressure, cardiovascular disease, hyperthyroidism, hypertension, seizure disorders. **Pregnancy Category B.**

INTERACTIONS

DRUG: **Alcohol, CNS depressants** may increase CNS depressant effects. **MAOIs** may increase anticholinergic, CNS depressant effects. **HERBAL:** None known. **FOOD:** None known. **LAB VALUES:** May suppress wheal, flare reactions to antigen skin testing, unless antihistamines discontinued 4 days prior to testing.

AVAILABILITY (Rx)

TABLETS: 4 mg. **SYRUP:** 2 mg/5 ml.

ADMINISTRATION/HANDLING

PO

- Give without regard to meals.
- Scored tablets may be crushed.

INDICATIONS/ROUTES/DOSAGE

ALLERGIC CONDITION

PO: ADULTS, CHILDREN ≥15 YRS: 4 mg 3 times/day. May increase dosage but do not exceed 0.5 mg/kg/day. CHILDREN 7–14 YRS: 4 mg 2–3 times/day, or 0.25 mg/kg daily in divided doses. CHILDREN 2–6 YRS: 2 mg 2–3 times/day, or 0.25 mg/kg daily in divided doses.

USUAL ELDERLY DOSAGE

PO: Initially, 4 mg 2 times/day.

Alert: Reduce dosage in pts with severe liver impairment.

SIDE EFFECTS

FREQUENT: Drowsiness, dizziness, muscular weakness, dry mouth/nose/throat/lips, urinary retention, thickening of bronchial secretions. Sedation, dizziness, hypotension more likely noted in elderly. **OCCASIONAL:** Epigastric distress, flushing of skin, visual disturbances, hearing disturbances, paresthesia, sweating, chills.

ADVERSE REACTIONS/ TOXIC EFFECTS

Children may experience dominant paradoxical reaction (restlessness, insomnia, euphoria, nervousness, tremors). Overdosage in children may result in hallucinations, convulsions, death. Hypersensitivity reaction (eczema, pruritus, rash, cardiac disturbances, angioedema, photosensitivity) may occur. Overdosage may vary from CNS depression (sedation, ap-

C

nea, cardiovascular collapse, death) to severe paradoxical reaction (hallucinations, tremor, seizures).

NURSING IMPLICATIONS

BASELINE ASSESSMENT

If pt is experiencing allergic reaction, obtain history of recently ingested foods, drugs, environmental exposure, recent emotional stress.

INTERVENTION/EVALUATION

Monitor B/P, esp. in elderly (increased risk of hypotension). Monitor children closely for paradoxical reaction.

PATIENT/FAMILY TEACHING

Tolerance to antihistaminic effect generally does not occur; tolerance to sedative effect may occur. Avoid tasks that require alertness, motor skills until response to drug is established. Dry mouth, drowsiness, dizziness may be an expected response of drug. Avoid alcoholic beverages during antihistamine therapy.

cytarabine

sigh-**tar**-ah-bean
(Ara-C, Cytosar, Cytosar-U)

Do not confuse with Cytadren, Cytovene, vidarabine.

CLASSIFICATION

PHARMACOTHERAPEUTIC: Antimetabolite. **CLINICAL:** Antineoplastic (see p. 71C).

ACTION

Converted intracellularly to nucleotide. Cell cycle–specific for S phase of cell division. Potent immunosuppressive activity. **Therapeutic Effect:** Appears to inhibit DNA synthesis.

PHARMACOKINETICS

Widely distributed; moderate amount crosses blood-brain barrier. Protein binding: 15%. Primarily excreted in urine. **Half-life:** 1–3 hrs.

USES

Treatment of acute and chronic myelocytic leukemia, acute lymphocytic leukemia, meningeal leukemia, non-Hodgkin's lymphoma in children. **Unlabeled:** Treatment of Hodgkin's lymphoma, myelodysplastic syndrome.

PRECAUTIONS

CONTRAINDICATIONS: None known. **CAUTIONS:** Impaired hepatic function.

LIFESPAN CONSIDERATIONS: Pregnancy/lactation: If possible, avoid use during pregnancy. May cause fetal malformations. Unknown if distributed in breast milk. Breast-feeding not recommended. **Pregnancy Category D. Children:** No age-related precautions noted. **Elderly:** Age-related renal impairment may require dosage adjustment.

INTERACTIONS

DRUG: May decrease effect of **antigout medications. Bone marrow depressants** may increase bone marrow depression. **Cyclophosphamide** may increase cardiomyopathy risk. **Live virus vaccines** may potentiate virus replication, increase vaccine side effects, decrease pt's antibody response to vaccine. **HERBAL:** None known. **FOOD:** None known. **LAB VALUES:** May increase SGOT (AST), bilirubin, alkaline phosphatase, uric acid.

AVAILABILITY (Rx)

POWDER FOR INJECTION: 100 mg, 1 g, 2 g.

C

ADMINISTRATION/HANDLING

Alert: May give by subcutaneous, IV push, IV infusion, or intrathecal routes. May be carcinogenic, mutagenic, or teratogenic (embryonic deformity). Handle with extreme care during preparation/administration.

SUBCUTANEOUS, IV, INTRATHECAL

Storage • Reconstituted solution is stable for 48 hrs at room temperature. • IV infusion solutions at concentration up to 0.5 mg/ml is stable for 7 days at room temperature. • Discard if slight haze develops.

Reconstitution • Reconstitute 100-mg vial with 5 ml Bacteriostatic Water for Injection with benzyl alcohol (10 ml for 500 mg vial) to provide concentration of 20 mg/ml and 50 mg/ml, respectively. • Dose may be further diluted with up to 1,000 ml D_5W or 0.9% NaCl for IV infusion. • For intrathecal use, reconstitute vial with preservative-free 0.9% NaCl or pt's spinal fluid. Dose usually administered in 5–15 ml of solution, after equivalent volume of CSF removed.

Rate of administration • For IV push, give over 1–3 min. • For IV infusion, give over 30 min to 24 hrs.

⊘ IV INCOMPATIBILITIES

Amphotericin B complex (AmBisome, Amphotec, Abelcet), ganciclovir (Cytovene), heparin, insulin (Regular).

IV COMPATIBILITIES

Dexamethasone (Decadron), diphenhydramine (Benadryl), filgrastim (Neupogen), granisetron (Kytril), heparin, hydromorphone (Dilaudid), lorazepam (Ativan), morphine, ondansetron (Zofran), potassium chloride, propofol (Diprivan).

INDICATIONS/ROUTES/DOSAGE

Alert: Dosage individualized based on clinical response, tolerance to adverse effects. When used in combination therapy, consult specific protocols for optimum dosage, sequence of drug administration. Modify dosage when serious hematologic depression occurs.

INDUCTION REMISSION

IV: ADULTS, ELDERLY, CHILDREN: 200 mg/m^2/day for 5 days at 2-wk intervals as a single agent. 100–200 mg/m^2/day for 5- to 10-day therapy course every 2–4 wks in combination therapy.

Intrathecal: ADULTS, ELDERLY, CHILDREN: 5–7.5 mg/m^2 q2–7days.

MAINTENANCE REMISSION

IV: ADULTS, ELDERLY, CHILDREN: 70–200 mg/m^2/day for 2–5 days every month.

IM, subcutaneous: ADULTS, ELDERLY, CHILDREN: 1–1.5 mg/m^2 as single dose at 1- to 4-wk intervals.

Intrathecal: ADULTS, ELDERLY, CHILDREN: 5–7.5 mg/m^2 q2–7days.

SIDE EFFECTS

FREQUENT: Subcutaneous, IV (16%–33%): Asthenia, fever, pain, change in taste/smell, nausea, vomiting (risk of nausea and vomiting greater with IV push than with continuous IV infusion). **Intrathecal (11%–28%):** Headache, asthenia, change in taste/smell, confusion, somnolence, nausea, vomiting. **OCCASIONAL: Subcutaneous, IV (7%–11%):** Abnormal gait, somnolence, constipation, back pain, urinary incontinence, peripheral edema, headache, confusion. **Intrathecal (3%–7%):** Peripheral edema, back pain, constipation, abnormal gait, urinary incontinence.

ADVERSE REACTIONS/ TOXIC EFFECTS

Major toxic effect is bone marrow depression resulting in blood dyscrasias (leukopenia, anemia, thrombocytopenia, megaloblastosis, reticulocytopenia), occurring minimally after single IV dose, but leukopenia, anemia, thrombocytopenia should be expected with daily or continuous IV therapy. Cytarabine syndrome (fever, myalgia, rash, conjunctivitis, malaise, chest pain), hyperuricemia may be noted. High-dose therapy may produce severe CNS, GI, pulmonary toxicity.

NURSING IMPLICATIONS

BASELINE ASSESSMENT

Leukocyte count decreases within 24 hrs after initial dose, continues to decrease for 7–9 days followed by brief rise at 12 days, decreases again at 15–24 days, then rises rapidly for next 10 days. Platelet count decreases 5 days after drug initiation to its lowest count at 12–15 days, then rises rapidly for next 10 days.

INTERVENTION/EVALUATION

Monitor CBC for evidence of bone marrow depression. Monitor for blood dyscrasias (fever, sore throat, signs of local infection, easy bruising, unusual bleeding from any site), symptoms of anemia (excessive tiredness, weakness). Monitor for signs of neuropathy (gait disturbances, handwriting difficulties, numbness).

PATIENT/FAMILY TEACHING

Increase fluid intake (may protect against hyperuricemia). Do not have immunizations without physician's approval (drug lowers body's resistance). Avoid contact with those who have recently received live virus vaccine. Promptly report fever, sore throat, signs of local infection, easy bruising, unusual bleeding from any site.

dacarbazine

day-**car**-bah-zeen
(DTIC ♣ DTIC-Dome)

Do not confuse with Dicarbosil, procarbazine.

◆CLASSIFICATION

PHARMACOTHERAPEUTIC: Alkylating agent. **CLINICAL:** Antineoplastic (see p. 71C).

ACTION

Forms methyldiazonium ions, which attack nucleophilic groups in DNA. Cross-links DNA strands. **Therapeutic Effect:** Inhibits DNA, RNA, protein synthesis.

PHARMACOKINETICS

Minimally crosses blood-brain barrier. Protein binding: 5%. Metabolized in liver. Excreted in urine. **Half-life:** 5 hrs (half-life increased with impaired renal function).

USES

Treatment of metastatic malignant melanoma, second-line therapy of Hodgkin's disease. **Unlabeled:** Treatment of soft tissue sarcoma, islet cell carcinoma, neuroblastoma.

PRECAUTIONS

CONTRAINDICATIONS: Demonstrated hypersensitivity to drug. **CAUTIONS:** Impaired hepatic function.

LIFESPAN CONSIDERATIONS: Pregnancy/lactation: If possible, avoid use during pregnancy, esp. first trimester. Breast-feeding not recommended. **Pregnancy Category C. Children:** Safety and efficacy not established. **Elderly:** Age-related renal impairment may require dosage adjustment.

INTERACTIONS

DRUG: Bone marrow depressants may enhance myelosuppression. **Live virus vaccines** may potentiate virus replication, increase vaccine side effects, decrease pt's antibody response to vaccine. **HERBAL:** None known. **FOOD:** None known. **LAB VALUES:** May increase SGOT (AST), SGPT (ALT), alkaline phosphatase, BUN.

AVAILABILITY (Rx)

POWDER FOR INJECTION: 100-mg, 200-mg vials.

ADMINISTRATION/HANDLING

Alert: May give by IV push or IV infusion. May be carcinogenic, mutagenic, or teratogenic. Handle with extreme care during preparation/administration.

IV

Storage • Protect from light; refrigerate vials. • Color change from ivory to pink indicates decomposition; discard. • Solution containing 10 mg/ml is stable for 8 hrs at room temperature or 72 hrs if refrigerated. • Solution diluted with up to 500 ml D_5W or 0.9% NaCl is stable for at least 8 hrs at room temperature or 24 hrs if refrigerated.

Reconstitution • Reconstitute 100-mg vial with 9.9 ml Sterile Water for Injection (19.7 ml for 200-mg vial) to provide concentration of 10 mg/ml.

Rate of administration • Give IV push over 2–3 min. • For IV infusion, further dilute with up to 250 ml D_5W or 0.9% NaCl. Infuse over 15–30 min. • Apply hot packs if local pain, burning sensation, irritation at injection site occurs. • Avoid extravasation (stinging, swelling, coolness, slight or no blood return at injection site).

IV INCOMPATIBILITIES
Allopurinol (Aloprim), cefepime (Maxipime), heparin, piperacillin/tazobactam (Zosyn).

IV COMPATIBILITIES
Etoposide (VePesid), granisetron (Kytril), ondansetron (Zofran), paclitaxel (Taxol).

INDICATIONS/ROUTES/DOSAGE

Alert: Dosage individualized based on clinical response, tolerance to adverse effects. When used in combination therapy, consult specific protocols for optimum dosage, sequence of drug administration.

MALIGNANT MELANOMA
IV: ADULTS, ELDERLY: 2–4.5 mg/kg/day for 10 days, repeated at 4-wk intervals, or 250 mg/m^2 daily for 5 days, repeated q3wks.

HODGKIN'S DISEASE
IV: ADULTS, ELDERLY: Combination therapy: 150 mg/m^2 daily for 5 days, repeated q4wks, or 375 mg/m^2 once, repeated q15days. CHILDREN: 375 mg/m^2 on days 1 and 15; repeat q28days.

SOLID TUMORS
IV: CHILDREN: 200–470 mg/m^2/day over 5 days q21–28days.

NEUROBLASTOMA
IV: CHILDREN: 800–900 mg/m^2 as single dose on day 1 of therapy q3–4wks in combination therapy.

SIDE EFFECTS

FREQUENT (90%): Nausea, vomiting, anorexia (occurs within 1 hr of initial dose, may last up to 12 hrs). **OCCASIONAL:** Facial flushing, paresthesia, alopecia, flulike syndrome (fever, myalgia, malaise), dermatologic reactions, CNS symptoms (confusion, blurred vision, headache, lethargy). **RARE:** Diarrhea, stomatitis (redness/burning of oral mucous membranes, gum/tongue inflammation), photosensitivity.

ADVERSE REACTIONS/ TOXIC EFFECTS

Bone marrow depression resulting in blood dyscrasias (leukopenia, thrombocytopenia) generally appears 2–4 wks after last drug dose. Hepatotoxicity occurs rarely.

NURSING IMPLICATIONS

BASELINE ASSESSMENT

Some clinicians recommend food/fluids be restricted 4–6 hrs before treatment; other clinicians believe good hydration to within 1 hr of treatment will avoid dehydration due to vomiting. Conflicting reports of effectiveness of administering antiemetics for nausea, vomiting.

INTERVENTION/EVALUATION

Monitor leukocyte, erythrocyte, platelet counts for evidence of bone marrow depression. Monitor for hematologic toxicity (fever, sore throat, signs of local infection, unusual bleeding/bruising from any site).

PATIENT/FAMILY TEACHING

Tolerance to GI effects occurs rapidly (generally after 1–2 days of treatment). Do not have immunizations without physician's approval (drug lowers body's resistance). Avoid contact with those who have recently received live virus vaccine. Promptly report fever, sore throat, signs of local infection, unusual bleeding/bruising from any site. Notify physician for persistent nausea, vomiting.

daclizumab

day-**cly**-zu-mab
(Zenapax)

CLASSIFICATION

PHARMACOTHERAPEUTIC: Monoclonal antibody. **CLINICAL:** Immunosuppressive (see p. 102C).

ACTION

Binds to and inhibits interleukin-2–mediated lymphocyte activation (critical pathway in cellular immune response involved in allograft rejection). **Therapeutic Effect:** Prevents organ rejection.

PHARMACOKINETICS

Half-life: 20 days (adults).

USES

Prophylaxis of acute organ rejection in pts receiving renal transplants (in combination with an immunosuppressive regimen). **Unlabeled:** Graft-vs-host disease.

PRECAUTIONS

CONTRAINDICATIONS: None known. **CAUTIONS:** Infection, history of malignancy.

LIFESPAN CONSIDERATIONS: Pregnancy/lactation: Unknown if crosses placenta or is distributed in breast milk. **Pregnancy Category C. Children/elderly:** No age-related precautions noted.

INTERACTIONS

DRUG: None known. **HERBAL:** None known. **FOOD:** None known. **LAB VALUES:** None known.

AVAILABILITY (Rx)

INJECTION: 25 mg/5 ml.

ADMINISTRATION/HANDLING

IV

Storage • Protect from light; refrigerate vials. • Once reconstituted, stable for 4 hrs at room temperature, 24 hrs if refrigerated.

Reconstitution • Dilute in 50 ml 0.9% NaCl. • Invert gently. • Avoid shaking.

Rate of administration • Infuse over 15 min.

⊘ **IV INCOMPATIBILITY**
Do not mix with any other medication.

INDICATIONS/ROUTES/DOSAGE

IV: ADULTS, CHILDREN: 1 mg/kg over 15 min. First dose no more than 24 hrs before transplantation, then q14days for total of 5 doses. **Maximum:** 100 mg.

SIDE EFFECTS

OCCASIONAL (>2%): Constipation, nausea, diarrhea, vomiting, abdominal pain, edema, headache, dizziness, fever, pain, fatigue, insomnia, weakness, arthralgia, myalgia, increased sweating.

ADVERSE REACTIONS/ TOXIC EFFECTS

None known.

NURSING IMPLICATIONS

BASELINE ASSESSMENT

Obtain baseline blood serum levels, vital signs, particularly B/P, pulse.

INTERVENTION/EVALUATION

Diligently monitor all blood serum levels, CBC. Assess B/P for hypertension/hypotension; pulse for evidence of tachycardia. Question for GI disturbances, urinary changes. Monitor for presence of wound infection, signs of systemic infection (fever, sore throat), unusual bleeding/bruising.

PATIENT/FAMILY TEACHING

Report difficulty in breathing or swallowing, tachycardia, rash, itching/swelling of lower extremities, weakness. Avoid pregnancy.

Dalmane

see flurazepam

dalteparin sodium

dawl-teh-pear-in
(Fragmin)

CLASSIFICATION

PHARMACOTHERAPEUTIC: Low-molecular-weight heparin. **CLINICAL:** Anticoagulant (see p. 28C).

ACTION

Antithrombin, in presence of low-molecular-weight heparin, inhibits factor Xa and thrombin. Only slightly influences platelet aggregation, prothrombin time (PT), activated partial thromboplastin time (aPTT). **Therapeutic Effect:** Produces anticoagulation.

PHARMACOKINETICS

	Onset	Peak	Duration
Subcutaneous	—	4 hrs	—

Protein binding: <10%. **Half-life:** 3–5 hrs.

USES

Treatment of unstable angina and non–Q-wave MI to prevent ischemic events. Prevention of deep vein thrombosis (DVT) in pts undergoing hip replacement or abdominal surgery who are at risk of thromboembolic complications. Those at risk are >40 yrs, obese, undergoing surgery under general anesthesia lasting >30 min, malignancy or history of DVT or pulmonary embolism.

PRECAUTIONS

CONTRAINDICATIONS: Active major bleeding, concurrent heparin therapy, thrombocytopenia associated with positive in vitro test for antiplatelet antibody, hypersensitivity to dalteparin, heparin, pork products. **CAUTIONS:** Conditions with increased risk of hemorrhage, bacterial endocarditis, history of heparin-induced thrombocytopenia, impaired renal/hepatic function, uncontrolled arterial hypertension, history of recent GI ulceration/hemorrhage, hypertensive or diabetic retinopathy.

D

LIFESPAN CONSIDERATIONS: Pregnancy/lactation: Use with caution, particularly during last trimester, immediate postpartum period (increased risk of maternal hemorrhage). Unknown if distributed in breast milk. **Pregnancy Category B. Children:** Safety and efficacy not established. **Elderly:** No age-related precautions noted.

INTERACTIONS

DRUG: Anticoagulants, platelet inhibitors may increase risk of bleeding. **HERBAL:** None known. **FOOD:** None known. **LAB VALUES:** Reversible increases in SGOT (AST), SGPT (ALT), alkaline phosphatase, LDH.

AVAILABILITY (Rx)

SYRINGE: 2,500 international units, 5,000 international units, 7,500 international units, 10,000 international units, 25,000 international units/ml. **VIAL:** 95,000 international units (10,000 international units/ml).

ADMINISTRATION/HANDLING

SUBCUTANEOUS

• Store at room temperature. • Instruct pt to sit/lie down before administering by deep subcutaneous injection. • Inject in U-shaped area around the navel, upper outer side of thigh, upper outer quadrangle of buttock. • Use a fine needle (25–26 gauge) to minimize tissue trauma. • Introduce entire length of needle (½ inch) into skin fold held between thumb and forefinger, holding needle during injection at a 45° to 90° angle. • Do not rub injection site after administration (prevents bruising). • Alternate the administration site with each injection.

INDICATIONS/ROUTES/DOSAGE

LOW- TO MODERATE-RISK ABDOMINAL SURGERY

Subcutaneous: ADULTS, ELDERLY: 2,500 international units 1–2 hrs before surgery, then daily for 5–10 days.

HIGH-RISK ABDOMINAL SURGERY

Subcutaneous: ADULTS, ELDERLY: 5,000 international units 1–2 hrs before surgery, then daily for 5–10 days.

TOTAL HIP SURGERY

Subcutaneous: ADULTS, ELDERLY: 2,500 international units 1–2 hrs before surgery, then 2,500 international units 6 hrs after surgery, then 5,000 international units/day for 7–10 days.

TREATMENT UNSTABLE ANGINA, NON–Q-WAVE MI

Subcutaneous: ADULTS, ELDERLY: 120 international units/kg q12h (**Maximum:** 10,000 international units/dose) with concurrent aspirin until clinically stable.

SIDE EFFECTS

OCCASIONAL (3%–7%): Hematoma at injection site. **RARE (<1%):** Hypersensitivity reaction (chills, fever, pruritus, urticaria, asthma, rhinitis, lacrimation, headache); mild, local skin irritation.

ADVERSE REACTIONS/ TOXIC EFFECTS

Accidental overdosage may lead to bleeding complications ranging from local ecchymoses to major hemorrhage. Thrombocytopenia occurs rarely.

NURSING IMPLICATIONS

BASELINE ASSESSMENT

Assess CBC, including platelet count. Determine initial B/P.

INTERVENTION/EVALUATION

Periodically monitor CBC, platelet count, stool for occult blood (no need for daily monitoring in pts with normal presurgical coagulation parameters). Assess for any sign of bleeding: bleeding at surgical site, hematuria, blood in stool, bleeding from gums, petechiae, bruising/bleeding from injection sites.

PATIENT/FAMILY TEACHING

Usual length of therapy is 5–10 days. Report any sign of bleeding. Do not take any OTC medication (esp. aspirin) without consulting physician. Report bleeding, bruising, dizziness/lightheadedness, rash, itching, fever, swelling, breathing difficulty. Rotate injection sites daily. Teach proper injection technique. Excessive bruising at injection site may be lessened by ice massage before injection.

danazol

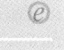

dan-ah-zole
(Cyclomen ✤, Danocrine)

CLASSIFICATION

PHARMACOTHERAPEUTIC: Testosterone derivative. **CLINICAL:** Androgen, hormone.

ACTION

Suppresses the pituitary-ovarian axis by inhibiting the output of pituitary gonadotropins. In endometriosis, causes atrophy of both normal and ectopic endometrial tissue. For fibrocystic breast disease, FSH and LH are depressed. Inhibits steroid synthesis and binding of steroids to their receptors in breast tissue. Increases serum levels of esterase inhibitor. **Therapeutic Effect:** Produces anovulation, amenorrhea. Reduces production of estrogen. Corrects biochemical deficiency as seen in hereditary angioedema.

USES

Palliative treatment of endometriosis, fibrocystic breast disease; prophylactic treatment of hereditary angioedema. **Unlabeled:** Treatment of gynecomastia, menorrhagia, precocious puberty.

PRECAUTIONS

CONTRAINDICATIONS: Severe cardiac/liver/renal function impairment. Active or history of thromboembolic disease, androgen tumor, abnormal vaginal bleeding. **CAUTIONS:** Renal function impairment, cardiac impairment, epilepsy, migraine headaches, diabetes. **Pregnancy Category X.**

INTERACTIONS

DRUG: May enhance effects of **anticoagulants.** May increase nephrotoxicity with **cyclosporine, tacrolimus. HERBAL:** None known. **FOOD:** None known. **LAB VALUES:** May increase liver function values.

AVAILABILITY (Rx)

CAPSULES: 50 mg, 100 mg, 200 mg.

INDICATIONS/ROUTES/DOSAGE

Alert: Initiate therapy during menstruation or when pt is not pregnant.

ENDOMETRIOSIS

PO: ADULTS: 200–800 mg/day in 2 divided doses for 3–9 mos.

FIBROCYSTIC BREAST DISEASE

PO: ADULTS: 100–400 mg/day in 2 divided doses.

HEREDITARY ANGIOEDEMA

PO: ADULTS: Initially, 200 mg 2–3 times/day. Decrease dosage by 50% or less at 1- to 3-mo intervals. If attack occurs, increase dosage by up to 200 mg/day.

D

SIDE EFFECTS

FREQUENT: Females: Amenorrhea, breakthrough bleeding/spotting, decreased breast size, increased weight, irregular menstrual period. **OCCASIONAL: Males/females:** Edema, rhabdomyolysis (muscle cramps, unusual fatigue), virilism (acne, oily skin), flushed skin, altered moods. **RARE: Males/females:** Hematuria, gingivitis, carpal tunnel syndrome, cataracts, severe headache, vomiting, rash, photosensitivity. **Females:** Enlarged clitoris, hoarseness, deepening voice, hair growth, monilial vaginitis. **Males:** Decreased testicle size.

ADVERSE REACTIONS/ TOXIC EFFECTS

Jaundice may occur in those receiving ≥400 mg/day. Liver dysfunction, eosinophilia, thrombocytopenia, pancreatitis occur rarely.

NURSING IMPLICATIONS

BASELINE ASSESSMENT

Inquire about menstrual cycle: Therapy should begin during menstruation. Establish baseline weight, B/P.

INTERVENTION/EVALUATION

Weigh 2–3 times/wk; report >5 lbs/wk gain or swelling of fingers/feet. Monitor B/P periodically. Check for jaundice (yellow sclera/skin, dark urine, clay-colored stools).

PATIENT/FAMILY TEACHING

Patient should use nonhormonal contraceptive during therapy. Do not take drug, check with physician if suspect pregnancy (risk to fetus). Stress importance of full length of therapy, regular visits to physician's office (hepatic function tests, CBC, amylase, lipase). Notify physician promptly of masculinizing effects (may not be reversible), weight gain, muscle cramps, fatigue. Spotting/bleeding may occur in first months of therapy for endometriosis (does not mean lack of efficacy). In fibrocystic breast disease, irregular menstrual periods and amenorrhea may occur with or without ovulation.

dantrolene sodium

dan-trow-lean

(Dantrium)

Do not confuse with Daraprim.

◆ CLASSIFICATION

CLINICAL: Skeletal muscle relaxant.

ACTION

Reduces muscle contraction by interfering with release of calcium ion. Reduces calcium ion concentration. **Therapeutic Effect:** Dissociates excitation-contraction coupling. Interferes with catabolic process associated with malignant hyperthermic crisis.

PHARMACOKINETICS

Poorly absorbed from GI tract. Protein binding: High. Metabolized in liver. Primarily excreted in urine. **Half-life:** IV: 4–8 hrs; PO: 8.7 hrs.

USES

PO: Relief of symptoms of spasticity due to spinal cord injuries, stroke, cerebral palsy, multiple sclerosis, esp. flexor spasms, concomitant pain, clonus, muscular rigidity. **Parenteral:** Management of fulminant hypermetabolism of skeletal muscle due to malignant hyperthermia crisis. **Unlabeled:** Treatment of neuroleptic malignant syndrome, relief of exercise-induced pain in pts with muscular dystrophy, treatment of flexor spasms.

PRECAUTIONS

CONTRAINDICATIONS: Active hepatic disease. **CAUTIONS:** Impaired cardiac/pulmonary function, history of previous liver disease.

LIFESPAN CONSIDERATIONS: Pregnancy/lactation: Readily crosses placenta. Do not use in breast-feeding mothers. **Pregnancy Category C. Children:** No age-related precautions noted in those >5 yrs. **Elderly:** No information available.

INTERACTIONS

DRUG: CNS depressants may increase CNS depression (short-term use). **Hepatotoxic medications** may increase risk of hepatotoxicity (chronic use). **HERBAL:** None known. **FOOD:** None known. **LAB VALUES:** May alter liver function tests.

AVAILABILITY (Rx)

CAPSULES: 25 mg, 50 mg, 100 mg. **POWDER FOR INJECTION:** 20-mg vial.

ADMINISTRATION/HANDLING

PO

- Give without regard to meals.

IV

Storage • Store at room temperature. • Use within 6 hrs after reconstitution. Solution is clear, colorless. Discard if cloudy, precipitate formed.

Reconstitution • Reconstitute 20-mg vial with 60 ml Sterile Water for Injection to provide concentration of 0.33 mg/ml.

Rate of administration • For IV infusion, administer over 1 hr. • Diligently monitor for extravasation (high pH of IV preparation). May produce severe complications.

IV INCOMPATIBILITY

None known.

INDICATIONS/ROUTES/DOSAGE

SPASTICITY

Alert: Begin with low-dose therapy, then increase gradually at 4- to 7-day intervals (reduces incidence of side effects).

PO: ADULTS, ELDERLY: Initially, 25 mg/day. Increase to 25 mg 2–4 times/day, then by 25-mg increments up to 100 mg 2–4 times/day. CHILDREN >5 YRS: Initially, 0.5 mg/kg 2 times/day. Increase to 0.5 mg/kg 3–4 times/day, then increase by 0.5 mg/kg/day up to 3 mg/kg 2–4 times/day. **Maximum:** 400 mg/day.

PREVENTION OF MALIGNANT HYPERTHERMIA CRISIS

PO: ADULTS, ELDERLY, CHILDREN: 4–8 mg/kg/day in 3–4 divided doses 1–2 days before surgery (give last dose 3–4 hrs before surgery).

IV infusion: ADULTS, ELDERLY, CHILDREN: 2.5 mg/kg about 1.25 hrs before surgery.

MANAGEMENT OF MALIGNANT HYPERTHERMIA CRISIS

IV: ADULTS, ELDERLY, CHILDREN: Initially (minimum), 1 mg/kg rapid IV; may repeat up to total maximum dose of 10 mg/kg. May follow with 4–8 mg/kg/day PO in 4 divided doses up to 3 days after crisis.

SIDE EFFECTS

FREQUENT: Drowsiness, dizziness, weakness, general malaise, diarrhea (may be severe). **OCCASIONAL:** Confusion, headache, insomnia, constipation, urinary frequency. **RARE:** Paradoxical CNS excitement/restlessness, paresthesia, tinnitus, slurred speech, tremor, blurred vision, dry mouth, diarrhea, nocturia, impotence.

ADVERSE REACTIONS/ TOXIC EFFECTS

Risk of hepatotoxicity, most notably in females, those >35 yrs, those taking other medications concurrently. Overt hepatitis noted most frequently between 3rd and 12th mo of therapy. Overdosage results in vomiting, muscular hypotonia, muscle twitching, respiratory depression, seizures.

D

NURSING IMPLICATIONS

BASELINE ASSESSMENT

Obtain baseline liver function tests (SGOT [AST], SGPT [ALT], alkaline phosphatase, total bilirubin). Record onset, type, location, duration of muscular spasm. Check for immobility, stiffness, swelling.

INTERVENTION/EVALUATION

Assist with ambulation. For those on long-term therapy, liver/renal function tests, blood counts should be performed periodically. Evaluate for therapeutic response: decreased intensity of skeletal muscle pain, spasm.

PATIENT/FAMILY TEACHING

Drowsiness usually diminishes with continued therapy. Avoid tasks that require alertness, motor skills until response to drug is established. Avoid alcohol/other depressants while taking medication. Report continued weakness, fatigue, nausea, diarrhea, skin rash, itching, bloody/tarry stools.

daptomycin

dap-toe-my-sin
(Cubicin)

CLASSIFICATION

PHARMACOTHERAPEUTIC: Lipopeptide antibacterial agent. **CLINICAL:** Antibiotic

ACTION

Binds to bacterial membranes and causes rapid depolarization of membrane potential. **Therapeutic Effect:** Inhibits protein synthesis, resulting in bacterial cell death.

PHARMACOKINETICS

Widely distributed. Protein binding: 90%. Primarily excreted unchanged in urine. Moderately removed by hemodialysis. **Half-life:** 7–8 hrs (half-life increased with impaired renal function).

USES

Treatment of complicated skin/skin structure infections caused by susceptible strains of gram-positive pathogens, including penicillin-resistant *Streptococcus pneumoniae,* methicillin-resistant *Staphyloccus aureus,* vancomycin-resistant enterococci.

PRECAUTIONS

CONTRAINDICATIONS: None known. **CAUTIONS:** Renal impairment, history of or current musculoskeletal disorders (risk of exacerbation), pregnancy.

LIFESPAN CONSIDERATIONS: Pregnancy/Lactation: Unknown if distributed in breast milk. **Pregnancy Category B. Children:** Safety and efficacy not established <18 yrs. **Elderly:** No age-related precautions noted.

INTERACTIONS

DRUG: Tobramycin increases serum concentration of **daptomycin.** Discontinue concurrent use with **HMG-CoA reductase inhibitors** (may cause myopathy). **HERBAL:** None known. **FOOD:** None known. **LAB VALUES:** May increase CPK levels. May alter liver function tests.

AVAILABILITY (Rx)

POWDER FOR INJECTION: 250-mg vial, 500-mg vial.

ADMINISTRATION/HANDLING

IV

Storage • Refrigerate. • Appears as pale yellow to light brown lyophilized cake. • Reconstituted solution is stable for 12 hrs at room temperature or up to 48 hrs if refrigerated. • Inspect for particulate matter.

Reconstitution • Reconstitute 250-mg vial with 5 ml 0.9% NaCl; reconstitute 500-mg vial with 10 ml 0.9% NaCl. Further dilute in 50 ml 0.9% NaCl.

Rate of administration • For intermittent IV infusion (piggyback), infuse over 30 min.

∅ IV INCOMPATIBILITIES

Incompatible with dextrose-containing diluents. If same IV line is used to administer different drugs, flush line with 0.9% NaCl.

INDICATIONS/ROUTES/DOSAGE

COMPLICATED SKIN/SKIN STRUCTURE INFECTIONS

IV infusion: ADULTS, ELDERLY: 4 mg/kg q24h for 7–14 days.

SEVERE RENAL FUNCTION IMPAIRMENT (creatinine clearance <30 ml/min)

IV infusion: ADULTS, ELDERLY: 4 mg/kg q48h for 7–14 days.

SIDE EFFECTS

FREQUENT (5%–6%): Constipation, nausea, peripheral injection site reactions, headache, diarrhea. **OCCASIONAL (3%–4%):** Insomnia, rash, vomiting. **RARE: (<2%–3%):** Pruritus, dizziness, hypotension.

ADVERSE REACTIONS/ TOXIC EFFECTS

Skeletal muscle myopathy characterized by muscle pain/weakness, particularly of the distal extremities, occurs rarely. Antibiotic-associated colitis (severe abdominal pain/tenderness; fever; watery/severe diarrhea) may result from altered bacterial balance.

NURSING IMPLICATIONS

BASELINE ASSESSMENT

Obtain culture/sensitivity test before first dose (therapy may begin before results are known).

INTERVENTION/EVALUATION:

Assess mouth for white patches on mucous membranes, tongue. Monitor bowel activity/stool consistency carefully; mild GI effects may be tolerable, but increasing severity may indicate onset of antibiotic-associated colitis. Be alert for superinfection: severe genital/anal pruritus, abdominal pain, severe mouth soreness, moderate to severe diarrhea. Monitor for dizziness, institute appropriate measures.

PATIENT/FAMILY TEACHING

Report rash, headache, nausea, any new symptom.

darbepoetin alfa

dar-bee-eh-poe-**ee**-tin alfa
(Aranesp)
Do not confuse with Aricept.

CLASSIFICATION

PHARMACOTHERAPEUTIC: Glycoprotein. **CLINICAL:** Hematopoietic.

ACTION

Stimulates formation of RBCs in bone marrow; increases serum half-life of epoetin. **Therapeutic Effect:** Induces erythropoiesis, release of reticulocytes from marrow.

PHARMACOKINETICS

Well absorbed after subcutaneous administration. **Half-life:** 48.5 hrs.

USES

Treatment of anemia associated with chronic renal failure. Treatment of chemotherapy-induced anemia.

D

PRECAUTIONS

CONTRAINDICATIONS: Uncontrolled hypertension, history of sensitivity to mammalian cell-derived products or human albumin. **CAUTIONS:** Pts with known porphyria (impairment of erythrocyte formation in bone marrow or responsible for liver impairment), hemolytic anemia, sickle cell anemia, thalassemia, history of seizures.

LIFESPAN CONSIDERATIONS: Pregnancy/lactation: Unknown if drug crosses placenta or is distributed in breast milk. **Pregnancy Category C. Children:** Safety and efficacy not established. **Elderly:** Age-related renal impairment may require dosage adjustment.

INTERACTIONS

DRUG: None known. **HERBAL:** None known. **FOOD:** None known. **LAB VALUES:** May decrease bleeding time, iron concentration, serum ferritin. May increase BUN, creatinine, phosphorus, potassium, sodium, uric acid.

AVAILABILITY (Rx)

INJECTION: 25 mcg/ml, 40 mcg/ml, 60 mcg/ml, 100 mcg/ml, 200 mcg/ml, 300 mcg/ml.

ADMINISTRATION/HANDLING

Alert: Avoid excessive agitation of vial; do not shake (will cause foaming).

SUBCUTANEOUS

• Use 1 dose per vial; do not reenter vial. Discard unused portion. May be mixed in a syringe with Bacteriostatic 0.9% NaCl with Benzyl Alcohol 0.9% (Bacteriostatic Saline) at a 1:1 ratio (benzyl alcohol acts as a local anesthetic; may reduce injection site discomfort).

IV

Storage • Refrigerate vials. Vigorous shaking may denature medication, rendering it inactive.

IV reconstitution • No reconstitution necessary.

Rate of IV administration • May be given as an IV bolus.

IV INCOMPATIBILITY

Do not mix with any other medications.

INDICATIONS/ROUTES/DOSAGE

ANEMIA IN CHRONIC RENAL FAILURE

Subcutaneous/IV bolus: ADULTS, ELDERLY: Initially, 0.45 mcg/kg once weekly. Adjust dosage to achieve and maintain a target Hgb not to exceed 12 g/dl. Do not increase dose more frequently than once monthly. Limit increases in Hgb to <1 g/dl over any 2-week period.

ANEMIA ASSOCIATED WITH CHEMOTHERAPY

IV/subcutaneous: ADULTS/ELDERLY: 2.25 mcg/kg/dose once weekly.

SIDE EFFECTS

FREQUENT: Myalgia, hypertension/hypotension, headache, diarrhea. **OCCASIONAL:** Fatigue, edema, vomiting, reaction at administration site, asthenia, dizziness.

ADVERSE REACTIONS/ TOXIC EFFECTS

Vascular access thrombosis, CHF, sepsis, arrhythmias, anaphylactic reaction occur rarely.

NURSING IMPLICATIONS

BASELINE ASSESSMENT

Assess B/P prior to drug administration (80% of pts with chronic renal failure have history of hypertension). B/P often rises during early therapy in those with history of hypertension. Assess serum iron (transferrin saturation should be >20%) and serum ferritin (>100 ng/ml) prior to and during therapy. Consider that all pts will eventually need supplemental iron therapy. Establish baseline CBC (esp. note Hct).

INTERVENTION/EVALUATION

Monitor Hct level diligently (if level increases >4 points in 2 wks, dosage should be reduced). Monitor Hgb, serum ferritin, CBC with differential, creatinine, BUN, potassium, phosphorus, reticulocyte count. Monitor B/P aggressively for increase (25% of pts taking medication require antihypertension therapy, dietary restrictions).

PATIENT/FAMILY TEACHING

Frequent blood tests needed to determine correct dose. Inform physician if any severe headache develops; avoid hazardous activities (e.g., driving) during first 90 days of therapy.

Darvocet-N

see propoxyphene

daunorubicin

dawn-oh-**rue**-bih-sin

(Cerubidine, DaunoXome)

Do not confuse with dactinomycin, doxorubicin

CLASSIFICATION

PHARMACOTHERAPEUTIC: Anthracycline antibiotic. **CLINICAL:** Antineoplastic (see p. 71C).

ACTION

Cell cycle–phase nonspecific. Most active in S phase of cell division. Appears to bind to DNA. **Therapeutic Effect:** Inhibits DNA, DNA-dependent RNA synthesis.

PHARMACOKINETICS

Widely distributed. Does not cross blood-brain barrier. Protein binding: High. Metabolized in liver to active metabolite. Excreted in urine, eliminated by biliary excretion. **Half-life:** 18.5 hrs; metabolite: 26.7 hrs.

USES

Treatment of leukemias (ALL, AML) in combination with other agents. DaunoXome: Advanced HIV-related Kaposi's sarcoma. **Unlabeled:** Treatment of neuroblastoma, non-Hodgkin's lymphoma, Ewing's sarcoma, Wilms' tumor, chronic myelocytic leukemia.

PRECAUTIONS

CONTRAINDICATIONS: CHF, left ventricular ejection fraction ≤40%, arrhythmias, preexisting bone marrow suppression. **CAUTIONS:** Those with liver, biliary, renal impairment.

LIFESPAN CONSIDERATIONS: Pregnancy/lactation: If possible, avoid use during pregnancy, esp. first trimester. May cause fetal harm. Breast-feeding not recommended. **Pregnancy Category D. Children:** Safety and efficacy not established. **Elderly:** Cardiotoxicity may be more frequent; reduced bone marrow reserves requires caution. Age-related renal impairment may require dosage adjustment.

INTERACTIONS

DRUG: May decrease effect of **antigout medications. Bone marrow depressants** may enhance myelosuppression. **Live virus vaccines** may potentiate virus replication, increase vaccine side effects, decrease pt's antibody response to vaccine. **HERBAL:** None known. **FOOD:** None known. **LAB VALUES:** May increase serum bilirubin, SGOT (AST), alkaline phosphatase levels. May raise blood uric acid level.

AVAILABILITY (Rx)

CERUBIDINE: **POWDER FOR INJECTION:** 20 mg. **SOLUTION FOR INJECTION:** 5 mg/ml.

D

DAUNOXOME: **INJECTION:** 2 mg/ml.

ADMINISTRATION/HANDLING

IV

Alert: Give by IV push or IV infusion. IV infusion not recommended due to vein irritation, risk of thrombophlebitis. Avoid small veins, swollen/edematous extremities, areas overlying joints/tendons. May be carcinogenic, mutagenic, or teratogenic. Handle with extreme care during preparation/administration.

Storage

CERUBIDINE

• Reconstituted solution is stable for 24 hrs at room temperature or 48 hrs if refrigerated. • Color change from red to blue-purple indicates decomposition; discard.

DAUNOXOME

• Refrigerate unopened vials. • Reconstituted solution is stable for 6 hrs refrigerated. • Do not use if opaque.

Reconstitution

CERUBIDINE

• Reconstitute each 20-mg vial with 4 ml Sterile Water for Injection to provide concentration of 5 mg/ml. • Gently agitate vial until completely dissolved.

DAUNOXOME

• Must dilute with equal part D_5W to provide concentration of 1 mg/ml. • Do not use any other diluent.

Rate of administration

CERUBIDINE

• For IV push, withdraw desired dose into syringe containing 10–15 ml 0.9% NaCl. Inject over 2–3 min into tubing of running IV solution of D_5W or 0.9% NaCl. • For IV infusion, further dilute with 100 ml D_5W or 0.9% NaCl. Infuse over 30–45 min. • Extravasation produces immediate pain, severe local tissue damage. Aspirate as much infiltrated drug as possible, then infiltrate area with hydrocortisone sodium succinate injection (50–100 mg hydrocortisone) and/or isotonic sodium thiosulfate injection or ascorbic acid injection (1 ml of 5% injection). Apply cold compresses.

DAUNOXOME

• Infuse over 60 min.

IV INCOMPATIBILITIES

Allopurinol (Aloprim), aztreonam (Azactam), cefepime (Maxipime), fludarabine (Fludara), piperacillin/tazobactam (Zosyn). **DAUNOXOME:** Do not mix with any other solution, esp. NaCl or bacteriostatic agents (e.g., benzyl alcohol).

IV COMPATIBILITIES

Cytarabine (Cytosar), etoposide (VePesid), filgrastim (Neupogen), granisetron (Kytril), ondansetron (Zofran).

INDICATIONS/ROUTES/DOSAGE

Alert: Dosage individualized based on clinical response, tolerance to adverse effects. When used in combination therapy, consult specific protocols for optimum dosage, sequence of drug administration. Do not exceed total dosage of 500–600 mg/m^2 in adults, 400–450 mg/m^2 in those who received irradiation of cardiac region, 300 mg/m^2 in children >2 yrs, 10 mg/kg in children <2 yrs (increases risk of cardiotoxicity). Reduce dosage in those with liver/renal impairment. Use body weight to calculate dose in children <2 yrs or surface area <0.5 m^2.

ALL

IV: ADULTS: 45 mg/m^2 on days 1–3 of induction course. CHILDREN: 25–45 mg/m^2 on days 1 and 8 of cycle.

AML

IV: ADULTS: 45 mg/m²/day for 3 days first cycle then for 2 days thereafter. CHILDREN: 30-60 mg/m² on days 1–3 of cycle.

KAPOSI'S SARCOMA (DaunoXome)

IV: ADULTS: 20–40 mg/m² over 1 hr. Repeat q2wks or 100 mg/m² q3wks.

SIDE EFFECTS

FREQUENT: Complete alopecia (scalp, axillary, pubic hair), nausea, vomiting begins a few hrs after administration, lasts 24–48 hrs. **DaunoXome:** Mild to moderate nausea, fatigue, fever. **OCCASIONAL:** Diarrhea, abdominal pain, esophagitis, stomatitis (redness/burning of oral mucous membranes, inflammation of gums/tongue), transverse pigmentation of fingernails/toenails. **RARE:** Transient fever, chills.

ADVERSE REACTIONS/ TOXIC EFFECTS

Bone marrow depression manifested as hematologic toxicity (generally severe leukopenia, anemia, thrombocytopenia). Decrease in platelet count, WBC occurs in 10–14 days, returns to normal level by third week. Cardiotoxicity noted as either acute, transient, abnormal EKG findings and/or cardiomyopathy manifested as CHF (risk increases when cumulative dose exceeds 550 mg/m² in adults and 300 mg/m² in children >2 yrs, or total dosage >10 mg/kg in children <2 yrs).

NURSING IMPLICATIONS

BASELINE ASSESSMENT

Obtain WBC, platelet, erythrocyte counts prior to and at frequent intervals during therapy. EKG should be obtained prior to therapy. Antiemetics may be effective in preventing, treating nausea.

INTERVENTION/EVALUATION

Monitor for stomatitis (burning, erythema of oral mucosa). May lead to ulceration within 2–3 days. Assess skin, nailbeds for hyperpigmentation. Monitor hematologic status, renal/hepatic function studies, serum uric acid level. Assess pattern of daily bowel activity/ stool consistency. Monitor for hematologic toxicity (fever, sore throat, signs of local infection, unusual bruising/ bleeding from any site), symptoms of anemia (excessive tiredness, weakness).

PATIENT/FAMILY TEACHING

Urine may turn reddish color for 1–2 days after beginning therapy. Alopecia is reversible, but new hair growth may have different color or texture. New hair growth resumes about 5 wks after last therapy dose. Maintain fastidious oral hygiene. Do not have immunizations without physician's approval (drug lowers body's resistance). Avoid contact with those who have recently received live virus vaccine. Promptly report fever, sore throat, signs of local infection, unusual bruising/bleeding from any site. Increase fluid intake (may protect against hyperuricemia). Contact physician for persistent nausea/vomiting.

DDAVP

see desmopressin

Decadron

see dexamethasone

deferoxamine mesylate

deaf-er-**ox**-ah-meen
(Desferal)
Do not confuse with cefuroxime, Disophrol.

CLASSIFICATION

CLINICAL: Antidote.

D

ACTION

Binds with iron to form complex. **Therapeutic Effect:** Promotes urine excretion of iron.

USES

Treatment of acute iron toxicity, chronic iron toxicity secondary to multiple transfusions associated with some chronic anemia (e.g., thalassemia). **Unlabeled:** Treatment/diagnosis of aluminum toxicity.

PRECAUTIONS

CONTRAINDICATIONS: Severe renal disease, anuria, primary hemochromatosis. **CAUTIONS:** Impaired renal function. **Pregnancy Category C.**

INTERACTIONS

DRUG: Vitamin C may increase effect. **HERBAL:** None known. **FOOD:** None known. **LAB VALUES:** May cause a falsely high total iron-binding capacity (TIBC).

AVAILABILITY (Rx)

INJECTION: 500 mg, 2 g.

ADMINISTRATION/HANDLING

Alert: Reconstitute each 500-mg vial with 2 ml Sterile Water for Injection to provide a concentration of 250 mg/ml.

SUBCUTANEOUS

- Administer subcutaneous very slowly; may give undiluted.

IM

- Inject deeply into upper outer quadrant of buttock; may give undiluted.

IV

- For IV infusion, further dilute with 0.9% NaCl, D_5W, and administer at maximum rate of 15 mg/kg/hr.
- A too rapid IV administration may produce skin flushing, urticaria, hypotension, shock.

IV INCOMPATIBILITY

Do not mix with any other IV medications.

INDICATIONS/ROUTES/DOSAGE

ACUTE IRON INTOXICATION

IM: ADULTS: Initially, 1 g, then 0.5 g q4h for 2 doses; may give additional doses of 0.5 g q4–12h. CHILDREN: 50 mg/kg/dose q6h. **Maximum:** 6 g/day.

IV: ADULTS: 15 mg/kg/hr. CHILDREN: 15 mg/kg/hr. **Maximum:** 6 g/day.

CHRONIC IRON OVERLOAD

Subcutaneous: ADULTS: 1–2 g/day over 8–24 hrs. CHILDREN: 20–50 mg/kg/day over 8–12 hrs. **Maximum:** 2 g/day.

IM: ADULTS: 0.5–1 g/day.

IV: ADULTS, CHILDREN: 15 mg/kg/hr. **Maximum:** 12 g/day.

SIDE EFFECTS

FREQUENT: Pain, induration at injection site, urine color change (to orange-rose). **OCCASIONAL:** Abdominal discomfort, diarrhea, leg cramps, impaired vision.

ADVERSE REACTIONS/TOXIC EFFECTS

High-frequency hearing loss, including tinnitus, has been noted.

NURSING IMPLICATIONS

BASELINE ASSESSMENT

Assess serum iron levels, iron-binding capacity prior to and during therapy.

INTERVENTION/EVALUATION

Question for evidence of hearing loss (neurotoxicity). Periodic slit-lamp ophthalmic exams should be obtained in those treated for chronic iron overload. For IV administration, monitor serum ferritin, iron, TIBC, body weight, growth, B/P. If using subcutaneous technique, monitor for pruritus, erythema, skin irritation, swelling.

PATIENT/FAMILY TEACHING

Inform pt medication may produce discomfort at IM or subcutaneous injection site. Urine will appear reddish. Discomfort may occur at site of injection.

delavirdine mesylate

dell-ah-**veer**-deen
(Rescriptor)

CLASSIFICATION

PHARMACOTHERAPEUTIC: Nonnucleoside reverse transcriptase inhibitor. **CLINICAL:** Antiretroviral (see pp. 58C, 99C).

ACTION

Inhibits catalytic reaction of HIV reverse transcriptase that is independent of nucleoside binding. **Therapeutic Effect:** Interrupts HIV replication, slows progression of HIV infection.

PHARMACOKINETICS

Rapidly absorbed after PO administration. Primarily distributed in blood plasma. Protein binding: 98%. Metabolized in the liver. Eliminated in feces and urine. **Half-life:** 2–11 hrs.

USES

Treatment of HIV infection (in combination with other antivirals).

PRECAUTIONS

CONTRAINDICATIONS: None known. **CAUTIONS:** Liver impairment.

LIFESPAN CONSIDERATIONS: Pregnancy/lactation: Unknown if drug crosses placenta or is distributed in breast milk. **Pregnancy Category C. Children:** Safe and efficacy not established in those <16 yrs. **Elderly:** Safety and efficacy not established.

INTERACTIONS

DRUG: Benzodiazepines, calcium channel blockers may cause life-threatening adverse effects. **Carbamazepine, phenobarbital, phenytoin** may decrease concentrations. **H_2 blockers** may decrease absorption. **Rifampin** may decrease concentrations. **HERBAL:** None known. **FOOD:** None known. **LAB VALUES:** May increase SGOT (AST), SGPT (ALT); may decrease neutrophil count.

AVAILABILITY (Rx)

TABLETS: 100 mg, 200 mg.

ADMINISTRATION/HANDLING

PO

• May disperse in water before consumption. • May give with or without food. • Patients with achlorhydria should take with orange juice, cranberry juice.

INDICATIONS/ROUTES/DOSAGE

HIV INFECTION

PO: ADULTS: 400 mg 3 times/day on empty stomach.

D

SIDE EFFECTS

FREQUENT (18%): Rash, pruritus. **OCCASIONAL (>2%):** Headache, nausea, diarrhea, fatigue, anorexia.

ADVERSE REACTIONS/ TOXIC EFFECTS

None known.

NURSING IMPLICATIONS

BASELINE ASSESSMENT

Obtain baseline laboratory testing, esp. liver function tests, prior to initiation of therapy and at periodic intervals during therapy. Offer emotional support.

INTERVENTION/EVALUATION

Assess skin for evidence of rash. Question if nausea is noted. Determine pattern of bowel activity/stool consistency. Assess eating pattern; monitor for weight loss. Monitor lab values carefully, particularly liver function.

PATIENT/FAMILY TEACHING

Do not take any medications, including OTC drugs, without consulting physician. Small, frequent meals may offset anorexia, nausea. Delavirdine is not a cure for HIV infection, nor does it reduce risk of transmission to others.

demecarium

(Humorsol)

See Classification section under: Antiglaucoma agents

demeclocycline hydrochloride

deh-meh-clo-**sigh**-clean
(Declomycin)

◆CLASSIFICATION

PHARMACOTHERAPEUTIC: Tetracycline. **CLINICAL:** Antibiotic.

ACTION

Bacteriostatic. Binds to ribosomal receptor sites; inhibits ADH-induced water reabsorption. **Therapeutic Effect:** Inhibits protein synthesis. Produces water diuresis.

USES

Treatment of acne, gonorrhea, pertussis, chronic bronchitis, urinary tract infections, syndrome of inappropriate ADH secretion (SIADH).

PRECAUTIONS

CONTRAINDICATIONS: Last half of pregnancy, infants, children ≤8 yrs. **CAUTIONS:** Renal impairment, sun/ultraviolet exposure (severe photosensitivity reaction). **Pregnancy Category D.**

INTERACTIONS

DRUG: **Antacids** containing aluminum/calcium/magnesium, **laxatives** containing magnesium, **oral iron** preparations, **dairy products** impair absorption of tetracyclines (give 1–2 hrs before or after tetracyclines). **Cholestyramine, colestipol** may decrease absorption. May decrease effect of **oral contraceptives. HERBAL:** None known. **FOOD:** **Milk, dairy products** may decrease absorption. **LAB VALUES:** May increase BUN, SGOT (AST), SGPT (ALT), alkaline phosphatase, amylase, bilirubin concentrations.

AVAILABILITY (Rx)

TABLETS: 150 mg, 300 mg.

INDICATIONS/ROUTES/DOSAGE

MILD TO MODERATE INFECTIONS

PO: ADULTS, ELDERLY: 600 mg/day in 2–4 divided doses. CHILDREN >8 YRS: 6–12 mg/kg/day in 2–4 divided doses.

UNCOMPLICATED GONORRHEA
PO: ADULTS: Initially, 600 mg, then 300 mg q12h for 4 days for total of 3 g.

CHRONIC FORM OF SIADH
PO: ADULTS, ELDERLY: 600 mg–1.2 g/day in 3–4 divided doses, or 3.25–3.75 mg/kg q6h.

SIDE EFFECTS

FREQUENT: Anorexia, nausea, vomiting, diarrhea, dysphagia, exaggerated sunburn reaction with moderate to high dosage. **OCCASIONAL:** Urticaria, rash. Long-term therapy may result in diabetes insipidus syndrome: polydipsia, polyuria, weakness.

ADVERSE REACTIONS/ TOXIC EFFECTS

Superinfection (esp. fungal), anaphylaxis, increased intracranial pressure occur rarely. Bulging fontanelles occur rarely in infants.

NURSING IMPLICATIONS

BASELINE ASSESSMENT

Question for history of allergies, esp. to tetracyclines.

INTERVENTION/EVALUATION

Determine pattern of bowel activity/stool consistency. Assess food intake, tolerance. Monitor I&O, renal function test results. Assess for rash. Be alert to superinfection: diarrhea, ulceration/changes of oral mucosa, tongue, anal/genital pruritus. Monitor B/P, LOC (potential for increased intracranial pressure.)

PATIENT/FAMILY TEACHING

Continue antibiotic for full length of treatment. Space doses evenly. Take oral doses on empty stomach with full glass of water. Avoid sun/ultraviolet light exposure.

Demedex

see torsemide

Demerol

see meperidine

denileukin diftitox

den-ee-**lew**-kin
(Ontak)

CLASSIFICATION

PHARMACOTHERAPEUTIC: Biologic response modifier. **CLINICAL:** Antineoplastic (see p. 71C).

ACTION

A cytotoxic fusion protein that targets cells expressing interleukin-2 (IL-2) receptors. After binding to IL-2 receptor, directs cytocidal action to malignant cutaneous T-cell lymphoma (CTCL) cells. **Therapeutic Effect:** Causes inhibition of protein synthesis and cell death.

USES

Treatment of persistent/recurrent T-cell lymphoma whose malignant cells express the CD25 component of the IL-2 receptor.

PRECAUTIONS

CONTRAINDICATIONS: None known. **CAUTIONS:** Preexisting cardiovascular disease, hypoalbuminemia. **Pregnancy Category C.**

INTERACTIONS

DRUG: None known. **HERBAL:** None known. **FOOD:** None known. **LAB VAL-**

UES: May decrease serum albumin, calcium, potassium, WBC count, Hgb, Hct. Increases transaminase level.

D

AVAILABILITY (Rx)

SOLUTION FOR INJECTION: 150 mcg/ml.

ADMINISTRATION/HANDLING

IV

Storage • Store frozen. • Solutions for IV infusion stable for 6 hrs.

Reconstitution • Thaw in refrigerator for up to 24 hrs or at room temperature for 1–2 hrs. • Inject calculated dose into empty infusion bag. No more than 9 ml 0.9% NaCl to be added to each ml denileukin.

Rate of administration • Infuse over 15 min.

IV INCOMPATIBILITY

Do not mix with any other IV medications.

INDICATIONS/ROUTES/DOSAGE

CTCL

IV infusion: ADULTS: 9 or 18 mcg/kg/day for 5 consecutive days q21 days. Infuse over at least 15 min.

SIDE EFFECTS

FREQUENT: Two distinct syndromes occur commonly: A hypersensitivity reaction (69%), consisting of 2 or more of the following: hypotension, back pain, dyspnea, vasodilation, vascular leak syndrome characterized by hypotension, edema, hypoalbuminemia, rash, chest tightness, tachycardia, dysphagia, syncope. Also, a flulike symptom complex (91%), consisting of 2 or more of the following: fever, chills, nausea, vomiting, diarrhea, myalgia, arthralgia. **OCCASIONAL (10%–25%):** Dizziness, chest pain, vasodilation, decreased weight, rhinitis, pruritus.

ADVERSE REACTIONS/ TOXIC EFFECTS

Pancreatitis, acute renal insufficiency, hematuria, hypothyroidism or hyperthyroidism occur rarely.

NURSING IMPLICATIONS

BASELINE ASSESSMENT

CBC, blood chemistries (including renal/hepatic function tests), chest x-ray should be performed prior to therapy and weekly thereafter. Assess serum albumin level before initiation of each treatment (should be ≥3 g/dl).

INTERVENTION/EVALUATION

Monitor serum albumin for hypoalbuminemia (generally occurs 1–2 wks after administration). Monitor for evidence of infection (lowered immune response: sore throat, fever, other vague symptoms).

PATIENT/FAMILY TEACHING

At home, increase fluid intake (protects against renal impairment). Do not have immunizations without physician's approval (drug lowers body resistance); avoid contact with those who have recently taken live virus vaccine.

Depacon

see valproic acid

Depakene

see valproic acid

Depakote

see valproic acid

Depo-Medrol

see methylprednisolone

Depo-Provera

see medroxyprogesterone

desipramine hydrochloride

deh-**sip**-rah-meen
(Apo-Desipramine✤, Norpramin, Novo-Desipramine✤)

Do not confuse with disopyramide, imipramine.

CLASSIFICATION

PHARMACOTHERAPEUTIC: Tricyclic. **CLINICAL:** Antidepressant (see p. 34C).

ACTION

Increases synaptic concentration of norepinephrine and/or serotonin (inhibits reuptake by presynaptic membrane). Strong anticholinergic activity. **Therapeutic Effect:** Produces antidepressant effect.

PHARMACOKINETICS

Rapidly, well absorbed from GI tract. Protein binding: 90%. Metabolized in liver. Primarily excreted in urine. Minimally removed by hemodialysis. **Half-life:** 12–27 hrs.

USES

Treatment of various forms of depression, often in conjunction with psychotherapy. **Unlabeled:** Treatment of panic disorder, neurogenic pain, attention deficit hyperactivity disorder, narcolepsy/cataplexy, bulimia nervosa, cocaine withdrawal.

PRECAUTIONS

CONTRAINDICATIONS: Use of MAOIs within 14 days, narrow-angle glaucoma. **CAUTIONS:** Cardiovascular disease, cardiac conduction disturbances, urinary retention, seizure disorders, hyperthyroidism, those taking thyroid replacement therapy.

LIFESPAN CONSIDERATIONS: Pregnancy/lactation: Crosses placenta. Minimally distributed in breast milk. **Pregnancy Category C. Children:** Not recommended in those <6 yrs. **Elderly:** Use lower dosages (higher dosages not tolerated, increases risk of toxicity).

INTERACTIONS

DRUG: Alcohol, CNS depressants may increase CNS, respiratory depression; hypotensive effects. **Antithyroid agents** may increase risk of agranulocytosis. **Phenothiazines** may increase sedative, anticholinergic effects. **Cimetidine** may increase concentration, toxicity. May decrease effects of **clonidine, guanadrel.** May increase cardiac effects with **sympathomimetics.** May increase risk of hypertensive crisis, hyperpyrexia, seizures with **MAOIs. Phenytoin** may decrease desipramine concentration. **HERBAL: St. John's wort** may have additive effects. **FOOD:** None known. **LAB VALUES:** May alter EKG readings, glucose serum level. Therapeutic blood serum level: 115–300 ng/ml; toxic blood serum level: >400 ng/ml.

AVAILABILITY (Rx)

TABLETS: 10 mg, 25 mg, 50 mg, 75 mg, 100 mg, 150 mg.

ADMINISTRATION/HANDLING

PO

- Give with food or milk if GI distress occurs.

INDICATIONS/ROUTES/DOSAGE

DEPRESSION

PO: ADULTS: 75 mg/day. May gradually increase to 150–200 mg/day. **Maximum:** 300 mg/day. ELDERLY: Initially, 10–25 mg/day. May gradually increase to 75–100 mg/day. **Maximum:** 300 mg/day. CHILDREN >12 YRS: Initially, 25–50 mg/day. May gradually increase to 100 mg/day. **Maximum:** 150 mg/day. CHILDREN 6–12 YRS: 1–3 mg/kg/day. **Maximum:** 5 mg/kg/day.

SIDE EFFECTS

FREQUENT: Drowsiness, fatigue, dry mouth, blurred vision, constipation, delayed micturition, postural hypotension, diaphoresis, disturbed concentration, increased appetite, urinary retention. **OCCASIONAL:** GI disturbances (nausea, GI distress, metallic taste sensation). **RARE:** Paradoxical reaction (agitation, restlessness, nightmares, insomnia), extrapyramidal symptoms (particularly fine hand tremor).

ADVERSE REACTIONS/ TOXIC EFFECTS

High dosage may produce confusion, seizures, severe drowsiness, arrhythmias, fever, hallucinations, agitation, shortness of breath, vomiting, unusual tiredness/weakness. Abrupt withdrawal from prolonged therapy may produce severe headache, malaise, nausea, vomiting, vivid dreams.

NURSING IMPLICATIONS

BASELINE ASSESSMENT

For those on long-term therapy, liver/renal function tests, blood counts should be performed periodically.

INTERVENTION/EVALUATION

Supervise suicidal-risk pt closely during early therapy (as depression lessens, energy level improves, increasing suicide potential). Assess appearance, behavior, speech pattern, level of interest, mood. Therapeutic blood serum level: 115–300 ng/ml; toxic blood serum level: >400 ng/ml.

PATIENT/FAMILY TEACHING

Change positions slowly to avoid hypotensive effect. Tolerance to postural hypotension, sedative, anticholinergic effects usually develops during early therapy. Maximum therapeutic effect may be noted in 2–4 wks. Do not abruptly discontinue medication.

desirudin

deh-**sear**-ew-din
(Iprivask)

CLASSIFICATION

PHARMACOTHERAPEUTIC: Antithrombin agent. **CLINICAL:** Anticoagulant.

ACTION

Binds specifically and directly to thrombin, inhibiting free circulating and clot-bound thrombin. **Therapeutic Effect:** Prolongs clotting time of human plasma.

PHARMACOKINETICS

Complete absorption. Distributed in extracellular space. Metabolized and eliminated by the kidney. **Half-life:** 2–3 hrs.

USES

Prophylaxis of deep vein thrombosis (DVT) in pts undergoing elective hip replacement surgery.

PRECAUTIONS

CONTRAINDICATIONS: Hypersensitivity to natural or recombinant hirudins (anticoagulation factors), pts with active bleeding and/or irreversible coagulation disorders. **CAUTIONS:** Pts with increased risk of hemorrhage (recent major surgery, organ biopsy, puncture of noncompressible vessel within last month, history of hemorrhagic stroke, intracranial/intraocular bleeding, severe uncontrolled hypertension, bacterial endocarditis, hemophilia, history of GI/pulmonary bleeding within past 3 mos), epidural/spinal anesthesia, renal impairment, hepatic function impairment.

LIFESPAN CONSIDERATIONS: Pregnancy/lactation: May be teratogenic. Unknown if drug is distributed in breast milk. **Pregnancy Category C. Children:** Safety and efficacy not established. **Elderly:** Age-related renal impairment may require dosage adjustment.

INTERACTIONS

DRUG: Dextran 40, systemic glucocorticoids, thrombolytics, anticoagulants increase risk of bleeding and should be discontinued prior to initiation of desirudin therapy. **HERBAL:** None known. **FOOD:** None known. **LAB VALUES:** May increase aPTT. May decrease Hgb, Hct.

AVAILABILITY (Rx)

POWDER FOR INJECTION: 15-mg vial with diluent, which includes 0.6 ml mannitol (3%) in Sterile Water for Injection.

ADMINISTRATION/HANDLING

SUBCUTANEOUS

Storage • Store vials at room temperature.

Reconstitution • Reconstitute each vial with 0.5 ml provided diluent. • Gently agitate or rotate. • Use reconstituted solution immediately but is stable for up to 24 hrs if stored at room temperature. • Discard unused portion.

Administration • Using a 26- or 27-gauge needle approx ½ inch long, withdraw reconstituted solution, inject by deep subcutaneous injection, alternating sites, between left and right anterolateral and left and right posterolateral abdominal wall. • Introduce entire length of needle into skinfold held between thumb and forefinger, holding skinfold during injection.

INDICATIONS/ROUTES/DOSAGE

PROPHYLAXIS OF DVT IN PTS UNDERGOING HIP REPLACEMENT SURGERY

Subcutaneous: ADULTS, ELDERLY: Initially, 15 mg q12h. Give initial dose 5–15 min prior to surgery, but following induction of regional block anesthesia, if used. May administer up to 12 days postop.

MODERATE RENAL FUNCTION IMPAIRMENT (≥ 31–60 ML/MIN)

Subcutaneous: ADULTS, ELDERLY: 5 mg q12h.

SEVERE RENAL FUNCTION IMPAIRMENT (<31 ML/MIN)

Subcutaneous: ADULTS, ELDERLY: 1.7 mg q12h.

SIDE EFFECTS

FREQUENT (6%): Hematoma. **OCCASIONAL (2%–4%):** Injection site mass, wound secretion, nausea, hypersensitivity reaction.

ADVERSE REACTIONS/ TOXIC EFFECTS

Serious/major hemorrhage, anaphylactic reaction occurs rarely.

D

NURSING IMPLICATIONS

BASELINE ASSESSMENT

Any medication that may enhance risk of hemorrhage should be discontinued prior to initiation of therapy. Obtain baseline aPTT. When monitoring B/P, avoid overinflation of cuff. Remove adhesive tape from any pressure dressing very carefully, slowly.

INTERVENTION/EVALUATION

Monitor aPTT, serum creatinine daily in pts with increased risk of bleeding, renal impairment. Dosage should be reduced if peak aPTT exceeds 2 times control. Assess for decrease in B/P and/or Hct, increase in pulse rate, complaint of abdominal/back pain, severe headache (may be evidence of hemorrhage). Question for increase in amount of discharge during menses. Check for excessive bleeding from minor cuts, scratches. Assess skin for bruises, gums for erythema, gingival bleeding, urine for hematuria.

PATIENT/FAMILY TEACHING

Use electric razor, soft toothbrush to prevent bleeding. Do not take any OTC medication (esp. aspirin) without consulting physician. Report any sign of red/dark urine, black/red stool, coffee-ground vomitus, red-speckled mucus from cough.

desloratidine

des-low-**rah**-tah-deen
(Clarinex)

CLASSIFICATION

PHARMACOTHERAPEUTIC: H_1 antagonist. **CLINICAL:** Nonsedating antihistamine.

ACTION

Exhibits selective peripheral histamine H_1 receptor blocking action. Competes with histamine at receptor site. Desloratidine has 2.5–4 times greater potency than its parent compound, loratadine. **Therapeutic Effect:** Prevents allergic response mediated by histamine (rhinitis, urticaria).

PHARMACOKINETICS

Rapidly, almost completely absorbed from GI tract. Distributed mainly in liver, lungs, GI tract, bile. Metabolized in liver to active metabolite (undergoes extensive first-pass metabolism). Excreted in urine, eliminated in feces. **Half-life:** 27 hrs (half-life increased in elderly, liver/renal disease).

USES

Relief of nasal symptoms of rhinitis (sneezing, rhinorrhea, itching/tearing of eyes, stuffiness), chronic idiopathic urticaria (hives); symptomatic relief of pruritus, urticaria.

PRECAUTIONS

CONTRAINDICATIONS: None known. **CAUTIONS:** Liver impairment. Safety in children <6 yrs unknown.

LIFESPAN CONSIDERATIONS: Pregnancy/lactation: Excreted in breast milk. **Pregnancy Category C. Children/elderly:** More sensitive to anticholinergic effects (e.g., dry mouth, nose, throat).

INTERACTIONS

DRUG: Ketoconazole, erythromycin may increase concentrations. **HERBAL:** None known. **FOOD:** None known. **LAB**

VALUES: May suppress wheal and flare reactions to antigen skin testing, unless antihistamines are discontinued 4 days before testing.

AVAILABILITY (Rx)

TABLETS: 5 mg. **REDITABS:** 5 mg.

ADMINISTRATION/HANDLING

PO

- Do not crush or break film-coated tablets.

INDICATIONS/ROUTES/DOSAGE

ALLERGIC RHINITIS, HIVES

PO: ADULTS, ELDERLY, CHILDREN >12 YRS: 5 mg once daily. RENAL/LIVER IMPAIRMENT: 5 mg every other day.

SIDE EFFECTS

FREQUENT (12%): Headache. **OCCASIONAL (3%):** Dry mouth, somnolence. **RARE (<3%):** Fatigue, dizziness, diarrhea, nausea.

ADVERSE REACTIONS/TOXIC EFFECTS

None known.

NURSING IMPLICATIONS

BASELINE ASSESSMENT

Assess lung sounds for wheezing; skin for urticaria, hives.

INTERVENTION/EVALUATION

For upper respiratory allergies, increase fluids to decrease viscosity of secretions, offset thirst, replace loss of fluids from diaphoresis. Monitor symptoms for therapeutic response.

PATIENT/FAMILY TEACHING

Does not cause drowsiness; however, if blurred vision or eye pain occurs, do not drive or perform activities requiring visual acuity. Avoid alcohol.

desmopressin

des-moe-**press**-in
(DDAVP, Octostim✤, Stimate)

CLASSIFICATION

PHARMACOTHERAPEUTIC: Synthetic pituitary hormone. **CLINICAL:** Antidiuretic.

ACTION

Increases reabsorption of water by increasing permeability of collecting ducts of the kidneys. Plasminogen activator. **Therapeutic Effect:** Decreases urinary output. Increases plasma factor VIII (antihemophilic factor).

PHARMACOKINETICS

Onset	Peak	Duration
PO		
1 hr	2–7 hrs	6–8 hrs
Intranasal		
15 min–1 hr	1–5 hrs	5–21 hrs
IV		
15–30 min	1.5–3 hrs	—

Poorly absorbed after PO/nasal administration. Metabolism: Unknown. **Half-life:** Oral: 1.5–2.5 hrs. Nasal: 3.3–3.5 hrs. IV: 0.4–4 hrs.

USES

DDAVP Intranasal: Primary nocturnal enuresis, central cranial diabetes insipidus. **Parenteral:** Central cranial diabetes insipidus, hemophilia A, von Willebrand's disease (type I). **Stimate Intranasal:** Hemophilia A, von Willebrand's disease (type I). **PO:** Central cranial diabetes insipidus.

PRECAUTIONS

CONTRAINDICATIONS: Severe type I, type IIB, platelet-type von Willebrand disease; hemophilia A with factor VIII levels <5% or hemophilia B. **CAUTIONS:** Predisposition to thrombus formation, conditions with fluid/electrolyte imbalance, coronary artery disease, hypertensive cardiovascular disease.

LIFESPAN CONSIDERATIONS: Pregnancy/lactation: Pregnancy Category B. Children: Caution in neonates, those <3 mos (increased risk of fluid balance problems). Careful fluid restrictions recommended in infants. **Elderly:** Increased risk of hyponatremia, water intoxication.

INTERACTIONS

DRUG: Carbamazepine, chlorpropamide, clofibrate may increase effect. **Demeclocycline, lithium, norepinephrine** may decrease effect. **HERBAL:** None known. **FOOD:** None known. **LAB VALUES:** None known.

AVAILABILITY (Rx)

TABLETS (DDAVP): 0.1 mg, 0.2 mg. **INJECTION (DDAVP):** 4 mcg/ml. **NASAL SOLUTION (DDAVP):** 100 mcg/ml. **NASAL SPRAY (Stimate):** 1.5 mg/ml (150 mcg/spray), **(DDAVP):** 100 mcg/ml (10 mcg/spray).

ADMINISTRATION/HANDLING

INTRANASAL

Refrigerate DDAVP nasal solution and Stimate nasal spray. Nasal solution and Stimate nasal spray are stable for 3 wks at room temperature if unopened. • DDAVP nasal spray is stable at room temperature. • A calibrated catheter (rhinyle) is used to draw up a measured quantity of desmopressin; with one end inserted in the nose, pt blows on the other end to deposit the solution deep in the nasal cavity. • For infants, young children, obtunded pts, an air-filled syringe may be attached to the catheter to deposit the solution.

SUBCUTANEOUS

• Estimate response by adequate sleep duration. • Morning and evening doses should be adjusted separately.

IV

Storage • Refrigerate. Stable for 2 wks at room temperature.

Reconstitution • For IV infusion, dilute in 10–50 ml 0.9% NaCl.

Rate of administration • Infuse over 15–30 min. • For preop use, administer 30 min before procedure. • Monitor B/P, pulse during IV infusion. • IV dose = 1/10 intranasal dose.

IV INCOMPATIBILITY

Information not available.

INDICATIONS/ROUTES/DOSAGE

PRIMARY NOCTURNAL ENURESIS

Intranasal: CHILDREN ≥6 YRS: Initially, 20 mcg (0.2 ml) at bedtime (1/2 dose each nostril). Adjust up to 40 mcg.

PO: CHILDREN >12 YRS: 0.2–0.6 mg once before bedtime.

CENTRAL CRANIAL DIABETES INSIPIDUS

PO: ADULTS, ELDERLY, CHILDREN ≥12 YRS: Initially, 0.05 mg 2 times/day. RANGE: 0.1–1.2 mg/day in 2–3 divided doses. CHILDREN <12 YRS: 0.05 mg initially, then 2 times/day. RANGE: 0.1–0.8 mg daily.

Intranasal: ADULTS, ELDERLY, CHILDREN >12 YRS: 5–40 mcg (0.05–0.4 ml) in 1–3 doses/day. CHILDREN 3 MOS–12 YRS: Initially, 5 mcg (0.05 ml)/day. RANGE: 5–30 mcg (0.05–0.3 ml)/day.

Subcutaneous/IV: ADULTS, ELDERLY, CHILDREN >12 YRS: 2–4 mcg/day in 2 divided doses or 1/10 of maintenance intranasal dose.

HEMOPHILIA A, VON WILLEBRAND'S DISEASE (type I)

IV infusion: ADULTS, ELDERLY, CHILDREN >10 KG: 0.3 mcg/kg diluted in 50 ml 0.9% NaCl. CHILDREN <10 KG: 0.3 mcg/kg diluted in 10 ml 0.9% NaCl.

Intranasal: ADULTS, ELDERLY, CHILDREN ≥12 YRS, >50 KG: 300 mcg (1 spray each nostril). ADULTS, ELDERLY, CHILDREN >12 YRS, <50 KG: 150 mcg as single spray.

SIDE EFFECTS

OCCASIONAL: IV: Pain/redness/swelling at injection site, headache, abdominal cramps, vulval pain, flushed skin; mild elevation of B/P; nausea with high dosages. **Nasal:** Rhinorrhea, nasal congestion; slight elevation of B/P.

ADVERSE REACTIONS/ TOXIC EFFECTS

Water intoxication or hyponatremia (headache, drowsiness, confusion, decreased urination, rapid weight gain, seizures, coma) may occur in overhydration. Elderly, infants, children are esp. at risk.

NURSING IMPLICATIONS

BASELINE ASSESSMENT

Establish baselines for B/P, pulse, weight, electrolytes, urine specific gravity. Check lab values for factor VIII coagulant concentration for hemophilia A, von Willebrand's disease; bleeding times.

INTERVENTION/EVALUATION

Check B/P, pulse with IV infusion. Monitor pt weight, fluid intake, urine volume, urine specific gravity, osmolality, electrolytes for diabetes insipidus. Assess factor VIII antigen levels, aPTT, factor VIII activity level for hemophilia.

PATIENT/FAMILY TEACHING

Avoid overhydration. Teach proper technique for intranasal administration. Inform physician if headache, shortness of breath, heartburn, nausea, abdominal cramps occur.

desonide

(Otic Tridesilon, Tridesilon)

See Classification section under: Corticosteroids: topical (p. 84C)

desoximetasone

(Topicort)

See Classification section under: Corticosteroids: topical (p. 84C)

D

Desyrel

see trazodone

Detrol

see tolterodine

dexamethasone

dex-a-**meth**-a-sone

(Decadron, Dexasone ✤, Maxidex)

Do not confuse with desoximetasone, dextromethorphan, Maxzide.

FIXED-COMBINATION(S)

Maxitrol, Dexacidin: dexamethasone/neomycin/polymyxin (anti-infectives): 0.1%/3.5 mg/10,000 U per g or ml. **Ciprodex Otic:** dextramethasone/ciprofloxacin (antibiotic): 0.1%/0.3%.

◆CLASSIFICATION

PHARMACOTHERAPEUTIC: Long-acting glucocorticoid. **CLINICAL:** Corticosteroid (see pp. 81C, 84C).

ACTION

Inhibits accumulation of inflammatory cells at inflammation sites, phagocytosis, lysosomal enzyme release and synthesis and/or release of mediators of inflammation. **Therapeutic Effect:** Prevents/suppresses cell and tissue immune reactions, inflammatory process.

PHARMACOKINETICS

Rapidly, completely absorbed from GI tract after PO administration. Widely distributed. Protein binding: High. Metabolized in liver. Primarily excreted in urine. Minimally removed by hemodialysis. **Half-life:** 3–4.5 hrs.

USES

Treatment of chronic inflammations; allergic, neoplastic, autoimmune diseases; management of cerebral edema, septic shock; adjuvant antiemetic in treatment of chemotherapy-induced emesis.

PRECAUTIONS

CONTRAINDICATIONS: Active untreated infections; viral, fungal, tuberculosis diseases of the eye. **CAUTIONS:** Respiratory tuberculosis, untreated systemic infections, ocular herpes simplex, hyperthyroidism, cirrhosis, ulcerative colitis, hypertension, osteoporosis pts at high thromboembolic risk, CHF, seizure disorders, peptic ulcer, diabetes. Prolonged use may result in cataracts, glaucoma.

LIFESPAN CONSIDERATIONS: Pregnancy/lactation: Crosses placenta. Distributed in breast milk. **Pregnancy Category C (D** if used in first trimester). **Children:** Prolonged treatment with high-dose therapy may decrease short-term growth rate, cortisol secretion. **Elderly:** Higher risk for developing hypertension, osteoporosis.

INTERACTIONS

DRUG: Amphotericin may increase hypokalemia. May decrease effect of **oral hypoglycemics, insulin, diuretics, potassium supplements.** May increase **digoxin** toxicity (due to hypokalemia). **Hepatic enzyme inducers** may decrease effect. **Live virus vaccines** may potentiate virus replication, increase vaccine side effects, decrease pt's antibody response to vaccine. **HERBAL:** None known. **FOOD:** None known. **LAB VALUES:** May decrease calcium, potassium, thyroxine. Increases cholesterol, glucose, lipids, sodium, amylase serum levels.

AVAILABILITY (Rx)

TABLETS: 0.25 mg, 0.5 mg, 0.75 mg, 1 mg, 1.5 mg, 2 mg, 4 mg, 6 mg. **ELIXIR:** 0.5 mg/5 ml, 1 mg/ml. **ORAL SOLUTION:** 0.5 mg/5 ml, 0.5 mg/0.5 ml. **INJECTION:** 4 mg/ml, 10 mg/ml. **INHALANT, INTRANASAL, OPHTHALMIC:** Solution, suspension, ointment. **TOPICAL:** Aerosol, cream.

ADMINISTRATION/HANDLING

PO

- Give with milk or food.

IM

- Give deep IM, preferably in gluteus maximus.

IV

Alert: Dexamethasone sodium phosphate may be given by IV push or IV infusion.

- For IV push, give over 1–4 min.
- For IV infusion, mix with 0.9% NaCl or D_5W and infuse over 15–30 min.
- For neonate, solution must be preservative free.
- IV solution must be used within 24 hrs.

OPHTHALMIC

- Place finger on lower eyelid and pull out until a pocket is formed between eye and lower lid. Hold dropper above pocket and place correct number of drops (¼–½ inch ointment) into pocket. Close eye gently. **Solution:** Apply digital pressure to lacrimal sac for 1–2 min (minimizes drainage into nose/throat, reducing risk of systemic effects). **Ointment:** Close eye for 1–2 min, rolling eyeball (increases contact area of drug to eye). Remove excess solution or ointment around eye with tissue. • Ointment may be used at night to reduce frequency of solution administration. • As with other corticosteroids, taper dosage slowly when discontinuing.

TOPICAL
• Gently cleanse area before application. • Use occlusive dressings only as ordered. • Apply sparingly and rub into area thoroughly.

⊘ IV INCOMPATIBILITIES
Daunorubicin (Cerubidine), ciprofloxacin (Cipro), idarubicin (Idamycin), midazolam (Versed).

IV COMPATIBILITIES
Aminophylline, cimetidine (Tagamet), cisplatin (Platinol), cyclophosphamide (Cytoxan), cytarabine (Cytosar), docetaxel (Taxotere), doxorubicin (Adriamycin), etoposide (VePesid), granisetron (Kytril), heparin, hydromorphone (Dilaudid), lorazepam (Ativan), morphine, ondansetron (Zofran), paclitaxel (Taxol), potassium chloride, propofol (Diprivan).

INDICATIONS/ROUTES/DOSAGE

ANTI-INFLAMMATORY
PO/IM/IV: ADULTS, ELDERLY: 0.75–9 mg/day in divided doses q6–12h. CHILDREN: 0.08–0.3 mg/kg/day in divided doses q6–12h.

CEREBRAL EDEMA
IV: ADULTS, ELDERLY: Initially, 10 mg, then 4 mg (IM/IV) q6h.

PO/IM/IV: CHILDREN: Loading dose of 1–2 mg/kg, then 1–1.5 mg/kg/day in divided doses q4–6h.

CHEMOTHERAPY ANTIEMETIC
IV: ADULTS, ELDERLY: 8–20 mg once, then 4 mg PO q4–6h or 8 mg q8h. CHILDREN: 10 mg/m^2/dose (**Maximum:** 20 mg), then 5 mg/m^2/dose q6h.

PHYSIOLOGIC REPLACEMENT
PO/IM/IV: ADULTS, ELDERLY: 0.03–0.15 mg/kg/day in divided doses q6–12h.

USUAL OPHTHALMIC DOSAGE
ADULTS, ELDERLY, CHILDREN: **Ointment:** Thin coating 3–4 times/day. **Suspension:** Initially, 2 drops q1h while awake and q2h at night for 1 day; then reduce to 3–4 times/day.

SIDE EFFECTS

FREQUENT: Inhalation: Cough, dry mouth, hoarseness, throat irritation. **Intranasal:** Burning, mucosal dryness. **Ophthalmic:** Blurred vision. **Systemic:** Insomnia, facial swelling ("moon face"), moderate abdominal distention, indigestion, increased appetite, nervousness, facial flushing, diaphoresis. **OCCASIONAL: Inhalation:** Localized fungal infection (thrush). **Intranasal:** Crusting inside nose, nosebleed, sore throat, ulceration of nasal mucosa. **Ophthalmic:** Decreased vision; watering of eyes; eye pain; burning, stinging, redness of eyes; nausea; vomiting. **Systemic:** Dizziness, decreased/blurred vision. **Topical:** Allergic contact dermatitis, purpura (blood-containing blisters), thinning of skin with easy bruising, telangiectasis (raised dark red spots on skin). **RARE: Inhalation:** Increased bronchospasm, esophageal candidiasis. **Intranasal:** Nasal/pharyngeal candidiasis, eye pain. **Systemic:** General allergic reaction (rash, hives); pain, redness, swelling at injection site; psychological changes; false sense of well-being; hallucinations; depression.

ADVERSE REACTIONS/ TOXIC EFFECTS

Long-term therapy: Muscle wasting (esp. arms, legs), osteoporosis, spontaneous fractures, amenorrhea, cataracts, glaucoma, peptic ulcer, CHF. **Abrupt withdrawal following long-term therapy:** Severe joint pain, severe headache, anorexia, nausea, fever, rebound inflammation, fatigue, weakness, lethargy, dizziness, orthostatic hypotension. **Ophthalmic:** Glaucoma, ocular hypertension, cataracts.

D

NURSING IMPLICATIONS

BASELINE ASSESSMENT

Question for hypersensitivity to any of the corticosteroids. Obtain baselines for height, weight, B/P, glucose, electrolytes.

INTERVENTION/EVALUATION

Monitor I&O, daily weight. Assess for edema. Evaluate food tolerance and bowel activity. Report hyperacidity promptly. Check vital signs at least 2 times/day. Be alert to infection: sore throat, fever, vague symptoms. Monitor electrolytes. Monitor for hypercalcemia (muscle twitching, cramps), hypokalemia (weakness, muscle cramps, numbness/tingling esp. lower extremities, nausea/vomiting, irritability). Assess emotional status, ability to sleep.

PATIENT/FAMILY TEACHING

Do not change dose/schedule or stop taking drug. **Must** taper off gradually under medical supervision. Notify physician of fever, sore throat, muscle aches, sudden weight gain/swelling. Severe stress (serious infection, surgery, trauma) may require increased dosage. Inform dentist, other physicians of dexamethasone therapy now or within past 12 mos. **Topical:** Apply after shower/bath for best absorption.

dexmedetomidine hydrochloride

decks-meh-deh-**tome**-ih-deen

(Precedex)

Do not confuse with Percocet, Peridex.

◆ CLASSIFICATION

PHARMACOTHERAPEUTIC: $Alpha_2$-agonist. **CLINICAL:** Nonbarbiturate sedative, hypnotic.

ACTION

Selective $alpha_2$-adrenergic agonist. **Therapeutic Effect:** Produces analgesic, hypnotic, sedative effects.

USES

Sedation of initially intubated and mechanically ventilated adults during treatment in intensive care setting.

PRECAUTIONS

CONTRAINDICATIONS: None known. **CAUTIONS:** Advanced heart block, severe CHF, impaired liver/renal function, hypovolemia. **Pregnancy Category C.**

INTERACTIONS

DRUG: Concurrent administration with **anesthetics, sedatives, hypnotics, opioids** may enhance effects. **HERBAL:** None known. **FOOD:** None known. **LAB VALUES:** May increase AST (SGOT), ALT (SGPT), potassium alkaline phosphatase.

AVAILABILITY (Rx)

INJECTION: 100 mcg/ml.

ADMINISTRATION/HANDLING

IV

Storage • Store at room temperature.

Reconstitution • Dilute 2 ml of dexmedetomidine with 48 ml 0.9 NaCl.

Rate of administration • Give as maintenance infusion.

IV INCOMPATIBILITY

Do not mix with any other medications.

INDICATIONS/ROUTES/DOSAGE

Alert: Must be diluted with 48 ml 0.9% NaCl prior to use. Do not infuse >24 hrs.

SEDATION

IV infusion: ADULTS: Loading dose of 1 mcg/kg over 10 min followed by maintenance dose of 0.2–0.7 mcg/kg/hr. ELDERLY: May decrease dosage. No guidelines available.

SIDE EFFECTS

FREQUENT: Hypotension (30%), nausea (11%). **OCCASIONAL (2%–3%):** Pain, fever, oliguria, thirst.

ADVERSE REACTIONS/ TOXIC EFFECTS

Bradycardia, atrial fibrillation, hypoxia, anemia, pain, pleural effusion may occur if IV is infused too rapidly.

NURSING IMPLICATIONS

INTERVENTION/EVALUATION

Monitor EKG for atrial fibrillation, pulse for bradycardia, B/P for hypotension, level of sedation. Assess respiratory rate, rhythm.

dexmethylphenidate hydrochloride

dex-meh-thyl-**fen**-ih-date
(Focalin)

CLASSIFICATION

PHARMACOTHERAPEUTIC: Piperidine derivative B **(Schedule II).** **CLINICAL:** CNS stimulant.

ACTION

Blocks reuptake mechanisms of norepinephrine, dopamine into presynaptic neurons. Increases release of these neurotransmitters into the synaptic cleft. **Therapeutic Effect:** Decreases motor restlessness, enhances attention span. Increases motor activity, mental alertness; diminishes sense of fatigue; enhances spirit.

PHARMACOKINETICS

Onset	Peak	Duration
PO		
—	—	4–5 hrs

Readily absorbed from GI tract. Plasma concentrations increase rapidly. Metabolized in liver. Excreted unchanged in urine. **Half-life:** 2.2 hrs.

USES

Adjunct in the treatment of attention deficit hyperactivity disorder (ADHD) with moderate to severe distractability, short attention spans, hyperactivity, emotional impulsivity in children >6 yrs.

PRECAUTIONS

CONTRAINDICATIONS: History of marked anxiety, tension, agitation; glaucoma; those with motor tics, family history/diagnosis of Tourette's syndrome; pts undergoing treatment with MAOIs or within 14 days following discontinuation of an MAOI. **CAUTIONS:** Cardiovascular disease, seizure disorders, psychosis. Avoid use in those with a history of substance abuse.

LIFESPAN CONSIDERATIONS: Pregnancy/lactation: Unknown if excreted in breast milk. **Pregnancy Category C. Children:** May be more susceptible to developing anorexia, insomnia, stomach pain, weight loss. Chronic use may inhibit growth. In psychotic children, may exacerbate symptoms of behavior disturbance, thought disorder. **Elderly:** No age-related precautions noted.

INTERACTIONS

DRUG: CNS stimulants may have additive effect. **MAOIs** may increase effects. Downward dosage adjustments of **phenobarbital, phenytoin, primidone, amitryptyline** may be necessary. May inhibit metabolism of **warfarin.** **HERBAL:** **Ma huang (ephedra)** may increase CNS stimulation. **FOOD:** None known. **LAB VALUES:** None known.

D

AVAILABILITY (Rx)

TABLETS: 2.5 mg, 5 mg, 10 mg.

ADMINISTRATION/HANDLING

PO

• Do not give drug in afternoon or evening (causes insomnia). • Tablets may be crushed. • May give with or without food.

INDICATIONS/ROUTES/DOSAGE

ATTENTION DEFICIT HYPERACTIVITY DISORDER

PO: PATIENTS NEW TO DEXMETHYLPHENIDATE, METHYLPHENIDATE: 2.5 mg twice daily (5 mg/day). May adjust dosage in 2.5- to 5-mg increments. **Maximum:** 20 mg/day. PATIENTS CURRENTLY TAKING METHYLPHENIDATE: Half the methylphenidate dosage. **Maximum:** 20 mg/day.

SIDE EFFECTS

FREQUENT: Abdominal discomfort. **OCCASIONAL:** Anorexia, fever, nausea. **RARE:** Blurred vision, difficulty with accommodation, motor/vocal tics, insomnia, tachycardia.

ADVERSE REACTIONS/ TOXIC EFFECTS

Withdrawal after chronic therapy may unmask symptoms of the underlying disorder. May lower the seizure threshold in those with history of seizures. Overdosage produces excessive sympathomimetic effects (vomiting, tremors, hyperreflexia, seizures, confusion, hallucinations, diaphoresis). Prolonged administration to children may produce temporary suppression of normal weight gain.

NURSING IMPLICATIONS

INTERVENTION/EVALUATION

CBC, differential, platelet count should be performed routinely during therapy. If paradoxical return of attention deficit occurs, dosage should be reduced or discontinued.

PATIENT/FAMILY TEACHING

Avoid tasks that require alertness, motor skills until response to drug is established. Report any increase in seizures. The last dose should be given several hours before retiring to prevent insomnia. Report nervousness, palpitations, fever, vomiting.

dexrazoxane

dex-rah-**zox**-ann
(Zinecard)

CLASSIFICATION

PHARMACOTHERAPEUTIC: Cytoprotective agent. **CLINICAL:** Antineoplastic adjunct.

ACTION

Rapidly penetrates myocardial cell membrane. Binds intracellular iron, prevents generation of oxygen free radicals by anthracyclines (thought to be responsible for anthracycline-induced cardiomyopathy). **Therapeutic Effect:** Protects against anthracycline-induced cardiomyopathy.

PHARMACOKINETICS

Rapidly distributed after IV administration. Not bound to plasma proteins. Primarily excreted in urine. Removed by peritoneal or hemodialysis. **Elimination half-life:** 2.1–2.5 hrs.

USES

Reduction of incidence, severity of cardiomyopathy associated with doxorubicin therapy in women with metastatic breast cancer. Not recommended with initiation of doxorubicin therapy.

PRECAUTIONS

CONTRAINDICATIONS: Chemotherapy regimens that do not contain an anthracycline. **CAUTIONS:** Chemotherapeutic agents that are additive to myelosuppression, concurrent FAC (fluorouracil, adriamycin, cyclophosphamide) therapy.

LIFESPAN CONSIDERATIONS: Pregnancy/lactation: May be embryotoxic, teratogenic. Unknown if distributed in breast milk. Breast-feeding not recommended. **Pregnancy Category C. Children:** Safety and efficacy not established. **Elderly:** Information not available.

INTERACTIONS

DRUG: Concurrent FAC **(fluorouracil, adriamycin, cyclophosphamide)** therapy may produce severe blood dyscrasias. **HERBAL:** None known. **FOOD:** None known. **LAB VALUES:** Concurrent FAC (fluorouracil, doxorubicin, cyclophosphamide) therapy may produce abnormal hepatic/renal function tests.

AVAILABILITY (Rx)

POWDER FOR INJECTION: 250 mg (10 mg/ml reconstituted in 25 ml single-use vial), 500 mg (10 mg/ml reconstituted in 50-ml single-use vial).

ADMINISTRATION/HANDLING

Alert: Do not mix with other drugs. Use caution in handling/preparation of reconstituted solution (glove use recommended).

IV

Storage • Store vials at room temperature. • Reconstituted solution is stable for 6 hrs at room temperature or if refrigerated. Discard unused solution.

Reconstitution • Reconstitute with 0.167 molar (M/6) sodium lactate injection to give concentration of 10 mg dexrazoxane for each ml of sodium lactate. • May further dilute with 0.9% NaCl or D_5W. Concentration should range from 1.3–5 mg/ml.

Rate of administration • Give reconstituted solution by slow IV push or IV infusion over 15–30 min. • After infusion is completed, and before a total elapsed time of 30 min from beginning of dexrazoxane infusion, give IV injection of doxorubicin.

IV INCOMPATIBILITY

Do not mix with other medications.

INDICATIONS/ROUTES/DOSAGE

Alert: Dexrazoxane should be used only in those who have received a cumulative doxorubicin dose of 300 mg/m^2 and are continuing with doxorubicin therapy.

CARDIOPROTECTIVE

IV: ADULTS, CHILDREN: Recommended dosage ratio of dexrazoxane to doxorubicin is 10:1 (e.g., 500 mg/m^2 dexrazoxane, 50 mg/m^2 doxorubicin).

SIDE EFFECTS

FREQUENT: Alopecia, nausea/vomiting, fatigue, malaise, anorexia, stomatitis, fever, infection, diarrhea. **OCCASIONAL:** Pain with injection, neurotoxicity, phlebitis, dysphagia, streaking/erythema. **RARE:** Urticaria, skin reaction.

ADVERSE REACTIONS/ TOXIC EFFECTS

FAC therapy with dexrazoxane may produce more severe leukopenia, granulocytopenia, thrombocytopenia than those receiving FAC without dexrazoxane. Overdosage removed by peritoneal or hemodialysis.

D

NURSING IMPLICATIONS

BASELINE ASSESSMENT

Use gloves when preparing solution. If powder/solution comes in contact with skin, wash immediately with soap and water. Antiemetics may be effective in preventing, treating nausea.

INTERVENTION/EVALUATION

Frequently monitor blood levels for evidence of blood dyscrasias. Assess for stomatitis (burning/erythema of oral mucosa at inner margin of lips, sore throat, difficulty swallowing). Monitor hematologic status, renal/hepatic function studies, cardiac function. Assess pattern of daily bowel activity/stool consistency. Monitor for hematologic toxicity (fever, signs of local infection, unusual bruising/bleeding from any site).

PATIENT/FAMILY TEACHING

Alopecia is reversible, but new hair growth may have different color/texture. New hair growth resumes 2–3 mos after last therapy dose. Maintain fastidious oral hygiene. Promptly report fever, sore throat, signs of local infection. Contact physician if persistent nausea/vomiting continues at home.

dextran, low molecular weight (dextran 40)

dex-tran

(Gentran, Rheomacrodex ✤)

dextran, high molecular weight (dextran 75)

(Macrodex)

◆CLASSIFICATION

PHARMACOTHERAPEUTIC: Branched polysaccharide. **CLINICAL:** Plasma volume expander.

ACTION

Produces plasma volume expansion due to high colloidal osmotic effect. Draws interstitial fluid into the intravascular space. May increase blood flow in microcirculation. **Therapeutic Effect:** Increases central venous pressure (CVP), cardiac output, stroke volume, B/P, urine output, capillary perfusion, pulse pressure. Decreases heart rate, peripheral resistance, blood viscosity. Corrects hypovolemia.

USES

Fluid replacement, blood volume expander in treatment of hypovolemia, shock, impending shock.

PRECAUTIONS

CONTRAINDICATIONS: Severe CHF, renal failure, severe thrombocytopenia, hypervolemia, severe bleeding disorders. **CAUTIONS:** Those with extreme dehydration, chronic liver disease. **Pregnancy Category C.**

INTERACTIONS

DRUG: None known. **HERBAL:** None known. **FOOD:** None known. **LAB VALUES:** Prolongs bleeding time, depresses platelet count. Decreases factors VIII, V, IX.

AVAILABILITY (Rx)

INJECTION: 10% dextran 40 in NaCl or D_5W, 6% dextran 75 in NaCl or D_5W.

ADMINISTRATION/HANDLING

IV

Storage • Store at room temperature. • Use only clear solutions. • Discard partially used containers.

Rate of administration • Give by IV infusion only. • Monitor pt closely during first min of infusion for anaphylactoid reaction. Monitor vital signs q5min. • Monitor urine flow rates during administration (if oliguria/anuria occurs, dextran 40 should be discontinued and osmotic diuretic given [minimizes vascular overloading]). • Monitor CVP when given by rapid infusion. If there is a precipitous rise in CVP, immediately discontinue drug (overexpansion of blood volume). • Monitor B/P diligently during infusion; if marked hypotension occurs, stop infusion immediately (imminent anaphylactic reaction). • If evidence of blood volume overexpansion occurs, discontinue drug until blood volume adjusts via diuresis.

∅ IV INCOMPATIBILITY

Do not add any medications to dextran solution.

INDICATIONS/ROUTES/DOSAGE

VOLUME EXPANSION/SHOCK

IV: ADULTS, ELDERLY: 500–1,000 ml at rate of 20–40 ml/min. **Maximum:** 20 ml/kg first 24 hrs, 10 ml/kg thereafter. CHILDREN: Total dose not to exceed 20 ml/kg day 1, 10 ml/kg/day thereafter.

Alert: Therapy should not continue >5 days.

SIDE EFFECTS

OCCASIONAL: Mild hypersensitivity reaction (urticaria, nasal congestion, wheezing).

ADVERSE REACTIONS/ TOXIC EFFECTS

Severe or fatal anaphylaxis (marked hypotension, cardiac/respiratory arrest) may occur, noted early during IV infusion, generally in those not previously exposed to IV dextran.

NURSING IMPLICATIONS

INTERVENTION/EVALUATION

Monitor urine output closely (increase in output generally occurs in oliguric pts after dextran administration). If no increase is observed after 500 ml dextran is infused, discontinue drug until diuresis occurs. Monitor for fluid overload (peripheral and/or pulmonary edema, impending CHF symptoms). Assess lung sounds for rales. Monitor CVP (detects overexpansion of blood volume). Monitor vital signs and observe closely for allergic reaction. Assess for bleeding, esp. following surgery or those on anticoagulant therapy (overt bleeding, esp. at surgical site, bruising, petechiae development).

dextroamphetamine sulfate

dex-tro-am-**fet**-ah-meen

(Dexedrine)

Do not confuse with Dextran, dextromethorphan, Excedrin.

CLASSIFICATION

PHARMACOTHERAPEUTIC: Amphetamine **(Schedule II). CLINICAL:** CNS stimulant.

ACTION

Enhances release, action of catecholamine (dopamine, norepinephrine) by blocking reuptake, inhibiting monoamine oxidase. **Therapeutic Effect:** Increases motor activity, mental alertness; decreases drowsiness, fatigue.

D

USES

Treatment of narcolepsy; treatment of attention deficit disorder (ADD) in hyperactive children; short-term treatment to assist caloric restriction in exogenous obesity.

PRECAUTIONS

CONTRAINDICATIONS: Hyperthyroidism, advanced arteriosclerosis, agitated states, moderate to severe hypertension, symptomatic cardiovascular disease, history of drug abuse, glaucoma, history of hypersensitivity to sympathomimetic amines, within 14 days following discontinuation of MAOI ingestion. **CAUTIONS:** Elderly, debilitated, tartrazine-sensitive pts. **Pregnancy Category C.**

INTERACTIONS

DRUG: **Tricyclic antidepressants** may increase cardiovascular effects. **Beta-blockers** may increase risk of hypertension, bradycardia, heart block. **CNS stimulants** may increase effects. May increase risk of arrhythmias with **digoxin. Meperidine** may increase risk of hypotension, respiratory depression, seizures, vascular collapse. **MAOIs** may prolong, intensify effects. May increase effects of **thyroid hormone. Thyroid hormones** may increase effects. **HERBAL:** None known. **FOOD:** None known. **LAB VALUES:** May increase plasma corticosteroid concentrations.

AVAILABILITY (Rx)

TABLETS: 5 mg, 10 mg. **CAPSULES (sustained-release):** 5 mg, 10 mg, 15 mg.

INDICATIONS/ROUTES/DOSAGE

NARCOLEPSY

PO: ADULTS, CHILDREN >12 YRS: Initially, 10 mg/day. Increase by 10 mg at weekly intervals until therapeutic response achieved. CHILDREN 6–12 YRS: Initially, 5 mg/day. Increase by 5 mg/day at weekly intervals until therapeutic response achieved. **Maximum:** 60 mg/day.

ATTENTION DEFICIT DISORDER (ADD)

PO: CHILDREN ≥6 YRS: Initially, 5 mg 1–2 times/day. Increase by 5 mg/day at weekly intervals until therapeutic response achieved. CHILDREN 3–5 YRS: Initially, 2.5 mg/day. Increase by 2.5 mg/day at weekly intervals until therapeutic response achieved. **Maximum:** 40 mg/day.

APPETITE SUPPRESSANT

PO: ADULTS: 5–30 mg daily in divided doses of 5–10 mg each dose, given 30–60 min before meals. **Extended-release:** 1 capsule in morning.

SIDE EFFECTS

FREQUENT: Irregular pulse. Increased motor activity, talkativeness, nervousness, mild euphoria, insomnia. **OCCASIONAL:** Headache, chills, dry mouth, GI distress, worsening depression in pts who are clinically depressed, tachycardia, palpitations, chest pain.

ADVERSE REACTIONS/ TOXIC EFFECTS

Overdose may produce skin pallor/flushing, arrhythmias, psychosis. Abrupt withdrawal following prolonged administration of high dosage may produce lethargy (may last for weeks). Prolonged administration to children with ADD may produce a temporary suppression of normal weight/height patterns.

NURSING IMPLICATIONS

INTERVENTION/EVALUATION

Monitor for CNS overstimulation, increase in B/P, weight loss.

PATIENT/FAMILY TEACHING

Normal dosage levels may produce tolerance to drug's anorexic mood-elevating effects within a few weeks. Avoid tasks that require alertness, motor skills until response to drug is established. Dry mouth may be relieved with sugarless gum, sips of tepid water. Take early in day. May mask extreme fatigue. Report pronounced nervousness, dizziness, decreased appetite, dry mouth.

DHEA

Also known as prasterone

CLASSIFICATION

HERBAL.

ACTION

Produced in adrenal glands and liver, metabolized to androstenedione, major precursor to androgens and estrogens. Also produced in the CNS and concentrated in the limbic regions; may function as an excitatory neuroregulator. **Effect:** Androgen or estrogen-like hormonal effects may be responsible for DHEA benefits.

USES

Used for increasing strength, energy, muscle mass; stimulation of immune system; improving cognitive function/memory; improving depressed mood/fatigue in HIV pts. Treatment of atherosclerosis, hyperglycemia, cancer; prevention of osteoporosis; to increase bone mineral density.

PRECAUTIONS

CONTRAINDICATIONS: None known. **CAUTIONS:** May increase risk of prostate, breast, hormone-sensitive cancers. Avoid use in those with breast, uterine, ovarian cancer; endometriosis; uterine fibroids; diabetes (can increase insulin resistance/sensitivity); depression (may increase risk of adverse psychiatric effects).

LIFESPAN CONSIDERATIONS: Pregnancy/lactation: May adversely effect pregnancy by increasing androgen levels; avoid use. **Children:** Safety and efficacy not established. **Elderly:** Age-related liver impairment may require caution.

INTERACTIONS

DRUG: Can increase **triazolam** concentration. May interfere with **estrogen/androgen** therapy. **HERBAL:** None known. **FOOD:** None known. **LAB VALUES:** None known.

AVAILABILITY (OTC)

CAPSULES: 25 mg. **TABLETS:** 25 mg.

INDICATIONS/ROUTES/DOSAGE

DEPRESSION

PO: ADULTS, ELDERLY: 30–90 mg/day.

USUAL ADULT DOSAGE

PO: ADULTS, ELDERLY: 25–50 mg/day.

SIDE EFFECTS

Acne, hair loss, hirsutism, voice deepening, insulin resistance, altered menstrual pattern, hypertension, abdominal pain, fatigue, headache, nasal congestion.

ADVERSE REACTIONS/ TOXIC EFFECTS

None known.

NURSING IMPLICATIONS

BASELINE ASSESSMENT

Assess for hormone-sensitive tumors (may stimulate growth). Use of hormone replacement therapy (avoid).

INTERVENTION/EVALUATION

Assess changes in mood, sleep pattern. Monitor changes in aggressiveness, irritability, restlessness.

PATIENT/FAMILY TEACHING

Avoid use in pregnancy/lactation; concurrent hormone replacement therapy. Lower dosage if acne develops.

D

Diabeta

see glyburide

diazepam

dye-**az**-eh-pam
(Apo-Diazepam🍁, Diastat, Diazemuls🍁, Dizac, Valium, Vivol🍁)

Do not confuse with diazoxide, Ditropan, Valcyte.

CLASSIFICATION

PHARMACOTHERAPEUTIC: Benzodiazepine **(Schedule IV). CLINICAL:** Antianxiety, skeletal muscle relaxant, anticonvulsant (see pp. 10C, 32C, 132C).

ACTION

Depresses all levels of the CNS by binding to the benzodiazepine receptor on the GABA receptor complex (major inhibitory neurotransmitter in the brain). **Therapeutic Effect:** Produces anxiolytic effect, elevates seizure threshold, produces skeletal muscle relaxation.

PHARMACOKINETICS

Onset	Peak	Duration
PO		
30 min	1–2 hrs	2–3 hrs
IM		
15 min	30–90 min	30–90 min
IV		
1–5 min	15 min	15–60 min

Well absorbed from GI tract. Widely distributed. Protein binding: 98%. Metabolized in liver to active metabolite. Excreted in urine. Minimally removed by hemodialysis. **Half-life:** 20–70 hrs (half-life increased in elderly, liver dysfunction).

USES

Short-term relief of anxiety symptoms, preanesthetic medication, relief of acute alcohol withdrawal. Adjunct for relief of acute musculoskeletal conditions, treatment of seizures (IV route used for termination of status epilepticus). **Gel:** Control of increased seizure activity in refractory epilepsy in those on stable regimens. **Unlabeled:** Treatment of panic disorders, tension headache, tremors.

PRECAUTIONS

CONTRAINDICATIONS: Comatose patient, preexisting CNS depression, respiratory depression, narrow-angle glaucoma, severe uncontrolled pain. **CAUTIONS:** Those receiving other CNS depressants, renal/liver impairment, hypoalbuminemia.

LIFESPAN CONSIDERATIONS: Pregnancy/lactation: Crosses placenta. Distributed in breast milk. May increase risk of fetal abnormalities if administered during first trimester of pregnancy. Chronic ingestion during pregnancy may produce withdrawal symptoms, CNS depression in neonates. **Pregnancy Category D. Children/elderly:** Use small initial doses with gradual increases to avoid ataxia, excessive sedation.

INTERACTIONS

DRUG: Alcohol, CNS depressants may increase CNS depressant effect. **HERBAL: Kava kava, valerian** may increase CNS depressant effects. **FOOD:** None known. **LAB VALUES:** May produce abnormal renal function tests; elevate SGOT (AST), SGPT (ALT), LDH, alkaline phosphatase, serum bilirubin. Therapeutic blood serum level: 0.5–2 mcg/ml; toxic blood serum level: >3 mcg/ml.

AVAILABILITY (Rx)

TABLETS: 2 mg, 5 mg, 10 mg. **CAPSULES (sustained-release):** 15 mg. **ORAL SOLUTION:** 5 mg/5 ml. **INJEC-**

TION: 5 mg/ml. **INJECTABLE EMULSION:** 5 mg/ml. **RECTAL GEL:** 2.5 mg, 10 mg, 15 mg, 20 mg.

ADMINISTRATION/HANDLING

PO

• Give without regard to meals. • Dilute oral concentrate with water, juice, carbonated beverages; may also be mixed in semisolid food (applesauce, pudding). • Tablets may be crushed. • Do not crush or break capsule.

IM

• Injection may be painful. Inject deeply into deltoid muscle.

IV

Storage • Store at room temperature.

Rate of administration • Give by IV push into tubing of a flowing IV solution as close to the vein insertion point as possible. • Administer directly into a large vein (reduces risk of thrombosis/phlebitis). Do not use small veins (e.g., wrist/dorsum of hand). • Administer IV at rate not exceeding 5 mg/min. For children, give over a 3-min period (a too rapid IV may result in hypotension, respiratory depression). • Monitor respirations q5–15min for 2 hours.

IV INCOMPATIBILITIES

Amphotericin B complex (AmBisome, Amphotec, Abelcet), cefepime (Maxipime), diltiazem (Cardizem), fluconazole (Diflucan), foscarnet (Foscavir), heparin, hydrocortisone (Solu-Cortef), hydromorphone (Dilaudid), meropenem (Merrem IV), potassium chloride, propofol (Diprivan), vitamins.

IV COMPATIBILITY

Dobutamine (Dobutrex), fentanyl, morphine.

INDICATIONS/ROUTES/DOSAGE

ANXIETY/SKELETAL MUSCLE RELAXANT

PO: ADULTS: 2–10 mg 2–4 times/day. ELDERLY: 2.5 mg 2 times/day. CHILDREN: 0.12–0.8 mg/kg/day in divided doses q6–8h.

IM/IV: ADULTS: 2–10 mg; repeat in 3–4 hrs. CHILDREN: 0.04–0.3 mg/kg/dose q2–4h. **Maximum:** 0.5 mg/kg in an 8-hr period.

PREANESTHESIA

IV: ADULTS, ELDERLY: 5–15 mg 5–10 min before procedure. CHILDREN: 0.2–0.3 mg/kg. **Maximum:** 10 mg.

ALCOHOL WITHDRAWAL

PO: ADULTS, ELDERLY: 10 mg 3–4 times during first 24 hrs, then reduce to 5–10 mg 3–4 times/day as needed.

IM/IV: ADULTS, ELDERLY: Initially, 10 mg, followed by 5–10 mg q3–4h.

STATUS EPILEPTICUS

IV: ADULTS, ELDERLY: 5–10 mg q10–15min up to 30 mg/8 hrs. CHILDREN ≥5 YRS: 0.05–0.3 mg/kg/dose q15–30min. **Maximum total dose:** 10 mg. CHILDREN >1 MO TO ≤5 YRS: 0.05–0.3 mg/kg/dose q15–30min. **Maximum total dose:** 5 mg.

Rectal gel: ADULTS, CHILDREN ≥12 YRS: 0.2 mg/kg. CHILDREN 6–11 YRS: 0.3 mg/kg. CHILDREN 2–5 YRS: 0.5 mg/kg. Dose may be repeated in 4–12 hrs.

Alert: Do not use more than 5 times/mo or more than once q5days.

SIDE EFFECTS

FREQUENT: Pain with IM injection, drowsiness, fatigue, ataxia (muscular incoordination). **OCCASIONAL:** Slurred speech, orthostatic hypotension, headache, hypoactivity, constipation, nausea, blurred vision. **RARE:** Paradoxical CNS hyperactivity/nervousness in children, excitement/restlessness in elderly/debilitated (generally noted during first 2 wks of therapy, particularly noted in presence of uncontrolled pain).

D

ADVERSE REACTIONS/ TOXIC EFFECTS

IV route may produce pain, swelling, thrombophlebitis, carpal tunnel syndrome. Abrupt or too rapid withdrawal may result in pronounced restlessness, irritability, insomnia, hand tremors, abdominal/muscle cramps, diaphoresis, vomiting, seizures. Abrupt withdrawal in pts with epilepsy may produce increase in frequency/severity of seizures. Overdosage results in somnolence, confusion, diminished reflexes, CNS depression, coma.

NURSING IMPLICATIONS

BASELINE ASSESSMENT

Assess B/P, pulse, respirations immediately prior to administration. Pt must remain recumbent for up to 3 hrs (individualized) after parenteral administration to reduce hypotensive effect. **Anxiety:** Assess autonomic response (cold, clammy hands, sweating), motor response (agitation, trembling, tension). **Musculoskeletal Spasm:** Record onset, type, location, duration of pain. Check for immobility, stiffness, swelling. **Seizures:** Review history of seizure disorder (length, intensity, frequency, duration, LOC). Observe frequently for recurrence of seizure activity. Initiate seizure precautions.

INTERVENTION/EVALUATION

Monitor heart rate, respiratory rate, B/P. Assess children, elderly for paradoxical reaction, particularly during early therapy. Evaluate for therapeutic response: a decrease in intensity/frequency of seizures; a calm, facial expression, decreased restlessness; decreased intensity of skeletal muscle pain. Therapeutic blood serum level: 0.5–2 mcg/ml; toxic blood serum level: >3 mcg/ml.

PATIENT/FAMILY TEACHING

Avoid alcohol. Limit caffeine. May cause drowsiness, impair ability to perform activities requiring mental alertness (e.g., driving). May be habit forming. Avoid abrupt discontinuation after prolonged use.

dibucaine

(Nupercainal)

See Classification section under: Anesthetics: local

diclofenac

dye-**klo**-feh-nak

(Cataflam, Diclotek✤, Novo-Difenac✤, Solaraze, Voltaren, Voltaren XR)

Do not confuse with Diflucan, Duphalac, Verelan.

FIXED-COMBINATION(S)

Arthrotec: diclofenac/misoprostol (an antisecretory gastric protectant): 50 mg/200 mcg; 75 mg/200 mcg.

✦CLASSIFICATION

PHARMACOTHERAPEUTIC: Nonsteroidal anti-inflammatory. **CLINICAL:** Analgesic, anti-inflammatory (see p. 110C).

ACTION

Inhibits prostaglandin synthesis, intensity of pain stimulus reaching sensory nerve endings. Constricts iris sphincter. **Therapeutic Effect:** Produces analgesic and anti-inflammatory effect. Prevents miosis during cataract surgery.

PHARMACOKINETICS

Onset	Peak	Duration
PO		
30 min	2–3 hrs	Up to 8 hrs

Completely absorbed from GI tract; penetrates cornea after ophthalmic administration (may be systemically absorbed). Widely distributed. Protein binding: >99%. Metabolized in liver. Primarily excreted in urine. Minimally removed by hemodialysis. **Half-life:** 1.2–2 hrs.

USES

Symptomatic treatment of acute and/or chronic rheumatoid arthritis, osteoarthritis, ankylosing spondylitis; postop inflammation of cataract extraction; analgesic, primary dysmenorrhea. Treatment of photophobia, relief of pain in incisional refractive surgery. **Solaraze:** Treatment of actinic keratoses. **Unlabeled:** Ophthalmic: Reduces occurrence/severity of cystoid macular edema post cataract surgery. **PO:** Treatment of vascular headaches.

PRECAUTIONS

CONTRAINDICATIONS: Hypersensitivity to diclofenac, aspirin, NSAIDs; porphyria. **CAUTIONS:** CHF, hypertension, impaired renal/liver function, history of GI disease. Avoid topical gel to open skin wounds, infections, exfoliative dermatitis, eyes, neonates, infants, children.

LIFESPAN CONSIDERATIONS: Pregnancy/lactation: Crosses placenta. Unknown if distributed in breast milk. Avoid use during last trimester (may adversely affect fetal cardiovascular system: premature closure of ductus arteriosus). **Pregnancy Category B** (**D** if used in third trimester or near delivery); ophthalmic: **C;** topical: **B. Children:** Safety and efficacy not established. **Elderly:** GI bleeding/ulceration more likely to cause serious adverse effects. Age-related renal impairment may increase risk of liver or renal toxicity; reduced dosage recommended.

INTERACTIONS

DRUG: May increase effects of **oral anticoagulants, heparin, thrombolytics.** May decrease effect of **antihypertensives, diuretics. Salicylates, aspirin** may increase risk of GI side effects, bleeding. **Bone marrow depressants** may increase risk of hematologic reactions. May increase concentration, toxicity of **lithium.** May increase **methotrexate** toxicity. **Probenecid** may increase concentration. **Ophthalmic:** May decrease effect of **acetylcholine, carbachol.** May decrease antiglaucoma effect of **epinephrine, other antiglaucoma medications. HERBAL: Ginkgo biloba** may increase risk of bleeding. **FOOD:** None known. **LAB VALUES:** May increase alkaline phosphatase, LDH, serum transaminase, potassium urine protein, BUN, serum creatinine. May decrease uric acid.

AVAILABILITY (Rx)

GEL: 3%. **TABLETS:** 50 mg (Cataflam). **TABLETS (delayed-release):** 25 mg, 50 mg, 75 mg. **TABLETS (extended-release):** 100 mg. **OPHTHALMIC SOLUTION:** 0.1%.

ADMINISTRATION/HANDLING

PO

• Do not crush or break enteric-coated form. • May give with food, milk, or antacids if GI distress occurs.

OPHTHALMIC

• Place finger on lower eyelid and pull out until pocket is formed between eye and lower lid. Hold dropper above pocket and place prescribed number of drops in pocket. • Close eye gently. Apply digital pressure to lacrimal sac for 1–2 min (minimized drainage into nose and throat, reducing risk of systemic effects). • Remove excess solution with tissue.

D

INDICATIONS/ROUTES/DOSAGE

OSTEOARTHRITIS

PO: ADULTS, ELDERLY: 100–150 mg/day in 2–3 divided doses. **Extended-release:** 100 mg/day as single dose.

RHEUMATOID ARTHRITIS

PO: ADULTS, ELDERLY: 150–200 mg/day in 2–4 divided doses. **Extended-release:** 100 mg/day. **Maximum:** 200 mg.

ANKYLOSING SPONDYLITIS

PO: ADULTS, ELDERLY: 100–125 mg/day in 4–5 divided doses.

ANALGESIC, PRIMARY DYSMENORRHEA

PO: ADULTS: 150 mg/day in 3 divided doses.

USUAL OPHTHALMIC DOSAGE

ADULTS, ELDERLY: Apply 1 drop to eye 4 times/day commencing 24 hrs after cataract surgery. Continue for 2 wks after surgery.

ACTINIC KERATOSES

Topical: ADULTS, ADOLESCENTS: Apply 2 times/day to lesion for 60–90 days.

USUAL PEDIATRIC DOSAGE

PO: 2–3 mg/kg/day in divided doses 2–4 times/day.

PHOTOPHOBIA

Ophthalmic: ADULTS, ELDERLY: 1 drop to affected eye 1 hr preop, within 15 min postop, then 4 times/day for 3 days.

SIDE EFFECTS

FREQUENT (3%–9%): PO: Headache, abdominal cramping, constipation, diarrhea, nausea, dyspepsia. **Ophthalmic:** Burning, stinging on instillation, ocular discomfort. **OCCASIONAL (1%–3%): PO:** Flatulence, dizziness, epigastric pain. **Ophthalmic:** Itching, tearing. **RARE (<1%): PO:** Rash, peripheral edema/fluid retention, visual disturbances, vomiting, drowsiness.

ADVERSE REACTIONS/TOXIC EFFECTS

Overdosage may result in acute renal failure. In those treated chronically, peptic ulcer, GI bleeding, gastritis, severe hepatic reaction (jaundice), nephrotoxicity (hematuria, dysuria, proteinuria); severe hypersensitivity reaction (bronchospasm, angiofacial edema) occur rarely.

NURSING IMPLICATIONS

BASELINE ASSESSMENT

Anti-inflammatory: Assess onset, type, location, duration of pain/inflammation. Inspect appearance of affected joints for immobility, deformities, skin condition.

INTERVENTION/EVALUATION

Monitor for headache, dyspepsia. Monitor pattern of daily bowel activity/stool consistency. Evaluate for therapeutic response: relief of pain, stiffness, swelling; increase in joint mobility; reduced joint tenderness; improved grip strength.

PATIENT/FAMILY TEACHING

Swallow tablet whole; do not crush or chew. Avoid aspirin, alcohol during therapy (increases risk of GI bleeding). If GI upset occurs, take with food, milk. Report skin rash, itching, weight gain, changes in vision, black stools, persistent headache. **Ophthalmic:** Do not use hydrogel soft contact lenses. **Topical:** Avoid exposure to sunlight/sun lamps. Inform physician if rash occurs.

dicloxacillin sodium

(Dycill, Dynapen, Pathocil)

See Classification section under: Antibiotic: penicillins (p. 26C)

dicyclomine hydrochloride

dye-**sigh**-clo-meen
(Bentyl, Bentylol✤, Formulex✤, Lomine✤)

Do not confuse with Aventyl, Benadryl, doxycycline, dyclonine.

CLASSIFICATION

CLINICAL: GI antispasmodic, anticholinergic.

ACTION

Direct relaxant action on smooth muscle. **Therapeutic Effect:** Reduces tone, motility of GI tract.

PHARMACOKINETICS

Onset	Peak	Duration
PO		
1–2 hrs	—	4 hrs

Readily absorbed from GI tract. Widely distributed. Metabolized in liver. **Half-life:** 9–10 hrs.

USES

Treatment of functional disturbances of GI motility (e.g., irritable bowel syndrome).

PRECAUTIONS

CONTRAINDICATIONS: Narrow-angle glaucoma, severe ulcerative colitis, toxic megacolon, obstructive disease of GI tract, paralytic ileus, intestinal atony, bladder neck obstruction due to prostatic hypertrophy, myasthenia gravis in those not treated with neostigmine, tachycardia secondary to cardiac insufficiency or thyrotoxicosis, cardiospasm, unstable cardiovascular status in acute hemorrhage. **EXTREME CAUTION:** Autonomic neuropathy, known or suspected GI infections, diarrhea, mild to moderate ulcerative colitis. **CAUTIONS:** Hyperthyroidism/hepatic or renal disease, hypertension, tachyarrhythmias, CHF, coronary artery disease, gastric ulcer, esophageal reflux or hiatal hernia associated with reflux esophagitis, infants, elderly, COPD.

LIFESPAN CONSIDERATIONS: Pregnancy/lactation: Unknown if drug crosses placenta or is distributed in breast milk. **Pregnancy Category B. Children:** Infants, young children more susceptible to toxic effects. **Elderly:** May cause excitement, agitation, drowsiness, confusion.

INTERACTIONS

DRUG: Antacids, antidiarrheals may decrease absorption. **Anticholinergics** may increase effects. May decrease absorption of **ketoconazole.** May increase severity of GI lesions with **potassium chloride (wax matrix). HERBAL:** None known. **FOOD:** None known. **LAB VALUES:** None known.

AVAILABILITY (Rx)

CAPSULES: 10 mg. **TABLETS:** 20 mg. **SYRUP:** 10 mg/5 ml. **INJECTION:** 10 mg/ml.

ADMINISTRATION/HANDLING

• Store capsules, tablets, syrup, parenteral form at room temperature.

PO

• Dilute oral solution with equal volume of water just before administration. • May give without regard to meals (food may slightly decrease absorption).

IM

• Injection should appear colorless. • Do not administer IV or subcutaneous. • Inject deep into large muscle mass. • Do not give for >2 days.

INDICATIONS/ROUTES/DOSAGE

FUNCTIONAL DISTURBANCES OF GI MOTILITY

PO: ADULTS: 10–20 mg 3–4 times/day up to 40 mg 4 times/day. CHILDREN 6

MOS–2 YRS: 5 mg 3–4 times/day. CHILDREN >2 YRS: 10 mg 3–4 times/day.

IM: ADULTS: 20 mg q4–6h.

D

USUAL ELDERLY DOSAGE

PO: 10–20 mg 4 times/day. May increase up to 160 mg/day.

SIDE EFFECTS

FREQUENT: Dry mouth (sometimes severe), constipation, decreased sweating ability. **OCCASIONAL:** Blurred vision, intolerance to light, urinary hesitancy, drowsiness (with high dosage), agitation/excitement/drowsiness noted in elderly (even with low dosages). IM may produce transient lightheadedness, irritation at injection site. **RARE:** Confusion, hypersensitivity reaction, increased intraocular pressure, nausea, vomiting, unusual tiredness.

ADVERSE REACTIONS/ TOXIC EFFECTS

Overdosage may produce temporary paralysis of ciliary muscle, pupillary dilation, tachycardia, palpitation, hot/dry/flushed skin, absence of bowel sounds, hyperthermia, increased respiratory rate, EKG abnormalities, nausea, vomiting, rash over face/upper trunk, CNS stimulation, psychosis (agitation, restlessness, rambling speech, visual hallucination, paranoid behavior, delusions), followed by depression.

NURSING IMPLICATIONS

BASELINE ASSESSMENT

Prior to giving medication, instruct pt to void (reduces risk of urinary retention).

INTERVENTION/EVALUATION

Monitor daily bowel activity/stool consistency. Assess for urinary retention. Monitor changes in B/P, temperature. Be alert for fever (increased risk of hyperthermia). Assess skin turgor, mucous membranes to evaluate hydration status (encourage adequate fluid intake), bowel sounds for peristalsis.

PATIENT/FAMILY TEACHING

Do not become overheated during exercise in hot weather (may result in heat stroke). Avoid hot baths, saunas. Avoid tasks that require alertness, motor skills until response to drug is established. Do not take antacids or antidiarrheals within 1 hr of taking this medication (decreased effectiveness).

didanosine

dye-**dan**-oh-sin
(Videx, Videx-EC)

CLASSIFICATION

PHARMACOTHERAPEUTIC: Purine nucleoside analogue. **CLINICAL:** Antiviral (see pp. 58C, 98C).

ACTION

Intracellularly converted into a triphosphate, interfering with RNA-directed DNA polymerase (reverse transcriptase). **Therapeutic Effect:** Virustatic, inhibiting replication of retroviruses, including HIV.

PHARMACOKINETICS

Variably absorbed from GI tract. Protein binding: <5%. Rapidly metabolized intracellularly to active form. Primarily excreted in urine. Partially (20%) removed by hemodialysis. **Half-life:** 1.5 hrs; metabolite: 8–24 hrs.

USES

Treatment of HIV infection in combination with other antiretroviral agents.

PRECAUTIONS

CONTRAINDICATIONS: Hypersensitivity to drug or any component of preparation. **CAUTIONS:** Renal/hepatic dysfunction, alcoholism, elevated triglycerides, T-cell counts <100 cells/mm^3; extreme caution with history of pancreatitis. Phenylketonuria and sodium-restricted diets due to phenylalanine, sodium content of preparations.

❖ **LIFESPAN CONSIDERATIONS: Pregnancy/lactation:** Use during pregnancy only if clearly needed. Discontinue nursing during didanosine therapy. **Pregnancy Category B. Children:** Well tolerated in children >3 mos. **Elderly:** Age-related renal impairment may require dosage adjustment.

INTERACTIONS

DRUG: May increase risk of pancreatitis, peripheral neuropathy with medications producing pancreatitis, peripheral neuropathy, respectively. May decrease absorption of **dapsone, itraconazole, ketoconazole, tetracyclines, fluoroquinolones. Stavudine** may increase risk of fatal lactic acidosis in pregnant women. **HERBAL:** None known. **FOOD:** Decreases absorption. **LAB VALUES:** May increase alkaline phosphatase, SGOT (AST), SGPT (ALT), bilirubin, amylase, lipase, triglycerides, uric acid. May decrease potassium.

AVAILABILITY (Rx)

TABLETS (chewable): 25 mg, 50 mg, 100 mg, 150 mg, 200 mg. **CAPSULES (delayed-release):** 125 mg, 200 mg, 250 mg, 400 mg. **POWDER FOR ORAL SOLUTION (single-dose packet):** 100 mg. **PEDIATRIC SOLUTION:** 10 mg/ml.

ADMINISTRATION/HANDLING

PO

• Store at room temperature. • Tablets dispersed in water are stable for 1 hr at room temperature; after reconstitution of buffered powder, oral solution is stable for 4 hrs at room temperature. • Pediatric powder for oral solution following reconstitution as directed, stable for 30 days refrigerated. • Give 1 hr before or 2 hrs after meals (food decreases rate and extent of absorption). • **Chewable tablets:** Thoroughly crush and disperse in at least 30 ml water prior to swallowing. Mixture should be stirred well (2–3 min) and swallowed immediately. • **Buffered powder for oral solution:** Reconstitute prior to administration by pouring contents of packet into about 4 oz water; stir until completely dissolved (up to 2–3 min). Do not mix with fruit juice or other acidic liquid because didanosine is unstable at acidic pH. • **Unbuffered pediatric powder:** Add 100–200 ml water to 2 or 4 g, respectively, to provide concentration of 20 mg/ml. Immediately mix with equal amount of antacid to provide concentration of 10 mg/ml. Shake thoroughly prior to removing each dose. • **Enteric-coated capsules:** Swallow whole, take on empty stomach.

INDICATIONS/ROUTES/DOSAGE

HIV

ADULTS, CHILDREN ≥13 YRS, ≥60 KG: 200 mg q12h or 400 mg once daily. **Oral solution:** 250 mg q12h. **Delayed-release capsules:** 400 mg once daily. ADULTS, CHILDREN ≥13 YRS, ≤60 KG: 125 mg q12h or 250 mg once daily. **Oral solution:** 167 mg q12h. **Delayed-release capsules:** 250 mg once daily. CHILDREN 3 MOS TO <13 YRS: 180–300 mg/m^2/day in divided doses q12h. CHILDREN <3 MOS: 50 mg/m^2/day in divided doses q12h.

DOSAGE IN RENAL IMPAIRMENT

PTS <60 KG:

Creatinine Clearance (ml/min)	Tablets	Oral Solution	Delayed-Release Capsules
30–59	75 mg 2 times/day	100 mg 2 times/day	125 mg once daily
10–29	100 mg once daily	100 mg once daily	125 mg once daily
<10	75 mg once daily	100 mg once daily	—

PTS ≥60 KG:

Creatinine Clearance (ml/min)	Tablets	Oral Solution	Delayed-Release Capsules
30–59	100 mg 2 times/day	100 mg 2 times/day	200 mg once daily
10–29	150 mg once daily	167 mg once daily	125 mg once daily
<10	100 mg once daily	100 mg once daily	125 mg once daily

SIDE EFFECTS

FREQUENT: Adults (>10%): Diarrhea, neuropathy, chills/fever. **Children (>25%):** Chills, fever, decreased appetite, pain, malaise, nausea, diarrhea, vomiting, abdominal pain, headache, nervousness, cough, rhinitis, dyspnea, asthenia, rash, itching. **OCCASIONAL: Adults (2%–9%):** Rash, itching, headache, abdominal pain, nausea, vomiting, pneumonia, myopathy, decreased appetite, dry mouth, dyspnea. **Children (10%–25%):** Failure to thrive, decreased weight, stomatitis, oral thrush, ecchymosis, arthritis, myalgia, insomnia, epistaxis, pharyngitis.

ADVERSE REACTIONS/ TOXIC EFFECTS

Pneumonia, opportunistic infection occur occasionally. Peripheral neuropathy, potentially fatal pancreatitis are the major toxicities.

NURSING IMPLICATIONS

BASELINE ASSESSMENT

Obtain baseline values for CBC, renal/hepatic function tests, vital signs, weight.

INTERVENTION/EVALUATION

In event of abdominal pain, nausea/vomiting, elevated serum amylase, triglycerides, contact physician prior to administering medication (potential for pancreatitis). Be alert to sensation of burning feet, "restless leg syndrome" (unable to find comfortable position for legs/feet), lack of coordination/other signs of peripheral neuropathy. Monitor consistency/frequency of stools. Check skin for rash, eruptions. Monitor blood chemistry, CBC. Assess for opportunistic infections: onset of fever, oral mucosa changes, cough, other respiratory symptoms. Check weight at least twice a week. Assess for visual/hearing difficulty; provide protection from light if photophobia develops.

PATIENT/FAMILY TEACHING

Avoid alcohol. Inform physician if numbness, tingling, persistent severe abdominal pain, nausea/vomiting occur. Shake oral suspension well before use, keep refrigerated. Discard solution after 30 days and obtain new supply.

Diflucan

see fluconazole

diflunisal

dye-**flew**-neh-sol
(Apo-Diflunisal ♣, Dolobid, Novo-Diflunisal ♣)

Do not confuse with Slo-bid.

CLASSIFICATION

PHARMACOTHERAPEUTIC: Nonsteroidal anti-inflammatory. **CLINICAL:** Antirheumatic, analgesic, vascular headache suppressant (see p. 110C).

ACTION

Inhibits prostaglandin synthesis, reducing inflammatory response and intensity of pain stimulus reaching sensory nerve endings. **Therapeutic Effect:** Produces analgesic and anti-inflammatory effect.

PHARMACOKINETICS

Onset	Peak	Duration
PO		
1 hr	2–3 hrs	8–12 hrs

Completely absorbed from GI tract. Widely distributed. Protein binding: >99%. Metabolized in liver. Primarily excreted in urine. Not removed by hemodialysis. **Half-life:** 8–12 hrs.

USES

Treatment of acute or long-term mild to moderate pain associated with acute and/or chronic rheumatoid arthritis, osteoarthritis. **Unlabeled:** Treatment of psoriatic arthritis, vascular headache.

PRECAUTIONS

CONTRAINDICATIONS: Hypersensitivity to NSAIDs, aspirin. Active GI bleeding, factor VII or IX deficiencies. **CAUTIONS:** Impaired renal/liver function, edema, elevated liver function tests, platelet/bleeding disorders, peptic ulcer disease, erosive gastritis, vitamin K deficiency.

LIFESPAN CONSIDERATIONS: Pregnancy/lactation: Crosses placenta. Distributed in breast milk. Avoid use during last trimester (may adversely affect fetal cardiovascular system: premature closure of ductus arteriosus). **Pregnancy Category C** (**D** if used in third trimester or near delivery). **Children:** Safety and efficacy not established. **Elderly:** GI bleeding/ulceration more likely to cause serious adverse effects. Age-related renal impairment may increase risk of liver/renal toxicity; decreased dosage recommended.

INTERACTIONS

DRUG: May increase effects of **oral anticoagulants, heparin, thrombolytics.** May decrease effect of **antihypertensives, diuretics. Salicylates, aspirin** may increase risk of GI side effects, bleeding. **Bone marrow depressants** may increase risk of hematologic reactions. May increase concentration, toxicity of **lithium.** May increase **methotrexate** toxicity. **Probenecid** may increase concentration. **HERBAL: Ginkgo biloba** may increase risk of bleeding. **FOOD:** None known. **LAB VALUES:** May increase serum transaminase activity. May decrease uric acid.

AVAILABILITY (Rx)

TABLETS: 250 mg, 500 mg.

ADMINISTRATION/HANDLING

PO

- May give with water, milk, or meals.
- Do not crush or break film-coated tablets.

INDICATIONS/ROUTES/DOSAGE

MILD TO MODERATE PAIN

PO: ADULTS, ELDERLY: Initially, 0.5–1 g, then 250–500 mg q8–12h. **Maximum:** 1.5 g/day.

RHEUMATOID ARTHRITIS, OSTEOARTHRITIS

PO: ADULTS, ELDERLY: 0.5–1 g/day in 2 divided doses. **Maximum:** 1.5 g/day.

SIDE EFFECTS

Side effects appear less frequently with short-term treatment. **OCCASIONAL (3%–9%):** Nausea, dyspepsia (heartburn, indigestion, epigastric pain), diarrhea, headache, rash. **RARE (1%–3%):** Vomiting, constipation, flatulence, dizziness, somnolence, insomnia, fatigue, tinnitus.

ADVERSE REACTIONS/ TOXIC EFFECTS

D

Overdosage may produce drowsiness, vomiting, nausea, diarrhea, hyperventilation, tachycardia, diaphoresis, stupor, coma. Peptic ulcer, GI bleeding, gastritis, severe hepatic reaction (cholestasis, jaundice) occur rarely. Nephrotoxicity (dysuria, hematuria, proteinuria, nephrotic syndrome), severe hypersensitivity reaction (bronchospasm, angiofacial edema) occur rarely.

NURSING IMPLICATIONS

BASELINE ASSESSMENT

Assess onset, type, location, duration of pain/inflammation. Inspect appearance of affected joints for immobility, deformities, skin condition.

INTERVENTION/EVALUATION

Monitor for nausea, dyspepsia. Assess skin for evidence of rash. Monitor pattern of daily bowel activity/stool consistency. Evaluate for therapeutic response: relief of pain, stiffness, swelling; increase in joint mobility; reduced joint tenderness; improved grip strength.

PATIENT/FAMILY TEACHING

Swallow tablet whole; do not crush or chew. If GI upset occurs, take with food, milk. Report GI distress, headache, rash.

digoxin

di-**jox**-in

(Lanoxicaps, Lanoxin)

Do not confuse with Desoxyn, doxepin, Levsinex, Lonox.

CLASSIFICATION

PHARMACOTHERAPEUTIC: Cardiac glycoside. **CLINICAL:** Antiarrhythmic, cardiotonic (see p. 78C).

ACTION

Increases influx of calcium from extracellular to intracellular cytoplasm. **Therapeutic Effect:** Potentiates the activity of the contractile heart muscle fibers and increases the force of myocardial contraction. Decreases conduction through the SA, AV nodes.

PHARMACOKINETICS

Onset	Peak	Duration
PO		
0.5–2 hrs	28 hrs	3–4 days
IV		
5–30 min	1–4 hrs	3–4 days

Readily absorbed from GI tract. Widely distributed. Protein binding: 30%. Partially metabolized in liver. Primarily excreted in urine. Minimally removed by hemodialysis. **Half-life:** 36–48 hrs (half-life increased with impaired renal function, elderly).

USES

Prophylactic management and treatment of CHF, control of ventricular rate in pts with atrial fibrillation. Treatment and prevention of recurrent paroxysmal atrial tachycardia.

PRECAUTIONS

CONTRAINDICATIONS: Ventricular fibrillation, ventricular tachycardia unrelated to CHF. **CAUTIONS:** Impaired renal function, impaired hepatic function, hypokalemia, advanced cardiac disease, acute MI, incomplete AV block, cor pulmonale, hypothyroidism, pulmonary disease.

LIFESPAN CONSIDERATIONS: Pregnancy/lactation: Crosses placenta. Distributed in breast milk. **Pregnancy Category C. Children:** Premature infants more susceptible to toxicity. **Elderly:** Age-related liver or renal function impairment may require adjusted dosage. Increased risk of loss of appetite.

INTERACTIONS

DRUG: Glucocorticoids, amphotericin, potassium-depleting diuretics may increase toxicity (due to hypokalemia). **Amiodarone** may increase concentration, toxicity; additive effect on SA, AV nodes. **Antiarrhythmics, parenteral calcium, sympathomimetics** may increase risk of arrhythmias. **Antidiarrheals, cholestyramine, colestipol, sucralfate** may decrease absorption. **Diltiazem, verapamil, fluoxetine, quinidine** may increase concentration. **Parenteral magnesium** may cause cardiac conduction changes, heart block. **HERBAL: Siberian ginseng** may increase serum levels. **FOOD:** None known. **LAB VALUES:** None known. Therapeutic blood serum level: 0.8–2 ng/ml; toxic blood serum level: >2 ng/ml.

AVAILABILITY (Rx)

TABLETS: 0.125 mg, 0.25 mg, 0.5 mg. **CAPSULES:** 0.05 mg, 0.1 mg, 0.2 mg. **ELIXIR:** 0.05 mg/ml. **INJECTION:** 0.25 mg/ml, 0.1 mg/ml.

ADMINISTRATION/HANDLING

Alert: IM rarely used (produces severe local irritation, erratic absorption). If no other route possible, give deep into muscle followed by massage. Give no more than 2 ml at any one site.

PO

- May give without regard to meals.
- Tablets may be crushed.

IV

- May give undiluted or dilute with at least a 4-fold volume of Sterile Water for Injection, or D_5W (less than this may cause a precipitate). Use immediately.
- Give IV slowly over at least 5 min.

IV INCOMPATIBILITIES

Amphotericin B complex (Abelcet, Amphotec, AmBisome), fluconazole (Diflucan), foscarnet (Foscavir), propofol (Diprivan).

IV COMPATIBILITIES

Cimetidine (Tagamet), diltiazem (Cardizem), furosemide (Lasix), heparin, insulin (Regular), lidocaine, midazolam (Versed), milrinone (Primacor), morphine, potassium chloride, propofol (Diprivan).

INDICATIONS/ROUTES/DOSAGE

Alert: Adjust dosage in elderly, pts with renal dysfunction. Larger doses often required for adequate control of ventricular rate in pts with atrial fibrillation/flutter. Administer loading dosage in several doses at 4- to 8-hr intervals.

USUAL DOSAGE FOR ADULTS
RAPID LOADING DOSAGE

IV: ADULTS, ELDERLY: 0.6–1 mg.

PO: ADULTS, ELDERLY: Initially, 0.5–0.75 mg, additional doses of 0.125–0.375 mg at 6- to 8-hr intervals. RANGE: 0.75–1.25 mg.

MAINTENANCE DOSAGE

PO/IV: ADULTS, ELDERLY: 0.125–0.375 mg/day.

USUAL DOSAGE FOR CHILDREN
RAPID LOADING DOSAGE

IV: CHILDREN >10 YRS: 8–12 mcg/kg; 5–10 YRS: 15–30 mcg/kg; 2–5 YRS: 25–35 mcg/kg; 1–24 MOS: 30–50 mcg/kg; FULL-TERM: 20–30 mcg/kg; PREMATURE: 15–25 mcg/kg.

PO: CHILDREN >10 YRS: 10–15 mcg/kg; 5–10 YRS: 20–35 mcg/kg; 2–5 YRS: 30–40 mcg/kg; 1–24 MOS: 35–60 mcg/kg; NEONATE: FULL-TERM: 25–35 mcg/kg; PREMATURE: 20–30 mcg/kg.

MAINTENANCE DOSAGE

PO/IV: CHILDREN: 25%–35% loading dose (20%–30% for premature).

DOSAGE IN RENAL IMPAIRMENT
Total digitalizing dose: decrease by 50% in end-stage renal disease.

Creatinine Clearance	Dosage
10–50 mg/min	25%–75% normal
<10 ml/min	10%–25% normal

SIDE EFFECTS

None known; however, there is a very narrow margin of safety between a therapeutic and toxic result. Chronic therapy may produce mammary gland enlargement in women but is reversible when drug is withdrawn.

ADVERSE REACTIONS/ TOXIC EFFECTS

The most common early manifestations of toxicity are GI disturbances (anorexia, nausea, vomiting), neurologic abnormalities (fatigue, headache, depression, weakness, drowsiness, confusion, nightmares). Facial pain, personality change, ocular disturbances (photophobia, light flashes, halos around bright objects, yellow or green color perception) may be noted.

NURSING IMPLICATIONS

BASELINE ASSESSMENT

Assess apical pulse for 60 sec (30 sec if on maintenance therapy). If pulse is ≤60/min (≤70/min for children), withhold drug, contact physician. Blood samples are best taken 6–8 hrs after dose or just before next dose.

INTERVENTION/EVALUATION

Monitor pulse for bradycardia, EKG for arrhythmias for 1–2 hrs after administration (excessive slowing of pulse may be a first clinical sign of toxicity). Assess for GI disturbances, neurologic abnormalities (signs of toxicity) q2–4h during digitalization (daily during maintenance). Monitor serum potassium, magnesium levels. Therapeutic blood serum level: 0.8–2 ng/ml; toxic blood serum level: >2 ng/ml.

PATIENT/FAMILY TEACHING

Stress importance of follow-up visits, tests. Teach pt to take apical pulse correctly and to report pulse <60/min (or as indicated by physician). Ensure pt understands signs of toxicity and need to notify physician if any occur. Wear/carry identification of digoxin therapy and inform dentist, other physician of taking digoxin. Do not increase or skip doses. Do not take OTC medications without consulting physician. Inform physician of decreased appetite, nausea/vomiting, diarrhea, visual changes.

digoxin immune FAB

(Digibind, DigiFab)

◆ **CLASSIFICATION**

CLINICAL: Antidote.

ACTION

Binds molecularly to digoxin in the extracellular space. **Therapeutic Effect:** Makes digoxin unavailable for binding at its site of action on cells in the body.

PHARMACOKINETICS

Onset	Peak	Duration
IV		
30 min	—	3–4 days

Widely distributed into extracellular space. Excreted in urine. **Half-life:** 15–20 hrs.

USES

Treatment of potentially life-threatening digoxin toxicity.

PRECAUTIONS

CONTRAINDICATIONS: None known. **CAUTIONS:** Impaired cardiac, renal function.

LIFESPAN CONSIDERATIONS: Pregnancy/lactation: Unknown if drug crosses placenta or is distributed in breast milk. **Pregnancy Category C. Children:** No age-related precautions noted. **Elderly:** Age-related renal impairment may require caution.

INTERACTIONS

DRUG: None known. **HERBAL:** None known. **FOOD:** None known. **LAB VALUES:** May alter potassium concentration. Serum digoxin concentration may increase precipitously and persist for up to 1 wk (until FAB/digoxin complex is eliminated from body).

AVAILABILITY (Rx)

POWDER FOR INJECTION: 38-mg vial, 40-mg vial (DigiFab).

ADMINISTRATION/HANDLING

IV

Storage • Refrigerate vials. • After reconstitution, is stable for 4 hrs if refrigerated. • Use immediately after reconstitution.

Reconstitution • Reconstitute each 38-mg vial with 4 ml Sterile Water for Injection to provide a concentration of 9.5 mg/ml. • Further dilute with 50 ml 0.9% NaCl.

Rate of administration • Infuse over 30 min (recommended that solution be infused through a 0.22-micron filter). • If cardiac arrest imminent, may give IV push.

IV INCOMPATIBILITY

None known.

INDICATIONS/ROUTES/DOSAGE

Dosage varies according to amount of digoxin to be neutralized. Refer to manufacturer's dosing guidelines.

SIDE EFFECTS

None known.

ADVERSE REACTIONS/ TOXIC EFFECTS

As result of digitalis toxicity, hyperkalemia may occur (diarrhea, paresthesia of extremities, heaviness of legs, decreased B/P, cold skin, grayish pallor, hypotension, mental confusion, irritability, flaccid paralysis, tented T waves, widening QRS, ST depression). When effect of digitalis is reversed, hypokalemia may develop rapidly (muscle cramping, nausea, vomiting, hypoactive bowel sounds, abdominal distention, difficulty breathing, postural hypotension). Rarely, low cardiac output, CHF may occur.

NURSING IMPLICATIONS

BASELINE ASSESSMENT

Obtain serum digoxin level before administering drug. If drawn <6 hrs before last digoxin dose, serum digoxin level may be unreliable. Those with impaired renal function may require >1 wk before serum digoxin assay is reliable. Assess muscle strength, mental status.

INTERVENTION/EVALUATION

Closely monitor temperature, B/P, EKG, potassium serum level during and after drug is administered. Watch for changes from initial assessment (hypokalemia may result in muscle strength changes, tremor, muscle cramps, change in mental status, cardiac arrhythmias; hyponatremia may result in confusion, thirst, cold/clammy skin).

dihydroergotamine

See ergotamine

D

dihydrotachysterol

See vitamin D

Dilacor XR

see diltiazem

Dilantin

see phenytoin

Dilaudid

see hydromorphone

diltiazem hydrochloride

dill-**tie**-ah-zem

(Apo-Diltiaz, Cardizem, Cardizem CD, Cardizem LA, Cartia XT, Dilacor XR, Novo-Diltiazem, Tiazac)

Do not confuse with Cardene, Ziac.

FIXED-COMBINATION(S)

Teczem: diltiazem/enalapril (ACE inhibitor): 180 mg/5 mg.

CLASSIFICATION

PHARMACOTHERAPEUTIC: Calcium channel blocker. **CLINICAL:** Antianginal, antihypertensive, antiarrhythmic (see pp. 15C, 67C).

ACTION

Inhibits calcium movement across cell membranes of cardiac, vascular smooth muscle (dilates coronary arteries, peripheral arteries/arterioles). **Therapeutic Effect:** Decreases heart rate, myocardial contractility; slows SA, AV conduction. Decreases total peripheral vascular resistance by vasodilation.

PHARMACOKINETICS

Onset	Peak	Duration
PO		
0.5–1 hr	—	—
Extended-release		
2–3 hrs	—	—
IV		
3 min	—	—

Well absorbed from GI tract. Protein binding: 70%–80%. Undergoes first-pass metabolism in liver. Metabolized in liver to active metabolite. Primarily excreted in urine. Not removed by hemodialysis. **Half-life:** 3–8 hrs.

USES

PO: Treatment of angina due to coronary artery spasm (Prinzmetal's variant angina), chronic stable angina (effort-associated angina). **Extended-Release:** Treatment of essential hypertension, angina. **Parenteral:** Temporary control of rapid ventricular rate in atrial fibrillation/flutter. Rapid conversion of PSVT to normal sinus rhythm.

PRECAUTIONS

CONTRAINDICATIONS: Sick sinus syndrome/second- or third-degree AV block (except in presence of pacemaker), severe hypotension (<90 mm Hg, systolic), acute MI, pulmonary congestion. **CAUTIONS:** Impaired renal/hepatic function, CHF.

LIFESPAN CONSIDERATIONS: Pregnancy/lactation: Distributed in breast milk. **Pregnancy Category C. Children:** No age-related precautions noted.

Elderly: Age-related renal impairment may require caution.

INTERACTIONS

DRUG: Beta-blockers may have additive effect. May increase **digoxin** concentration. **Procainamide, quinidine** may increase risk of QT interval prolongation. **Carbamazepine, quinidine, theophylline** may increase concentration, toxicity. **HERBAL:** None known. **FOOD:** None known. **LAB VALUES:** PR interval may be increased.

AVAILABILITY (Rx)

TABLETS: 30 mg, 60 mg, 90 mg, 120 mg. **CAPSULES (sustained-release):** 60 mg, 90 mg, 120 mg, 180 mg, 240 mg, 300 mg, 360 mg, 420 mg. **INJECTION:** 5 mg/ml vials. **READY-TO-HANG INFUSION:** 1 mg/ml.

ADMINISTRATION/HANDLING

PO

• Give before meals and at bedtime. • Tablets may be crushed. • Do not crush sustained-release capsules.

IV

Storage • Refrigerate vials. • After dilution, stable for 24 hrs.

Reconstitution • Add 125 mg to 100 ml D_5W, 0.9% NaCl to provide a concentration of 1 mg/ml. Add 250 mg to 250 or 500 ml diluent to provide a concentration of 0.83 mg/ml or 0.45 mg/ml, respectively. Maximum concentration: 1.25 g/250 ml (5 mg/ml).

Rate of administration • Infuse per dilution/rate chart provided by manufacturer.

IV INCOMPATIBILITIES

Acetazolamide (Diamox), acyclovir (Zovirax), aminophylline, ampicillin, ampicillin/sulbactam (Unasyn), cefoperazone (Cefobid), diazepam (Valium), furosemide (Lasix), heparin, insulin, nafcillin, phenytoin (Dilantin), rifampin (Rifadin), sodium bicarbonate.

IV COMPATIBILITIES

Albumin, aztreonam (Azactam), bumetanide (Bumex), cefazolin (Ancef), cefotaxime (Claforan), ceftazidime (Fortaz), ceftriaxone (Rocephin), cefuroxime (Zinacef), cimetidine (Tagamet), ciprofloxacin (Cipro), clindamycin (Cleocin), digoxin (Lanoxin), dobutamine (Dobutrex), dopamine (Intropin), gentamicin, hydromorphone (Dilaudid), lidocaine, lorazepam (Ativan), metoclopramide (Reglan), metronidazole (Flagyl), midazolam (Versed), morphine, multivitamins, nitroglycerin, norepinephrine (Levophed), potassium chloride, potassium phosphate, tobramycin (Nebcin), vancomycin (Vancocin).

INDICATIONS/ROUTES/DOSAGE

ANGINA

PO: ADULTS, ELDERLY: Initially, 30 mg 4 times/day. Increase up to 180–360 mg/day in 3–4 divided doses at 1- to 2-day intervals.

CD capsules: ADULTS, ELDERLY: Initially, 120–180 mg/day; titrate over 7–14 days. RANGE: Up to 480 mg/day.

ESSENTIAL HYPERTENSION

PO: Extended-release: ADULTS, ELDERLY: Initially, 60–120 mg 2 times/day. **CD capsules:** ADULTS, ELDERLY: Initially, 180–240 mg/day. RANGE: 240–360 mg in 2 divided doses. **Dilacor XR:** ADULTS, ELDERLY: Initially, 180–240 mg/day. RANGE: 180–480 mg/day.

USUAL PARENTERAL DOSAGE

IV push: ADULTS, ELDERLY: Initially, 0.25 mg/kg actual body weight over 2 min. May repeat in 15 min at dose of 0.35 mg/kg actual body weight. Subsequent doses individualized.

IV infusion: ADULTS, ELDERLY: After initial bolus injection, 5–10 mg/hr, may increase at 5 mg/hr up to 15 mg/hr. Maintain over 24 hrs.

Alert: Refer to manufacturer's information for dose concentration/infusion rates.

D

SIDE EFFECTS

FREQUENT (5%–10%): Peripheral edema, dizziness, lightheadedness, headache, bradycardia, asthenia (loss of strength, weakness). **OCCASIONAL (2%–5%):** Nausea, constipation, flushing, altered EKG. **RARE (<2%):** Rash, micturition disorder (polyuria, nocturia, dysuria, frequency of urination), abdominal discomfort, somnolence.

ADVERSE REACTIONS/ TOXIC EFFECTS

Abrupt withdrawal may increase frequency/duration of angina. CHF, second- and third-degree AV block occur rarely. Overdosage produces nausea, drowsiness, confusion, slurred speech, profound bradycardia.

NURSING IMPLICATIONS

BASELINE ASSESSMENT

Concurrent therapy of sublingual nitroglycerin may be used for relief of anginal pain. Record onset, type (sharp, dull, squeezing), radiation, location, intensity, duration of anginal pain, and precipitating factors (exertion, emotional stress). Assess baseline renal/liver function tests. Assess B/P, apical pulse immediately before drug is administered.

INTERVENTION/EVALUATION

Assist with ambulation if dizziness occurs. Assess for peripheral edema behind medial malleolus (sacral area in bedridden pts). Monitor pulse rate for bradycardia. With IV therapy, assess B/P, renal/liver function tests, EKG. Question for asthenia, headache.

PATIENT/FAMILY TEACHING

Do not abruptly discontinue medication. Compliance with therapy regimen is essential to control anginal pain. To avoid hypotensive effect, rise slowly from lying to sitting position, wait momentarily before standing. Avoid tasks that require alertness, motor skills until response to drug is established. Contact physician/nurse if irregular heartbeat, shortness of breath, pronounced dizziness, nausea, or constipation occurs.

dimenhydrinate

(Dramamine)

See Classification section under: Antihistamines (p. 48C)

dinoprostone

dye-noe-**pros**-tone

(Cervidil, Prepidil Gel, Prostin E_2)

Do not confuse with bepridil.

◆ CLASSIFICATION

PHARMACOTHERAPEUTIC: Prostaglandin. **CLINICAL:** Oxytocic, abortifacient, antihemorrhagic.

ACTION

Direct action on myometrium. Direct softening, dilation effect on cervix. **Therapeutic Effect:** Stimulates myometrial contractions in gravid uterus.

PHARMACOKINETICS

Undergoes rapid enzymatic deactivation primarily in maternal lungs. Protein binding: 73%. Primarily excreted in urine.

USES

Suppository: To induce abortion from the 12th wk of pregnancy through the second trimester; to evacuate uterine contents in missed abortion or intrauterine fetal death up to 28 wks gestational age (as calculated from the first day of the last normal menstrual period), benign hydatidiform mole. Treatment of postpartum/postabortion hemorrhage, induction labor at or near term. **Gel:** Ripening unfavorable cervix in pregnant women at or near term with medical/obstetric need for labor induction. Induction of labor at or near term.

PRECAUTIONS

CONTRAINDICATIONS: Hypersensitivity to dinoprostone or other prostaglandins; acute pelvic inflammatory disease; active cardiac/renal/hepatic/pulmonary disease, fetal malpresentation or significant cephalopelvic disproportion. **CAUTIONS:** Cervicitis, infected endocervical lesions or acute vaginitis, history of asthma, hypotension/hypertension, anemia, jaundice, diabetes, epilepsy, uterine fibroids, compromised (scarred) uterus, cardiovascular/renal/hepatic disease.

LIFESPAN CONSIDERATIONS: Pregnancy/lactation: SUPPOSITORY: Teratogenic, therefore abortion must complete. GEL: Sustained uterine hyperstimulation may affect fetus (e.g., abnormal heart rate). **Pregnancy Category C. Children/elderly:** Not used in these pt populations.

INTERACTIONS

DRUG: Oxytocics may cause uterine hypertonus, possibly causing uterine rupture or cervical laceration. **HERBAL:** None known. **FOOD:** None known. **LAB VALUES:** None known.

AVAILABILITY (Rx)

VAGINAL SUPPOSITORY: 20 mg. **VAGINAL GEL:** 0.5 mg (Prepidil). **VAGINAL INSERTS:** 10 mg (Cervidil).

ADMINISTRATION/HANDLING

SUPPOSITORY

• Keep frozen (<4°F); bring to room temperature just before use. • Administer only in hospital setting with emergency equipment available. • Warm suppository to room temperature before removing foil wrapper. • Avoid skin contact due to risk of absorption. • Insert high in vagina. • Pt should remain supine for 10 min after administration.

GEL

• Refrigerate. • Use caution in handling, prevent skin contact. Wash hands thoroughly with soap and water following administration. • Bring to room temperature just before use (avoid forcing the warming process). • Assemble dosing apparatus as described in manufacturer insert. • Have pt in dorsal position with cervix visualized using a speculum. • Introduce gel into cervical canal just below level of internal os. • Have pt remain in supine position at least 15–30 min (minimizes leakage from cervical canal).

INDICATIONS/ROUTES/DOSAGE

ABORTIFACIENT

Intravaginal: ADULTS: 20 mg (one suppository) high into vagina. May repeat at 3- to 5-hr intervals until abortion occurs. Do not administer >2 days.

RIPENING UNFAVORABLE CERVIX

Intracervical: (Prepidil): ADULTS: Initially, 0.5 mg (2.5 ml); if no cervical/uterine response, may repeat 0.5-mg dose in 6 hrs. **Maximum:** 1.5 mg (7.5 ml) for a 24-hr period. **(Cervidil):** ADULTS: 10 mg over 12-hr period. Remove upon onset of active labor or 12 hrs following insertion.

SIDE EFFECTS

FREQUENT: Vomiting (66%), diarrhea (40%), nausea (33%). **OCCASIONAL:** Headache (10%), chills/shivering (10%), hives, bradycardia, increased uterine pain accompanying abortion, peripheral vasoconstriction. **RARE:** Flushing, vulvae edema.

D

ADVERSE REACTIONS/ TOXIC EFFECTS

Excessive dosage may cause uterine hypertonicity with spasm/tetanic contraction, leading to cervical laceration/perforation, uterine rupture, hemorrhage.

NURSING IMPLICATIONS

BASELINE ASSESSMENT

Offer emotional support. **Suppository:** Obtain orders for antiemetics, antidiarrheals, meperidine, other pain medication for abdominal cramps. Assess any uterine activity, vaginal bleeding. **Gel:** Assess Bishop score. Assess degree of effacement (determines size of shielded endocervical catheter).

INTERVENTION/EVALUATION

Suppository: Check strength, duration, frequency of contractions and monitor vital signs q15min until stable, then hourly until abortion complete. Check resting uterine tone. Administer medications for relief of GI effects if indicated or for abdominal cramps. **Gel:** Monitor uterine activity (onset of uterine contractions), fetal status (heart rate), character of cervix (dilation, effacement). Have pt remain recumbent 12 hrs after application with continuous electronic monitoring of fetal heart rate and uterine activity. Record maternal vital signs at least hourly in presence of uterine activity. Reassess Bishop score.

PATIENT/FAMILY TEACHING

Suppository: Report fever, chills, foul-smelling/increased vaginal discharge, uterine cramps/pain promptly.

Diovan

see valsartan

diphenhydramine hydrochloride

dye-phen-**high**-dra-meen
(Allerdryl ✤, Benadryl, Nytol ✤)

Do not confuse with benazepril, Bentyl, Benylin, calamine, dimenhydrinate.

FIXED-COMBINATION(S)

With calamine, an astringent, and camphor, a counterirritant **(Caladryl).**

◆CLASSIFICATION

PHARMACOTHERAPEUTIC: Ethanolamine. **CLINICAL:** Antihistamine, anticholinergic, antipruritic, antitussive, antiemetic, antidyskinetic (see p. 48C).

ACTION

Competes with histamine at histaminic receptor sites. Inhibits central acetylcholine. **Therapeutic Effect:** Results in anticholinergic, antipruritic, antitussive, antiemetic effects. Produces antidyskinetic, sedative effect.

PHARMACOKINETICS

Onset	Peak	Duration
PO		
15–30 min	1–4 hrs	4–6 hrs
IM/IV		
<15 min	1–4 hrs	4–6 hrs

Well absorbed after PO, parenteral administration. Widely distributed. Protein binding: 98%–99%. Metabolized in liver.

Primarily excreted in urine. **Half-life:** 1–4 hrs.

USES

Treatment of allergic reactions, parkinsonism; prevention/treatment of nausea, vomiting, vertigo due to motion sickness; antitussive; short-term management of insomnia. Topical form used for relief of pruritus, insect bites, skin irritations.

PRECAUTIONS

CONTRAINDICATIONS: Acute asthmatic attack, those receiving MAOIs. **CAUTIONS:** Narrow-angle glaucoma, peptic ulcer, prostatic hypertrophy, pyloroduodenal or bladder neck obstruction, asthma, COPD, increased intraocular pressure, cardiovascular disease, hyperthyroidism, hypertension, seizure disorders.

LIFESPAN CONSIDERATIONS: Pregnancy/lactation: Crosses placenta. Detected in breast milk (may produce irritability in nursing infants). Increased risk of seizures in neonates, premature infants if used during third trimester of pregnancy. May prohibit lactation. **Pregnancy Category B. Children:** Not recommended in newborns or premature infants (increased risk of paradoxical reaction). **Elderly:** Increased risk for dizziness, sedation, confusion, hypotension, hyperexcitability.

INTERACTIONS

DRUG: Alcohol, CNS depressants may increase CNS depressant effects. **MAOIs** may increase anticholinergic, CNS depressant effects. **Anticholinergics** may increase anticholinergic effects. **HERBAL:** None known. **FOOD:** None known. **LAB VALUES:** May suppress wheal and flare reactions to antigen skin testing unless antihistamines are discontinued 4 days before testing.

AVAILABILITY (OTC)

CAPSULES: 25 mg, 50 mg. **TABLETS:** 25 mg, 50 mg. **TABLETS (chewable):** 12.5 mg. **SYRUP:** 12.5 mg/5 ml. **ELIXIR:** 12.5 mg/5 ml. **INJECTION (Rx):** 50 mg/ml. **CREAM:** 2%. **SPRAY:** 2%.

D

ADMINISTRATION/HANDLING

PO

• Give without regard to meals. • Scored tablets may be crushed. • Do not crush capsules or film-coated tablets.

IM

• Give deep IM into large muscle mass.

IV

• May be given undiluted. • Give IV injection over at least 1 min.

IV INCOMPATIBILITIES

Allopurinol (Aloprim), amphotericin B complex (Abelcet, AmBisome, Amphotec), cefepime (Maxipime), dexamethasone (Decadron), foscarnet (Foscavir).

IV COMPATIBILITIES

Atropine, cisplatin (Platinol), cyclophosphamide (Cytoxan), cytarabine (Cytosar), droperidol (Inapsine), fentanyl, glycopyrrolate (Robinul), heparin, hydrocortisone (Solu-Cortef), hydromorphone (Dilaudid), hydroxyzine (Vistaril), lidocaine, metoclopramide (Reglan), midazolam (Versed), morphine, ondansetron (Zofran), potassium chloride, promethazine (Phenergan), propofol (Diprivan).

INDICATIONS/ROUTES/DOSAGE

MODERATE TO SEVERE ALLERGIC REACTION, DYSTONIC REACTION

PO/IM/IV: ADULTS, ELDERLY: 25–50 mg q4h. **Maximum:** 400 mg/day. CHILDREN: 5 mg/kg/day in divided doses q6–8h. **Maximum:** 300 mg/day.

MOTION SICKNESS, MINOR ALLERGIC RHINITIS

PO/IM/IV: ADULTS, ELDERLY, CHILDREN >12 YRS: 25–50 mg q4–6h. **Maximum:** 300 mg/day. CHILDREN 6–12 YRS: 12.5–

25 mg q4–6h. **Maximum:** 150 mg/day. CHILDREN 2–6 YRS: 6.25 mg q4–6h. **Maximum:** 37.5 mg/day.

ANTITUSSIVE
PO: ADULTS, ELDERLY, CHILDREN >12 YRS: 25 mg q4h. **Maximum:** 150 mg/day. CHILDREN 6–12 YRS: 12.5 mg q4h. **Maximum:** 75 mg/day. CHILDREN 2–6 YRS: 6.25 mg q4h. **Maximum:** 37.5 mg/day.

NIGHTTIME SLEEP AID
PO: ADULTS, ELDERLY, CHILDREN >12 YRS: 50 mg qhs. CHILDREN 2–12 YRS: 1 mg/kg/dose. **Maximum:** 50 mg.

PRURITUS RELIEF
Topical: ADULTS, ELDERLY, CHILDREN >12 YRS: 1% OR 2% STRENGTH: Apply 3–4 times/day. CHILDREN 2–12 YRS: 1% STRENGTH: Apply 3–4 times/day.

SIDE EFFECTS

FREQUENT: Drowsiness, dizziness, muscular weakness, hypotension, dry mouth/nose/throat/lips, urinary retention, thickening of bronchial secretions. Sedation, dizziness, hypotension more likely noted in elderly. **OCCASIONAL:** Epigastric distress, flushing, visual or hearing disturbances, paresthesia, diaphoresis, chills.

ADVERSE REACTIONS/ TOXIC EFFECTS

Children may experience dominant paradoxical reactions (restlessness, insomnia, euphoria, nervousness, tremors). Overdosage in children may result in hallucinations, seizures, death. Hypersensitivity reaction (eczema, pruritus, rash, cardiac disturbances, photosensitivity) may occur. Overdosage may vary from CNS depression (sedation, apnea, hypotension, cardiovascular collapse, death) to severe paradoxical reaction (hallucinations, tremor, seizures).

NURSING IMPLICATIONS

BASELINE ASSESSMENT

If pt is having acute allergic reaction, obtain history of recently ingested foods, drugs, environmental exposure, recent emotional stress. Monitor rate, depth, rhythm, type of respiration, quality/rate of pulse. Assess lung sounds for rhonchi, wheezing, rales.

INTERVENTION/EVALUATION

Monitor B/P, esp. in elderly (increased risk of hypotension). Monitor children closely for paradoxical reaction.

PATIENT/FAMILY TEACHING

Tolerance to antihistaminic effect generally does not occur; tolerance to sedative effect may occur. Avoid tasks that require alertness, motor skills until response to drug is established. Dry mouth, drowsiness, dizziness may be an expected response of drug. Avoid alcohol.

diphenoxylate hydrochloride with atropine sulfate

dye-phen-**ox**-e-late
(Lomotil, Lonox)
Do not confuse with Lamictal, Lanoxin, Loprox, Lovenox.

FIXED COMBINATION(S)

Lomotil: diphenoxylate/atropine (anticholinergic, antispasmodic): 2.5 mg/0.025 mg.

◆ CLASSIFICATION

PHARMACOTHERAPEUTIC: Meperidine derivative. **CLINICAL:** Antidiarrheal (see p. 41C).

ACTION

Acts locally, centrally. **Therapeutic Effect:** Reduces intestinal motility.

PHARMACOKINETICS

Well absorbed from GI tract. Metabolized in liver to active metabolite. Primarily eliminated in feces. **Half-life:** 2.5 hrs; metabolite: 12–24 hrs.

USES

Adjunctive treatment of acute, chronic diarrhea.

PRECAUTIONS

CONTRAINDICATIONS: Severe liver disease, jaundice, dehydration, narrow-angle glaucoma, children <2 yrs. **CAUTIONS:** Cirrhosis, renal/liver disease, renal impairment, acute ulcerative colitis.

LIFESPAN CONSIDERATIONS: Pregnancy/lactation: Unknown if drug crosses placenta or is distributed in breast milk. **Pregnancy Category C. Children:** Not recommended (increased susceptibility to toxicity, including respiratory depression). **Elderly:** More susceptible to anticholinergic effects, confusion, respiratory depression.

INTERACTIONS

DRUG: Alcohol, CNS depressants may increase effect. **Anticholinergics** may increase effect of atropine. **MAOIs** may precipitate hypertensive crisis. **HERBAL:** None known. **FOOD:** None known. **LAB VALUES:** May increase amylase.

AVAILABILITY (Rx)

TABLETS: 2.5 mg. **LIQUID:** 2.5 mg/5 ml.

ADMINISTRATION/HANDLING

PO

- Give without regard to meals. If GI irritation occurs, give with food or meals.
- Use liquid for children 2–12 yrs (use graduated dropper for administration of liquid medication).

INDICATIONS/ROUTES/DOSAGE

ANTIDIARRHEAL

PO: ADULTS, ELDERLY: Initially, 15–20 mg/day in 3–4 divided doses, then 5–15 mg/day in 2–3 divided doses. CHILDREN 9–12 YRS: 2 mg 5 times/day. CHILDREN 6–8 YRS: 2 mg 4 times/day. CHILDREN 2–5 YRS: 2 mg 3 times/day.

SIDE EFFECTS

FREQUENT: Drowsiness, lightheadedness, dizziness, nausea. **OCCASIONAL:** Headache, dry mouth. **RARE:** Flushing, tachycardia, urinary retention, constipation, paradoxical reaction (restlessness, agitation), blurred vision.

ADVERSE REACTIONS/ TOXIC EFFECTS

Dehydration may predispose to toxicity. Paralytic ileus, toxic megacolon (constipation, decreased appetite, stomach pain with nausea/vomiting) occur rarely. Severe anticholinergic reaction (severe lethargy, hypotonic reflexes, hyperthermia) may result in severe respiratory depression, coma.

NURSING IMPLICATIONS

BASELINE ASSESSMENT

Check baseline hydration status: skin turgor, mucous membranes for dryness, urinary status.

INTERVENTION/EVALUATION

Encourage adequate fluid intake. Assess bowel sounds for peristalsis. Monitor daily bowel activity, stool consistency (watery, loose, soft, semisolid, solid), record time of evacuation. Assess for abdominal disturbances. Discontinue medication if abdominal distention occurs.

D

PATIENT/FAMILY TEACHING

Avoid tasks that require alertness, motor skills until response to drug is established. Avoid alcohol, barbiturates. Contact physician if fever, palpitations occur or diarrhea persists. Report abdominal distention.

dipivefrin

(Propine)

See Classification section under: Antiglaucoma agents (p. 45C)

Diprivan

see propofol

dipyridamole

die-pie-**rid**-ah-mole

(Apo-Dipyridamole✤, Novodipiradol✤, Persantine)

Do not confuse with Aggrastat, disopyramide, Periactin.

FIXED-COMBINATION(S)

Aggrenox: dipyridamole/aspirin (antiplatelet): 200 mg/25 mg.

◆ CLASSIFICATION

PHARMACOTHERAPEUTIC: Blood modifier, platelet aggregation inhibitor. **CLINICAL:** Antiplatelet, antianginal, diagnostic agent (see p. 29C).

ACTION

Inhibits activity of adenosine deaminase and phosphodiesterase, enzymes causing accumulation of adenosine, cyclic AMP. **Therapeutic Effect:** Inhibits platelet aggregation, may cause coronary vasodilation.

PHARMACOKINETICS

Slowly, variably absorbed from GI tract. Widely distributed. Protein binding: 91%–99%. Metabolized in liver. Primarily eliminated via biliary excretion. **Half-life:** 10–15 hrs.

USES

Adjunct to warfarin (Coumadin) anticoagulant therapy in prevention of postop thromboembolic complications of cardiac valve replacement. **IV:** Alternative to exercise in thallium myocardial perfusion imaging for evaluation of coronary artery disease. **Unlabeled:** Prophylaxis of myocardial reinfarction, treatment of transient ischemic attacks (TIAs).

PRECAUTIONS

CONTRAINDICATIONS: None known. **CAUTIONS:** Hypotension.

LIFESPAN CONSIDERATIONS: Pregnancy/lactation: Distributed in breast milk. **Pregnancy Category C. Children:** Safety and efficacy not established. **Elderly:** No age-related precautions noted.

INTERACTIONS

DRUG: May increase risk of bleeding with **anticoagulants, heparin, thrombolytics, aspirin, salicylates. HERBAL:** None known. **FOOD:** None known. **LAB VALUES:** None known.

AVAILABILITY (Rx)

TABLETS: 25 mg, 50 mg, 75 mg. **INJECTION:** 5 mg/ml.

ADMINISTRATION/HANDLING

PO

- Best taken on empty stomach with full glass of water.

IV

- Dilute to at least 1:2 ratio with 0.9%

NaCl or D_5W for total volume of 20–50 ml (undiluted may cause irritation). • Infuse over 4 min. • Inject thallium within 5 min after dipyridamole infusion.

IV INCOMPATIBILITY

No information available via Y-site administration.

INDICATIONS/ROUTES/DOSAGE

PREVENTION OF THROMBOEMBOLIC DISORDERS

PO: ADULTS, ELDERLY: 75–100 mg 4 times/day in combination with other medications. CHILDREN: 3–6 mg/kg/day in 3 divided doses.

DIAGNOSTIC

IV: ADULTS, ELDERLY (BASED ON WEIGHT): 0.142 mg/kg/min infused over 4 min; doses >60 mg not needed for any pt.

SIDE EFFECTS

FREQUENT (14%): Dizziness. **OCCASIONAL (2%–6%):** Abdominal distress, headache, rash. **RARE (<2%):** Diarrhea, vomiting, flushing, pruritus.

ADVERSE REACTIONS/ TOXIC EFFECTS

Overdosage produces peripheral vasodilation, resulting in hypotension.

NURSING IMPLICATIONS

BASELINE ASSESSMENT

Assess for presence of chest pain. Obtain baseline B/P, pulse. When used as antiplatelet, check hematologic levels.

INTERVENTION/EVALUATION

Assist with ambulation if dizziness occurs. Monitor heart sounds by auscultation. Assess B/P for hypotension. Assess skin for flushing, rash.

PATIENT/FAMILY TEACHING

Avoid alcohol. If nausea occurs, cola, unsalted crackers, dry toast may relieve effect. Therapeutic response may not be achieved before 2–3 mos of continuous therapy. Use caution when getting up suddenly from lying or sitting position.

D

dirithromycin

dih-**rith**-row-my-sin

(Dynabac)

Do not confuse with Dynacin, DynaCirc.

CLASSIFICATION

PHARMACOTHERAPEUTIC: Macrolide. **CLINICAL:** Antibiotic (see p. 24C).

ACTION

Binds to ribosomal receptor sites of susceptible organisms. **Therapeutic Effect:** Inhibits protein synthesis.

PHARMACOKINETICS

Rapidly absorbed from GI tract. Widely distributed into tissues and within cells. Protein binding: 15%–30%. Eliminated primarily unchanged via biliary excretion. Not removed by hemodialysis. **Half-life:** 30–44 hrs.

USES

Treatment of mild to moderate infections of upper respiratory tract (pharyngitis, tonsillitis), acute bronchitis, chronic bronchitis, uncomplicated skin/skin structure infections, community-acquired pneumonia.

PRECAUTIONS

CONTRAINDICATIONS: Hypersensitivity to dirithromycin, erythromycins, any macrolide antibiotic. **CAUTIONS:** Hepatic/renal dysfunction.

LIFESPAN CONSIDERATIONS: Pregnancy/lactation: Unknown if distributed in breast milk. **Pregnancy Category C. Children:** Safety and efficacy not established in those <12 yrs. **Elderly:** No age-related precautions noted.

D

INTERACTIONS

DRUG: **H_2 antagonists** increase **dirithromycin** absorption. **Aluminum/magnesium-containing antacids** may decrease concentration (give 1 hr prior to or 2 hrs following antacid). **HERBAL:** None known. **FOOD:** None known. **LAB VALUES:** May increase platelet count, potassium CPK, eosinophils, neutrophils.

AVAILABILITY (Rx)

TABLETS (enteric-coated): 250 mg.

ADMINISTRATION/HANDLING

PO

• Administer with food or within 1 hr of having eaten (food increases absorption). • Swallow whole (tablets not to be cut, crushed, or chewed).

INDICATIONS/ROUTES/DOSAGE

PHARYNGITIS/TONSILLITIS

PO: ADULTS, ELDERLY, CHILDREN ≥12 YRS: 500 mg once daily for 10 days.

ACUTE BRONCHITIS, CHRONIC BRONCHITIS

PO: ADULTS, ELDERLY, CHILDREN ≥12 YRS: 500 mg once daily for 7 days.

COMMUNITY-ACQUIRED PNEUMONIA

PO: ADULTS, ELDERLY, CHILDREN ≥12 YRS: 500 mg once daily for 14 days.

SKIN, SKIN STRUCTURE INFECTIONS

PO: ADULTS, ELDERLY, CHILDREN ≥12 YRS: 500 mg once daily for 7 days.

SIDE EFFECTS

FREQUENT (8%–10%): Abdominal pain, headache, nausea, diarrhea. **OCCASIONAL (2%–3%):** Vomiting, dyspepsia, dizziness, nonspecific pain, asthenia. **RARE (<2%):** Increased cough, flatulence, rash, dyspnea, pruritus/urticaria, insomnia.

ADVERSE REACTIONS/TOXIC EFFECTS

Superinfections, esp. antibiotic-associated colitis (abdominal cramps, watery severe diarrhea, fever), may result from altered bacterial balance.

NURSING IMPLICATIONS

BASELINE ASSESSMENT

Question for history of allergies to dirithromycin, erythromycins.

INTERVENTION/EVALUATION

Monitor for improvement in signs/symptoms of infection, WBC. Check for GI discomfort, nausea, headache, diarrhea. Determine pattern of bowel activity/stool consistency. Evaluate for superinfection: genital/anal pruritus, sore mouth/tongue, moderate to severe diarrhea.

PATIENT/FAMILY TEACHING

Continue therapy for full length of treatment. Take medication with food or within 1 hr of having eaten. Do not take with aluminum/magnesium-containing antacids.

disopyramide phosphate

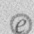

dye-so-**peer**-ah-myd

(Norpace, Norpace CR, Rythmodan)

Do not confuse with desipramine, dipyridamole, Rythmol.

CLASSIFICATION

CLINICAL: Antiarrhythmic (see p. 12C).

ACTION

Prolongs refractory period of cardiac cell by direct effect, decreasing myocardial excitability and conduction velocity. **Therapeutic Effect:** Depresses myocardial contractility. Has anticholinergic, negative inotropic effects.

USES

Suppression and prevention of ventricular ectopy, unifocal/multifocal premature ventricular contractions, episodes of ventricular tachycardia. **Unlabeled:** Prophylaxis/treatment of supraventricular tachycardia.

PRECAUTIONS

CONTRAINDICATIONS: Preexisting urinary retention, preexisting second- or third-degree AV block, cardiogenic shock, narrow-angle glaucoma, unless pt is undergoing cholinergic therapy. **CAUTIONS:** CHF, myasthenia gravis, prostatic hypertrophy, sick sinus syndrome (bradycardia/tachycardia), Wolff-Parkinson-White syndrome, bundle-branch block, impaired renal/hepatic function. **Pregnancy Category C.**

INTERACTIONS

DRUG: **Other antiarrhythmics (e.g., propranolol, diltiazem, verapamil)** may prolong conduction, decrease cardiac output. **Pimozide** may increase cardiac arrhythmias. **HERBAL:** None known. **FOOD:** None known. **LAB VALUES:** May decrease glucose. May cause EKG changes. May increase cholesterol, triglycerides. Therapeutic blood serum level: 2–8 mcg/ml; toxic blood serum level: >8 mcg/ml.

AVAILABILITY (Rx)

CAPSULES: 100 mg, 150 mg. **CAPSULES (extended-release):** 100 mg, 150 mg.

INDICATIONS/ROUTES/DOSAGE

USUAL DOSAGE

PO: ADULTS, ELDERLY >50 KG: 150 mg q6h (300 mg q12h with extended-release). ADULTS, ELDERLY <50 KG: 100 mg q6h (200 mg q12h with extended-release). CHILDREN 12–18 YRS: 6–15 mg/kg/day in divided doses q6h. CHILDREN 5–11 YRS: 10–15 mg/kg/day in divided doses q6h. CHILDREN 1–4 YRS: 10–20 mg/kg/day in divided doses q6h. CHILDREN <1 YR: 10–30 mg/kg/day in divided doses q6h.

RAPID CONTROL OF ARRHYTHMIAS

Alert: Do not use extended-release capsules.

PO: ADULTS, ELDERLY >50 KG: Initially, 300 mg, then 150 mg q6h. ADULTS, ELDERLY <50 KG: Initially, 200 mg, then 100 mg q6h.

SEVERE REFRACTORY ARRHYTHMIAS

PO: ADULTS, ELDERLY: Up to 400 mg q6h.

USUAL PEDIATRIC DOSAGE

PO: CHILDREN 12–18 YRS: 6–15 mg/kg/day. CHILDREN 5–11 YRS: 10–15 mg/kg/day. CHILDREN 1–4 YRS: 10–20 mg/kg/day. CHILDREN <1 YR: 10–30 mg/kg/day.

DOSAGE IN RENAL IMPAIRMENT

With or without loading dose of 150 mg:

Creatinine Clearance	Dosage
>40 ml/min	100 mg q6h (extended-release 200 mg q12h)
30–40 ml/min	100 mg q8h
15–29 ml/min	100 mg q12h
<15 ml/min	100 mg q24h

DOSAGE IN HEPATIC IMPAIRMENT

100 mg q6h (200 mg q12h with extended-release).

DOSAGE IN CARDIOMYOPATHY, CARDIAC DECOMPENSATION

No loading dose; 100 mg q6–8h with gradual dosage adjustments.

D

SIDE EFFECTS

FREQUENT (>9%): Dry mouth (32%), urinary hesitancy, constipation. **OCCASIONAL** (3%–9%): Blurred vision; dry eyes, nose, throat; urinary retention; headache; dizziness; fatigue; nausea. **RARE** (<1%): Impotence, hypotension, edema, weight gain, shortness of breath, syncope, chest pain, nervousness, diarrhea, vomiting, decreased appetite, rash, itching.

ADVERSE REACTIONS/ TOXIC EFFECTS

May produce or aggravate CHF. May produce severe hypotension, shortness of breath, chest pain, syncope (esp. in those with primary cardiomyopathy or CHF). Hepatic toxicity occurs rarely.

NURSING IMPLICATIONS

BASELINE ASSESSMENT

Before giving medication, instruct pt to void (reduces risk of urinary retention).

INTERVENTION/EVALUATION

Monitor EKG for cardiac changes, particularly widening of QRS complex, prolongation of PR and QT intervals. Monitor B/P, EKG, serum potassium, glucose, liver enzymes. Monitor I&O (be alert to urinary retention). Assess for evidence of CHF (cough, dyspnea [particularly on exertion], rales at base of lungs, fatigue). Assist with ambulation if dizziness occurs. Therapeutic blood serum level: 2–8 mcg/ml; toxic blood serum level: >8 mcg/ml.

PATIENT/FAMILY TEACHING

Report shortness of breath, productive cough. Do not use nasal decongestants, OTC cold preparations (stimulants) without physician approval. Restrict salt, alcohol intake.

Dipropan

see oxybutynin

dobutamine hydrochloride

do-**byew**-ta-meen
(Dobutrex)
Do not confuse with Dopamine.

CLASSIFICATION

PHARMACOTHERAPEUTIC: Sympathomimetic. **CLINICAL**: Cardiac stimulant (see p. 133C).

ACTION

Direct-acting inotropic agent acting primarily on $beta_1$-adrenergic receptors. Decreases preload, afterload. **Therapeutic Effect:** Enhances myocardial contractility, stroke volume, cardiac output. Excessive doses increase heart rate. Improves renal blood flow, urine output.

PHARMACOKINETICS

Onset	Peak	Duration
IV		
1–2 min	10 min	Length of infusion

Metabolized in liver. Primarily excreted in urine. Not removed by hemodialysis. **Half-life:** 2 min.

USES

Short-term management of cardiac decompensation.

PRECAUTIONS

CONTRAINDICATIONS: Idiopathic hypertrophic subaortic stenosis, hypovolemic pts, sulfite sensitivity. **CAUTIONS:** Atrial fibrillation, hypertension.

LIFESPAN CONSIDERATIONS: Pregnancy/lactation: Unknown if drug crosses placenta or is distributed in breast milk. Has not been administered to pregnant women. **Pregnancy Category B. Children/elderly:** No age-related precautions noted.

INTERACTIONS

DRUG: Tricyclic antidepressants, MAOIs, oxytocics may increase effect (arrhythmias, hypertension); **beta-blockers** may antagonize effects; **digoxin** may increase risk of arrhythmias, additional inotropic effect. **HERBAL:** None known. **FOOD:** None known. **LAB VALUES:** Decreases potassium serum levels.

AVAILABILITY (Rx)

INJECTION: 12.5 mg/ml vial. **INFUSION:** Ready to use: 1 mg/ml, 2 mg/ml, 4 mg/ml.

ADMINISTRATION/HANDLING

Alert: Correct hypovolemia with volume expanders before dobutamine infusion. Those with atrial fibrillation should be digitalized before infusion. Administer by IV infusion only.

IV

Storage • Store at room temperature. Freezing produces crystallization. • Pink discoloration of solution (due to oxidation) does not indicate loss of potency if used within recommended time period. • Further diluted solution for infusion must be used within 24 hrs.

Reconstitution • Dilute 250-mg ampoule with 10 ml Sterile Water for Injection or D_5W for injection. Resulting solution: 25 mg/ml. Add additional 10 ml of diluent if not completely dissolved (resulting solution: 12.5 mg/ml). • Further dilute 250-mg vial with D_5W or 0.9% NaCl. Maximum concentration: 3.125 g/250 ml (12.5 mg/ml).

Rate of administration • Use infusion pump to control flow rate. • Titrate dosage to individual response. Infiltration causes local inflammatory changes. Extravasation may cause dermal necrosis.

IV INCOMPATIBILITIES

Acyclovir (Zovirax), alteplase (Activase), amphotericin B complex (Abelcet, AmBisome, Amphotec), bumetanide (Bumex), cefepime (Maxipime), foscarnet (Foscavir), furosemide (Lasix), heparin, piperacillin/tazobactam (Zosyn).

IV COMPATIBILITIES

Amiodarone (Cordarone), calcium chloride, calcium gluconate, diltiazem (Cardizem), dopamine (Intropin), enalaprilal (Vasotec), famotidine (Pepcid), hydromorphone (Dilaudid), insulin (Regular), lidocaine, lorazepam (Ativan), magnesium sulfate, midazolam (Versed), milrinone (Primacor), morphine, nitroglycerin, norepinephrine (Levophed), potassium chloride, propofol (Diprivan).

INDICATIONS/ROUTES/DOSAGE

Alert: Dosage determined by pt response.

IV infusion: ADULTS, ELDERLY, CHILDREN: 2.5–15 mcg/kg/min. Rarely, infusion rate up to 40 mcg/kg/min to increase cardiac output. NEONATES: 2–15 mcg/kg/min.

SIDE EFFECTS

FREQUENT (5%): Increased heart rate, blood pressure. **OCCASIONAL (3%–5%):** Pain at injection site. **RARE (1%–3%):** Nausea, headache, anginal pain, shortness of breath, fever.

ADVERSE REACTIONS/ TOXIC EFFECTS

Overdosage may produce marked increase in heart rate (≥30 beats/min), marked increase in systolic B/P (≥50 mm Hg), anginal pain, premature ventricular beats.

D

NURSING IMPLICATIONS

BASELINE ASSESSMENT

Pt must be on continuous cardiac monitoring. Determine weight (for dosage calculation). Obtain initial B/P, heart rate, respirations. Correct hypovolemia before drug therapy.

INTERVENTION/EVALUATION

Continuously monitor for cardiac rate, arrhythmias. With physician, establish parameters for adjusting rate or stopping infusion. Maintain accurate I&O; measure urine output frequently. Assess potassium levels and dobutamine plasma level (therapeutic range: 40–190 ng/ml). Monitor B/P continuously (hypertension greater risk in pts with preexisting hypertension). Check cardiac output and pulmonary wedge pressure or central venous pressure frequently. Immediately notify physician of decreased urine output, cardiac arrhythmias, significant increase in B/P, heart rate, or less commonly hypotension.

Dobutrex

see dobutamine

docetaxel

dox-eh-**tax**-el
(Taxotere)
Do not confuse with Taxol.

CLASSIFICATION

PHARMACOTHERAPEUTIC: Antimitotic agent, taxoid. **CLINICAL:** Antineoplastic (see p. 71C).

ACTION

Disrupts the microtubular cell network, essential for cellular function. **Therapeutic Effect:** Inhibits cell mitosis.

PHARMACOKINETICS

Distributed into peripheral compartments. Protein binding: 94%. Extensively metabolized. Excreted primarily in feces with lesser amount in urine. **Half-life:** 11.1 hrs.

USES

Treatment of locally advanced or metastatic breast carcinoma after the failure of any prior chemotherapy. Treatment of metastatic non–small cell lung cancer. **Unlabeled:** Treatment of small cell lung, ovarian, head and neck, prostate, bladder cancer.

PRECAUTIONS

CONTRAINDICATIONS: Neutrophil count <1,500 cells/mm^3, history of severe hypersensitivity to docetaxel or other drugs formulated with polysorbate 80. **CAUTIONS:** Impaired liver function, bone marrow depression, herpes zoster, chickenpox, preexisting pleural effusion, infection, chemotherapy/radiation.

LIFESPAN CONSIDERATIONS: Pregnancy/lactation: May cause fetal harm. Unknown if distributed in breast milk; do not breast-feed. **Pregnancy Category D. Children:** Safety and efficacy not established in those <16 yrs. **Elderly:** No age-related precautions noted.

INTERACTIONS

DRUG: Cyclosporine, ketoconazole, erythromycin may significantly modify **docetaxel** metabolism. **Live virus vac-**

cines may potentiate replication, increase side effects and/or decrease antibody responses of vaccine virus. **HERBAL:** None known. **FOOD:** None known. **LAB VALUES:** May significantly increase bilirubin, BUN, serum creatinine, transaminase, alkaline phosphatase. Reduces neutrophils, thrombocytes, WBC count.

AVAILABILITY (Rx)

INJECTION: 20 mg in 0.5 ml with diluent, 80 mg in 2 ml with diluent.

ADMINISTRATION/HANDLING

Alert: Dilution is required prior to administration. Pt should be premedicated with oral corticosteroids (e.g., dexamethasone 16 mg/day for 5 days beginning day 1 before docetaxel therapy; reduces severity of fluid retention, hypersensitivity reaction).

IV

Storage • Refrigerate vial. Freezing does not adversely affect drug. • Protect from bright light. • Stand vial at room temperature for 5 min before administering (do not store in PVC bags). • Premixed solution is stable for 8 hrs either at room temperature or if refrigerated.

Reconstitution • Withdraw contents of diluent (provided by manufacturer) and add to vial of docetaxel. • Gently rotate to ensure thorough mixing to provide a solution of 10 mg/ml. • Withdraw dose and add to 250 ml 0.9% NaCl or D_5W in glass or polyolefin container to provide a final concentration of 0.3–0.9 mg/ml.

Rate of administration • Administer as a 1-hr infusion. • Monitor closely for hypersensitivity reaction (i.e., flushing, localized skin reaction, bronchospasm [may occur within a few mins after beginning infusion]).

∅ IV INCOMPATIBILITIES

Amphotericin (Fungizone), doxorubicin liposome (DaunoXome), methylprednisolone (Solu-Medrol), nalbuphine (Nubain).

IV COMPATIBILITIES

Bumetanide (Bumex), calcium gluconate, dexamethasone (Decadron), diphenhydramine (Benadryl), dobutamine (Dobutrex), dopamine (Intropin), furosemide (Lasix), granisetron (Kytril), heparin, hydromorphone (Dilaudid), lorazepam (Ativan), magnesium sulfate, mannitol, morphine, ondansetron (Zofran), potassium chloride.

INDICATIONS/ROUTES/DOSAGE

BREAST CARCINOMA

IV infusion: ADULTS: 60–100 mg/m^2 given over 1 hr q3wks. Those dosed initially at 100 mg/m^2 who experience febrile neutropenia, neutrophils <500 cells/mm^3 for >1 wk, severe/cumulative cutaneous reactions, severe peripheral neuropathy during therapy should have dose adjusted from 100 to 75 mg/m^2. If reaction continues, lower dose from 75 to 55 mg/m^2 or stop therapy. Those dosed at 60 mg/m^2 and do not experience symptoms just listed may tolerate increased dose.

NON–SMALL CELL LUNG CARCINOMA

IV infusion: ADULTS: 75 mg/m^2 q3wks. Adjust dosage if toxicity occurs.

SIDE EFFECTS

FREQUENT: Alopecia (80%), asthenia (i.e., loss of strength) (62%), hypersensitivity reaction (i.e., dermatitis) (59%). Hypersensitivity reaction decreases to 16% in those treated with premedicated oral corticosteroids. Fluid retention (49%), stomatitis (redness/burning of oral mucous membranes, gum/tongue inflammation) (43%); nausea, diarrhea (40%), fever (30%); nail changes (28%), vomiting (24%); myalgia (19%). **OCCASIONAL:** Hypotension, edema, anorexia, headache, weight gain, infection

D

(urinary tract, injection site, catheter tip), dizziness. **RARE:** Dry skin, sensory disorders (vision, speech, taste), arthralgia, myalgia, weight loss, conjunctivitis, hematuria, proteinuria.

D

ADVERSE REACTIONS/ TOXIC EFFECTS

In those with normal liver function tests, neutropenia (<2,000 cells/mm^3), leukopenia (<4,000 cells/mm^3) occurs in 96% of pts. Anemia (<11 g/dl) occurs in 90%. Thrombocytopenia (<100,000 cells/mm^3) occurs in 8%. Infection occurs in 28%. Neurosensory, neuromotor (distal extremity paresthesias, weakness) occur in 54% and 13%, respectively.

NURSING IMPLICATIONS

BASELINE ASSESSMENT

Offer emotional support to pt/family. Antiemetics may be effective in preventing, treating nausea, vomiting. Pt should be pretreated with corticosteroids before therapy to reduce fluid retention, hypersensitivity reaction.

INTERVENTION/EVALUATION

Frequent monitoring of blood counts is essential, particularly neutrophil count (<1,500 cells/mm^3 requires discontinuation of therapy). Monitor renal/hepatic function studies; serum uric acid levels. Observe for cutaneous reactions characterized by rash with eruptions, mainly on hands/feet. Assess for extravascular fluid accumulation: rales in lungs, dependent edema, dyspnea at rest, pronounced abdominal distention (due to ascites).

PATIENT/FAMILY TEACHING

Alopecia is reversible, but new hair growth may have different color or texture. New hair growth resumes 2–3 mos after last therapy dose. Maintain fastidious oral hygiene. Do not have immunizations without physician approval (drug lowers body's resistance). Avoid those who have recently taken live virus vaccine.

docosanol

dough-**coe**-san-all
(Abreva)

◆ CLASSIFICATION

PHARMACOTHERAPEUTIC: Anti-infective. **CLINICAL:** Topical antiviral.

ACTION

Inhibits fusion between plasma membrane and the herpes simplex virus envelope. **Therapeutic Effect:** Reduces viral replication and activity.

USES

Treatment of cold sores/fever blisters due to either herpes simplex virus type 1 or type 2.

AVAILABILITY (OTC)

CREAM: 10%.

INDICATIONS/ROUTES/DOSAGE

COLD SORES, FEVER BLISTERS

Topical: ADULTS, ELDERLY: Apply to lesions 5 times/day at onset of symptoms, continuing until lesions are healed, up to a maximum of 10 days.

PRECAUTIONS

CONTRAINDICATIONS: None known. **CAUTIONS:** None known. **Pregnancy Category B.**

INTERACTIONS

DRUG: None known. **HERBAL:** None known. **FOOD:** None known. **LAB VALUES:** None known.

SIDE EFFECTS

RARE (1%–5%): Headache, mild erythema.

ADVERSE REACTIONS/ TOXIC EFFECTS

None known.

NURSING IMPLICATIONS

BASELINE ASSESSMENT

Use only on lips/face. Do not apply to oral mucous membranes. Avoid application in, near eyes (produces irritation).

PATIENT/FAMILY TEACHING

Avoid exposure of cold sores to direct sunlight.

docusate

dock-cue-sate
(Pro-Cal-Sof, Surfak)

docusate sodium

(Colace, Diocto, Selax✤, SoFlax✤, Surfak)

◆CLASSIFICATION

PHARMACOTHERAPEUTIC: Bulk-producing laxative. **CLINICAL:** Stool softener (see p. 104C).

ACTION

Decreases surface film tension by mixing liquid and bowel contents. **Therapeutic Effect:** Increases infiltration of liquid to form a softer stool.

PHARMACOKINETICS

Minimal absorption from GI tract. Acts in small/large intestine. Results occur 1–2 days after first dose (may take 3–5 days).

USES

Stool softener for those who need to avoid straining during defecation; constipation associated with hard, dry stools.

CONTRAINDICATIONS: Concomitant use of mineral oil; intestinal obstruction, nausea, vomiting, acute abdominal pain. **CAUTIONS:** None known.

LIFESPAN CONSIDERATIONS: Pregnancy/lactation: Unknown if drug is distributed in breast milk. **Pregnancy Category C. Children:** Not recommended in children <6 yrs. **Elderly:** No age-related precautions noted.

INTERACTIONS

DRUG: May increase absorption of **mineral oil, danthron. HERBAL:** None known. **FOOD:** None known. **LAB VALUES:** None known.

AVAILABILITY (OTC)

CALCIUM: **CAPSULES:** 240 mg.

SODIUM: **TABLETS:** 100 mg. **CAPSULES:** 50 mg, 100 mg, 250 mg. **SYRUP:** 50 mg/15 ml, 60 mg/15 ml. **LIQUID:** 150 mg/15 ml. **SOLUTION:** 50 mg/ml. **ELIXIR:** 60 mg/15 ml.

ADMINISTRATION/HANDLING

- Drink 6–8 glasses of water/day (aids stool softening).
- Give each dose with full glass of water or fruit juice.
- Administer docusate liquid with milk, fruit juice, or infant formula (masks bitter taste).

INDICATIONS/ROUTES/DOSAGE

Stool softener: ADULTS, ELDERLY, CHILDREN >12 YRS: 50–500 mg/day in 1–4 divided doses. CHILDREN 6–12 YRS: 40–150 mg/day in 1–4 divided doses. CHILDREN 3–5 YRS: 20–60 mg/day in 1–4 divided doses. CHILDREN <3 YRS: 10–40 mg in 1–4 divided doses.

SIDE EFFECTS

OCCASIONAL: Mild GI cramping, throat irritation (liquid preparation). **RARE:** Rash.

ADVERSE REACTIONS/ TOXIC EFFECTS

None known.

D

NURSING IMPLICATIONS

INTERVENTION/EVALUATION

Encourage adequate fluid intake. Assess bowel sounds for peristalsis. Monitor daily bowel activity/stool consistency (watery, loose, soft, semisolid, solid), record time of evacuation.

PATIENT/FAMILY TEACHING

Institute measures to promote defecation: increase fluid intake, exercise, high-fiber diet.

dofetilide

doe-**fet**-ill-ide
(Tikosyn)

◆CLASSIFICATION

PHARMACOTHERAPEUTIC: Potassium channel blocker. **CLINICAL:** Antiarrhythmic: Class III (see p. 15C).

ACTION

A selective potassium channel blocker; prolongs repolarization without affecting conduction velocity by blocking one or more time-dependent potassium currents. No effect on sodium channels, adrenergic alpha, beta receptors. **Therapeutic Effect:** Terminates reentrant tachyarrhythmias, preventing reinduction.

USES

Maintenance of normal sinus rhythm (NSR) in pts with atrial fibrillation/flutter of >1 wk duration who have been converted to NSR.

PRECAUTIONS

CONTRAINDICATIONS: Paroxysmal atrial fibrillation; congenital or acquired long QT syndrome; severe renal impairment; concurrent use with verapamil, prochlorperazine, megestrol; concurrent use of drugs that prolong QT interval; hypokalemia; hypomagnesemia; concurrent amiodarone. **CAUTIONS:** None known. **Pregnancy Category C.**

INTERACTIONS

DRUG: **Amiloride, metformin, megestrol, prochlorperazine, triamterene** increase dofetilide serum levels. **Bepridil, phenothiazines, tricyclic antidepressants** may increase QT interval. **Cimetidine, verapamil** increase dofetilide serum plasma levels. **Ketoconazole, trimethoprim** increase maximum plasma concentration. **HERBAL:** None known. **FOOD:** **Grapefruit juice** can increase dofetilide levels. **LAB VALUES:** None known.

AVAILABILITY (Rx)

CAPSULES: 125 mcg, 250 mcg, 500 mcg.

INDICATIONS/ROUTES/DOSAGE

ANTIARRHYTHMIAS

PO: ADULTS, ELDERLY: Individualized using a seven-step dosing algorithm dependent upon calculated creatinine clearance, QT measurements.

SIDE EFFECTS

OCCASIONAL (<5%): Headache, chest pain, dizziness, dyspnea, nausea, insomnia, back/abdominal pain, diarrhea, rash.

ADVERSE REACTIONS/ TOXIC EFFECTS

Angioedema, bradycardia, cerebral ischemia, facial paralysis, serious arrhythmias (ventricular, various forms of heart block) may be noted.

NURSING IMPLICATIONS

BASELINE ASSESSMENT

Have cardiac monitoring equipment and personnel for constant cardiac, B/P monitoring.

INTERVENTION/EVALUATION

Monitor EKG with attention to QT interval occurrence of ventricular arrhythmias. Monitor for changes in serum creatinine.

PATIENT/FAMILY TEACHING

May take without regard to food. Compliance is essential; follow dosing instructions diligently. Report dizziness, tachycardia, severe diarrhea, diaphoresis, vomiting, loss of appetite, increased thirst.

dolasetron

dole-**ah**-seh-tron
(Anzemet)
Do not confuse with Aldomet.

CLASSIFICATION

PHARMACOTHERAPEUTIC: Selective receptor antagonist. **CLINICAL:** Antiemetic.

ACTION

Exhibits selective 5-HT_3 receptor antagonism. Action may be central (CTZ) or peripheral (vagus nerve termina). **Therapeutic Effect:** Prevents nausea/vomiting.

PHARMACOKINETICS

Oral form readily absorbed from GI tract. Protein binding: 69%–77%. Metabolized in liver. Primarily excreted in urine. Unknown if removed by hemodialysis. **Half-life:** 5–10 hrs.

USES

Oral: Prevention of nausea/vomiting associated with cancer chemotherapy, including high-dose cisplatin; prevention of postop nausea/vomiting. **Injection:** Treatment of postop nausea/vomiting. **Unlabeled:** Radiation therapy–induced nausea/vomiting.

D

PRECAUTIONS

CONTRAINDICATIONS: None known. **CAUTIONS:** Those who have or may have prolongation of cardiac conduction intervals, hypokalemia, hypomagnesemia, those taking diuretics with potential for inducing electrolyte disturbances, congenital QT syndrome, those taking antiarrhythmics that may lead to QT prolongation and cumulative high-dose anthracycline therapy.

LIFESPAN CONSIDERATIONS: Pregnancy/lactation: Unknown if distributed in breast milk. **Pregnancy Category B. Children:** Safety and efficacy not established in those <2 yrs. **Elderly:** No age-related precautions noted.

INTERACTIONS

DRUG: None known. **HERBAL:** None known. **FOOD:** None known. **LAB VALUES:** May alter liver function tests.

AVAILABILITY (Rx)

TABLETS: 50 mg, 100 mg. **INJECTION:** 20 mg/ml.

ADMINISTRATION/HANDLING

PO

• Do not cut, break, or chew film-coated tablets. • For children 2–16 yrs, injection form may be mixed in apple or apple-grape juice for oral dosing at 1.8 mg/kg up to a maximum of 100 mg.

IV

Storage • Store vials at room temperature. • After dilution, solution is stable for 24 hrs at room temperature or 48 hrs if refrigerated.

Reconstitution • May dilute in 0.9% NaCl, D_5W, D_5W with 0.45% NaCl, D_5W with lactated Ringer's, lactated Ringer's, or 10% mannitol injection to 50 ml.

Rate of administration • Can be given as IV push as rapidly as 100 mg/30 sec. • Intermittent IV infusion (piggyback) may be infused over 15 min.

IV INCOMPATIBILITY

No information available via Y-site administration.

INDICATIONS/ROUTES/DOSAGE

PREVENTION OF CHEMOTHERAPY-INDUCED NAUSEA/VOMITING

IV: ADULTS, CHILDREN 1–16 YRS: 1.8 mg/kg as a single dose 30 min before chemotherapy. **Maximum:** 100 mg.

PO: ADULTS: 100 mg within 1 hr of chemotherapy. CHILDREN 2–16 YRS: 1.8 mg/kg within 1 hr of chemotherapy. **Maximum:** 100 mg.

TREATMENT/PREVENTION OF POSTOP NAUSEA/VOMITING

IV: ADULTS: 12.5 mg. CHILDREN 2–16 YRS: 0.35 mg/kg. **Maximum:** 12.5 mg. Give approximately 15 min before cessation of anesthesia or as soon as nausea presents.

PO: ADULTS: 100 mg. CHILDREN 2–16 YRS: 1.2 mg/kg. **Maximum:** 100 mg within 2 hrs of surgery.

SIDE EFFECTS

FREQUENT (5%–10%): Headache, diarrhea, fatigue. **OCCASIONAL (1%–5%):** Fever, dizziness, tachycardia, dyspepsia.

ADVERSE REACTIONS/ TOXIC EFFECTS

Overdose may produce combination of CNS stimulation, depressant effects.

NURSING IMPLICATIONS

BASELINE ASSESSMENT

Assess for dehydration if excessive vomiting occurs (poor skin turgor, dry mucous membranes, longitudinal furrows in tongue). Provide emotional support.

INTERVENTION/EVALUATION

Monitor for therapeutic relief from nausea/vomiting, EKG in high-risk pts. Maintain quiet, supportive atmosphere.

Dolobid

see diflunisal

Dolopine

see methadone

donepezil hydrochloride

doh-**neh**-peh-zil

(Aricept)

Do not confuse with Aciphex, Ascriptin.

CLASSIFICATION

PHARMACOTHERAPEUTIC: Cholinesterase inhibitor. **CLINICAL:** Cholinergic.

ACTION

Enhances cholinergic function by increasing the concentration of acetylcholine through inhibition of the hydrolysis of acetylcholine by the enzyme acetylcholinesterase. **Therapeutic Effect:** Slows the progression of Alzheimer's disease.

PHARMACOKINETICS

Well absorbed following PO administration. Protein binding: 96%. Extensively metabolized. Eliminated in urine and feces. **Half-life:** 70 hrs.

USES

Treatment of mild to moderate dementia of Alzheimer's disease.

PRECAUTIONS

CONTRAINDICATIONS: History of hypersensitivity to donepezil or piperidine derivatives. **CAUTIONS:** Asthma, COPD, bladder outflow obstruction, history of ulcer disease, those on concurrent NSAIDs, "sick sinus syndrome" or other supraventricular cardiac conduction conditions, seizures.

LIFESPAN CONSIDERATIONS: Pregnancy/lactation: Unknown if distributed in breast milk. **Pregnancy Category C. Children:** Safety and efficacy not established. **Elderly:** No age-related precautions noted.

INTERACTIONS

DRUG: Ketoconazole, quinidine inhibit metabolism of donepezil. Decreases effect of **anticholinergics.** Increases gastric acid secretion of **NSAIDs,** synergistic effects of **succinylcholine, neuromuscular blocking agents, cholinergic agonists. Paroxetine** may decrease metabolism, increase concentration. **HERBAL:** None known. **FOOD:** None known. **LAB VALUES:** May decrease potassium, increase creatine kinase, blood sugar, LDH.

AVAILABILITY (Rx)

TABLETS: 5 mg, 10 mg.

ADMINISTRATION/HANDLING

PO

- May be given without regard to meals or time of administration (morning vs. evening dose), although it is suggested dose be given in the evening, just before bedtime.

INDICATIONS/ROUTES/DOSAGE

ALZHEIMER'S DISEASE

PO: ADULTS, ELDERLY: 5–10 mg/day as a single dose. If initial dose is 5 mg, do not increase to 10 mg for 4–6 wks.

SIDE EFFECTS

FREQUENT (8%–11%): Nausea, diarrhea, headache, insomnia, nonspecific pain, dizziness. **OCCASIONAL (3%–6%):** Mild muscle cramps, fatigue, vomiting, anorexia, ecchymosis. **RARE (2%–3%):** Depression, abnormal dreams, weight loss, arthritis, somnolence, syncope, frequent urination.

ADVERSE REACTIONS/ TOXIC EFFECTS

Overdosage may result in cholinergic crisis, characterized by severe nausea, increased salivation, diaphoresis, bradycardia, hypotension, flushed skin, stomach pain, respiratory depression, seizures, cardiorespiratory collapse. Increasing muscle weakness may occur, resulting in death if respiratory muscles are involved. **ANTIDOTE:** 1–2 mg IV atropine sulfate with subsequent doses based on therapeutic response.

NURSING IMPLICATIONS

BASELINE ASSESSMENT

Obtain baseline vital signs. Assess history for peptic ulcer, urinary obstruction, asthma, COPD, seizure disorder, cardiac conduction disturbances.

INTERVENTION/EVALUATION

Monitor for cholinergic reaction: GI discomfort/cramping, feeling of facial warmth, excessive salivation and diaphoresis, lacrimation, pallor, urinary urgency, dizziness. Monitor for nausea, diarrhea, headache, insomnia.

PATIENT/FAMILY TEACHING

Report nausea, vomiting, diarrhea, diaphoresis, increased salivary secretions, severe abdominal pain, dizziness. May take without regard to food. Not a cure for Alzheimer's disease but may slow the progression of symptoms.

dong quai

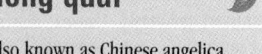

Also known as Chinese angelica, dang gui, tang kuei, toki

CLASSIFICATION

HERBAL

ACTION

Competitively inhibits estradiol binding to estrogen receptors. Has vasodilation, antispasmodic, CNS stimulant activity. **Effect:** Reduces symptoms of menopause.

USES

Gynecologic ailments, including menstrual cramps, menopause symptoms; uterine stimulant. Also used to control hypertension and as anti-inflammatory, vasodilator, immunosuppressant, analgesic, antipyretic.

PRECAUTIONS

CONTRAINDICATIONS: Pregnancy due to uterine stimulant effect, bleeding disorders, excessive menstrual flow. **CAUTIONS:** Lactation; breast, ovarian, uterine cancer.

LIFESPAN CONSIDERATIONS: Pregnancy/lactation: Contraindicated. **Children:** Safety and efficacy not established. **Elderly:** No age-related precautions noted.

INTERACTIONS

DRUG: Increases anticoagulant effect, risk of bleeding with **warfarin. HERBAL: Feverfew, garlic, ginger, ginkgo, ginseng** may increase risk of bleeding. **FOOD:** None known. **LAB VALUES:** May increase prothrombin time/INR.

AVAILABILITY

DONG QUAI SOFTGEL: 200 mg, 530 mg, 565 mg.

INDICATIONS/ROUTES/DOSAGE

GYNECOLOGIC AILMENTS, OTHER PURPORTED USES

PO: ADULTS, ELDERLY: 3–4 g/day in divided doses with meals.

SIDE EFFECTS

Diarrhea, photosensitivity, nausea, vomiting, anorexia, increased menstrual flow.

ADVERSE REACTIONS/ TOXIC EFFECTS

None known.

NURSING IMPLICATIONS

BASELINE ASSESSMENT

Assess if pt is pregnant/breast-feeding, taking other medications, esp. those that increase risk of bleeding.

INTERVENTION/EVALUATION

Assess for hypersensitivity reaction.

PATIENT/FAMILY TEACHING

Inform physician if pregnant or planning to become pregnant. Do not breast-feed. May cause photosensitivity reaction; sunscreen or protective clothing should be worn.

dopamine hydrochloride

dope-a-meen
(Intropin)
Do not confuse with dobutamine, Dopram, Isoptin.

CLASSIFICATION

PHARMACOTHERAPEUTIC: Sympathomimetic (adrenergic agonist). **CLINICAL:** Cardiac stimulant, vasopressor (see p. 133C).

ACTION

Stimulates adrenergic receptors; effects are dose dependent. **Low Dosages (1–5 mcg/kg/min):** Stimulates dopaminergic receptors causing renal vasodilation. **Therapeutic Effect:** Increases renal blood flow, urine flow, sodium excretion. **Low to Moderate Dosages (5–15 mcg/kg/min):** Positive inotropic effect by direct action, release of norepinephrine. **Therapeutic Effect:** Increases myocardial contractility, stroke volume, cardiac output. **High Dosages (>15 mcg/kg/min):** Stimulates alpha-receptors. **Therapeutic Effect:** Increases peripheral resistance, renal vasoconstriction, increases systolic, diastolic B/P.

PHARMACOKINETICS

Onset	Peak	Duration
IV		
1–2 min	—	<10 min

Widely distributed. Does not cross blood-brain barrier. Metabolized in liver, kidney, plasma. Primarily excreted in urine. Not removed by hemodialysis. **Half-life:** 2 min.

USES

Prophylaxis/treatment of acute hypotension, shock (associated with MI, trauma, renal failure, cardiac decompensation, open heart surgery), treatment of low cardiac output, CHF.

PRECAUTIONS

CONTRAINDICATIONS: Pheochromocytoma, uncorrected tachyarrhythmias, ventricular fibrillation, sulfite sensitivity. **CAUTIONS:** Ischemic heart disease, occlusive vascular disease.

LIFESPAN CONSIDERATIONS: Pregnancy/lactation: Unknown if drug crosses placenta or is distributed in breast milk. **Pregnancy Category C. Children:** Recommended close hemodynamic monitoring (gangrene due to extravasation reported). **Elderly:** No age-related precautions noted.

INTERACTIONS

DRUG: Tricyclic antidepressants may increase cardiovascular effects. **Beta-blockers** may decrease effects. May increase risk of arrhythmias with **digoxin. Ergot alkaloids** may increase vasoconstriction. **MAOIs** may increase cardiac stimulation, vasopressor effects. **HERBAL:** None known. **FOOD:** None known. **LAB VALUES:** None known.

AVAILABILITY (Rx)

INJECTION: 40 mg/ml, 80 mg/ml, 160 mg/ml. **INJECTION (Premix with Dextrose):** 80 mg/100 ml, 160 mg/100 ml, 320 mg/100 ml.

ADMINISTRATION/HANDLING

Alert: Blood volume depletion must be corrected before administering dopamine (may be used concurrently with fluid replacement).

IV

Storage • Do not use solutions darker than slightly yellow or discolored to yellow, brown, or pink to purple (indicates decomposition of drug). • Stable for 24 hrs after dilution.

D

Reconstitution • Available prediluted in 250 or 500 ml D_5W or dilute each 5-ml (200-mg) ampoule in 250–500 ml 0.9% NaCl, D_5W/0.45 NaCl, D_5W/0.45 NaCl, D_5W/lactated Ringer's or lactated Ringer's (concentration is dependent on dosage and fluid requirement of pt); 250 ml solution yields 800 mcg/ml; 500 ml solution yields 400 mcg/ml. Maximum concentration: 3.2 g/250 ml (12.8 mg/ml).

Rate of administration • Administer into large vein (antecubital fossa or central line) to prevent extravasation. • Use infusion pump to control rate of flow. • Titrate each pt to the desired hemodynamic or renal response (optimum urine flow determines dosage).

∅ IV INCOMPATIBILITIES

Acyclovir (Zovirax), amphotericin B complex (Abelcet, AmBisome, Amphotec), cefepime (Maxipime), furosemide (Lasix), insulin.

IV COMPATIBILITIES

Amiodarone (Cordarone), calcium chloride, diltiazem (Cardizem), dobutamine (Dobutrex), enalapril (Vasotec), heparin, hydromorphone (Dilaudid), labetalol (Trandate), levofloxacin (Levaquin), lidocaine, lorazepam (Ativan), methylprednisolone (Solu-Medrol), midazolam (Versed), milrinone (Primacor), morphine, nicardipine (Cardene), nitroglycerin, norepinephrine (Levophed), piperacillin/tazobactam (Zosyn), potassium chloride, propofol (Diprovan).

INDICATIONS/ROUTES/DOSAGE

IV: ADULTS, ELDERLY: 1 mcg/kg/min up to 50 mcg/kg/min titrated to desired response. CHILDREN: 1–20 mcg/kg/min. **Maximum:** 50 mcg/kg/min. NEONATES: 1–20 mcg/kg/min.

SIDE EFFECTS

FREQUENT: Headache, ectopic beats, tachycardia, anginal pain, palpitations, vasoconstriction, hypotension, nausea, vomiting, dyspnea. **OCCASIONAL:** Piloerection (goose bumps), bradycardia, widening of QRS complex.

ADVERSE REACTIONS/ TOXIC EFFECTS

High dosages may produce ventricular arrhythmias. Pts with occlusive vascular disease are high-risk candidates for further compromise of circulation to extremities, which may result in gangrene. Extravasation resulting in tissue necrosis with sloughing may occur with IV administration.

NURSING IMPLICATIONS

BASELINE ASSESSMENT

Check for MAOI therapy within last 2–3 wks (requires dosage reduction). Pt must be on continuous cardiac monitoring. Determine weight (for dosage calculation). Obtain initial B/P, heart rate, respirations.

INTERVENTION/EVALUATION

Continuously monitor for cardiac arrhythmias. Measure urine output frequently. If extravasation occurs, immediately infiltrate the affected tissue with 10–15 ml 0.9% NaCl solution containing 5–10 mg phentolamine mesylate. Monitor B/P, heart rate, respirations q15min during administration (or more often if indicated). Assess cardiac output, pulmonary wedge pressure, or central venous pressure frequently. Assess peripheral circulation (palpate pulses, note color/temperature of extremities). Immediately notify physician of decreased urine output, cardiac arrhythmias, significant changes in B/P or heart rate (or failure to respond to increase/decrease in infusion rate), decreased peripheral circulation (cold, pale, or mottled extremities). Taper dosage prior to discontinuing because abrupt cessation of therapy may result in marked hypotension. Be alert to excessive vasoconstriction (as evidenced by decreased urine output, increased heart rate or arrhythmias, a disproportionate increase in diastolic B/P, decrease in pulse pressure); slow or temporarily stop the infusion, notify physician.

dorzolamide

(Trusopt)

See Classification section under: Antiglaucoma agents (p. 46C)

doxacurium chloride

(Nuromax)

See Classification section under: Neuromuscular blockers (p. 106C)

doxazosin mesylate

docks-ah-**zoe**-sin

(Cardura)

Do not confuse with Cardene, Cordarone, Coumadin, doxapram, doxepin, doxorubicin, K-Dur, Ridaura.

CLASSIFICATION

PHARMACOTHERAPEUTIC: Alpha-adrenergic blocker. **CLINICAL:** Antihypertensive (see p. 53C).

ACTION

Selectively blocks $alpha_1$-adrenergic receptors, decreasing peripheral vascular resistance. **Therapeutic Effect:** Results in peripheral vasodilation, lowering B/P, relaxes smooth muscle of bladder/prostate.

PHARMACOKINETICS

Onset	Peak	Duration
PO		
—	2–6 hrs	24 hrs

Well absorbed from GI tract. Protein binding: 98%–99%. Metabolized in liver. Primarily eliminated in feces. Not removed by hemodialysis. **Half-life:** 19–22 hrs.

USES

Treatment of mild to moderate hypertension. Used alone or in combination with other antihypertensives. Treatment of benign prostatic hyperplasia.

PRECAUTIONS

CONTRAINDICATIONS: None known. **CAUTIONS:** Chronic renal failure, impaired hepatic function.

LIFESPAN CONSIDERATIONS: Pregnancy/lactation: Unknown if drug crosses placenta or is distributed in breast milk. **Pregnancy Category C. Children:** Safety and efficacy not established. **Elderly:** May be more sensitive to hypotensive effects.

INTERACTIONS

DRUG: NSAIDs, estrogen may decrease effect. **Hypotension-producing medications** may increase effect. **HERBAL:** None known. **FOOD:** None known. **LAB VALUES:** None known.

AVAILABILITY (Rx)

TABLETS: 1 mg, 2 mg, 4 mg, 8 mg.

ADMINISTRATION/HANDLING

PO

- Give without regard to food.

D

INDICATIONS/ROUTES/DOSAGE

HYPERTENSION

PO: ADULTS: Initially, 1 mg once daily. May increase up to 16 mg/day. ELDERLY: Initially, 0.5 mg once daily.

BENIGN PROSTATIC HYPERPLASIA

PO: ADULTS, ELDERLY: Initially, 1 mg/day. May increase q1–2 wks. **Maximum:** 8 mg/day.

SIDE EFFECTS

FREQUENT (10%–20%): Dizziness, asthenia, headache, edema. **OCCASIONAL (3%–9%):** Nausea, pharyngitis, rhinitis, pain in extremities, somnolence. **RARE (1%–3%):** Palpitations, diarrhea, constipation, dyspnea, muscle pain, altered vision, dizziness, nervousness.

ADVERSE REACTIONS/ TOXIC EFFECTS

First-dose syncope (hypotension with sudden loss of consciousness) generally occurs 30–90 min following initial dose of 2 mg or greater, a too rapid increase in dose, or addition of another antihypertensive agent to therapy. May be preceded by tachycardia (120–160 beats/min).

NURSING IMPLICATIONS

BASELINE ASSESSMENT

Give first dose at bedtime. If initial dose is given during daytime, pt must remain recumbent for 3–4 hrs. Assess B/P, pulse immediately prior to each dose, and q15–30min until B/P is stabilized (be alert to fluctuations).

INTERVENTION/EVALUATION

Monitor pulse diligently (first-dose syncope may be preceded by tachycardia). Assess for edema, headache. Assist with ambulation if dizziness, lightheadedness occurs.

PATIENT/FAMILY TEACHING

Full therapeutic effect may not occur for 3–4 wks. May cause syncope (fainting). Avoid driving for 12–24 hrs after first dose or increase in dosage. Use caution driving or operating machinery or when rising from sitting or lying position.

doxepin hydrochloride

dox-eh-pin

(Novo-Doxepin✱, Prudoxin, Sinequan, Zonalon)

Do not confuse with doxapram, doxazosin, Doxidan, saquinavir.

◆ CLASSIFICATION

PHARMACOTHERAPEUTIC: Tricyclic. **CLINICAL:** Antidepressant, antianxiety, antineuralgic, antiulcer, antipruritic (see p. 35C).

ACTION

Increases synaptic concentrations of norepinephrine and/or serotonin. **Therapeutic Effect:** Produces antidepressant, anxiolytic effect.

PHARMACOKINETICS

Rapidly, well absorbed from GI tract. Protein binding: 80%–85%. Metabolized in liver to active metabolite. Primarily excreted in urine. Not removed by hemodialysis. **Half-life:** 6–8 hrs. **Topical:** Absorbed through skin, distributed to body tissues, metabolized to active metabolite, eliminated renally.

USES

Treatment of various forms of depression, often in conjunction with psychotherapy. Treatment of anxiety. **Topical:** Treatment of pruritus associated with eczema. **Unlabeled:** Treatment of panic disorder, neurogenic pain, prophylaxis for vascular headache, pruritus in idiopathic urticaria.

PRECAUTIONS

CONTRAINDICATIONS: Hypersensitivity to other tricyclic antidepressants, narrow-angle glaucoma, urinary retention. **CAUTIONS:** Prostatic hypertrophy, history of urinary retention/obstruction, glaucoma, diabetes mellitus, seizures, hyperthyroidism, cardiac/hepatic/renal disease, schizophrenia, increased intraocular pressure, hiatal hernia.

LIFESPAN CONSIDERATIONS: Pregnancy/lactation: Crosses placenta. Distributed in breast milk. **Pregnancy Category C. Topical: Pregnancy Category B. Children:** Safety and efficacy not established. **Elderly:** Increased risk of toxicity (lower dosages recommended).

INTERACTIONS

DRUG: Alcohol, CNS depressants may increase CNS, respiratory depression; hypotensive effects. **Antithyroid agents** may increase risk of agranulocytosis. **Phenothiazines** may increase sedative, anticholinergic effects. **Cimetidine** may increase concentration, toxicity. May decrease effects of **clonidine, guanadrel.** May increase cardiac effects with **sympathomimetics.** May increase risk of hypertensive crisis, hyperthermia, seizures with **MAOIs. HERBAL:** None known. **FOOD:** None known. **LAB VALUES:** May alter EKG readings, glucose. Therapeutic blood serum level: 110–250 ng/ml; toxic blood serum level: >300 ng/ml.

AVAILABILITY (Rx)

CAPSULES: 10 mg, 25 mg, 50 mg, 75 mg, 100 mg, 150 mg. **ORAL CONCENTRATE:** 10 mg/ml. **CREAM:** 5%.

ADMINISTRATION/HANDLING

PO

• Give with food or milk if GI distress occurs. • Dilute concentrate in 8-oz glass of water, milk, orange, grapefruit, tomato, prune, pineapple juice. Incompatible with carbonated drinks.

D

INDICATIONS/ROUTES/DOSAGE

DEPRESSION/ANXIETY

PO: ADULTS: 30–150 mg/day at bedtime or in 2–3 divided doses. May increase to 300 mg/day. ADOLESCENTS: Initially, 25–50 mg/day as single or divided doses. May increase to 100 mg/day. CHILDREN <12 YRS: 1–3 mg/kg/day.

USUAL ELDERLY DOSAGE

PO: Initially, 10–25 mg at bedtime. May increase by 10–25 mg/day q3–7days. **Maximum:** 75 mg/day.

USUAL TOPICAL DOSAGE

Topical: ADULTS, ELDERLY: Apply thin layer 4 times/day.

SIDE EFFECTS

FREQUENT: PO: Orthostatic hypotension, drowsiness, dry mouth, headache, increased appetite/weight, nausea, unusual tiredness, unpleasant taste. **Topical:** Edema at application site, increased itching/eczema, burning, stinging of skin, altered taste, dizziness, drowsiness, dry skin, dry mouth, fatigue, headache, thirst. **OCCASIONAL: PO:** Blurred vision, confusion, constipation, hallucinations, difficult urination, eye pain, irregular heartbeat, fine muscle tremors, nervousness, impaired sexual function, diarrhea, increased diaphoresis, heartburn, insomnia. **Topical:** Anxiety, skin irritation/cracking, nausea. **RARE:** Allergic reaction, alopecia, tinnitus, breast enlargement. **Topical:** Fever.

ADVERSE REACTIONS/ TOXIC EFFECTS

High dosage may produce confusion, seizures, severe drowsiness, arrhythmias, fever, hallucinations, agitation, shortness of breath, vomiting, unusual tiredness/weakness. Abrupt withdrawal from prolonged therapy may produce headache, malaise, nausea, vomiting, vivid dreams.

NURSING IMPLICATIONS

BASELINE ASSESSMENT

Assess B/P, pulse, EKG (those with history of cardiovascular disease).

INTERVENTION/EVALUATION

Monitor B/P, pulse, weight. Supervise suicidal-risk pt closely during early therapy (as depression lessens, energy level improves, increasing suicide potential). Assess appearance, behavior, speech pattern, level of interest, mood. Therapeutic blood serum level: 110–250 ng/ml; toxic blood serum level: >300 ng/ml.

PATIENT/FAMILY TEACHING

May cause drowsiness or decrease ability to perform tasks requiring mental alertness, physical coordination. Avoid tasks that require alertness, motor skills until response to drug is established. May cause dry mouth. Avoid alcohol, limit caffeine. May increase appetite. Avoid exposure to sunlight/artificial light source. Therapeutic effect may be noted within 2–5 days, maximum effect within 2–3 wks.

doxercalciferol

(Hectorol)

See vitamin D

doxorubicin

dox-o-**roo**-bi-sin

(Adriamycin, Caelyx✤, Doxil)

Do not confuse with Daunorubicin, Idamycin, Idarubicin.

◆CLASSIFICATION

PHARMACOTHERAPEUTIC: Anthracycline antibiotic. **CLINICAL:** Antineoplastic (see p. 71C).

ACTION

Inhibits DNA, DNA-dependent RNA synthesis by binding with DNA strands. Liposomal encapsulation increases uptake by tumors, prolongs action, may decrease toxicity. **Therapeutic Effect:** Prevents cellular division.

PHARMACOKINETICS

Widely distributed. Does not cross blood-brain barrier. Protein binding: 74%–76%. Metabolized rapidly in liver to active metabolite. Primarily eliminated via biliary system. Not removed by hemodialysis. **Half-life:** 16 hrs; metabolite: 32 hrs.

USES

Produces regression in breast, ovarian, thyroid, transitional cell bladder, bronchogenic, gastric carcinoma; soft tissue, bone sarcomas; neuroblastoma; Wilms' tumor; lymphomas of Hodgkin's and non-Hodgkin's type; acute lymphoblastic and myeloblastic leukemia; primary liver cancer. **Doxil:** Treatment of AIDS-related Kaposi's sarcoma, metastatic ovarian cancer. **Unlabeled:** Treatment of head/neck, cervical, liver, pancreatic, prostatic, testicular, endometrial carcinoma; treatment of germ cell tumors, multiple myeloma.

PRECAUTIONS

CONTRAINDICATIONS: Severe CHF; cardiomyopathy; preexisting myelosuppression; previous or concomitant treatment with idarubicin mitoxantrone, cyclophosphamide, irradiation of the cardiac region. **CAUTIONS:** Impaired liver function.

LIFESPAN CONSIDERATIONS: Pregnancy/lactation: If possible, avoid use during pregnancy, esp. first trimester. Breast-feeding not recommended. **Pregnancy Category D. Children/elderly:** Cardiotoxicity may be more frequent in those <2 yrs or >70 yrs.

INTERACTIONS

DRUG: May decrease effect of **antigout medication. Bone marrow depressants** may increase bone marrow depression. May increase cardiotoxicity with **daunorubicin. Live virus vaccines** may potentiate virus replication, increase vaccine side effects, decrease pt's antibody response to vaccine. **HERBAL:** None known. **FOOD:** None known. **LAB VALUES:** May cause EKG changes. May increase uric acid. **Doxil:** May reduce neutrophil, RBC count.

AVAILABILITY (Rx)

POWDER FOR INJECTION: 10 mg, 20 mg, 50 mg, 200 mg. **LIPID COMPLEX (Doxil):** 2 mg/ml.

ADMINISTRATION/HANDLING

Alert: Wear gloves. If powder/solution comes in contact with skin, wash thoroughly. Avoid small veins; swollen/edematous extremities; areas overlying joints, tendons. **Doxil:** Do not use with in-line filter or mix with any diluent except D_5W. May be carcinogenic, mutagenic, or teratogenic. Handle with extreme care during preparation/administration.

IV

Storage • Store at room temperature. • Reconstituted solution is stable for 24 hrs at room temperature or 48 hrs if refrigerated. • Protect from prolonged exposure to sunlight; discard unused solution.

DOXIL

• Refrigerate unopened vials. • After solution is diluted, use within 24 hrs.

Reconstitution • Reconstitute each 10-mg vial with 5 ml preservative-free 0.9% NaCl (10 ml for 20 mg; 25 ml for 50 mg) to provide concentration of 2 mg/ml. • Shake vial; allow contents to dissolve. • Withdraw appropriate volume of air from vial during reconstitution (avoids excessive pressure buildup). • May be further diluted with 50 ml D_5W or 0.9% NaCl and give as a continuous infusion through a central venous line.

DOXIL

• Dilute each dose in 250 ml D_5W.

Rate of administration • For IV push, administer into tubing of freely running IV infusion of D_5W or 0.9% NaCl, preferably via butterfly needle, at rate no faster than 3–5 min (avoids local erythematous streaking along vein and facial flushing). • Must test for flashback q30sec to be certain needle remains in vein during injection. • Extravasation produces immediate pain, severe local tissue damage. Terminate administration immediately; withdraw as much medication as possible, obtain extravasation kit, follow protocol.

DOXIL

• Give as infusion over >30 min. • Do not use in-line filters.

IV INCOMPATIBILITIES

DOXORUBICIN: Allopurinol (Aloprim), amphotericin B complex (Abelcet, AmBisome, Amphotec), cefepime (Maxipime), furosemide (Lasix), ganciclovir (Cytovene), heparin, piperacillin/tazobactam (Zosyn), propofol (Diprivan).

DOXIL: Do not mix with any other medications.

IV COMPATIBILITIES

Dexamethasone (Decadron), diphenhydramine (Benadryl), etoposide (VePesid), granisetron (Kytril), hydromorphone (Dilaudid), lorazepam (Ativan), morphine, ondansetron (Zofran), paclitaxel (Taxol), propofol (Diprivan).

INDICATIONS/ROUTES/DOSAGE

Alert: Dosage individualized based on clinical response, tolerance to adverse effects. When used in combination therapy, consult specific protocols for optimum dosage, sequence of drug administration.

USUAL DOSE

IV: ADULTS: 60–75 mg/m^2 single dose q21 days, 20 mg/m^2 once weekly, or 25–30 mg/m^2 daily on 2–3 successive days q4wks. Due to cardiotoxicity, do not exceed cumulative dose of 550 mg/m^2 (400–450 mg/m^2 for those whose previous therapy included related compounds or irradiation of cardiac region). CHILDREN: 35–75 mg/m^2 as single dose q3wks or 20–30 mg/m^2 weekly or 60–90 mg/m^2 as continuous infusion over 96 hrs q3–4wks.

KAPOSI'S SARCOMA: (Doxil)

IV infusion: ADULTS: 20 mg/m^2 q3wks (infuse over 30 min).

OVARIAN CANCER: (Doxil)

IV infusion: ADULTS: 50 mg/m^2 q4wks.

DOSAGE IN HEPATIC IMPAIRMENT

Serum Bilirubin Concentration	Dosage
1.2–3 mg/dl	50% usual dose
>3 mg/dl	25% usual dose

SIDE EFFECTS

FREQUENT: Complete alopecia (scalp, axillary, pubic hair), nausea, vomiting, stomatitis, esophagitis (esp. if drug given daily on several successive days), reddish urine. **Doxil:** Nausea. **OCCASIONAL:** Anorexia, diarrhea, hyperpigmentation of nailbeds, phalangeal, dermal creases. **RARE:** Fever, chills, conjunctivitis, lacrimation.

ADVERSE REACTIONS/ TOXIC EFFECTS

Bone marrow depression manifested as hematologic toxicity (principally leukopenia and, to lesser extent, anemia, thrombocytopenia). Generally occurs within 10–15 days, returns to normal levels by third week. Cardiotoxicity noted as either acute, transient abnormal EKG findings and/or cardiomyopathy manifested as CHF.

NURSING IMPLICATIONS

BASELINE ASSESSMENT

Obtain WBC, platelet, erythrocyte counts prior to and at frequent intervals during therapy. Obtain EKG prior to therapy, liver function studies prior to each dose. Antiemetics may be effective in preventing, treating nausea.

INTERVENTION/EVALUATION

Monitor for stomatitis (burning/erythema of oral mucosa at inner margin of lips, difficulty swallowing). May lead to ulceration of mucous membranes within 2–3 days. Assess skin, nailbeds for hyperpigmentation. Monitor hematologic status, renal/hepatic function studies, serum uric acid levels. Assess pattern of daily bowel activity/stool consistency. Monitor for hematologic toxicity (fever, sore throat, signs of local infection, unusual bruising/bleeding from any site), symptoms of anemia (excessive tiredness, weakness).

PATIENT/FAMILY TEACHING

Alopecia is reversible, but new hair growth may have different color, texture. New hair growth resumes 2–3 mos after last therapy dose. Maintain fastidious oral hygiene. Do not have immunizations without physician's approval (drug lowers body's resistance). Avoid contact with those who have recently received live virus vaccine. Promptly report fever, sore throat, signs of local infection, unusual bruising/bleeding from any site. Contact physician for persistent nausea/vomiting. Avoid alcohol.

doxycycline

dock-see-**sigh**-clean
(Adoxa, Apo-Doxy✤, Doryx, Doxycin✤, Periostat, Vibra-Tabs, Vibramycin)

Do not confuse with Dicyclomine, doxylamine.

CLASSIFICATION

PHARMACOTHERAPEUTIC: Tetracycline. **CLINICAL:** Antibiotic.

ACTION

Inhibits protein synthesis by binding to ribosomes. **Therapeutic Effect:** Prevents bacterial cell growth.

USES

Treatment of periodontitis; respiratory, skin/soft tissue, urinary tract infections; syphilis; uncomplicated gonorrhea; pelvic inflammatory disease; rheumatic fever prophylaxis; brucellosis; trachoma; Rocky Mountain spotted fever; typhus; Q fever; rickettsia; smallpox; psittacosis; ornithosis; granuloma inguinale; lymphogranuloma venereum; adjunctive treatment of intestinal amebiasis. **Adoxa:** Treatment of severe acne. **Unlabeled:** Treatment of gonorrhea, malaria, atypical mycobacterial infections, prophylaxis/treatment of traveler's diarrhea, rheumatoid arthritis, prevention of Lyme disease.

PRECAUTIONS

CONTRAINDICATIONS: Hypersensitivity to tetracyclines, sulfite, last half of pregnancy, children <8 yrs, severe liver dysfunction. **CAUTIONS:** Sun/ultraviolet light exposure (severe photosensitivity reaction). **Pregnancy Category D.**

INTERACTIONS

DRUG: **Antacids** containing aluminum/calcium/magnesium, **laxatives** containing magnesium decrease absorption. **Oral iron preparations** impair absorption of tetracyclines (give 1–2 hrs before or after tetracyclines). **Barbiturates, phenytoin, carbamazepine** may decrease doxycycline concentrations. **Cholestyramine, colestipol** may decrease absorption. May decrease effect of **oral contraceptives. HERBAL:** None known. **FOOD:** None known. **LAB VALUES:** May increase SGOT (AST), SGPT (ALT), alkaline phosphatase, amylase, bilirubin concentrations; may alter CBC.

AVAILABILITY (Rx)

CAPSULES: 50 mg, 100 mg. **TABLETS:** 20 mg, 100 mg. **POWDER FOR ORAL SUSPENSION:** 50 mg/5 ml. **SYRUP:** 50 mg/5 ml. **POWDER FOR INJECTION:** 100 mg, 200 mg. **CAPSULES (EXTENDED RELEASE):** 75 mg, 100 mg.

ADMINISTRATION/HANDLING

Alert: Do not administer IM or subcutaneous. Space doses evenly around clock.

PO

• Store capsules, tablets at room temperature. • Oral suspension is stable for 2 wks at room temperature. Give with full glass of fluid. • May take with food or milk.

IV

Storage • After reconstitution, IV infusion (piggyback) is stable for 12 hrs at room temperature, 72 hrs if refrigerated.

• Protect from direct sunlight. Discard if precipitate forms.

Reconstitution • Reconstitute each 100-mg vial with 10 ml Sterile Water for Injection for concentration of 10 mg/ml. • Further dilute each 100 mg with at least 100 ml D_5W, 0.9% NaCl, lactated Ringer's.

Rate of administration • Give by intermittent IV infusion (piggyback). • Infuse >1–4 hrs.

IV INCOMPATIBILITIES
Allopurinol (Aloprim), heparin, piperacillin/tazobactam (Zosyn).

IV COMPATIBILITY
Amiodarone (Cordarone), diltiazem (Cardizem), hydromorphone (Dilaudid), magnesium sulfate, morphine, propofol (Diprivan).

INDICATIONS/ROUTES/DOSAGE

USUAL DOSAGE
PO: ADULTS, ELDERLY: Initially, 200 mg (100 mg q12h), then 100 mg/day as single dose or in 2 divided doses (100 mg q12h in severe infections). CHILDREN >8 YRS, >45 KG: 2–4 mg/kg/day divided q12–24h. **Maximum:** 200 mg/day.

IV: ADULTS, ELDERLY: Initially, 200 mg as 1–2 infusions; then 100–200 mg/day (200 mg as 12 infusions). CHILDREN ≥8 YRS: 2–4 mg/kg/day divided q12–24h. **Maximum:** 200 mg/day.

ACUTE GONOCOCCAL INFECTIONS
PO: ADULTS: Initially, 200 mg, then 100 mg at bedtime on first day; then 100 mg 2 times/day for 14 days.

SYPHILIS
PO/IV: ADULTS: 200 mg/day in divided doses for 14–28 days.

TRAVELER'S DIARRHEA
PO: ADULTS, ELDERLY: 100 mg daily during a period of risk (up to 14 days) and for 2 days after returning home.

PERIODONTITIS
PO: ADULTS: 20 mg 2 times/day.

SIDE EFFECTS

FREQUENT: Anorexia, nausea, vomiting, diarrhea, dysphagia, photosensitivity (may be severe). **OCCASIONAL:** Rash, urticaria.

ADVERSE REACTIONS/ TOXIC EFFECTS

Superinfection (esp. fungal), benign intracranial hypertension (headache, visual changes). Liver toxicity, fatty degeneration of liver, pancreatitis occur rarely.

NURSING IMPLICATIONS

BASELINE ASSESSMENT

Question for history of allergies, esp. to tetracyclines, sulfites.

INTERVENTION/EVALUATION

Determine pattern of bowel activity/ stool consistency. Assess skin for rash. Monitor LOC due to potential for increased intracranial pressure. Be alert for superinfection: diarrhea, ulceration or changes of oral mucosa, anal/ genital pruritus.

PATIENT/FAMILY TEACHING

Avoid unnecessary exposure to sunlight. Do not take with antacids, iron products, dairy products. Complete full course of therapy. After application of dental gel, avoid tooth brushing, flossing the treated areas for 7 days.

dronabinol

drow-**nab**-in-all
(Marinol)
Do not confuse with droperidol.

◆ **CLASSIFICATION**

PHARMACOTHERAPEUTIC: Controlled substance **(Schedule III). CLINICAL:** Antinausea, antiemetic, appetite stimulant.

ACTION

Inhibits vomiting control mechanisms in medulla oblongata. **Therapeutic Effect:** Inhibits vomiting.

USES

Prevention, treatment of nausea, vomiting due to cancer chemotherapy; appetite stimulant in AIDS, cancer pts.

PRECAUTIONS

CONTRAINDICATIONS: Nausea, vomiting other than due to chemotherapy. **CAUTIONS:** Hypertension, heart disease; manic, depressive, or schizophrenic pts. Not recommended in children. **Pregnancy Category C.**

INTERACTIONS

DRUG: **CNS depressants** may enhance sedative effects. **HERBAL:** None known. **FOOD:** None known. **LAB VALUES:** None known.

AVAILABILITY (Rx)

CAPSULES, GELATIN: 2.5 mg, 5 mg, 10 mg.

INDICATIONS/ROUTES/DOSAGE

NAUSEA, VOMITING

PO: ADULTS, CHILDREN: Initially, 5 mg/m^2, 1–3 hrs before chemotherapy, then q2–4h after chemotherapy for total of 4–6 doses/day. May increase by 2.5 mg/m^2 up to 15 mg/m^2 dose.

APPETITE STIMULANT

PO: ADULTS: Initially, 2.5 mg 2 times/day (before lunch, dinner). RANGE: 2.5–20 mg/day.

SIDE EFFECTS

FREQUENT (3%–24%): Euphoria, dizziness, paranoid reaction, somnolence. **OCCASIONAL (1%–3%):** Asthenia, ataxia, confusion, abnormal thinking, depersonalization. **RARE (<1%):** Diarrhea, depression, nightmares, speech difficulties, headache, anxiety, ringing in ears, flushed skin.

ADVERSE REACTIONS/ TOXIC EFFECTS

Mild intoxication may produce increased sensory awareness (e.g., taste, smell, sound), altered time perception, reddened conjunctiva, dry mouth, tachycardia. Moderate intoxication may produce memory impairment, urinary retention. Severe intoxication may produce lethargy, decrease motor coordination, slurred speech, postural hypotension.

NURSING IMPLICATIONS

BASELINE ASSESSMENT

Assess dehydration status if excessive vomiting occurs (skin turgor, mucous membranes, urine output).

INTERVENTION/EVALUATION

Supervise closely for serious mood, behavior responses. Monitor B/P, heart rate.

PATIENT/FAMILY TEACHING

Report visual disturbances. Relief from nausea/vomiting generally occurs within 15 min of drug administration. Avoid alcohol, barbiturates. Avoid tasks that require alertness, motor skills until response to drug is established. For appetite stimulation take before lunch and dinner.

droperidol

droe-**pear**-ih-dall

(Inapsine)

D

D

◆ CLASSIFICATION

PHARMACOTHERAPEUTIC: General anesthetic. **CLINICAL:** Anesthesia adjunct, antiemetic.

ACTION

Antagonizes dopamine neurotransmission at synapses by blocking postsynaptic dopamine receptor sites; partially blocks adrenergic receptor binding sites. **Therapeutic Effect:** Produces tranquilization, antiemetic effect.

PHARMACOKINETICS

Onset	Peak	Duration
IM		
3–10 min	30 min	2–4 hrs
IV		
3–10 min	30 min	2–4 hrs

Well absorbed after IM administration. Crosses blood-brain barrier. Metabolized in liver. Primarily excreted in urine. **Half-life:** 2.3 hrs.

USES

Adjunct for general anesthesia. Treatment of nausea/vomiting associated with surgical and diagnostic procedures.

PRECAUTIONS

CONTRAINDICATIONS: Known or suspected QT prolongation, congenital long QT syndrome. **CAUTIONS:** Impaired hepatic/renal/cardiac function (may cause cardiac arrhythmias during administration).

LIFESPAN CONSIDERATIONS: Pregnancy/lactation: Crosses placenta. Unknown if drug is distributed in breast milk. **Pregnancy Category C. Children:** Dystonias more likely. **Elderly:** May be more sensitive to sedative, hypotensive effects.

INTERACTIONS

DRUG: CNS depressants may increase CNS depressant effect. **Antihypertensives** may increase hypotension. **HERBAL:** None known. **FOOD:** None known. **LAB VALUES:** None known.

AVAILABILITY (Rx)

INJECTION: 2.5 mg/ml.

ADMINISTRATION/HANDLING

Alert: Pt must remain recumbent for 30–60 min in head-low position with legs raised, to minimize hypotensive effect.

Storage • Store parenteral form at room temperature.

IM

• Inject slowly, deep IM into upper outer quadrant of gluteus maximus.

IV

• May give undiluted as IV push over 2–5 min. • Dose for high-risk pts should be added to D_5W or lactated Ringer's injection to a concentration of 1 mg/50 ml and given as an IV infusion.

IV INCOMPATIBILITIES

Allopurinol (Aloprim), amphotericin B complex (Abelcet, AmBisome, Amphotic), cefepime (Maxipime), foscarnet (Foscavir), heparin, methotrexate, piperacillin/tazobactam (Zosyn).

IV COMPATIBILITIES

Atropine, diphenhydramine (Benadryl), glycopyrrolate (Robinul), metoclopramide (Reglan), midazolam (Versed), morphine, potassium chloride, promethazine (Phenergan).

INDICATIONS/ROUTES/DOSAGE

PREOP

IM/IV: ADULTS, ELDERLY: 2.5–10 mg 30–60 min before induction of general anesthesia. CHILDREN 2–12 YRS: 0.088–0.165 mg/kg.

ADJUNCT FOR INDUCTION OF GENERAL ANESTHESIA

IV: ADULTS, ELDERLY: 0.22–0.275 mg/

kg. CHILDREN 2–12 YRS: 0.088–0.165 mg/kg.

ADJUNCT FOR MAINTENANCE OF GENERAL ANESTHESIA
IV: ADULTS, ELDERLY: 1.25–2.5 mg.

DIAGNOSTIC PROCEDURES WITHOUT GENERAL ANESTHESIA
IM: ADULTS, ELDERLY: 2.5–10 mg 30–60 min before procedure. If needed, may give additional doses of 1.25–2.5 mg (usually by IV injection).

ADJUNCT TO REGIONAL ANESTHESIA
IM/IV: ADULTS, ELDERLY: 2.5–5 mg.

POSTOP NAUSEA/VOMITING
IV/IM: ADULTS, ELDERLY: Initially, 2.5 mg. May repeat with 1.25 mg to achieve desired effect. CHILDREN 2–12 YRS: 0.05–0.06 mg/kg. **Maximum:** 0.1 mg/kg.

NAUSEA/VOMITING
IM/IV: ADULTS, ELDERLY: Initially, 2.5 mg. Additional doses of 1.25 mg may be given to achieve desired effect. CHILDREN 2–12 YRS: 0.05–0.06 mg/kg (maximum initial dose of 0.1 mg/kg). Additional dose may be given to achieve desired effect.

SIDE EFFECTS

FREQUENT: Mild to moderate hypotension. **OCCASIONAL:** Tachycardia, postop drowsiness, dizziness, chills, shivering. **RARE:** Postop nightmares, facial sweating, bronchospasm.

ADVERSE REACTIONS/ TOXIC EFFECTS

May produce cardiac arrhythmias. Extrapyramidal symptoms may appear as akathisia (motor restlessness), dystonias: torticollis (neck muscle spasm), opisthotonos (rigidity of back muscles), oculogyric crisis (rolling back of eyes).

NURSING IMPLICATIONS

BASELINE ASSESSMENT

Assess vital signs. Have pt void. Raise side rails. Instruct to remain recumbent.

INTERVENTION/EVALUATION

Monitor B/P, pulse diligently for hypotensive reaction during and after procedure. Assess pulse for tachycardia. Monitor for extrapyramidal symptoms. Evaluate for therapeutic response from anxiety: a calm facial expression, decreased restlessness. Monitor for decreased nausea, vomiting.

drotrecogin alfa

dro-trae-**coe**-gin alfa
(Xigris)

CLASSIFICATION

PHARMACOTHERAPEUTIC: Activated protein C. **CLINICAL:** Antisepsis agent.

ACTION

Recombinant-produced preparation of human-activated protein C. Possesses profibrinolytic, antithrombotic, anti-inflammatory effects. **Therapeutic Effect:** Interferes with some of the body's harmful responses to severe infection, including the formation of blood clots that can lead to organ failure, death.

PHARMACOKINETICS

Inactivated by endogenous plasma protease inhibitors. Clearance occurs within 2 hrs of initiating infusion. **Half-life:** 1.6 hrs.

USES

Treatment of severe sepsis or septic shock with evidence of organ dysfunction in pts who have a high risk of death.

D

PRECAUTIONS

CONTRAINDICATIONS: Active internal bleeding, recent (≤3 mos) hemorrhagic stroke, recent (≤2 mos) intracranial or intraspinal surgery or severe head trauma, trauma with an increased risk of life-threatening bleeding, presence of an epidural catheter, intracranial neoplasm or mass lesion or evidence of cerebral herniation. **CAUTIONS:** Concurrent use of heparin, platelet count <30,000/mm^3, prolonged prothrombin time, recent (≤6 wks) GI bleeding, recent (≤3 days) thrombolytic therapy, recent (≤7 days) anticoagulant or aspirin therapy, intracranial aneurysm, chronic severe hepatic disease.

LIFESPAN CONSIDERATIONS **Pregnancy/lactation:** Unknown if the drug can cause fetal harm. Unknown if excreted in breast milk. **Pregnancy Category C.** **Children/elderly:** Safety and efficacy not established.

INTERACTIONS

DRUG: None known. Use caution when used with other drugs that affect hemostasis. **HERBAL:** None known. **FOOD:** None known. **LAB VALUES:** May variably prolong PTT.

AVAILABILITY (Rx)

POWDER FOR INFUSION: 5 mg, 20 mg.

ADMINISTRATION/HANDLING

IV

Storage • Store unreconstituted vials at room temperature. • Start infusion within 3 hrs after reconstitution.

Reconstitution • Reconstitute 5-mg vials with 2.5 ml Sterile Water for Injection and 20-mg vials with 10 ml Sterile Water for Injection. Resulting concentration is 2 mg/ml. • Slowly add the Sterile Water for Injection by swirling; do not shake or invert vial. • Further dilute with 0.9% NaCl. • Withdraw amount from vial and add to infusion bag containing 0.9% NaCl for a final concentration of between 100 and 200 mcg/ml; direct the stream to the side of the bag (minimizes agitation). • Invert infusion bag to mix solution.

Rate of administration • Administer via a dedicated IV line or a dedicated lumen of a multilumen CVL. • Administer infusion rate of 24 mcg/kg/hr for 96 hrs. • If infusion is interrupted, restart drug at 24 mcg/kg/hr.

⊘ IV INCOMPATIBILITY

Do not mix with other medications.

IV COMPATIBILITY

0.9% NaCl, lactated Ringer's, dextrose are the only solutions that can be administered through the same line.

INDICATIONS/ROUTES/DOSAGE

SEVERE SEPSIS

IV infusion: ADULTS, ELDERLY: 24 mcg/kg/hr given for 96 hrs.

SIDE EFFECTS

None known.

ADVERSE REACTIONS/ TOXIC EFFECTS

RARE (2%): Bleeding (intrathoracic, retroperitoneal, GU, GI, intra-abdominal, intracranial).

NURSING IMPLICATIONS

BASELINE ASSESSMENT

Criteria that must be met before initiating drug therapy: age >18 yrs, no pregnancy or breast-feeding, actual body weight <135 kg, ≥3 systemic inflammatory response criteria (fever, heart rate >90 beats/min, respiratory rate >20 breaths/min, increased WBC count), and at least one sepsis-induced organ or system failure (cardiovascular, renal, respiratory, hematologic, or unexplained metabolic acidosis).

INTERVENTION/EVALUATION

Monitor closely for hemorrhagic complication.

Dulcolax

see bisacodyl

DuoNeb

see albuterol or ipratropium

Duragesic

see fentanyl

Duramorph

see morphine

dutasteride

do-tah-**stir**-eyed

(Avodart)

CLASSIFICATION

PHARMACOTHERAPEUTIC: Androgen hormone inhibitor. **CLINICAL:** Benign prostatic hyperplasia agent.

ACTION

Inhibits steroid 5-alpha reductase, an intracellular enzyme that converts testosterone into dihydrotestosterone (DHT) in the prostate gland, providing a reduction in serum DHT. **Therapeutic Effect:** Regresses enlarged prostate gland.

PHARMACOKINETICS

Onset	Peak	Duration
PO		
24 hrs	—	3–8 wks

Moderately absorbed after PO administration. Widely distributed. Protein binding: 99%. Metabolized in the liver. Primarily excreted via the feces. **Half-life:** Up to 5 wks.

USES

Treatment of benign prostatic hyperplasia (BPH). **Unlabeled:** Treatment of hair loss.

PRECAUTIONS

CONTRAINDICATIONS: Physical handling of tablet in those who may become or are pregnant. Avoid use in women. **CAUTIONS:** Impaired liver disease, obstructive uropathy, preexisting sexual dysfunction (e.g., reduced male libido, impotence). **Pregnancy Category X.**

INTERACTIONS

DRUG: None known. **HERBAL:** None known. **FOOD:** None known. **LAB VALUES:** Produces decrease in serum prostate-specific antigen (PSA) levels.

AVAILABILITY (Rx)

TABLETS: 0.5 mg.

ADMINISTRATION/HANDLING

PO

• Do not crush or break film-coated tablets. • Give without regards to meals.

INDICATIONS/ROUTES/DOSAGE

BENIGN PROSTATIC HYPERPLASIA

PO: ADULTS, ELDERLY: 0.5 mg once daily.

SIDE EFFECTS

OCCASIONAL: Gynecomastia, sexual dysfunction (decreased libido, impotence, ejaculatory disturbances).

E

ADVERSE REACTIONS/ TOXIC EFFECTS

Toxicity manifested as rash, diarrhea, abdominal pain.

NURSING IMPLICATIONS

BASELINE ASSESSMENT

Serum PSA determination should be performed in pts with BPH prior to beginning therapy and periodically thereafter.

INTERVENTION/EVALUATION

Diligently monitor I&O. Assess for signs/symptoms of BPH (hesitancy, reduced force of urinary stream, postvoid dribbling, sensation of incomplete bladder emptying).

PATIENT/FAMILY TEACHING

Discuss potential for impotence; volume of ejaculate may be decreased during treatment. May not notice improved urinary flow for up to 6 mos after treatment. Women who may be or are pregnant should not handle tablets (Pregnancy Category X).

Dyazide

see hydrochlorothiazide or triamterene

DynaCirc

see isradipine

echinacea

Also known as black susans, comb flower, red sunflower, scurvy root

CLASSIFICATION

HERBAL.

ACTION

Stimulates immune system. Possesses antiviral/immune stimulatory effects. Increases phagocytosis, lymphocyte activity (possibly by releasing tumor necrosis factor, interleukin-1, interferon). **Effect:** Prevents/reduces symptoms associated with upper respiratory infections.

USES

Immune system stimulant used for treatment/prevention of the common cold and other upper respiratory infections. Also used for urinary tract infections, vaginal candidiasis.

PRECAUTIONS

CONTRAINDICATIONS: Pregnancy/lactation, children <2 yrs, those with autoimmune disease (e.g., multiple sclerosis, SLE, HIV/AIDS), tuberculosis, history of allergic conditions. **CAUTIONS:** Diabetes (may alter control of blood sugar). Do not use for >8 wks (may decrease effectiveness).

LIFESPAN CONSIDERATIONS: Pregnancy/lactation: Contraindicated. **Pregnancy Category C. Children:** Safety and efficacy not established in those <2 yrs. **Elderly:** No age-related precautions noted.

INTERACTIONS

DRUG: May interfere with immunosuppressant therapy **(e.g., corticosteroids, cyclosporine, mycophenolate).** Topical **econazole** may reduce recurring vaginal candida infections. **HERBAL:** None known. **FOOD:** None known. **LAB VALUES:** None known.

AVAILABILITY (OTC)

CAPSULES: 200 mg, 380 mg, 400 mg, 500 mg. **POWDER:** 25 g, 100 g, 500 g. **LIQUID.**

INDICATIONS/ROUTES/DOSAGE

USUAL ADULT DOSAGE

PO: ADULTS, ELDERLY: 6–9 ml herbal juice for a maximum of 8 wks.

Alert: A variety of doses have been used depending on the preparation.

SIDE EFFECTS

Well tolerated. May cause allergic reaction (urticaria, acute asthma/dyspnea, angioedema), fever, nausea, vomiting, diarrhea, unpleasant taste, abdominal pain, dizziness.

ADVERSE REACTIONS/ TOXIC EFFECTS

None known.

NURSING IMPLICATIONS

BASELINE ASSESSMENT

Assess if pregnant/breast-feeding, history of autoimmune disease, receiving immunosuppressant therapy.

INTERVENTION/EVALUATION

Assess for hypersensitivity reaction, improvement in infection.

PATIENT/FAMILY TEACHING

Do not use during pregnancy/lactation, children <2 yrs. Do not use for >8 wks without at least 1-wk rest.

echothiophate

(Phospholine Iodide)

See Classification section under: Antiglaucoma agents (p. 44C)

Ecotrin

see aspirin

edetate calcium

See Appendix A: Antidotes

EES

see erythromycin

efavirenz

eh-fah-**vir**-enz
(Sustiva)

◆ CLASSIFICATION

PHARMACOTHERAPEUTIC: Nonnucleoside reverse transcriptase inhibitor. **CLINICAL:** Antiretroviral (see pp. 59C, 99C).

ACTION

Inhibits activity of HIV-1 reverse transcriptase (RT). **Therapeutic Effect:** Interrupts HIV replication, slowing progression of HIV infection.

PHARMACOKINETICS

Rapidly absorbed after PO administration. Protein binding: 99%. Metabolized to major isoenzymes in liver. Eliminated in urine and feces. **Half-life:** 40–55 hrs.

USES

Treatment of HIV infection in combination with other appropriate antiretroviral agents.

E

PRECAUTIONS

CONTRAINDICATIONS: History of hypersensitivity to efavirenz, monotherapy, concurrent administration with midazolam, triazolam, ergot derivatives. **CAUTIONS:** History of mental illness, substance abuse, liver impairment.

LIFESPAN CONSIDERATIONS: Pregnancy/lactation: Breast-feeding not recommended. **Pregnancy Category C. Children:** Safety and efficacy not established in those <3 yrs; may have increased incidence of rash. **Elderly:** No age-related precautions noted.

INTERACTIONS

DRUG: Midazolam, triazolam, ergot derivatives may create serious or life-threatening events (cardiac arrhythmias, prolonged sedation, respiratory depression). **Alcohol, psychoactive drugs** may produce additive CNS effects. **Phenobarbital, rifampin, rifabutin** lowers efavirenz plasma concentration. Decreases **clarithromycin** plasma levels. Decreases **indinavir, saquinavir** plasma concentrations; increases **nelfinavir, ritonavir** plasma concentrations; alters **warfarin** plasma concentrations. **HERBAL:** None known. **FOOD:** None known. **LAB VALUES:** May produce false-positive urine test results for cannabinoid, increases total cholesterol, triglycerides, increases SGOT (AST), SGPT (ALT) liver enzymes.

AVAILABILITY (Rx)

CAPSULES: 50 mg, 100 mg, 200 mg. **TABLETS:** 600 mg.

ADMINISTRATION/HANDLING

PO

- Give without regard to meals.
- High-fat meal may increase absorption and should be avoided.

INDICATIONS/ROUTES/DOSAGE

HIV INFECTION

PO: ADULTS, ELDERLY: 600 mg once daily in combination. Bedtime dosing is recommended during first 2–4 wks (due to temporary CNS side effects). CHILDREN >3 YRS, >40 KG: 600 mg once daily. 32.5–40 KG: 400 mg once daily. 25–32.5 KG: 350 mg once daily. 20–25 KG: 300 mg once daily. 15–20 KG: 250 mg once daily. 10–15 KG: 200 mg once daily.

SIDE EFFECTS

FREQUENT (52%) mild to severe symptoms: Dizziness, vivid dreams, insomnia, confusion, impaired concentration, amnesia, agitation, depersonalization, hallucinations, euphoria. **OCCASIONAL:** Mild to moderate maculopapular rash (27%); nausea, fatigue, headache, diarrhea, fever, cough (<26%).

ADVERSE REACTIONS/ TOXIC EFFECTS

None known.

NURSING IMPLICATIONS

BASELINE ASSESSMENT

Offer emotional support to pt/family. Obtain baseline SGOT (AST), SGPT (ALT) in pts with history of hepatitis B or C; cholesterol; triglycerides prior to initiating therapy and at intervals during therapy. Obtain history of all prescription and OTC medication (high level of drug interaction).

INTERVENTION/EVALUATION

Monitor for CNS, psychological symptoms: severe acute depression, including suicidal ideation/attempts, dizziness, impaired concentration, somnolence, abnormal dreams, insomnia (begins during first or second day of therapy, generally resolves in 2–4 wks). Assess for evidence of rash (common side effect). Monitor liver enzyme studies for abnormalities. Assess for headache, nausea, diarrhea.

PATIENT/FAMILY TEACHING

Avoid high-fat meals during therapy. If rash appears, contact physician immediately. CNS, psychological symptoms occur in more than half the pts and may cause dizziness, impaired concentration, delusions, depression. Take medication every day as prescribed. Do not alter dose or discontinue medication without informing physician. Avoid tasks that require alertness, motor skills until response to drug is established. Drug is not a cure for HIV infection, nor does it reduce risk of transmission to others.

Effexor

see venlafaxine

Efudex

see fluorouracil

Elavil

see amitriptyline

eletriptan

el-eh-**trip**-tan
(Relpax)

CLASSIFICATION

PHARMACOTHERAPEUTIC: Serotonin receptor agonist. **CLINICAL:** Antimigraine.

PHARMACOKINETICS

Well absorbed following PO administration. Metabolized by the liver to inactive metabolite. Eliminated in urine. **Half-life:** 4.4 hrs (half-life increased in hepatic impairment, elderly >65 yrs).

ACTION

Binds selectively to vascular receptors producing a vasoconstrictive effect on cranial blood vessels. **Therapeutic Effect:** Produces relief of migraine headache.

USES

Treatment of acute migraine headache with or without aura.

PRECAUTIONS

CONTRAINDICATIONS: Severe hepatic impairment, coronary artery disease, uncontrolled hypertension, ischemic heart disease, arrhythmias associated with cardiac conduction pathways. **CAUTIONS:** Mild to moderate renal/hepatic impairment, controlled hypertension, history of cerebrovascular accident.

LIFESPAN CONSIDERATIONS: Pregnancy/lactation: May decrease possibility of ovulation. Distributed in breast milk. **Pregnancy Category C. Children:** Safety and efficacy not established in pts <18 yrs. **Elderly:** Increased risk of hypertension in pts >65 yrs.

INTERACTIONS

DRUG: Ergotamine-containing drugs may produce vasospastic reaction. Avoid taking **ketoconazole, itraconazole, nefazodone, clarithromycin, ritonivir, nelfinavir** within 72 hrs prior to initiation of therapy. Concurrent use with **sibutramine** may produce "serotonin syndrome" (motor weakness, shivering, myoclonus, altered consciousness, CNS irritability). **HERBAL:** None known. **FOOD:** None known. **LAB VALUES:** None known.

AVAILABILITY (Rx)

TABLETS: 20 mg, 40 mg.

ADMINISTRATION/HANDLING

PO

- Do not crush or break film-coated tablets.

E

INDICATIONS/ROUTES/DOSAGE

MIGRAINE

PO: ADULTS, ELDERLY: 20–40 mg. If headache improves but then returns, a repeat dose may be given at least 2 hrs following the initial dose. **Maximum daily dose:** 80 mg.

SIDE EFFECTS

OCCASIONAL (5%–6%): Dizziness, somnolence, asthenia (loss of strength, energy), nausea. **RARE (2%–3%):** Paresthesia, headache, dry mouth, warm/hot temperature sensation, dyspepsia (heartburn, epigastric distress), dysphagia (including throat tightness, difficulty swallowing).

ADVERSE REACTIONS/ TOXIC EFFECTS

Cardiac ischemia, coronary artery vasospasm, MI, noncardiac vasospasm-related reactions (hemorrhage, stroke) occur rarely but particularly in pts with hypertension, obesity, diabetes, strong family history of coronary artery disease; smokers; males >40 yrs; postmenopausal women.

NURSING CONSIDERATIONS

BASELINE ASSESSMENT

Question pt regarding onset, location, duration of migraine, possible precipitating symptoms. Obtain baseline B/P for evidence of uncontrolled hypertension (contraindication).

INTERVENTION/EVALUATION

Assess for relief of migraine headache, potential for photophobia, phonophobia (sound sensitivity, nausea, vomiting).

PATIENT/FAMILY TEACHING

Take a single dose as soon as symptoms of an actual migraine attack appear. Medication is intended to relieve migraine headaches, not to prevent or reduce number of attacks. Avoid tasks that require alertness, motor skills until response to drug is established. If heart throbbing, pain/tightness in chest or throat, sudden/severe abdominal pain, pain/weakness of extremities occurs, contact physician immediately.

emtricitabine

em-trih-**sit**-ah-bean
(Emtriva)

CLASSIFICATION

PHARMACOTHERAPEUTIC: Nucleoside reverse transcriptase inhibitor. **CLINICAL:** Antiretroviral agent.

ACTION

Inhibits HIV-1 reverse transcriptase by incorporating into viral DNA, resulting in chain termination. **Therapeutic Effect:** Slows HIV replication, reducing progression of HIV infection.

PHARMACOKINETICS

Rapidly and extensively absorbed from GI tract. Primarily excreted in urine (86%) with a lesser amount excreted in feces (14%). 30% removed by hemodialysis. Unknown if removed by peritoneal dialysis. **Half-life:** 10 hrs.

USES

Used in combination with other antiretroviral agents for treatment of HIV-1 infection in adults.

PRECAUTIONS

CONTRAINDICATIONS: None known. **CAUTIONS:** Impaired hepatic/renal function.

LIFESPAN CONSIDERATIONS: Pregnancy/lactation: Breast-feeding not recommended. **Pregnancy Category B. Children:** Safety and effectiveness have not been established. **Elderly:** Age-related decreased renal function may require dosage adjustment.

INTERACTIONS

DRUG: None known. **HERBAL:** None known. **FOOD:** None known. **LAB VALUES:** May elevate lipase, amylase, triglycerides, SGPT (ALT), SGOT (AST). May alter blood glucose.

AVAILABILITY (Rx)

CAPSULES: 200 mg.

ADMINISTRATION/HANDLING

PO

- Give without regard to food.

INDICATIONS/ROUTES/DOSAGE

HIV INFECTION

PO: ADULTS, ELDERLY: 200 mg once daily.

DOSAGE IN RENAL IMPAIRMENT

Creatinine Clearance	Dosage
30–49 ml/min	200 mg q48h
15–29 ml/min	200 mg q72h
<15 ml/min, hemodialysis pts	200 mg q96h

SIDE EFFECTS

FREQUENT (13%–23%): Headache, rhinitis, rash, diarrhea, nausea. **OCCASIONAL (4%–14%):** Cough, vomiting, abdominal pain, insomnia, depression, paresthesia, dizziness, peripheral neuropathy, dyspepsia (heartburn, epigastric distress), myalgia. **RARE (2%–3%):** Arthralgia, abnormal dreams.

ADVERSE REACTIONS/ TOXIC EFFECTS

Lactic acidosis, hepatomegaly with steatosis (excess fat in liver) occur rarely; may be severe.

NURSING IMPLICATIONS

BASELINE ASSESSMENT

Obtain baseline laboratory testing, esp. liver function tests, triglycerides prior to beginning and at periodic intervals during emtricitabine therapy. Offer emotional support.

INTERVENTION/EVALUATION

Monitor stool frequency/consistency (watery, loose, soft). Question for evidence of nausea, pruritus (itching). Assess skin for rash, urticaria (hives). Monitor clinical chemistry tests for marked lab abnormalities.

PATIENT/FAMILY TEACHING

May cause redistribution of body fat. Continue therapy for full length of treatment. Emtricitabine is not a cure for HIV infection, nor does it reduce risk of transmission to others: Pt needs to continue practices to prevent HIV transmission. Pts may continue to acquire illnesses associated with advanced HIV infection.

enalapril maleate

en-**al**-ah-prill

(Apo-Enalapril ✤, Vasotec)

Do not confuse with Anafranil, Eldepryl, ramipril.

FIXED-COMBINATION(S)

Lexxel: enalapril/felodipine (calcium channel blocker): 5 mg/2.5 mg; 5 mg/5 mg. **Teczem:** enalapril/diltiazem (calcium channel blocker): 5 mg/180 mg. **Vaseretic:** enalapril/

hydrochlorothiazide (diuretic): 5 mg/12.5 mg; 10 mg/25 mg.

CLASSIFICATION

PHARMACOTHERAPEUTIC: Angiotensin-converting enzyme (ACE) inhibitor. **CLINICAL:** Antihypertensive, vasodilator (see p. 6C).

ACTION

Suppresses renin-angiotensin-aldosterone system (prevents conversion of angiotensin I to angiotensin II, a potent vasoconstrictor; may inhibit angiotensin II at local vascular, renal sites). Decreases plasma angiotensin II, increases plasma renin activity, decreases aldosterone secretion. **Therapeutic Effect:** In hypertension, reduces peripheral arterial resistance. In CHF, increases cardiac output; decreases peripheral vascular resistance, B/P, pulmonary capillary wedge pressure, heart size.

PHARMACOKINETICS

Onset	Peak	Duration
PO		
1 hr	4–6 hrs	24 hrs
IV		
15 min	1–4 hrs	6 hrs

Readily absorbed from GI tract (not affected by food). Protein binding: 50%–60%. Converted to active metabolite. Primarily excreted in urine. Removed by hemodialysis. **Half-life:** 11 hrs (half-life increased with impaired renal function).

USES

Treatment of hypertension alone or in combination with other antihypertensives. Adjunctive therapy for CHF. **Unlabeled:** Treatment of diabetic nephropathy, renal crisis in scleroderma.

PRECAUTIONS

CONTRAINDICATIONS: History of angioedema with previous treatment with ACE inhibitors. **CAUTIONS:** Renal impairment, those with sodium depletion or on diuretic therapy, dialysis, hypovolemia, coronary/cerebrovascular insufficiency.

LIFESPAN CONSIDERATIONS: Pregnancy/lactation: Crosses placenta. Distributed in breast milk. May cause fetal/neonatal mortality/morbidity. **Pregnancy Category D** (**C** if used in first trimester). **Children:** Safety and efficacy not established. **Elderly:** May be more susceptible to hypotensive effects.

INTERACTIONS

DRUG: Alcohol, diuretics, hypotensive agents may increase effects. **HERBAL:** None known. **FOOD:** None known. **LAB VALUES:** May increase potassium, SGOT (AST), SGPT (ALT), alkaline phosphatase, bilirubin, BUN, creatinine. May decrease sodium. May cause positive ANA titer.

AVAILABILITY (Rx)

TABLETS: 2.5 mg, 5 mg, 10 mg, 20 mg.
INJECTION: 1.25 mg/ml.

ADMINISTRATION/HANDLING

PO

• Give without regard to food. • Tablets may be crushed.

IV

Storage • Store parenteral form at room temperature. • Use only clear, colorless solution. • Diluted IV solution is stable for 24 hrs at room temperature.

Reconstitution • May give undiluted or dilute with D_5W or 0.9% NaCl.

Rate of administration • For IV push, give undiluted over 5 min. • For IV piggyback, infuse over 10–15 min.

IV INCOMPATIBILITIES
Amphotericin (Fungizone), amphotericin B complex (Abelcet, AmBisome, Amphotec), cefepime (Maxipime), phenytoin (Dilantin).

IV COMPATIBILITIES
Calcium gluconate, dobutamine (Dobutrex), dopamine (Intropin), fentanyl (Sublimaze), heparin, lidocaine, magnesium sulfate, morphine, nitroglycerin, potassium chloride, potassium phosphate, propofol (Diprivan).

INDICATIONS/ROUTES/DOSAGE

HYPERTENSION
PO: ADULTS, ELDERLY: Initially, 2.5–5 mg/day. RANGE: 10–40 mg/day in 1–2 divided doses.

IV: ADULTS, ELDERLY: 0.625–1.25 mg q6h up to 5 mg q6h.

CHF
PO: ADULTS, ELDERLY: Initially, 2.5–5 mg/day. RANGE: 5–20 mg/day in 2 divided doses.

USUAL PEDIATRIC DOSE
PO: CHILDREN: 0.1 mg/kg/day in 1–2 divided doses. **Maximum:** 0.5 mg/kg/day. NEONATES: 0.1 mg/kg/day q24h.

IV: CHILDREN, NEONATES: 5–10 mcg/kg/dose q8–24h.

DOSAGE IN RENAL IMPAIRMENT

Creatinine Clearance	% Usual Dose
10–50 ml/min	75–100
<10 ml/min	50

SIDE EFFECTS
FREQUENT (5%–7%): Postural hypotension, headache, dizziness. **OCCASIONAL (2%–3%):** Orthostatic hypotension, fatigue, diarrhea, cough, syncope. **RARE (<2%):** Angina, abdominal pain, vomiting, nausea, rash, asthenia (loss of strength/energy), syncope.

ADVERSE REACTIONS/ TOXIC EFFECTS
Excessive hypotension ("first-dose syncope") may occur in those with CHF, severely salt/volume depleted. Angioedema (swelling of face, lips), hyperkalemia occur rarely. Agranulocytosis, neutropenia may be noted in pts with impaired renal function, collagen vascular disease (systemic lupus erythematosus, scleroderma). Nephrotic syndrome may be noted in those with history of renal disease.

NURSING IMPLICATIONS

BASELINE ASSESSMENT
Obtain B/P immediately prior to each dose (be alert to fluctuations). In pts with renal impairment, autoimmune disease, or taking drugs that affect leukocytes/immune response, CBC should be performed prior to beginning therapy, q2wks for 3 mos, then periodically thereafter.

INTERVENTION/EVALUATION
Assist with ambulation if dizziness occurs. Monitor serum potassium, BUN, serum creatinine levels, B/P. Monitor pattern of daily bowel activity/stool consistency.

PATIENT/FAMILY TEACHING
To reduce hypotensive effect, rise slowly from lying to sitting position, permit legs to dangle from bed momentarily before standing. Several weeks may be needed for full therapeutic effect of B/P reduction. Skipping doses or voluntarily discontinuing drug may produce severe, rebound hypertension. Limit alcohol. Inform physician if vomiting, diarrhea, excessive perspiration occurs or if swelling of face, lips, tongue, difficulty in breathing is noted.

E

enfuvirtide

en-**few**-vir-tide
(Fuzeon)

CLASSIFICATION

PHARMACOTHERAPEUTIC: Fusion inhibitor. **CLINICAL:** Antiretroviral agent.

ACTION

Interferes with the entry of HIV-1 into CD4+ cells by inhibiting fusion of viral, cellular membranes. **Therapeutic Effect:** Slows HIV replication, reducing progression of HIV infection.

PHARMACOKINETICS

Comparable absorption when injected into subcutaneous tissue of abdomen, thigh, arm. Protein binding: 92%. Undergoes catabolism to amino acids. **Half-life:** 3.8 hrs.

USES

Used in combination with other antiretroviral agents for treatment of HIV-1 infection in treatment-experienced pts with evidence of HIV-1 replication.

PRECAUTIONS

CONTRAINDICATIONS: None known. **CAUTIONS:** None known.

LIFESPAN CONSIDERATIONS: Pregnancy/lactation: Breast-feeding not recommended. **Pregnancy Category B. Children:** Safety and effectiveness have not been established <6 yrs. **Elderly:** No age-related precautions noted.

INTERACTIONS

DRUG: None known. **HERBAL:** None known. **FOOD:** None known. **LAB VALUES:** May elevate lipase, amylase, triglycerides, SGPT (ALT), SGOT (AST), creatine phosphokinase, blood glucose. May decrease hemoglobin, WBCs.

AVAILABILITY (Rx)

POWDER FOR INJECTION: 108-mg (approx. 90 mg/ml when reconstituted) vials.

ADMINISTRATION/HANDLING

SUBCUTANEOUS

Storage • Store at room temperature. • Refrigerate reconstituted solution; use within 24 hrs. Bring reconstituted solution to room temperature before injection.

Reconstitution • Reconstitute with 1.1 ml Sterile Water for Injection. • Visually inspect vial for particulate matter. Solution should appear clear, colorless. • Discard unused portion.

Subcutaneous administration • Administer into the upper arm, anterior thigh, abdomen. Administer each subcutaneous injection at a different site than the preceding injection site.

INDICATIONS/ROUTES/DOSAGE

HIV INFECTION

Subcutaneous: ADULTS, ELDERLY: 90 mg (1 ml) twice daily. CHILDREN 6–16 YRS: 2 mg/kg twice daily up to a maximum dose of 90 mg twice daily.

PEDIATRIC DOSING GUIDELINES

Weight [kg (lbs)]	Dose [mg (ml)]
11–15.5 (24–34)	27 (0.3)
15.6–20 (>34–44)	36 (0.4)
20.1–24.5 (>44–54)	45 (0.5)
24.6–29 (>54–64)	54 (0.6)
29.1–33.5 (>64–74)	63 (0.7)
33.6–38 (>74–84)	72 (0.8)
38.1–42.5 (>84–94)	81 (0.9)
>42.5 (>94)	90 (1)

SIDE EFFECTS

COMMON (98%): Local injection site reactions (pain, discomfort, induration, erythema, nodules, cysts, pruritus, ecchymosis). **FREQUENT (16%–26%):** Diarrhea, nausea, fatigue. **OCCASIONAL (4%–11%):** Insomnia, peripheral neuropathy, depression, cough, weight/appetite decrease, sinusitis, anxiety, asthenia (loss of strength, energy), myalgia, cold sores. **RARE (2%–3%):** Constipation, influenza, upper abdominal pain, anorexia, conjunctivitis.

ADVERSE REACTIONS/ TOXIC EFFECTS

May potentiate bacterial pneumonia. Hypersensitivity (rash, fever, chills, rigors, hypotension), thrombocytopenia, neutropenia, renal insufficiency/failure occur rarely.

NURSING IMPLICATIONS

BASELINE ASSESSMENT

Obtain baseline laboratory testing, esp. liver function tests, triglycerides prior to beginning enfuvirtide therapy and at periodic intervals during therapy. Offer emotional support.

INTERVENTION/EVALUATION

Assess skin for local injection site/hypersensitivity reaction. Question for evidence of nausea, fatigue. Assess sleep pattern. Monitor for insomnia, signs/symptoms of depression. Monitor clinical chemistry tests for marked laboratory abnormalities.

PATIENT/FAMILY TEACHING

Advise pt that an increased rate of bacterial pneumonia has occurred with enfuvirtide and to seek medical attention if cough with fever, rapid breathing, shortness of breath occurs. Continue therapy for full length of treatment. Enfuvirtide is not a cure for HIV infection, nor does it reduce risk of transmission to others: Pt needs to continue practices to prevent HIV transmission.

enoxacin

(Penetrex)

See Classification section under: Antibiotic: fluoroquinolones (p. 23C)

enoxaparin sodium

en-**ox**-ah-pear-in

(Klexane✤, Lovenox)

Do not confuse with Lotronex.

◆ CLASSIFICATION

PHARMACOTHERAPEUTIC: Low-molecular-weight heparin. **CLINICAL:** Anticoagulant (see p. 28C).

ACTION

Potentiates the action of antithrombin III and inactivates coagulation factor Xa. **Therapeutic Effect:** Produces anticoagulation. Does not significantly influence bleeding time, prothrombin time (PT), activated partial thromboplastin time (aPTT).

PHARMACOKINETICS

	Onset	Peak	Duration
Subcutaneous	—	3–5 hrs	12 hrs

Well absorbed following subcutaneous administration. Eliminated primarily in urine. Not removed by hemodialysis. **Half-life:** 4.5 hrs.

USES

Prevention of postop deep vein thrombosis (DVT) following hip/knee replacement surgery, abdominal surgery. Long-term DVT prevention following hip replacement surgery, nonsurgical acute illness. Treatment of unstable angina, non–Q-wave MI, acute DVT (with warfarin). **Unlabeled:** Prevents DVT following general surgical procedures.

PRECAUTIONS

CONTRAINDICATIONS: Active major bleeding, concurrent heparin therapy, thrombocytopenia associated with positive in vitro test for antiplatelet antibody, hypersensitivity to heparin, pork products. **CAUTIONS:** Conditions with increased risk of hemorrhage, history of heparin-induced thrombocytopenia, impaired renal function, elderly, uncontrolled arterial hypertension, history of recent GI ulceration/hemorrhage.

LIFESPAN CONSIDERATIONS: Pregnancy/lactation: Use with caution, particularly during last trimester, immediate postpartum period (increased risk of maternal hemorrhage). Unknown if excreted in breast milk. **Pregnancy Category B. Children:** Safety and efficacy not established. **Elderly:** May be more susceptible to bleeding.

INTERACTIONS

DRUG: Anticoagulants, platelet inhibitors may increase bleeding. **HERBAL:** None known. **FOOD:** None known. **LAB VALUES:** Reversible increases in SGOT (AST), SGPT (ALT), alkaline phosphatase, LDH.

AVAILABILITY (Rx)

INJECTION: 30 mg/0.3 ml, 40 mg/0.4 ml, 60 mg/0.6 ml, 80 mg/0.8 ml, 100 mg/1 ml, 120 mg/0.8 ml, 150 mg/1 ml, prefilled syringes.

ADMINISTRATION/HANDLING

Alert: Do not mix with other injections or infusions. Do not give IM.

SUBCUTANEOUS

• Parenteral form appears clear and colorless to pale yellow. • Store at room temperature. • Instruct pt to lie down before administering by deep subcutaneous injection. • Inject between left and right anterolateral and left and right posterolateral abdominal wall. • Introduce entire length of needle (½ inch) into skin fold held between thumb and forefinger, holding skin fold during injection.

INDICATIONS/ROUTES/DOSAGE

Alert: Give initial dose as soon as possible after surgery but not more than 24 hrs after surgery.

PREVENTION OF DVT (hip, knee surgery)
Subcutaneous: ADULTS, ELDERLY: 30 mg twice daily, generally for 7–10 days.

PREVENTION OF DVT ABDOMINAL SURGERY
Subcutaneous: ADULTS, ELDERLY: 40 mg daily for 7–10 days.

PREVENTION OF LONG-TERM DVT, NONSURGICAL ACUTE ILLNESS
Subcutaneous: ADULTS, ELDERLY: 40 mg once daily for 3 wks.

ANGINA, MI
Subcutaneous: ADULTS, ELDERLY: 1 mg/kg q12h (treatment).

ACUTE DVT
Subcutaneous: ADULTS, ELDERLY: 1 mg/kg q12h or 1.5 mg/kg once daily.

USUAL DOSAGE FOR CHILDREN
Subcutaneous: 0.5 mg/kg q12h (prophylaxis); 1 mg/kg q12h (treatment).

DOSAGE IN RENAL IMPAIRMENT
Clearance decreased when creatinine clearance <30 ml/min. Monitor, adjust dosage.

SIDE EFFECTS

OCCASIONAL (1%–4%): Injection site hematoma, nausea, peripheral edema.

ADVERSE REACTIONS/ TOXIC EFFECTS

Accidental overdosage may lead to bleeding complications ranging from local ecchymoses to major hemorrhage. **ANTIDOTE:** Effects of enoxaparin may generally be stopped by IV injection of protamine sulfate (1% solution) at a dose of 1 mg per 1 mg enoxaparin. A second dose of protamine sulfate at a dose of 0.5 mg per 1 mg of enoxaparin may be given if aPTT tested 2–4 hrs after the first injection remains prolonged.

NURSING IMPLICATIONS

BASELINE ASSESSMENT

Assess CBC, including platelet count.

INTERVENTION/EVALUATION

Periodically monitor CBC, platelet count, stool for occult blood (no need for daily monitoring in pts with normal presurgical coagulation parameters). Assess for any sign of bleeding: bleeding at surgical site, hematuria, blood in stool, bleeding from gums, petechiae, bruising, bleeding from injection sites.

PATIENT/FAMILY TEACHING

Usual length of therapy is 7–10 days. Do not take any OTC medication (esp. aspirin) without consulting physician.

entacapone

en-tah-cah-**pone**
(Comtan)

FIXED-COMBINATION(S)

Stavelo: entacapone/carbidopa-levodopa (antiparkinson agent) 200 mg/12.5 mg/50 mg; 200 mg/25 mg/100 mg; 200 mg/37.5 mg/150 mg.

◆ CLASSIFICATION

PHARMACOTHERAPEUTIC: Enzyme inhibitor. **CLINICAL:** Antiparkinson agent.

ACTION

Inhibits the enzyme, catechol-*O*-methyltransferase (COMT), potentiating dopamine activity and increasing the duration of action of levodopa. **Therapeutic Effect:** Decreases signs/symptoms of Parkinson's disease.

PHARMACOKINETICS

Rapidly absorbed after PO administration. Protein binding: 98%. Metabolized in the liver. Primarily eliminated via biliary excretion. Not removed by hemodialysis. **Half-life:** 2.4 hrs.

USES

In conjunction with levodopa/carbidopa, improves quality of life in pts with Parkinson's disease.

PRECAUTIONS

CONTRAINDICATIONS: Hypersensitivity, concomitant use of MAOIs (see Interactions). **CAUTIONS:** Renal/liver impairment. May increase risk of orthostatic hypotension and syncope, exacerbate dyskinesias.

LIFESPAN CONSIDERATIONS: Pregnancy/lactation: Unknown if distributed in breast milk. **Pregnancy Category C. Children:** N/A. **Elderly:** No age-related precautions noted.

INTERACTIONS

DRUG: Other CNS depressants may have additive effect. **Nonselective MAOIs (e.g., phenelzine)** may result in inhibiting pathway for normal catecholamine metabolism. **Probenecid, cholestyramine, erythromycin, ampicillin** may decrease excretion of entacapone. **Isoproterenol, epinephrine, norepinephrine, dopamine, dobutamine, methyldopa, isoetharine, bitolterol** may increase risk of arrhythmias, changes in B/P. **HERBAL:** None known. **FOOD:** None known. **LAB VALUES:** None known.

AVAILABILITY (Rx)

TABLETS: 200 mg.

ADMINISTRATION/HANDLING

PO

- Give without regard to food.

INDICATIONS/ROUTES/DOSAGE

Alert: Always administer with levodopa/carbidopa.

PARKINSON'S DISEASE

PO: ADULTS, ELDERLY: 200 mg concomitantly with each dose of levodopa/carbidopa to maximum of 8 times/daily (1,600 mg).

SIDE EFFECTS

FREQUENT (>10%): Dyskinesia (uncontrolled body movements), nausea, urine discoloration (dark yellow, orange), diarrhea. **OCCASIONAL** (3%–9%): Abdominal pain, vomiting, constipation, dry mouth, fatigue, back pain. **RARE** (<2%): Anxiety, somnolence, agitation, dyspepsia, flatulence, diaphoresis, asthenia, dyspnea.

ADVERSE REACTIONS/ TOXIC EFFECTS

None known.

NURSING IMPLICATIONS

INTERVENTION/EVALUATION

Monitor for evidence of dyskinesia (difficulty with movement). Assess for clinical reversal of symptoms (improvement of tremor of head/hands at rest, masklike facial expression, shuffling gait, muscular rigidity). Monitor B/P. Assess for orthostatic hypotension, diarrhea.

PATIENT/FAMILY TEACHING

Avoid tasks that require alertness, motor skills until response to drug is established. May cause color change in urine/sweat (dark yellow, orange). Report any uncontrolled movement of face, eyelids, mouth, tongue, arms, hands, legs.

ephedra

Also known as ma huang, sea grape, teamsters tea, yellow horse

Do not confuse with ephedrine.

CLASSIFICATION

HERBAL/CNS STIMULANT.

ACTION

A nonselective alpha- and beta-receptor agonist that stimulates the sympathetic nervous system. **Effect:** Increases B/P, heart rate; causes peripheral vasoconstriction, bronchodilation.

USES

Weight loss, cardiovascular/CNS stimulant. Also used for allergic disorders, nasal congestion, bronchospasm, asthma, bronchitis.

PRECAUTIONS

CONTRAINDICATIONS: Angina, anorexia, bulimia, cerebral insufficiency. Heart disease (may cause tachycardia, arrhythmias), hyperthyroidism, uncontrolled hypertension, pregnancy/lactation. **CAUTIONS:** Anxiety, benign prostate hypertrophy (BPH), diabetes, glaucoma, those with urinary retention.

LIFESPAN CONSIDERATIONS: Pregnancy/lactation: Contraindicated. **Children:** Safety and efficacy not established; avoid use. **Elderly:** Safety and efficacy not established.

INTERACTIONS

DRUG: May decrease effects of **beta-blockers.** May increase toxicity with **MAOIs, theophylline, decongestants. HERBAL: Caffeine** can increase risk of side effects. **FOOD: Coffee, tea** can increase risk of stimulatory effects.

LAB VALUES: May increase blood glucose.

AVAILABILITY

TABLETS: 25 mg. **TEA, TINCTURE, EXTRACT.**

INDICATIONS/ROUTES/DOSAGE

USUAL ADULT DOSAGE

PO: ADULTS, ELDERLY: 25 mg 3 times/day.

Alert: Dosages as low as 12–36 mg/day associated with severe adverse effects.

SIDE EFFECTS

Most common include dizziness, restlessness, anxiety, insomnia, headache, anorexia, nausea, vomiting, flushing, tingling, tachycardia, increased B/P.

ADVERSE REACTIONS/ TOXIC EFFECTS

Psychosis, myalgia, cardiomyopathy, rhabdomyolysis, MI, stroke have been reported.

NURSING IMPLICATIONS

BASELINE ASSESSMENT

Assess medication history (esp. decongestants, theophylline, MAOIs, beta-blockers). Assess if pregnant/breast-feeding (contraindicated), history of cardiovascular/cerebrovascular disease, glaucoma, seizures, hyperthyroidism, hypertension, psychosis.

INTERVENTION/EVALUATION

Assess for hypersensitivity reactions, dermatitis, increase in cardiovascular side effects (e.g., hypertension, palpitations, chest pain), CNS stimulation (e.g., insomnia, anxiety, nervousness, tremors, hallucinations).

PATIENT/FAMILY TEACHING

Do not use if pregnant/breast-feeding, history of cardiovascular/cerebrovascular disease, diabetes, hypertension, glaucoma, thyroid disorders. Avoid use longer than 1 wk. Avoid use in combination with other stimulants such as caffeine.

epinephrine

eh-pih-**nef**-rin

(Adrenalin, EpiPen, Primatene)

Do not confuse with ephedrine.

CLASSIFICATION

PHARMACOTHERAPEUTIC: Sympathomimetic (adrenergic agonist). **CLINICAL:** Antiglaucoma, bronchodilator, cardiac stimulant, antiallergic, antihemorrhagic, priapism reversal agent (see pp. 45C, 134C).

ACTION

Stimulates alpha-adrenergic receptors (vasoconstriction, pressor effects), beta$_1$-adrenergic receptors (cardiac stimulation), and beta$_2$-adrenergic receptors (bronchial dilation, vasodilation). **Therapeutic Effect:** Relaxes smooth muscle of the bronchial tree, produces cardiac stimulation, dilates skeletal muscle vasculature. **Ophthalmic:** Increases outflow of aqueous humor from anterior eye chamber. **Therapeutic Effect:** Dilates pupils (constricts conjunctival blood vessels).

PHARMACOKINETICS

Onset	Peak	Duration
Subcutaneous		
5–10 min	20 min	1–4 hrs
IM		
5–10 min	20 min	1–4 hrs
Inhalation		
3–5 min	20 min	1–3 hrs
Ophthalmic		
1 hr	4–8 hrs	12–24 hrs

Minimal absorption after inhalation, well absorbed after parenteral administration. Metabolized in liver, other tissues, sympathetic nerve endings. Excreted in urine. **Ophthalmic:** May have systemic absorption from drainage into nasal pharyngeal passages. Mydriasis occurs within several minutes, persists for several hours; vasoconstriction occurs within 5 min, lasts <1 hr.

USES

Treatment of acute exacerbation of bronchial asthma attacks, reversible bronchospasm in pts with chronic bronchitis, emphysema, hypersensitivity reactions. Restores cardiac rhythm in cardiac arrest. **Ophthalmic:** Management of chronic open-angle glaucoma. **Unlabeled: Systemic:** Treatment of gingival/pulpal hemorrhage, priapism. **Ophthalmic:** Treatment of conjunctival congestion during surgery, secondary glaucoma.

PRECAUTIONS

CONTRAINDICATIONS: Hypertension, hyperthyroidism, ischemic heart disease, cardiac arrhythmias, cerebrovascular insufficiency, narrow-angle glaucoma, shock. **CAUTIONS:** Elderly, diabetes mellitus, angina pectoris, tachycardia, MI, severe renal/hepatic impairment, psychoneurotic disorders, hypoxia.

LIFESPAN CONSIDERATIONS: Pregnancy/lactation: Crosses placenta. Distributed in breast milk. **Pregnancy Category C. Children/elderly:** No age-related precautions noted.

INTERACTIONS

DRUG: Tricyclic antidepressants, MAOIs may increase cardiovascular effects. May decrease effects of **beta-blockers. Ergonovine, methergine, oxytocin** may increase vasoconstriction. **Digoxin, sympathomimetics** may increase risk of arrhythmias. **HERBAL:** None known. **FOOD:** None known. **LAB VALUES:** May decrease serum potassium levels.

AVAILABILITY (Rx)

INJECTION IN PREFILLED INJECTOR: 0.3 mg/0.3 ml, 0.15 mg/0.3 ml. **INJECTION:** 0.1 mg/ml, 1 mg/ml. **SOLUTION FOR ORAL INHALATION:** 2.25%, 1.125%. **OPHTHALMIC SOLUTION:** 0.5%, 1%, 2%.

ADMINISTRATION/HANDLING

SUBCUTANEOUS

• Shake ampoule thoroughly. • Use tuberculin syringe for subcutaneous into lateral deltoid region. • Massage rejection site (minimizes vasoconstriction effect).

IV

Storage • Store parenteral forms at room temperature. • Do not use if solution appears discolored or contains a precipitate.

Reconstitution • For injection, dilute each 1 mg of 1:1,000 solution with 10 ml 0.9 NaCl to provide 1:10,000 solution and inject each 1 mg or fraction thereof >1 min. • For infusion, further dilute with 250–500 D_5W. Maximum concentration: 64 mg/250 ml.

Rate of administration • For IV infusion, give at 1–10 mcg/min (titrate to desired response).

IV INCOMPATIBILITY

Ampicillin (Omnipen, Polycillin).

IV COMPATIBILITIES

Calcium chloride, calcium gluconate, diltiazem (Cardizem), dobutamine (Dobutrex), dopamine (Intropin), fentanyl (Sublimaze), heparin, hydromorphone (Dilaudid), lorazepam (Ativan), midazolam (Versed), milrinone (Primacor), morphine, nitroglycerin, norepinephrine (Levophed), potassium chloride, propofol (Diprivan).

INDICATIONS/ROUTES/DOSAGE

ASYSTOLE

IV: ADULTS, ELDERLY: 1 mg q3–5min up to 0.1 mg/kg q3–5min. CHILDREN: 0.01 mg/kg (0.1 ml/kg of 1:10,000 solution).

May repeat q3–5min. Subsequent doses 0.1 mg/kg (0.1 ml/kg) of a 1:1,000 solution q3–5min.

BRADYCARDIA

IV infusion: ADULTS, ELDERLY: 1–10 mcg/min titrated to desired effect.

IV: CHILDREN: 0.01 mg/kg (0.1 ml/kg of 1:10,000 solution q3–5min. **Maximum:** 1 mg/10 ml.

BRONCHODILATOR

IM/subcutaneous: ADULTS, ELDERLY 0.1–0.5 mg (1:1,000) q10–15 min to 4 hrs.

Subcutaneous: CHILDREN: 10 mcg/kg (0.01 ml/kg of 1:1,000) **Maximum:** 0.5 mg, or suspension (1:200) 0.005 ml/kg/dose (0.025 mg/kg/dose) to a maximum of 0.15 ml (0.75 mg for single dose) q8–12h.

HYPERSENSITIVITY REACTION

IM/subcutaneous: ADULTS, ELDERLY: 0.3–0.5 mg q15–20 min.

Subcutaneous: CHILDREN: 0.01 mg/kg q15min for 2 doses, then q4h. **Maximum single dose:** 0.5 mg.

USUAL INHALATION DOSAGE

Inhalation: ADULTS, ELDERLY, CHILDREN >4 YRS: 1 inhalation, may repeat in at least 1 min; subsequent doses no sooner than 3 hrs.

Nebulizer: ADULTS, ELDERLY, CHILDREN >4 YRS: 1–3 deep inhalations; subsequent doses no sooner than 3 hrs.

GLAUCOMA

Ophthalmic: ADULTS, ELDERLY: 1–2 drops 1–2 times/day.

SIDE EFFECTS

FREQUENT: Systemic: Tachycardia, palpitations, nervousness. **Ophthalmic:** Headache, stinging, burning, other eye irritation, watering of eyes. **OCCASIONAL: Systemic:** Dizziness, lightheadedness, facial flushing, headache, diaphoresis, increased B/P, nausea, trembling, insomnia, vomiting, weakness. **Ophthalmic:** Blurred/decreased vision, eye pain. **RARE: Systemic:** Chest discomfort/pain, arrhythmias, bronchospasm, dry mouth/throat.

ADVERSE REACTIONS/ TOXIC EFFECTS

Excessive doses may cause acute hypertension, arrhythmias. Prolonged/excessive use may result in metabolic acidosis (due to increased serum lactic acid concentrations). Observe for disorientation, weakness, hyperventilation, headache, nausea, vomiting, diarrhea.

NURSING IMPLICATIONS

INTERVENTION/EVALUATION

Monitor for vital sign changes. Assess lung sounds for rhonchi, wheezing, rales. Monitor ABGs. In cardiac arrest, monitor EKG, B/P, pulse.

PATIENT/FAMILY TEACHING

Avoid excessive use of caffeine derivatives (chocolate, coffee, tea, cola, cocoa). **Ophthalmic:** Slight burning, stinging may occur on initial instillation. Report any new symptoms (tachycardia, shortness of breath, dizziness) immediately: may be systemic effects.

epirubicin

eh-pea-**rew**-bih-sin
(Ellence)

◆CLASSIFICATION

PHARMACOTHERAPEUTIC: Anthracycline antibiotic. **CLINICAL:** Antineoplastic (see p. 71C).

ACTION

Exact mechanism unknown but may include formation of a complex with DNA by intercalation of its planar rings with consequent inhibition of DNA, RNA, protein synthesis. Inhibits DNA helicase activity, preventing enzymatic separation of double-stranded DNA and interfering with replication and transcription. **Therapeutic Effect:** Produces antiproliferative and cytotoxic activity.

E

PHARMACOKINETICS

Widely distributed into tissues. Protein binding: 77%. Metabolized in liver, RBCs. Primarily eliminated through biliary excretion. Not removed by hemodialysis. **Half-life:** 33 hrs.

USES

Component of adjuvant therapy in pts with evidence of axillary node tumor involvement following resection of primary breast cancer. **Unlabeled:** Lung, ovarian carcinoma; non-Hodgkin's lymphoma; sarcomas.

PRECAUTIONS

CONTRAINDICATIONS: Baseline neutrophil count <1,500 cells/mm^3. Severe myocardial insufficiency, recent MI. Previous treatment with anthracyclines up to maximum cumulative dose. Hypersensitivity to epirubicin. Severe liver impairment. **CAUTIONS:** Renal/liver function impairment.

LIFESPAN CONSIDERATIONS: Pregnancy/lactation: May cause fetal harm. Unknown if distributed in breast milk. **Pregnancy Category D. Children:** Safety and efficacy not established. **Elderly:** No age-related precautions noted but monitor for toxicity.

INTERACTIONS

DRUG: Cimetidine may increase serum concentrations. **HERBAL:** None known. **FOOD:** None known. **LAB VALUES:** None known.

AVAILABILITY (Rx)

INJECTION: 2 mg/ml single-use vial.

ADMINISTRATION/HANDLING

Alert: Exclude pregnant staff from working with epirubicin; wear protective clothing. If accidental contact with skin/eyes occurs, flush area immediately with copious amounts of water.

IV

Storage • Refrigerate vial. • Protect from light. • Use within 24 hrs of first penetration of rubber stopper. • Discard unused portion.

Reconstitution • Ready-to-use vials require no reconstitution.

Rate of administration • Infuse medication into tubing of free-flowing IV of 0.9% NaCl or D_5W over 3–5 min.

IV INCOMPATIBILITIES

Heparin, 5-fluorouracil (5-FU). Do not mix with other medications in same syringe.

INDICATIONS/ROUTES/DOSAGE

BREAST CANCER

IV infusion: ADULTS: (in combination with 5-FU and Cytoxan). Initially, 100–120 mg/m^2 in repeated cycles of 3–4 wks. Total dose may be given day 1 of each cycle or divided equally on days 1 and 8 of each cycle.

Alert: Dosage adjustment necessary for pts with bone marrow, liver dysfunction; hematologic toxicities; severe renal impairment.

SIDE EFFECTS

Alert: Venous sclerosis may result if infused into a small vein. **FREQUENT (70%–83%):** Nausea, vomiting, alopecia, amenorrhea. **OCCASIONAL (5%–9%):** Stomatitis (burning/erythema of oral mucosa, oral ulceration of mucous membranes, difficulty swallowing), diarrhea, hot flashes. **RARE (1%–2%):** Rash, pruritus, fever, lethargy, conjunctivitis.

ADVERSE REACTIONS/ TOXIC EFFECTS

Cardiotoxicity noted as either acute, transient abnormal EKG findings and/or cardiomyopathy manifested as CHF. Risk increased with total cumulative dose in excess of 900 mg/m^2. Extravasation during administration causes severe local tissue necrosis. Bone marrow depression manifested as hematologic toxicity (principally leukopenia and, to lesser extent, anemia, thrombocytopenia).

NURSING IMPLICATIONS

BASELINE ASSESSMENT

Obtain WBC, platelet, erythrocyte counts prior to and at frequent intervals during therapy. Obtain EKG before therapy, liver function studies prior to each dose. Antiemetics may be effective in preventing, treating nausea.

INTERVENTION/EVALUATION

Monitor for stomatitis (may lead to ulceration of mucous membranes within 2–3 days). Monitor blood counts for evidence of myelosuppression, renal/hepatic function studies, cardiac function. Assess pattern of daily bowel activity, stool consistency. Monitor for hematologic toxicity (fever, sore throat, signs of local infection, unusual bruising/bleeding from any site), symptoms of anemia (excessive tiredness, weakness).

PATIENT/FAMILY TEACHING

Alopecia is reversible, but new hair growth may have different color, texture. New hair growth resumes 2–3 mos after last therapy dose. Maintain fastidious oral hygiene. Do not have immunizations without physician's approval (drug lowers body's resistance). Avoid contact with those who have recently received live virus vaccine. Promptly report fever, sore throat, signs of local infection, easy unusual bruising/bleeding from any site.

Epivir

see lamivudine

eplerenone

(eh-**pleh**-reh-known)
(Inspra)

◆CLASSIFICATION

PHARMACOTHERAPEUTIC: Aldosterone receptor antagonist. **CLINICAL:** Antihypertensive.

ACTION

Binds to the mineralocorticoid receptors in the kidney, heart, blood vessels, brain, blocking the binding of aldosterone. **Therapeutic Effect:** Reduces B/P.

PHARMACOKINETICS

Absorption unaffected by food. Protein binding: 50%. No active metabolites. Not removed by hemodialysis. Excreted in the urine with a lesser amount eliminated in the feces. **Half-life:** 4–6 hrs.

USES

Treatment of hypertension alone or in combination with other antihypertensive agents.

PRECAUTIONS

CONTRAINDICATIONS: Pts with serum potassium >5.5 mEq/L, type 2 diabetes with microalbuminuria, serum creatinine >2 mg/dl in males or >1.8 mg/dl in females, creatinine clearance <50 ml/

min, concurrent use of potassium supplements or potassium-sparing diuretics (amiloride, spironolactone, triamterene), strong inhibitors (ketoconazole, itraconazole). **CAUTIONS:** Hepatic function impairment, hyperkalemia.

E

LIFESPAN CONSIDERATIONS Pregnancy/lactation: Unknown if drug crosses placenta or is distributed in breast milk. **Pregnancy Category B. Children:** Safety and efficacy not established. **Elderly:** No age-related precautions noted.

INTERACTIONS

DRUG: ACE inhibitors, angiotensin II antagonists, erythromycin, saquinavir, verapamil, fluconazole increases risk of hyperkalemia. **HERBAL: St. John's wort** decreases drug effectiveness. **FOOD: Grapefruit juice** produces small increase in potassium level. **LAB VALUES:** May increase potassium. May decrease sodium.

AVAILABILITY (Rx)

TABLETS: 25 mg, 50 mg, 100 mg.

ADMINISTRATION/HANDLING

- Do not break, crush, or chew film-coated tablets.

INDICATION/ROUTES/DOSAGE

HYPERTENSION

PO: ADULTS, ELDERLY: 50 mg once daily. If 50 mg once daily presents an inadequate B/P response, may increase dosage to 50 mg twice daily. If pt is on concurrent erythromycin, saquinavir, verapamil, or fluconazole, reduce initial dose to 25 mg once daily.

SIDE EFFECTS

RARE (1%–3%): Dizziness, diarrhea, cough, fatigue, influenza-like symptoms, abdominal pain.

ADVERSE REACTIONS/TOXIC EFFECTS

Hyperkalemia may occur, particularly in pts with type 2 diabetes and microalbuminuria.

NURSING IMPLICATIONS

BASELINE ASSESSMENT

Obtain B/P, apical pulse immediately before each dose, in addition to regular monitoring (be alert to fluctuations). If excessive reduction in B/P occurs, place pt in supine position, feet slightly elevated.

INTERVENTION/EVALUATION

Assist with ambulation if dizziness occurs. Monitor serum potassium levels. Assess B/P for hypertension/hypotension. Monitor pattern of daily bowel activity, stool consistency. Assess for evidence of flulike symptoms.

PATIENT/FAMILY TEACHING

Avoid tasks that require alertness, motor skills until response to drug is established (possible dizziness effect). Need for lifelong control. Caution against exercising during hot weather (risk of dehydration, hypotension).

epoetin alfa

eh-po-**ee**-tin
(Epogen, Eprex, Procrit)
Do not confuse with Neupogen.

CLASSIFICATION

PHARMACOTHERAPEUTIC: Glycoprotein. **CLINICAL:** Erythropoietin.

ACTION

Stimulates division, differentiation of erythroid progenitor cells in bone marrow. **Therapeutic Effect:** Induces erythropoiesis, releases reticulocytes from marrow.

PHARMACOKINETICS

Well absorbed following subcutaneous administration. Following administration, an increase in reticulocyte count seen within 10 days, increases in Hgb, Hct, RBC count within 2–6 wks. **Half-life:** 4–13 hrs.

USES

Treatment of anemia in pts receiving or who have received chemotherapy, those with chronic renal failure, HIV-infected pts on zidovudine (AZT) therapy, those scheduled for elective nonvascular surgery, reducing need for allogenic blood transfusions. **Unlabeled:** Prevents anemia in pts donating blood before elective surgery, autologous transfusion; treatment of anemia associated with neoplastic diseases.

PRECAUTIONS

CONTRAINDICATIONS: Uncontrolled hypertension, history of sensitivity to mammalian cell-derived products or human albumin. **CAUTIONS:** Pts with known porphyria (impairment of erythrocyte formation in bone marrow); history of seizures.

LIFESPAN CONSIDERATIONS: Pregnancy/lactation: Unknown if drug crosses placenta or is distributed in breast milk. **Pregnancy Category C. Children:** Safety and efficacy not established in those <12 yrs. **Elderly:** No age-related precautions noted.

INTERACTIONS

DRUG: May need to increase **heparin** (increase in RBC volume may enhance blood clotting). **HERBAL:** None known. **FOOD:** None known. **LAB VALUES:** May decrease bleeding time, iron concentration, serum ferritin. May increase BUN, creatinine, phosphorus, potassium, sodium, uric acid.

AVAILABILITY (Rx)

INJECTION: 2,000 units/ml, 3,000 units/ml, 4,000 units/ml, 10,000 units/ml, 20,000 units/ml, 40,000 units/ml.

E

ADMINISTRATION/HANDLING

Alert: Avoid excessive agitation of vial; do not shake (foaming).

SUBCUTANEOUS

• Use 1 dose per vial; do not reenter vial. Discard unused portion. May be mixed in a syringe with Bacteriostatic 0.9% NaCl with benzyl alcohol 0.9% (Bacteriostatic Saline) at a 1:1 ratio (benzyl alcohol acts as a local anesthetic; may reduce injection site discomfort).

IV

Storage • Refrigerate. • Vigorous shaking may denature medication, rendering it inactive.

IV reconstitution: • No reconstitution necessary.

Rate of administration: • May be given as an IV bolus.

IV INCOMPATIBILITY

Do not mix with any other medications.

INDICATIONS/ROUTES/DOSAGE

CHEMOTHERAPY PATIENTS

IV/subcutaneous: ADULTS, ELDERLY, CHILDREN: 150 units/kg/dose 3 times/wk. **Maximum:** 1,200 units/kg/wk.

REDUCTION OF ALLOGENIC BLOOD TRANSFUSIONS IN ELECTIVE SURGERY

Subcutaneous: ADULTS, ELDERLY: 300 units/kg/day 10 days before, on day of, and 4 days after surgery.

CHRONIC RENAL FAILURE

Subcutaneous/IV bolus: ADULTS, ELDERLY: Initially, 50–100 units/kg 3 times/wk. TARGET HCT RANGE: 30%–

36%. Dosage adjustments not earlier than 1-mo intervals unless clinically indicated. DECREASE DOSE: Hct increasing and approaching 36% (temporarily hold doses if Hct continues to rise, reinstate lower dose when Hct begins to decrease); Hct increases by >4 points in 2 wks (monitor Hct 2 times/wk for 2–6 wks). INCREASE DOSE: Hct does not increase 5–6 points after 8 wks (with iron stores adequate) and Hct below target range. MAINTENANCE: *(Dialysis):* 75 units/kg 3 times/wk. RANGE: 12.5–525 units/kg. *(Nondialysis):* 75–150 units/kg/wk.

AZT-TREATED, HIV-INFECTED PTS

Alert: Pts receiving AZT with serum erythropoietin levels >500 milliunits likely not to respond to therapy.

Subcutaneous/IV: ADULTS: Initially, 100 units/kg 3 times/wk for 8 wks; may increase by 50–100 units/kg 3 times/wk. Evaluate response q4–8wks thereafter; adjust dose by 50–100 units/kg 3 times/wk. If doses >300 units/kg 3 times/wk are not eliciting response, unlikely pt will respond. MAINTENANCE: Titrate to maintain desired Hct.

SIDE EFFECTS

CANCER PTS ON CHEMOTHERAPY: **FREQUENT (17%–20%):** Fever, diarrhea, nausea, vomiting, edema. **OCCASIONAL (11%–13%):** Asthenia (loss of strength, energy), shortness of breath, paresthesia. **RARE (3%–5%):** Dizziness, trunk pain.

CHRONIC RENAL FAILURE PTS: **FREQUENT (11%–24%):** Hypertension, headache, nausea, arthralgia. **OCCASIONAL (7%–9%):** Fatigue, edema, diarrhea, vomiting, chest pain, skin reactions at administration site, asthenia (loss of strength, energy), dizziness.

AZT-TREATED HIV-INFECTED PTS: **FREQUENT (15%–38%):** Fever, fatigue, headache, cough, diarrhea, rash, nausea. **OCCASIONAL (9%–14%):** Shortness of breath, asthenia (loss of strength, weakness), skin reaction at injection site, dizziness.

ADVERSE REACTIONS/ TOXIC EFFECTS

Hypertensive encephalopathy, thrombosis, cerebrovascular accident, MI, seizures have occurred rarely. Hyperkalemia occurs occasionally in pts with chronic renal failure, usually in those who do not conform to medication compliance, dietary guidelines, frequency of dialysis.

NURSING IMPLICATIONS

BASELINE ASSESSMENT

Assess B/P prior to drug initiation (80% of pts with chronic renal failure have history of hypertension). B/P often rises during early therapy in pts with history of hypertension. Consider that all pts will eventually need supplemental iron therapy. Assess serum iron (should be >20%) and serum ferritin (should be >100 ng/ml) prior to and during therapy. Establish baseline CBC (esp. note Hct). Monitor aggressively for increased B/P (25% of pts on medication require antihypertensive therapy, dietary restrictions).

INTERVENTION/EVALUATION

Monitor Hct level diligently (if level increases >4 points in 2 wks, dosage should be reduced); assess CBC routinely. Monitor temperature, esp. in cancer pts on chemotherapy and zidovudine-treated HIV pts, and BUN, uric acid, creatinine, phosphorus, potassium, esp. in chronic renal failure pts.

PATIENT/FAMILY TEACHING

Frequent blood tests needed to determine correct dosage. Inform physician if any severe headache develops. Avoid potentially hazardous activity during first 90 days of therapy (increased risk of seizures in renal pts during first 90 days).

Epogen

see epoetin alfa

epoprostenol sodium, PG_2, PGX, prostacyclin

ep-oh-**pros**-ten-awl
(Flolan)

◆CLASSIFICATION

PHARMACOTHERAPEUTIC: Vasodilator. **CLINICAL:** Antihypertensive.

ACTION

Directly vasodilates pulmonary, systemic arterial vascular beds and inhibits platelet aggregation. **Therapeutic Effect:** Reduces right and left ventricular afterload; increases cardiac output, stroke volume.

USES

Long-term treatment of primary pulmonary hypertension in class III and IV pts (New York Heart Association). **Unlabeled:** Pulmonary hypertension associated with adult respiratory distress syndrome (ARDS), systemic lupus erythematosus, congenital heart disease; neonatal pulmonary hypertension; cardiopulmonary bypass surgery; hemodialysis; refractory CHF; severe community-acquired pneumonia.

PRECAUTIONS

CONTRAINDICATIONS: Chronic use in those with CHF (severe ventricular systolic dysfunction). **CAUTIONS:** Elderly. **Pregnancy Category B.**

INTERACTIONS

DRUG: Hypotensive effects may be increased by **other vasodilators** or using acetate in dialysis fluids. **Anticoagulants, antiplatelets** may increase risk of bleeding. **Vasoconstrictors** may decrease effect. **HERBAL:** None known. **FOOD:** None known. **LAB VALUES:** None known.

AVAILABILITY (Rx)

POWDER FOR RECONSTITUTION: 0.5 mg, 1.5 mg.

ADMINISTRATION/HANDLING

IV

Storage • Store unopened vial at room temperature. • Do not freeze. • Reconstituted solutions may be refrigerated for ≤48 hrs.

Reconstitution • Must use diluent provided by manufacturer. • Follow instructions of manufacturer for dilution to specific concentrations.

Rate of administration • Give as a pump infusion only

∅ IV INCOMPATIBILITY

Do not mix with any other medications.

INDICATIONS/ROUTES/DOSAGE

PULMONARY HYPERTENSION

Alert: Infused continuously through permanent indwelling central venous catheter using an infusion pump. May give through peripheral vein on temporary basis.

IV infusion: ADULTS, ELDERLY: (ACUTE DOSE-RANGING PROCEDURE): Initially, 2 ng/kg/min increased in increments of 2 ng/kg/min q15min until dose-limiting adverse effects occur. (CHRONIC INFUSION): Start at 4 ng/kg/min less than the maximum dose rate tolerated during acute dose ranging (or ½ maximum rate if rate was <5 ng/kg/min).

SIDE EFFECTS

ACUTE PHASE: **FREQUENT:** Flushing (58%), headache (49%), nausea (32%), vomiting (32%), hypotension (16%), anxiety (11%), chest pain (11%), dizziness (8%). **OCCASIONAL (2%–5%):** Bradycardia, abdominal pain, muscle pain, dyspnea, back pain. **RARE (<2%):** Diaphoresis, dyspepsia, paresthesia, tachycardia.

CHRONIC PHASE: **FREQUENT (>20%):** Dyspnea, asthenia, dizziness, headache, chest pain, nausea, vomiting, palpitations, edema, jaw pain, tachycardia, flushing, myalgia, nonspecific muscle pain, paresthesia, diarrhea, anxiety, chills/fever/flu-like symptoms. **OCCASIONAL (10%–20%):** Rash, depression, hypotension, pallor, syncope, bradycardia, ascites.

ADVERSE REACTIONS/ TOXIC EFFECTS

Overdose may cause hyperglycemia/ ketoacidosis (increased urination, thirst, fruitlike breath). Angina, MI, thrombocytopenia occur rarely. Abrupt withdrawal (including large reduction in dosage, interruption in drug delivery) may produce rebound pulmonary hypertension (dyspnea, dizziness, asthenia).

NURSING IMPLICATIONS

INTERVENTION/EVALUATION

Monitor standing/supine B/P for several hours after any dosage adjustment. Assess for therapeutic response: improvement in pulmonary function, decreased dyspnea on exertion (DOE), fatigue, syncope, chest pain, pulmonary vascular resistance, pulmonary arterial pressure.

PATIENT/FAMILY TEACHING

Instruct pt on drug reconstitution, drug administration, care of the permanent central venous catheter. Brief interruptions in drug delivery may result in rapid, deteriorating symptoms. Drug therapy will be necessary for a prolonged period, possibly years.

eprosartan

eh-pro-**sar**-tan
(Teveten)

FIXED COMBINATION(S)

Teveten HCT: eprosartan/hydrochlorothiazide (a diuretic) 400 mg/12.5 mg.

◆ CLASSIFICATION

PHARMACOTHERAPEUTIC: Angiotensin II receptor antagonist. **CLINICAL:** Antihypertensive (see p. 7C).

ACTION

Potent vasodilator. Blocks vasoconstrictor and aldosterone-secreting effects of angiotensin II, inhibiting the binding of angiotensin II to the ATI receptors. **Therapeutic Effect:** Causes vasodilation, decreased peripheral resistance, decrease in B/P.

PHARMACOKINETICS

Rapidly absorbed after PO administration. Protein binding: 98%. Undergoes first-pass metabolism in liver to active metabolites. Excreted in urine and biliary system. Minimally removed by hemodialysis. **Half-life:** 5–9 hrs.

USES

Treatment of hypertension.

PRECAUTIONS

CONTRAINDICATIONS: Hyperaldosteronism, bilateral renal artery stenosis.

CAUTIONS: Unilateral renal artery stenosis, preexisting renal insufficiency, significant aortic/mitral stenosis.

LIFESPAN CONSIDERATIONS: Pregnancy/lactation: Has caused fetal/neonatal morbidity, mortality. Potential for adverse effects on nursing infant. Do not breast-feed. **Pregnancy Category C** (**D** if used in second or third trimester). **Children:** Safety and efficacy not established. **Elderly:** No age-related precautions noted.

INTERACTIONS

DRUG: None known. **HERBAL:** None known. **FOOD:** None known. **LAB VALUES:** May increase BUN, serum creatinine, SGOT (AST), SGPT (ALT), alkaline phosphatase, bilirubin. May decrease Hgb, Hct.

AVAILABILITY (Rx)

TABLETS: 400 mg, 600 mg.

ADMINISTRATION/HANDLING

PO

• Give without regard to food. • Do not crush or break tablets.

INDICATIONS/ROUTES/DOSAGE

HYPERTENSION

PO: ADULTS, ELDERLY: Initially, 600 mg/day. RANGE: 400–800 mg/day.

SIDE EFFECTS

OCCASIONAL (2%–5%): Headache, cough, dizziness. **RARE (<2%):** Muscle pain, fatigue, diarrhea, upper respiratory infection, dyspepsia.

ADVERSE REACTIONS/ TOXIC EFFECTS

Overdosage may manifest as hypotension and tachycardia; bradycardia occurs less often.

NURSING IMPLICATIONS

BASELINE ASSESSMENT

Obtain B/P, apical pulse immediately prior to each dose, in addition to regular monitoring (be alert to fluctuations). Question for possibility of pregnancy (see Pregnancy Category), history of hepatic/renal impairment, renal artery stenosis. Assess medication history (esp. diuretic).

INTERVENTION/EVALUATION

Monitor supine B/P, electrolytes, serum creatinine, BUN, urinalysis, pulse for tachycardia.

PATIENT/FAMILY TEACHING

Inform female pt regarding consequences of second and third trimester exposure to medication. Avoid tasks that require alertness, motor skills (possible dizziness effect). Restrict sodium, alcohol intake. Follow diet, control weight. Do not stop taking medication. Need for lifelong control. Caution against exercising during hot weather (risk of dehydration, hypotension). Check B/P regularly.

eptifibatide

ep-tih-**fye**-bah-tide
(Integrilin)

CLASSIFICATION

PHARMACOTHERAPEUTIC: Glycoprotein IIb/IIIa inhibitor. **CLINICAL:** Antiplatelet, antithrombotic (see p. 29C).

ACTION

Produces rapid inhibition of platelet aggregation by preventing binding of fibrinogen to receptor sites on platelets. **Therapeutic Effect:** Prevents closure of treated coronary arteries. Prevents acute cardiac ischemic complications.

USES

Treatment of pts with acute coronary syndrome (ACS), including those managed medically and those undergoing percutaneous coronary intervention (PCI).

E

PRECAUTIONS

CONTRAINDICATIONS: Active internal bleeding, recent (≤6 wks) GI/GU bleeding, history of CVA <2 yrs or CVA with residual neurologic defect, oral anticoagulants <7 days unless prothrombin time <1.22 × control, thrombocytopenia (<100,000 cells/mcl), recent surgery/trauma (≤6 wks), intracranial neoplasm, AV malformation/aneurysm, severe uncontrolled hypertension, history of vasculitis, prior IV dextran use prior to or during PTCA. **CAUTIONS:** Pts who weigh <75 kg; those >65 yrs; history of GI disease; pts receiving thrombolytics, heparin, aspirin, PTCA <12 hrs of onset of symptoms for acute MI, prolonged PTCA (>70 min), failed PTCA.

LIFESPAN CONSIDERATIONS: Pregnancy/lactation: Unknown if drug causes fetal harm or can affect reproduction capacity. Unknown if distributed in breast milk. **Pregnancy Category B. Children:** Safety and efficacy not established. **Elderly:** Major bleeding risk increased.

INTERACTIONS

DRUG: Anticoagulants, heparin may increase risk of hemorrhage. **Platelet aggregation inhibitors (e.g., aspirin, dextran, thrombolytic agents)** may increase risk of bleeding. **HERBAL:** None known. **FOOD:** None known. **LAB VALUES:** Increases clotting time (ACT), prothrombin time (PT), activated partial thromboplastin time (aPTT); decreases platelet count.

ADMINISTRATION/HANDLING

IV

Storage • Store vials in refrigerator. Solution appears clear, colorless. Do not shake. Discard any unused portion left in vial or if preparation contains *any* opaque particles.

Reconstitution • Withdraw bolus dose from 10-ml vial (2 mg/ml); for IV infusion withdraw from 100-ml vial (0.75/ml). IV push and infusion administration may be given undiluted.

Rate of administration • Give IV push over 1–2 min.

IV INCOMPATIBILITY

Administer in separate line; no other medication should be added to infusion solution.

AVAILABILITY (Rx)

INJECTION: 0.75 mg/ml, 2 mg/ml.

INDICATIONS/ROUTES/DOSAGE

ADJUNCT PCI

IV bolus/IV infusion: ADULTS, ELDERLY: 180 mcg/kg before PCI initiation, then continuous drip of 2 mcg/kg/min and a second 180 mcg/kg bolus 10 min after the first.

ACS

IV bolus/IV infusion: ADULTS, ELDERLY: 180 mcg/kg bolus then 2 mcg/kg/min until discharge or CABG, up to 72 hrs.

SIDE EFFECTS

OCCASIONAL (7%): Hypotension.

ADVERSE REACTIONS/TOXIC EFFECTS

Minor to major bleeding complications may occur, most commonly at arterial access site for cardiac catheterization.

NURSING IMPLICATIONS

BASELINE ASSESSMENT

Assess platelet count, Hgb, Hct before treatment. If platelet count <90,000/mm^3, additional platelet counts should be obtained routinely to avoid thrombocytopenia.

INTERVENTION/EVALUATION

Diligently monitor for potential bleeding, particularly at other arterial, venous puncture sites. If possible, urinary catheters, nasogastric tubes should be avoided.

ergoloid mesylates

ur-go-loyd mess-**ah**-lates

CLASSIFICATION

PHARMACOTHERAPEUTIC: Ergot alkaloid. **CLINICAL:** Psychotherapeutic.

ACTION

Central action decreases vascular tone, slows heart rate. Peripheral action blocks alpha-adrenergic receptors. **Therapeutic Effect:** Improves O_2 uptake, improves cerebral metabolism.

USES

Treatment of age-related (those >60 yrs) mental capacity decline (cognitive/interpersonal skills, mood, self-care, apparent motivation).

PRECAUTIONS

CONTRAINDICATIONS: Acute or chronic psychosis, regardless of etiology. **CAUTIONS:** None known. **Pregnancy Category C.**

INTERACTIONS

DRUG: None known. **HERBAL:** None known. **FOOD:** None known. **LAB VALUES:** None known.

AVAILABILITY (Rx)

TABLETS (sublingual): 1 mg. **TABLETS (oral):** 1 mg.

INDICATIONS/ROUTES/DOSAGE

AGE-RELATED DECLINE IN MENTAL CAPACITY

PO/sublingual: ADULTS, ELDERLY: Initially, 1 mg 3 times/day. RANGE: 1.5–12 mg/day.

SIDE EFFECTS

OCCASIONAL: GI distress, transient nausea, sublingual irritation.

ADVERSE REACTIONS/TOXIC EFFECTS

Overdose may produce blurred vision, dizziness, syncope, headache, flushed face, nausea, vomiting, decreased appetite, stomach cramps, stuffy nose.

NURSING IMPLICATIONS

BASELINE ASSESSMENT

Exclude possibility that pt's signs/symptoms arise from a possibly reversible, treatable condition secondary to systemic disease, neurologic disease, primary disturbance of mood prior to administering medication.

INTERVENTION/EVALUATION

Monitor BP pulse, peripheral circulation. Assess for relief of symptoms.

PATIENT/FAMILY TEACHING

Elimination of symptoms appears gradual; results may not be noted for 3–4 wks. May cause nausea, GI upset. Allow sublingual tablets to dissolve completely under tongue.

ergotamine tartrate

er-**got**-a-meen
(Ergomar, Medihaler Ergotamine✤)

dihydroergotamine

(D.H.E., Ergomar✤, Migranal)

FIXED-COMBINATION(S)

Cafergot, Wigraine: ergotamine/caffeine (stimulant): 1 mg/100 mg; 2 mg/100 mg. **Bellergal-S:** ergotamine/belladonna (anticholinergic)/phenobarbital (sedative-hypnotic): 0.6 mg/0.2 mg/40 mg.

CLASSIFICATION

PHARMACOTHERAPEUTIC: Ergotamine derivative. **CLINICAL:** Antimigraine.

ACTION

Alpha-adrenergic blocker that directly stimulates vascular smooth muscle. May also have antagonist effects on serotonin. **Therapeutic Effect:** Vasoconstricts peripheral and cerebral blood vessels.

PHARMACOKINETICS

Slow, incomplete absorption from GI tract; rapid, extensive absorption rectally. Protein binding: >90%. Undergoes extensive first-pass metabolism in liver. Metabolized to active metabolite. Eliminated in feces via biliary system. **Half-life:** 21 hrs.

USES

Ergotamine: Prevents or aborts vascular headaches (e.g., migraine, cluster headaches). **Dihydroergotamine:** Treatment of migraine headache with or without aura; injection also used to treat cluster headache.

PRECAUTIONS

CONTRAINDICATIONS: Peripheral vascular disease (thromboangiitis obliterans, syphilitic arteritis, severe arteriosclerosis, thrombophlebitis, Raynaud's disease), impaired renal/hepatic function, severe pruritus, coronary artery disease, hypertension, sepsis, malnutrition. **CAUTIONS:** None known.

LIFESPAN CONSIDERATIONS: Pregnancy/lactation: Contraindicated in pregnancy (produces uterine stimulant action, resulting in possible fetal death or retarded fetal growth); increases vasoconstriction of placental vascular bed. Drug distributed in breast milk. May produce diarrhea, vomiting in neonate. May prohibit lactation. **Pregnancy Category X. Children:** No precautions in those >6 yrs, but only use when unresponsive to other medication. **Elderly:** Age-related occlusive peripheral vascular disease increases risk of peripheral vasoconstriction. Age-related renal impairment may require caution.

INTERACTIONS

DRUG: Beta-blockers, erythromycin may increase risk of vasospasm. May decrease effect of **nitroglycerin. Ergot alkaloids, systemic vasoconstrictors** may increase pressor effect. **HERBAL:** None known. **FOOD:** None known. **LAB VALUES:** None known.

AVAILABILITY (Rx)

TABLETS (sublingual): 2 mg. **INJECTION:** 1 mg/ml. **NASAL SPRAY:** 0.5 mg/spray. **SUPPOSITORY:** 2 mg (with 100 mg caffeine).

ADMINISTRATION/HANDLING

SUBLINGUAL

- Place under tongue; do not swallow.

INDICATIONS/ROUTES/DOSAGE

VASCULAR HEADACHES

ERGOTAMINE

PO: ADULTS, ELDERLY: *Cafergot:* 2 mg at

onset of headache, then 1–2 mg q30min. **Maximum:** 6 mg/episode; 10 mg/wk.

Sublingual: ADULTS, ELDERLY: *Ergomar:* 1 tablet at onset of headache, then 1 tablet q30min. **Maximum:** 3 tablets/24 hrs; 5 tabs/wk.

PO/sublingual: CHILDREN: 1 mg at onset of headache, then 1 mg q30min. **Maximum:** 3 mg/episode.

Rectal: ADULTS, ELDERLY: 1 suppository at onset of headache, then second dose in 1 hr. **Maximum:** 2/episode; 5/wk

DIHYDROERGOTAMINE

IM/subcutaneous: ADULTS, ELDERLY: 1 mg at onset of headache; repeat hourly. **Maximum:** 3 mg/day; 6 mg/wk.

IV: ADULTS, ELDERLY: 1 mg at onset of headache; repeat hourly. **Maximum:** 2 mg/day; 6 mg/wk.

Intranasal: ADULTS, ELDERLY: 1 spray (0.5 mg) into each nostril; repeat in 15 min. **Maximum:** 4 sprays/day; 8 sprays/wk.

SIDE EFFECTS

OCCASIONAL (2%–5%): Cough, dizziness. **RARE (<2%):** Muscle pain, fatigue, diarrhea, upper respiratory infection, dyspepsia.

ADVERSE REACTIONS/ TOXIC EFFECTS

Prolonged administration or excessive dosage may produce ergotamine poisoning: nausea, vomiting, weakness of legs, pain in limb muscles, numbness/tingling of fingers/toes, precordial pain, tachycardia/bradycardia, hypertension/hypotension. Localized edema, itching due to vasoconstriction of peripheral arteries/arterioles. Feet, hands will become cold, pale, numb. Muscle pain occurs when walking and later, even at rest. Gangrene may occur. Occasionally confusion, depression, drowsiness, seizures occur.

NURSING IMPLICATIONS

BASELINE ASSESSMENT

Question for history of peripheral vascular disease, renal/hepatic impairment, possibility of pregnancy. Question regarding onset, location, duration of migraine, possible precipitating symptoms.

INTERVENTION/EVALUATION

Monitor closely for evidence of ergotamine overdosage as result of prolonged administration or excessive dosage (see Adverse Reactions/Toxic Effects).

PATIENT/FAMILY TEACHING

Initiate therapy at first sign of migraine headache. Report if there is need to progressively increase dose to relieve vascular headaches or if irregular heartbeat, nausea, vomiting, numbness/tingling of fingers/toes, pain/weakness of extremities is noted. Discuss contraception with physician; report suspected pregnancy immediately (Pregnancy Category X).

ertapenem

er-tah-**pen**-em
(Invanz)

CLASSIFICATION

PHARMACOTHERAPEUTIC: Carbapenem. **CLINICAL:** Antibiotic.

ACTION

Penetrates bacterial cell wall of microorganisms, inhibiting cell wall synthesis. **Therapeutic Effect:** Produces bacterial cell death.

PHARMACOKINETICS

Almost completely absorbed following IM administration. Protein binding: 85%–95%. Widely distributed. Primarily excreted in urine with smaller amount eliminated in feces. Removed by hemodialysis. **Half-life:** 4 hrs.

USES

Treatment of moderate to severe intra-abdominal, skin/skin structure infections; community-acquired pneumonia; complicated urinary tract infection; acute pelvic infection.

PRECAUTIONS

CONTRAINDICATIONS: History of hypersensitivity to beta-lactams (meropenem, imipenem-cilastin). **IM:** Hypersensitivity to local anesthetics of amide type. **CAUTIONS:** Hypersensitivity to penicillins, cephalosporins, other allergens; impaired renal function; CNS disorders, esp. brain lesions or history of seizures.

LIFESPAN CONSIDERATIONS: Pregnancy/lactation: Distributed in breast milk. **Pregnancy Category B. Children:** Safety and efficacy not established in those <18 yrs. **Elderly:** Advanced/end-stage renal insufficiency may require dosage adjustment.

INTERACTIONS

DRUG: Probenecid reduces renal excretion of **ertapenem** (do not use concurrently). **HERBAL:** None known. **FOOD:** None known. **LAB VALUES:** May increase SGOT (AST), SGPT (ALT), alkaline phosphatase. May decrease Hgb, Hct, platelet count, potassium.

AVAILABILITY (Rx)

LYOPHILIZED POWDER: 1-g vial.

ADMINISTRATION/HANDLING

IM

Reconstitution • Reconstitute with 3.2 ml 1% lidocaine HCl injection (without epinephrine). • Shake vial thoroughly. • Inject deep in large muscle mass (gluteal or lateral part of thigh). • Administer suspension within 1 hr after preparation.

IV

Storage • Solution appears colorless to yellow (variation in color does not affect potency). • Discard if solution contains precipitate. • Reconstituted solution is stable for 6 hrs at room temperature, 24 hrs if refrigerated.

Reconstitution • Dilute 1-g vial with 10 ml 0.9% NaCl or Bacteriostatic Water for Injection. • Shake well to dissolve. • Further dilute with 50 ml 0.9% NaCl.

Rate of administration • Give by intermittent IV infusion (piggyback). Do not give IV push. • Infuse over 20–30 min.

IV INCOMPATIBILITIES

Do not mix or infuse with any other medications. Do not use diluents or IV solutions containing dextrose.

IV COMPATIBILITIES

Compatible with Water for Injection, 0.9% NaCl.

INDICATIONS/ROUTES/DOSAGE

INFECTION

IM: ADULTS, ELDERLY: 1 g given once/day for up to 7 days.

IV: ADULTS, ELDERLY: 1 g given once/day for up to 14 days.

RENAL IMPAIRMENT

IM/IV: ADULTS, ELDERLY WITH CREATININE CLEARANCE <30 ML/MIN: 500 mg daily.

SIDE EFFECTS

FREQUENT (6%–10%): Diarrhea, nausea, headache. **OCCASIONAL (2%–5%):** Altered mental status, insomnia, rash, abdominal pain, constipation, vomiting, edema/swelling, fever. **RARE (<2%):** Dizziness, cough, oral candidiasis, anxiety, tachycardia, phlebitis at IV site.

ADVERSE REACTIONS/ TOXIC EFFECTS

Antibiotic-associated colitis, other superinfections may occur. Anaphylactic reactions in those receiving beta-lactams have occurred. Seizures may occur in those with CNS disorders (brain lesions, history of seizures), bacterial meningitis, or severely impaired renal function.

NURSING IMPLICATIONS

BASELINE ASSESSMENT

Question for history of allergies, particularly to beta-lactams, penicillins, cephalosporins. Inquire about history of seizures.

INTERVENTION/EVALUATION

Monitor daily bowel activity, stool consistency (watery, loose, soft). Monitor for nausea, vomiting. Evaluate hydration status. Evaluate for inflammation at IV injection site. Assess skin for rash. Check mental status; be alert to tremors, possible seizures. Assess sleep pattern for evidence of insomnia.

PATIENT/FAMILY TEACHING

Notify physician in event of tremors, seizures, rash, diarrhea, other new symptoms.

Eryc

see erythromycin

Erythrocin

see erythromycin

erythromycin

eh-rith-row-**my**-sin
(Akne-Mycin, Apo-Erythro Base✤, EES, Erybid✤, Eryc, EryDerm, EryPed, Ery-Tab, Erythrocin, Erythromid✤, PCE)

FIXED-COMBINATION(S)

Eryzole, Pediazole: erythromycin/sulfisoxazole (sulfonamide): 200 mg/600 mg per 5 ml.

◆ CLASSIFICATION

PHARMACOTHERAPEUTIC: Macrolide. **CLINICAL:** Antibiotic, antiacne (see p. 25C).

ACTION

Bacteriostatic. Penetrates bacterial cell membrane and reversibly binds to bacterial ribosomes. **Therapeutic Effect:** Inhibits protein synthesis.

PHARMACOKINETICS

Variably absorbed from GI tract (affected by dosage form used). Widely distributed. Protein binding: 70%–90%. Metabolized in liver. Primarily eliminated in feces via bile. Not removed by hemodialysis. **Half-life:** 1.4–2 hrs (half-life increased with impaired renal function).

USES

Respiratory infections, otitis media, pertussis, inflammatory acne vulgaris, diphtheria (adjunctive therapy), Legionnaires' disease, intestinal amebiasis, preop intestinal antisepsis. Prophylaxis for rheumatic fever, bacterial endocarditis, respiratory tract surgery/invasive procedures, gonococcal ophthalmia neonatorum (if penicillin, tetracycline is contraindicated), gonorrheal pelvic inflammatory disease, coexisting chlamydial infections, uncomplicated urogenital infections, Lyme disease (<9 yrs). **Top-**

ical: Treatment of acne vulgaris. **Ophthalmic:** Treatment of ocular infections, prophylaxis for neonatal conjunctivitis, ophthalmia neonatorium. **Unlabeled: Systemic:** Treatment of acne vulgaris, chancroid, *Campylobacter* enteritis, gastroparesis, Lyme disease. **Topical:** Treatment of minor bacterial skin infections. **Unlabeled: Ophthalmic:** Treatment of blepharitis, conjunctivitis, keratitis, chlamydial trachoma.

PRECAUTIONS

CONTRAINDICATIONS: Hypersensitivity to erythromycins, preexisting liver disease, history of hepatitis due to erythromycins. Do not administer Pediazole to infants <2 mos. **CAUTIONS:** Hepatic dysfunction. If combination therapy is used (Pediazole), consider precautions of sulfonamides. IV may cause tachycardia, prolonged QT interval.

LIFESPAN CONSIDERATIONS: Pregnancy/lactation: Crosses placenta. Distributed in breast milk. Erythromycin estolate may increase liver function enzymes in pregnant women. **Pregnancy Category B. Children/elderly:** No age-related precautions noted. High dosage in those with decreased liver/renal function increases risk of hearing loss.

INTERACTIONS

DRUG: May inhibit metabolism of **carbamazepine.** May decrease effects of **chloramphenicol, clindamycin.** May increase concentration, toxicity of **buspirone, cyclosporine, felodipine, lovastatin, simvastatin. Hepatotoxic medications** may increase hepatotoxicity. May increase risk of toxicity with **theophylline.** May increase effect of **warfarin. HERBAL:** None known. **FOOD:** None known. **LAB VALUES:** May increase SGOT (AST), SGPT (ALT), alkaline, phosphatase, bilirubin.

AVAILABILITY (Rx)

POWDER FOR INJECTION: 500 mg, 1 g.

BASE: **TABLETS:** 250 mg, 333 mg, 500 mg. **TABLETS (delayed-release):** 333 mg. **CAPSULES (delayed-release):** 250 mg.

ESTOLATE: **TABLETS:** 500 mg. **CAPSULES:** 250 mg. **ORAL SUSPENSION:** 125 mg/5 ml, 250 mg/5 ml.

ETHYLSUCCINATE: **TABLETS (chewable):** 200 mg. **TABLETS:** 400 mg. **ORAL SUSPENSION:** 200 mg/5 ml, 400 mg/5 ml. **ORAL DROPS:** 100 mg /2.5 ml.

STEARATE: **TABLETS:** 250 mg, 500 mg.

OPHTHALMIC OINTMENT: 5%. **TOPICAL SOLUTION:** 1.5%, 2%. **TOPICAL GEL:** 2%. **TOPICAL OINTMENT:** 2%.

ADMINISTRATION/HANDLING

PO

• Store capsules, tablets at room temperature. • Oral suspension is stable for 14 days at room temperature. • Administer erythromycin base, stearate 1 hr prior to or 2 hrs following food. Erythromycin estolate, ethylsuccinate may be given without regard to meals, but optimal absorption occurs when given on empty stomach. • Give with 8 oz water. • If swallowing difficulties exist, sprinkle capsule contents on teaspoon of applesauce, follow with water. • Do not swallow chewable tablets whole.

IV

Storage • Store parenteral form at room temperature. • Initial reconstituted solution in vial is stable for 2 wks refrigerated or 24 hrs at room temperature. • Diluted IV solutions stable for 8 hrs at room temperature, 24 hrs if refrigerated. • Discard if precipitate forms.

Reconstitution • Reconstitute each 500 mg with 10 ml Sterile Water for Injection without preservative to provide a concentration of 50 mg/ml. • Further dilute with 100–250 ml D_5W or 0.9% NaCl.

Rate of administration • For intermittent IV infusion (piggyback), infuse over 20–60 min. • For continuous infusion, infuse over 6–24 hrs.

Ophthalmic: • Place finger on lower eyelid, pull out until a pocket is formed between eye and lower lid. Place ¼–½ inch layer of ointment into pocket. • Have pt close eye gently for 1–2 min, rolling eyeball (increases contact area of drug to eye). • Remove excess ointment around eye with tissue.

⊘ IV INCOMPATIBILITY

Fluconazole (Diflucan).

IV COMPATIBILITIES

Aminophylline, amiodarone (Cordarone), diltiazem (Cardizem), heparin, hydromorphone (Dilaudid), lidocaine, lorazepam (Ativan), magnesium sulfate, midazolam (Versed), morphine, multivitamins, potassium chloride.

INDICATIONS/ROUTES/DOSAGE

USUAL PARENTERAL DOSAGE

IV: ADULTS, ELDERLY, CHILDREN: 15–20 mg/kg/day in divided doses. **Maximum:** 4 g/day.

USUAL ORAL DOSAGE

PO: ADULTS, ELDERLY: 250 mg q6h; 500 mg q12h; or 333 mg q8h. Increase up to 4 g/day. CHILDREN: 30–50 mg/kg/day in divided doses up to 60–100 mg/kg/day for severe infections. NEONATES: 20–40 mg/kg/day in divided doses q6–12h.

PREOP INTESTINAL ANTISEPSIS

PO: ADULTS, ELDERLY: Give 1 g at 1 PM, 2 PM, and 11 PM on day before surgery (with neomycin). CHILDREN: 20 mg/kg; same regimen as above.

ACNE VULGARIS

Topical: ADULTS: Apply thin layer to affected area 2 times/day.

GONOCOCCAL OPHTHALMIA NEONATORUM

Ophthalmic: NEONATES: 0.5–2 cm no later than 1 hr after delivery.

SIDE EFFECTS

FREQUENT: Abdominal discomfort/cramping, phlebitis/thrombophlebitis with IV administration. **Topical:** Dry skin (50%). **OCCASIONAL:** Nausea, vomiting, diarrhea, rash, urticaria. **RARE: Ophthalmic:** Sensitivity reaction with increased irritation, burning, itching, inflammation. **Topical:** Urticaria.

ADVERSE REACTIONS/ TOXIC EFFECTS

Superinfections, esp. antibiotic-associated colitis (genital/anal pruritus, sore mouth/tongue, moderate to severe diarrhea), reversible cholestatic hepatitis may occur. High dosage in pts with renal impairment may lead to reversible hearing loss. Anaphylaxis occurs rarely.

NURSING IMPLICATIONS

BASELINE ASSESSMENT

Question for history of allergies (particularly erythromycins), hepatitis.

INTERVENTION/EVALUATION

Determine pattern of bowel activity, stool consistency. Assess skin for rash. Assess for hepatotoxicity: malaise, fever, abdominal pain, GI disturbances. Evaluate for superinfection. Check for phlebitis (heat, pain, red streaking over vein). Monitor for high-dose hearing loss.

PATIENT/FAMILY TEACHING

Continue therapy for full length of treatment. Doses should be evenly spaced. Do *not* swallow chewable tablets whole. Take medication with 8 oz water 1 hr prior to or 2 hrs following food/beverage. **Ophthalmic:** Report burning, itching, inflammation: **Topical:** Report excessive dryness, itching, burning. Improvement of acne may not occur for 1–2 mos; maximum benefit may take 3 mos; therapy may last months or years. Use caution if using other topical acne preparations containing peeling or abrasive agents, medicated or abrasive soaps, cosmetics containing alcohol (e.g., astringents, aftershave lotion).

E

escitalopram

es-sih-**tail**-oh-pram
(Lexapro)

CLASSIFICATION

PHARMACOTHERAPEUTIC: Serotonin reuptake inhibitor. **CLINICAL:** Antidepressant (see p. 35C).

ACTION

Blocks uptake of the neurotransmitter serotonin at CNS neuronal presynaptic membranes, increasing availability at postsynaptic receptor sites. **Therapeutic Effect:** Resulting enhancement of postsynaptic activity produces antidepressant effect.

PHARMACOKINETICS

Well absorbed after PO administration. Primarily metabolized in the liver. Primarily excreted in the feces with a lesser amount eliminated in the urine. **Half-life:** 35 hrs.

USES

Treatment of major depressive disorder exhibited as persistent, prominent dysphoria (occurring nearly every day for at least 2 wks) manifested by 4 of 8 symptoms: appetite change, sleep pattern change, increased fatigue, impaired concentration, feelings of guilt or worthlessness, loss of interest in usual activities, psychomotor agitation or retardation, suicidal tendencies.

PRECAUTIONS

CONTRAINDICATIONS: Concurrent use of MAOIs, breast-feeding. **CAUTIONS:** Liver/renal impairment; history of seizures, mania, hypomania; concurrent use of CNS depressants.

LIFESPAN CONSIDERATIONS: Pregnancy/lactation: Distributed in breast milk. **Pregnancy Category C. Children:** May cause increased anticholinergic effects or hyperexcitability. **Elderly:** More sensitive to anticholinergic effects (e.g., dry mouth), more likely to experience dizziness, sedation, confusion, hypotension, hyperexcitability.

INTERACTIONS

DRUG: MAOIs may cause serotonergic syndrome (excitement, diaphoresis, rigidity, hyperthermia, autonomic hyperactivity, coma). **Antifungals, macrolide antibiotics, cimetidine** may increase plasma levels; **carbamazepine** may decrease plasma levels. Increases **metoprolol** plasma levels. **HERBAL:** None known. **FOOD:** None known. **LAB VALUES:** May reduce serum sodium.

AVAILABILITY (Rx)

TABLETS: 5 mg, 10 mg, 20 mg. **ORAL SOLUTION:** 5 mg/5 ml.

ADMINISTRATION/HANDLING

PO

• Give without regard to food. • Do not crush film-coated tablets.

INDICATIONS/ROUTES/DOSAGE

ANTIDEPRESSANT

PO: ADULTS: Initially, 10 mg once daily in the morning or evening. May increase to 20 mg after a minimum of 1 wk. EL-

DERLY, IMPAIRED HEPATIC FUNCTION: 10 mg/day.

SIDE EFFECTS

FREQUENT (11%–21%): Nausea, dry mouth, somnolence, insomnia, excessive sweating. **OCCASIONAL (4%–8%):** Tremor, diarrhea/loose stools, abnormal ejaculation, dyspepsia, fatigue, anxiety, vomiting, anorexia. **RARE (2%–3%):** Sinusitis, sexual dysfunction, menstrual disorder, abdominal pain, agitation, decreased libido.

ADVERSE REACTIONS/ TOXIC EFFECTS

Overdosage manifested as dizziness, drowsiness, tachycardia, severe somnolence, confusion, seizures.

NURSING IMPLICATIONS

BASELINE ASSESSMENT

For pts on long-term therapy, liver/renal function tests, blood counts should be performed periodically. Observe/record behavior. Assess psychological status, thought content, sleep pattern, appearance, interest in environment.

INTERVENTION/EVALUATION

Supervise suicidal-risk pt closely during early therapy (as energy level improves, suicide potential increases). Assess appearance, behavior, speech pattern, level of interest, mood.

PATIENT/FAMILY TEACHING

Do not stop taking medication or increase dosage. Avoid use of alcohol. Avoid tasks that require alertness, motor skills until response to drug is established.

Eskalith

see lithium carbonate

esmolol hydrochloride

ez-moe-lol
(Brevibloc)

◆ CLASSIFICATION

PHARMACOTHERAPEUTIC: $Beta_1$-adrenergic blocker. **CLINICAL:** Antiarrhythmic (see pp. 14C, 62C).

ACTION

Selectively blocks $beta_1$-adrenergic receptors. **Therapeutic Effect:** Slows sinus heart rate, decreases cardiac output, decreasing B/P.

USES

Rapid, short-term control of ventricular rate in those with supraventricular arrhythmias, sinus tachycardia. Intraop/postop control of tachycardia/hypertension.

PRECAUTIONS

CONTRAINDICATIONS: Overt cardiac failure, cardiogenic shock, heart block greater than first degree, sinus bradycardia. **CAUTIONS:** History of allergy, bronchial asthma, emphysema, bronchitis, CHF, diabetes, impaired renal function. **Pregnancy Category C.**

INTERACTIONS

DRUG: Sympathomimetics, xanthines may mutually inhibit effects. May mask symptoms of hypoglycemia, prolong hypoglycemic effect of **insulin, oral hypoglycemics. MAOIs** may cause significant hypertension. **HERBAL:** None known. **FOOD:** None known. **LAB VALUES:** None known.

AVAILABILITY (Rx)

INJECTION: 10 mg/ml, 250 mg/ml.

ADMINISTRATION/HANDLING

Alert: Give by IV infusion. Avoid butterfly needles, very small veins.

IV

Storage • Use only clear and colorless to light yellow solution. • After dilution, solution is stable for 24 hrs. • Discard solution if it is discolored or if precipitate forms.

Reconstitution • The 250 mg/ml ampoule is not for direct IV injection but must be diluted to a final concentration not to exceed 10 mg/ml (prevents vein irritation). • For IV infusion, remove 20 ml from 500-ml container of D_5W, D_5W/Ringer's, D_5W/lactated Ringer's, D_5W/0.9% NaCl, D_5W/0.45% NaCl, 0.9% NaCl, lactated Ringer's or 0.45% NaCl and dilute 5-g vial esmolol to remaining 480 ml of solution to provide concentration of 10 mg/ml. Maximum concentration: 10 g/250 ml (40 mg/ml).

Rate of administration • Administer by controlled infusion device; titrate to tolerance and response. • Infuse IV loading dose over 1–2 min. • Hypotension (systolic B/P <90 mm Hg) is greatest during first 30 min of IV infusion.

IV INCOMPATIBILITIES
Amphotericin B complex (Abelcet, AmBisome, Amphotec), furosemide (Lasix).

IV COMPATIBILITIES
Amiodarone (Cordarone), diltiazem (Cardizem), dopamine (Intropin), heparin, magnesium, midazolam (Versed), potassium chloride, propofol (Diprivan).

INDICATIONS/ROUTES/DOSAGE

IV: ADULTS, ELDERLY: Initially, loading dose of 500 mcg/kg/min for 1 min, followed by 50 mcg/kg/min for 4 min. If optimum response is not attained in 5 min, give second loading dose of 500 mcg/kg/min for 1 min, followed by infusion of 100 mcg/kg/min for 4 min. Additional loading doses can be given and infusion increased by 50 mcg/kg/min (up to 200 mcg/kg/min) for 4 min. Once desired response is attained, cease loading dose and increase infusion by no more than 25 mcg/kg/min. Interval between doses may be increased to 10 min. Infusion usually administered over 24–48 hrs in most pts. RANGE: 50–200 mcg/kg/min with average dose of 100 mcg/kg/min.

SIDE EFFECTS

Generally well tolerated, with transient and mild side effects. **FREQUENT:** Hypotension (systolic B/P <90 mm Hg) manifested as dizziness, nausea, diaphoresis, headache, cold extremities, fatigue. **OCCASIONAL:** Anxiety, drowsiness, flushed skin, vomiting, confusion, inflammation at injection site, fever.

ADVERSE REACTIONS/ TOXIC EFFECTS

Excessive dosage may produce profound hypotension, bradycardia, dizziness, syncope, drowsiness, breathing difficulty, bluish fingernails/palms of hands, seizures. May potentiate insulin-reduced hypoglycemia in diabetic pts.

NURSING IMPLICATIONS

BASELINE ASSESSMENT

Assess B/P, apical pulse immediately before drug is administered (if pulse is ≤60/min or systolic B/P is <90 mm Hg, withhold medication, contact physician).

INTERVENTION/EVALUATION

Monitor B/P for hypotension, EKG, heart rate, respiratory rate, development of diaphoresis, dizziness (usually first sign of impending hypotension). Assess pulse for quality, irregular rate, bradycardia, extremities for coldness. Assist with ambulation if dizziness occurs. Assess for nausea, diaphoresis, headache, fatigue.

esomeprazole

es-oh-**mep**-rah-zole
(Nexium)

CLASSIFICATION

PHARMACOTHERAPEUTIC: Proton pump inhibitor. **CLINICAL:** Gastric acid inhibitor (see p. 128C).

ACTION

Converted to active metabolites that irreversibly bind to and inhibit H^+, K^+, ATPase (an enzyme on surface of gastric parietal cells). Inhibits hydrogen ion transport into gastric lumen. **Therapeutic Effect:** Increases gastric pH, reducing gastric acid production.

PHARMACOKINETICS

Well absorbed after PO administration. Protein binding: 97%. Extensively metabolized by the liver. Primarily excreted in urine. **Half-life:** 1–1.5 hrs.

USES

Short-term treatment (4–8 wks) of erosive esophagitis (diagnosed by endoscopy); symptomatic gastroesophageal reflux disease (GERD). Used in triple therapy with amoxicillin and clarithromycin for treatment of *H. pylori* infection in pts with duodenal ulcer.

PRECAUTIONS

CONTRAINDICATIONS: None known. **CAUTIONS:** None known.

LIFESPAN CONSIDERATIONS: Pregnancy/lactation: Unknown if drug crosses placenta or is distributed in breast milk. **Pregnancy Category B. Children:** Safety and efficacy not established. **Elderly:** No age-related precautions noted.

INTERACTIONS

DRUG: May decrease concentration of **ketoconazole, iron, digoxin. HERBAL:** None known. **FOOD:** None known. **LAB VALUES:** None known.

AVAILABILITY (Rx)

CAPSULES (delayed-release): 20 mg, 40 mg.

ADMINISTRATION/HANDLING

PO

- Give ≥1 hr before eating.
- Do not crush or chew capsule; swallow whole. For those with difficulty swallowing capsules, open capsule and mix pellets with 1 tbsp applesauce. Swallow spoonful without chewing.

INDICATIONS/ROUTES/DOSAGE

EROSIVE ESOPHAGITIS

PO: ADULTS, ELDERLY: 20–40 mg once daily for 4–8 wks.

MAINTENANCE HEALING OF EROSIVE ESOPHAGITIS

PO: ADULTS, ELDERLY: 20 mg/day.

GERD

PO: ADULTS, ELDERLY: 20 mg once daily for 4 wks.

***H. PYLORI* DUODENAL ULCER**

PO: ADULTS, ELDERLY: **Esomeprazole:** 40 mg once daily, with amoxicillin 1,000 mg and clarithromycin 500 mg twice daily for 10 days.

SIDE EFFECTS

FREQUENT (7%): Headache. **OCCASIONAL (2%–3%):** Diarrhea, abdominal pain, nausea. **RARE (<2%):** Dizziness, asthenia (loss of strength), vomiting, constipation, rash, cough.

E

ADVERSE REACTIONS/ TOXIC EFFECTS

None known.

NURSING IMPLICATIONS

INTERVENTION/EVALUATION

Evaluate for therapeutic response (i.e., relief of GI symptoms). Question if GI discomfort, nausea, diarrhea occur.

PATIENT/FAMILY TEACHING

Report headache. Take ≥1 hr prior to eating. For pts with difficulty swallowing capsules, open capsule and mix pellets with 1 tbsp applesauce. Swallow spoonful without chewing.

estazolam

es-**tay**-zoe-lam
(ProSom)

Do not confuse with Proscar, Prozac, Psorcon.

◆ CLASSIFICATION

PHARMACOTHERAPEUTIC: Benzodiazepine **(Schedule IV). CLINICAL:** Sedative-hypnotic (see p. 129C).

ACTION

Enhances action of inhibitory neurotransmitter gamma-aminobutyric acid (GABA). **Therapeutic Effect:** Depressant effects occur at all levels of CNS.

USES

Short-term treatment of insomnia (up to 6 wks). Reduces sleep induction time, number of nocturnal awakenings; increases length of sleep.

PRECAUTIONS

CONTRAINDICATIONS: Sensitivity to other benzodiazepines, pregnancy (Pregnancy Category X). **CAUTIONS:** Impaired renal/hepatic function. Pts with potential for drug abuse. **Pregnancy Category X.**

INTERACTIONS

DRUG: **Alcohol, CNS depressants** may increase CNS depressant effect. **HERBAL:** **Kava kava, valerian** may increase CNS depression. **FOOD:** None known. **LAB VALUES:** None known.

AVAILABILITY (Rx)

TABLETS: 1 mg, 2 mg.

INDICATIONS/ROUTES/DOSAGE

Alert: Use smallest effective dosage in those with liver disease, low serum albumin.

INSOMNIA

PO: ADULTS >18 YRS: 1–2 mg at bedtime. ELDERLY/DEBILITATED: 0.5–1 mg at bedtime.

SIDE EFFECTS

FREQUENT: Drowsiness, sedation, rebound insomnia (may occur for 1–2 nights after drug is discontinued), dizziness, confusion, euphoria. **OCCASIONAL:** Weakness, anorexia, diarrhea. **RARE:** Paradoxical CNS excitement, restlessness (particularly noted in elderly/debilitated).

ADVERSE REACTIONS/ TOXIC EFFECTS

Overdosage results in somnolence, confusion, diminished reflexes, respiratory depression, coma.

NURSING IMPLICATIONS

BASELINE ASSESSMENT

Raise bed rails. Provide environment conducive to sleep (back rub, quiet environment, low lighting). Question for possibility of pregnancy (Pregnancy Category X).

INTERVENTION/EVALUATION

Assess sleep pattern of pt. Assess elderly/debilitated for paradoxical reaction, particularly during early therapy. Evaluate for therapeutic response: decrease in number of nocturnal awakenings, increase in length of sleep.

PATIENT/FAMILY TEACHING

Smoking reduces drug effectiveness. Rebound insomnia may occur when drug is discontinued after short-term therapy. Do not use during pregnancy. Avoid alcohol.

Estrace

see estradiol

Estraderm

see estradiol

estradiol

ess-tra-**dye**-ole
(Estrace)

estradiol cypionate

(Depo Estradiol, Depogen)

estradiol transdermal

(Alora, Climara, Esclim, Estraderm, Vivelle, Vivelle Dot)

estradiol valerate

(Delestrogen, Valogen)
Do not confuse with Testoderm.

FIXED-COMBINATION(S)

Activella: estradiol/norethindrone (hormone): 1 mg/0.5 mg. **Combipatch:** estradiol/norethindrone (hormone): 0.05 mg/0.14 mg; 0.05 mg/0.25 mg. **Femhrt:** estradiol/norethindrone (hormone): 5 mcg/1 mg/. **Lunelle:** estradiol/medroxyprogesterone (progestin): 5 mg/25 mg per 0.5 ml.

◆ CLASSIFICATION

PHARMACOTHERAPEUTIC: Estrogen. **CLINICAL:** Estrogen, antineoplastic.

ACTION

Increases synthesis of DNA, RNA, proteins in target tissues; reduces release of gonadotropin-releasing hormone from hypothalamus; reduces FSH and LH release from the pituitary. **Therapeutic Effect:** Promotes normal growth, development of female sex organs, maintaining GU function, vasomotor stability. Prevents accelerated bone loss by inhibiting bone resorption, restoring balance of bone resorption and formation. Inhibits LH, decreases serum concentration of testosterone.

PHARMACOKINETICS

Well absorbed from GI tract. Widely distributed. Protein binding: 50%–80%. Metabolized in liver. Primarily excreted in urine. **Half-life:** Unknown.

USES

Management of atrophic vaginitis, atrophic dystrophy of vulva, menopausal symptoms, female hypogonadism, primary ovarian failure, hypoestrogenism, prevention of postmenopausal osteoporosis. **Unlabeled:** Treatment of Turner's syndrome.

PRECAUTIONS

CONTRAINDICATIONS: Thrombophlebitis or thromboembolic disorders, active arterial thrombosis, thyroid dysfunction, abnormal vaginal bleeding, estrogen-dependent cancer, known or suspected breast cancer, blood dyscrasias, pregnancy. **CAUTIONS:** Renal/liver insufficiency, diseases that may be exacerbated by fluid retention, children in whom bone growth is not complete.

LIFESPAN CONSIDERATIONS: Pregnancy/lactation: Distributed in breast milk. May be harmful to offspring. Not for use during lactation. **Pregnancy Category X.** **Children:** Caution in those whom bone growth not complete (may accelerate epiphyseal closure). **Elderly:** No age-related precautions noted.

INTERACTIONS

DRUG: May interfere with effects of **bromocriptine.** May increase concentration of **cyclosporine,** increasing hepatic/toxicity, nephrotoxicity. **Hepatotoxic medications** may increase hepatotoxicity. **HERBAL: Saw palmetto** effects increased. **FOOD:** None known. **LAB VALUES:** May affect metapyrone, thyroid function tests. May decrease cholesterol, LDH. May increase calcium, glucose, HDL, triglycerides.

AVAILABILITY (Rx)

TABLETS: (Estrace): 0.5 mg, 1 mg, 2 mg. **INJECTION: (Cypionate):** 5 mg/ml; **(Valerate):** 10 mg/ml, 20 mg/ml, 40 mg/ml. **TRANSDERMAL:** 0.025 mg, 0.0375 mg, 0.05 mg, 0.075 mg, 0.1 mg. **VAGINAL CREAM:** 100 mcg/g. **VAGINAL RING:** 0.05 mg, 0.1 mg, 2 mg.

Alert: Transdermal Climara is administered once weekly; others are twice weekly.

ADMINISTRATION/HANDLING

PO

- Administer at the same time each day.

IM

- Rotate vial to disperse drug in solution.
- Inject deep IM in gluteus maximus.

VAGINAL

- Apply at bedtime for best absorption.
- Insert end of filled applicator into vagina, directed slightly toward sacrum; push plunger down completely.
- Avoid skin contact with cream (prevents skin absorption).

TRANSDERMAL

- Remove old patch; select new site (buttocks an alternative application site).
- Peel off protective strip to expose adhesive surface.
- Apply to clean, dry, intact skin on the trunk of the body (area with as little hair as possible).
- Press in place for at least 10 sec (do not apply to the breasts or waistline).

INDICATIONS/ROUTES/DOSAGE

FEMALE HYPOGONADISM

IM (Cypionate): 1.5–2 mg/mo. **(Valerate):** 10–20 mg/mo.

PO: 0.5–2 mg/day cyclically (3 wks on, 1 wk off).

Transdermal (Climara): Once weekly 0.025–0.05 mg. Other transdermals: Twice weekly: 0.05 mg 2 times/wk cyclically in pts with intact uterus, continuous in pts without a uterus.

VAGINAL/VULVAE ATROPHY

Intravaginal: Initially, 200–400 mcg/day (2–4 g of cream) estradiol daily for 1–2 wks; then 100–200 mcg (1–2 g) daily for 1–2 wks. MAINTENANCE: After vaginal mucosa restored: 100 mcg 1–3 times/wk for 3 wks, off 1 wk per cycle.

MENOPAUSAL SYMPTOMS

IM (Cypionate): 1–5 mg/day cyclically (3 wks on, 1 wk off). **(Valerate):** 10–20 mg q4wks.

PO: 0.5–2 mg/day cyclically or continuously.

Transdermal: 25–50 mcg 1–2 times/wk depending on product used.

BREAST CANCER
PO: 10 mg 3 times/day for at least 3 mos.

PROSTATE CANCER
PO: 1–2 mg 3 times/day.

IM (Valerate): 30 mg q1–2wks.

PREVENTION OF POSTMENOPAUSAL OSTEOPOROSIS
PO: 0.5 mg/day, cyclically (23 days on, 5 days off).

Transdermal (Alora, Climara, Vivelle): 25–100 mcg/day.

SIDE EFFECTS

FREQUENT: Anorexia, nausea, swelling of breasts, peripheral edema evidenced by swollen ankles, feet. **Transdermal route:** Skin irritation, redness. **OCCASIONAL:** Vomiting (esp. with high dosages), headache (may be severe), intolerance to contact lenses, increased B/P, glucose intolerance, brown spots on exposed skin. **Vaginal route:** Local irritation, vaginal discharge, changes in vaginal bleeding (spotting, breakthrough, prolonged bleeding). **RARE:** Chorea (involuntary movements), hirsutism (abnormal hairiness), loss of scalp hair, depression.

ADVERSE REACTIONS/ TOXIC EFFECTS

Prolonged administration increases risk of gallbladder disease, thromboembolic disease, breast, cervical, vaginal, endometrial, liver carcinoma. Cholestatic jaundice occurs rarely.

NURSING IMPLICATIONS

BASELINE ASSESSMENT

Question for hypersensitivity to estrogen; previous jaundice or thromboembolic disorders associated with pregnancy; estrogen therapy. Question for possibility of pregnancy (Pregnancy Category X).

INTERVENTION/EVALUATION

Monitor B/P, weight, serum calcium, glucose, liver enzymes.

PATIENT/FAMILY TEACHING

Limit alcohol, caffeine. Inform physician if sudden headache, vomiting, disturbance of vision/speech, numbness/weakness of extremity, chest pain, calf pain, shortness of breath, severe abdominal pain, mental depression, unusual bleeding occurs.

estramustine phosphate sodium

es-trah-**mew**-steen
(Emcyt)
Do not confuse with Eryc.

◆CLASSIFICATION

PHARMACOTHERAPEUTIC: Alkylating agent, estrogen/nitrogen mustard. **CLINICAL:** Antineoplastic (see p. 72C).

ACTION

Binds to microtubule-associated proteins, causing their disassembly. **Therapeutic Effect:** Reduces serum testosterone concentration.

PHARMACOKINETICS

Well absorbed from GI tract. Highly localized in prostatic tissue. Rapidly dephosphorylated during absorption into peripheral circulation. Metabolized in liver. Primarily eliminated in feces via biliary system. **Half-life:** 20 hrs.

USES

Treatment of metastatic/ progressive carcinoma of prostate gland.

E

PRECAUTIONS

CONTRAINDICATIONS: Hypersensitivity to estradiol or nitrogen mustard, active thrombophlebitis or thrombolic disorders unless tumor is cause for thrombolic disorders and benefits outweigh risk. **CAUTIONS:** History of thrombophlebitis, thrombosis, thromboembolic disorders; cerebrovascular, coronary artery disease; impaired hepatic function; metabolic bone disease in those with hypercalcemia, renal insufficiency.

LIFESPAN CONSIDERATIONS: Pregnancy/lactation, Pregnancy Category C. Children: Not used in these populations. **Elderly:** Age-related renal impairment and/or peripheral vascular disease may require caution.

INTERACTIONS

DRUG: Hepatotoxic drugs may increase risk of hepatotoxicity. **HERBAL:** None known. **FOOD:** None known. **LAB VALUES:** May increase SGOT (AST), LDH, bilirubin, cortisol, glucose, phospholipids, prolactin, prothrombin, sodium, triglycerides. May decrease antithrombin 3, folate, pregnanediol excretion, phosphate. May alter thyroid function tests.

AVAILABILITY (Rx)

CAPSULES: 140 mg.

ADMINISTRATION/HANDLING

PO

• Refrigerate capsules (may remain at room temperature for 24–48 hrs without loss of potency). • Give with water 1 hr before or 2 hrs after meals.

INDICATIONS/ROUTES/DOSAGE

PROSTATIC CARCINOMA

PO: ADULTS, ELDERLY: 10–16 mg/kg/day (140 mg for each 10 kg weight) in 3–4 doses/day.

SIDE EFFECTS

FREQUENT: Peripheral edema of lower extremities, breast tenderness/enlargement, diarrhea, flatulence, nausea. **OCCASIONAL:** Increase in B/P, thirst, dry skin, easy bruising, flushing, thinning hair, night sweats. **RARE:** Headache, rash, fatigue, insomnia, vomiting.

ADVERSE REACTIONS/ TOXIC EFFECTS

May exacerbate CHF, increased risk of pulmonary emboli, thrombophlebitis, cerebrovascular accident.

NURSING IMPLICATIONS

INTERVENTION/EVALUATION

Monitor B/P periodically.

PATIENT/FAMILY TEACHING

Do not take with milk, milk products, calcium-rich food, calcium-containing antacids. Use contraceptive measures during therapy. If headache (migraine or severe), vomiting, disturbed speech/vision, dizziness, numbness, shortness of breath, calf pain, heaviness in chest, unexplained cough occurs, contact physician.

estropipate

ess-troe-**pie**-pate
(Ogen)

CLASSIFICATION

PHARMACOTHERAPEUTIC: Estrogen. **CLINICAL:** Hormone.

ACTION

Increases synthesis of DNA, RNA, various proteins in responsive tissues. Reduces release of gonadotropin-releasing hormone, reducing follicle-stimulating hormone (FSH), luteinizing hormone (LH). **Therapeutic Effect:** Promotes normal growth, development of female sex organs, maintaining GU function, vasomotor stability. Prevents accelerated bone loss by inhibiting bone resorption, restoring balance of bone resorption/formation.

USES

Management of moderate to severe vasomotor symptoms associated with menopause. Treatment of atrophic vaginitis, kraurosis vulvae, female hypogonadism, castration, primary ovarian failure. Prevention of osteoporosis.

PRECAUTIONS

CONTRAINDICATIONS: Thrombophlebitis or thromboembolic disorders, active arterial thrombosis, thyroid dysfunction, abnormal vaginal bleeding, estrogen-dependent cancer, known/suspected breast cancer, blood dyscrasias, pregnancy. **CAUTIONS:** Renal/liver insufficiency, diseases that may be exacerbated by fluid retention. **Pregnancy Category X.**

INTERACTIONS

DRUG: May interfere with effects of **bromocriptine.** May increase concentration of **cyclosporine,** increasing hepatic nephrotoxicity. **Hepatotoxic medications** may increase hepatotoxicity. **HERBAL: Saw palmetto** effects increased. **FOOD:** None known. **LAB VALUES:** May affect metapyrone, thyroid function tests. May decrease cholesterol, LDH. May increase calcium, glucose, HDL, triglycerides.

AVAILABILITY (Rx)

TABLETS: 0.625 mg, 0.75 mg, 1.25 mg, 1.5 mg, 2.5 mg, 3 mg.

INDICATIONS/ROUTES/DOSAGE

VASOMOTOR SYMPTOMS, ATROPHIC VAGINITIS, KRAUROSIS VULVAE

PO: ADULTS, ELDERLY: 0.625–5 mg/day cyclically.

ATROPHIC VAGINITIS, KRAUROSIS VULVAE

Intravaginal: ADULTS, ELDERLY: 2–4 g/day cyclically.

FEMALE HYPOGONADISM, CASTRATION, PRIMARY OVARIAN FAILURE

PO: ADULTS, ELDERLY: 1.25–7.5 mg/day for 21 days; off 8–10 days. Repeat if bleeding does not occur by end of off cycle.

OSTEOPOROSIS PREVENTION

PO: ADULTS, ELDERLY: 0.625 mg/day (25 days of 31-day cycle/mo).

SIDE EFFECTS

FREQUENT: Anorexia, nausea, swelling of breasts, peripheral edema evidenced by swollen ankles, feet. **OCCASIONAL:** Vomiting (esp. with high dosages), headache (may be severe), intolerance to contact lenses, increased B/P, glucose intolerance, brown spots on exposed skin. **Vaginal route:** Local irritation, vaginal discharge, changes in vaginal bleeding (spotting, breakthrough, prolonged bleeding). **RARE:** Chorea (involuntary movements), hirsutism (abnormal hairiness), loss of scalp hair, depression.

ADVERSE REACTIONS/TOXIC EFFECTS

Prolonged administration increases risk of gallbladder disease, thromboembolic disease, breast, cervical, vaginal, endometrial, liver carcinoma. Cholestatic jaundice occurs rarely.

NURSING IMPLICATIONS

BASELINE ASSESSMENT

Question for hypersensitivity to estrogen; previous jaundice; thromboembolic disorders associated with pregnancy; estrogen therapy. Question for possibility of pregnancy (Pregnancy Category X).

INTERVENTION/EVALUATION

Promptly report signs/symptoms of thromboembolic or thrombotic disorders: sudden severe headache, shortness of breath, vision/speech disturbance, numbness of an extremity.

PATIENT/FAMILY TEACHING

Avoid smoking due to increased risk of heart attack/blood clots. Notify physician of abnormal vaginal bleeding, depression. With vaginal application, remain recumbent at least 30 min after application; do not use tampons. Stop taking the medication and contact physician at once if pregnancy is suspected.

etanercept

ee-**tan**-er-cept
(Enbrel)

CLASSIFICATION

PHARMACOTHERAPEUTIC: Protein. **CLINICAL:** Antiarthritic.

ACTION

Binds to tumor necrosis factor (TNF), blocking its interaction with cell surface receptors (TNF is involved in inflammatory and immune responses; elevated TNF is found in synovial fluid of rheumatoid arthritis pts). **Therapeutic Effects:** Reduces rheumatoid arthritis effects.

PHARMACOKINETICS

Well absorbed after subcutaneous administration. Blocks interactions with cell surface tumor necrosis factor receptors (TNFR). **Half-life:** 115 hrs.

USES

Reduces signs/symptoms of moderately to severely active rheumatoid arthritis (RA). Treatment of active juvenile RA, ankylosing spondylitis, psoriatic arthritis. **Unlabeled:** Crohn's disease.

PRECAUTIONS

CONTRAINDICATIONS: Serious active infection, sepsis. **CAUTIONS:** History of recurrent infections, illnesses that predispose to infection (e.g., diabetes).

LIFESPAN CONSIDERATIONS: Pregnancy/lactation: Unknown if excreted in breast milk. **Pregnancy Category B. Children:** No age-related precautions noted in those >4 yrs. **Elderly:** No age-related precautions noted.

INTERACTIONS

DRUG: None known. **HERBAL:** None known. **FOOD:** None known. **LAB VALUES:** None known.

AVAILABILITY (Rx)

POWDER FOR INJECTION: 25 mg.

ADMINISTRATION/HANDLING

Alert: Do not add other medications to solution. Do not use filter during reconstitution or administration.

SUBCUTANEOUS

• Reconstitute with 1 ml of sterile Bacteriostatic Water for Injection (0.9% benzyl alcohol). Do not reconstitute with other diluents. • Slowly inject the diluent into the vial. Some foaming will occur. To avoid excessive foaming, slowly swirl contents until powder is dissolved (<5 min). • Visually inspect solution for particles, discoloration. Reconstituted solution should appear clear, colorless. If discolored, cloudy, or particles remain, discard solution; do not use. • Withdraw all the solution into syringe. Final volume should be approx. 1 ml. • Inject into thigh, abdomen, or upper arm. Rotate injection sites. • Give new injection at least 1 inch from an old site and never into area when skin is tender, bruised, red, hard. • Refrigerate. • Once reconstituted, may be stored under refrigeration for up to 6 hrs.

INDICATIONS/ROUTES/DOSAGE

RHEUMATOID ARTHRITIS

Subcutaneous: ADULTS, ELDERLY: 25 mg twice weekly given 72–96 hrs apart. CHILDREN 4–17 YRS: 0.4 mg/kg (**Maximum:** 25 mg dose) twice weekly given 72–96 hrs apart.

SIDE EFFECTS

FREQUENT (37%): Injection site reaction (erythema, itching, pain, swelling). Incidence of abdominal pain, vomiting is higher in children than in adults. **OCCASIONAL (4%–16%):** Headache, rhinitis, dizziness, pharyngitis, cough, asthenia, abdominal pain, dyspepsia. **RARE (<3%):** Sinusitis, allergic reaction.

ADVERSE REACTIONS/ TOXIC EFFECTS

Infection (pyelonephritis, cellulitis, osteomyelitis, wound infection, leg ulcer, septic arthritis, diarrhea), upper respiratory tract infection (bronchitis, pneumonia) occur frequently (29%–38%). Formation of autoimmune antibodies may occur. Serious adverse effects occur rarely (heart failure, hypertension/hypotension, pancreatitis, GI hemorrhage, dyspnea).

NURSING IMPLICATIONS

BASELINE ASSESSMENT

Assess onset, type, location, duration of pain/inflammation. If a significant exposure to varicella virus has occurred during treatment, therapy should be temporarily discontinued and treatment with varicella-zoster immune globulin be considered.

INTERVENTION/EVALUATION

Assess for joint swelling, pain, tenderness; ESR or C-reactive protein level; CBC with differential; platelet count.

PATIENT/FAMILY TEACHING

Instruct in subcutaneous injection, including areas of the body acceptable as injection sites. Injection site reaction generally occurs in first month of treatment and decreases in frequency during continued therapy. Do not receive live vaccines during treatment. Inform physician if there is persistent fever, bruising, bleeding, pallor.

ethacrynic acid

eth-ah-**krin**-ick

(Edecrin)

Do not confuse with Ecotrin.

CLASSIFICATION

PHARMACOTHERAPEUTIC: Diuretic. **CLINICAL:** Loop diuretic (see p. 87C).

ACTION

Enhances excretion of sodium, chloride, potassium at ascending limb of loop of Henle and distal renal tubule. **Therapeutic Effect:** Produces diuretic effect.

USES

Treatment of edema associated with CHF, severe renal impairment, nephrotic syndrome, hepatic cirrhosis; short-term management of ascites, children with CHF. **Unlabeled:** Treatment of hypertension, hypercalcemia.

PRECAUTIONS

CONTRAINDICATIONS: Anuria, severe renal impairment. **CAUTIONS:** Hepatic cirrhosis, ascites, history of gout, pancreatitis, systemic lupus erythematosus, diabetes mellitus, elderly, debilitated. **Pregnancy Category B** (**D** if used in pregnancy-induced hypertension).

INTERACTIONS

DRUG: **Amphotericin, ototoxic, and nephrotoxic agents** may increase toxicity. May decrease effect of **anticoagulants, heparin.** Hypokalemia-causing agents may increase risk of hypokalemia. May increase risk of lithium toxicity. **HERBAL:** None known. **FOOD:** None known. **LAB VALUES:** May increase glucose, BUN, uric acid, urinary phosphate. May decrease calcium, chloride, magnesium, potassium, sodium.

ADMINISTRATION/HANDLING

PO

• Give with food to avoid GI upset, preferably with breakfast (may prevent nocturia).

IV

Storage • Store vials at room temperature. • Discard if parenteral form appears hazy or opalescent. • Discard unused reconstituted solution after 24 hrs.

Reconstitution • For IV infusion, reconstitute each 50 mg ethacrynate sodium with 50 ml D_5W or 0.9% NaCl.

Rate of administration • For IV push, administer slowly over several minutes. • For IV infusion, infuse over 20–30 min.

IV INCOMPATIBILITY

No information available via Y-site administration.

IV COMPATIBILITIES

Heparin, potassium chloride.

AVAILABILITY (Rx)

TABLETS: 25 mg, 50 mg. **POWDER FOR INJECTION:** 50 mg.

INDICATIONS/ROUTES/DOSAGE

EDEMA

PO: ADULTS, ELDERLY: 25–400 mg/day in 1–2 divided doses. CHILDREN: 1 mg/kg/dose once daily. May increase at 2- to 3-day intervals. **Maximum:** 3 mg/kg/day.

IV: ADULTS, ELDERLY: 0.5–1 mg/kg/dose. **Maximum:** 100 mg/dose. CHILDREN: 1 mg/kg/dose.

SIDE EFFECTS

FREQUENT: Expected: Increase in urine frequency/volume. **OCCASIONAL:** Nausea, gastric upset with cramping, diarrhea, headache, fatigue, apprehension. **RARE:** Severe, watery diarrhea.

ADVERSE REACTIONS/ TOXIC EFFECTS

Vigorous diuresis may lead to profound water loss and electrolyte depletion, resulting in hypokalemia, hyponatremia, dehydration, coma, circulatory collapse. Acute hypotensive episodes may occur, sometimes several days after beginning of therapy. Ototoxicity may occur, esp. in those with severe renal impairment. Can exacerbate diabetes, systemic lupus erythematosus, gout, pancreatitis. Blood dyscrasias have been reported.

NURSING IMPLICATIONS

BASELINE ASSESSMENT

Check B/P for hypotension prior to administration. Obtain baseline electrolytes (particularly check for low potassium). Assess for edema, skin turgor, mucous membranes for hydration status. Monitor I&O.

INTERVENTION/EVALUATION

Monitor B/P, vital signs, electrolytes, I&O, weight. Note extent of diuresis. Watch for changes from initial assessment (hypokalemia may result in muscle strength changes, tremor, muscle cramps, change in mental status, cardiac arrhythmias; hyponatremia may result in confusion, thirst, cold/clammy skin).

PATIENT/FAMILY TEACHING

Expect increased frequency, volume of urination. Eat foods high in potassium, such as whole grains (cereals), legumes, meat, bananas, apricots, orange juice, potatoes (white, sweet), raisins.

ethambutol

eth-**am**-byoo-toll

(Etibi ✱, Myambutol)

Do not confuse with Nembutal.

CLASSIFICATION

PHARMACOTHERAPEUTIC: Isonicotinic acid derivative. **CLINICAL:** Antitubercular.

ACTION

Interferes with RNA synthesis. **Therapeutic Effect:** Suppresses mycobacterial multiplication.

PHARMACOKINETICS

Rapidly, well absorbed from GI tract. Widely distributed. Protein binding: 20%–30%. Metabolized in liver. Primarily excreted in urine. Removed by hemodialysis. **Half-life:** 3–4 hrs (half-life increased with impaired renal function).

USES

In conjunction with at least one other antitubercular agent for initial treatment and retreatment of clinical tuberculosis. **Unlabeled:** Treatment of atypical mycobacterial infections.

PRECAUTIONS

CONTRAINDICATIONS: Optic neuritis. **CAUTIONS:** Renal dysfunction, gout, ocular defects: diabetic retinopathy, cataracts, recurrent ocular inflammatory conditions. Not recommended for children <13 yrs.

LIFESPAN CONSIDERATIONS: Pregnancy/lactation: Crosses placenta. Excreted in breast milk. **Pregnancy Category B. Children:** Safety and efficacy not established in those <13 yrs. **Elderly:** Age-related renal impairment may require dosage adjustment.

INTERACTIONS

DRUG: Neurotoxic medications may increase risk of neurotoxicity. **HERBAL:** None known. **FOOD:** None known. **LAB VALUES:** May increase uric acid.

AVAILABILITY (Rx)

TABLETS: 100 mg, 400 mg.

ADMINISTRATION/HANDLING

PO

- Give with food (decreases GI upset).

INDICATIONS/ROUTES/DOSAGE

TUBERCULOSIS

PO: ADULTS, ELDERLY, CHILDREN: 15–25 mg/kg/day as single dose or 50 mg/kg 2 times/wk. **Maximum:** 2.5 g/dose.

NONTUBERCULOSIS MYCOBACTERIUM

PO: ADULTS, ELDERLY, CHILDREN: 15 mg/kg/day. **Maximum:** 1 g/day.

DOSAGE IN RENAL IMPAIRMENT

Creatinine Clearance	Dosage Interval
10–50 ml/min	q24–36h
<10 ml/min	q48h

SIDE EFFECTS

OCCASIONAL: Acute gouty arthritis (chills, pain, swelling of joints with hot skin), confusion, abdominal pain, nausea, vomiting, anorexia, headache. **RARE:** Rash, fever, blurred vision, eye pain, red-green color blindness.

ADVERSE REACTIONS/ TOXIC EFFECTS

Optic neuritis (occurs more often with high dosage, long-term therapy), peripheral neuritis, thrombocytopenia, anaphylactoid reaction occur rarely.

NURSING IMPLICATIONS

BASELINE ASSESSMENT

Evaluate initial CBC, renal/hepatic test results.

INTERVENTION/EVALUATION

Assess for vision changes (altered color perception, decreased visual acuity may be first signs): Discontinue drug and notify physician immediately. Give with food if GI distress occurs. Monitor serum uric acid. Assess for hot/painful/swollen joints, esp. big toe, ankle, knee (gout). Report numbness, tingling, burning of extremities (peripheral neuritis).

PATIENT/FAMILY TEACHING

Do not skip doses; take for full length of therapy (may take months or years). Notify physician immediately of any visual problem (visual effects generally reversible with discontinuation of ethambutol, but in rare cases may take up to a year to disappear or may be permanent); promptly report swelling/pain of joints, numbness/tingling/burning of hands/feet.

ethosuximide

(Zarontin)

See Classification section under: Anticonvulsants

etidronate disodium

eh-**tye**-droe-nate

(Didronel)

Do not confuse with etidocaine, etomidate.

◆CLASSIFICATION

PHARMACOTHERAPEUTIC: Bisphosphonate. **CLINICAL:** Calcium regulator.

ACTION

Inhibits osteocystic osteolysis, decreases mineral release and matrix in bone. **Therapeutic Effect:** Decreases bone resorption.

USES

PO: Treatment of symptomatic Paget's disease of the bone, prevention/treatment of heterotopic ossification following hip replacement or due to spinal injury. **IV:** Treatment of hypercalcemia associated with malignant neoplasms inadequately managed by dietary modification, oral hydration; treatment of hypercalcemia of malignancy persisting after adequate hydration has been restored.

PRECAUTIONS

CONTRAINDICATIONS: Clinically overt osteomalacia. **CAUTIONS:** Those with restricted calcium, vitamin D intake, impaired renal function, hyperphosphatemia. **Pregnancy Category C** (parenteral). **Pregnancy Category B** (oral).

INTERACTIONS

DRUG: Antacids with **calcium, magnesium, aluminum,** foods with **calcium, mineral supplements** may decrease absorption. **HERBAL:** None known. **FOOD:** None known. **LAB VALUES:** None known.

AVAILABILITY (Rx)

TABLETS: 200 mg, 400 mg. **INJECTION:** 300-mg amps (50 mg/ml).

ADMINISTRATION/HANDLING

IV

Storage • Store at room temperature.

Reconstitution • Must dilute with at least 250 ml 0.9% NaCl or D_5W.

Rate of administration • Infuse over at least 2 hrs.

IV INCOMPATIBILITY

Do not mix with other medications.

INDICATIONS/ROUTES/DOSAGE

PAGET'S DISEASE

PO: ADULTS, ELDERLY: Initially, 5–10 mg/kg/day not to exceed 6 mos or 11–20 mg/kg/day not to exceed 3 mos. Repeat only after drug-free period of at least 90 days.

HETEROTOPIC OSSIFICATION (due to spinal cord injury)

PO: ADULTS, ELDERLY: 20 mg/kg/day for 2 wks; then 10 mg/kg/day for 10 wks.

HETEROTOPIC OSSIFICATION (complicating total hip replacement)

PO: ADULTS, ELDERLY: 20 mg/kg/day for 1 mo preop; follow with 20 mg/kg/day for 3 mos postop.

HYPERCALCEMIA ASSOCIATED WITH MALIGNANCY

IV: ADULTS, ELDERLY: 7.5 mg/kg/day for 3 days; retreatment no sooner than 7-day intervals between courses. Follow with oral therapy on day after last infusion (20 mg/kg/day for 30 days; may extend up to 90 days).

SIDE EFFECTS

FREQUENT: Nausea, diarrhea, continuing or more frequent bone pain in those with Paget's disease. **OCCASIONAL:** Bone fractures (esp. femur). **Parenteral:** Metallic, altered, loss of taste. **RARE:** Hypersensitivity reaction.

ADVERSE REACTIONS/ TOXIC EFFECTS

Nephrotoxicity (hematuria, dysuria, proteinuria) noted with parenteral route.

NURSING IMPLICATIONS

BASELINE ASSESSMENT

Obtain lab baselines, esp. electrolytes, renal function.

INTERVENTION/EVALUATION

Assess for diarrhea. Monitor electrolytes. Check I&O, BUN, creatinine in pts with impaired renal function. Evaluate pain in pts with Paget's disease.

PATIENT/FAMILY TEACHING

May take up to 3 mos for therapeutic response. Ensure milk, dairy products in diet for calcium, vitamin D. Take medication on empty stomach, 2 hrs after food, vitamins, antacids.

etodolac

eh-**toe**-doe-lack

(Apo-Etodolac ♣, Lodine, Lodine XL, Ultradol ♣)

Do not confuse with codeine, iodine.

CLASSIFICATION

PHARMACOTHERAPEUTIC: NSAID. **CLINICAL:** Nonsteroidal anti-inflammatory, analgesic (see p. 110C).

ACTION

Produces analgesic, anti-inflammatory effect by inhibiting prostaglandin synthesis. **Therapeutic Effect:** Reduces inflammatory response, intensity of pain stimulus reaching sensory nerve endings.

PHARMACOKINETICS

Onset	Peak	Duration
PO analgesic		
30 min	—	4–12 hrs

Completely absorbed from GI tract. Widely distributed. Protein binding: >99%. Metabolized in liver. Primarily excreted in urine. Not removed by hemodialysis. **Half-life:** 6–7 hrs.

USES

Acute and long-term treatment of osteoarthritis, management of pain, treatment of rheumatoid arthritis. **Unlabeled:** Treatment of acute gouty arthritis, vascular headache.

PRECAUTIONS

CONTRAINDICATIONS: Active peptic ulcer, GI ulceration, chronic inflammation of GI tract, GI bleeding disorders, history of hypersensitivity to aspirin/NSAIDs. **CAUTIONS:** Impaired renal/hepatic function, history of GI tract disease, predisposition to fluid retention.

LIFESPAN CONSIDERATIONS: Pregnancy/lactation: Unknown if drug crosses placenta or is distributed in breast milk. Avoid use during last trimester (may adversely affect fetal cardiovascular system: premature closure of ductus arteriosus). **Pregnancy Category C** (**D** if used in third trimester or near delivery). **Children:** Safety and efficacy not established. **Elderly:** GI bleeding, ulceration more likely to cause serious adverse effects. Age-related renal impairment may increase risk of liver/renal toxicity; decreased dosage recommended.

INTERACTIONS

DRUG: May increase effects of **oral anticoagulants, heparin, thrombolytics.** May decrease effect of **antihypertensives, diuretics. Salicylates, aspirin** may increase risk of GI side effects, bleeding. **Bone marrow depressants** may increase risk of hematologic reactions. May increase concentration, toxicity of **lithium.** May increase **methotrexate** toxicity. **Probenecid** may increase concentration. **HERBAL: Feverfew, Ginkgo biloba** may increase risk of bleeding. **FOOD:** None known. **LAB VALUES:** May increase bleeding time, creatinine, liver function tests. May decrease uric acid.

AVAILABILITY (Rx)

CAPSULES: 200 mg, 300 mg. **TABLETS:** 400 mg, 500 mg. **TABLETS: (extended-release):** 400 mg, 500 mg, 600 mg.

ADMINISTRATION/HANDLING

PO

• Do not crush or break capsules, extended-release capsules. • May give with food, milk, antacids if GI distress occurs.

INDICATIONS/ROUTES/DOSAGE

Alert: Reduce dosage in elderly; maximum dose for pts weighing <60 kg: 20 mg/kg.

OSTEOARTHRITIS

PO: ADULTS, ELDERLY: Initially, 800–1,200 mg/day in 2–4 divided doses. MAINTENANCE: 600–1,200 mg/day.

RHEUMATOID ARTHRITIS

PO: ADULTS, ELDERLY: Initially, 300 mg 2–3 times/day or 400–500 mg 2 times/day. MAINTENANCE: 600–1,200 mg/day.

ANALGESIA

PO: ADULTS, ELDERLY: 200–400 mg q6–8h as needed. **Maximum:** 1,200 mg/day.

SIDE EFFECTS

OCCASIONAL (3%–9%): Dizziness, headache, abdominal pain/cramps, bloated feeling, diarrhea, nausea, indigestion. **RARE (1%–3%):** Constipation, rash, itching, visual changes, ringing in ears.

ADVERSE REACTIONS/ TOXIC EFFECTS

Overdosage may result in acute renal failure. In those treated chronically, peptic ulcer, GI bleeding, gastritis, severe hepatic reaction (jaundice), nephrotoxicity (hematuria, dysuria, proteinuria), severe hypersensitivity reaction (bronchospasm, angiofacial edema) occur rarely.

NURSING IMPLICATIONS

BASELINE ASSESSMENT

Assess onset, type, location, duration of pain/inflammation. Inspect appearance of affected joints for immobility, deformities, skin condition.

INTERVENTION/EVALUATION

Monitor CBC, liver/renal function. Observe for bleeding/bruising. Evaluate for therapeutic response: relief of pain, stiffness, swelling; increase in joint mobility; reduced joint tenderness; improved grip strength.

PATIENT/FAMILY TEACHING

Swallow capsule whole; do not crush or chew. Avoid aspirin, alcohol during therapy (increases risk of GI bleeding). Report GI distress, visual disturbances, rash, edema, headache. Report any signs of bleeding. Take with food, milk, antacid if GI distress occurs. Use caution performing tasks that require alertness.

etoposide, VP-16

eh-**toe**-poe-side
(Etopophos, VePesid)
Do not confuse with Pepcid, Versed.

◆ CLASSIFICATION

PHARMACOTHERAPEUTIC: Epipodophyllotoxin. **CLINICAL:** Antineoplastic (see p. 72C).

ACTION

Induces single- and double-stranded breaks in DNA. Cell cycle–dependent and phase specific with maximum effect on S, G_2 phase of cell division. **Therapeutic Effect:** Inhibits or alters DNA synthesis.

PHARMACOKINETICS

Variably absorbed from GI tract. Rapidly distributed. Low concentrations in CSF. Protein binding: 97%. Metabolized in liver. Primarily excreted in urine. Not removed by hemodialysis. **Half-life:** 3–12 hrs.

USES

Treatment of refractory testicular tumors, small cell lung carcinoma. **Unlabeled:** Treatment of bladder carcinoma; Hodgkin's, non-Hodgkin's lymphoma; acute myelocytic leukemia; Ewing's sarcoma; AIDS-associated Kaposi's sarcoma.

PRECAUTIONS

CONTRAINDICATIONS: Pregnancy. **CAUTIONS:** Liver/renal impairment, bone marrow suppression.

LIFESPAN CONSIDERATIONS: Pregnancy/lactation: If possible, avoid use during pregnancy, esp. first trimester. May cause fetal harm. Breast-feeding not recommended. **Pregnancy Category D. Children:** Safety and efficacy not established. **Elderly:** Age-related renal impairment may require dosage adjustment.

INTERACTIONS

DRUG: Bone marrow depressants may increase bone marrow depression. **Live virus vaccines** may potentiate virus replication, increase vaccine side effects, decrease pt's antibody response to vaccine. **HERBAL:** None known. **FOOD:** None known. **LAB VALUES:** None known.

AVAILABILITY (Rx)

CAPSULES: 50 mg. **INJECTION:** 20 mg/ml. **INJECTION (water soluble). Etopophos:** 100 mg/ml.

E

ADMINISTRATION/HANDLING

Alert: Administer by slow IV infusion. Wear gloves when preparing solution. If powder/solution comes in contact with skin, wash immediately and thoroughly with soap, water. May be carcinogenic, mutagenic, or teratogenic. Handle with extreme care during preparation/administration.

PO

Storage • Refrigerate gelatin capsules.

IV

VEPESID

• Store injection at room temperature before dilution. • Concentrate for injection is clear, yellow. • Diluted solution is stable at room temperature for 96 hrs at 0.2 mg/ml, 48 hrs at 0.4 mg/ml. • Discard if crystallization occurs.

ETOPOPHOS

• Refrigerate vials. • Stable for 24 hrs after reconstitution.

Reconstitution

VEPESID

• Dilute each 100 mg (5 ml) with at least 250 ml D_5W or 0.9% NaCl to provide concentration of 0.4 mg/ml (500 ml for concentration of 0.2 mg/ml).

ETOPOPHOS

• Reconstitute each 100 mg with 5–10 ml Sterile Water for Injection, D_5W, or 0.9% NaCl to provide concentration of 20 mg/ml or 10 mg/ml, respectively. • May give without further dilution or further dilute to concentration as low as 0.1 mg/ml with 0.9% NaCl or D_5W.

Rate of Administration

VEPESID

• Infuse slowly, over 30–60 min (rapid IV may produce marked hypotension). • Monitor for anaphylactic reaction during infusion (chills, fever, dyspnea, sweating, lacrimation, sneezing, throat/back/chest pain).

ETOPOPHOS

• May give over as little as 5 min up to 210 min.

⊘ IV INCOMPATIBILITIES

Cefepime (Maxipime), filgrastim (Neupogen), idarubicin (Idamycin). **ETOPOPHOS:** amphotericin (Fungizone), cefepime (Maxipime), chlorpromazine (Thorazine), methylprednisolone (Solu-Medrol), prochlorperazine (Compazine).

IV COMPATIBILITIES

Carboplatin (Paraplatin), cisplatin (Platinol), cytarabine (Cytosar), daunorubicin (Cerubidine), doxorubicin (Adriamycin), granisetron (Kytril), mitoxantrone (Novatrone), ondansetron (Zofran).

ETOPOPHOS

Carboplatin (Paraplatin), cisplatin (Platinol), cytarabine (Cytosar), dacarbazine (DTIC-Dome), daunorubicin (Cerubidine), dexamethasone (Decadron), diphenydramine (Benadryl), doxorubicin (Adriamycin), granisetron (Kytril), magnesium sulfate, mannitol, mitoxantron (Novantrone), ondansetron (Zofran), potassium chloride.

INDICATIONS/ROUTES/DOSAGE

Alert: Dosage individualized based on clinical response, tolerance to adverse effects. Treatment repeated at 3- to 4-wk intervals.

REFRACTORY TESTICULAR TUMORS

IV: ADULTS: Combination therapy: 50–100 mg/m²/day on days 1 to 5 or 100 mg/m^2/day on days 1, 3, 5. Given q3–4 wks for 3–4 courses

SMALL CELL LUNG CARCINOMA

PO: ADULTS: 2 times IV dose rounded to nearest 50 mg. Given once daily for doses ≤400 mg or in divided doses for doses >400 mg.

IV: ADULTS: COMBINATION THERAPY: 35 mg/m^2 daily for 4 consecutive days up to 50 mg/m^2 daily for 5 consecutive days. Given q3–4 wks.

USUAL DOSE FOR CHILDREN

IV: 60–150 mg/m^2/day for 2–5 days q3–6wks.

SIDE EFFECTS

FREQUENT (43%–66%): Mild to moderate nausea/vomiting, alopecia. **OCCASIONAL (6%–13%):** Diarrhea, anorexia, stomatitis (redness/burning of oral mucous membranes, gum/tongue inflammation). **RARE (≤2%):** Hypotension, peripheral neuropathy.

ADVERSE REACTIONS/ TOXIC EFFECTS

Bone marrow depression manifested as hematologic toxicity (principally leukopenia, thrombocytopenia, anemia, and, to lesser extent, pancytopenia). Leukopenia occurs within 7–14 days after drug administration; thrombocytopenia occurs within 9–16 days after administration. Bone marrow recovery occurs by day 20. Hepatotoxicity occurs occasionally.

NURSING IMPLICATIONS

BASELINE ASSESSMENT

Obtain hematology tests prior to and at frequent intervals during therapy. Antiemetics readily control nausea, vomiting.

INTERVENTION/EVALUATION

Monitor Hgb, Hct, WBC, platelet count. Assess pattern of daily bowel activity/stool consistency. Monitor for hematologic toxicity (fever, sore throat, signs of local infection, unusual bruising/bleeding from any site), symptoms of anemia (excessive tiredness, weakness). Assess for paresthesias (peripheral neuropathy). Monitor for stomatitis (redness/burning of oral mucous membranes, gum/tongue inflammation).

PATIENT/FAMILY TEACHING

Alopecia is reversible, but new hair growth may have different color, texture. Do not have immunizations without physician's approval (drug lowers body's resistance). Avoid contact with those who have recently received live virus vaccine. Promptly report fever, sore throat, signs of local infection, unusual bruising/bleeding from any site.

Eulexin

see flutamide

Evista

see raloxifene

Execlon

see rivastigmine

exemestane

x-eh-**mess**-tane

(Aromasin)

◆CLASSIFICATION

PHARMACOTHERAPEUTIC: Hormone. **CLINICAL:** Antineoplastic (see p. 72C).

E

ACTION

An irreversible, steroidal aromatase inactivator (aromatase is the principal enzyme that converts androgens to estrogens in both premenopausal and postmenopausal women); acts as false substrate for aromatase enzyme; binds irreversibly to active site of enzyme, causing its inactivation. **Therapeutic Effect:** Lowers circulating estrogens in those with breast cancers in which tumor growth is estrogen dependent.

PHARMACOKINETICS

Rapidly absorbed following PO administration. Distributed extensively into tissues. Protein binding: 90%. Metabolized in liver; eliminated in urine and feces. **Half-life:** 24 hrs.

USES

Treatment of advanced breast cancer in postmenopausal women whose disease has progressed following tamoxifen therapy. **Unlabeled:** Prevention of prostate cancer.

PRECAUTIONS

CONTRAINDICATIONS: Hypersensitivity to exemestane. **CAUTIONS:** Do not give to premenopausal women.

LIFESPAN CONSIDERATIONS: Pregnancy/lactation: Indicated for postmenopausal women. **Pregnancy Category D. Children:** N/A. **Elderly:** No age-related precautions noted.

INTERACTIONS

DRUG: None known. **HERBAL:** None known. **FOOD:** None known. **LAB VALUES:** May increase SGOT (AST), SGPT (ALT), alkaline phosphatase.

AVAILABILITY (Rx)

TABLETS: 25 mg.

ADMINISTRATION/HANDLING

PO

- Give after a meal.

INDICATIONS/ROUTES/DOSAGE

BREAST CANCER

PO: ADULTS, ELDERLY: 25 mg once daily after a meal.

SIDE EFFECTS

FREQUENT (10%–22%): Fatigue, nausea, depression, hot flashes, pain, insomnia, anxiety, dyspnea. **OCCASIONAL (5%–8%):** Headache, dizziness, vomiting, edema (peripheral, leg), abdominal pain, anorexia, flulike symptoms, diaphoresis, constipation, hypertension. **RARE (4%):** Diarrhea.

ADVERSE REACTIONS/ TOXIC EFFECTS

None known.

NURSING IMPLICATIONS

INTERVENTION/EVALUATION

Monitor for onset of depression. Assess sleep pattern. Monitor for and assist with ambulation if dizziness occurs. Assess for headache. Offer antiemetic for nausea/vomiting.

PATIENT/FAMILY TEACHING

Notify physician if nausea, hot flashes become unmanageable. Avoid tasks that require alertness, motor skills until response to drug is established. Best taken after meals and at the same time each day.

ezetimibe

eh-**zeh**-tih-myb
(Zetia)

CLASSIFICATION

PHARMACOTHERAPEUTIC: Antihyperlipidemic. **CLINICAL:** Anticholesterol agent.

ACTION

Inhibits cholesterol absorption in the small intestine, leading to a decrease in the delivery of intestinal cholesterol to the liver. **Therapeutic Effect:** Reduces total cholesterol, LDL cholesterol, triglycerides; increases HDL cholesterol.

PHARMACOKINETICS

Well absorbed following PO administration. Protein binding: >90%. Metabolized in the small intestine and liver. Excreted by the kidneys and bile. **Half-life:** 22 hrs.

USES

Adjunct to diet therapy for reduction of elevated total cholesterol, LDL cholesterol, apolipoprotein B. Used in combination with HMG-CoA reductase inhibitors.

PRECAUTIONS

CONTRAINDICATIONS: Concurrent use of an HMG-CoA reductase inhibitor (atorvastatin, cerivastatin, fluvastatin, lovastatin, pravastatin, simvastatin) in pts with active liver disease, unexplained persistent elevations in serum transaminases, moderate or severe hepatic insufficiency. **CAUTIONS:** Diabetes, hypothyroidism, obstructive liver disease, chronic renal failure, hepatic function impairment.

LIFESPAN CONSIDERATIONS: Pregnancy/lactation: Unknown if drug crosses placenta or is distributed in breast milk. **Pregnancy Category C. Children:** Safety and efficacy not established in pts <10 yrs. **Elderly:** Age-related mild hepatic impairment may require dosage adjustment. Not recommended in pts with moderate or severe haptic impairment.

E

INTERACTIONS

DRUG: Aluminum and magnesium-containing antacids, fenofibrate, gemfibrozil, cyclosporine increases **ezetimibe** plasma concentration. **Cholestyramine** decreases drug effectiveness. **HERBAL:** None known. **FOOD:** None known. **LAB VALUES:** May increase SGOT (AST), SGPT (ALT), alkaline phosphatase, bilirubin.

AVAILABILITY (Rx)

TABLETS: 10 mg.

ADMINISTRATION/HANDLING

- Give without regard to food.

INDICATION/ROUTES/DOSAGE

HYPERCHOLESTEROLEMIA

PO: ADULTS, ELDERLY: Initially, 10 mg once daily, given with or without food.

COADMINISTRATION WITH BILE ACID SEQUESTRANTS

PO: ADULTS, ELDERLY: Dosing of ezetimibe should occur at least 2 hrs prior to or at least 4 hrs following administration of a bile acid dequestrant.

SIDE EFFECTS

OCCASIONAL (3%–4%): Back pain, diarrhea, arthralgia, sinusitis, abdominal pain. **RARE (2%):** Cough, pharyngitis, fatigue.

ADVERSE REACTIONS/ TOXIC EFFECTS

None known.

NURSING IMPLICATIONS

BASELINE ASSESSMENT

Obtain lipid cholesterol, triglycerides, liver function tests, including serum ALT, blood counts during initial therapy and periodically during treatment. Treatment should be discontinued if liver enzyme levels persist >3 times normal limit.

INTERVENTION/EVALUATION

Monitor daily bowel activity, stool consistency. Question pt for signs/symptoms of back pain, abdominal disturbances. Monitor cholesterol, triglyceride concentrations for therapeutic response.

PATIENT/FAMILY TEACHING

Periodic lab tests are essential part of therapy. Do not stop medication without consulting physician.

famciclovir

fam-**sigh**-klo-vir
(Famvir)

CLASSIFICATION

PHARMACOTHERAPEUTIC: Synthetic nucleoside. **CLINICAL:** Antiviral (see p. 59C).

ACTION

Inhibits viral DNA synthesis. **Therapeutic Effect:** Suppresses herpes simplex virus and varicella-zoster virus replication.

PHARMACOKINETICS

Rapidly, extensively absorbed following PO administration. Protein binding: 20%–25%. Rapidly metabolized to penciclovir by enzymes in gut wall, plasma, liver. Eliminated unchanged in urine. Removed by hemodialysis. **Half-life:** 2 hrs.

USES

Management of acute herpes zoster (shingles), treatment/suppression of recurrent genital herpes, treatment of recurrent mucocutaneous herpes simplex in HIV pts.

PRECAUTIONS

CONTRAINDICATIONS: None known. **CAUTIONS:** Renal/liver function impairment.

LIFESPAN CONSIDERATIONS: Pregnancy/lactation: Increase in mammary adenocarcinoma in animals. Unknown if excreted in breast milk. **Pregnancy Category B. Children:** Safety and efficacy not established. **Elderly:** Age-related renal function impairment may require dosage adjustment.

INTERACTIONS

DRUG: None known. **HERBAL:** None known. **FOOD:** None known. **LAB VALUES:** None known.

AVAILABILITY (Rx)

TABLETS: 125 mg, 250 mg, 500 mg.

ADMINISTRATION/HANDLING

PO

- Give without regard to meals.

INDICATIONS/ROUTES/DOSAGE

HERPES ZOSTER

PO: ADULTS: 500 mg q8h for 7 days.

RECURRENT GENITAL HERPES

PO: ADULTS: 125 mg twice daily for 5 days.

SUPPRESSION OF RECURRENT GENITAL HERPES

PO: ADULTS: 250 mg twice daily for up to 1 yr.

RECURRENT HERPES SIMPLEX

PO: ADULTS: 500 mg twice daily for 7 days.

DOSAGE IN RENAL IMPAIRMENT

Dosage based on creatinine clearance (ml/min):

Creatinine Clearance	Herpes Zoster	Genital Herpes
40–59	500 mg q12h	125 mg q12h
20–39	500 mg q24h	125 mg q24h
<20	250 mg q24h	125 mg q24h

HEMODIALYSIS PTS

PO: ADULTS: 250 mg (herpes zoster) or 125 mg (genital herpes) after each dialysis treatment.

SIDE EFFECTS

FREQUENT: Headache (23%), nausea (12%). **OCCASIONAL (2%–10%):** Dizziness, somnolence, numbness of feet, diarrhea, vomiting, constipation, decreased appetite, fatigue, fever, pharyngitis, sinusitis, pruritus. **RARE (<2%):** Inability to sleep, abdominal pain, dyspepsia, flatulence, back pain, arthralgia.

ADVERSE REACTIONS/ TOXIC EFFECTS

None known.

NURSING IMPLICATIONS

INTERVENTION/EVALUATION

Evaluate cutaneous lesions. Be alert to neurologic effects: headache, dizziness. Provide analgesics, comfort measures; esp. exhausting in elderly.

PATIENT/FAMILY TEACHING

Drink adequate fluids. Fingernails should be kept short, hands clean. Do not touch lesions with fingers to avoid spreading infection to new site. **Genital herpes:** Continue therapy for full length of treatment. Space doses evenly. Avoid sexual intercourse during duration of lesions to prevent infecting partner. Notify physician if lesions do not improve or recur.

famotidine

fah-**mow**-tih-deen

(Mylanta AR, Novo-Famotidine ✦ Pepcid, Pepcid AC, Pepcid RPD, Ulcidine ✦)

FIXED-COMBINATION(S)

Pepcid Complete: famotidine/calcium chloride/magnesium hydroxide (antacids): 10 mg/800 mg/165 mg.

◆CLASSIFICATION

PHARMACOTHERAPEUTIC: H_2 receptor antagonist. **CLINICAL:** Antiulcer, gastric acid secretion inhibitor (see p. 92C).

ACTION

Inhibits histamine action at H_2 receptors of parietal cells. **Therapeutic Effect:** Inhibits gastric acid secretion (fasting, nocturnal, or when stimulated by food, caffeine, insulin).

PHARMACOKINETICS

Onset	Peak	Duration
PO		
1 hr	1–4 hrs	10–12 hrs
IV		
1 hr	0.5–3 hrs	10–12 hrs

Rapidly, incompletely absorbed from GI tract. Protein binding: 15%–20%. Partially metabolized in liver. Primarily excreted in urine. Not removed by hemodialysis. **Half-life:** 2.5–3.5 hrs (half-life increased with impaired renal function).

USES

Short-term treatment of active duodenal ulcer. Prevention of duodenal ulcer recurrence. Treatment of active benign gastric ulcer, pathologic GI hypersecretory conditions. Short-term treatment of gastroesophageal reflux disease, including erosive esophagitis. OTC formulation for relief of heartburn, acid indigestion, sour stomach. **Unlabeled:** Prophylaxis for aspiration pneumonitis. Autism.

PRECAUTIONS

CONTRAINDICATIONS: None known. **CAUTIONS:** Impaired renal/hepatic function.

LIFESPAN CONSIDERATIONS: Pregnancy/lactation: Unknown if drug crosses placenta or is distributed in breast milk. **Pregnancy Category B. Children:** No age-related precautions noted. **Elderly:** Confusion more likely to occur, esp. in those with impaired renal/liver function.

INTERACTIONS

DRUG: Antacids may decrease absorption (do not give within ½–1 hr). May decrease absorption of **ketoconazole** (give at least 2 hrs after). **HERBAL:** None known. **FOOD:** None known. **LAB VALUES:** Interferes with skin tests using allergen extracts. May increase liver enzymes.

AVAILABILITY (Rx)

TABLETS: 10 mg (OTC), 20 mg, 40 mg. **TABLET (chewable):** 10 mg (OTC). **POWDER FOR ORAL SUSPENSION:** 40 mg/5 ml. **INJECTION:** 10 mg/ml, 20 mg/50 ml NaCl infusion.

ADMINISTRATION/HANDLING

PO

• Store tablets, suspension at room temperature. • Following reconstitution, oral suspension is stable for 30 days at room temperature. • Give without regard to meals. Best given after meals or at bedtime. • Shake suspension well before use. • Pepcid RPD dissolves under tongue; does not require water for dosing.

IV

Storage • Refrigerate unreconstituted vials. • IV solution appears clear, colorless. • After dilution, IV solution is stable for 48 hrs at room temperature.

Reconstitution • For IV push, dilute 20 mg with 5–10 ml 0.9% NaCl, D_5W, $D_{10}W$, lactated Ringer's, or 5% sodium bicarbonate. • For intermittent IV infusion (piggyback), dilute with 50–100 ml D_5W, or 0.9% NaCl.

Rate of administration • IV push given over at least 2 min. • Infuse piggyback over 15–30 min.

IV INCOMPATIBILITIES

Amphotericin B complex (Abelcet, Amphotec, AmBisome), cefepime (Maxipime), furosemide (Lasix), piperacillin/tazobactam (Zosyn).

IV COMPATIBILITIES

Calcium gluconate, dobutamine (Dobutrex), dopamine (Intropin), heparin, hydromorphone (Dilaudid), insulin (Regular), lidocaine, lorazepam (Ativan), magnesium sulfate, midazolam (Versed), morphine, nitroglycerin, norepinephrine (Levophed), potassium chloride, potassium phosphate, propofol (Diprivan).

INDICATIONS/ROUTES/DOSAGE

ACUTE THERAPY—DUODENAL ULCER

PO: ADULTS, ELDERLY: 40 mg at bedtime or 20 mg q12h. MAINTENANCE: 20 mg at bedtime. CHILDREN 1–6 YRS: 0.5 mg/kg/day. **Maximum:** 40 mg.

ACUTE THERAPY—BENIGN GASTRIC ULCER

PO: ADULTS, ELDERLY: 40 mg at bedtime.

GASTROESOPHAGEAL REFLUX DISEASE (GERD)

PO: ADULTS, ELDERLY: 20 mg 2 times/day up to 6 wks; 20–40 mg 2 times/day up to 12 wks in pts with esophagitis (including erosions, ulcerations). CHILDREN 1–16 YRS: 1 mg/kg/day in 2 divided doses. **Maximum:** 80 mg/day.

PATHOLOGIC HYPERSECRETORY CONDITIONS

PO: ADULTS, ELDERLY: Initially, 20 mg q6h up to 160 mg q6h.

ACID INDIGESTION, HEARTBURN, SOUR STOMACH

PO: ADULTS, ELDERLY: 10 mg 15–60 min before eating. **Maximum:** 2 tablets/day.

USUAL PARENTERAL DOSAGE

IV: ADULTS, ELDERLY: 20 mg q12h. CHILDREN: 0.25 mg/kg q12h. **Maximum:** 40 mg/day.

DOSAGE IN RENAL IMPAIRMENT

Creatinine Clearance (ml/min)	Dosing Frequency
10–50	q24h
<10	q36–48h

SIDE EFFECTS

OCCASIONAL (5%): Headache. **RARE (≤2%):** Constipation, diarrhea, dizziness.

ADVERSE REACTIONS/ TOXIC EFFECTS

None known.

NURSING IMPLICATIONS

INTERVENTION/EVALUATION

Monitor daily bowel activity/stool consistency. Monitor for diarrhea/constipation, headache.

PATIENT/FAMILY TEACHING

May take without regard to meals or antacids. Report headache. Avoid excessive amounts of coffee, aspirin. If symptoms of heartburn, acid indigestion, sour stomach persist with medication, consult physician.

Famvir

see famciclovir

Faslodex

see fulvestrant

felodipine

feh-**low**-dih-peen
(Plendil, Renedil✱)

Do not confuse with pindolol, Pletal, Prinivil.

FIXED-COMBINATION(S)

Lexxel: felodipine/enalapril (ACE inhibitor): 2.5 mg/5 mg; 5 mg/5 mg.

◆CLASSIFICATION

PHARMACOTHERAPEUTIC: Calcium channel blocker. **CLINICAL:** Antihypertensive, antianginal (see p. 67C).

ACTION

Inhibits calcium movement across cardiac, vascular smooth muscle. Potent peripheral vasodilator (does not depress SA, AV nodes). **Therapeutic Effect:** Increases myocardial contractility, heart rate, cardiac output; decreases peripheral vascular resistance, B/P.

PHARMACOKINETICS

Onset	Peak	Duration
PO		
2–5 hrs	—	—

Rapidly, completely absorbed from GI tract. Protein binding: >99%. Undergoes first-pass metabolism in liver. Metabolized in liver. Primarily excreted in urine. Not removed by hemodialysis. **Half-life:** 11–16 hrs.

USES

Management of hypertension. May be used alone or with other antihypertensives. **Unlabeled:** Treatment of chronic angina pectoris, Raynaud's phenomena, CHF.

PRECAUTIONS

CONTRAINDICATIONS: None known. **CAUTIONS:** Severe left ventricular dysfunction, CHF, liver/renal impairment, hypertrophic cardiomyopathy, edema, concomitant administration with beta-blockers/digoxin.

F

LIFESPAN CONSIDERATIONS: Pregnancy/lactation: Unknown if drug crosses placenta or is distributed in breast milk. **Pregnancy Category C. Children:** Safety and efficacy not established. **Elderly:** May experience greater hypotension response. Constipation may be more problematic.

INTERACTIONS

DRUG: Beta-blockers may have additive effect. May increase **digoxin** concentration. **Procainamide, quinidine** may increase risk of QT interval prolongation. **Erythromycin** may increase concentration/toxicity. **Hypokalemia-producing agents** may increase risk of arrhythmias. **HERBAL: DHEA** may increase concentrations. **FOOD: Grapefruit/grapefruit juice** may increase absorption, concentrations. **LAB VALUES:** None known.

AVAILABILITY (Rx)

TABLETS (extended-release): 2.5 mg, 5 mg, 10 mg.

ADMINISTRATION/HANDLING

PO

• Give without regard to food. • Do not crush or break tablets.

INDICATIONS/ROUTES/DOSAGE

HYPERTENSION

PO: ADULTS: Initially, 5 mg/day as single dose. ELDERLY, PTS WITH IMPAIRED LIVER FUNCTION: Initially, 2.5 mg/day. Adjust dosage at no less than 2-wk intervals. MAINTENANCE: 2.5–10 mg/day.

SIDE EFFECTS

FREQUENT (18%–22%): Headache, peripheral edema. **OCCASIONAL (4%–6%):** Flushing, respiratory infection, dizziness, lightheadedness, asthenia (loss of strength, weakness). **RARE (<3%):** Paresthesia, abdominal discomfort, nervousness, muscle cramping, cough, diarrhea, constipation.

ADVERSE REACTIONS/ TOXIC EFFECTS

Overdosage produces nausea, drowsiness, confusion, slurred speech, hypotension, bradycardia.

NURSING IMPLICATIONS

BASELINE ASSESSMENT

Assess B/P, apical pulse immediately prior to drug administration (if pulse is ≤60/min or systolic B/P is <90 mm Hg, withhold medication, contact physician).

INTERVENTION/EVALUATION

Assist with ambulation if lightheadedness, dizziness occur. Assess for peripheral edema behind media/malleolus (sacral area in bedridden pts). Monitor pulse rate for bradycardia. Assess skin for flushing. Monitor liver enzyme tests. Question for headache, asthenia.

PATIENT/FAMILY TEACHING

Do not abruptly discontinue medication. Compliance with therapy regimen is essential to control hypertension. To avoid hypotensive effect, rise slowly from lying to sitting position. Wait momentarily before standing. Avoid tasks that require alertness, motor skills until response to drug is established. Contact physician/nurse if irregular heartbeat, shortness of breath, pronounced dizziness, nausea occurs. Swallow whole; do not crush or chew. Avoid grapefruit juice.

fenofibrate

fen-oh-**figh**-brate
(Apo-Fenofibrate ✤, Tricor)

◆CLASSIFICATION

CLINICAL: Antihyperlipidemic (see p. 51C).

ACTION

Enhances synthesis of lipoprotein lipase (VLDL). **Therapeutic Effect:** Increases VLDL catabolism, reduces total plasma triglycerides.

PHARMACOKINETICS

Well absorbed from GI tract. Absorption increased when given with food. Protein binding: 99%. Rapidly metabolized in liver to active metabolite. Excreted primarily in urine, lesser amount in feces. Not removed by hemodialysis. **Half-life:** 20 hrs.

USES

Adjunct to diet therapy in adult pts with very high serum triglyceride levels who are at risk of pancreatitis and who do not respond adequately to a determined dietary effort to control triglyceride levels. Increases HDL.

PRECAUTIONS

CONTRAINDICATIONS: Hypersensitivity to fenofibrate, severe renal/hepatic dysfunction (including primary biliary cirrhosis, unexplained persistent liver function abnormality), gallbladder disease. **CAUTIONS:** Anticoagulant therapy, history of liver disease, substantial alcohol consumption.

LIFESPAN CONSIDERATIONS: Pregnancy/lactation: Safety in pregnancy not established. Avoid use in nursing mothers. **Pregnancy Category C. Children:** Safety and efficacy not established. **Elderly:** No age-related precautions noted.

INTERACTIONS

DRUG: Potentiates effects of **anticoagulants.** Concurrent administration with **cyclosporine** increases risk of nephrotoxicity. Increased risk of severe myopathy, rhabdomyolysis, acute renal failure may occur with **HMG-CoA reductase inhibitors. Bile acid sequestrants** impede **fenofibrate** absorption (give fenofibrate 1 hr prior to or 4–6 hrs following bile acid sequestrant administration). **HERBAL:** None known. **FOOD:** Food increases drug absorption. **LAB VALUES:** May increase serum transaminase (SGOT [AST], SGPT [ALT]), creatinine kinase (CK), blood urea levels. May decrease Hgb, Hct, WBC, uric acid.

AVAILABILITY (Rx)

CAPSULES: 67 mg, 134 mg, 200 mg. **TABLETS:** 54 mg, 160 mg.

ADMINISTRATION/HANDLING

PO

- Give with meals.

INDICATIONS/ROUTES/DOSAGE

HYPERTRIGLYCERIDEMIA

PO: ADULTS, ELDERLY: **Capsule:** Initially, 67 mg/day. May increase to 200 mg/day. **Tablet:** Initially, 54 mg/day. May increase to 160 mg/day.

HYPERCHOLESTEROLEMIA

PO: ADULTS, ELDERLY: **Capsule:** 200 mg/day with meals. **Tablet:** 160 mg/day with meals.

SIDE EFFECTS

FREQUENT (4%–8%): Pain, rash, headache, asthenia/fatigue, flu syndrome, dyspepsia, nausea/vomiting, rhinitis. **OCCA-**

SIONAL (2%–3%): Diarrhea, abdominal pain, constipation, flatulence, arthralgia, decreased libido, dizziness, pruritus. **RARE (<2%):** Increased appetite, insomnia, polyuria, cough, blurred vision, eye floaters, earache.

ADVERSE REACTIONS/ TOXIC EFFECTS

May increase cholesterol excretion into bile, leading to cholelithiasis. Pancreatitis, hepatitis, thrombocytopenia, agranulocytosis occur rarely.

NURSING IMPLICATIONS

BASELINE ASSESSMENT

Obtain lipid cholesterol, triglycerides, liver function tests (including serum SGPT [ALT]), blood counts during initial therapy and periodically during treatment. Treatment should be discontinued if liver enzyme levels persist >3 times normal limit.

INTERVENTION/EVALUATION

For pts on concurrent therapy with HMG-CoA reductase inhibitors, monitor for complaints of myopathy (muscle pain, weakness). Monitor serum creatine kinase levels. Monitor cholesterol, triglyceride concentrations for therapeutic response.

PATIENT/FAMILY TEACHING

Take with food. Inform physician if diarrhea, constipation, nausea becomes severe. Report skin rash/irritation, insomnia, muscle pain, tremors/dizziness.

fenoldopam

phen-**ole**-doe-pam
(Corlopam)

CLASSIFICATION

PHARMACOTHERAPEUTIC: Vasodilator (dopamine receptor agonist). **CLINICAL:** Antihypertensive.

ACTION

Rapid-acting vasodilator. An agonist for D_1-like dopamine receptor, produces vasodilation in coronary, renal, mesenteric, peripheral arteries. **Therapeutic Effect:** Reduces systolic, diastolic B/P; increases heart rate.

PHARMACOKINETICS

After IV administration, metabolized in the liver. Primarily excreted in urine. Unknown if removed by hemodialysis. **Half-life:** Approx. 5 min.

USES

Short-term (≤48 hrs) management of severe hypertension when rapid, but quickly reversible, emergency reduction of B/P is clinically indicated, including malignant hypertension with deteriorating end-organ function.

PRECAUTIONS

CONTRAINDICATIONS: None known. **CAUTIONS:** Glaucoma, intraocular hypertension, tachycardia, hypotension, hypokalemia, sulfite sensitivity.

LIFESPAN CONSIDERATIONS: Pregnancy/lactation: Unknown if distributed in breast milk. **Pregnancy Category B. Children:** Safety and efficacy not established. **Elderly:** No age-related precautions noted.

INTERACTIONS

DRUG: Concurrent use of **beta-blockers** may produce excessive hypotension. **HERBAL:** None known. **FOOD:** None known. **LAB VALUES:** May elevate BUN, glucose, transaminase, LDH. May decrease potassium.

AVAILABILITY (Rx)

INJECTION: 10 mg/ml.

ADMINISTRATION/HANDLING

Alert: Must give by continuous IV infusion, not as a bolus injection.

IV

Storage • Store ampoules at room temperature. • Diluted solution is stable for 24 hrs. Discard any solution not used within 24 hrs.

Reconstitution • Each 10 mg (1 ml) must be diluted with 250 ml 0.9% NaCl or D_5W to provide a concentration of 40 mcg/ml.

Rate of administration • Administer as IV infusion at initial rate of 0.1 mcg/kg/min. • Use infusion pump.

IV INCOMPATIBILITIES

Do not mix with any other medication. Specific IV incompatibilities not available.

INDICATIONS/ROUTES/DOSAGE

HYPERTENSION

IV infusion (continuous): ADULTS: Initially, 0.1 mcg/kg/min. **Maximum:** 1.7 mcg/kg/min. Titrate dose up or down in increments of 0.05–0.1 mcg/kg/min no more frequently than q15min. May discontinue gradually or abruptly.

SIDE EFFECTS

Alert: Avoid beta-blockers (may cause unexpected hypotension).

OCCASIONAL: Headache (7%), flushing (3%), nausea (4%), hypotension (2%). **RARE (≤2%):** Nervousness/anxiety, vomiting, constipation, nasal congestion, diaphoresis, back pain.

ADVERSE REACTIONS/TOXIC EFFECTS

Excessive hypotension occurs occasionally; B/P must be monitored diligently during infusion. Substantial tachycardia may lead to ischemic cardiac events, worsened heart failure. Allergic-type reactions, including anaphylaxis and life-threatening asthmatic exacerbation in those with sulfite sensitivity.

NURSING IMPLICATIONS

BASELINE ASSESSMENT

Determine initial B/P, apical pulse. It is essential to diligently monitor B/P, EKG during infusion to avoid hypotension and too rapid decrease of B/P. Assess medication history (esp. beta-blockers). Obtain baseline serum electrolytes, particularly potassium, and periodically thereafter during infusion. Question asthmatic pts for history of sulfite sensitivity. Check with physician for desired B/P range level.

INTERVENTION/EVALUATION

Monitor rate of infusion frequently. Monitor EKG for tachycardia (may lead to ischemic heart disease, MI, angina, extrasystoles, worsening heart failure). Monitor closely for symptomatic hypotension.

fenoprofen calcium

fen-oh-**pro**-fen

(Nalfon)

Do not confuse with Naldecon.

◆CLASSIFICATION

PHARMACOTHERAPEUTIC: NSAID. **CLINICAL:** Nonsteroidal anti-inflammatory, analgesic, antigout, vascular headache prophylactic/suppressant (see p. 110C).

ACTION

Produces analgesic, anti-inflammatory effect by inhibiting prostaglandin synthesis. **Therapeutic Effect:** Reduces inflammatory response, intensity of pain stimulus reaching sensory nerve endings.

USES

Treatment of acute or long-term mild to moderate pain, symptomatic treatment of acute and/or chronic rheumatoid arthritis, osteoarthritis. **Unlabeled:** Treatment of vascular headaches, ankylosing spondylitis, psoriatic arthritis.

F

PRECAUTIONS

CONTRAINDICATIONS: Active peptic ulcer, GI ulceration, chronic inflammation of GI tract, GI bleeding disorders, history of hypersensitivity to aspirin/NSAIDs, history of significantly impaired renal function. **CAUTIONS:** Impaired renal/hepatic function, history of GI tract diseases, predisposition to fluid retention. **Pregnancy Category B** (**D** if used in third trimester or near delivery).

INTERACTIONS

DRUG: May increase effects of **oral anticoagulants, heparin, thrombolytics.** May decrease effect of **antihypertensives, diuretics. Salicylates, aspirin** may increase risk of GI side effects, bleeding. **Bone marrow depressants** may increase risk of hematologic reactions. May increase concentration, toxicity of **lithium.** May increase **methotrexate** toxicity. **Probenecid** may increase concentrations. **HERBAL:** None known. **FOOD:** None known. **LAB VALUES:** May increase serum transaminase, LDH, alkaline phosphatase, BUN, creatinine, potassium, glucose, protein, bleeding time.

AVAILABILITY (Rx)

CAPSULES: 200 mg, 300 mg. **TABLETS:** 600 mg.

INDICATIONS/ROUTES/DOSAGE

Alert: Do not exceed 3.2 g/day.

MILD TO MODERATE PAIN

PO: ADULTS, ELDERLY: 200 mg q4–6h as needed.

RHEUMATOID ARTHRITIS, OSTEOARTHRITIS

PO: ADULTS, ELDERLY: 300–600 mg 3–4 times/day.

SIDE EFFECTS

FREQUENT (3%–9%): Headache, somnolence/drowsiness, dyspepsia (heartburn, indigestion, epigastric pain), nausea, vomiting, constipation. **OCCASIONAL (1%–2%):** Dizziness, pruritus, nervousness, asthenia (loss of strength), diarrhea, abdominal cramps, flatulence, tinnitus, blurred vision, peripheral edema/fluid retention.

ADVERSE REACTIONS/ TOXIC EFFECTS

Overdosage may result in acute hypotension, tachycardia. Peptic ulcer, GI bleeding, nephrotoxicity (dysuria, cystitis, hematuria, proteinuria, nephrotic syndrome), gastritis, severe hepatic reaction (cholestasis, jaundice), severe hypersensitivity reaction (bronchospasm, angiofacial edema) occur rarely.

NURSING IMPLICATIONS

BASELINE ASSESSMENT

Assess onset, type, location, duration of pain/inflammation. Inspect appearance of affected joints for immobility, deformities, skin condition.

INTERVENTION/EVALUATION

Assist with ambulation if somnolence/drowsiness/dizziness occurs. Monitor for evidence of dyspepsia. Monitor pattern of daily bowel activity, stool consistency. Check behind medial malleolus for fluid retention (usually first area noted). Evaluate for therapeutic response: relief of pain, stiffness, swelling; increase in joint mobility; reduced joint tenderness; improved grip strength.

PATIENT/FAMILY TEACHING

Swallow capsule whole; do not crush or chew. Avoid tasks that require alertness, motor skills until response to drug is established. If GI upset occurs, take with food, milk. Avoid aspirin, alcohol during therapy (increases risk of GI bleeding).

fentanyl

fen-**tah**-nil

(Actig, Duragesic, Sublimaze)

Do not confuse with alfentanil.

CLASSIFICATION

PHARMACOTHERAPEUTIC: Opioid, narcotic agonist **(Schedule II). CLINICAL:** Analgesic (see p. 120C).

ACTION

Binds at opiate receptor sites within CNS, reducing stimuli from sensory nerve endings. **Therapeutic Effect:** Increases pain threshold, alters pain reception, inhibits ascending pain pathways.

PHARMACOKINETICS

Onset	Peak	Duration
IM		
7–15 min	20–30 min	1–2 hrs
IV		
1–2 min	3–5 min	0.5–1 hr
Transdermal		
6–8 hrs	24 hrs	72 hrs
Transmucosal		
5–15 min	20–30 min	1–2 hrs

Well absorbed after topical, IM administration. Transmucosal absorbed through mucosal tissue of mouth, GI tract. Protein binding: 80%–85%. Metabolized in liver. Primarily eliminated via biliary system. **Half-life:** IV: 2–4 hrs. Transdermal: 17 hrs. Transmucosal: 6.6 hrs.

USES

For sedation, relief of pain, preop medication; adjunct to general or regional anesthesia. Management of chronic pain *(transdermal)*. **Actig:** Treatment breakthrough for pain in chronic cancer or AIDS-related pain.

PRECAUTIONS

CONTRAINDICATIONS: Increased intracranial pressure, severe respiratory depression, severe renal/liver impairment. **CAUTIONS:** Bradycardia; renal, liver, respiratory disease; head injuries; impaired consciousness; use of MAOI within 14 days; transdermal not recommended in those <12 yrs or <18 yrs and <50 kg.

LIFESPAN CONSIDERATIONS: Pregnancy/lactation: Readily crosses placenta. Unknown if distributed in breast milk. May prolong labor if administered in latent phase of first stage of labor or before cervical dilation of 4–5 cm has occurred. Respiratory depression may occur in neonate if mother received opiates during labor. **Pregnancy Category C (D** if used for prolonged periods or at high dosages at term). **Children:** PATCH: Safety and efficacy not established in those <12 yrs. Neonates more susceptible to respiratory depressant effects. **Elderly:** May be more susceptible to respiratory depressant effects. Age-related renal impairment may require dosage adjustment.

INTERACTIONS

DRUG: Benzodiazepines may increase risk of hypotension, respiratory depression. **Buprenorphine** may decrease effect. **CNS depressants** may increase respiratory depression, hypotension. **HERBAL:** None known. **FOOD:** None known. **LAB VALUES:** May increase amylase, lipase plasma concentrations.

AVAILABILITY (Rx)

INJECTION: 50 mcg/ml. **TRANSDERMAL PATCH:** 25 mcg/hr, 50 mcg/hr, 75 mcg/hr, 100 mcg/hr. **LOZENGES:** 200 mcg, 400 mcg, 600 mcg, 800 mcg, 1,200 mcg, 1,600 mcg.

F

ADMINISTRATION/HANDLING

IV

Storage • Store parenteral form at room temperature.

Rate of administration • For initial anesthesia induction dosage, give small amount, via tuberculin syringe. • Give by slow IV injection (over 1–2 min). • Too rapid IV increases risk of severe adverse reactions (skeletal, thoracic muscle rigidity resulting in apnea, laryngospasm, bronchospasm, peripheral circulatory collapse, anaphylactoid effects, cardiac arrest). • Opiate antagonist (naloxone) should be readily available.

TRANSDERMAL

• Apply to nonhairy area of intact skin of upper torso. • Use flat, nonirritated site. • Firmly press evenly for 10–20 sec, ensuring adhesion is in full contact with skin and edges are completely sealed. • Use only water to cleanse site before application (soaps, oils, etc., may irritate skin). • Rotate sites of application. • Used patches are carefully folded so that system adheres to itself; discard in toilet.

TRANSMUCOSAL

• Suck lozenge vigorously.

∅ IV INCOMPATIBILITY

Phenytoin (Dilantin).

IV COMPATIBILITIES

Atropine, bupivacaine (Marcaine, Sensorcaine), clonidine (Duraclon), diltiazem (Cardizem), diphenhydramine (Benadryl), dobutamine (Dobutrex), dopamine (Intropin), droperidol (Inapsine), heparin, hydromorphone (Dilaudid), ketorolac (Toradol), lorazepam (Ativan), metoclopramide (Reglan), midazolam (Versed), milrinone (Primacor), morphine, nitroglycerin, norepinephrine (Levophed), ondansetrone (Zofran), potassium chloride, propofol (Diprivan).

INDICATIONS/ROUTES/DOSAGE

SEDATION (minor procedures/analgesia)

IM/IV: ADULTS, ELDERLY, CHILDREN >12 YRS: 0.5–1 mcg/kg/dose; may repeat after 30–60 min. CHILDREN 1–12 YRS: 1–2 mcg/kg/dose. CHILDREN <1 YR: 1–4 mcg/kg/dose.

PREOP SEDATION, ADJUNCT REGIONAL ANESTHESIA, POSTOP PAIN

IM/IV: ADULTS, ELDERLY, CHILDREN >12 YRS: 50–100 mcg/dose.

ADJUNCT TO GENERAL ANESTHESIA

IV: ADULTS, ELDERLY, CHILDREN >12 YRS: 2–50 mcg/kg.

TRANSDERMAL DOSE

ADULTS, ELDERLY, CHILDREN >12 YRS: Initially, 25 mcg/hr system. May increase after 3 days.

TRANSMUCOSAL DOSE

ADULTS, CHILDREN: 200–400 mcg for breakthrough cancer pain.

USUAL EPIDURAL DOSE

Alert: May be combined with local anesthetic (e.g., bupivacaine).

ADULTS, ELDERLY: Bolus of 100 mcg, then continuous infusion rate of 4–12 ml/hr of a 10 mcg/ml concentration.

CONTINUOUS ANALGESIA

IV: ADULTS, ELDERLY, CHILDREN 1–12 YRS: Bolus of 1–2 mcg/kg, then 1 mcg/kg/hr. RANGE: 1–5 mcg/kg/hr. CHILDREN <1 YR: Bolus of 1–2 mcg/kg, then 0.5–1 mcg/kg/hr.

USUAL TRANSMUCOSAL DOSAGE

Transmucosal: ADULTS, CHILDREN: 200–400 mcg for breakthrough cancer pain.

DOSAGE IN RENAL IMPAIRMENT

Creatinine Clearance	Dosage
10–50 ml/min	75% of dose
<10 ml/min	50% of dose

SIDE EFFECTS

FREQUENT: Transdermal (3%–10%): Headache, itching skin, nausea, vomiting, sweating, difficulty breathing, confusion, dizziness, drowsiness, diarrhea, constipation, decreased appetite. **IV:** Postop drowsiness, nausea, vomiting. **OCCASIONAL: Transdermal (1%–3%):** Chest pain, irregular heartbeat, redness/itching/swelling/tingling/burning of skin, fainting, agitation. **IV:** Postop confusion, blurred vision, chills, orthostatic hypotension, constipation, difficulty urinating.

ADVERSE REACTIONS/ TOXIC EFFECTS

Overdosage or too rapid IV results in severe respiratory depression, skeletal/thoracic muscle rigidity resulting in apnea, laryngospasm, bronchospasm, cold/clammy skin, cyanosis, coma. Tolerance to analgesic effect may occur with repeated use.

NURSING IMPLICATIONS

BASELINE ASSESSMENT

Resuscitative equipment, opiate antagonist (naloxone 0.5 mcg/kg) must be available. Establish baseline B/P, respirations. Assess type, location, intensity, duration of pain.

INTERVENTION/EVALUATION

Assist with ambulation. Encourage pt to turn, cough, deep breathe q2h. Monitor respiratory rate, B/P, heart rate, oxygen saturation. Assess for relief of pain.

PATIENT/FAMILY TEACHING

Avoid alcohol; do not take other medications without consulting physician. Do not drive, perform other activities requiring alertness, coordination. Teach pt proper transdermal application. Use as directed to avoid overdosage; potential for physical dependence with prolonged use. After long-term use, must be discontinued slowly.

F

Feosol

see ferrous sulfate

Fergon

see ferrous gluconate

Fer-In-Sol

see ferrous sulfate

ferrous fumarate

fair-us **fume**-ah-rate
(Femiron, Feostat, Palafer✤)

ferrous gluconate

fair-us **glue**-kuh-nate
(Apo-Ferrous Gluconate✤, Fergon, Ferralet, Simron)

ferrous sulfate

fair-us **sul**-fate
(Apo-Ferrous Sulfate✤, Feosol, Fer-In-Sol, Slow-Fe)

F

FIXED-COMBINATION(S)

Ferro-Sequels: ferrous fumarate/ docusate (stool softener): 150 mg/ 100 mg.

◆ CLASSIFICATION

PHARMACOTHERAPEUTIC: Enzymatic mineral. **CLINICAL:** Iron preparation (see p. 93C).

ACTION

Essential component in formation of Hgb, myoglobin, enzymes. **Therapeutic Effect:** Necessary for effective erythropoiesis, transport/utilization of O_2.

PHARMACOKINETICS

Absorbed in duodenum, upper jejunum; 10% absorbed in those with normal iron stores, increased to 20%–30% in those with inadequate iron stores. Primarily bound to serum transferrin. Excreted in urine, sweat, sloughing of intestinal mucosa, menses. **Half-life:** 6 hrs.

USES

Prevention/treatment of iron deficiency anemia due to inadequate diet, malabsorption, pregnancy, blood loss.

PRECAUTIONS

CONTRAINDICATIONS: Hemochromatosis, hemosiderosis, hemolytic anemias, peptic ulcer, regional enteritis, ulcerative colitis. **CAUTIONS:** Bronchial asthma, iron hypersensitivity.

LIFESPAN CONSIDERATIONS: Pregnancy/lactation: Crosses placenta. Excreted in breast milk. **Pregnancy Category A. Children/elderly:** No age-related precautions noted.

INTERACTIONS

DRUG: **Antacids, calcium supplements, pancreatin, pancrelipase** may decrease absorption. May decrease absorption of **quinolones, etidronate, tetracyclines.** **HERBAL:** None known. **FOOD:** None known. **LAB VALUES:** May increase bilirubin. May decrease calcium. May obscure occult blood in stools.

AVAILABILITY (OTC)

FERROUS FUMARATE: **TABLETS:** 63 mg, 195 mg, 200 mg, 324 mg, 350 mg. **TABLETS (chewable):** 100 mg. **CAPSULES (controlled-release):** 325 mg. **SUSPENSION:** 100 mg/5 ml. **ORAL DROPS:** 45 mg/0.6 ml.

FERROUS GLUCONATE: **TABLETS:** 300 mg, 320 mg. **TABLETS (sustained-release):** 320 mg.

FERROUS SULFATE: **TABLETS:** 195 mg, 300 mg, 324 mg. **CAPSULES:** 250 mg. **TABLETS (timed-release):** 325 mg. **SYRUP:** 90 mg/5 ml. **ELIXIR:** 220 mg/5 ml. **ORAL DROPS:** 125 mg/ml.

FERROUS SULFATE (exsiccated): **TABLETS:** 200 mg. **CAPSULES:** 190 mg. **CAPSULES (timed-release):** 159 mg, 250 mg. **TABLETS (slow-release):** 160 mg.

ADMINISTRATION/HANDLING

PO

• Store all forms (tablets, capsules, suspension, drops) at room temperature. • Ideally, give between meals with water but may give with meals if GI discomfort occurs. • Transient staining of mucous membranes, teeth will occur with liquid iron preparation. To avoid this, place liquid on back of tongue with dropper or straw. • Avoid simultaneous administration of antacids or tetracycline. • Do not crush sustained-release preparations.

INDICATIONS/ROUTES/DOSAGE

Alert: Dosage expressed in terms of elemental iron. Elemental iron content: ferrous fumarate: 33% (99 mg iron/300 mg tablet); ferrous gluconate: 11.6% (35 mg iron/300 mg tablet); ferrous sulfate: 20% (60 mg iron/300 mg tablet).

DEFICIENCY

PO: ADULTS, ELDERLY: 2–3 mg/kg/day or 50–100 mg elemental iron 2 times/day up to 100 mg 4 times/day. CHILDREN: 3 mg/kg/day elemental iron in 1–3 divided doses.

PROPHYLAXIS

PO: ADULTS, ELDERLY: 60–100 mg elemental iron/day. CHILDREN: 1–2 mg/kg/day elemental iron. **Maximum:** 15 mg elemental iron/day.

SIDE EFFECTS

OCCASIONAL: Mild, transient nausea. **RARE:** Heartburn, anorexia, constipation, diarrhea.

ADVERSE REACTIONS/ TOXIC EFFECTS

Large doses may aggravate existing GI tract disease (peptic ulcer, regional enteritis, ulcerative colitis). Severe iron poisoning occurs mostly in children and is manifested as vomiting, severe abdominal pain, diarrhea, dehydration, followed by hyperventilation, pallor/cyanosis, cardiovascular collapse.

NURSING IMPLICATIONS

BASELINE ASSESSMENT

To prevent mucous membrane and teeth staining with liquid preparation, use dropper/straw and allow solution to drop on back of tongue. Eggs, milk inhibit absorption.

INTERVENTION/EVALUATION

Monitor serum iron, total iron-binding capacity, reticulocyte count, Hgb, ferritin. Monitor daily pattern of bowel activity, stool consistency. Assess for clinical improvement, record relief of iron deficiency symptoms (fatigue, irritability, pallor, paresthesia of extremities, headache).

PATIENT/FAMILY TEACHING

Expect stools to darken in color. If GI discomfort occurs, take after meals or with food. Do not take within 2 hrs of antacids (prevents absorption).

feverfew

Also known as bachelor's button, featherfew, midsummer daisy, Santa Maria

CLASSIFICATION

HERBAL.

ACTION

Exact mechanism unknown. May inhibit platelet aggregation, serotonin release from platelets, leukocytes. Also inhibits/blocks prostaglandin synthesis. **Effect:** Reduces pain intensity, vomiting, noise sensitivity with severe migraine headaches.

USES

Fever, headache, prevention of migraine and menstrual irregularities, arthritis, psoriasis, allergies, asthma, vertigo.

PRECAUTIONS

CONTRAINDICATIONS: Pregnancy/lactation (may cause uterine contraction/abortion). Allergies to ragweed, chrysanthemums, marigolds, daisies. **CAUTIONS:** None known.

LIFESPAN CONSIDERATIONS: Pregnancy/lactation: Contraindicated. **Children:** Safety and efficacy not established; avoid use. **Elderly:** No age-related precautions noted.

INTERACTIONS

DRUG: May increase risk of bleeding with **anticoagulants, antiplatelets. NSAIDs** may decrease effectiveness of feverfew. **HERBAL: Garlic, ginger,**

see also www.elsevierhealth.com/EVOLVE/SaundersNDH

F

ginkgo may increase risk of bleeding. **FOOD:** None known. **LAB VALUES:** None known.

AVAILABILITY

CAPSULES: 100 mg. **FEVERFEW LEAF:** 380 mg.

INDICATIONS/ROUTES/DOSAGE

F

MIGRAINE HEADACHE

PO: ADULTS, ELDERLY: 50–100 mg extract/day. **Leaf:** 50–125 mg/day.

SIDE EFFECTS

ORAL: Abdominal pain, muscle stiffness, pain, indigestion, diarrhea, flatulence, nausea, vomiting. **CHEWING LEAF:** Mouth ulceration, inflammation of oral mucosa and tongue, swelling of lips, loss of taste.

ADVERSE REACTIONS/ TOXIC EFFECTS

Hypersensitivity reaction.

NURSING IMPLICATIONS

BASELINE ASSESSMENT

Assess if pregnant/breast-feeding (contraindicated).

INTERVENTION/EVALUATION

Assess for hypersensitivity reaction, mouth ulcers, muscle/joint pain.

PATIENT/FAMILY TEACHING

Do not use during pregnancy/lactation. Avoid use in children.

fexofenadine hydrochloride

fecks-**oh**-fen-ah-deen
(Allegra)

FIXED-COMBINATION(S)

Allegra-D: fexofenadine/pseudoephedrine (sympathomimetic): 60 mg/120 mg.

CLASSIFICATION

PHARMACOTHERAPEUTIC: Piperidine. **CLINICAL:** Antihistamine (see p. 48C).

ACTION

Prevents, antagonizes most histamine effects (e.g., urticaria, pruritus). **Therapeutic Effect:** Relieves allergic rhinitis symptoms.

PHARMACOKINETICS

Rapidly absorbed after PO administration. Does not cross blood-brain barrier. Protein binding: 60%–70%. Minimally metabolized. Eliminated in feces, excreted in urine. Not removed by hemodialysis. **Half-life:** 14.4 hrs (half-life increased with impaired renal function).

USES

Relief of symptoms associated with seasonal allergic rhinitis (sneezing, rhinorrhea, itching of throat/eyes) in adults, children >12 yrs.

PRECAUTIONS

CONTRAINDICATIONS: None known. **CAUTIONS:** Severe renal impairment.

LIFESPAN CONSIDERATIONS: Pregnancy/lactation: Unknown if drug crosses placenta or is distributed in breast milk. **Pregnancy Category C. Children:** Safety and efficacy not established in those <12 yrs. **Elderly:** No age-related precautions noted.

INTERACTIONS

DRUG: None known. **HERBAL:** None known. **FOOD:** None known. **LAB VALUES:** May suppress wheal and flare reactions to antigen skin testing. Discontinue at least 4 days before testing.

AVAILABILITY (Rx)

CAPSULES: 60 mg. **TABLETS:** 30 mg, 60 mg, 180 mg.

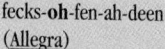

ADMINISTRATION/HANDLING

PO

- Give without regard to food.

INDICATIONS/ROUTES/DOSAGE

ALLERGIC RHINITIS

PO: ADULTS, ELDERLY, CHILDREN >12 YRS: 60 mg 2 times/day or 180 mg once daily. CHILDREN, 6–11 YRS: 30 mg 2 times/day.

DOSAGE IN RENAL IMPAIRMENT

PO: ADULTS, ELDERLY, CHILDREN >12 YRS: 60 mg once daily. CHILDREN, 6–11 YRS: 30 mg once daily.

SIDE EFFECTS

RARE (<2%): Drowsiness, headache, fatigue, nausea, vomiting, abdominal distress, dysmenorrhea.

ADVERSE REACTIONS/ TOXIC EFFECTS

None known.

NURSING IMPLICATIONS

BASELINE ASSESSMENT

If pt is having an allergic reaction, obtain history of recently ingested foods, drugs, environmental exposure, recent emotional stress. Monitor rate, depth, rhythm, type of respiration; quality, rate of pulse. Assess lung sounds for rhonchi, wheezing, rales.

INTERVENTION/EVALUATION

Assess for therapeutic response; relief from allergy: itching, red, watery eyes, rhinorrhea, sneezing.

PATIENT/FAMILY TEACHING

Avoid tasks that require alertness, motor skills until response to drug is established. Avoid alcohol during antihistamine therapy. Coffee, tea may help reduce drowsiness.

filgrastim

fill-**grass**-tim

(Neupogen)

Do not confuse with Epogen, Nutramigen.

◆ CLASSIFICATION

PHARMACOTHERAPEUTIC: Biologic modifier. **CLINICAL:** Granulocyte colony-stimulating factor (GCSF).

ACTION

Stimulates production, maturation, activation of neutrophils. **Therapeutic Effect:** Activates neutrophils to increase their migration and cytotoxicity.

PHARMACOKINETICS

Readily absorbed after subcutaneous administration. Not removed by hemodialysis. **Half-life:** 3.5 hrs.

USES

Decrease infection incidence in pts with nonmyeloid malignancies receiving myelosuppressive therapy associated with severe neutropenia, fever. Reduce neutropenia duration (and sequelae) in pt with nonmyeloid malignancies having myeloablative therapy followed by bone marrow transplant (BMT). Mobilization of hematopoietic progenitor cells into peripheral blood for collection by leukapheresis. Improve neutrophil recovery, reduce fever duration following chemotherapy for acute myeloid leukemia (AML). **Unlabeled:** Treatment of AIDS-related neutropenia; chronic, severe neutropenia, drug-induced neutropenia; myelodysplastic syndrome.

PRECAUTIONS

CONTRAINDICATIONS: Hypersensitivity to *Escherichia coli*–derived proteins, 24 hrs before or after cytotoxic chemotherapy, use with other drugs that may result in lowered platelet count. **CAUTIONS:** Malignancy with myeloid characteristics due to G-CSF's potential to act as a growth factor; gout, psoriasis, preexisting cardiac conditions.

LIFESPAN CONSIDERATIONS: Pregnancy/lactation: Unknown if drug crosses placenta or is distributed in breast milk. **Pregnancy Category C. Children/elderly:** No age-related precautions noted.

F

INTERACTIONS

DRUG: None known. **HERBAL:** None known. **FOOD:** None known. **LAB VALUES:** May increase alkaline phosphatase, LDH, uric acid, leukocyte (LAP) scores.

AVAILABILITY (Rx)

INJECTION: 300 mcg/ml, 480 mcg/0.8 ml.

ADMINISTRATION/HANDLING

Alert: May be given by subcutaneous injection, short IV infusion (15–30 min), or continuous IV infusion.

SUBCUTANEOUS

Storage • Store in refrigerator, but remove before use and allow to warm to room temperature. • Aspirate syringe before injection (avoid intra-arterial administration).

IV

Storage • Refrigerate vials. • Stable for up to 24 hrs at room temperature (provided vial contents are clear, containing no particulate matter). Remains stable if accidentally exposed to freezing temperature.

Reconstitution • Use single-dose vial, do not reenter vial. Do not shake. • Dilute with 10–50 ml D_5W to concentration of ≥15 mcg/ml. For concentration from 5–15 mcg/ml, add 2 ml of 5% albumin to each 50 ml D_5W to provide a final concentration of 2 mg/ml. Do not dilute to a final concentration of <5 mcg/ml.

Rate of administration • For intermittent infusion (piggyback), infuse over 15–30 min. • For continuous infusion, give single dose over 4–24 hrs. • In all situations, flush IV line with D_5W before and after administration.

IV INCOMPATIBILITIES

Amphotericin (Fungizone), cefepime (Maxipime), cefotaxime (Claforan), cefoxitin (Mefoxin), ceftizoxime (Cefizox), ceftriaxone (Rocephin), cefuroxime (Zinacef), clindamycin (Cleocin), dactinomycin (Cosmegen), etoposide (VePesid), fluorouracil, furosemide (Lasix), heparin, mannitol, methylprednisolone (Solu-Medrol), mitomycin (Mutamycin), prochlorperazine (Compazine).

IV COMPATIBILITIES

Bumetanide (Bumex), calcium gluconate, hydromorphone (Dilaudid), lorazepam (Ativan), morphine, potassium chloride.

INDICATIONS/ROUTES/DOSAGE

Alert: Begin at least 24 hrs after last dose of chemotherapy; discontinue at least 24 hrs before next dose of chemotherapy.

MYELOSUPPRESSIVE

Subcutaneous/IV or subcutaneous infusion: ADULTS, ELDERLY: Initially, 5 mcg/kg/day. May increase by 5 mcg/kg for each chemotherapy cycle based on duration/severity of absolute neutrophil count (ANC) nadir.

Alert: Begin at least 24 hrs after last dose of chemotherapy and at least 24 hrs after bone marrow infusion.

BMT

IV or subcutaneous infusion: ADULTS, ELDERLY: 5–10 mcg/kg/day. Adjust dose daily during period of neutrophil recovery based on neutrophil response.

MOBILIZE PROGENITOR CELLS

IV/subcutaneous: ADULTS: 10 mcg/kg/day beginning at least 4 days before first leukapheresis and continuing until last leukapheresis.

SIDE EFFECTS

FREQUENT: Nausea/vomiting (57%), mild-to-severe bone pain (22%) (occurs more frequently in those receiving high dose via IV form, less frequently in low-dose, subcutaneous form); alopecia (18%), diarrhea (14%), fever (12%), fatigue (11%). **OCCASIONAL (5%–9%):** Anorexia, dyspnea, headache, cough, skin rash. **RARE (<5%):** Psoriasis, hematuria/proteinuria, osteoporosis.

ADVERSE REACTIONS/ TOXIC EFFECTS

Chronic administration occasionally produces chronic neutropenia, splenomegaly. Thrombocytopenia, MI, arrhythmias occur rarely. Adult respiratory distress syndrome may occur in septic pts.

NURSING IMPLICATIONS

BASELINE ASSESSMENT

CBC, platelet count (differential) should be obtained prior to therapy initiation and twice weekly thereafter.

INTERVENTION/EVALUATION

In septic pts, be alert to adult respiratory distress syndrome. Closely monitor those with preexisting cardiac conditions. Monitor B/P (transient decrease in B/P may occur), temperature, CBC with differential, platelet count, Hct, uric acid, liver function tests.

PATIENT/FAMILY TEACHING

Inform physician of fever, chills, severe bone pain, chest pain, palpitations.

finasteride

fin-**ah**-stir-eyd

(Propecia, Proscar)

Do not confuse with Posicor, ProSom, Prozac, Psorcon.

◆CLASSIFICATION

PHARMACOTHERAPEUTIC: Androgen hormone inhibitor. **CLINICAL:** Benign prostatic hyperplasia agent.

ACTION

Inhibits steroid 5-alpha reductase, an intracellular enzyme that converts testosterone into dihydrotestosterone (DHT) in the prostate gland, providing a reduction in serum DHT. **Therapeutic Effect:** Regresses the enlarged prostate gland.

PHARMACOKINETICS

Onset	Peak	Duration
PO		
24 hrs	1–2 days	5–7 days

Protein binding: 90%. Rapidly absorbed from GI tract. Widely distributed. Metabolized in liver. **Half-life:** 6–8 hrs. Onset of clinical effect: 3–6 mos of continued therapy.

USES

Reduces risk of acute urinary retention, need for surgery in symptomatic benign prostatic hypertrophy (BPH). Most improvement noted in hesitancy, feeling of incomplete bladder emptying, interruption of urinary stream, difficulty initiating flow, dysuria, impaired size and force of urinary stream. Treatment for hair loss. **Unlabeled:** Adjuvant monotherapy after radical prostatectomy in treatment of prostate cancer.

PRECAUTIONS

CONTRAINDICATIONS: Physical handling of tablet or in those who may become or are pregnant, exposure to semen in those who may become pregnant. **CAUTIONS:** Liver function abnormalities.

LIFESPAN CONSIDERATIONS: Pregnancy/lactation: Physical handling of tablet in those who may become or are pregnant. May produce abnormalities of external genitalia of male fetus. **Pregnancy Category X. Children:** Not indicated in children. **Elderly:** Efficacy not established.

INTERACTIONS

DRUG: None known. **HERBAL:** None known. **FOOD:** None known. **LAB VALUES:** Produces decrease in serum prostate-specific antigen (PSA) levels (even in presence of prostate cancer).

AVAILABILITY (Rx)

TABLETS: 1 mg, 5 mg.

ADMINISTRATION/HANDLING

PO

• Do not break or crush film-coated tablets. • Give without regard to meals.

INDICATIONS/ROUTES/DOSAGE

BENIGN PROSTATIC HYPERTROPHY

PO: ADULTS, ELDERLY: 5 mg once daily (minimum 6 mos).

HAIR LOSS

PO: ADULTS: 1 mg daily.

SIDE EFFECTS

OCCASIONAL (2%–4%): Impotence, decreased libido, gynecomastia, decreased volume of ejaculate.

ADVERSE REACTIONS/ TOXIC EFFECTS

None known.

NURSING IMPLICATIONS

BASELINE ASSESSMENT

Digital rectal exam, serum PSA determination should be performed in those with BPH prior to initiating therapy and periodically thereafter.

INTERVENTION/EVALUATION

Diligent monitoring of I&O, esp. in those with large residual urinary volume, severely diminished urinary flow for obstructive uropathy.

PATIENT/FAMILY TEACHING

Pt should be aware of potential for impotence. May not notice improved urinary flow even if prostate gland shrinks. Need to take medication >6 mos, and it is unknown if medication decreases need for surgery. Because of potential risk to male fetus, women who are or may become pregnant should not handle tablets or be exposed to pt's semen. Volume of ejaculate may be decreased during treatment.

Fioricet

see acetaminophen

Fiorinal

see aspirin

Flagyl

see metronidazole

flavoxate

flay-**vocks**-ate
(Urispas)
Do not confuse with Urised.

◆ **CLASSIFICATION**

PHARMACOTHERAPEUTIC: Anticholinergic. **CLINICAL:** Antispasmodic.

ACTION

Relaxes detrusor, other smooth muscle by cholinergic blockade, counteracting muscle spasm of urinary tract. **Therapeutic Effect:** Produces anticholinergic, local anesthetic, analgesic effect, relieving urinary symptoms.

USES

Symptomatic relief of dysuria, urgency, nocturia, frequency, incontinence associated with cystitis, prostatitis, urethritis, urethrocystitis, urethrotrigonitis.

PRECAUTIONS

CONTRAINDICATIONS: Pyloric/duodenal obstruction, GI hemorrhage/obstruction, ileus, obstructions of lower urinary tract. **CAUTIONS:** Glaucoma. **Pregnancy Category B.**

INTERACTIONS

DRUG: None known. **HERBAL:** None known. **FOOD:** None known. **LAB VALUES:** None known.

AVAILABILITY (Rx)

TABLETS: 100 mg.

INDICATIONS/ROUTES/DOSAGE

URINARY ANTISPASMODIC

PO: ADULTS, ELDERLY, ADOLESCENTS: 100–200 mg 3–4 times/day.

SIDE EFFECTS

Generally well tolerated. Side effects usually mild, transient. **FREQUENT:** Drowsiness, dry mouth, throat. **OCCASIONAL:** Constipation, difficult urination, blurred vision, dizziness, headache, increased light sensitivity, nausea, vomiting, stomach pain. **RARE:** Confusion (primarily in elderly), hypersensitivity, increase intraocular pressure, leukopenia.

ADVERSE REACTIONS/ TOXIC EFFECTS

Anticholinergic effect with overdose (unsteadiness, severe dizziness, drowsiness, fever, flushed face, shortness of breath, nervousness, irritability).

NURSING IMPLICATIONS

BASELINE ASSESSMENT

Assess for dysuria, urgency, frequency, incontinence, suprapubic pain.

INTERVENTION/EVALUATION

Monitor for symptomatic relief. Observe elderly, esp. for mental confusion.

PATIENT/FAMILY TEACHING

Avoid driving, other tasks requiring alertness, coordination, manual dexterity (blurred vision, drowsiness).

flecainide

(Tambocor)
See Classification section under: Antiarrhythmics (p. 14C)

Flexeril

see cyclobenzaprine

F

Flomax

see tamsulosin

Flonase

see fluticasone

Flovent

see fluticasone

fluconazole

flu-**con**-ah-zole
(Apo-Fluconazole✱, Diflucan)
Do not confuse with diclofenac.

CLASSIFICATION

CLINICAL: Antifungal.

ACTION

Interferes with cytochrome (necessary for ergosterol formation). Fungistatic. **Therapeutic Effect:** Directly damages fungal membrane, altering membrane function.

PHARMACOKINETICS

Well absorbed from GI tract. Widely distributed (including CSF). Protein binding: 11%. Partially metabolized in liver. Primarily excreted unchanged in urine. Partially removed by hemodialysis. **Half-life:** 20–30 hrs (half-life increased with impaired renal function).

USES

Treatment of oropharyngeal, esophageal, vaginal candidiasis; serious systemic candida infections (e.g., urinary tract infections, peritonitis, pneumonia); *Cryptococcus neoformans* meningitis. Prevention of candidiasis in bone marrow transplants. **Unlabeled:** Treatment of coccidioidomycosis, cryptococcosis, onychomycosis, fungal pneumonia/septicemia, ringworm of the hand.

PRECAUTIONS

CONTRAINDICATIONS: None known. **CAUTIONS:** Hepatic/renal impairment, hypersensitivity to other triazoles (e.g., itraconazole, terconazole), imidazoles (e.g., butoconazole, ketoconazole).

LIFESPAN CONSIDERATIONS: Pregnancy/lactation: Unknown if excreted in breast milk. **Pregnancy Category C. Children:** No age-related precautions noted. **Elderly:** Age-related renal impairment may require dosage adjustment.

INTERACTIONS

DRUG: May increase concentration, effects of **oral hypoglycemics.** High doses increase **cyclosporine** concentration. May decrease metabolism of **phenytoin, warfarin. Rifampin** may increase metabolism. **HERBAL:** None known. **FOOD:** None known. **LAB VALUES:** May increase SGOT (AST), SGPT (ALT), alkaline phosphatase, bilirubin.

AVAILABILITY (Rx)

TABLETS: 50 mg, 100 mg, 150 mg, 200 mg. **POWDER FOR ORAL SUSPENSION:** 10 mg/ml, 40 mg/ml. **INJECTION:** 2 mg/ml (in 100- or 200-ml containers).

ADMINISTRATION/HANDLING

PO

• Give without regard to meals. • PO and IV therapy equally effective; IV therapy for pt intolerant of the drug or unable to take orally.

IV

Storage • Store at room temperature. • Do not remove from outer wrap until ready to use. • Squeeze inner bag to check for leaks. • Do not use parenteral form if solution is cloudy, precipitate forms, seal is not intact, or it is discolored. • Do not add supplementary medication.

Rate of administration • Do not exceed maximum flow rate 200 mg/hr.

⊘ IV INCOMPATIBILITIES
Amphotericin (Fungizone), amphotericin B complex (Abelcet, Amphotec, AmBisome), ampicillin (Polycillin), calcium gluconate, cefotaxime (Claforan), ceftazidime (Fortaz), ceftriaxone (Rocephin), cefuroxime (Zinacef), chloramphenicol (Chloromycetin), clindamycin (Cleocin), diazepam (Valium), digoxin (Lanoxin), erythromycin (Erythrocin), furosemide (Lasix), haloperidol (Haldol), hydroxyzine (Vistaril), imipenem/cilastatin (Primaxin), sulfamethoxazole-trimethoprim (Bactrim).

IV COMPATIBILITIES
Diltiazem (Cardizem), dobutamine (Dobutrex), dopamine (Intropin), heparin, lorazepam (Ativan), midazolam (Versed), propofol (Diprivan).

INDICATIONS/ROUTES/DOSAGE

OROPHARYNGEAL CANDIDIASIS
PO/IV: ADULTS, ELDERLY: Initially, 200 mg once, then 100 mg/day for at least 14 days. CHILDREN: Initially, 6 mg/kg/day once, then 3 mg/kg/day.

ESOPHAGEAL CANDIDIASIS
PO/IV: ADULTS, ELDERLY: 200 mg once, then 100 mg/day (up to 400 mg/day) for 21 days and at least 14 days following resolution of symptoms. CHILDREN: 6 mg/kg/day once, then 3 mg/kg/day (up to 12 mg/kg/day).

VAGINAL CANDIDIASIS
PO: ADULTS: 150 mg once.

CANDIDIASIS PREVENTION
PO: ADULTS: 400 mg/day.

SYSTEMIC CANDIDIASIS
PO/IV: ADULTS, ELDERLY: Initially, 400 mg once, then 200 mg/day (up to 400 mg/day) for at least 28 days and at least 14 days following resolution of symptoms. CHILDREN: 6–12 mg/kg/day.

CRYPTOCOCCAL MENINGITIS
PO/IV: ADULTS, ELDERLY: Initially, 400 mg once, then 200 mg/day (up to 800 mg/day). Continue for 10–12 wks after CSF becomes negative (200 mg/day for suppression of relapse in pts with AIDS). CHILDREN: 12 mg/kg/day once, then 6–12 mg/kg/day; 6 mg/kg/day for suppression.

ONYCHOMYCOSIS
PO: ADULTS: 150 mg weekly.

DOSAGE IN RENAL IMPAIRMENT
After loading dose of 400 mg, daily dose based on creatinine clearance:

Creatinine Clearance	% of Recommended Dose
>50	100
21–50	50
11–20	25
Dialysis	Dose after dialysis

SIDE EFFECTS

OCCASIONAL (1%–4%): Hypersensitivity reaction (fever, chills, rash, pruritus), dizziness, drowsiness, headache, constipation, diarrhea, nausea, vomiting, abdominal pain.

ADVERSE REACTIONS/ TOXIC EFFECTS

Exfoliative skin disorders, serious hepatic effects, blood dyscrasias (eosinophilia, thrombocytopenia, anemia, leukopenia) have been reported rarely.

NURSING IMPLICATIONS

BASELINE ASSESSMENT
Establish baselines for CBC, potassium, hepatic function studies.

INTERVENTION/EVALUATION

Assess for hypersensitivity reaction (chills, fever). Monitor liver/renal function tests, potassium, CBC, platelet count. Report rash, itching promptly. Monitor temperature at least daily. Determine pattern of bowel activity, stool consistency. Assess for dizziness; provide assistance as needed.

F

PATIENT/FAMILY TEACHING

Do not drive car, use machinery if dizziness/drowsiness occurs. Notify physician of dark urine, pale stool, yellow skin/eyes, rash with or without itching. Pts with oropharyngeal infections should be taught good oral hygiene. Consult physician before taking any other medication.

fludarabine phosphate

flew-**dare**-ah-bean
(Fludara)
Do not confuse with FUDR.

CLASSIFICATION

PHARMACOTHERAPEUTIC: Antimetabolite. **CLINICAL:** Antineoplastic (see p. 72C).

ACTION

Interferes with DNA polymerase alpha, ribonucleotide reductase, DNA primase. **Therapeutic Effect:** Inhibits DNA synthesis, induces cell death.

PHARMACOKINETICS

Rapidly dephosphorylated in serum, then phosphorylated intracellularly to active triphosphate. Primarily excreted in urine. **Half-life:** 7–20 hrs.

USES

Treatment of chronic lymphocytic leukemia in those who have not responded to or have not progressed with another standard alkylating agent.

PRECAUTIONS

CONTRAINDICATIONS: Concomitant administration with pentostatin. **CAUTIONS:** Preexisting neurologic problems, renal insufficiency, bone marrow suppression.

LIFESPAN CONSIDERATIONS: Pregnancy/lactation: If possible, avoid use during pregnancy, esp. first trimester. May cause fetal harm. Not known whether distributed in breast milk. Breast-feeding not recommended. **Pregnancy Category D. Children:** Safety and efficacy not established. **Elderly:** Age-related renal impairment may require dosage adjustment.

INTERACTIONS

DRUG: May decrease effect of **antigout** medications. **Bone marrow depressants** may increase risk of bone marrow depression. **Live virus vaccines** may potentiate virus replication, increase vaccine side effects, decrease pt's antibody response to vaccine. **HERBAL:** None known. **FOOD:** None known. **LAB VALUES:** May increase uric acid, alkaline phosphatase, SGOT (AST).

AVAILABILITY (Rx)

INJECTION: 50 mg.

ADMINISTRATION/HANDLING

Alert: Give by IV infusion. Do not add to other IV infusions. Avoid small veins; swollen/edematous extremities; areas overlying joints, tendons.

IV

Storage • Store in refrigerator. • Handle with extreme care during preparation/administration. If contact with skin or mucous membranes occurs, wash thoroughly with soap and water; rinse eyes profusely with plain water. • After reconstitution, use within 8 hrs; discard unused portion.

Reconstitution • Reconstitute 50-mg vial with 2 ml Sterile Water for Injection to provide a concentration of 25 mg/ml. • Further dilute with 100–125 ml 0.9% NaCl or D_5W.

Rate of administration • Infuse over 30 min.

⌀ IV INCOMPATIBILITIES
Acyclovir (Zovirax), amphotericin (Fungizone), hydroxyzine (Vistaril), prochlorperazine (Compazine).

IV COMPATIBILITIES
Heparin, hydromorphone (Dilaudid), lorazepam (Ativan), magnesium sulfate, morphine, multivitamins, potassium chloride.

INDICATIONS/ROUTES/DOSAGE

Alert: Dosage is individualized based on clinical response, tolerance to adverse effects. When used in combination therapy, consult specific protocols for optimum dosage, sequence of drug administration. Dosage based on pt's actual weight. Use ideal body weight in obese/edematous pts.

CHRONIC LYMPHOCYTIC LEUKEMIA
IV: ADULTS: 25 mg/m^2 daily for 5 consecutive days. Continue up to 3 additional cycles. Begin each course of treatment q28days.

ACUTE LEUKEMIA
IV: CHILDREN: 10 mg/m^2 bolus (over 15 min), then IV infusion of 30.5 mg/m^2/day.

SOLID TUMORS
IV: CHILDREN: 9 mg/m^2 bolus, then 27 mg/m^2/day for 5 days as continuous infusion.

NON-HODGKIN'S LYMPHOMA
IV: ADULTS, ELDERLY: Initially, 20 mg/m^2, then 30 mg/m^2/day for 48 hrs.

DOSAGE IN RENAL IMPAIRMENT

Creatinine Clearance	Dosage
30–70 ml/min	Decrease dose by 20%
<30 ml/min	Not recommended

SIDE EFFECTS

FREQUENT: Fever (60%), nausea/vomiting (36%), chills (11%). **OCCASIONAL (10%–20%):** Fatigue, generalized pain, rash, diarrhea, cough, weakness, stomatitis (burning/erythema of oral mucosa, sore throat, difficulty swallowing), dyspnea, weakness, peripheral edema. **RARE (3%–7%):** Anorexia, sinusitis, dysuria, myalgia, paresthesia, headaches, visual disturbances.

ADVERSE REACTIONS/ TOXIC EFFECTS

Pneumonia occurs frequently. Severe bone marrow toxicity (anemia, thrombocytopenia, neutropenia) may occur. Tumor lysis syndrome may occur with onset of flank pain, hematuria. This syndrome may include hypercalcemia, hyperphosphatemia, hyperuricemia, and result in renal failure. GI bleeding may occur. High dosage may produce acute leukemia, blindness, coma.

NURSING IMPLICATIONS

BASELINE ASSESSMENT

Assess baseline CBC, platelet, serum creatinine. Drug should be discontinued if intractable vomiting, diarrhea, stomatitis, GI bleeding occurs.

INTERVENTION/EVALUATION

Assess for weakness, visual disturbances, peripheral edema. Assess for onset of pneumonia. Monitor for dyspnea, cough, rapidly falling WBC, intractable diarrhea, GI bleeding (bright red/tarry stool). Assess oral mucosa for mucosal erythema, ulceration at inner margin of lips, sore throat, difficulty swallowing (stomatitis). Assess skin for rash. Be alert to possible tumor lysis syndrome (onset of flank pain, hematuria).

PATIENT/FAMILY TEACHING

Avoid crowds, exposure to infection. Maintain fastidious oral hygiene. Promptly report fever, sore throat, signs of local infection, unusual bruising/bleeding from any site. Contact physician if nausea/vomiting continues.

F

fludrocortisone

floo-droe-**kor**-tih-sone

(Florinef)

Do not confuse with Fioricet, Fiorinal.

CLASSIFICATION

PHARMACOTHERAPEUTIC: Mineralocorticoid. **CLINICAL:** Glucocorticosteroid (see p. 81C).

ACTION

Acts at distal tubules. **Therapeutic Effect:** Increases potassium, hydrogen ion excretion, sodium reabsorption, water retention.

PHARMACOKINETICS

Well absorbed from GI tract. Protein binding: 42%. Widely distributed. Metabolized in liver, kidney. Primarily excreted in urine. **Half-life:** 3.5 hrs.

USES

Partial replacement therapy for primary and secondary adrenocortical insufficiency in Addison's disease. Adjunctive treatment of salt-losing forms of congenital adrenogenital syndrome. **Unlabeled:** Treatment of idiopathic orthostatic hypotension, acidosis in renal tubular disorders.

PRECAUTIONS

CONTRAINDICATIONS: CHF, systemic fungal infection. **CAUTIONS:** Hypertension, edema, impaired renal function.

LIFESPAN CONSIDERATIONS: Pregnancy/lactation: Unknown whether drug crosses placenta or is distributed in breast milk. **Pregnancy Category C. Children:** May cause growth suppression, inhibition of endogenous steroid production. **Elderly:** Studies not performed.

INTERACTIONS

DRUG: May increase **digoxin** toxicity (hypokalemia). **Hepatic enzyme inducers (e.g., phenytoin)** may increase metabolism. **Hypokalemia-causing medications** may increase effect. **Sodium-containing medication** may increase sodium, edema, B/P. **HERBAL:** None known. **FOOD:** None known. **LAB VALUES:** May increase sodium. May decrease potassium, Hct.

AVAILABILITY (Rx)

TABLETS: 0.1 mg.

ADMINISTRATION/HANDLING

PO

- Give with food or milk.

INDICATIONS/ROUTES/DOSAGE

ADDISON'S DISEASE

PO: ADULTS, ELDERLY: 0.05–0.1 mg/day. RANGE: 0.1 mg 3 times/wk–0.2 mg/day. Administration with cortisone/hydrocortisone preferred.

SALT-LOSING ADRENOGENITAL SYNDROME

PO: ADULTS, ELDERLY: 0.1–0.2 mg/day.

USUAL PEDIATRIC DOSAGE

PO: 0.05–0.1 mg/day.

SIDE EFFECTS

FREQUENT: Increased appetite, exaggerated sense of well-being, abdominal distention, weight gain, insomnia, mood swings. **High-dose, prolonged therapy, too rapid withdrawal:** Increased susceptibility to infection (signs/symptoms masked); delayed wound healing, hypokalemia, hypocalcemia, GI distress, diarrhea/constipation, hypertension. **OCCASIONAL:** Headache (frontal, occipital), dizziness, menstrual difficulty/amenorrhea, gastric ulcer development. **RARE:** Hypersensitivity reaction.

ADVERSE REACTIONS/ TOXIC EFFECTS

LONG-TERM THERAPY: Muscle wasting (esp. arms, legs), osteoporosis, spontaneous fractures, amenorrhea, cataracts, glaucoma, peptic ulcer, CHF. **ABRUPT WITHDRAWAL AFTER LONG-TERM THERAPY:** Anorexia, nausea, fever, headache, joint pain, rebound inflammation, fatigue, weakness, lethargy, dizziness, orthostatic hypotension.

NURSING IMPLICATIONS

BASELINE ASSESSMENT

Obtain baselines for weight, B/P, blood glucose, electrolytes, chest x-ray, EKG.

INTERVENTION/EVALUATION

Monitor serum electrolytes, glucose, B/P, serum renin. Taper dosage slowly if medication is to be discontinued.

PATIENT/FAMILY TEACHING

Do not change dose/schedule or stop taking drug; must taper off gradually. Report fever, sore throat, muscle aches, sudden weight gain/swelling, continuing headaches. Maintain careful personal hygiene, avoid exposure to disease, trauma. Severe stress (serious infection, surgery, trauma) may require increased dosage.

flumazenil

flew-**maz**-ah-nil
(Anexate ✤, Romazicon)

◆ CLASSIFICATION

PHARMACOTHERAPEUTIC: Benzodiazepine receptor antagonist. **CLINICAL:** Antidote.

ACTION

Antagonizes the effect of benzodiazepines on the GABA receptor complex in the CNS. **Therapeutic Effect:** Reverses sedative effect of benzodiazepines.

PHARMACOKINETICS

Onset	Peak	Duration
IV		
1–2 min	6–10 min	<1 hr

Duration, degree of benzodiazepine reversal related to dosage, plasma concentration. Protein binding: 50%. Metabolized by liver; excreted in urine.

USES

Complete or partial reversal of sedative effects of benzodiazepines when general anesthesia has been induced and/or maintained with benzodiazepines, when sedation has been produced with benzodiazepines for diagnostic and therapeutic procedures, management of benzodiazepine overdosage.

PRECAUTIONS

CONTRAINDICATIONS: History of hypersensitivity to benzodiazepines, those who have been given a benzodiazepine for control of a potentially life-threatening condition (control of intracranial pressure, status epilepticus), those showing signs of serious cyclic antidepressant overdose manifested by motor abnormalities, arrhythmias, anticholinergic signs, cardiovascular collapse. **CAUTIONS:** Head injury, impaired hepatic function, alcoholism, drug dependency.

LIFESPAN CONSIDERATIONS: Pregnancy/lactation: Unknown whether drug crosses placenta or is distributed in breast milk. Not recommended during labor, delivery. **Pregnancy Category C. Children:** No age-related precautions noted. **Elderly:** Benzodiazepine-induced sedation tends to be deeper, more prolonged requiring careful monitoring.

INTERACTIONS

DRUG: Toxic effects (seizures, arrhythmias) of other drugs taken in overdose (esp. **tricyclic antidepressants**) may emerge with reversal of sedative effect of **benzodiazepines**. **HERBAL:** None known. **FOOD:** None known. **LAB VALUES:** None known.

AVAILABILITY (Rx)

INJECTION: 0.1 mg/ml.

ADMINISTRATION/HANDLING

Alert: Compatible with D_5W, lactated Ringer's, 0.9% NaCl.

IV

Storage • Store parenteral form at room temperature. • Discard after 24 hrs once medication is drawn into syringe, is mixed with any solutions, or if particulate/discoloration is noted. • Rinse spilled medication from skin with cool water.

Rate of administration • **Reverse conscious sedation or general anesthesia:** Give over 15 sec. • **Benzodiazepine overdose:** Give over 30 sec. • Administer through freely running IV infusion into large vein (local injection produces pain, inflammation at injection site).

IV INCOMPATIBILITY

No information available via Y-site administration.

IV COMPATIBILITIES

Aminophylline, cimetidine (Tagamet), dobutamine (Dobutrex), dopamine (Intropin), famotidine (Pepcid), heparin, lidocaine, procainamide (Pronestyl), ranitidine (Zantac).

INDICATIONS/ROUTES/DOSAGE

REVERSAL OF CONSCIOUS SEDATION, IN GENERAL ANESTHESIA

IV: ADULTS, ELDERLY: Initially, 0.2 mg (2 ml) over 15 sec; may repeat 0.2-mg dose in 45 sec; then at 60-sec intervals. **Maximum:** 1 mg (10 ml total dose). CHILDREN, NEONATES: Initially, 0.01 mg/kg. **Maximum:** 0.2 mg. May repeat after 45 sec and then every minute. **Maximum cumulative dose:** 0.05 mg/kg or 1 mg.

Alert: If resedation occurs, repeat dose at 20-min intervals. **Maximum:** 1 mg (given as 0.2 mg/min) at any one time, 3 mg in any 1 hr.

BENZODIAZEPINE OVERDOSE

IV: ADULTS, ELDERLY: Initially, 0.2 mg (2 ml) over 30 sec; may repeat after 30 sec with 0.3 mg (3 ml) over 30 sec if desired LOC not achieved. Further doses of 0.5 mg (5 ml) over 30 sec may be administered at 60-sec intervals. **Maximum:** 3 mg (30 ml) total dose. CHILDREN, NEONATES: Initially 0.01 mg/kg. **Maximum:** 0.2 mg. May repeat every minute. **Maximum cumulative dose:** 1 mg.

Alert: If resedation occurs, repeat dose at 20-min intervals. **Maximum:** 1 mg (given as 0.5 mg/min) at any one time, 3 mg in any 1 hr.

USUAL DOSAGE FOR CHILDREN

IV: Initially, 0.01 mg/kg. **Maximum:** 2

mg. May repeat in 45 seconds, then at 60-sec intervals. **Maximum cumulative dose:** 1 mg.

SIDE EFFECTS

FREQUENT (3%–11%): Agitation, anxiety, dry mouth, dyspnea, insomnia, palpitations, tremors, headache, blurred vision, dizziness, ataxia, nausea, vomiting, pain at injection site, diaphoresis. **OCCASIONAL (1%–3%):** Fatigue, flushing, auditory disturbances, thrombophlebitis, skin rash. **RARE (<1%):** Hives, itching, hallucinations.

ADVERSE REACTIONS/ TOXIC EFFECTS

Toxic effects (seizures, arrhythmias) of other drugs taken in overdose (esp. tricyclic antidepressants) may emerge with reversal of sedative effect of benzodiazepines. May provoke panic attack in those with history of panic disorder.

NURSING IMPLICATIONS

BASELINE ASSESSMENT

ABGs should be obtained prior to and at 30-min intervals during IV administration. Prepare to intervene in reestablishing airway, assisting ventilation (drug may not fully reverse ventilatory insufficiency induced by benzodiazepines). Note that effects of flumazenil may wear off before effects of benzodiazepines.

INTERVENTION/EVALUATION

Properly manage airway, assisted breathing, maintain circulatory access and support, perform internal decontamination by lavage and charcoal, provide adequate clinical evaluation. Monitor for reversal of benzodiazepine effect. Assess for possible resedation, respiratory depression, hypoventilation. Assess closely for return of unconsciousness (narcosis) for at least 1 hr after pt is fully alert.

PATIENT/FAMILY TEACHING

Avoid ingestion of alcohol, tasks that require alertness, motor skills or taking nonprescription drugs until at least 18–24 hrs after discharge.

flunisolide

flew-**nis**-oh-lide

(AeroBid, Nasalide, Nasarel, Rhinalar✤)

Do not confuse with fluocinonide, Nasalcrom.

CLASSIFICATION

PHARMACOTHERAPEUTIC: Adrenocorticosteroid. **CLINICAL:** Antiasthmatic, anti-inflammatory (see pp. 65C, 81C).

ACTION

Controls rate of protein synthesis, depresses migration of polymorphonuclear leukocytes, reverses capillary permeability, stabilizes lysosomal membranes. **Therapeutic Effect:** Prevents or controls inflammation.

USES

Inhalation: Control of bronchial asthma in those requiring chronic steroid therapy. **Intranasal:** Relief of symptoms of seasonal/perennial rhinitis. **Unlabeled:** Prevents recurrence of postsurgical nasal polyps.

PRECAUTIONS

CONTRAINDICATIONS: Hypersensitivity to any corticosteroid, primary treatment of status asthmaticus, systemic fungal infections, persistently positive sputum cultures for *Candida albicans.* **CAUTIONS:** Adrenal insufficiency. **Pregnancy Category C.**

INTERACTIONS

DRUG: None known. **HERBAL:** None known. **FOOD:** None known. **LAB VALUES:** None known.

AVAILABILITY (Rx)

AEROSOL: 250 mcg/activation. **NASAL SPRAY:** 25 mcg/activation.

F

ADMINISTRATION/HANDLING

INHALATION

• Shake container well; exhale as completely as possible. • Place mouthpiece fully into mouth; holding inhaler upright, inhale deeply, slowly while pressing the top of the canister and hold breath as long as possible before exhaling; then exhale slowly. • Wait 1 min between inhalations when multiple inhalations ordered (allows for deeper bronchial penetration). • Rinse mouth with water immediately after inhalation (prevents mouth/throat dryness).

INTRANASAL

• Clear nasal passages before use (topical nasal decongestants may be needed 5–15 min before use). • Tilt head slightly forward. • Insert spray tip up in one nostril, pointing toward inflamed nasal turbinates, away from nasal septum. • Pump medication into one nostril while holding other nostril closed and concurrently inspire through nose. • Discard opened nasal solution after 3 mos.

INDICATIONS/ROUTES/DOSAGE

USUAL INHALATION DOSAGE

Inhalation: ADULTS, ELDERLY: 2 inhalations 2 times/day, morning and evening. **Maximum:** 4 inhalations 2 times/day. CHILDREN 6–15 YRS: 2 inhalations 2 times/day.

USUAL INTRANASAL DOSAGE

Alert: Improvement seen within few days; may take up to 3 wks. Do not continue beyond 3 wks if no significant improvement occurs.

Intranasal: ADULTS, ELDERLY: Initially, 2 sprays each nostril 2 times/day, may increase to 2 sprays 3 times/day. **Maximum:** 8 sprays each nostril/day. CHILDREN 6–14 YRS: Initially, 1 spray 3 times/day or 2 sprays 2 times/day. **Maximum:** 4 sprays each nostril/day. MAINTENANCE: Smallest amount to control symptoms.

SIDE EFFECTS

FREQUENT: Inhalation (10%–25%): Unpleasant taste, nausea, vomiting, sore throat, diarrhea, upset stomach, cold symptoms, nasal congestion. **OCCASIONAL: Inhalation (3%–9%):** Dizziness, irritability, nervousness, shakiness, abdominal pain, heartburn, fungal infection in mouth/pharynx/larynx, edema. **Intranasal:** Mild nasopharyngeal irritation, dryness, rebound congestion, bronchial asthma, rhinorrhea, loss of sense of taste.

ADVERSE REACTIONS/ TOXIC EFFECTS

Acute hypersensitivity reaction (urticaria, angioedema, severe bronchospasm) occurs rarely. Transfer from systemic to local steroid therapy may unmask previously suppressed bronchial asthma condition.

NURSING IMPLICATIONS

BASELINE ASSESSMENT

Establish baseline assessment of asthma, rhinitis.

INTERVENTION/EVALUATION

Advise pts receiving bronchodilators by inhalation concomitantly with steroid inhalation therapy to use bronchodilator several minutes before corticosteroid aerosol (enhances penetration of steroid into bronchial tree). Monitor rate, depth, rhythm, type of respiration; quality/rate of pulse. Assess lung sounds for rhonchi, wheezing, rales. Monitor ABGs.

PATIENT/FAMILY TEACHING

Do not change dose schedule or stop taking drug; must taper off gradually under medical supervision. Maintain careful mouth hygiene. Rinse mouth with water immediately after inhalation (prevents mouth/throat dryness, fungal infection of mouth). Increase fluid intake (decreases lung secretion viscosity). **Intranasal:** Teach proper use of nasal spray. Clear nasal passages before use. Contact physician if no improvement in symptoms, sneezing/nasal irritation occurs. Improvement usually noted in several days.

fluocinolone acetonide

(Flurosyn, Synalar, Synemol)

fluocinonide

(Lidex, Vasoderm)

See Classification section under: Corticosteroids: topical (p. 84C)

fluoride

flur-eyd

(Fluor-A-Day, Fluoritab, Fluotic✱, Luride)

CLASSIFICATION

PHARMACOTHERAPEUTIC: Trace element. **CLINICAL:** Dietary supplement.

ACTION

Increases tooth resistance to acid dissolution. **Therapeutic Effect:** Promotes remineralization of decalcified enamel, inhibits dental plaque bacteria, increases resistance to development of caries. Maintains bone strength.

USES

Dietary supplement for prevention of dental caries in children.

PRECAUTIONS

CONTRAINDICATIONS: Arthralgia, GI ulceration, severe renal insufficiency. **CAUTIONS:** None known.

INTERACTIONS

DRUG: Aluminum hydroxide, calcium may decrease absorption. **HERBAL:** None known. **FOOD:** None known. **LAB VALUES:** May increase SGOT (AST), alkaline phosphatase.

AVAILABILITY (Rx)

TOPICAL CREAM: 1.1%. **GEL-DROPS:** 1.1%. **TOPICAL GEL:** 0.4%, 1.1%. **LOZENGE:** 2.2 mg. **ORAL SOLUTION DROPS:** 1.1 mg/ml. **ORAL SOLUTION RINSE:** 0.05%, 0.2%, 0.44%. **TABLETS (chewable):** 0.58 mg, 1.1 mg, 2.2 mg.

INDICATIONS/ROUTES/DOSAGE

DIETARY SUPPLEMENT

Water Fluoride	Age	mg/day
<0.3 ppm	<2 yrs	0.25 mg/day
	2–3 yrs	0.5 mg/day
	>3–13 yrs	1 mg/day
0.3–0.7 ppm	<2 yrs	None
	2–3 yrs	0.25 mg/day
	>3–13 yrs	0.5 mg/day
>0.7 ppm	None	None

SIDE EFFECTS

RARE: Oral mucous membrane ulceration.

ADVERSE REACTIONS/ TOXIC EFFECTS

Hypocalcemia, tetany, bone pain (esp. ankles, feet), electrolyte disturbances, arrhythmias occur rarely. May cause skeletal fluorosis, osteomalacia, osteosclerosis.

NURSING IMPLICATIONS

PATIENT/FAMILY TEACHING

Do not take with milk, other dairy products (decreases absorption). Rinses, gels should be used at bedtime after brushing, flossing. Expectorate excess—do not swallow. Do not eat, drink, rinse mouth after application.

fluorouracil

phlur-oh-**your**-ah-sill
(Adrucil, Efudex, Fluoroplex)
Do not confuse with Efidac.

CLASSIFICATION

PHARMACOTHERAPEUTIC: Antimetabolite. **CLINICAL:** Antineoplastic (see p. 72C).

ACTION

Blocks formation of thymidylic acid. **Therapeutic Effect:** Inhibits DNA, RNA synthesis. **Topical:** Destroys rapidly proliferating cells. Cell cycle–specific for S phase of cell division.

PHARMACOKINETICS

Crosses blood-brain barrier. Widely distributed. Rapidly metabolized in tissues to active metabolite, which is localized intracellularly. Primarily excreted via lungs as CO_2. Removed by hemodialysis. **Half-life:** 20 hrs.

USES

Parenteral: Treatment of carcinoma of colon, rectum, breast, stomach, pancreas. Used in combination with levamisole after surgical resection in pts with Duke's stage C colon cancer. **Topical:** Treatment of multiple actinic, solar keratoses, superficial basal cell carcinomas. **Unlabeled: Parenteral:** Treatment of bladder, prostate, ovarian, cervical, endometrial, lung, liver, head/neck carcinomas; treatment of pericardial, peritoneal, pleural effusions. **Topical:** Treatment of actinic cheilitis, radiodermatitis.

PRECAUTIONS

CONTRAINDICATIONS: Poor nutritional status, depressed bone marrow function, potentially serious infections, major surgery within previous month. **CAUTIONS:** History of high-dose pelvic irradiation, metastatic cell infiltration of bone marrow, impaired hepatic/renal function.

LIFESPAN CONSIDERATIONS: Pregnancy/lactation: If possible, avoid use during pregnancy, esp. first trimester. May cause fetal harm. Unknown whether distributed in breast milk. Breast-feeding not recommended. **Pregnancy Category D. Children:** No age-related precautions noted. **Elderly:** Age-related renal impairment may require dosage adjustment.

INTERACTIONS

DRUG: Bone marrow depressants may increase risk of bone marrow depression. **Live virus vaccines** may potentiate virus replication, increase vaccine side effects, decrease pt's antibody response to vaccine. **HERBAL:** None known. **FOOD:** None known. **LAB VALUES:** May decrease albumin. May increase excretion of 5-HIAA in urine. **Topical:** May cause eosinophilia, leukocytosis, thrombocytopenia, toxic granulation.

AVAILABILITY (Rx)

INJECTION: 50 mg/ml. **CREAM:** 1%, 5%. **TOPICAL SOLUTION:** 1%, 2%, 5%.

ADMINISTRATION/HANDLING

Alert: Give by IV injection or IV infusion. Do not add to other IV infusions. Avoid small veins, swollen/edematous extremities, areas overlying joints, tendons.

May be carcinogenic, mutagenic, or teratogenic. Handle with extreme care during preparation/administration.

IV

Storage • Solution appears colorless to faint yellow. Slight discoloration does not adversely affect potency or safety. • If precipitate forms, redissolve by heating, shaking vigorously; allow to cool to body temperature.

Reconstitution • IV push does not need to be diluted or reconstituted. Inject through Y-tube or 3-way stopcock of free-flowing solution. • For IV infusion, further dilute with D_5W or 0.9% NaCl.

Rate of administration • Give IV push slowly over 1–2 min. • IV infusion is administered over 30 min–24 hrs. • Extravasation produces immediate pain, severe local tissue damage. Follow protocol.

∅ IV INCOMPATIBILITIES

Amphotericin B complex (Abelcet, Amphotec, AmBisome), droperidol (Inapsine), filgrastim (Neupogen), ondansetron (Zofran), vinorelbine (Navelbine).

IV COMPATIBILITIES

Granisetron (Kytril), heparin, hydromorphone (Dilaudid), leucovorin, morphine, ondansetron (Zofran), potassium chloride, propofol (Diprivan).

INDICATIONS/ROUTES/DOSAGE

Alert: Dosage is individualized based on clinical response, tolerance to adverse effects. When used in combination therapy, consult specific protocols for optimum dosage, sequence of drug administration. Dosage based on pt's actual weight. Use ideal body weight in obese/edematous pts.

INITIAL COURSE

IV: ADULTS, ELDERLY, CHILDREN: Initially, 12 mg/kg/day for 4–5 days. **Maximum:** 800 mg/day. MAINTENANCE: 6 mg/kg every other day for 4 doses. Repeat in 4 wks or 15 mg/kg as a single bolus dose. Or, 5–15 mg/kg/wk as a single dose, not to exceed 1 g.

USUAL TOPICAL DOSAGE

ADULTS: Apply 2 times/day to cover lesions.

F

SIDE EFFECTS

OCCASIONAL: Anorexia, diarrhea, minimal alopecia, fever, dry skin, fissuring, scaling, erythema. **Topical:** Pain, pruritus, hyperpigmentation, irritation, inflammation, burning at application site. **RARE:** Nausea, vomiting, anemia, esophagitis, proctitis, GI ulcer, confusion, headache, lacrimation, visual disturbances, angina, allergic reactions.

ADVERSE REACTIONS/ TOXIC EFFECTS

Earliest sign of toxicity (4–8 days after beginning of therapy) is stomatitis (dry mouth, burning sensation, mucosal erythema, ulceration at inner margin of lips). Most common dermatologic toxicity is pruritic rash (generally appears on extremities, less frequently on trunk). Leukopenia generally occurs within 9–14 days after drug administration (may occur as late as 25th day). Thrombocytopenia occasionally occurs within 7–17 days after administration. Hematologic toxicity may manifest itself as pancytopenia, agranulocytosis.

NURSING IMPLICATIONS

BASELINE ASSESSMENT

Obtain CBC with differential, platelet count, renal/liver function tests.

INTERVENTION/EVALUATION

Monitor for rapidly falling WBC, intractable diarrhea, GI bleeding (bright red/tarry stool). Assess oral mucosa for mucosal erythema, ulceration of inner margin of lips, sore throat, difficulty swallowing (stomatitis). Drug should be discontinued if intractable diarrhea, stomatitis, GI bleeding occurs. Assess skin for rash.

PATIENT/FAMILY TEACHING

Maintain fastidious oral hygiene. Inform physician of signs/symptoms of infection, bleeding, bruising, visual changes, nausea, vomiting, diarrhea, chest pain, palpitations. Avoid sunlight/artificial light sources; wear protective clothing, sunglasses, sunscreen. **Topical:** Apply only to affected area. Do not use occlusive coverings. Be careful near eyes, nose, mouth. Wash hands thoroughly after application. Treated areas may be unsightly for several weeks after therapy.

fluoxetine hydrochloride

flew-**ox**-eh-teen

(Novo-Fluoxetine✱, Prozac, Prozac Weekly, Sarafem)

Do not confuse with fluvastatin, Prilosec, Proscar, ProSom, Serophene.

CLASSIFICATION

PHARMACOTHERAPEUTIC: Psychotherapeutic. **CLINICAL:** Antidepressant, antiobsessional agent, antibulimic (see p. 35C).

ACTION

Selectively inhibits serotonin uptake in CNS, enhancing serotonergic function. **Therapeutic Effect:** Resulting enhancement of synaptic activity produces antidepressant, antiobsessional, antibulimic effect.

PHARMACOKINETICS

Well absorbed from GI tract. Crosses blood-brain barrier. Protein binding: 94%. Metabolized in liver to active metabolite. Primarily excreted in urine. Not removed by hemodialysis. **Half-life:** 2–3 days; metabolite: 7–9 days.

USES

Treatment of clinical depression, obsessive-compulsive disorder (OCD), bulimia nervosa, premenstrual dysphoric disorder (PMDD). **Unlabeled:** Treatment of hot flashes.

PRECAUTIONS

CONTRAINDICATIONS: Within 14 days of MAOI ingestion. **CAUTIONS:** Seizure disorder, cardiac dysfunction, diabetes, those at high risk for suicide.

LIFESPAN CONSIDERATIONS: Pregnancy/lactation: Unknown whether drug crosses placenta or is distributed in breast milk. **Pregnancy Category C. Children:** May be more sensitive to behavioral side effects (e.g., insomnia, restlessness). **Elderly:** No age-related precautions noted.

INTERACTIONS

DRUG: **Alcohol, CNS depressants** antagonize CNS depressant effect. May displace **highly protein-bound medications** from protein-binding sites **(e.g., oral anticoagulants). MAOIs** may produce serotonin syndrome. May increase **phenytoin** concentration, toxicity. **HERBAL:** **St. John's wort** may have additive effect. **FOOD:** None known. **LAB VALUES:** None known.

AVAILABILITY (Rx)

CAPSULES: 10 mg, 20 mg, 40 mg, 90 mg. **LIQUID:** 20 mg/5 ml. **TABLETS:** 10 mg, 20 mg.

ADMINISTRATION/HANDLING

PO

• Give with food or milk if GI distress occurs.

INDICATIONS/ROUTES/DOSAGE

Alert: Use lower or less frequent doses in those with renal/hepatic impairment, elderly, those with concurrent disease or on multiple medications.

DEPRESSION, OCD

PO: ADULTS: Initially, 20 mg each morning. If therapeutic improvement does not occur after 2 wks, gradually increase dose to maximum 80 mg/day in 2 equally divided doses in morning, noon. ELDERLY: Initially, 10 mg/day. May increase by 10–20 mg q2wks. Avoid administration at night. CHILDREN 7–17 YRS: Initially, 5–10 mg/day. Titrate upward as needed (20 mg/day usual dosage). **Prozac Weekly:** ADULTS: 90 mg/wk begin 7 days after last dose of 20 mg.

BULIMIA

PO: ADULTS: 60 mg once daily in morning.

PREMENSTRUAL DYSPHORIC DISORDER

PO: ADULTS: 20 mg/day.

SIDE EFFECTS

FREQUENT (>10%): Headache, asthenia (loss of strength), inability to sleep, anxiety, nervousness, drowsiness, nausea, diarrhea, decreased appetite. **OCCASIONAL (2%–9%):** Dizziness, tremor, fatigue, vomiting, constipation, dry mouth, abdominal pain, nasal congestion, diaphoresis. **RARE (<2%):** Flushed skin, lightheadedness, decreased ability to concentrate.

ADVERSE REACTIONS/ TOXIC EFFECTS

Overdosage may produce seizures, nausea, vomiting, excessive agitation, restlessness.

NURSING IMPLICATIONS

BASELINE ASSESSMENT

For pts on long-term therapy, baseline liver/renal function tests, blood counts should be performed periodically thereafter.

INTERVENTION/EVALUATION

Supervise suicidal-risk pt closely during early therapy (as energy level improves, suicide potential increases). Assess appearance, behavior, speech pattern, level of interest, mood. Monitor stool frequency/consistency. Assess skin for appearance of rash. Monitor liver function tests, weight, glucose, sodium.

PATIENT/FAMILY TEACHING

Maximum therapeutic response may require ≥4 wks of therapy. Do not abruptly discontinue medication. Avoid tasks that require alertness, motor skills until response to drug is established. Avoid alcohol. To avoid insomnia take last dose of drug before 4 PM.

F

fluoxymesterone

floo-ox-ih-**mes**-teh-rone
(Halotestin)

Do not confuse with Halotex, halothane.

CLASSIFICATION

PHARMACOTHERAPEUTIC: Androgen. **CLINICAL:** Sex hormone, antineoplastic.

ACTION

Stimulates RNA polymerase activity, increasing protein production. Synthetic anabolic steroid. **Therapeutic Effect:** Responsible for normal growth, development of male sex organs, maintenance of secondary sex characteristics.

USES

Replacement of endogenous testicular hormone, palliative treatment of breast cancer in women, postpartum breast engorgement. **Unlabeled:** Treatment of anemia.

PRECAUTIONS

CONTRAINDICATIONS: Serious cardiac, renal, hepatic dysfunction. Do not use for men with carcinomas of the breast, prostate. **CAUTIONS:** Decreased renal/liver function, benign prostate hypertrophy, hypercalcemia (may be aggravated in pts with metastatic breast cancer), history of MI, diabetes mellitus. **Pregnancy Category X.**

F

INTERACTIONS

DRUG: May increase effect of **oral anticoagulants. Hepatotoxic medications** may increase hepatotoxicity. **HERBAL:** None known. **FOOD:** None known. **LAB VALUES:** May increase alkaline phosphatase, SGOT (AST), bilirubin, calcium, potassium, sodium, Hgb, Hct, LDL. May decrease HDL.

AVAILABILITY (Rx)

TABLETS: 2 mg, 10 mg.

INDICATIONS/ROUTES/DOSAGE

MALES (hypogonadism)
PO: ADULTS: 5–20 mg/day.

MALES (delayed puberty)
PO: ADULTS: 2.5–20 mg/day for 4–6 mos.

FEMALES (inoperable breast cancer)
PO: ADULTS: 10–40 mg/day in divided doses for 1–3 mos.

FEMALES (prevent postpartum breast pain/engorgement)
PO: ADULTS: Initially, 2.5 mg shortly after delivery, then 5–10 mg/day in divided doses for 4–5 days.

SIDE EFFECTS

FREQUENT: Females: Amenorrhea, virilism (e.g., acne, decreased breast size, enlarged clitoris, male pattern baldness), deepening voice. **Males:** UTI, breast soreness, gynecomastia, priapism, virilism (e.g., acne, early pubic hair growth). **OCCASIONAL:** Edema, nausea, vomiting, mild acne, diarrhea, stomach pain. **Males:** Impotence, testicular atrophy.

ADVERSE REACTIONS/ TOXIC EFFECTS

Peliosis hepatitis (liver, spleen replaced with blood-filled cysts), hepatic neoplasms, and hepatocellular carcinoma have been associated with prolonged high dosage.

NURSING IMPLICATIONS

BASELINE ASSESSMENT

Establish baseline weight, B/P, Hgb, Hct. Check liver function test results, electrolytes, cholesterol if ordered. Wrist x-rays may be ordered to determine bone maturation in children.

INTERVENTION/EVALUATION

Assess electrolytes, cholesterol, Hgb, Hct (periodically for high dosage), liver function test results. With breast cancer or immobility, check for hypercalcemia (lethargy, muscle weakness, confusion, irritability). Be alert to signs of virilization. Monitor sleep patterns.

PATIENT/FAMILY TEACHING

Weigh daily, report weekly gain of ≥5 lbs. Notify physician if jaundice, nausea, vomiting, acne, ankle swelling occurs. **Female:** Promptly report menstrual irregularities, hoarseness, deepening of voice. **Male:** Report frequent erections, difficulty urinating, gynecomastia.

fluphenazine hydrochloride (oral) fluphenazine decanoate (injection)

flew-**phen**-ah-zeen
(Moditen ✱, Prolixin)

CLASSIFICATION

PHARMACOTHERAPEUTIC: Phenothiazine. **CLINICAL:** Antipsychotic (see p. 56C).

ACTION

Antagonizes dopamine neurotransmission at synapses by blocking postsynaptic dopaminergic receptors in brain. **Therapeutic Effect:** Decreases psychotic behavior. Produces weak anticholinergic, sedative, antiemetic effects; strong extrapyramidal activity.

USES

Management of psychotic disturbances (schizophrenia, delusions, hallucinations). **Unlabeled:** Treatment of neurogenic pain (adjunct to tricyclic antidepressants).

PRECAUTIONS

CONTRAINDICATIONS: Narrow-angle glaucoma, bone marrow suppression, severe liver/cardiac disease, severe hypotension/hypertension, subcortical brain damage. **CAUTIONS:** Seizures, Parkinson's disease. **Pregnancy Category C.**

INTERACTIONS

DRUG: **Alcohol, CNS depressants** may increase respiratory depression, hypotensive effects. **Tricyclic antidepressants, MAOIs** may increase sedative, anticholinergic effects. **Antithyroid agents** may increase risk of agranulocytosis. Extrapyramidal symptoms (EPS) may increase with **EPS-producing medications. Hypotensives** may increase hypotension. May decrease **levodopa** effects. **Lithium** may decrease absorption, produce adverse neurologic effects. **HERBAL:** None known. **FOOD:** None known. **LAB VALUES:** May produce false-positive pregnancy or PKU test. EKG changes may occur, including QT interval and T-wave disturbances.

AVAILABILITY (Rx)

TABLETS: 1 mg, 2.5 mg, 5 mg, 10 mg. **ELIXIR:** 2.5 mg/5 ml. **CONCENTRATE:** 5 mg/ml. **INJECTION:** 25 mg/ml.

INDICATIONS/ROUTES/DOSAGE

PSYCHOTIC DISORDERS

PO: ADULTS: Initially, 2.5–10 mg/day in divided doses q6–8h. MAINTENANCE: 1–5 mg/day. ELDERLY: 1–2.5 mg/day; increase gradually as needed. CHILDREN: 0.25–0.75 mg 1–4 times/day.

DECANOATE FORMULATION

IM/subcutaneous: ADULTS: 12.5–25 mg, may repeat q1–3wks. MAINTENANCE: Up to 50 mg q1–4wks. **Maximum:** 100 mg/dose. CHILDREN >12 YRS: 6.25–18.75 mg/wk, may increase to 12.5–25 mg q1–3 wks. CHILDREN 5–12 YRS: 3.125–12.5 mg, may repeat q1–3wks.

SIDE EFFECTS

FREQUENT: Hypotension, dizziness, fainting occur frequently after first injection, occasionally after subsequent injections, rarely with oral dosage. **OCCASIONAL:** Drowsiness during early therapy, dry mouth, blurred vision, lethargy, constipation/diarrhea, nasal congestion, peripheral edema, urinary retention. **RARE:** Ocular changes, skin pigmentation (in pts on high doses for prolonged periods).

ADVERSE REACTIONS/ TOXIC EFFECTS

Extrapyramidal symptoms appear dose related (particularly high dosage), divided into 3 categories: akathisia (inability to sit still, tapping of feet, urge to move around), parkinsonian symptoms (masklike face, tremors, shuffling gait, hypersalivation), acute dystonias (torticollis [neck muscle spasm], opisthotonos [rigidity of back muscles], oculogyric crisis [rolling back of eyes]). Dystonic reaction may produce profuse diaphoresis, pallor. Tardive dyskinesia (protrusion of tongue, puffing of cheeks, chewing/puckering of the mouth) occurs rarely (may be irreversible). Abrupt withdrawal after long-term therapy may precipitate nausea, vomiting, gastritis, dizziness, tremors. Blood dyscrasias, particularly agranulocytosis, mild leukopenia (sore mouth/gums/throat) may occur. May lower seizure threshold.

NURSING IMPLICATIONS

BASELINE ASSESSMENT

Avoid skin contact with solution (contact dermatitis). Assess behavior, appearance, emotional status, response to environment, speech pattern, thought content.

INTERVENTION/EVALUATION

Monitor B/P for hypotension. Monitor CBC for blood dyscrasias. Monitor for fine tongue movement (may be early sign of tardive dyskinesia). Supervise suicidal-risk pt closely during early therapy (as depression lessens, energy level improves, increasing suicide potential). Assess for therapeutic response (interest in surroundings, improvement in self-care, increased ability to concentrate, relaxed facial expression).

PATIENT/FAMILY TEACHING

Full therapeutic effect may take up to 6 wks. Urine may darken. Do not abruptly withdraw from long-term drug therapy. Drowsiness generally subsides during continued therapy. Avoid tasks that require alertness, motor skills until response to drug is established.

flurandrenolide

(Cordran)

See Classification section under: Corticosteroids: topical (p. 84C)

flurazepam hydrochloride

flur-**ah**-zah-pam

(Apo-Flurazepam✦, Dalmane)

Do not confuse with Dialume.

◆ CLASSIFICATION

PHARMACOTHERAPEUTIC: Benzodiazepine **(Schedule IV). CLINICAL:** Sedative-hypnotic (see p. 129C).

ACTION

Enhances action of inhibitory neurotransmitter gamma-aminobutyric acid (GABA). **Therapeutic Effect:** Produces hypnotic effect due to CNS depression.

PHARMACOKINETICS

Onset	Peak	Duration
PO		
15–20 min	3–6 hrs	7–8 hrs

Well absorbed from GI tract. Protein binding: 97%. Crosses blood-brain barrier. Widely distributed. Metabolized in liver to active metabolite. Primarily excreted in urine. Not removed by hemodialysis. **Half-life:** 2.3 hrs; metabolite: 40–114 hrs.

USES

Short-term treatment of insomnia (≤4 wks). Reduces sleep-induction time, number of nocturnal awakenings; increases length of sleep.

PRECAUTIONS

CONTRAINDICATIONS: Acute narrow-angle glaucoma, acute alcohol intoxication. **CAUTIONS:** Impaired renal/hepatic function.

LIFESPAN CONSIDERATIONS: Pregnancy/lactation: Crosses placenta. May be distributed in breast milk. Chronic ingestion during pregnancy may produce withdrawal symptoms, CNS depression in neonates. **Pregnancy Category X. Children:** Safety and efficacy not established in those <15 yrs. **Elderly:** Use small initial doses with gradual dose increases to avoid ataxia, excessive sedation.

INTERACTIONS

DRUG: **Alcohol, CNS depressants** may increase CNS depressant effect. **HERBAL:** **Kava kava, valerian** may increase CNS depression. **FOOD:** None known. **LAB VALUES:** None known.

AVAILABILITY (Rx)

CAPSULES: 15 mg, 30 mg.

ADMINISTRATION/HANDLING

PO

- Give without regard to meals. • Capsules may be emptied and mixed with food.

INDICATIONS/ROUTES/DOSAGE

INSOMNIA

PO: ADULTS: 15–30 mg at bedtime. ELDERLY/DEBILITATED/LIVER DISEASE/LOW SERUM ALBUMIN, CHILDREN >15 YRS: 15 mg at bedtime.

SIDE EFFECTS

FREQUENT: Drowsiness, dizziness, ataxia, sedation. Morning drowsiness may occur initially. **OCCASIONAL:** GI disturbances, nervousness, blurred vision, dry mouth, headache, confusion, skin rash, irritability, slurred speech. **RARE:** Paradoxical CNS excitement/restlessness (particularly noted in elderly/debilitated).

ADVERSE REACTIONS/ TOXIC EFFECTS

Abrupt or too rapid withdrawal after long-term use may result in pronounced restlessness/irritability, insomnia, hand tremors, abdominal/muscle cramps, sweating, vomiting, seizures. Overdosage results in somnolence, confusion, diminished reflexes, coma.

NURSING IMPLICATIONS

BASELINE ASSESSMENT

Assess B/P, pulse, respirations immediately prior to administration. Raise bed rails. Provide environment conducive to sleep (back rub, quiet environment, low lighting).

INTERVENTION/EVALUATION

Assess for paradoxical reaction, particularly during early therapy. Evaluate for therapeutic response: decrease in number of nocturnal awakenings, increase in length of sleep duration.

PATIENT/FAMILY TEACHING

Smoking reduces drug effectiveness. Do not abruptly withdraw medication after long-term use. May have disturbed sleep 1–2 nights after discontinuing. Notify physician if pregnant or planning to become pregnant (Pregnancy Category X). Avoid alcohol, other CNS depressants. May be habit forming.

flurbiprofen

fleur-bih-pro-fen
(Ansaid, Froben✦, Ocufen)

◆CLASSIFICATION

PHARMACOTHERAPEUTIC: Phenylalkanoic acid. **CLINICAL:** Nonsteroidal anti-inflammatory, antidysmenorrheal (see p. 110C).

ACTION

Produces analgesic, anti-inflammatory effect by inhibiting prostaglandin synthesis. Relaxes iris sphincter. **Therapeutic Effect:** Reduces inflammatory response, intensity of pain stimulus reaching sensory nerve endings. Prevents, reduces miosis.

PHARMACOKINETICS

Well absorbed from GI tract, penetrates cornea after ophthalmic administration (may be systemically absorbed). Widely distributed. Protein binding: 99%. Metabolized in liver. Primarily excreted in urine. **Half-life:** 3–4 hrs.

USES

Symptomatic treatment of acute and/or chronic rheumatoid arthritis, osteoarthritis, dysmenorrhea, pain; inhibits intraoperative miosis.

PRECAUTIONS

CONTRAINDICATIONS: Active peptic ulcer, GI ulceration, chronic inflammation of GI tract, GI bleeding disorders, history of hypersensitivity to aspirin/NSAIDs. **CAUTIONS:** Impaired renal/hepatic function, history of GI tract disease, predisposition to fluid retention, soft contact lens wearers, surgical pts with bleeding tendencies.

LIFESPAN CONSIDERATIONS: Pregnancy/lactation: Crosses placenta. Unknown whether distributed in breast milk. Avoid use during last trimester (may adversely affect fetal cardiovascular system: premature closure of ductus arteriosus). **Pregnancy Category B (D** if used in third trimester or near delivery). **Ophthalmic: Pregnancy Category C. Children:** Safety and efficacy not established. **Elderly:** GI bleeding/ulceration more likely to cause serious adverse effects. Age-related renal impairment may increase risk of liver/renal toxicity, decreased dosage recommended.

INTERACTIONS

DRUG: May increase effects of **oral anticoagulants, heparin, thrombolytics.** May decrease effect of **antihypertensives, diuretics. Salicylates, aspirin** may increase risk of GI side effects, bleeding. **Bone marrow depressants** may increase risk of hematologic reactions. May increase concentration, toxicity of **lithium.** May increase **methotrexate** toxicity. **Probenecid** may increase concentration. **Ophthalmic:** May decrease effect of **acetylcholine, carbachol.** May decrease antiglaucoma effect of **epinephrine, other antiglaucoma medications. HERBAL: Feverfew** may have decreased effect. **Ginkgo biloba** may increase risk of bleeding. **FOOD:** None known. **LAB VALUES:** May increase serum transaminase, alkaline phosphatase, LDH, bleeding time.

AVAILABILITY (Rx)

TABLETS: 50 mg, 100 mg. **OPHTHALMIC SOLUTION:** 0.03%.

ADMINISTRATION/HANDLING

PO

• Do not crush or break enteric-coated form. • May give with food, milk, antacids if GI distress occurs.

OPHTHALMIC

• Place finger on lower eyelid, pull out until pocket is formed between eye and lower lid. • Hold dropper above pocket, place prescribed number of drops into pocket. Close eye gently. • Apply digital pressure to lacrimal sac for 1–2 min (minimizes drainage into nose/throat, reducing risk of systemic effects). • Remove excess solution with tissue.

INDICATIONS/ROUTES/DOSAGE

RHEUMATOID ARTHRITIS, OSTEOARTHRITIS

PO: ADULTS, ELDERLY: 200–300 mg/day in 2–4 divided doses. Do not give >100 mg/dose or 300 mg/day.

DYSMENORRHEA

PO: ADULTS: 50 mg 4 times/day.

USUAL OPHTHALMIC DOSAGE

Ophthalmic: ADULTS, ELDERLY, CHILDREN: 1 drop q30min starting 2 hrs before surgery for total of 4 doses.

SIDE EFFECTS

OCCASIONAL: PO (3%–9%): Headache, abdominal pain, diarrhea, indigestion, nausea, fluid retention. **Ophthalmic:** Burning, stinging on instillation, keratitis, elevated intraocular pressure. **RARE (<3%):** Blurred vision, flushed skin, dizziness, drowsiness, nervousness, insomnia, unusual weakness, constipation, decreased appetite, vomiting, confusion.

ADVERSE REACTIONS/ TOXIC EFFECTS

Overdosage may result in acute renal failure. In those treated chronically, peptic ulcer, GI bleeding, gastritis, severe hepatic reaction (jaundice), nephrotoxicity (hematuria, dysuria, proteinuria), severe hypersensitivity reaction (bronchospasm, angiofacial edema), cardiac arrhythmias occur rarely.

NURSING IMPLICATIONS

BASELINE ASSESSMENT

Anti-inflammatory: Assess onset, type, location, duration of pain/inflammation. Inspect appearance of affected joints for immobility, deformities, skin condition.

INTERVENTION/EVALUATION

Monitor for headache, dyspepsia, dizziness. Monitor pattern of daily bowel activity, stool consistency. **Systemic Use:** CBC, platelets, BUN, serum creatinine, liver function tests, occult blood loss. **Ocular:** Periodic eye exams. **Anti-inflammatory:** Evaluate for therapeutic response: relief of pain, stiffness, swelling; increase in joint mobility; reduced joint tenderness; improved grip strength.

PATIENT/FAMILY TEACHING

Swallow tablet whole; do not crush or chew. Avoid aspirin, alcohol (increases risk of GI bleeding). If GI upset occurs, take with food, milk. Report GI distress, visual disturbances, rash, edema, headache. **Ophthalmic:** Eye burning may occur with instillation.

flutamide

flew-tah-myd
(Euflex♣, Eulexin, Novo-Flutamide♣)
Do not confuse with Flumadine.

◆CLASSIFICATION

PHARMACOTHERAPEUTIC: Antiandrogen, hormone. **CLINICAL:** Antineoplastic (see p. 72C).

ACTION

Inhibits androgen uptake and/or binding of androgen in tissues. Interferes with testosterone at cellular level (complements leuprolide). **Therapeutic Effect:** Suppresses testicular androgen production.

PHARMACOKINETICS

Completely absorbed from GI tract. Protein binding: 94%–96%. Metabolized in liver to active metabolite. Primarily excreted in urine. Not removed by hemodialysis. **Half-life:** 6 hrs (half-life increased in elderly).

USES

F

Treatment of metastatic carcinoma of prostate (in combination with LHRH analogues, e.g., leuprolide). Management of locally confined stages B_2-C, D_2 carcinoma.

PRECAUTIONS

CONTRAINDICATIONS: Severe liver impairment. **CAUTIONS:** None known.

LIFESPAN CONSIDERATIONS: Pregnancy/lactation: Not used in this pt population. **Pregnancy Category D. Children:** Not used in children. **Elderly:** No age-related precautions noted.

INTERACTIONS

DRUG: None known. **HERBAL:** None known. **FOOD:** None known. **LAB VALUES:** May increase estradiol, testosterone, SGOT (AST), SGPT (ALT), bilirubin, creatinine, glucose.

AVAILABILITY (Rx)

CAPSULES: 125 mg.

ADMINISTRATION/HANDLING

PO

- Give without regard to food.

INDICATIONS/ROUTES/DOSAGE

PROSTATIC CARCINOMA

PO: ADULTS, ELDERLY: 250 mg q8h.

SIDE EFFECTS

FREQUENT: Hot flashes (50%); loss of libido, impotence, diarrhea (24%); generalized pain (23%); asthenia (loss of strength, energy) (17%); constipation (12%); nausea; nocturia (11%). **OCCASIONAL (6%–8%):** Dizziness, paresthesia, insomnia, impotence, peripheral edema, gynecomastia. **RARE (4%–5%):** Rash, sweating, hypertension, hematuria, vomiting, urinary incontinence, headache, flu syndrome, photosensitivity.

ADVERSE REACTIONS/ TOXIC EFFECTS

Hepatotoxicity, including hepatic encephalopathy, hemolytic anemia may be noted.

NURSING IMPLICATIONS

INTERVENTION/EVALUATION

Periodically monitor hepatic function tests in long-term therapy.

PATIENT/FAMILY TEACHING

Do not stop taking medication (both drugs must be continued). Urine color may change to amber/yellow-green. Avoid prolonged exposure to sun/tanning beds. Wear clothing to protect from ultraviolet exposure until tolerance is determined.

fluticasone propionate

flew-**tih**-cah-sewn
(Cutivate, Flonase, Flovent)

FIXED-COMBINATION(S)

Advair: fluticasone/salmeterol (bronchodilator): 100 mcg/50 mcg; 250 mcg/50 mcg; 500 mcg/50 mcg.

CLASSIFICATION

PHARMACOTHERAPEUTIC: Corticosteroid. **CLINICAL:** Anti-inflammatory, antipruritic (see pp. 65C, 81C, 84C).

ACTION

Controls rate of protein synthesis, depresses migration of polymorphonuclear leukocytes, reverses capillary permeability, stabilizes lysosomal membranes. **Therapeutic Effect:** Prevents or controls inflammation.

PHARMACOKINETICS

Inhalation/intranasal: Protein binding: 91%. Undergoes extensive first-pass metabolism in liver. Excreted in urine. **Half-life:** 3–7.8 hrs. **Topical:** Amount absorbed depends on drug, area, skin condition (absorption increased with elevated skin temperature, hydration, inflamed/denuded skin).

USES

Nasal: Relief of seasonal/perennial allergic rhinitis. **Topical:** Relief of inflammation/pruritus associated with steroid-responsive disorders (e.g., contact dermatitis, eczema). **Inhalation:** Maintenance treatment of asthma for those requiring oral corticosteroid therapy. **Powder:** Maintenance of asthma treatment in children ≥4 yrs.

PRECAUTIONS

CONTRAINDICATIONS: Untreated localized infection of nasal mucosa. **Inhalation:** Primary treatment of status asthmaticus, other acute asthma episodes. **CAUTIONS:** Active or quiescent tuberculosis, untreated fungal, bacterial, or systemic ocular herpes simplex viral infection.

LIFESPAN CONSIDERATIONS: Pregnancy/lactation: Unknown if drug crosses placenta or is distributed in breast milk. **Pregnancy Category C. Children:** Safety and efficacy not established in those <4 yrs. Children ≥4 yrs may experience growth suppression with prolonged or high doses. **Elderly:** No age-related precautions noted.

INTERACTIONS

DRUG: None known. **HERBAL:** None known. **FOOD:** None known. **LAB VALUES:** None known.

AVAILABILITY (Rx)

AEROSOL FOR ORAL INHALATION (Flovent): 44 mcg/inhalation, 110 mcg/inhalation 220 mcg/inhalation. **TOPICAL CREAM (Cultivate):** 0.05%. **TOPICAL OINTMENT (Cultivate):** 0.005%. **POWDER FOR ORAL INHALATION (Flovent Diskus, Flovent Rotadisk):** 50 mcg, 100 mcg, 250 mcg. **INTRANASAL SPRAY (Flonase):** 50 mcg/inhalation.

ADMINISTRATION/HANDLING

INHALATION

• Shake container well; exhale as completely as possible. • Place mouthpiece fully into mouth; holding inhaler upright, inhale deeply, slowly while pressing the top of the canister; hold breath as long as possible before exhaling, then exhale slowly. • Wait 1 min between inhalations when multiple inhalations ordered (allows for deeper bronchial penetration). • Rinse mouth with water immediately after inhalation (prevents mouth/throat dryness).

INTRANASAL

• Clear nasal passages before use (topical nasal decongestants may be needed 5–15 min before use). • Tilt head slightly forward. • Insert spray tip up in 1 nostril, pointing toward inflamed nasal turbinates, away from nasal septum. • Pump medication into 1 nostril while holding other nostril closed, concurrently inspire through nose.

INDICATIONS/ROUTES/DOSAGE

ALLERGIC RHINITIS

Intranasal: ADULTS, ELDERLY: Initially, 200 mcg (2 sprays each nostril once daily or 1 spray each nostril q12h).

F

MAINTENANCE: 1 spray each nostril once daily. **Maximum:** 200 mcg/day. CHILDREN >4 YRS: Initially, 100 mcg (1 spray each nostril once daily). **Maximum:** 200 mcg/day.

USUAL TOPICAL DOSAGE

Topical: ADULTS, ELDERLY, CHILDREN >3 MOS: Apply sparingly to affected area 1–2 times/day.

F

USUAL INHALATION DOSAGE (dry powder formulation)

Inhalation: CHILDREN 4–11 YRS: 50–100 mcg twice daily.

PREVIOUS TREATMENT: BRONCHODILATORS

Inhalation: ADULTS, ELDERLY, CHILDREN >12 YRS: Initially, 100 mcg q12h. **Maximum:** 500 mcg/day.

PREVIOUS TREATMENT: INHALED STEROIDS

Inhalation: ADULTS, ELDERLY, CHILDREN >12 YRS: Initially, 100–250 mcg q12h. **Maximum:** 500 mcg q12h.

PREVIOUS TREATMENT: ORAL STEROIDS

Inhalation: ADULTS, ELDERLY, CHILDREN >12 YRS: DISKUS: 500–1,000 mcg 2 times/day. ROTADISK: 1,000 mcg 2 times/day.

SIDE EFFECTS

FREQUENT: Inhalation: Throat irritation, hoarseness, dry mouth, coughing, temporary wheezing, localized fungal infection in mouth, pharynx, larynx (particularly if mouth is not rinsed with water following each administration). **Intranasal:** Mild nasopharyngeal irritation; nasal irritation, burning, stinging, dryness, rebound congestion, rhinorrhea, loss of sense of taste. **OCCASIONAL: Intranasal:** Nasal/pharyngeal candidiasis, headache. **Inhalation:** Oral candidiasis. **Topical:** Burning/itching of skin.

ADVERSE REACTIONS/ TOXIC EFFECTS

None known.

NURSING IMPLICATIONS

BASELINE ASSESSMENT

Establish baseline history of skin disorder, asthma, rhinitis.

INTERVENTION/EVALUATION

Monitor rate, depth, rhythm, type of respiration; quality/rate of pulse. Assess lung sounds for rhonchi, wheezing, rales. Monitor ABGs. Assess oral mucous membranes for evidence of candidiasis. Monitor growth in pediatric pts. **Topical:** Assess involved area for therapeutic response to irritation.

PATIENT/FAMILY TEACHING

Advise pts receiving bronchodilators by inhalation concomitantly with steroid inhalation therapy to use bronchodilator several minutes before corticosteroid aerosol (enhances penetration of steroid into bronchial tree). Do not change dose schedule or stop taking drug; must taper off gradually under medical supervision. Maintain careful oral hygiene. Rinse mouth with water immediately after inhalation (prevents mouth/throat dryness, fungal infection of mouth). Increase fluid intake (decreases lung secretion viscosity). **Intranasal:** Teach proper use of nasal spray. Clear nasal passages before use. Contact physician if no improvement in symptoms or sneezing/nasal irritation occurs. Improvement noted in several days. **Topical:** Rub thin film gently into affected area. Use only for prescribed area and no longer than ordered. Avoid contact with eyes.

fluvastatin

flu-vah-**stah**-tin

(Lescol, Lescol XL)

Do not confuse with fluoxetine.

◆ **CLASSIFICATION**

PHARMACOTHERAPEUTIC: HMG-CoA reductase inhibitor. **CLINICAL:** Antihyperlipidemic (see p. 50C).

ACTION

Inhibits HMG-CoA reductase, the enzyme that catalyzes the early step in cholesterol synthesis. **Therapeutic Effect:** Decreases LDL cholesterol, VLDL, plasma triglycerides. Increases HDL cholesterol concentration slightly.

PHARMACOKINETICS

Well absorbed from GI tract (unaffected by food). Does not cross blood-brain barrier. Protein binding: >98%. Primarily eliminated in feces. **Half-life:** 1.2 hrs.

USES

Adjunct to diet therapy to decrease elevated total, LDL cholesterol concentrations in those with primary hypercholesterolemia (types IIa, IIb), those with combined hypercholesterolemia, hypertriglyceridemia. Treatment of elevated triglycerides, apolipoprotein, secondary prevention of coronary events.

PRECAUTIONS

CONTRAINDICATIONS: Active liver disease, unexplained increased serum transaminase. **CAUTIONS:** Anticoagulant therapy, history of liver disease, substantial alcohol consumption. Withholding/discontinuing fluvastatin may be necessary when pt at risk for renal failure (secondary to rhabdomyolysis); major surgery; severe acute infection; trauma; hypotension; severe metabolic, endocrine, electrolyte disorders; uncontrolled seizures.

LIFESPAN CONSIDERATIONS: Pregnancy/lactation: Contraindicated in pregnancy (suppression of cholesterol biosynthesis may cause fetal toxicity), lactation. Unknown whether drug is distributed in breast milk. **Pregnancy Category X. Children:** Safety and efficacy not established. **Elderly:** No age-related precautions noted.

INTERACTIONS

DRUG: Increased risk of rhabdomyolysis, acute renal failure with **cyclosporine, erythromycin, gemfibrozil, niacin, other immunosuppressants. HERBAL:** None known. **FOOD:** None known. **LAB VALUES:** May increase creatinine kinase (CK) levels, serum transaminase concentrations.

AVAILABILITY (Rx)

CAPSULES: 20 mg, 40 mg. **TABLETS (extended-release):** 80 mg.

ADMINISTRATION/HANDLING

PO

- Give without regard to food.

INDICATIONS/ROUTES/DOSAGE

HYPERLIPOPROTEINEMIA

PO: ADULTS, ELDERLY: Initially, 20 mg/day in the evening. May increase up to 40 mg/day. MAINTENANCE: 20–40 mg/day in single or divided doses. PTS REQUIRING >25% DECREASE IN LDL-C: 40 mg 1–2 times/day (may use 80-mg tablets once daily).

SIDE EFFECTS

FREQUENT (5%–8%): Headache, dyspepsia, back pain, myalgia, arthralgia, diarrhea, abdominal cramping, rhinitis. **OCCASIONAL (2%–4%):** Nausea, vomiting, insomnia, constipation, flatulence, rash, fatigue, cough, dizziness.

ADVERSE REACTIONS/ TOXIC EFFECTS

Myositis (inflammation of voluntary muscle), with or without increased CK, muscle weakness, occurs rarely. May progress to frank rhabdomyolysis, renal impairment.

NURSING IMPLICATIONS

BASELINE ASSESSMENT

Question for possibility of pregnancy before initiating therapy (Pregnancy Category X). Assess baseline lab results: cholesterol, triglycerides, liver function tests.

INTERVENTION/EVALUATION

Determine pattern of bowel activity. Check for headache, dizziness, blurred vision. Assess for rash, pruritus. Monitor cholesterol, triglyceride lab results for therapeutic response. Be alert for malaise, muscle cramping/weakness.

PATIENT/FAMILY TEACHING

Follow special diet (important part of treatment). Periodic lab tests are essential part of therapy. Report promptly any muscle pain/weakness, esp. if accompanied by fever, malaise.

fluvoxamine maleate

flew-**vox**-ah-meen

CLASSIFICATION

PHARMACOTHERAPEUTIC: Serotonin reuptake inhibitor. **CLINICAL:** Antidepressant, antiobsessional (see p. 36C).

ACTION

Selectively inhibits serotonin neuronal uptake in CNS. **Therapeutic Effect:** Produces antidepressant, antiobsessive effects.

USES

Treatment of obsessive-compulsive disorder (OCD). **Unlabeled:** Treatment of depression.

PRECAUTIONS

CONTRAINDICATIONS: Within 14 days of MAOI ingestion. **CAUTIONS:** Impaired renal/hepatic function, elderly. **Pregnancy Category C.**

INTERACTIONS

DRUG: **MAOIs** may produce serious reactions (hyperthermia, rigidity, myoclonus). **Tryptophan, lithium** may enhance serotonergic effects. **Tricyclic antidepressants** may increase concentration. Fluvoxamine may increase concentration/toxicity of **benzodiazepines, carbamazepine, clozapine, theophylline.** May increase effects of **warfarin.** **HERBAL:** **St. John's wort** may have additive effect. **FOOD:** None known. **LAB VALUES:** None known.

AVAILABILITY (Rx)

TABLETS: 25 mg, 50 mg, 100 mg.

INDICATIONS/ROUTES/DOSAGE

Alert: Use lower or less frequent dosing in impaired hepatic function, elderly.

OCD

PO: ADULTS: 50 mg at bedtime; increase by 50 mg q4–7days. Doses >100 mg/day in 2 divided doses. **Maximum:** 300 mg/day. CHILDREN 8–17 YRS: 25 mg at bedtime; increase by 25 mg q4–7days. Doses >50 mg/day in 2 divided doses. **Maximum:** 200 mg/day.

SIDE EFFECTS

FREQUENT: Nausea (40%); headache, somnolence, insomnia (21%–22%). **OCCASIONAL (8%–14%):** Nervousness, dizziness, diarrhea/loose stools, dry mouth, asthenia (loss of strength, weakness), dyspepsia, constipation, abnormal ejaculation. **RARE (3%–6%):** Anorexia, anxiety, tremor, vomiting, flatulence, urinary frequency, sexual dysfunction, taste change.

ADVERSE REACTIONS/ TOXIC EFFECTS

Overdosage may produce seizures, nausea, vomiting, excessive agitation, extreme restlessness.

NURSING IMPLICATIONS

INTERVENTION/EVALUATION

Supervise suicidal-risk pt closely during early therapy (as energy level improves, suicide potential increases). Assess appearance, behavior, speech pattern, level of interest, mood. Assist with ambulation if dizziness, somnolence occurs. Monitor stool frequency/consistency.

PATIENT/FAMILY TEACHING

Maximum therapeutic response may require ≥4 wks of therapy. Dry mouth may be relieved by sugarless gum, sips of tepid water. Do not abruptly discontinue medication. Avoid tasks that require alertness, motor skills until response to drug is established.

folic acid (vitamin B_9)

foe-lick
(Apo-Folic ♣, Folvite)
Do not confuse with Florvite.

sodium folate

(Folvite-parenteral)

CLASSIFICATION

PHARMACOTHERAPEUTIC: Coenzyme. **CLINICAL:** Nutritional supplement.

ACTION

Stimulates production of RBCs, WBCs, platelets. **Therapeutic Effect:** Essential for nucleoprotein synthesis, maintenance of normal erythropoiesis.

PHARMACOKINETICS

Oral form almost completely absorbed from GI tract (upper duodenum). Protein binding: High. Metabolized in liver, plasma to active form. Excreted in urine. Removed by hemodialysis.

USES

Treatment of megaloblastic, macrocytic anemia associated with pregnancy, infancy, childhood, inadequate dietary intake. **Unlabeled:** Decreases risk of colon cancer.

PRECAUTIONS

CONTRAINDICATIONS: Anemias (pernicious, aplastic, normocytic, refractory). **CAUTIONS:** None known.

LIFESPAN CONSIDERATIONS: Pregnancy/lactation: Distributed in breast milk. **Pregnancy Category A** (**C** if more than RDA). **Children/elderly:** No age-related precautions noted.

INTERACTIONS

DRUG: May decrease effects of **hydantoin anticonvulsants. Analgesics, anticonvulsants, carbamazepine, estrogens** may increase folic acid requirements. **Antacids, cholestyramine** may decrease absorption. **Methotrexate, triamterene, trimethoprim** may antagonize effects. **HERBAL:** None known. **FOOD:** None known. **LAB VALUES:** May decrease vitamin B_{12} concentration.

AVAILABILITY (Rx)

TABLETS (OTC): 0.4 mg, 0.8 mg. **TABLETS (Rx):** 1 mg. **INJECTION (Rx):** 5 mg/ml.

ADMINISTRATION/HANDLING

Alert: Parenteral form used in acutely ill, parenteral/enteral alimentation, those unresponsive to oral route in GI malabsorption syndrome. Dosage >0.1 mg daily may conceal pernicious anemia.

INDICATIONS/ROUTES/DOSAGE

F

DEFICIENCY

IV/IM/subcutaneous/PO: ADULTS, ELDERLY, CHILDREN >10 YRS: Initially, 1 mg/day. MAINTENANCE: 0.5 mg/day. CHILDREN 1–10 YRS: Initially, 1 mg/day. MAINTENANCE: 0.1–0.4 mg/day. INFANTS: 50 mcg/day.

SUPPLEMENT

PO/IM/IV/subcutaneous: ADULTS, ELDERLY, CHILDREN ≥4 YRS: 0.4 mg/day. CHILDREN <4 YRS: 0.3 mg/day. CHILDREN <1 YR: 0.1 mg/day. PREGNANCY: 0.8 mg/day.

SIDE EFFECTS

None known.

ADVERSE REACTIONS/ TOXIC EFFECTS

Allergic hypersensitivity occurs rarely with parenteral form. Oral folic acid is nontoxic.

NURSING IMPLICATIONS

BASELINE ASSESSMENT

Pernicious anemia should be ruled out with Schilling test and vitamin B_{12} blood level prior to therapy is initiated (may produce irreversible neurologic damage). Resistance to treatment may occur if decreased hematopoiesis, alcoholism, antimetabolic drugs, deficiency of vitamin B_6, B_{12}, C, E is evident.

INTERVENTION/EVALUATION

Assess for therapeutic improvement: improved sense of well-being, relief from iron deficiency symptoms (fatigue, shortness of breath, sore tongue, headache, pallor).

PATIENT/FAMILY TEACHING

Eat foods rich in folic acid, including fruits, vegetables, organ meats.

follitropin alpha

(Gonal-F)

See Classification section under: Fertility agents (p. 89C)

fomepizole

(Antizol)

See Appendix A: Antidotes

fondaparinux sodium

fond-dah-**pear**-in-ux

(Arixtra)

◆ **CLASSIFICATION**

PHARMACOTHERAPEUTIC: Factor Xa inhibitor, pentasaccharide. **CLINICAL:** Antithrombotic.

ACTION

Selectively binds to antithrombin and increases its affinity for factor Xa (inhibition of factor Xa stops the blood coagulation cascade). **Therapeutic Effect:** Indirectly prevents formation of thrombin and subsequently the fibrin clot.

PHARMACOKINETICS

Well absorbed following subcutaneous administration. Undergoes minimal, if any, metabolism. Highly bound to antithrombin III. Distributed mainly in blood and to a minor extent in extravascular fluid. Excreted unchanged in urine. Removed by hemodialysis. **Half-life:** 17–21 hrs (half-life prolonged in those with impaired renal function).

USES

Prevention of venous thromboembolism in pts undergoing total hip replacement, hip fracture surgery, knee replacement surgery.

PRECAUTIONS

CONTRAINDICATIONS: Active bleeding (risk of uncontrollable hemorrhage, severe renal impairment, weight <50 kg, bacterial endocarditis, thrombocytopenia associated with fondaparinux). **CAUTIONS:** Conditions with increased risk of hemorrhage (GI ulceration, hemophilia, concurrent use of antiplatelet agents, severe uncontrolled hypertension, history of cerebrovascular accident), history of heparin-induced thrombocytopenia, impaired renal function, elderly, neuraxial anesthesia, indwelling epidural catheter use.

LIFESPAN CONSIDERATIONS: Pregnancy/lactation: Use with caution, particularly during last trimester, immediate postpartum period (increased risk of maternal hemorrhage). Unknown if excreted in breast milk. **Pregnancy Category B. Children:** Safety and efficacy not established. **Elderly:** Age-related decreased renal function may increase risk of bleeding.

INTERACTIONS

DRUG: Anticoagulants, platelet inhibitors may increase bleeding. **HERBAL:** None known. **FOOD:** None known. **LAB VALUES:** Reversible increases in SGOT (AST), SGPT (ALT), serum creatinine. May decrease Hgb, Hct, platelet count.

ADMINISTRATION/HANDLING

SUBCUTANEOUS

• Parenteral form appears clear, colorless. Discard if discoloration/particulate matter is noted. • Store at room temperature. • Do not expel the air bubble from the prefilled syringe before injection. Pinch a fold of skin at the injection site between thumb and forefinger. Introduce entire length of subcutaneous needle into skin fold during injection. Inject into fatty tissue between left and right anterolateral or left and right posterolateral abdominal wall. Rotate injection sites.

F

INDICATIONS/ROUTES/DOSAGE

PREVENTION OF VENOUS THROMBOEMBOLISM

Subcutaneous: ADULTS: 2.5 mg once daily for 5–9 days after surgery. Initial dose should be given 6–8 hrs after surgery. Dosage should be adjusted in elderly, those with renal impairment.

AVAILABILITY (Rx)

PREFILLED SYRINGE: 2.5 mg.

SIDE EFFECTS

OCCASIONAL (14%): Fever. **RARE (1%–4%):** Injection site hematoma, nausea, peripheral edema.

ADVERSE REACTIONS/TOXIC EFFECTS

Accidental overdosage may lead to bleeding complications ranging from local ecchymoses to major hemorrhage. Thrombocytopenia occurs rarely.

NURSING IMPLICATIONS

BASELINE ASSESSMENT

Assess CBC, including platelet count, baseline BUN, creatinine clearance.

F

INTERVENTION/EVALUATION

Periodically monitor CBC, platelet count, stool for occult blood (no need for daily monitoring in pts with normal presurgical coagulation parameters). Assess for any signs of bleeding: bleeding at surgical site, hematuria, blood in stool, bleeding from gums, petechiae, bruising, bleeding from injection sites. Monitor B/P; hypotension may indicate bleeding.

PATIENT/FAMILY TEACHING

Usual length of therapy is 5–9 days. Do not take any OTC medication (esp. aspirin, NSAIDs). Consult physician if swelling in hands, feet is noted or unusual back pain, unusual bleeding/bruising, weakness, sudden/severe headache occurs.

formoterol fumarate

four-**moh**-tur-all
(Foradil Aerolizer)

◆CLASSIFICATION

PHARMACOTHERAPEUTIC: Sympathomimetic (beta$_2$-adrenergic agonist). **CLINICAL:** Bronchodilator (see p. 64C).

ACTION

Long-acting bronchodilator. Stimulates beta$_2$-adrenergic receptors in the lungs, resulting in relaxation of bronchial smooth muscle. Also inhibits release of mediators from various cells in the lungs, including mast cells, with little effect on heart rate. **Therapeutic Effect:** Relieves bronchospasm, reduces airway resistance. Produces improved bronchodilation, improved nighttime asthma control, improved peak flow rates.

PHARMACOKINETICS

Onset	Peak	Duration
Inhalation		
1–3 min	0.5–1 hr	12 hrs

Absorbed from bronchi following inhalation. Metabolized in liver. Primarily excreted in urine. Unknown if removed by hemodialysis. **Half-life:** 10 hrs.

USES

For long-term maintenance treatment of asthma, prevention of exercise-induced bronchospasm, treatment of bronchoconstriction in pts with COPD. Can be used concomitantly with short-acting beta-agonists, inhaled or systemic corticosteroids, theophylline therapy.

PRECAUTIONS

CONTRAINDICATIONS: None known. **CAUTIONS:** Hypertension, cardiovascular disease, convulsive disorder, thyrotoxicosis.

LIFESPAN CONSIDERATIONS: Pregnancy/lactation: Unknown if drug crosses placenta or is distributed in breast milk. **Pregnancy Category C. Children:** Safety and efficacy not established in children <5 yrs. **Elderly:** May be more sensitive to tremor or tachycardia due to age-related increased sympathetic sensitivity.

INTERACTIONS

DRUG: Beta-adrenergic blocking agents (beta-blockers) can antagonize bronchodilating effects. May potentiate cardiovascular effects with **MAOIs, tricyclic antidepressants,** drugs that can prolong QT interval **(erythromycin, thioridazine, quinidine). Diuretics, xanthine derivatives, steroids** can increase risk of hypokalemia. **HERBAL:** None known. **FOOD:** None known. **LAB VALUES:** May reduce serum potassium level, increase blood glucose level.

AVAILABILITY (Rx)

INHALATION POWDER IN CAPSULES: 12 mcg.

ADMINISTRATION/HANDLING

Storage • Maintain capsules in individual blister pack until immediately before use. Do not swallow capsules. Do not use with a spacer.

Inhalation: • Pull off Aerolizer Inhaler cover, twisting mouthpiece in direction of the arrow to open. • Place capsule in chamber. Capsule is pierced by pressing and releasing buttons on the side of the Aerolizer, once only. • Exhale completely; place mouthpiece into mouth, close lips. • Inhale quickly, deeply through mouth (this causes capsule to spin, dispensing the drug). Hold breath as long as possible before exhaling slowly. • Check capsule to make sure all the powder is gone. If not, inhale again to receive rest of the dose. Rinse mouth with water immediately after inhalation (prevents mouth/throat dryness).

INDICATIONS/ROUTES/DOSAGE

MAINTENANCE TREATMENT OF ASTHMA

Inhalation: ADULTS, ELDERLY, CHILDREN >5 YRS: Inhale contents of 1 capsule every 12 hrs.

EXERCISE-INDUCED ASTHMA

Inhalation: ADULTS, ELDERLY, CHILDREN >12 YRS: Inhale contents of 1 capsule at least 15 min before exercise.

SIDE EFFECTS

OCCASIONAL: Tremor, cramps, tachycardia, insomnia, headache, irritability, irritation of mouth/throat.

ADVERSE REACTIONS/ TOXIC EFFECTS

Excessive sympathomimetic stimulation may produce palpitations, extrasystoles, chest pain.

NURSING IMPLICATIONS

INTERVENTION/EVALUATION

Monitor rate, depth, rhythm, type of respiration; quality/rate of pulse; EKG, serum potassium, ABG determinations. Assess lung sounds for wheezing (bronchoconstriction), rales.

PATIENT/FAMILY TEACHING

Instruct on proper use of inhaler. Increase fluid intake (decreases lung secretion viscosity). Rinsing mouth with water immediately after inhalation may prevent mouth/throat irritation. Avoid excessive use of caffeine derivatives (chocolate, coffee, tea, cola).

Fortaz

see ceftazidime

Fortovase

see saquinavir

Fosamax

see alendronate

foscarnet sodium

fos-**car**-net

(Foscavir)

CLASSIFICATION

CLINICAL: Antiviral (see p. 59C).

ACTION

Provides selective inhibition at binding site on virus-specific DNA polymerases and reverse transcriptases. **Therapeutic Effect:** Inhibits replication of herpes virus.

PHARMACOKINETICS

F

Sequestered into bone, cartilage. Protein binding: 14%–17%. Primarily excreted unchanged in urine. Removed by hemodialysis. **Half-life:** 3.3–6.8 hrs (half-life increased with impaired renal function).

USES

Alternative to ganciclovir for treatment of cytomegalovirus (CMV) infections, CMV retinitis in patients with AIDS, treatment of acyclovir-resistant mucocutaneous herpes simplex infections in immunocompromised patients, acyclovir-resistant herpes zoster infections.

PRECAUTIONS

CONTRAINDICATIONS: None known. **CAUTIONS:** Neurologic/cardiac abnormalities, history of renal impairment, altered calcium, other electrolyte levels.

LIFESPAN CONSIDERATIONS: Pregnancy/lactation: Unknown if distributed in breast milk. **Pregnancy Category C. Children:** Safety and efficacy not established. **Elderly:** Age-related renal impairment may require dosage adjustment.

INTERACTIONS

DRUG: Nephrotoxic medications may increase risk of renal toxicity. **Pentamidine (IV)** may cause reversible hypocalcemia, hypomagnesemia, nephrotoxicity. **Zidovudine** may increase anemia. **HERBAL:** None known. **FOOD:** None known. **LAB VALUES:** May increase SGOT (AST), SGPT (ALT), alkaline phosphatase, bilirubin, creatinine. May decrease magnesium, potassium. May alter calcium, phosphate concentrations.

AVAILABILITY (Rx)

INJECTION: 24 mg/ml.

ADMINISTRATION/HANDLING

IV

Storage • Store parenteral vials at room temperature. • After dilution, stable for 24 hrs at room temperature. • Do not use if solution is discolored or contains particulate material.

Reconstitution • The standard 24 mg/ml solution may be used without dilution when central venous catheter is used for infusion; 24 mg/ml solution *must* be diluted to 12 mg/ml when peripheral vein catheter is being used. • Only D_5W or 0.9% NaCl solution for injection should be used for dilution.

Rate of administration • Because dosage is calculated on body weight, unneeded quantity may be removed before start of infusion to avoid overdosage. Aseptic technique must be used and solution administered within 24 hrs of first entry into sealed bottle. • Do not give by IV injection or rapid infusion (increases toxicity). • Administer by IV infusion at a rate not faster than 1 hr for doses up to 60 mg/kg and 2 hrs for doses >60 mg/kg. • To minimize toxicity and phlebitis, use central venous lines or veins with adequate bloodflow to permit rapid dilution, dissemination of foscarnet. • Use IV infusion pump to prevent accidental overdose.

IV INCOMPATIBILITIES

Acyclovir (Zovirax), amphotericin (Fungizone), diazepam (Valium), digoxin (Lanoxin), diphenhydramine (Benadryl), dobutamine (Dobutrex), droperidol (Inapsine), ganciclovir (Cytovene), haloperidol (Haldol), leucovorin, midazolam (Versed), pentamidine (Pentam IV), prochlorperazine (Compazine), trimethoprim-sulfamethoxazole (Bactrim), vancomycin (Vancocin).

IV COMPATIBILITIES

Dopamine (Intropin), heparin, hydromorphone (Dilaudid), lorazepam (Ativan), morphine, potassium chloride.

INDICATIONS/ROUTES/DOSAGE

CMV RETINITIS

IV: ADULTS, ELDERLY: Initially, 60 mg/kg q8h (may dose as 100 mg q12h) for 2–3 wks. MAINTENANCE: 90–120 mg/kg/day as a single IV infusion.

HERPES SIMPLEX

IV: ADULTS: 40 mg/kg q8–12h for 2–3 wks or until healed.

DOSAGE IN RENAL IMPAIRMENT

Dosage individualized according to pt's creatinine clearance. Refer to dosing guide provided by manufacturer.

SIDE EFFECTS

FREQUENT: Fever (65%); nausea (47%); vomiting, diarrhea (30%). **OCCASIONAL (≥5%):** Anorexia, pain/inflammation at injection site, fever, rigors, malaise, hypertension/hypotension, headache, paresthesia, dizziness, rash, diaphoresis, nausea, vomiting, abdominal pain. **RARE (1%–5%):** Back/chest pain, edema, hypertension/hypotension, flushing, pruritus, constipation, dry mouth.

ADVERSE REACTIONS/ TOXIC EFFECTS

Renal impairment is a major toxicity that occurs to some extent in most pts. Seizures, mineral/electrolyte imbalances may be life threatening.

NURSING IMPLICATIONS

BASELINE ASSESSMENT

Obtain baseline mineral and electrolyte levels, vital signs, CBC values, renal function tests. Risk of renal impairment can be reduced by sufficient fluid intake to assure diuresis prior to and during therapy.

INTERVENTION/EVALUATION

Monitor serum creatinine, calcium, phosphorus, potassium, magnesium, Hgb, Hct, ophthalmologic exams. Assess for signs of electrolyte imbalance, esp. hypocalcemia (perioral tingling, numbness/paresthesia of extremities), hypokalemia (weakness, muscle cramps, numbness/tingling of extremities, irritability). Monitor renal function tests. Assess for tremors; provide safety measures for potential seizures. Assess for bleeding, anemia, developing superinfections.

PATIENT/FAMILY TEACHING

Important to report perioral tingling, numbness in the extremities, paresthesias during or following infusion (may indicate electrolyte abnormalities). Tremors should be reported promptly due to potential for seizures.

fosfomycin tromethamine

foss-foe-**my**-sin

(Monurol)

Do not confuse with Monopril.

◆ CLASSIFICATION

PHARMACOTHERAPEUTIC: Antibiotic. **CLINICAL:** Urinary tract infection agent.

ACTION

Inhibits synthesis of peptidoglycan. **Therapeutic Effect:** Prevents bacterial cell wall synthesis. Bactericidal.

USES

Single-dose treatment for uncomplicated urinary tract infections (UTI) in women.

PRECAUTIONS

CONTRAINDICATIONS: None known. **CAUTIONS:** None known. **Pregnancy Category B.**

INTERACTIONS

DRUG: **Metoclopramide** lowers serum concentration, urinary excretion of **fosfomycin**. **HERBAL:** None known. **FOOD:** None known. **LAB VALUES:** May increase eosinophil count, bilirubin, SGOT (AST), SGPT (ALT), alkaline phosphatase. May alter WBC, platelet count. May decrease Hct, Hgb.

AVAILABILITY (Rx)

POWDER: 3 g.

ADMINISTRATION/HANDLING

- Give without regard to food.

INDICATIONS/ROUTES/DOSAGE

UTI

PO: FEMALES: 3 g in 4 oz water as a single dose. MALES (COMPLICATED UTI): 3 g daily for 2–3 days.

SIDE EFFECTS

OCCASIONAL (3%–9%): Diarrhea, nausea, headache, back pain. **RARE (<2%):** Dysmenorrhea, pharyngitis, abdominal pain, rash.

ADVERSE REACTIONS/ TOXIC EFFECTS

None known.

NURSING IMPLICATIONS

PATIENT/FAMILY TEACHING

Symptoms should improve in 2–3 days. Always mix medication with water before taking.

fosinopril

foh-**sin**-oh-prill
(Monopril)
Do not confuse with Monurol.

◆CLASSIFICATION

PHARMACOTHERAPEUTIC: Angiotensin-converting enzyme (ACE) inhibitor. **CLINICAL:** Antihypertensive (see p. 6C).

ACTION

Suppresses renin-angiotensin-aldosterone system (prevents conversion of angiotensin I to angiotensin II, a potent vasoconstrictor; may inhibit angiotensin II at local vascular and renal sites). Decreases plasma angiotensin II, increases plasma renin activity, decreases aldosterone secretion. **Therapeutic Effect:** Reduces peripheral arterial resistance, pulmonary capillary wedge pressure; improves cardiac output, exercise tolerance.

PHARMACOKINETICS

Onset	Peak	Duration
PO		
1 hr	2–6 hrs	24 hrs

Slowly absorbed from GI tract. Protein binding: 97%–98%. Metabolized in liver, GI mucosa to active metabolite. Primarily excreted in urine. Minimal removal by hemodialysis. **Half-life:** 11.5 hrs.

USES

Treatment of hypertension. Used alone or in combination with other antihypertensives. Treatment of heart failure. **Unlabeled:** Treatment of post-MI left ventricular dysfunction, diabetic/nondiabetic nephropathy. Treatment of renal crisis in scleroderma.

PRECAUTIONS

CONTRAINDICATIONS: History of angioedema with previous treatment with ACE inhibitors. **CAUTIONS:** Renal impairment, those with sodium depletion or on diuretic therapy, dialysis, hypovolemia, coronary/cerebrovascular insufficiency.

LIFESPAN CONSIDERATIONS: Pregnancy/lactation: Crosses placenta. Distributed in breast milk. May cause fetal/neonatal mortality/morbidity. **Pregnancy Category C** (**D** if used in second or third trimester). **Children:** Safety and efficacy not established. Neonates, infants may be at increased risk for oliguria, neurologic abnormalities. **Elderly:** May be more sensitive to hypotensive effects.

INTERACTIONS

DRUG: Alcohol, diuretics, hypotensive agents may increase effects. **NSAIDs** may decrease effect. **Potassium-sparing diuretics, potassium supplements** may cause hyperkalemia. May increase **lithium** concentration, toxicity. **HERBAL:** None known. **FOOD:** None known. **LAB VALUES:** May increase potassium, SGOT (AST), SGPT (ALT), alkaline phosphatase, bilirubin, BUN, creatinine. May decrease sodium. May cause positive ANA titer.

AVAILABILITY (Rx)

TABLETS: 10 mg, 20 mg, 40 mg.

ADMINISTRATION/HANDLING

PO

• Give without regard to food. • Tablets may be crushed.

INDICATIONS/ROUTES/DOSAGE

HYPERTENSION (used alone)

PO: ADULTS, ELDERLY: Initially, 10 mg/day. MAINTENANCE: 20–40 mg/day. **Maximum:** 80 mg/day.

HYPERTENSION (with diuretic)

Alert: Discontinue diuretic 2–3 days before initiation of fosinopril therapy.

PO: ADULTS, ELDERLY: Initially, 10 mg/day titrated to pt's needs.

HEART FAILURE

PO: ADULTS, ELDERLY: Initially, 5–10 mg. MAINTENANCE: 20–40 mg/day.

SIDE EFFECTS

FREQUENT (9%–12%): Dizziness, cough. **OCCASIONAL (2%–4%):** Hypotension, nausea, vomiting, upper respiratory infection.

ADVERSE REACTIONS/ TOXIC EFFECTS

Excessive hypotension ("first-dose syncope") may occur in pts with CHF, severely salt/volume depleted. Angioedema (swelling of face/lips), hyperkalemia occur rarely. Agranulocytosis, neutropenia may be noted in those with impaired renal function, collagen vascular disease (systemic lupus erythematosus, scleroderma). Nephrotic syndrome may be noted in those with history of renal disease.

NURSING IMPLICATIONS

BASELINE ASSESSMENT

Obtain B/P immediately prior to each dose, in addition to regular monitoring (be alert to fluctuations). Renal function tests should be performed prior to beginning therapy. In pts with renal impairment, autoimmune disease, or taking drugs that affect leukocytes or immune response, CBC, differential count should be performed before therapy begins and q2wks for 3 mos, then periodically thereafter.

INTERVENTION/EVALUATION

If excessive reduction in B/P occurs, place pt in supine position with legs elevated. Assist with ambulation if dizziness occurs. Assess for urinary frequency. Auscultate lung sounds for rales, wheezing in those with CHF. Monitor urinalysis for proteinuria. Monitor serum potassium levels in those on concurrent diuretic therapy.

PATIENT/FAMILY TEACHING

Report any sign of infection (sore throat, fever). Several weeks may be needed for full therapeutic effect of B/P reduction. Skipping doses or voluntarily discontinuing drug may produce severe, rebound hypertension. To reduce hypotensive effect, rise slowly from lying to sitting position, permit legs to dangle from bed momentarily before standing. Inform physician if vomiting, excessive perspiration, persistent cough develops.

fosphenytoin

fos-**phen**-ih-twon
(Cerebyx)
Do not confuse with Celebrex.

CLASSIFICATION

PHARMACOTHERAPEUTIC: Hydantoin. **CLINICAL:** Anticonvulsant (see p. 32C).

ACTION

Stabilizes neuronal membranes, limits spread of seizure activity. Decreases sodium, calcium, ion influx in neurons. Decreases posttetanic potentiation, repetitive afterdischarge. **Therapeutic Effect:** Decreases seizure activity.

PHARMACOKINETICS

Completely absorbed after IM administration. Protein binding: 95%–99%. After IM or IV administration, rapidly/completely hydrolyzed to phenytoin. **Time of complete conversion to phenytoin:** IM: 4 hrs after injection; IV: 2 hrs after the end of infusion. **Half-life for conversion to phenytoin:** 8–15 min.

USES

Acute treatment, control of generalized convulsive status epilepticus; prevention, treatment of seizures occurring during neurosurgery; short-term substitution of oral phenytoin.

PRECAUTIONS

CONTRAINDICATIONS: Hypersensitivity to fosphenytoin, phenytoin, severe bradycardia, SA block, second- or third-degree AV block, Adams-Stokes syndrome. **CAUTIONS:** Porphyria, hypotension, severe myocardial insufficiency, renal/hepatic disease, hypoalbuminemia.

LIFESPAN CONSIDERATIONS: Pregnancy/lactation: May increase frequency of seizures during pregnancy. Increased risk of congenital malformations. Unknown if excreted in breast milk. **Pregnancy Category D. Children:** Safety not established. **Elderly:** Lower dosage recommended.

INTERACTIONS

DRUG: May decrease effect of **glucocorticoids. Alcohol, CNS depressants** may increase CNS depression. **Antacids** may decrease absorption. **Amiodarone, anticoagulants, cimetidine, disulfiram, fluoxetine, isoniazid, sulfonamides** may increase fosphenytoin concentration, effects, toxicity. **Fluconazole, ketoconazole, miconazole** may increase concentration. **Lidocaine, propranolol** may increase cardiac depressant effects. **Valproic acid** may increase concentration, decrease metabolism. May increase **xanthine** metabolism. **HERBAL:** None known. **FOOD:**

None known. **LAB VALUES:** May increase alkaline phosphatase, GGT, glucose.

AVAILABILITY (Rx)

INJECTION: 75 mg/ml (equivalent to 50 mg/ml phenytoin). **PE:** phenytoin equivalent.

ADMINISTRATION/HANDLING

IV

Storage • Refrigerate. Do not store at room temperature >48 hrs. • After dilution, solution is stable for 8 hrs at room temperature or 24 hrs if refrigerated.

Reconstitution • Dilute in D_5W or 0.9% NaCl to a concentration ranging from 1.5–25 mg PE/ml.

Rate of administration • Administer at rate of ≤150 mg PE/min (decreases risk of hypotension).

∅ IV INCOMPATIBILITY

Midazolam (Versed).

IV COMPATIBILITIES

Lorazepam (Ativan), phenobarbital, potassium chloride.

INDICATIONS/ROUTES/DOSAGE

Alert: 150 mg fosphenytoin yields 100 mg phenytoin. Dose, concentration solution, infusion rate of fosphenytoin expressed in terms of PE. Lower, less frequent dosing in elderly may be required. Not approved for pediatric use.

STATUS EPILEPTICUS

IV: ADULTS: LOADING DOSE: 15–20 mg PE/kg infused at rate of 100–150 mg PE/min.

NONEMERGENT SEIZURES

IV: ADULTS: LOADING DOSE: 10–20 mg PE/kg. MAINTENANCE: 4–6 mg PE/kg/day.

SIDE EFFECTS

FREQUENT: Dizziness, paresthesia, tinnitus, pruritus, headache, somnolence. **OCCASIONAL:** Morbilliform rash.

ADVERSE REACTIONS/ TOXIC EFFECTS

Too high fosphenytoin blood concentration may produce ataxia (muscular incoordination), nystagmus (rhythmic oscillation of eyes), double vision, lethargy, slurred speech, nausea, vomiting, hypotension. As level increases, extreme lethargy to comatose states occur.

NURSING IMPLICATIONS

BASELINE ASSESSMENT

Review history of seizure disorder (intensity, frequency, duration, LOC). Initiate seizure precautions. Obtain vital signs, medication history (esp. use of phenytoin, other anticonvulsants). Observe clinically.

INTERVENTION/EVALUATION

Measure cardiac function, EKG, respiratory function, B/P during and immediately following infusion (10–20 min). Discontinue if skin rash appears. Interrupt or decrease rate if hypotension, arrhythmias are detected. Assess pt postinfusion (may feel dizzy, ataxic, drowsy). Assess blood levels of fosphenytoin (2 hrs post IV infusion or 4 hrs post IM injection).

PATIENT/FAMILY TEACHING

Teach pts about their seizure condition and role in its management. If noncompliance is an issue in causing acute seizures, discuss and address reasons for noncompliance.

Fragmin

see dalteparin

frovatriptan

fro-vah-**trip**-tan
(Frovan)

◆CLASSIFICATION

PHARMACOTHERAPEUTIC: Serotonin receptor agonist. **CLINICAL:** Antimigraine (see p. 54C).

F

ACTION

Binds selectively to vascular receptors, producing a vasoconstrictive effect on cranial blood vessels. **Therapeutic Effect:** Produces relief of migraine headache.

PHARMACOKINETICS

Well absorbed after PO administration. Metabolized by the liver to inactive metabolite. Eliminated in urine. **Half-life:** 26 hrs (half-life increased in hepatic impairment).

USES

Treatment of acute migraine attack with or without aura in adults.

PRECAUTIONS

CONTRAINDICATIONS: Coronary artery disease, uncontrolled hypertension, severe hepatic impairment (Child-Pugh grade C), cerebrovascular/peripheral vascular syndromes, ischemic heart disease (angina pectoris, history of MI, silent ischemia), Prinzmetal's angina, concurrent use (or within 24 hrs) of ergotamine-containing preparations, concurrent (or within 2 wks) of MAO therapy, hemiplegic/basilar migraine, within 24 hrs of another serotonin receptor agonist. **CAUTIONS:** Mild to moderate hepatic impairment, pt profile suggesting cardiovascular risks.

LIFESPAN CONSIDERATIONS: Pregnancy/lactation: Unknown if excreted in breast milk. **Pregnancy Category C. Children:** Safety and efficacy not established. **Elderly:** Not recommended in the elderly.

INTERACTIONS

DRUG: Ergotamine-containing drugs may produce vasospastic reaction. **Oral contraceptives** reduce **frovatriptan** clearance, volume of distribution. Combined use of **fluoxetine, fluvoxamine, paroxetine, sertraline** may produce weakness, hyperreflexia, uncoordination. **Propranolol** may dramatically increase plasma concentration of frovatriptan. **HERBAL:** None known. **FOOD:** None known. **LAB VALUES:** None known.

AVAILABILITY (Rx)

TABLETS: 2.5 mg.

ADMINISTRATION/HANDLING

PO

• Do not crush or chew film-coated tablets.

INDICATION/ROUTE/DOSAGE

MIGRAINE

PO: ADULTS, ELDERLY: Initially, 2.5 mg. Second dose may be given if headache recurs (provided first dose gave some relief) but not sooner than 2 hrs from the first dose. **Maximum:** 7.5 mg/day.

SIDE EFFECTS

OCCASIONAL (4%–8%): Dizziness, paresthesia, fatigue, flushing. **RARE (2%–3%):** Hot/cold sensation, dry mouth, dyspepsia (heartburn, epigastric distress).

ADVERSE REACTIONS/ TOXIC EFFECTS

Cardiac events (ischemia, coronary artery vasospasm, MI), noncardiac vasospasm-related reactions (hemorrhage, stroke) occur rarely but particularly in those with hypertension, obesity; smokers; diabetics; those with strong family history of coronary artery disease; male >40 yrs; postmenopausal women.

NURSING CONSIDERATIONS

BASELINE ASSESSMENT

Question for history of peripheral vascular disease, renal/hepatic impairment, possibility of pregnancy. Question regarding onset, location, duration of migraine, possible precipitating symptoms.

INTERVENTION/EVALUATION

Assess for relief of migraine headache, potential for photophobia, phonophobia (sound sensitivity, nausea, vomiting).

PATIENT/FAMILY TEACHING

Take a single dose as soon as symptoms of an actual migraine attack appear. Medication is intended to relieve migraine headaches, not to prevent or reduce number of attacks. Avoid tasks that require alertness, motor skills until response to drug is established. If palpitations/pain/tightness in chest or throat, sudden/severe abdominal pain, pain/weakness of extremities occurs, contact physician immediately.

fulvestrant

full-**ves**-trant
(Faslodex)

CLASSIFICATION

PHARMACOTHERAPEUTIC: Estrogen antagonist. **CLINICAL:** Antineoplastic (see p. 72C).

ACTION

Competes with endogenous estrogen at estrogen receptor binding sites. **Therapeutic Effect:** Inhibits tumor growth.

PHARMACOKINETICS

Extensively and rapidly distributed after IM administration. Protein binding: 99%. Metabolized in the liver. Eliminated by hepatobiliary route; excreted in the feces. **Half-life:** 40 days in postmenopausal women. Peak serum levels occur in 7–9 days.

USES

Treatment of hormone receptor–positive metastatic breast cancer in postmenopausal women with disease progression following antiestrogen therapy.

PRECAUTIONS

CONTRAINDICATIONS: Suspected or known pregnancy. **CAUTIONS:** Thrombocytopenia, bleeding diathesis, anticoagulant therapy, liver disease, reduced hepatic blood flow, estrogen receptor–negative breast cancer.

LIFESPAN CONSIDERATIONS: Pregnancy/lactation: Do not administer to pregnant women. Unknown if excreted in breast milk. **Pregnancy Category D. Children:** Not for use in children. **Elderly:** No age-related precautions noted.

INTERACTIONS

DRUG: None known. **HERBAL:** None known. **FOOD:** None known. **LAB VALUES:** None known.

AVAILABILITY (Rx)

PREFILLED SYRINGE: 50 mg/ml in 5- and 2.5-ml syringes.

ADMINISTRATION/HANDLING

IM

Administer slowly into the buttock as a single 5-ml injection or 2 concurrent 2.5-ml injections.

INDICATIONS/ROUTES/DOSAGE

BREAST CANCER

IM: ADULTS, ELDERLY: 250 mg given once monthly.

SIDE EFFECTS

FREQUENT (13%–26%): Nausea, hot flashes, pharyngitis, asthenia (loss of strength/energy), vomiting, vasodilatation, headache. **OCCASIONAL (5%–12%):** Injection site pain, constipation, diarrhea, abdominal pain, anorexia, dizziness, insomnia, paresthesia, bone/back pain, depression, anxiety, peripheral edema, rash, sweating, fever. **RARE (1%–2%):** Vertigo, weight gain.

ADVERSE REACTIONS/ TOXIC EFFECTS

Urinary tract infection occurs occasionally. Vaginitis, anemia, thromboembolic phenomena, leukopenia occur rarely.

NURSING IMPLICATIONS

BASELINE ASSESSMENT

An estrogen receptor assay should be done prior to beginning therapy. Baseline CT should be performed initially and periodically thereafter for evidence of tumor regression.

INTERVENTION/EVALUATION

Monitor blood chemistry, plasma lipids. Be alert to increased bone pain, ensure adequate pain relief. Check for edema, esp. of dependent areas. Monitor for and assist with ambulation if asthenia/dizziness occurs. Assess for headache. Offer antiemetic for nausea/vomiting.

PATIENT/FAMILY TEACHING

Notify physician if nausea, asthenia, hot flashes become unmanageable.

furosemide

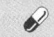

feur-**oh**-sah-mide
(Apo-Furosemide, Lasix)
Do not confuse with Torsemide.

CLASSIFICATION

PHARMACOTHERAPEUTIC: Loop. **CLINICAL:** Diuretic (see p. 87C).

ACTION

Enhances excretion of sodium, chloride, potassium by direct action at ascending limb of loop of Henle. **Therapeutic Effect:** Produces diuretic effect.

PHARMACOKINETICS

Onset	Peak	Duration
PO		
30–60 min	1–2 hrs	6–8 hrs
IM		
30 min	—	—
IV		
5 min	20–60 min	2 hrs

Well absorbed from GI tract. Protein binding: 91%–97%. Partially metabolized in liver. Primarily excreted in urine (in severe renal impairment, nonrenal clearance increases). Not removed by hemodialysis. **Half-life:** 30–90 min (half-life increased with impaired renal/liver function, in neonates).

USES

Treatment of edema associated with CHF, chronic renal failure (including nephrotic syndrome), hepatic cirrhosis, acute pulmonary edema. Treatment of hypertension, either alone or in combination with other antihypertensives. **Unlabeled:** Treatment of hypercalcemia.

PRECAUTIONS

CONTRAINDICATIONS: Anuria, hepatic coma, severe electrolyte depletion. **CAUTIONS:** Hepatic cirrhosis.

LIFESPAN CONSIDERATIONS: Pregnancy/lactation: Crosses placenta. Distributed in breast milk. **Pregnancy Category C (D** if used in pregnancy-induced hypertension). **Children:** Half-life increased in neonates; may require increased dosage interval. **Elderly:** May be more sensitive to hypotensive, electrolyte effects, developing circulatory collapse, thromboembolic effect. Age-related renal function impairment may require dosage adjustment.

INTERACTIONS

DRUG: **Amphotericin, ototoxic, nephrotoxic agents** may increase toxicity. May decrease effect of **anticoagulants, heparin. Hypokalemia-causing agents** may increase risk of hypokalemia. May increase risk of **lithium** toxicity. **Probenecid** may increase concentrations. **HERBAL:** None known. **FOOD:** None known. **LAB VALUES:** May increase glucose, BUN, uric acid. May decrease calcium, chloride, magnesium, potassium, sodium.

AVAILABILITY (Rx)

TABLETS: 20 mg, 40 mg, 80 mg. **ORAL SOLUTION:** 10 mg/ml, 40 mg/5 ml. **INJECTION:** 10 mg/ml.

ADMINISTRATION/HANDLING

PO

• Give with food to avoid GI upset, preferably with breakfast (may prevent nocturia).

IM

• Temporary pain at injection site may be noted.

IV

Storage • Solution appears clear, colorless. • Discard yellow solutions.

Rate of administration • May give undiluted but is compatible with D_5W, 0.9% NS, or lactated Ringer's solutions. • Administer each 40 mg or fraction by IV push over 1–2 min. Do not exceed administration rate of 4 mg/min in those with renal impairment.

IV INCOMPATIBILITIES

Ciprofloxacin (Cipro), diltiazem (Cardizem), dobutamine (Dobutrex), dopamine (Intropin), doxorubicin (Adriamycin), droperidol (Inapsine), esmolol (Brevibloc), famotidine (Pepcid), filgrastim (Neupogen), fluconazole (Diflucan), gemcitabine (Gemzar), gentamicin (Garamycin), idarubicin (Idamycin), labetalol (Trandate), meperidine (Demerol), metoclopramide (Reglan), midazolam (Versed), milrinone (Primacor), nicardipine (Cardene), ondansetron (Zofran), quinidine, thiopental (Pentothal), vecuronium (Norcuron), vinblastine (Velban), vincristine (Oncovin), vinorelbine (Navelbine).

IV COMPATIBILITIES

Aminophylline, amiodarone (Cordarone), bumetanide (Bumex), calcium gluconate, cimetidine (Tagamet), heparin, hydromorphone (Dilaudid), lidocaine, morphine, nitroglycerin, norepinephrine (Levophed), potassium chloride, propofol (Diprivan).

INDICATIONS/ROUTES/DOSAGE

EDEMA/HYPERTENSION

PO: ADULTS, ELDERLY: Initially, 20–80 mg/dose; may increase by 20–40 mg/dose at 6- to 8-hr intervals. May titrate up to 600 mg/day in severe edematous states. CHILDREN: 1–6 mg/kg/day in divided doses q6–12h.

IM/IV: ADULTS, ELDERLY: 20–40 mg/dose; may repeat in 1–2 hrs and increase by 20 mg/dose. CHILDREN: 1–2 mg/kg/dose q6–12h. NEONATES: 1–2 mg/kg/dose q12–24h.

IV infusion: ADULTS, ELDERLY: Bolus of 0.1 mg/kg, then 0.1 mg/kg/hr; may double q2h. **Maximum:** 0.4 mg/kg/hr. CHILDREN: 0.05 mg/kg/hr; titrate to desired effect.

SIDE EFFECTS

EXPECTED: Increase in urinary frequency/volume. **FREQUENT:** Nausea, gastric upset with cramping, diarrhea, constipation, electrolyte disturbances. **OCCASIONAL:** Dizziness, lightheadedness, headache, blurred vision, par-

F

esthesia, photosensitivity, rash, weakness, urinary frequency/bladder spasm, restlessness, diaphoresis. **RARE:** Flank/loin pain.

ADVERSE REACTIONS/ TOXIC EFFECTS

Vigorous diuresis may lead to profound water loss/electrolyte depletion, resulting in hypokalemia, hyponatremia, dehydration. Sudden volume depletion may result in increased risk of thrombosis, circulatory collapse, sudden death. Acute hypotensive episodes may occur, sometimes several days after beginning of therapy. Ototoxicity manifested as deafness, vertigo, tinnitus (ringing/roaring in ears) may occur, esp. in pts with severe renal impairment. Can exacerbate diabetes mellitus, systemic lupus erythematosus, gout, pancreatitis. Blood dyscrasias have been reported.

NURSING IMPLICATIONS

BASELINE ASSESSMENT

Check vital signs, esp. B/P for hypotension prior to administration. Assess baseline electrolytes, particularly check for low potassium. Assess edema, skin turgor, mucous membranes for hydration status. Assess muscle strength, mental status. Note skin temperature, moisture. Obtain baseline weight. Initiate I&O monitoring.

INTERVENTION/EVALUATION

Monitor B/P, vital signs, electrolytes, I&O, weight. Note extent of diuresis. Watch for changes from initial assessment (hypokalemia may result in changes in muscle strength, tremor, muscle cramps, change in mental status, cardiac arrhythmias). Hyponatremia may result in confusion, thirst, cold/clammy skin.

PATIENT/FAMILY TEACHING

Expect increased frequency and volume of urination. Report irregular heartbeat, signs of electrolyte imbalances (noted previously), hearing abnormalities (e.g., sense of fullness in ears, ringing/roaring in ears). Eat foods high in potassium such as whole grains (cereals), legumes, meat, bananas, apricots, orange juice, potatoes (white, sweet), raisins. Avoid sun/sunlamps.

gabapentin

gah-bah-**pen**-tin
(Neurontin)
Do not confuse with Noroxin.

◆ CLASSIFICATION

CLINICAL: Anticonvulsant, antineuralgic (see p. 33C).

ACTION

Exact mechanism unknown. May be due to increased gamma-aminobutyric acid (GABA) synthesis rate, increased GABA accumulation, or binding to as yet undefined receptor sites in brain tissue. **Therapeutic Effect:** Produces anticonvulsant activity, reduces neuropathic pain.

PHARMACOKINETICS

Well absorbed from GI tract (not affected by food). Protein binding: <5%. Widely distributed. Crosses blood-brain barrier. Primarily excreted unchanged in urine. Removed by hemodialysis. **Half-life:** 5–7 hrs (half-life increased with impaired renal function, elderly).

USES

Adjunct in treatment of partial seizures in children >12 yrs and adults (with or without secondary generalized seizures, partial seizures in children 3–12 yrs); adjunct in treatment of neuropathic pain, postherpetic neuralgia. **Unlabeled:** Treatment of migraines, essential tremors, hot flashes, psychiatric disorders, hyperhidrosis.

PRECAUTIONS

CONTRAINDICATIONS: None known. **CAUTIONS:** Renal impairment.

LIFESPAN CONSIDERATIONS: Pregnancy/lactation: Unknown whether it is distributed in breast milk. **Pregnancy Category C. Children:** Safety and efficacy not established in those <3 yrs. **Elderly:** Age-related renal impairment may require dosage adjustment.

INTERACTIONS

DRUG: None known. **HERBAL:** None known. **FOOD:** None known. **LAB VALUES:** May decrease WBCs.

AVAILABILITY (Rx)

CAPSULES: 100 mg, 300 mg, 400 mg. **ORAL SOLUTION:** 250 mg/5 ml. **TABLETS:** 600 mg, 800 mg.

ADMINISTRATION/HANDLING

PO

- Give without regard to meals; may give with food to avoid or reduce GI upset.
- If treatment is discontinued or anticonvulsant therapy is added, do so gradually over at least 1 wk (reduces risk of loss of seizure control).

INDICATIONS/ROUTES/DOSAGE

SEIZURE CONTROL

Alert: Maximum time between doses should not exceed 12 hrs.

PO: ADULTS, ELDERLY, CHILDREN >12 YRS: Initially, 300 mg 3 times/day. May titrate. RANGE: 900–1,800 mg/day in 3 divided doses. **Maximum:** 3,600 mg/day. CHILDREN 3–12 YRS: Initially, 10–15 mg/kg/day in 3 divided doses. May titrate up to 25–35 mg/kg/day (Children 5–12 yrs) and 40 mg/kg/day (Children 3–4 yrs). **Maximum:** 50 mg/kg/day.

NEUROPATHIC PAIN

PO: ADULTS, ELDERLY: Initially, 100 mg 3 times/day; may increase by 300 mg/day at weekly intervals. **Maximum:** Up to 3,600 mg/day in 3 divided doses. CHILDREN: Initially, 5 mg/kg/dose at bedtime, then 5 mg/kg/dose for 2 doses on day 2, then 5 mg/kg/dose for 3 doses on day 3. RANGE: 8–35 mg/kg/day in 3 divided doses.

POSTHERPETIC NEURALGIA

PO: ADULTS, ELDERLY: 300 mg day 1, 300 mg 2 times/day on day 2, 300 mg 3 times/day on day 3. Titrate up to 1,800 mg/day.

RENAL FUNCTION IMPAIRMENT

Based on creatinine clearance:

Creatinine Clearance	Dosage
>60 ml/min	400 mg q8h
30–60 ml/min	300 mg q12h
15–29 ml/min	300 mg daily
<15 ml/min	300 mg every other day
Hemodialysis	200–300 mg after each 4-hr hemodialysis

SIDE EFFECTS

FREQUENT (11%–19%): Fatigue, somnolence, dizziness, ataxia. **OCCASIONAL (3%–8%):** Nystagmus (rapid eye movements), tremor, diplopia (double vision), rhinitis, weight gain. **RARE (<2%):** Nervousness, dysarthria (speech difficulty), memory loss, dyspepsia, pharyngitis, myalgia.

ADVERSE REACTIONS/ TOXIC EFFECTS

Abrupt withdrawal may increase seizure frequency. Overdosage may result in double vision, slurred speech, drowsiness, lethargy, diarrhea.

NURSING IMPLICATIONS

BASELINE ASSESSMENT

Review history of seizure disorder (type, onset, intensity, frequency, duration, LOC). Routine laboratory monitoring of blood serum levels unnecessary for safe use.

INTERVENTION/EVALUATION

Provide safety measures as needed. Monitor seizure frequency/duration, renal function, weight, behavior in children.

PATIENT/FAMILY TEACHING

Take gabapentin only as prescribed; do not abruptly stop taking drug (may increase seizure frequency). Do not drive, operate machinery, perform activities requiring mental acuity due to potential dizziness, somnolence. Avoid alcohol. Carry identification card/bracelet to note seizure disorder/anticonvulsant therapy.

G

galantamine

gal-**an**-tah-mine
(Reminyl)

Do not confuse with Remeron, Remicade.

CLASSIFICATION

PHARMACOTHERAPEUTIC: Cholinesterase inhibitor. **CLINICAL:** Antidementia.

ACTION

Elevates acetylcholine concentrations in cerebral cortex by slowing degeneration of acetylcholine released by still intact cholinergic neurons (Alzheimer's disease involves degeneration of cholinergic neuronal pathways). **Therapeutic Effect:** Slows progression of Alzheimer's disease.

PHARMACOKINETICS

Rapidly absorbed from GI tract. Protein binding: 18%. Distributed to blood cells; binds to plasma proteins, mainly albumin. Metabolized in the liver. Excreted in the urine. Plasma concentration increases in pts with moderate to severe hepatic impairment. **Half-life:** 7 hrs.

USES

Treatment of mild to moderate dementia of Alzheimer's type.

PRECAUTIONS

CONTRAINDICATIONS: Severe hepatic, renal impairment. **CAUTIONS:** Moderately impaired renal/hepatic function, history of ulcer disease, those on concurrent NSAIDs, asthma, COPD, bladder outflow obstruction, supraventricular cardiac conduction conditions.

LIFESPAN CONSIDERATIONS: Pregnancy/lactation: Unknown if drug crosses placenta or is distributed in breast milk. **Pregnancy Category B. Children:** Not prescribed for this pt population. **Elderly:** No age-related precautions noted, but use is not recommended in those with severe hepatic, renal impairment (creatinine clearance <9 ml/min).

INTERACTIONS

DRUG: Cimetidine, ketoconazole, paroxetine, erythromycin may increase galantamine concentration; may interfere with **succinylcholine, bethanechol** effects. **HERBAL:** None known. **FOOD:** None known. **LAB VALUES:** None known.

AVAILABILITY (Rx)

TABLETS: 4 mg, 8 mg, 12 mg. **ORAL SOLUTION:** 4 mg/ml.

ADMINISTRATION/HANDLING

PO

- Give with morning and evening meals.

INDICATIONS/ROUTES/DOSAGE

ALZHEIMER'S DISEASE

PO: ADULTS, ELDERLY: Initially, 4 mg twice daily (8 mg/day). If well tolerated and after a minimum of 4 wks, may increase to 8 mg twice daily (16 mg/day). After a minimum of 4 wks, may increase to 12 mg twice daily (24 mg/day). **Range:** 16–24 mg/day in 2 divided doses.

DOSAGE IN RENAL/LIVER IMPAIRMENT

Moderate impairment: Maximum of 16 mg/day. **Severe impairment:** Not recommended.

Alert: If therapy is interrupted for several days or longer, must retitrate as noted.

SIDE EFFECTS

FREQUENT (5%–17%): Nausea, vomiting, diarrhea, anorexia, weight loss. **OCCASIONAL (4%–9%):** Abdominal pain, insomnia, depression, headache, dizziness, fatigue, rhinitis. **RARE (<3%):** Tremors, constipation, confusion, cough, anxiety, urinary incontinence.

ADVERSE REACTIONS/ TOXIC EFFECTS

Overdose can cause cholinergic crises (increased salivation, lacrimation, urination, defecation, bradycardia, hypotension, increased muscle weakness). Treatment aimed at general supportive measures, use of anticholinergics (e.g., atropine).

NURSING IMPLICATIONS

BASELINE ASSESSMENT

Assess cognitive, behavioral, functional deficits of pt. Assess liver, renal function.

INTERVENTION/EVALUATION

Monitor cognitive, behavioral, functional status of pt. Evaluate EKG, periodic rhythm strips in pts with underlying arrhythmias. Monitor for symptoms of ulcer, GI bleeding.

PATIENT/FAMILY TEACHING

Take with morning and evening meals (reduces risk of nausea). Avoid tasks that require alertness, motor skills until response to drug is established. Report persistent GI disturbances, excessive salivation, diaphoresis, or excessive tearing; excessive fatigue; insomnia; depression, dizziness; increased muscle weakness.

ganciclovir sodium

gan-**sye**-klo-vir

(Cytovene, Vitrasert)

Do not confuse with Cytosar.

CLASSIFICATION

PHARMACOTHERAPEUTIC: Synthetic nucleoside. **CLINICAL:** Antiviral (see p. 59C).

ACTION

Converted intracellularly, competes with viral DNA polymerases and direct incorporation into growing viral DNA chains. **Therapeutic Effect:** Interferes with DNA synthesis, viral replication.

PHARMACOKINETICS

Widely distributed. Protein binding: 1%–2%. Undergoes minimal metabolism. Primarily excreted unchanged in urine. Removed by hemodialysis. **Half-life:** 2.5–3.6 hrs (half-life increased with impaired renal function).

USES

Treatment of cytomegalovirus (CMV) retinitis in immunocompromised patients, CMV GI infections and pneumonitis; prevention of CMV disease in transplant patients. Possesses antiviral activity against herpes simplex. **Unlabeled:** Treatment of other CMV infections (e.g., pneumonitis, gastroenteritis, hepatitis).

PRECAUTIONS

CONTRAINDICATIONS: Hypersensitivity to ganciclovir or acyclovir. Not for use in immunocompetent persons or those with congenital or neonatal CMV disease. Absolute neutrophil count <500/mm^3, platelet count <25,000/mm^3. **CAUTIONS:** Patients with neutropenia, thrombocytopenia, impaired renal function; children (long-term safety not determined due to potential for long-term carcinogenic and adverse reproductive effects).

G

LIFESPAN CONSIDERATIONS: Pregnancy/lactation: Effective contraception should be used during therapy; ganciclovir should not be used during pregnancy. Nursing should be discontinued; may be resumed no sooner than 72 hrs after the last dose of ganciclovir. **Pregnancy Category C. Children:** Safety and efficacy not established in those <12 yrs. **Elderly:** Age-related renal impairment may require dosage adjustment.

INTERACTIONS

DRUG: Bone marrow depressants may increase bone marrow depression. May increase risk of seizures with **imipenem-cilastatin.** May increase hematologic toxicity with **zidovudine. HERBAL:** None known. **FOOD:** None known. **LAB VALUES:** May increase SGOT (AST), SGPT (ALT), alkaline phosphatase, bilirubin.

AVAILABILITY (Rx)

CAPSULES: 250 mg, 500 mg. **POWDER FOR INJECTION:** 500 mg. **IMPLANT:** 4.5 mg.

ADMINISTRATION/HANDLING

PO

- Give with food.

IV

Storage • Store vials at room temperature. Do not refrigerate. • Reconstituted solution in vial is stable for 12 hrs at room temperature. • After dilution, refrigerate, use within 24 hrs. • Discard if precipitate forms, discoloration occurs. • Avoid exposure to skin, eyes, mucous membranes. • Latex gloves and safety glasses should be used during preparation/handling of solution. • Avoid inhalation. • If solution contacts skin/mucous membranes, wash thoroughly with soap and water; rinse eyes thoroughly with plain water.

Reconstitution • Reconstitute 500-mg vial with 10 ml Sterile Water for Injection to provide a concentration of 50 mg/ml; do **not** use Bacteriostatic Water (contains parabens, which is incompatible with ganciclovir). • Further dilute with 100 ml D_5W, 0.9% NaCl, lactated Ringer's, or any combination thereof to provide a concentration of 5 mg/ml.

Rate of administration • Administer only by IV infusion over 1 hr. • Do not give by IV push or rapid IV infusion (increases risk of toxicity); protect from infiltration (high pH causes severe tissue irritation). • Use large veins to permit rapid dilution and dissemination of ganciclovir (minimizes phlebitis); central venous ports may reduce catheter-associated infection.

IV INCOMPATIBILITIES

Aldesleukin (Proleukin), amifostine (Ethyol), aztreonam (Azactam), cefepime (Maxipime), cytarabine (ARA-C), doxorubicin (Adriamycin), fludarabine (Fludara), foscarnet (Foscavir), gemcitabine (Gemzar), ondansetron (Zofran), piperacillin/tazobactam (Zosyn), sargramostim (Leukine), vinorelbine (Navelbine).

IV COMPATIBILITIES

Amphotericin, enalapril (Vasotec), filgrastim (Neupogen), fluconazole (Diflucan), propofol (Diprivan).

INDICATIONS/ROUTES/DOSAGE

RETINITIS

IV: ADULTS, CHILDREN >3 MOS: 10 mg/kg/day in divided doses q12h for 14–21 days, then 5 mg/kg/day as a single daily dose.

PREVENTION OF CMV IN TRANSPLANT PTS

IV: ADULTS, CHILDREN: 10 mg/kg/day in divided doses q12h for 7–14 days, then 5 mg/kg/day as a single daily dose.

OTHER CMV INFECTIONS

IV: ADULTS, CHILDREN: Initially, 10 mg/kg/day in divided doses q12h for 14–21 days, then 5 mg/kg/day as a single daily dose.

MAINTENANCE

PO: ADULTS: 1,000 mg 3 times/day or 500 mg q3h (6 times/day). CHILDREN: 30 mg/kg/dose q8h.

INTRAVITREAL IMPLANT

ADULTS: 1 implant q6–9mos plus ganciclovir orally. CHILDREN >9 YRS: 1 implant q6–9mos plus ganciclovir orally (30 mg/dose q8h).

ADULT DOSAGE IN RENAL IMPAIRMENT

Creatinine Clearance (ml/min)	IV Indications	IV Maintenance	Oral
50–69	2.5 mg/kg q12h	2.5 mg/kg q24h	1,500 mg/day
25–49	2.5 mg/kg q24h	1.25 mg/kg q24h	1,000 mg/day
10–24	1.25 mg/kg q24h	0.625 mg/kg q24h	500 mg/day
<10	1.25 mg/kg 3 times/wk	0.625 mg 3 times/wk	500 mg 3 times/wk

SIDE EFFECTS

FREQUENT: Diarrhea (41%), fever (40%), nausea (25%), abdominal pain (17%), vomiting (13%). **OCCASIONAL (6%–11%):** Diaphoresis, infection, paresthesia, flatulence, pruritus. **RARE (2%–4%):** Headache, stomatitis, dyspepsia, vomiting, phlebitis.

ADVERSE REACTIONS/ TOXIC EFFECTS

Hematologic toxicity occurs commonly: leukopenia (29%–41%), anemia (19%–25%). Intraocular insert produces visual acuity loss, vitreous hemorrhage, retinal detachment occasionally. GI hemorrhage occurs rarely.

G

NURSING IMPLICATIONS

BASELINE ASSESSMENT

Evaluate hematologic baseline. Obtain specimens for support of differential diagnosis (urine, feces, blood, throat) because retinal infection is usually due to hematogenous dissemination.

INTERVENTION/EVALUATION

Monitor I&O, ensure adequate hydration (minimum 1,500 ml/24 hrs). Diligently evaluate hematology reports for neutropenia, thrombocytopenia, decreased platelets. Question pt regarding vision, therapeutic improvement, complications. Assess for rash, pruritus.

PATIENT/FAMILY TEACHING

Ganciclovir provides suppression, not cure of CMV retinitis. Frequent blood tests, eye exams are necessary during therapy because of toxic nature of drug. It is essential to report any new symptom promptly. May temporarily or permanently inhibit sperm production in men, suppress fertility in women. Barrier contraception should be used during and for 90 days after therapy because of mutagenic potential.

ganirelix

(Antagon)
See Classification section under: Fertility agents (p. 89C)

garlic

Also known as ail, allium, nectar of the gods, poor man's treacle, stinking rose

CLASSIFICATION

HERBAL.

ACTION

Possesses antithrombotic properties, can increase fibrinolytic activity, decrease platelet aggregation, increase prothrombin time. Acts as an HMG-CoA reductase inhibitor (statins). **Therapeutic Effect:** Lowers cholesterol levels. Causes smooth muscle relaxation/vasodilation, reducing B/P. Reduces oxidative stress and LDL oxidation, preventing age-related vascular changes, atherosclerosis. Prevents endothelial cell depletion, producing antioxidant effect.

USES

Treatment of hypertension, hyperlipidemia; prevention of coronary artery disease, age-related vascular changes, atherosclerosis.

PRECAUTIONS

CONTRAINDICATIONS: Pts with bleeding disorders. **CAUTIONS:** Diabetes (may decrease blood sugar levels), inflammatory GI conditions (may irritate the GI tract). Hypothyroidism (may reduce iodine uptake). May prolong bleeding time (discontinue 1–2 wks before surgery).

LIFESPAN CONSIDERATIONS: Pregnancy/lactation: Caution: May stimulate labor and cause colic in infants. **Children:** Safety and efficacy not established (may be beneficial in children with hypercholesterolemia). **Elderly:** No age-related precautions noted.

INTERACTIONS

DRUG: May increase hypoglycemic effect of **insulin, oral antidiabetic agents.** May enhance effects of **anticoagulants/antiplatelets (e.g., warfarin, aspirin, clopidogrel, enoxaparin).** May decrease effects of **cyclosporine, oral contraceptives.** May decrease concentration/effects of **saquinavir, other HIV antiretrovirals.** **HERBAL:** **Feverfew, ginger, ginkgo, ginseng** may increase risk of bleeding. **FOOD:** None known. **LAB VALUES:** May decrease blood glucose, cholesterol, increase INR.

AVAILABILITY (OTC)

CAPSULES: 100 mg, 300 mg, 500 mg, 1,000 mg, 1.5 g. **TABLETS:** 400 mg, 1,250 mg. **TEA. EXTRACT. OIL. POWDER.**

INDICATIONS/ROUTES/DOSAGE

HYPERLIPIDEMIA, HYPERTENSION

PO (capsules, powder, tea): ADULTS, ELDERLY: 600–1,200 mg/day in divided doses 3 times/day.

Alert: Appropriate doses for other conditions vary depending on the preparation used.

SIDE EFFECTS

Breath/body odor, mouth/GI burning, heartburn, nausea, vomiting, diarrhea, allergic reactions (e.g., rhinitis, urticaria, angioedema).

ADVERSE REACTIONS/ TOXIC EFFECTS

None known.

NURSING IMPLICATIONS

BASELINE ASSESSMENT

Assess lipid levels, determine whether pt is taking anticoagulants/antiplatelets. Assess if diabetic, taking insulin or oral hypoglycemic agents.

INTERVENTION/EVALUATION

Monitor CBC, coagulation studies, lipid levels, glucose levels. Assess for hypersensitivity reaction, contact dermatitis.

PATIENT/FAMILY TEACHING

Avoid use in pregnancy/breast-feeding. Inform all health care providers of garlic use. Discontinue 1–2 wks before any procedure in which bleeding may occur.

gatifloxacin

gat-ih-**flocks**-ah-sin
(Tequin, Zymar)

CLASSIFICATION

PHARMACOTHERAPEUTIC: Fluoroquinolone. **CLINICAL:** Antibiotic (see p. 23C).

ACTION

Inhibits two enzymes, topoisomerase II and IV, in susceptible microorganisms. **Therapeutic Effect:** Interferes with bacterial DNA replication. Prevents, delays resistance emergence. Bactericidal.

PHARMACOKINETICS

Well absorbed from GI tract following PO administration. Protein binding: 20%. Widely distributed. Metabolized in liver. Primarily excreted in urine. **Half-life:** 7–14 hrs.

USES

Treatment of infections due to acute bacterial exacerbation of chronic bronchitis, acute sinusitis, community-acquired pneumonia, uncomplicated skin/skin structure infections, cystitis, complicated urinary tract infections, pyelonephritis, urethral gonorrhea in men/women, endocervical and rectal gonorrhea in women. **Ophthalmic:** Topical treatment of bacterial conjunctivitis due to susceptible strains of bacteria.

PRECAUTIONS

CONTRAINDICATIONS: Hypersensitivity to quinolones. **CAUTIONS:** Renal/hepatic impairment, CNS disorders, cerebral atherosclerosis, seizures, those with prolonged QT interval. Other medications known to prolong the QT interval (e.g., erythromycin, tricyclic antidepressants), uncorrected hypokalemia, those receiving quinidine, procainamide, amiodarone, sotalol.

LIFESPAN CONSIDERATIONS: Pregnancy/lactation: Unknown if distributed in breast milk. **Pregnancy Category C. Children:** Safety and efficacy not established. **Elderly:** Age-related renal impairment may require dosage adjustment.

INTERACTIONS

DRUG: Probenecid may increase plasma concentration, half-life of **gatifloxacin. Antacids, iron preparations, digoxin** may decrease plasma concentration, half-life. **HERBAL:** None known. **FOOD:** None known. **LAB VALUES:** None known.

AVAILABILITY (Rx)

TABLETS: 200 mg, 400 mg. **INJECTION:** 200-mg, 400-mg vials. **OPHTHALMIC SOLUTION:** 0.3%.

ADMINISTRATION/HANDLING

PO

• Give without regard to meals. • Oral gatifloxacin should be administered 4 hrs before giving antacids, multivitamins, ferrous sulfate, buffered tablets or solutions.

OPHTHALMIC: Tilt head backward, have pt look up. Gently pull lower eyelid down until pocket formed. Hold dropper above pocket and without touching eyelid or conjunctival sac place drops into center of pocket. Close eyes gently, apply gentle finger pressure to lacrimal sac at inner canthus. Remove excess solution around eye with a tissue.

G

IV

Storage • Available prediluted and ready for use. • Also available in 20- and 40-ml vials, which must be diluted in 100–200 ml D_5W, 0.9% NaCl.

Rate of administration • Infuse over 60 min. • Do not give by rapid or bolus IV.

IV INCOMPATIBILITIES

Amphotericin (Fungizone), potassium phosphate.

IV COMPATIBILITIES

Aminophylline, calcium gluconate, hydromorphone (Dilaudid), lidocaine, lorazepam (Ativan), magnesium sulfate, methylprednisolone (SoluMedrol), metoclopramide (Reglan), midazolam (Versed), morphine, nitroglycerin, potassium chloride, sodium phosphate.

INDICATIONS/ROUTES/DOSAGE

CHRONIC BRONCHITIS, COMPLICATED URINARY TRACT INFECTIONS, PYELONEPHRITIS

PO/IV: ADULTS >18 YRS, ELDERLY: 400 mg/day for 7–10 days (5 days for chronic bronchitis).

SINUSITIS

PO/IV: ADULTS >18 YRS, ELDERLY: 400 mg/day for 10 days.

PNEUMONIA

PO/IV: ADULTS >18 YRS, ELDERLY: 400 mg/day for 7–14 days.

CYSTITIS

PO/IV: ADULTS >18 YRS, ELDERLY: 400 mg as a single dose or 200 mg/day for 3 days.

URETHRAL GONORRHEA IN MEN/ WOMEN, ENDOCERVICAL AND RECTAL GONORRHEA IN WOMEN

PO/IV: ADULTS >18 YRS, ELDERLY: 400 mg as a single dose.

DOSAGE IN RENAL IMPAIRMENT

Creatinine Clearance	Dosage
40 ml/min	400 mg/day
<40 ml/min	Initially, 400 mg/day then 200 mg/day
Hemodialysis	Initially, 400 mg/day then 200 mg/day
Peritoneal dialysis	Initially, 400 mg/day then 200 mg/day

USUAL OPHTHALMIC DOSAGE: ADULTS, ELDERLY, CHILDREN >1 YR: 1 drop q2h while awake for 2 days, then 1 drop up to 4 times a day for days 3–7.

SIDE EFFECTS

OCCASIONAL (3%–8%): Nausea, vaginitis, diarrhea, headache, dizziness. **Ophthalmic:** Conjunctival irritation, increased tearing, corneal inflammation. **RARE (0.1%–3%):** Abdominal pain, constipation, dyspepsia, stomatitis, edema, insomnia, abnormal dreams, diaphoresis, change in taste, rash. **Ophthalmic:** Swelling around cornea, dry eye, eye pain, eyelid swelling, headache, red eye, reduced visual acuity, altered taste.

ADVERSE REACTIONS/ TOXIC EFFECTS

Pseudomembranous colitis (severe abdominal pain/cramps, severe watery diarrhea, fever) may occur. Superinfection (genital/anal pruritus, ulceration/changes in oral mucosa, moderate to severe diarrhea) may occur.

NURSING IMPLICATIONS

BASELINE ASSESSMENT

Question for history of hypersensitivity to gatifloxacin, quinolones.

INTERVENTION/EVALUATION

Determine pattern of bowel activity. Assist with ambulation if dizziness occurs. Assess for headache, nausea, vaginitis. Monitor WBC, signs of infection, mental status.

PATIENT/FAMILY TEACHING

Do not skip dose; take full course of therapy. Take with 8 oz water; drink several glasses of water between meals. Do not take antacids within 4 hrs of medication (reduces/destroys effectiveness). Avoid exposure to direct sunlight during therapy and for several days following treatment.

gefitinib

geh-**fih**-tih-nib
(Iressa)

CLASSIFICATION

PHARMACOTHERAPEUTIC: Epidermal growth factor receptor antibody. **CLINICAL:** Antineoplastic.

ACTION

Blocks the signaling pathway that binds to a receptor (epidermal growth factor receptor [EGFR]) on the surface of cells. The purpose of EGFR is to activate an enzyme, tyrosine kinase, to send signals inside the cell, instructing the cell to grow. **Therapeutic Effect:** Inhibits activation of tyrosine kinase, effectively inhibiting signaling at the receptor, preventing growth signal within the cancer cell.

PHARMACOKINETICS

Slowly absorbed, extensively distributed throughout the body. Protein binding: 90%. Undergoes extensive hepatic metabolism. Excreted in the feces. **Half-life:** 48 hrs.

USES

Treatment in pts with locally advanced or metastatic non–small cell lung cancer after failure of platinum-based and docetaxel chemotherapies.

PRECAUTIONS

CONTRAINDICATIONS: None known. **CAUTIONS:** Severe renal impairment, impaired hepatic function.

LIFESPAN CONSIDERATIONS: Pregnancy/lactation: Has potential to cause fetal harm, potential for loss of the pregnancy. Substitute formula feedings for breast-feedings. Those with child-bearing potential should use contraceptive methods during treatment and up to 12 mos following therapy. **Pregnancy Category D. Children:** Safety and efficacy not established. **Elderly:** No age-related precautions noted.

INTERACTIONS

DRUG: Rifampin, phenytoin, ranitidine, cimetidine, sodium bicarbonate may decrease gefitinib concentration, effectiveness. **Ketoconazole, itaconazole** increases gefitinib concentration. Increases **metoprolol** effect. Increases bleeding potential with **warfarin. HERBAL:** None known. **FOOD:** None known. **LAB VALUES:** May increase bilirubin, alkaline phosphatase, SGOT (AST), SGPT (ALT).

AVAILABILITY (Rx)

TABLETS: 250 mg.

ADMINISTRATION/HANDLING

• Give without regard to food. Do not crush or break film-coated tablet.

INDICATIONS/ROUTES/DOSAGE

NON–SMALL CELL LUNG CANCER

PO: ADULTS, ELDERLY: Give one 250-mg tablet daily. In those receiving rifampin or phenytoin, may increase dose to 500 mg daily.

G

SIDE EFFECTS

FREQUENT (25%–48%): Diarrhea, rash, acne. **OCCASIONAL (8%–13%):** Dry skin, nausea, vomiting, pruritus. **RARE (2%–7%):** Anorexia, asthenia (loss of strength, energy), weight loss, peripheral edema, eye pain.

ADVERSE REACTIONS/ TOXIC EFFECTS

Pancreatitis, ocular hemorrhage occur rarely. Hypersensitivity reaction produces angioedema, urticaria.

NURSING IMPLICATIONS

BASELINE ASSESSMENT

Antiemetics, antidiarrheals may be effective in preventing/treating nausea, vomiting, diarrhea. Patients with poorly tolerated diarrhea may be helped by briefly interrupting drug therapy (up to 14 days) followed by reinstatement.

INTERVENTION/EVALUATION

Encourage adequate fluid intake. Assess bowel sounds for hyperactivity. Monitor daily bowel activity/stool consistency (watery, loose, soft, semisolid, solid). Assess skin for evidence of rash.

PATIENT/FAMILY TEACHING

Do not have immunizations without physician's approval (drug lowers body's resistance). Avoid crowds, persons with known infections. Report signs of infection at once (fever, flulike symptoms). Contact physician if severe/persistent diarrhea, nausea, vomiting, anorexia occurs. Avoid pregnancy during therapy.

gemcitabine hydrochloride

gem-**cih**-tah-bean
(Gemzar)

◆ CLASSIFICATION

PHARMACOTHERAPEUTIC: Antimetabolite. **CLINICAL:** Antineoplastic (see p. 72C).

ACTION

Inhibits ribonucleotide reductase, the enzyme necessary for catalyzing DNA synthesis. **Therapeutic Effect:** Produces cell death in those cells undergoing DNA synthesis.

PHARMACOKINETICS

After IV infusion, not extensively distributed (increased with length of infusion). Protein binding: <10%. Excreted primarily in urine as metabolite. **Half-life:** 42–94 min (influenced by gender/duration of infusion).

USES

Treatment of locally advanced (stage II, III) or metastatic (stage IV) adenocarcinoma of pancreas. Indicated for pts previously treated with 5-fluorouracil. Monotherapy or in combination with cisplatin for treatment for locally advanced/ metastatic non–small cell lung cancer.

PRECAUTIONS

CONTRAINDICATIONS: None known. **CAUTIONS:** Impaired renal function, hepatic insufficiency.

LIFESPAN CONSIDERATIONS: Preg-

nancy/lactation: If possible, avoid use during pregnancy, esp. first trimester. May cause fetal harm. Unknown if distributed in breast milk. Breast-feeding not recommended. **Pregnancy Category D. Children:** Safety and efficacy not established. **Elderly:** Increased risk of hematologic toxicity.

INTERACTIONS

DRUG: Bone marrow depressants may increase risk of bone marrow depression. **Live virus vaccines** may potentiate virus replication, increase vaccine side effects, decrease pt's antibody response to vaccine. **HERBAL:** None known. **FOOD:** None known. **LAB VALUES:** May increase SGOT (AST), SGPT (ALT), alkaline phosphatase, bilirubin, creatinine, BUN.

AVAILABILITY (Rx)

POWDER FOR RECONSTITUTION: 200-mg, 1-g vial.

ADMINISTRATION/HANDLING

IV

Storage • Store at room temperature (refrigeration may cause crystallization). • Reconstituted solution is stable for 24 hrs at room temperature.

Reconstitution • Use gloves when handling/preparing gemcitabine. • Reconstitute 200-mg or 1-g vial with 0.9% NaCl injection without preservative (5 ml or 25 ml, respectively) to provide a concentration of 40 mg/ml. • Shake to dissolve.

Rate of administration • May give without further dilution. • May be further diluted with 0.9% NaCl to a concentration as low as 0.1 mg/ml. • Infuse over 30 min (do not exceed rate over 1 hr—increases toxicity).

IV INCOMPATIBILITIES
Acyclovir (Zovirax), amphotericin (Fungizone), cefoperazone (Cefobid), furosemide (Lasix), ganciclovir (Cytovene), imipenem/cilastatin (Primaxin), irinotecan (Camptosar), methotrexate, methylprednisolone (Solu-Medrol), mitomycin (Mutamycin), piperacillin/tazobactam (Zosyn), prochlorperazine (Compazine).

IV COMPATIBILITIES
Bumetanide (Bumex), calcium gluconate, dexamethasone (Decadron), diphenhydramine (Benadryl), dobutamine (Dobutrex), dopamine (Intropin), granisetron (Kytril), heparin, hydrocortisone (Solu-Cortef), lorazepam (Ativan), ondansetron (Zofran), potassium.

G

INDICATIONS/ROUTES/DOSAGE

Alert: Dosage is individualized on basis of clinical response and tolerance to adverse effects. When used in combination therapy, consult specific protocols for optimum dosage, sequence of drug administration.

NON–SMALL CELL LUNG CANCER
IV: ADULTS, ELDERLY, CHILDREN: (In combination with cisplatin) 1,000 mg/m^2 days 1, 8, 15. Repeat q28days or 1,250 mg/m^2 days 1 and 8. Repeat q21days.

PANCREATIC CANCER
IV infusion: ADULTS: 1,000 mg/m^2 once weekly for up to 7 wks (or until toxicity necessitates decreasing/holding the dose), followed by 1 wk of rest. Subsequent cycles should consist of once weekly for 3 consecutive wks out of every 4 wks. Pts completing cycles at 1,000 mg/m^2 may increase dose to 1,250 mg/m^2 as tolerated. Dose for next cycle may be increased to 1,500 mg/m^2.

Alert: May increase dose provided the absolute granulocyte count (AGC) and platelet nadirs exceed 1,500 × 10^6/L and 100,000 × 10^6/L, respectively.

DOSE REDUCTION GUIDELINES

AGC (10^6/L)		Platelets (10^6/L)	% Full Dose
1,000	and	100,000	100
500–999	or	50,000–99,000	75
<500	or	<50,000	Hold

SIDE EFFECTS

FREQUENT: Nausea/vomiting (69%), generalized pain (48%), fever (41%), mild to moderate pruritic rash (30%), mild to moderate dyspnea, constipation (23%), peripheral edema (20%). **OCCASIONAL (10%–19%):** Diarrhea, petechiae, alopecia, stomatitis (burning/erythema of oral mucosa, sore throat, difficulty swallowing), infection, somnolence, paresthesia. **RARE:** Diaphoresis, rhinitis, insomnia, malaise.

ADVERSE REACTIONS/ TOXIC EFFECTS

Severe bone marrow suppression evidenced by anemia, thrombocytopenia, leukopenia occurs commonly.

NURSING IMPLICATIONS

BASELINE ASSESSMENT

CBC, renal/hepatic function tests should be performed prior to starting therapy and periodically thereafter. Drug should be suspended or dosage modified if bone marrow suppression is detected.

INTERVENTION/EVALUATION

Assess all lab results prior to giving each dose. Monitor for dyspnea, fever, pruritic rash, dehydration due to vomiting. Assess oral mucosa for erythema, ulceration at inner margin of lips, sore throat, difficulty swallowing (stomatitis). Assess skin for rash. Monitor for and report diarrhea. Provide antiemetics as needed.

PATIENT/FAMILY TEACHING

Avoid crowds/exposure to infection. Maintain fastidious oral hygiene. Promptly report fever, sore throat, signs of local infection, easy bruising, rash. Contact physician if nausea/vomiting continues at home.

gemfibrozil

gem-**fie**-bro-zill
(Apo-Gemfibrozil✤, Lopid, Novo-Gemfibrozil✤)

◆ CLASSIFICATION

PHARMACOTHERAPEUTIC: Fibric acid derivative. **CLINICAL:** Antihyperlipoproteinemic (see p. 51C).

ACTION

Inhibits lipolysis of fat in adipose tissue; decreases liver uptake of free fatty acids (reduces hepatic triglyceride production). Inhibits synthesis of VLDL carrier apolipoprotein B. **Therapeutic Effect:** Lowers serum cholesterol, triglycerides (decreases VLDL, LDL; increases HDL).

PHARMACOKINETICS

Well absorbed from GI tract. Protein binding: 99%. Metabolized in liver. Primarily excreted in urine. Not removed by hemodialysis. **Half-life:** 1.5 hrs.

USES

Treatment of hyperlipidemia, decreases risk of coronary heart disease in pts with type IIB hyperlipidemia. Treatment of severe primary hyperlipidemia (types IV, V).

PRECAUTIONS

CONTRAINDICATIONS: Hepatic dysfunction (including primary biliary cirrhosis), severe renal dysfunction, preexisting gallbladder disease. **CAUTIONS:** Hypothyroidism, diabetes mellitus, estrogen or anticoagulant therapy.

LIFESPAN CONSIDERATIONS: Pregnancy/lactation: Unknown if drug crosses placenta or is distributed in breast milk. Decision to discontinue nursing or drug should be based on potential for serious adverse effects. **Pregnancy Category C. Children:** Not recommended in those <2 yrs (cholesterol necessary for normal development). **Elderly:** Age-related renal impairment may require dosage adjustment.

INTERACTIONS

DRUG: May increase effect of **warfarin, repaglinide.** May cause rhabdomyolysis, leading to acute renal failure, with **lovastatin. HERBAL:** None known. **FOOD:** None known. **LAB VALUES:** May increase SGOT (AST), SGPT (ALT), alkaline phosphatase, bilirubin, creatinine kinase, LDH. May decrease Hgb, Hct, potassium, leukocyte counts.

AVAILABILITY (Rx)

TABLETS: 600 mg. **CAPSULES:** 300 mg.

ADMINISTRATION/HANDLING

PO

- Give 30 min before morning and evening meals.

INDICATIONS/ROUTES/DOSAGE

HYPERLIPIDEMIA

PO: ADULTS, ELDERLY: 900 mg to 1.5 g/day in 2 divided doses.

SIDE EFFECTS

FREQUENT (20%): Dyspepsia. **OCCASIONAL (2%–10%):** Abdominal pain, diarrhea, nausea, vomiting, fatigue. **RARE (<2%):** Constipation, acute appendicitis, vertigo, headache, rash, altered taste.

ADVERSE REACTIONS/ TOXIC EFFECTS

Cholelithiasis, cholecystitis, acute appendicitis, pancreatitis, malignancy occur rarely.

NURSING IMPLICATIONS

BASELINE ASSESSMENT

Assess baseline lab results: serum glucose, triglyceride, cholesterol levels; liver function tests; CBC.

INTERVENTION/EVALUATION

Determine pattern of bowel activity. Monitor LDL, VLDL, serum triglyceride, cholesterol lab results for therapeutic response. Assess for rash, pruritus. Check for headache, dizziness, blurred vision. Monitor liver function, hematology tests. Assess for pain, esp. right upper quadrant/epigastric pain suggestive of adverse gallbladder effects. Monitor serum glucose for those receiving insulin, oral antihyperglycemics.

PATIENT/FAMILY TEACHING

Follow special diet (important part of treatment). Take before meals. Periodic lab tests are essential part of therapy. Notify physician if dizziness, blurred vision, abdominal pain, diarrhea, nausea, vomiting becomes pronounced.

gemifloxacin mesylate

gem-ih-**flocks**-ah-sin
(Factive)

CLASSIFICATION

PHARMACOTHERAPEUTIC: Fluoroquinolone. **CLINICAL:** Antibacterial.

ACTION

Interferes with DNA-gyrase in susceptible microorganisms. **Therapeutic Effect:** Inhibits DNA replication, repair. Bactericidal.

PHARMACOKINETICS

Rapidly, well absorbed from GI tract. Widely distributed. Penetrates well into lung tissue and fluid. Protein binding: 70%. Undergoes limited liver metabolism. Primarily excreted in feces with a lesser amount eliminated in the urine. Partially removed by hemodialysis. **Half-life:** 4–12 hrs.

USES

Treatment of acute bacterial exacerbation of chronic bronchitis, community-acquired pneumonia of mild to moderate severity.

G

PRECAUTIONS

CONTRAINDICATIONS: History of prolongation of QTc interval, uncorrected electrolyte disorders (hypokalemia, hypomagnesemia), those receiving quinidine, procainamide, amiodarone, sotalol, history of hypersensitivity to fluoroquinolone antibiotic agents. **CAUTIONS:** Impaired hepatic/renal function, clinically significant bradycardia, acute myocardial ischemia.

LIFESPAN CONSIDERATIONS: Pregnancy/lactation: Has potential for teratogenic effects. Substitute formula feedings for breast feedings. **Pregnancy Category C. Children:** Safety and efficacy not established <18 yrs. **Elderly:** Age-related renal impairment may require dosage adjustment.

INTERACTIONS

DRUG: Concurrent use of Class IA and Class III **antiarrhythmics, antipsychotics, tricyclic antidepressants, erythromycin** may increase risk of QTc prolongation, life-threatening arrhythmias. **Magnesium- and aluminum-containing antacids, iron salts, bismuth subsalicylate, sucralfate, didanosine, zinc salts, other metals** may decrease absorption. **Cyclosporine** increases risk of nephrotoxicity. **Probenecid** increases gemifloxacin serum concentration. **HERBAL:** None known. **FOOD:** None known. **LAB VALUES:** May increase SGOT (AST), SGPT (ALT), alkaline phosphatase, LDH, bilirubin, BUN, creatinine.

AVAILABILITY (Rx)

TABLETS: 320 mg.

ADMINISTRATION/HANDLING

PO

- Give without regard to meals. Do not crush or break tablet. Do not administer antacids with or within 2 hrs of gemifloxacin.

INDICATIONS/ROUTES/DOSAGE

ACUTE BACTERIAL EXACERBATION OF CHRONIC BRONCHITIS

PO: ADULTS, ELDERLY: 320 mg once daily for 5 days.

COMMUNITY-ACQUIRED PNEUMONIA

PO: ADULTS, ELDERLY: 320 mg once daily for 7 days.

DOSAGE IN RENAL IMPAIRMENT

Dose and/or frequency is modified based on degree of renal impairment.

Creatinine Clearance	Dosage
>40 ml/min	320 mg once daily
≤40 ml/min	160 mg once daily

SIDE EFFECTS

OCCASIONAL (2%–4%): Diarrhea, rash, nausea. **RARE (≤1%):** Headache, abdominal pain, dizziness.

ADVERSE REACTIONS/ TOXIC EFFECTS

Antibiotic-associated colitis (severe abdominal pain/tenderness, watery, severe diarrhea), fungal overgrowth may result from altered bacterial balance.

NURSING IMPLICATIONS

BASELINE ASSESSMENT

Question for history of hypersensitivity to fluoroquinolone antibiotics.

INTERVENTION/EVALUATION

Monitor signs/symptoms of infection, WBC count, liver function tests. Encourage adequate fluid intake. Monitor daily bowel activity/stool consistency (watery, loose, soft, semisolid, solid). Assess skin for evidence of rash. Be alert for superinfection (oral candidiasis, genital pruritus).

PATIENT/FAMILY TEACHING

Take with 8 oz of water, without regard to food. Drink several glasses of water between meals. Complete full course of therapy. Do not take antacids with or within 2 hrs of gemifloxacin dose (reduces/destroys effectiveness).

gemtuzumab ozogamicin

gem-**too**-zoo-mab
(Mylotarg)

CLASSIFICATION

PHARMACOTHERAPEUTIC: Monoclonal antibody. **CLINICAL:** Antineoplastic (see p. 73C).

ACTION

Composed of an antibody conjoined with a cytotoxic antitumor antibody. The antibody portion binds to an antigen expressed on surface of leukemic blast cells in >80% of pts with acute myeloid leukemia (AML), resulting in formation of a complex. This releases the antibiotic inside the lysosomes of the myeloid cells. **Therapeutic Effect:** Binds to DNA, resulting in DNA double-strand breaks and cell death. Produces inhibition of colony formation in cultures of adult leukemic bone marrow cells.

PHARMACOKINETICS

After first infusion, elimination half-life is 45 hrs; after second dose, elimination half-life increased to 60 hrs.

USES

Treatment of pts with CD33 AML in first relapse who are >60 yrs and not considered candidates for cytotoxic chemotherapy.

PRECAUTIONS

CONTRAINDICATIONS: None known. **CAUTIONS:** Liver impairment.

LIFESPAN CONSIDERATIONS: Pregnancy/lactation: May cause fetal harm. Unknown if excreted in breast milk. **Pregnancy Category D. Children:** Safety and efficacy not established. **Elderly:** No age-related precautions noted.

INTERACTIONS

DRUG: None known. **HERBAL:** None known. **FOOD:** None known. **LAB VALUES:** May decrease WBCs, Hgb, Hct, platelet count, potassium, magnesium. May increase bilirubin, SGOT (AST), SGPT (ALT), transaminase.

AVAILABILITY (Rx)

POWDER FOR INJECTION: 5 mg.

ADMINISTRATION/HANDLING

IV

Storage • Protect from direct and indirect sunlight and unshielded fluorescent light during preparation/administration. • Refrigerate, do not freeze. • Following reconstitution in vial, stable for 8 hrs if refrigerated and protected from light. • Once diluted with 100 ml 0.9% NaCl, use immediately.

Reconstitution • Prepare in a biologic safety hood with fluorescent light off. • Allow vials to come to room temperature. • Reconstitute each vial with 5 ml Sterile Water for Injection using sterile syringes to provide concentration of 1 mg/ml. • Gently swirl; inspect for particulate matter/discoloration. • Withdraw desired volume from each vial and inject into 100 ml 0.9% NaCl and place into a UV protectant bag.

Rate of administration • Do not give IV push or bolus. • Infuse over 2 hrs. • Use separate line equipped with a low protein binding 1.2-micron filter. • May give through peripheral or central line.

IV INCOMPATIBILITY
Do not mix with any other medications.

G

INDICATIONS/ROUTES/DOSAGE

AML

IV infusion: ADULTS ≥60 YRS: 9 mg/m^2; repeat in 14 days for total of 2 doses.

Alert: Diphenhydramine 50 mg and acetaminophen 650–1,000 mg given 1 hr before administering; follow by acetaminophen 650–1,000 mg q4h for 2 doses, then q4h as needed. Full recovery from hematologic toxicities is not a requirement for giving second dose.

SIDE EFFECTS

Alert: Most pts experience a postinfusion symptom complex of fever (85%), chills (73%), nausea (70%), vomiting (63%) that resolves within 2–4 hrs with supportive therapy.

FREQUENT (31%–44%): Asthenia (loss of strength, energy), diarrhea, abdominal pain, headache, stomatitis (burning/erythema of oral mucosa, ulceration, sore throat, difficulty swallowing), dyspnea, epistaxis. **OCCASIONAL (15%–25%):** Constipation, neutropenic fever, nonspecific rash, herpes simplex infection, hypertension, hypotension, petechiae, peripheral edema, dizziness, insomnia, back pain. **RARE (10%–14%):** Pharyngitis, ecchymosis, dyspepsia, tachycardia, hematuria, rhinitis.

ADVERSE REACTIONS/ TOXIC EFFECTS

Severe myelosuppression occurs in 98% of all pts, characterized as neutropenia, anemia, thrombocytopenia. Sepsis occurs in 25% of pts. Hepatotoxicity may occur.

NURSING IMPLICATIONS

BASELINE ASSESSMENT

Obtain baseline CBC. Hepatic function studies, blood serum chemistry for comparison to expected myelosuppression. Use strict aseptic technique to protect pt from infection.

INTERVENTION/EVALUATION

Monitor CBC, blood chemistries, WBC, hepatic function studies. Monitor for myelosuppression (fever, sore throat, signs of local infection, unusual bruising/bleeding from any site), symptoms of anemia (excessive tiredness, weakness). Assess for impending stomatitis. Monitor B/P for hypertension/hypotension.

PATIENT/FAMILY TEACHING

Do not have immunizations without physician's approval (drug lowers body's resistance). Avoid contact with those who have recently received live virus vaccine. Promptly report fever, sore throat, signs of local infection, unusual bruising/bleeding from any site.

Gemzar

see gemtuzumab

gentamicin sulfate

jen-tah-**my**-sin
(Alcomicin, Cidomycin, Garamycin, Genoptic, Gentacidin)

◆CLASSIFICATION

PHARMACOTHERAPEUTIC: Aminoglycoside. **CLINICAL:** Antibiotic (see p. 18C).

ACTION

Irreversibly binds to protein of bacterial ribosomes. **Therapeutic Effect:** Interferes in protein synthesis of susceptible microorganisms. Bactericidal.

PHARMACOKINETICS

Rapid, complete absorption after IM administration. Protein binding: <30%. Widely distributed (does not cross blood-brain barrier, low concentrations in CSF). Excreted unchanged in urine. Removed by hemodialysis. **Half-life:** 2–4 hrs (half-life increased with impaired renal function, neonates; decreased in cystic fibrosis, burn or febrile pts).

USES

Parenteral: Treatment of skin/skin structure, bone, joint, respiratory tract, intra-abdominal, complicated urinary tract, acute pelvic infections; postop; burns; septicemia; meningitis. **Ophthalmic:** Ointment/solution for superficial eye infections. **Topical:** Cream/ointment for superficial skin infections. Ophthalmic or topical applications may be combined with systemic administration for serious, extensive infections. **Unlabeled: Topical:** Prophylaxis of minor bacterial skin infections, treatment of dermal ulcer.

PRECAUTIONS

CONTRAINDICATIONS: Hypersensitivity to gentamicin, other aminoglycosides (cross-sensitivity). Sulfite sensitivity may result in anaphylaxis, esp. in asthmatics. **CAUTIONS:** Elderly, neonates because of renal insufficiency/immaturity; neuromuscular disorders (potential for respiratory depression), prior hearing loss, vertigo, renal impairment. Cumulative effects may occur with concurrent systemic administration and topical application to large areas.

LIFESPAN CONSIDERATIONS: Pregnancy/lactation: Readily crosses placenta; unknown if distributed in breast milk. **Pregnancy Category C. Children:** Caution in neonates: Immature renal function increases half-life and toxicity. **Elderly:** Age-related renal impairment may require dosage adjustment.

INTERACTIONS

DRUG: Other aminoglycosides, nephrotoxic, ototoxic-producing medications may increase toxicity. May increase effects of **neuromuscular blocking agents. HERBAL:** None known. **FOOD:** None known. **LAB VALUES:** May increase BUN, SGOT (AST), SGPT (ALT), bilirubin, creatinine, LDH concentrations; may decrease serum calcium, magnesium, potassium, sodium concentrations. Therapeutic blood serum level: Peak 6–10 mcg/ml; trough: 0.5–2 mcg/ml. Toxic blood serum level: Peak: >10 mcg/ml; trough: >2 mcg/ml.

AVAILABILITY (Rx)

INJECTION: 10 mg/ml, 40 mg/ml, 2 mg/ml (Intrathecal). **OPHTHALMIC SOLUTION:** 3 mg/ml. **OPHTHALMIC OINTMENT:** 3 mg/g. **CREAM:** 0.5%. **OINTMENT:** 0.1%.

ADMINISTRATION/HANDLING

IM

• To minimize discomfort, give deep IM slowly. • Less painful if injected into gluteus maximus rather than lateral aspect of thigh.

IV

Storage • Store vials at room temperature. • Solution appears clear or slightly yellow. • Intermittent IV infusion (piggyback) is stable for 24 hrs at room temperature. • Discard if precipitate forms.

Reconstitution • Dilute with 50–200 ml D_5W or 0.9% NaCl. Amount of diluent for infants, children depends on individual needs.

Rate of administration • Infuse over 30–60 min for adults, older children; over 60–120 min for infants, young children.

G

INTRATHECAL

• Use only 2 mg/ml intrathecal preparation without preservative. • Mix with 10% estimated CSF volume or NaCl. • Use intrathecal forms immediately after preparation. Discard unused portion. • Give over 3–5 min.

OPHTHALMIC

• Place finger on lower eyelid, pull out until a pocket is formed between eye and lower lid • Hold dropper above pocket, place correct number of drops (¼–½ inch ointment) into pocket. Close eye gently. • **Solution:** Apply digital pressure to lacrimal sac for 1–2 min (minimizes drainage into nose/throat, reducing risk of systemic effects). • **Ointment:** Close eye for 1–2 min, rolling eyeball (increases contact area of drug to eye). • Remove excess solution or ointment around eye with tissue.

∅ IV INCOMPATIBILITIES

Allopurinol (Aloprim), amphotericin B complex (Abelcet, AmBisome, Amphotec), furosemide (Lasix), heparin, hetastarch (Hespan), idarubicin (Idamycin), indomethacin (Indocin), propofol (Diprivan).

IV COMPATIBILITIES

Amiodarone (Cordarone), diltiazem (Cardizem), enalapril (Vasotec), filgrastim (Neupogen), hydromorphone (Dilaudid), insulin, lorazepam (Ativan), magnesium sulfate, midazolam (Versed), morphine, multivitamins.

INDICATIONS/ROUTES/DOSAGE

Alert: Space parenteral doses evenly around the clock. Dosage based on ideal body weight. Peak, trough level determined periodically to maintain desired serum concentrations (minimizes risk of toxicity). **Recommended peak level:** 4–10 mcg/ml; **trough level:** 1–2 mcg/ml.

USUAL DOSAGE

IM/IV: ADULTS, ELDERLY: 3–6 mg/kg/day in divided doses q8h or 4–6.6 mg/kg once daily. CHILDREN 5–12 YRS: 2–2.5 mg/kg/dose q8h. CHILDREN <5 YRS: 2.5 mg/kg/dose q8h. NEONATES: 2.5–3.5 mg/kg/dose q8–12h.

HEMODIALYSIS

IM/IV: ADULTS, ELDERLY: 0.5–0.7 mg/kg/dose postdialysis. CHILDREN: 1.25–1.75 mg/kg/dose postdialysis.

INTRATHECAL

ADULTS: 4–8 mg/day. CHILDREN 3 MOS–12 YRS: 1–2 mg/day. NEONATES: 1 mg/day.

USUAL OPHTHALMIC DOSAGE

Ointment: ADULTS, ELDERLY: Thin strip to conjunctiva 2–3 times/day. **Solution:** 1–2 drops q2–4h up to 2 drops qh.

USUAL TOPICAL DOSAGE

ADULTS, ELDERLY: Apply 3–4 times/day.

SIDE EFFECTS

OCCASIONAL: Pain, induration at IM injection site; phlebitis, thrombophlebitis with IV administration; hypersensitivity reactions: rash, fever, urticaria, pruritus. **Ophthalmic:** Burning, tearing, itching, blurred vision. **Topical:** Redness, itching. **RARE:** Alopecia, hypertension, weakness.

ADVERSE REACTIONS/ TOXIC EFFECTS

Nephrotoxicity (evidenced by increased BUN and serum creatinine, decreased creatinine clearance) may be reversible if drug stopped at first sign of symptoms; irreversible ototoxicity (tinnitus, dizziness, ringing/roaring in ears, reduced hearing), neurotoxicity (headache, dizziness, lethargy, tremors, visual disturbances) occur occasionally. Risk is greater with higher dosages, prolonged therapy, or if solution is applied directly to mucosa. Superinfections, particularly with fungi, may result from bacterial imbalance via any route of administration. Ophthalmic application may cause paresthesia of conjunctiva, mydriasis.

NURSING IMPLICATIONS

BASELINE ASSESSMENT

Dehydration must be treated prior to beginning parenteral therapy. Establish baseline hearing acuity. Question for history of allergies, esp. to aminoglycosides and sulfites (and parabens for topical/ophthalmic routes).

INTERVENTION/EVALUATION

Monitor I&O (maintain hydration), urinalysis (casts, RBCs, WBCs, decrease in specific gravity). Be alert to ototoxic, neurotoxic symptoms (see Adverse Reactions/Toxic Effects). Check IM injection site for induration. Evaluate IV site for phlebitis (heat, pain, red streaking over vein). Assess for rash (**ophthalmic:** redness, burning, itching, tearing; **topical:** redness, itching). Be alert for superinfection, particularly genital/anal pruritus, changes in oral mucosa, diarrhea. When treating pts with neuromuscular disorders, assess respiratory response carefully. Therapeutic blood serum level: Peak 6–10 mcg/ml; trough: 0.5–2 mcg/ml. Toxic blood serum level: Peak: >10 mcg/ml; trough: >2 mcg/ml.

PATIENT/FAMILY TEACHING

Discomfort may occur with IM injection. Blurred vision, tearing may occur briefly after each ophthalmic dose. Notify physician in event of any hearing, visual, balance, urinary problems, even after therapy is completed. **Ophthalmic:** Contact physician if tearing, redness, irritation continues. **Topical:** Cleanse area gently before applying; notify physician if redness, itching occurs.

G

Geodon

see ziprasidone

ginger

Also known as black ginger, race ginger, zingiber

CLASSIFICATION

HERBAL.

ACTION

Possesses antipyretic, analgesic, antitussive, sedative properties. Increases GI motility; may act on serotonin receptors, primarily 5-HT_3. **Effect:** Reduces nausea/vomiting.

USES

Prevention of nausea/vomiting caused by motion sickness, early pregnancy, dyspepsia; treatment of rheumatoid arthritis.

PRECAUTIONS

CONTRAINDICATIONS: None known. **CAUTIONS:** Pregnancy; pts with bleeding conditions, diabetes (may cause hypoglycemia).

LIFESPAN CONSIDERATIONS: Pregnancy/lactation: Use during pregnancy is controversial (large amounts act as an abortifacient). **Children:** Safety and efficacy not established. **Elderly:** No age-related precautions noted.

INTERACTIONS

DRUG: Large amounts may increase risk of bleeding with **anticoagulants, antiplatelets. HERBAL: Feverfew, garlic, ginkgo, ginseng** may increase risk of bleeding. **FOOD:** None known. **LAB VALUES:** None known.

AVAILABILITY

CAPSULES: 470 mg, 550 mg. **ROOT:** 470 mg, 550 mg. **EXTRACT. POWDER. TABLETS. TEA. TINCTURE.**

INDICATIONS/ROUTES/DOSAGE

MORNING SICKNESS

PO: ADULTS: 250 mg 4 times/day. **Maximum:** 4 g/day.

MOTION SICKNESS

PO: ADULTS: 1 g (dried powder root) 30 min before travel.

NAUSEA

PO: ADULTS: 550–1,100 mg 3 times/day.

SIDE EFFECTS

Abdominal discomfort, heartburn, diarrhea, hypersensitivity reaction, nausea.

ADVERSE REACTIONS/ TOXIC EFFECTS

CNS depression, arrhythmias.

NURSING IMPLICATIONS

BASELINE ASSESSMENT

Assess for use of anticoagulants, antiplatelets (may increase risk of bleeding).

INTERVENTION/EVALUATION

Monitor for hypersensitivity reaction.

PATIENT/FAMILY TEACHING

Use cautiously during pregnancy/breastfeeding.

ginkgo biloba

Also known as fossil tree, maidenhair tree, tanakan

CLASSIFICATION

HERBAL.

ACTION

Possesses antioxidant, free radical scavenging properties. **Effect:** Protects tissues from oxidative damage, prevents progression of tissue degeneration in pts with dementia. Inhibits platelet-activating factor bonding at numerous cells, decreasing platelet aggregation, smooth muscle contraction; may increase cardiac contractility and coronary blood flow. Decreases blood viscosity, improving circulation by relaxing vascular smooth muscle. Increases cerebral and peripheral blood flow, reduces vascular permeability. May influence neurotransmitter system (e.g., cholinergic).

USES

Dementia syndromes, including Alzheimer's. Improves cerebral and peripheral circulation. Improves conditions associated with cerebral vascular insufficiency (e.g., memory loss, difficulty concentrating, vertigo, tinnitus). Improves cognitive behavior/sleep patterns in pts with depression. Acts as an antioxidant.

PRECAUTIONS

CONTRAINDICATIONS: Pregnancy/lactation. **CAUTIONS:** Pts with bleeding disorders, diabetes; epileptic pts or those prone to seizures. Avoid use in couples having difficulty conceiving.

LIFESPAN CONSIDERATIONS: Pregnancy/lactation: Contraindicated. **Children:** Safety and efficacy not established. Avoid use. **Elderly:** No age-related precautions noted.

INTERACTIONS

DRUG: May increase effect of **MAOIs.** May increase bleeding with **anticoagulants, antiplatelets (e.g., warfarin, aspirin, heparin, clopidogrel). HERBAL: Feverfew, ginger, garlic, ginseng** may increase risk of bleeding. **FOOD:** None known. **LAB VALUES:** May alter blood glucose levels.

AVAILABILITY (OTC)

CAPSULES: 40 mg, 60 mg. **TABLETS:** 40 mg, 60 mg. **FLUID EXTRACT. TINCTURE.**

INDICATIONS/ROUTES/DOSAGE

DEMENTIA

PO: ADULTS, ELDERLY: 120–240 mg/day (extract) in 2–3 doses.

VERTIGO, TINNITUS

PO: ADULTS, ELDERLY: 120–160 mg/day.

SIDE EFFECTS

Headache, dizziness, palpitations, constipation, allergic skin reactions. Large doses may cause nausea, vomiting, diarrhea, weakness, lack of muscle tone.

ADVERSE REACTIONS/ TOXIC EFFECTS

None known.

NURSING IMPLICATIONS

BASELINE ASSESSMENT

Assess for use of anticoagulants/antiplatelets, MAOIs. Assess for history of bleeding disorders, diabetes, seizures.

INTERVENTION/EVALUATION

Monitor for hypersensitivity reaction, blood glucose levels.

PATIENT/FAMILY TEACHING

Avoid use with anticoagulants/antiplatelets. May take up to 6 mos before it becomes effective. Do not use during pregnancy/breast-feeding. Avoid use in children.

ginseng

Also known as Asian ginseng, Chinese ginseng, red ginseng

CLASSIFICATION

HERBAL.

ACTION

Affects the hypothalamic-pituitary-adrenal axis. Appears to stimulate natural killer cell action. **Effect:** Reduces stress. Affects immune function.

USES

Increases resistance to stress. Boosts energy level. Enhances brain activity. Increases physical endurance. Aids in blood sugar control. Improves cognitive function, concentration, memory, work efficiency.

PRECAUTIONS

CONTRAINDICATIONS: Pts with bleeding tendencies, thrombosis. Avoid use during pregnancy/lactation. **CAUTIONS:** Pts with cardiac disorders, diabetes, hormone-sensitive cancers (e.g., breast, uterine, ovarian), endometriosis, uterine fibroids.

LIFESPAN CONSIDERATIONS: Pregnancy/lactation: Insufficient information. Do not use. **Children:** Safety and efficacy not established. **Elderly:** No age-related precautions noted.

INTERACTIONS

DRUG: May increase bleeding with **anticoagulants, antiplatelets (e.g., aspi-**

rin, clopidogrel, enoxaparin, heparin, warfarin). May increase effect of **oral antidiabetic agents, insulin.** May decrease effect of **furosemide.** May interfere with immunosuppressant drugs **(e.g., cyclosporine, prednisone).** **HERBAL: Chamomile, feverfew, garlic, ginger, ginkgo** may increase risk of bleeding. **FOOD: Coffee, tea** may increase effect. **LAB VALUES:** May prolong aPTT, decrease glucose.

G

AVAILABILITY (OTC)

CAPSULES: 100 mg, 250 mg, 410 mg, 500 mg. **TABLETS:** 250 mg, 1,000 mg. **DRIED ROOT. EXTRACT. POWDER. TEA (usually 1,500 mg/bag). TINCTURE.**

INDICATIONS/ROUTES/DOSAGE

USUAL DOSAGE

PO: ADULTS, ELDERLY: (Tablets/capsules): 200–600 mg/day. (Powder root): 0.6–3 g 1–3 times/day. (Tea—1,500 mg): 1–3 times/day.

SIDE EFFECTS

FREQUENT: Insomnia. **OCCASIONAL:** Vaginal bleeding, amenorrhea, palpitations, hypertension, diarrhea, headache, allergic reactions.

ADVERSE REACTIONS/ TOXIC EFFECTS

None known.

NURSING IMPLICATIONS

BASELINE ASSESSMENT

Determine whether pt is pregnant/ breast-feeding. Assess if pt is diabetic, taking oral hypoglycemic agents, insulin. Assess for anticoagulant, immunosuppressant use. Determine baseline blood glucose.

INTERVENTION/EVALUATION

Monitor coagulation studies, glucose levels. Assess for hypersensitivity reaction, rash.

PATIENT/FAMILY TEACHING

Avoid use in pregnancy/breast-feeding, children. Avoid continuous use for >3 mos.

glatiramer

glah-**tie**-rah-mir

(Copaxone)

Do not confuse with Compazine.

CLASSIFICATION

PHARMACOTHERAPEUTIC: Immunosuppressive. **CLINICAL:** Neurologic agent.

ACTION

Exact mechanism unknown. May act by modifying immune processes thought to be responsible for pathogenesis of multiple sclerosis. **Therapeutic Effect:** Slows progression of multiple sclerosis.

PHARMACOKINETICS

Substantial fraction of glatiramer is hydrolyzed locally. Some fraction of injected material enters lymphatic circulation, reaching regional lymph nodes; some may enter systemic circulation intact.

USES

Treatment of relapsing, remitting multiple sclerosis.

PRECAUTIONS

CONTRAINDICATIONS: Hypersensitivity to glatiramer, mannitol. **CAUTIONS:** Immediate postinjection reaction (flushing, chest pain, palpitations, anxiety, dyspnea, urticaria).

LIFESPAN CONSIDERATIONS: Pregnancy/lactation: Unknown if distributed in breast milk. **Pregnancy Category B. Children:** Safety and efficacy not established. **Elderly:** Information not available.

INTERACTIONS

DRUG: None known. **HERBAL:** None known. **FOOD:** None known. **LAB VALUES:** None known.

AVAILABILITY (Rx)

INJECTION: 20 mg/ml, prefilled syringes.

ADMINISTRATION/HANDLING

SUBCUTANEOUS

- Refrigerate syringes.

INDICATIONS/ROUTES/DOSAGE

MULTIPLE SCLEROSIS

Subcutaneous: ADULTS, ELDERLY: 20 mg once daily.

SIDE EFFECTS

COMMON (40%–73%): Pain, erythema, inflammation, pruritus at injection site, asthenia (loss of strength, energy). **FREQUENT (18%–27%):** Arthralgia, vasodilation, anxiety, hypertonia, nausea, transient chest pain, dyspnea, flu syndrome, rash, pruritus. **OCCASIONAL (10%–17%):** Palpitations, back pain, diaphoresis, rhinitis, diarrhea, urinary urgency. **RARE (6%–8%):** Anorexia, fever, neck pain, peripheral edema, ear pain, facial edema, vertigo, vomiting.

ADVERSE REACTIONS/ TOXIC EFFECTS

Infection occurs commonly. Lymphadenopathy occurs occasionally.

NURSING IMPLICATIONS

INTERVENTION/EVALUATION

Assess injection site for reaction. Monitor for fever, chills (evidence of infection); treat accordingly.

PATIENT/FAMILY TEACHING

Report difficulty in breathing/swallowing, rash, itching, swelling of lower extremities, weakness. Avoid pregnancy.

Gleevec

see imatinib

glimepiride

glim-**eh**-purr-eyd

(Amaryl)

Do not confuse with glipizide.

CLASSIFICATION

PHARMACOTHERAPEUTIC: Second-generation sulfonylurea. **CLINICAL:** Hypoglycemic (see p. 39C).

ACTION

Promotes release of insulin from beta cells of pancreas, increases insulin sensitivity at peripheral sites. **Therapeutic Effect:** Lowers blood glucose concentration.

PHARMACOKINETICS

Onset	Peak	Duration
PO		
—	2–3 hrs	24 hrs

Completely absorbed from GI tract. Protein binding: >99%. Metabolized in liver. Excreted in urine and eliminated in feces. **Half-life:** 5–9.2 hrs.

USES

Adjunct to diet/exercise in management of non–insulin dependent diabetes mellitus (type 2, NIDDM). Use in combination with insulin or metformin in pts whose diabetes is not controlled by diet/exercise in conjunction with oral hypoglycemic agent.

PRECAUTIONS

CONTRAINDICATIONS: Sole therapy for type 1 diabetes mellitus, diabetic complications (ketosis, acidosis, diabetic coma), stress situations (severe infection, trauma, surgery), severe renal/hepatic impairment. **CAUTIONS:** Severe diarrhea, intestinal obstruction, prolonged vomiting, liver disease, hyperthyroidism (uncontrolled), impaired renal function, adrenal insufficiency, debilitation, malnutrition, pituitary insufficiency.

LIFESPAN CONSIDERATIONS: Pregnancy/lactation: Not recommended for use during pregnancy. Unknown if distributed in breast milk. **Pregnancy Category C. Children:** Safety and efficacy not established. **Elderly:** Hypoglycemia may be difficult to recognize. Age-related renal impairment may increase sensitivity to glucose lowering effect.

INTERACTIONS

DRUG: May increase effect of **oral anticoagulants. Fluconazole, cimetidine, ranitidine, ciprofloxacin, MAOIs, quinidine, salicylates** (large doses) may increase effect. **Beta-blockers** may increase hypoglycemic effect, mask signs of hypoglycemia. **Corticosteroids, thiazide diuretics, lithium** may decrease effect. **HERBAL:** None known. **FOOD:** None known. **LAB VALUES:** May increase alkaline phosphatase, SGOT (AST), LDH, creatinine, BUN.

AVAILABILITY (Rx)

TABLETS: 1 mg, 2 mg, 4 mg.

ADMINISTRATION/HANDLING

PO

- Give with breakfast or first main meal.

INDICATIONS/ROUTES/DOSAGE

DIABETES MELLITUS

PO: ADULTS, ELDERLY: Initially, 1–2 mg once daily, with breakfast or first main meal. MAINTENANCE: 1–4 mg once daily. After dose of 2 mg is reached, dosage should be increased in increments of up to 2 mg q1–2wks, based on blood glucose response. **Maximum:** 8 mg/day.

RENAL FUNCTION IMPAIRMENT

PO: ADULTS: 1 mg once/day.

SIDE EFFECTS

FREQUENT: Altered taste sensation, dizziness, drowsiness, weight gain, constipation, diarrhea, heartburn, nausea, vomiting, stomach fullness, headache. **OCCASIONAL:** Increased sensitivity of skin to sunlight, peeling of skin, itching, rash.

ADVERSE REACTIONS/ TOXIC EFFECTS

Hypoglycemia may occur due to overdosage, insufficient food intake (esp. with increased glucose demands). GI hemorrhage, cholestatic hepatic jaundice, leukopenia, thrombocytopenia, pancytopenia, agranulocytosis, aplastic or hemolytic anemia occurs rarely.

NURSING IMPLICATIONS

BASELINE ASSESSMENT

Check blood glucose level. Discuss lifestyle to determine extent of learning, emotional needs. Ensure follow-up instruction if pt/family do not thoroughly understand diabetes management or glucose-testing technique.

INTERVENTION/EVALUATION

Monitor blood glucose, food intake. Assess for hypoglycemia (cool, wet skin tremors, dizziness, anxiety, headache, tachycardia, numbness in mouth, hunger, diplopia), hyperglycemia (polyuria, polyphagia, polydipsia, nausea, vomiting, dim vision, fatigue, deep/rapid breathing). Be alert to conditions that alter glucose requirements: fever, increased activity/stress, surgical procedure.

PATIENT/FAMILY TEACHING

Prescribed diet is principal part of treatment; do not skip/delay meals. Carry candy, sugar packets, other sugar supplements for immediate response to hypoglycemia. Wear medical alert identification. Check with physician when glucose demands are altered (e.g., fever, infection, trauma, stress, heavy physical activity).

glipizide

glip-ih-zide
(Glucotrol, Glucotrol XL)
Do not confuse with glimepiride, glyburide.

FIXED-COMBINATION(S)

Metaglip: glipizide/metformin (an antidiabetic): 2.5 mg/250 mg; 2.5 mg/500 mg; 5 mg/500 mg.

CLASSIFICATION

PHARMACOTHERAPEUTIC: Second-generation sulfonylurea. **CLINICAL:** Hypoglycemic (see p. 39C).

ACTION

Promotes release of insulin from beta cells of pancreas, increases insulin sensitivity at peripheral sites. **Therapeutic Effect:** Lowers blood glucose concentration.

PHARMACOKINETICS

Onset	Peak	Duration
PO		
15–30 min	2–3 hrs	12–24 hrs
Extended-release		
2–3 hrs	6–12 hrs	24 hrs

Well absorbed from GI tract. Protein binding: 99%. Metabolized in liver. Excreted in urine. **Half-life:** 2–4 hrs.

USES

Adjunct to diet/exercise in management of stable, mild to moderately severe non–insulin dependent diabetes mellitus (type 2, NIDDM). May be used to supplement insulin in those with type 1 diabetes mellitus.

PRECAUTIONS

CONTRAINDICATIONS: Type 1 diabetes mellitus, diabetic ketoacidosis with or without coma. **CAUTIONS:** Adrenal/pituitary insufficiency, hypoglycemic reactions, impaired liver/renal function.

LIFESPAN CONSIDERATIONS: Pregnancy/lactation: Insulin is drug of choice during pregnancy; glipizide given within 1 mo of delivery may produce neonatal hypoglycemia. Drug crosses placenta. Distributed in breast milk. **Pregnancy Category C. Children:** Safety and efficacy not established. **Elderly:** Hypoglycemia may be difficult to recognize. Age-related renal impairment may increase sensitivity to glucose-lowering effect.

INTERACTIONS

DRUG: May increase effect of **oral anticoagulants. Fluconazole, cimetidine, ranitidine, ciprofloxacin, MAOIs, quinidine, salicylates** (large doses) may increase effect. **Beta-blockers** may increase hypoglycemic effect, mask signs of hypoglycemia. **Corticosteroids, thiazide diuretics, lithium** may decrease effect. **HERBAL:** None known. **FOOD:** None known. **LAB VALUES:** May increase alkaline phosphatase, SGOT (AST), LDH, creatinine, BUN.

AVAILABILITY (Rx)

TABLETS: 5 mg, 10 mg. **TABLETS (extended-release):** 2.5 mg, 5 mg, 10 mg.

ADMINISTRATION/HANDLING

PO

- May give with food (response better if

taken 15–30 min before meals). • Do not crush extended-release tablets.

INDICATIONS/ROUTES/DOSAGE

DIABETES MELLITUS

PO: ADULTS: Initially, 5 mg/day (2.5 mg in geriatric or those with liver disease). Adjust dosage in 2.5- to 5-mg increments at intervals of several days. **Maximum single dose:** 15 mg. **Maximum dose/day:** 40 mg. **Maximum (ER tablet):** 20 mg/day.

G

USUAL ELDERLY DOSAGE

PO: Initially, 2.5–5 mg/day. May increase by 2.5–5 mg/day q1–2wks.

SIDE EFFECTS

FREQUENT: Altered taste sensation, dizziness, drowsiness, weight gain, constipation, diarrhea, heartburn, nausea, vomiting, stomach fullness, headache. **OCCASIONAL:** Increased sensitivity of skin to sunlight, peeling of skin, itching, rash.

ADVERSE REACTIONS/ TOXIC EFFECTS

Hypoglycemia may occur because of overdosage, insufficient food intake (esp. with increased glucose demands). GI hemorrhage, cholestatic hepatic jaundice, leukopenia, thrombocytopenia, pancytopenia, agranulocytosis, aplastic or hemolytic anemia occurs rarely.

NURSING IMPLICATIONS

BASELINE ASSESSMENT

Check blood glucose level. Discuss lifestyle to determine extent of learning, emotional needs. Ensure follow-up instruction if pt/family do not thoroughly understand diabetes management or glucose-testing technique.

INTERVENTION/EVALUATION

Monitor blood glucose and food intake. Assess for hypoglycemia (cool, wet skin, tremors, dizziness, anxiety, headache, tachycardia, numbness in mouth, hunger, diplopia), hyperglycemia (polyuria, polyphagia, polydipsia, nausea, vomiting, dim vision, fatigue, deep/rapid breathing). Be alert to conditions that alter glucose requirements: fever, increased activity/stress, surgical procedure.

PATIENT/FAMILY TEACHING

Prescribed diet is principal part of treatment; do not skip/delay meals. Carry candy, sugar packets, other sugar supplements for immediate response to hypoglycemia. Wear medical alert identification. Check with physician when glucose demands are altered (e.g., fever, infection, trauma, stress, heavy physical activity).

glucagon hydrochloride

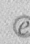

glue-ka-gon
(Glucagon Emergency Kit)
Do not confuse with Glaucon.

CLASSIFICATION

PHARMACOTHERAPEUTIC: Glucose elevating agent. **CLINICAL:** Antihypoglycemic, antispasmodic, antidote.

ACTION

Promotes hepatic glycogenolysis, gluconeogenesis. Stimulates enzyme to increase production of cAMP. **Therapeutic Effect:** Increases plasma glucose concentration, relaxant effect on smooth muscle, and exerts inotropic myocardial effect.

USES

Treatment of severe hypoglycemia in diabetic pts. Not for use in chronic hypoglycemia or hypoglycemia due to starvation, adrenal insufficiency (liver glycogen unavailable). Diagnostic aid in radiographic examination of GI tract. **Unlabeled:** Treatment of toxicity associated with beta-blockers, calcium channel blockers; esophageal obstruction due to foreign bodies.

PRECAUTIONS

CONTRAINDICATIONS: Pheochromocytoma, hypersensitivity to glucagon (protein). **CAUTIONS:** History of insulinoma, pheochromocytoma. **Pregnancy Category B.**

INTERACTIONS

DRUG: May increase **anticoagulant** effect. **HERBAL:** None known. **FOOD:** None known. **LAB VALUES:** May decrease potassium.

AVAILABILITY (Rx)

POWDER FOR INJECTION: 1 mg.

ADMINISTRATION/HANDLING

Alert: Place pt on side to prevent aspiration (glucagon, hypoglycemia may produce nausea/vomiting).

SUBCUTANEOUS/IM/IV

• Store vial at room temperature. • After reconstitution, is stable for 48 hrs if refrigerated. If reconstituted with Sterile Water for Injection, use immediately. Do not use glucagon solution unless clear. • Reconstitute powder with manufacturer's diluent when preparing doses of ≤2 mg. For doses >2 mg, dilute with Sterile Water for Injection. • To provide 1 mg glucagon/ml, use 1 ml diluent. For 1-mg vial of glucagon, use 10 ml diluent for 10-mg vial. • Pt will usually awaken in 5–20 min. Although 1–2 additional doses may be administered, concern for effects of continuing cerebral hypoglycemia requires consideration of parenteral glucose. • When pt awakens, give supplemental carbohydrate to restore liver glycogen and prevent secondary hypoglycemia. If pt fails to respond to glucagon, IV glucose is necessary.

∅ IV INCOMPATIBILITY

Do not mix with any other medications.

INDICATIONS/ROUTES/DOSAGE

Alert: Administer IV dextrose if pt fails to respond to glucagon.

HYPOGLYCEMIA

Subcutaneous/IM/IV: ADULTS, ELDERLY: 0.5–1 mg. May repeat 1–2 additional doses if response is delayed. CHILDREN <20 KG: 0.5 mg.

DIAGNOSTIC AID

IM/IV: ADULTS, ELDERLY: 0.25–2 mg.

SIDE EFFECTS

OCCASIONAL: Nausea, vomiting. **RARE:** Allergic reaction (urticaria, respiratory distress, hypotension).

ADVERSE REACTIONS/ TOXIC EFFECTS

Overdose may produce persistent nausea/vomiting, hypokalemia (severe weakness, decreased appetite, irregular heartbeat, muscle cramps).

NURSING IMPLICATIONS

BASELINE ASSESSMENT

Obtain immediate assessment, including history, clinical signs/symptoms. If hypoglycemic coma is established, give glucagon promptly.

INTERVENTION/EVALUATION

Monitor response time carefully. Have IV dextrose readily available in event pt does not awaken within 5–20 min. Assess for possible allergic reaction (urticaria, respiratory difficulty, hypotension). When pt is conscious, give carbohydrate.

PATIENT/FAMILY TEACHING

Recognize significance of identifying symptoms of hypoglycemia: pale, cool skin; anxiety, difficulty concentrating, headache, hunger, nausea, nervousness, shakiness, diaphoresis, unusual tiredness, weakness, unconsciousness. If symptoms of hypoglycemia develop, instruct pt/family/friend to give sugar form first (orange juice, honey, hard candy, sugar cubes, table sugar dissolved in water or juice) followed by cheese and crackers, half a sandwich, or glass of milk.

G

glucosamine/ chondroitin

◆ **CLASSIFICATION**

HERBAL.

ACTION

Glucosamine: Necessary for synthesis of mucopolysaccharides, which comprise the body's tendons, ligaments, cartilage, synovial fluid. May decrease glucose-induced insulin secretion. **Effect:** Relieves symptoms of osteoarthritis. **Chondroitin:** Endogenously found in cartilage tissue, substrate for forming joint matrix structure. May have some anticoagulant properties. **Effect:** Relieves symptoms of osteoarthritis.

USES

Treatment of osteoarthritis.

PRECAUTIONS

CONTRAINDICATIONS: None known. **CAUTIONS: Glucosamine:** Diabetes (may increase insulin resistance). **Chondroitin:** None known.

LIFESPAN CONSIDERATIONS: Pregnancy/lactation: Avoid use. **Children:** Safety and efficacy not established. **Elderly:** No age-related precautions noted.

INTERACTIONS

DRUG: Glucosamine: None known. **Chondroitin:** Monitor anticoagulant therapy. **HERBAL:** None known. **FOOD:** None known. **LAB VALUES: Glucosamine:** May increase glucose. **Chondroitin:** May increase antifactor Xa level.

AVAILABILITY (OTC)

GLUCOSAMINE: **CAPSULES:** 500 mg. **TABLETS:** 500 mg.

CHONDROITIN: **CAPSULES:** 250 mg.

Alert: Many combination products are available.

INDICATIONS/ROUTES/DOSAGE

OSTEOARTHRITIS

PO: ADULTS, ELDERLY: (Glucosamine): 500 mg 3 times/day or 1–2 g/day. (Chondroitin): 200–400 mg 2–3 times/day.

SIDE EFFECTS

GLUCOSAMINE: Mild GI symptoms (e.g., gas, bloating, cramps). **CHONDROITIN:** Well tolerated. May cause nausea, diarrhea, constipation, edema, alopecia, allergic reactions.

ADVERSE REACTIONS/ TOXIC EFFECTS

None known.

NURSING IMPLICATIONS

BASELINE ASSESSMENT

Determine whether pt is taking anticoagulants/antiplatelets, antidiabetic drugs. Determine whether pt is pregnant/breast-feeding.

EVALUATION/INTERVENTION

Monitor effectiveness of therapy in relieving osteoarthritis symptoms, blood glucose levels.

PATIENT/FAMILY TEACHING

Avoid use in pregnancy/breast-feeding, children. May take several mos of therapy to be effective. Glucosamine may alter glucose levels.

Glucophage

see metformin

Glucotrol

see glipizide

glyburide

glye-byoo-ride
(Daonil ✤, DiaBeta, Euglucon ✤, Glynase, Micronase)

Do not confuse with Micro-K, Micronor, Zebeta.

FIXED-COMBINATION(S)

Glucovance: glyburide/metformin (an antidiabetic): 1.25 mg/250 mg; 2.5 mg/500 mg; 5 mg/500 mg.

CLASSIFICATION

PHARMACOTHERAPEUTIC: Second-generation sulfonylurea. **CLINICAL:** Hypoglycemic (see p. 39C).

ACTION

Promotes release of insulin from beta cells of pancreas, increases insulin sensitivity at peripheral sites. **Therapeutic Effect:** Lowers blood glucose concentration.

PHARMACOKINETICS

Onset	Peak	Duration
PO		
0.25–1 hr	1–2 hrs	12–24 hrs

Well absorbed from GI tract. Protein binding: 99%. Metabolized in liver to weakly active metabolite. Primarily excreted in urine. Not removed by hemodialysis. **Half-life:** 1.4–1.8 hrs.

USES

Adjunct to diet/exercise in management of stable, mild to moderately severe non–insulin dependent diabetes mellitus (type 2, NIDDM). May be used to supplement insulin in those with type 1 diabetes mellitus.

PRECAUTIONS

CONTRAINDICATIONS: Sole therapy for type 1 diabetes mellitus, diabetic ketoacidosis with or without coma. **CAUTIONS:** Adrenal/pituitary insufficiency, hypoglycemic reactions, impaired liver/renal function.

LIFESPAN CONSIDERATIONS: Pregnancy/lactation: Crosses placenta. Distributed in breast milk. May produce neonatal hypoglycemia if given within 2 wks of delivery. **Pregnancy Category C. Children:** Safety and efficacy not established. **Elderly:** Hypoglycemia may be difficult to recognize. Age-related renal impairment may increase sensitivity to glucose-lowering effect.

INTERACTIONS

DRUG: May increase effect of **oral anticoagulants. Fluconazole, cimetidine, ranitidine, ciprofloxacin, MAOIs, quinidine, salicylates** (large doses) may increase effect. **Beta-blockers** may increase hypoglycemic effect, mask signs of hypoglycemia. **Corticosteroids, thiazide diuretics, lithium** may decrease effect. **HERBAL:** None known. **FOOD:** None known. **LAB VALUES:** May increase alkaline phosphatase, SGOT (AST), LDH, creatinine, BUN.

AVAILABILITY (Rx)

TABLETS: 1.25 mg, 2.5 mg, 5 mg. **(Glynase):** 1.5 mg, 3 mg, 6 mg.

ADMINISTRATION/HANDLING

PO

• May give with food (response better if taken 15–30 min before meals).

INDICATIONS/ROUTES/DOSAGE

DIABETES MELLITUS

PO: ADULTS: Initially, 2.5–5 mg. May increase by 2.5 mg/day at weekly intervals. MAINTENANCE: 1.25–20 mg/day. **Maximum:** 20 mg/day. ELDERLY: Initially, 1.25–2.5 mg/day. May increase by 1.25–2.5 mg/day at 1–3-wk intervals.

MICRONIZED TABLETS (GLYNASE)

PO: ADULTS, ELDERLY: Initially, 0.75–3 mg/day. May increase by 1.5 mg/day at weekly intervals. MAINTENANCE: 0.75–12 mg/day as single dose or in divided doses.

DOSAGE IN RENAL IMPAIRMENT

Not recommended in pts with creatinine clearance <50 ml/min.

SIDE EFFECTS

FREQUENT: Altered taste sensation, dizziness, drowsiness, weight gain, constipation, diarrhea, heartburn, nausea, vomiting, stomach fullness, headache. **OCCASIONAL:** Increased sensitivity of skin to sunlight, peeling of skin, itching, rash.

ADVERSE REACTIONS/ TOXIC EFFECTS

Overdosage, insufficient food intake may produce hypoglycemia, esp. with increased glucose demands. Cholestatic jaundice, leukopenia, thrombocytopenia, pancytopenia, agranulocytosis, aplastic or hemolytic anemia occurs rarely.

NURSING IMPLICATIONS

BASELINE ASSESSMENT

Check blood glucose level. Discuss lifestyle to determine extent of learning, emotional needs. Ensure follow-up instruction if pt/family do not thoroughly understand diabetes management or glucose-testing technique.

INTERVENTION/EVALUATION

Monitor blood glucose, food intake. Assess for hypoglycemia (cool, wet skin; tremors, dizziness, anxiety, headache, tachycardia, numbness in mouth, hunger, diplopia) hyperglycemia (polyuria, polyphagia, polydipsia, nausea, vomiting, dim vision, fatigue, deep/rapid breathing). Be alert to conditions that alter glucose requirements: fever, increased activity/stress, surgical procedure.

PATIENT/FAMILY TEACHING

Prescribed diet is principal part of treatment; do not skip/delay meals. Carry candy, sugar packets, other sugar supplements for immediate response to hypoglycemia. Wear medical alert identification. Check with physician when glucose demands are altered (e.g., fever, infection, trauma, stress, heavy physical activity).

glycopyrrolate

gly-ko-**pie**-roll-ate
(Robinul, Robinul Forte ✦)

◆CLASSIFICATION

PHARMACOTHERAPEUTIC: Quaternary anticholinergic. **CLINICAL:** Antimuscarinic, antiarrhythmic, cholinergic adjunct.

ACTION

Inhibits action of acetylcholine at postganglionic parasympathetic sites in smooth muscle, secretory glands, CNS. **Therapeutic Effect:** Reduces salivation/excessive secretions of respiratory tract; reduces gastric secretions, acidity.

USES

Inhibits salivation/excessive secretions of the respiratory tract. Reverses the muscarinic effects of cholinergic agents (e.g., neostigmine).

PRECAUTIONS

CONTRAINDICATIONS: Narrow-angle glaucoma, acute hemorrhage, tachycardia, ulcerative colitis, obstructive uropathy, paralytic ileus, myasthenia gravis. **CAUTIONS:** Those with fever, hyperthyroidism, liver/renal disease, hypertension, CHF, GI infections, diarrhea, reflux esophagitis. **Pregnancy Category B.**

INTERACTIONS

DRUG: **Antacids, antidiarrheals** may decrease absorption. **Anticholinergics** may increase effects. May decrease absorption of **ketoconazole.** May increase severity of GI lesions with **potassium chloride** (wax matrix). **HERBAL:** None known. **FOOD:** None known. **LAB VALUES:** May decrease uric acid.

AVAILABILITY (Rx)

INJECTION: 0.2 mg/ml.

∅ IV INCOMPATIBILITY

None known.

IV COMPATIBILITIES

Diphenhydramine (Benadryl), droperidol (Inapsine), hydromorphone (Dilaudid), hydroxyzine (Vistaril), lidocaine, midazolam (Versed), morphine, promethazine (Phenergan).

INDICATIONS/ROUTES/DOSAGE

PREOP

IM: ADULTS, ELDERLY: 4.4 mcg/kg 30–60 min before procedure. CHILDREN ≥2 YRS: 4.4 mcg/kg. CHILDREN <2 YRS: 4.4–8.8 mcg/kg.

BLOCK EFFECTS OF ANTICHOLINESTERASE AGENTS

IV: ADULTS, ELDERLY: 0.2 mg for each 1 mg neostigmine or 5 mg pyridostigmine.

SIDE EFFECTS

FREQUENT: Dry mouth (sometimes severe), decreased sweating, constipation. **OCCASIONAL:** Blurred vision, bloated feeling, urinary hesitancy, drowsiness (with high dosage), headache, intolerance to light, loss of taste, nervousness, flushing, insomnia, impotence, mental confusion/excitement (particularly in elderly, children). Parenteral form may produce temporary lightheadedness, local irritation. **RARE:** Dizziness, faintness.

ADVERSE REACTIONS/ TOXIC EFFECTS

Overdosage may produce temporary paralysis of ciliary muscle, pupillary dilation, tachycardia, palpitation, hot/dry/ flushed skin, absence of bowel sounds, hyperthermia, increased respiratory rate, EKG abnormalities, nausea, vomiting, rash over face/upper trunk, CNS stimulation, psychosis (agitation, restlessness, rambling speech, visual hallucination, paranoid behavior, delusions), followed by depression.

NURSING IMPLICATIONS

BASELINE ASSESSMENT

Before giving medication, instruct pt to void (reduces risk of urinary retention).

INTERVENTION/EVALUATION

Monitor daily bowel activity/stool consistency. Palpate bladder for urinary retention. Monitor heart rate, changes in B/P, temperature. Assess skin turgor, mucous membranes to evaluate hydration status (encourage adequate fluid intake), bowel sounds for peristalsis. Be alert for fever (increased risk of hyperthermia).

PATIENT/FAMILY TEACHING

May cause dry mouth. Take 30 min before meals (food decreases absorption

G

of medication). Use care not to become overheated during exercise in hot weather (may result in heat stroke). Avoid hot baths, saunas. Avoid tasks that require alertness, motor skills until response to drug is established. Do not take antacids or medicine for diarrhea within 1 hr of taking this medication (decreased effectiveness).

gold sodium thiomalate

gold sodium thigh-oh-**mal**-ate (Myochrysine)

CLASSIFICATION

PHARMACOTHERAPEUTIC: Gold compound. **CLINICAL:** Antirheumatic, anti-inflammatory.

ACTION

Unknown. May decrease prostaglandin synthesis or alter cellular mechanisms by inhibiting sulfhydryl systems. **Therapeutic Effect:** Decreases synovial inflammation, retards cartilage/bone destruction (suppresses or prevents, but does not cure, arthritis, synovitis).

USES

Treatment of progressive rheumatoid arthritis. **Unlabeled:** Treatment of psoriatic arthritis.

PRECAUTIONS

CONTRAINDICATIONS: Severe liver/renal impairment, systemic lupus erythematosus, history of blood dyscrasias, CHF, exfoliative dermatitis, colitis. Concurrent use of antimalarials, immunosuppressive agents, penicillamine, phenylbutazone. **CAUTIONS:** None known. **Pregnancy Category C.**

INTERACTIONS

DRUG: Bone marrow depressants, hepatotoxic, nephrotoxic medications may increase toxicity. **Penicillamine** may increase risk of adverse hematologic/renal effects. **HERBAL:** None known. **FOOD:** None known. **LAB VALUES:** May decrease Hgb, Hct, platelets, WBCs. May alter liver function tests. May increase urine protein.

AVAILABILITY (Rx)

INJECTION: 50 mg/ml.

INDICATIONS/ROUTES/DOSAGE

RHEUMATOID ARTHRITIS

Alert: Give as weekly injections.

IM: ADULTS, ELDERLY: Initially, 10 mg, then 25 mg for second dose. Follow with 25–50 mg/wk until improvement noted or total of 1 g administered. MAINTENANCE: 25–50 mg q2wks for 2–20 wks; if stable, may increase to q3–4wk intervals. CHILDREN: Initially, 10 mg, then 1 mg/kg/wk. **Maximum single dose:** 50 mg. MAINTENANCE: 1 mg/kg/dose at 2 to 4-wk intervals.

DOSAGE IN RENAL IMPAIRMENT

Creatinine Clearance	Dosage
50–80 ml/min	50% of usual dose
<50 ml/min	Not recommended

SIDE EFFECTS

FREQUENT: Pruritic dermatitis, stomatitis (erythema, redness, shallow ulcers of oral mucous membranes, sore throat, difficulty swallowing), diarrhea/loose stools, abdominal pain, nausea. **OCCASIONAL:** Vomiting, anorexia, flatulence, dyspepsia, conjunctivitis, photosensitivity. **RARE:** Constipation, urticaria, rash.

ADVERSE REACTIONS/ TOXIC EFFECTS

Signs of gold toxicity: decreased Hgb, leukopenia (WBC <4,000 mm^3), reduced granulocyte counts (<150,000/mm^3), proteinuria, hematuria, blood dyscrasias (anemia, leukopenia, thrombocytopenia, eosinophilia), glomerulonephritis, nephrotic syndrome, cholestatic jaundice.

NURSING IMPLICATIONS

BASELINE ASSESSMENT

Rule out pregnancy prior to beginning treatment; CBC, urinalysis, renal/liver function tests should be performed before therapy begins.

INTERVENTION/EVALUATION

Monitor daily bowel activity/stool consistency. Assess urine tests for proteinuria, hematuria. Monitor CBC, renal/hepatic function studies. Assess skin daily for rash, purpura, ecchymoses. Assess oral mucous membranes, borders of tongue, palate, pharynx for ulceration, complaint of metallic taste sensation (signs of stomatitis). Evaluate for therapeutic response: relief of pain, stiffness, swelling; increase in joint mobility; reduced joint tenderness; improved grip strength.

PATIENT/FAMILY TEACHING

Therapeutic response may take ≥6 mos. Avoid exposure to sunlight (gray to blue pigment may appear). Maintain diligent oral hygiene.

gonadorelin

go-nad-oh-**rell**-in

(Factrel, Lutrepulse, Relisom✤)

Do not confuse with gonadotropin, guanadrel, Sectral.

◆CLASSIFICATION

PHARMACOTHERAPEUTIC: Gonadotropin-releasing hormone. **CLINICAL:** Diagnostic agent.

ACTION

Stimulates release of luteinizing hormone (LH) from the anterior pituitary gland. **Therapeutic Effect:** Stimulates release of gonadotropin-releasing hormone from hypothalamus.

USES

Evaluation of hypothalamic pituitary gonadotropic function, evaluation of abnormal gonadotropin regulation as in precocious or delayed puberty, treatment of primary hypothalamic amenorrhea.

PRECAUTIONS

CONTRAINDICATIONS: None known. **CAUTIONS:** None known. **Pregnancy Category B.**

INTERACTIONS

DRUG: None known. **HERBAL:** None known. **FOOD:** None known. **LAB VALUES:** None known.

AVAILABILITY (Rx)

POWDER FOR INJECTION: (Factrel): 100 mcg **(Lutrepulse):** 0.8 mg, 3.2 mg.

INDICATIONS/ROUTES/DOSAGE

Alert: Test should be conducted in the absence of other drugs that affect pituitary secretion of gonadotropins.

GONADORELIN ACETATE

PRIMARY HYPOTHALAMIC AMENORRHEA

IV (Lutrepulse) pump: ADULTS: 5 mcg q90min (range 1–20 mcg); treatment interval 21 days. Refer to manufacturer's manual for proper dilutions/settings on pump. Response usually occurs 2–3 wks after initiation. Continue additional 2 wks after ovulation occurs (maintains corpus luteum). **Note:** Pump will pulsate q90 min for 7 days.

GONADORELIN HYDROCHLORIDE

DIAGNOSTIC AGENT

IV/subcutaneous: ADULTS: 100 mcg. In females, perform test in early follicular phase of menstrual cycle.

G

SIDE EFFECTS

OCCASIONAL: Swelling, pain, or itching at injection site with subcutaneous administration. Local or generalized skin rash with chronic subcutaneous administration. **RARE:** Headache, nausea, lightheadedness, abdominal discomfort, hypersensitivity reactions (bronchospasm, tachycardia, flushing, urticaria), induration at injection site.

ADVERSE REACTIONS/ TOXIC EFFECTS

Anaphylactic reaction occurs rarely.

NURSING IMPLICATIONS

BASELINE ASSESSMENT

Prior to starting test ensure that pt understands procedure. **Gonadorelin Acetate:** Pt instructions included with kit from manufacturer. **Gonadorelin Hydrochloride:** Venous blood sample (for LH) to be drawn immediately prior to administration.

INTERVENTION/EVALUATION

Gonadorelin Acetate: With baseline pelvic ultrasound, perform follow-up studies. **Gonadorelin Hydrochloride:** Change cannula, IV site at 48-hr intervals. Ensure that protocol for test is maintained: usually venous blood samples (for LH) drawn after administration at intervals of 15, 30, 45, 60, 120 min.

goserelin acetate

gos-**er**-ah-lin
(Zoladex, Zoladex LA✱)

◆CLASSIFICATION

PHARMACOTHERAPEUTIC: Gonadotropin-releasing hormone analogue. **CLINICAL:** Antineoplastic (see pp. 73C, 89C).

ACTION

Synthetic luteinizing hormone–releasing hormone analogue. Stimulates release of luteinizing hormone (LH), follicle-stimulating hormone (FSH) from anterior pituitary. **Therapeutic Effect:** Increases testosterone concentrations. After initial increase, decreases release of LH, FSH, testosterone.

USES

Treatment of advanced carcinoma of prostate as alternative when orchiectomy, estrogen therapy is either not indicated or unacceptable to pt. In combination with flutamide before and during radiation therapy for early stages of prostate cancer. Management of endometriosis. Treatment of advanced breast cancer in premenopausal and perimenopausal women. Endometrial thinning before ablation for dysfunctional uterine bleeding.

PRECAUTIONS

CONTRAINDICATIONS: Pregnancy. **CAUTIONS:** None known. **Pregnancy Category D** (advanced breast cancer). **Category X** (endometriosis, endometrial thinning).

INTERACTIONS

DRUG: None known. **HERBAL:** None known. **FOOD:** None known. **LAB VAL-**

UES: May increase serum acid phosphatase, testosterone concentrations.

AVAILABILITY (Rx)

IMPLANT: 3.6 mg, 10.8 mg.

INDICATIONS/ROUTES/DOSAGE

PROSTATIC CARCINOMA

Subcutaneous/implant: ADULTS >18 YRS, ELDERLY: 3.6 mg q28days or 10.8 mg q12wks into upper abdominal wall.

BREAST CARCINOMA, ENDOMETRIOSIS

Subcutaneous/implant: ADULTS: 3.6 mg q28 days into upper abdominal wall.

ENDOMETRIAL THINNING

Subcutaneous: ADULTS: 3.6 mg once or 4 wks apart in 2 doses.

SIDE EFFECTS

FREQUENT: Headache (60%), hot flashes (55%), depression (54%), diaphoresis (45%), sexual dysfunction (21%), decreased erection (18%), lower urinary tract symptoms (13%). **OCCASIONAL (5%–10%):** Nausea, pain, lethargy, dizziness, insomnia, anorexia, nausea, rash, upper respiratory infection, hair growth, abdominal pain. **RARE:** Pruritus.

ADVERSE REACTIONS/ TOXIC EFFECTS

Arrhythmias, CHF, hypertension occur rarely. Ureteral obstruction, spinal cord compression observed (immediate orchiectomy may be necessary).

NURSING IMPLICATIONS

INTERVENTION/EVALUATION

Monitor pt closely for worsening signs/symptoms of prostatic cancer, esp. during first month of therapy.

PATIENT/FAMILY TEACHING

Use contraceptive measures during therapy. Inform physician if pt becomes pregnant or regular menstruation persists. Breakthrough menstrual bleeding may occur if dose is missed. Use nonhormonal methods of contraception.

granisetron

gran-**is**-eh-tron
(Kytril)

♦CLASSIFICATION

PHARMACOTHERAPEUTIC: Serotonin receptor antagonist. **CLINICAL:** Antiemetic.

ACTION

Selectively blocks serotonin stimulation at receptor sites on abdominal vagal afferent nerve and chemoreceptor trigger zone. **Therapeutic Effect:** Prevents nausea, vomiting.

PHARMACOKINETICS

Onset	Peak	Duration
IV		
1–3 min	—	24 hrs

Rapidly, widely distributed to tissues. Protein binding: 65%. Metabolized in liver to active metabolite. Excreted in urine, eliminated in feces. **Half-life:** 10–12 hrs (half-life increased in elderly).

USES

Prevents nausea, vomiting associated with emetogenic cancer therapy (includes high-dose cisplatin). Prevention/treatment of postop nausea/vomiting. **Unlabeled:** Prophylaxis of nausea/vomiting associated with cancer radiotherapy. **PO:** Prevention of nausea/vomiting associated with radiation therapy.

PRECAUTIONS

CONTRAINDICATIONS: None known. **CAUTIONS:** Safety in children <2 yrs not established.

LIFESPAN CONSIDERATIONS: Pregnancy/lactation: Unknown if drug is distributed in breast milk. **Pregnancy Category B. Children:** Safety and efficacy not established in pts <2 yrs. **Elderly:** No age-related precautions noted.

G

INTERACTIONS

DRUG: Hepatic enzyme inducers may decrease effect. **HERBAL:** None known. **FOOD:** None known. **LAB VALUES:** May increase SGOT (AST), SGPT (ALT).

AVAILABILITY (Rx)

TABLETS: 1 mg. **INJECTION:** 1 mg/ml. **ORAL SOLUTION:** 1 mg/5 ml.

ADMINISTRATION/HANDLING

IV

Storage • Appears as a clear, colorless solution. • Store at room temperature. • After dilution, is stable for at least 24 hrs at room temperature. • Inspect for particulates, discoloration.

Reconstitution • May be given undiluted or dilute with 20–50 ml 0.9% NaCl or D_5W. Do not mix with other medications.

Rate of administration • May give undiluted as IV push over 30 sec. • For IV piggyback, infuse over 5–20 min depending on volume of diluent used.

IV INCOMPATIBILITY

Amphotericin B (Fungizone).

IV COMPATIBILITIES

Allopurinol (Aloprim), bumetanide (Bumex), calcium gluconate, carboplatin (Paraplatin), cisplatin (Platinol), cyclophosphamide (Cytoxan), cytarabine (ARA-C), dacarbazine (DTIC), dexamethasone (Decadron), diphenhydramine (Benadryl), docetaxel (Taxotere), doxorubicin (Adriamycin), etoposide (VePesid), gemcitabine (Gemzar), magnesium, mitoxantrone (Novantrone), paclitaxel (Taxol), potassium.

INDICATIONS/ROUTES/DOSAGE

PROPHYLAXIS OF CHEMOTHERAPY INDUCED NAUSEA/VOMITING

IV: ADULTS, ELDERLY, CHILDREN >2 YRS: 10 mcg/kg/dose (or 1 mg/dose) given within 30 min of chemotherapy. **PO:** ADULTS, ELDERLY: 2 mg once daily up to 1 hr prior to chemotherapy or 1 mg 2 times/day.

Alert: Administer on days of chemotherapy.

PROPHYLAXIS OF RADIATION-INDUCED NAUSEA/VOMITING

PO: ADULTS, ELDERLY: 2 mg once daily given 1 hr prior to radiation therapy.

POSTOPERATIVE NAUSEA/VOMITING

IV: ADULTS/ELDERLY: 1 mg as a single dose.

SIDE EFFECTS

FREQUENT (14%–21%): Headache, constipation, asthenia (loss of strength). **OCCASIONAL (6%–8%):** Diarrhea, abdominal pain. **RARE (<2%):** Altered taste, hypersensitivity reaction.

ADVERSE REACTIONS/ TOXIC EFFECTS

None known.

NURSING IMPLICATIONS

BASELINE ASSESSMENT

Ensure that granisetron is given within 30 min of start of chemotherapy.

INTERVENTION/EVALUATION

Monitor for therapeutic effect. Assess for headache. Monitor frequency/consistency of stools.

PATIENT/FAMILY TEACHING

Granisetron is effective shortly following administration; prevents nausea, vomiting. Explain that transitory taste disorder may occur.

griseofulvin

griz-ee-oh-**full**-vin
(Fulvicin P/G, Fulvicin U/F, Grifulvin V, Gris-PEG)

✦CLASSIFICATION

CLINICAL: Antifungal.

ACTION

Inhibits fungal cell mitosis by disrupting mitotic spindle structure. **Therapeutic Effect:** Fungistatic.

USES

Treatment of tinea (ringworm): t. capitis, t. corporis, t. cruris, t. pedis, t. unguium.

PRECAUTIONS

CONTRAINDICATIONS: Porphyria, hepatocellular failure. **CAUTIONS:** Exposure to sun/ultraviolet light (photosensitivity), hypersensitivity to penicillins. **Pregnancy Category C.**

INTERACTIONS

DRUG: May decrease effects of **warfarin, oral contraceptives. HERBAL:** None known. **FOOD:** None known. **LAB VALUES:** None known.

AVAILABILITY (Rx)

TABLETS (microsize): 250 mg, 500 mg. **ORAL SUSPENSION:** 125 mg/5 ml. **TABLETS (ultramicrosize):** 125 mg, 250 mg, 330 mg.

INDICATIONS/ROUTES/DOSAGE

USUAL DOSAGE

Alert: Duration depends on the site of infection.

Microsize: ADULTS: 500–1,000 mg as single or divided doses. CHILDREN: 10–20 mg/kg/day.

Ultramicrosize: ADULTS: 330–750 mg/day as single or divided doses. CHILDREN >2 YRS: 5–10 mg/kg/day.

SIDE EFFECTS

OCCASIONAL: Hypersensitivity reaction (rash, pruritus, urticaria), headache, nausea, diarrhea, excessive thirst, flatulence, oral thrush, dizziness, insomnia. **RARE:** Paresthesia of hands/feet, proteinuria, photosensitivity reaction.

ADVERSE REACTIONS/ TOXIC EFFECTS

Granulocytopenia should cause discontinuation of drug.

NURSING IMPLICATIONS

BASELINE ASSESSMENT

Question for history of allergies, esp. to griseofulvin, penicillins.

INTERVENTION/EVALUATION

Assess skin for rash, response to therapy. Determine pattern of bowel activity/stool consistency. Question presence of headache: onset, location, type of discomfort. Assess for dizziness.

PATIENT/FAMILY TEACHING

Prolonged therapy (weeks or months) is usually necessary. Do not miss a dose; continue therapy as long as ordered. Avoid alcohol (may produce tachycardia, flushing). May cause photosensitivity reaction; avoid exposure to sunlight. Maintain good hygiene (prevents superinfection). Separate personal items in direct contact with affected areas. Keep affected areas dry; wear light clothing for ventilation. Take with foods high in fat such as milk, ice cream (reduces GI upset and assists absorption).

guaifenesin (glyceryl guaiacolate)

guay-**fen**-ah-sin
(Balminil, Benylin E, Humibid, Mucinex, Robitussin)

FIXED-COMBINATION(S)

Robitussin AC: guaifenesin/codeine (a narcotic analgesic): 100 mg/10 mg; 75 mg/2.5 mg per 5 ml. **Robitussin DM:** guaifenesin/dextromethorphan (a cough suppressant): 100 mg/10 mg per 5 ml.

CLASSIFICATION

CLINICAL: Expectorant.

G

ACTION

Stimulates respiratory tract secretion by decreasing phlegm adhesiveness, viscosity, fluid volume. **Therapeutic Effect:** Promotes removal of viscous mucus.

PHARMACOKINETICS

Well absorbed from GI tract. Metabolized in liver. Excreted in urine.

USES

Symptomatic relief of cough in presence of mucus in respiratory tract. Not for use with persistent cough due to smoking, asthma, emphysema, cough accompanied by excessive secretions.

PRECAUTIONS

CONTRAINDICATIONS: None known. **CAUTIONS:** None known.

LIFESPAN CONSIDERATIONS: Pregnancy/lactation: Unknown if drug crosses placenta or is distributed in breast milk. **Pregnancy Category C. Children/elderly:** No age-related precautions noted. Caution advised in pts <2 yrs with persistent cough.

INTERACTIONS

DRUG: None known. **HERBAL:** None known. **FOOD:** None known. **LAB VALUES:** None known.

AVAILABILITY (OTC)

TABLETS: 100 mg, 200 mg. **TABLETS (sustained-release):** 600 mg. **CAPSULES:** 200 mg. **CAPSULES (sustained-release):** 300 mg. **SYRUP:** 100 mg/5 ml. **LIQUID:** 200 mg/5 ml, 100 mg/5 ml.

ADMINISTRATION/HANDLING

PO

• Store syrup, liquid, capsules at room temperature. • Give without regard to meals. • Do not crush or break sustained-release capsule. May sprinkle contents on soft food, then swallow without crushing/chewing.

INDICATIONS/ROUTES/DOSAGE

Alert: Give extended-release capsules at 12-hr intervals.

EXPECTORANT

PO: ADULTS, ELDERLY, CHILDREN >12 YRS: 200–400 mg q4h. **Maximum:** 2.4 g/day. CHILDREN 6–12 YRS: 100–200 mg q4h. **Maximum:** 1.2 g/day. CHILDREN 2–5 YRS: 50–100 mg q4h. **Maximum:** 600 mg/day. CHILDREN <2 YRS: 12 mg/kg/day in 6 divided doses.

SIDE EFFECTS

RARE: Dizziness, headache, rash, diarrhea, nausea, vomiting, stomach pain.

ADVERSE REACTIONS/TOXIC EFFECTS

Excessive dosage may produce nausea, vomiting.

NURSING IMPLICATIONS

BASELINE ASSESSMENT

Assess type, severity, frequency of cough. Increase fluid intake, environmental humidity to lower viscosity of lung secretions.

INTERVENTION/EVALUATION

Initiate deep breathing, coughing exercises, particularly in pts with impaired pulmonary function. Assess for clinical improvement; record onset of relief of cough.

PATIENT/FAMILY TEACHING

Avoid tasks that require alertness, motor skills until response to drug is established. Do not take for chronic cough. Inform physician if cough persists or if fever, rash, headache, sore throat is present with cough. Maintain adequate hydration.

guanabenz

(Wytensin)
See Classification section under: Antihypertensives (p. 52C)

guanadrel

(Hylorel)
See Classification section under: Antihypertensives

guanfacine

(Tenex)
See Classification section under: Antihypertensives (p. 52C)

halcinonide

(Halog)
See Classification section under: Corticosteroids: topical

Haldol

see haloperidol

halobetasol

(Ultravate)
See Classification section under: Corticosteroids: topical (p. 85C)

haloperidol

hal-oh-**pear**-ih-dawl
(Apo-Haloperidol✤, Haldol, Novo-peridol✤, Peridol✤)

Do not confuse with Halcion, Halog, Stadol.

CLASSIFICATION

CLINICAL: Antipsychotic, antiemetic, antidyskinetic (see p. 56C).

ACTION

Competitively blocks postsynaptic dopamine receptors, interrupts nerve impulse movement, increases turnover of brain dopamine. **Therapeutic Effect:** Produces tranquilizing effect. Strong extrapyramidal, antiemetic effects; weak anticholinergic, sedative effects.

PHARMACOKINETICS

Readily absorbed from GI tract. Protein binding: 92%. Extensively metabolized in liver. Primarily excreted in urine. Not removed by hemodialysis. **Half-life:** PO: 12–37 hrs; IM: 17–25 hrs, IV: 10–19 hrs.

USES

Treatment of psychoses, Tourette's disorder, severe behavioral problems in children, emergency sedation of severely agitated/delirious pts. **Unlabeled:** Treatment of infantile autism, Huntington's chorea, nausea/vomiting associated with cancer chemotherapy.

H

PRECAUTIONS

CONTRAINDICATIONS: Narrow-angle glaucoma, bone marrow suppression, CNS depression, severe liver/cardiac disease, parkinsonism. **CAUTIONS:** Renal/liver dysfunction, cardiovascular disease, history of seizures.

LIFESPAN CONSIDERATIONS: Pregnancy/lactation: Crosses placenta. Distributed in breast milk. **Pregnancy Category C. Children:** More susceptible to dystonias; not recommended in those <3 yrs. **Elderly:** More susceptible to orthostatic hypotension, anticholinergic effects/sedation, increased risk for extrapyramidal effects. Decreased dosage recommended.

INTERACTIONS

DRUG: Alcohol, CNS depressants may increase CNS depression. **Epinephrine** may block alpha-adrenergic effects. **Extrapyramidal symptom (EPS)-producing medications** may increase EPS. **Lithium** may increase neurologic toxicity. **HERBAL:** None known. **FOOD:** None known. **LAB VALUES:** None known. Therapeutic blood serum level: 0.2–1 mcg/ml; toxic blood serum level: >1 mcg/ml.

AVAILABILITY (Rx)

TABLETS: 0.5 mg, 1 mg, 2 mg, 5 mg, 10 mg, 20 mg. **ORAL CONCENTRATE:** 2 mg/ml. **INJECTION:** 5 mg/ml. **INJECTION (Decanoate):** 50 mg/ml, 100 mg/ml.

ADMINISTRATION/HANDLING

PO

- Give without regard to meals.
- Scored tablets may be crushed.

IM

Parenteral administration: Pt must remain recumbent for 30–60 min in head-low position with legs raised to minimize hypotensive effect. • Prepare Decanoate IM injection using 21-gauge needle. • Do not exceed maximum volume of 3 ml per IM injection site. • Inject slow, deep IM into upper outer quadrant of gluteus maximus.

IV

Alert: Only haloperidol lactate is given IV.

Storage • Discard if precipitate forms, discoloration occurs. • Store at room temperature. • Protect from light, do not freeze.

Reconstitution • May give undiluted. • Flush with at least 2 ml 0.9% NaCl before and after administration. • May add to 30–50 ml most solutions (D_5W preferred).

Rate of administration • Give IV push at rate of 5 mg/min. • Infuse IV piggyback over 30 min. • For IV infusion, up to 25 mg/hr has been used (titrated to pt response).

IV INCOMPATIBILITIES

Allopurinol (Aloprim), amphotericin B complex (Abelcet, AmBisome, Amphotec), cefepime (Maxipime), fluconazole (Diflucan), foscarnet (Foscavir), heparin, nitroprusside (Nipride), piperacillin-tazobactam (Zosyn).

IV COMPATIBILITIES

Dobutamine (Dobutrex), dopamine (Intropin), fentanyl (Sublimaze), hydromorphone (Dilaudid), lidocaine, lorazepam (Ativan), midazolam (Versed), morphine, nitroglycerin, norepinephrine (Levophed), propofol (Diprivan).

INDICATIONS/ROUTES/DOSAGE

USUAL ADULT DOSAGE

PO: 0.5–5 mg 2–3 times/day. **Maximum:** 100 mg/day.

IM/IV (lactate): 2–5 mg q4–8h as needed.

IM (decanoate): 10–15 times stabilized oral dose given at 3- to 4-wk intervals.

USUAL ELDERLY DOSAGE

PO: Initially, 0.25–0.5 mg 1–2 times/day. May increase by 0.25–0.5 mg/day at weekly intervals.

USUAL DOSAGE FOR CHILDREN

PO: 3–12 YRS, 15–40 KG: Initially, 0.25–0.5 mg/day in divided doses. May increase by 0.25–0.5 mg q5–7days. **Maximum:** 0.15 mg/kg/day.

IM (lactate): 6–12 YRS: 1–3 mg/dose q4–8h. **Maximum:** 0.15 mg/kg/day.

SIDE EFFECTS

FREQUENT: Blurred vision, constipation, orthostatic hypotension, dry mouth, swelling/soreness of female breasts, peripheral edema. **OCCASIONAL:** Allergic reaction, difficulty urinating, decreased thirst, dizziness, decreased sexual function, drowsiness, nausea, vomiting, photosensitivity, lethargy.

ADVERSE REACTIONS/ TOXIC EFFECTS

EPS appear to be dose related and may be noted in first few days of therapy. Marked drowsiness/lethargy, excessive salivation, fixed stare may be mild to severe in intensity. Less frequently seen are severe akathisia (motor restlessness), acute dystonias: torticollis (neck muscle spasm), opisthotonos (rigidity of back muscles), oculogyric crisis (rolling back of eyes). Tardive dyskinesia (protrusion of tongue, puffing of cheeks, chewing/puckering of the mouth) may occur during long-term administration or after drug discontinuance and may be irreversible. Risk is greater in female geriatric pts. Abrupt withdrawal after long-term therapy may provoke transient dyskinesia signs.

NURSING IMPLICATIONS

BASELINE ASSESSMENT

Assess behavior, appearance, emotional status, response to environment, speech pattern, thought content.

INTERVENTION/EVALUATION

Supervise suicidal-risk pt closely during early therapy (as depression lessens, energy level improves, causing increased suicide potential). Monitor for rigidity, tremor, mask-like facial expression, fine tongue movement. Assess for therapeutic response (interest in surroundings, improvement in self-care, increased ability to concentrate, relaxed facial expression). Therapeutic blood serum level: 0.2–1 mcg/ml. Toxic blood serum level: >1 mcg/ml.

PATIENT/FAMILY TEACHING

Full therapeutic effect may take up to 6 wks. Do not abruptly withdraw from long-term drug therapy. Sugarless gum, sips of tepid water may relieve dry mouth. Drowsiness generally subsides during continued therapy. Avoid tasks that require alertness, motor skills until response to drug is established. Avoid alcohol. Report muscle stiffness. Avoid exposure to sunlight, overheating, dehydration (increased risk of heat stroke).

haloprogin

(Halotex)

See Classification section under: Antifungals: topical

heparin sodium

hep-ah-rin

(Hepalean ✦, Heparin Leo ✦)

Do not confuse with Hespan.

CLASSIFICATION

PHARMACOTHERAPEUTIC: Blood modifier. **CLINICAL:** Anticoagulant (see p. 29C).

ACTION

Interferes with blood coagulation by blocking conversion of prothrombin to thrombin and fibrinogen to fibrin. **Therapeutic Effect:** Prevents further extension of existing thrombi or new clot formation. No effect on existing clots.

PHARMACOKINETICS

Well absorbed following subcutaneous administration. Protein binding: Very high. Metabolized in liver, removed from circulation via uptake by reticuloendothelial system. Primarily excreted in urine. Not removed by hemodialysis. **Half-life:** 1–6 hrs.

USES

Prophylaxis and/or treatment of venous thrombosis, pulmonary embolism, peripheral arterial embolism, atrial fibrillation with embolism. Prevention of thromboembolus in cardiac and vascular surgery, dialysis procedures, blood transfusions, blood sampling for laboratory purposes. Adjunct in treatment of coronary occlusion with acute MI. Maintains patency of indwelling intravascular devices. Diagnosis/treatment of acute/chronic consumptive coagulation pathology (e.g., disseminated intravascular coagulation [DIC]). Prevents cerebral thrombosis in progressive strokes.

PRECAUTIONS

CONTRAINDICATIONS: Severe thrombocytopenia, subacute bacterial endocarditis, intracranial hemorrhage, severe hypotension, uncontrolled bleeding. **CAUTIONS:** IM injections, peptic ulcer disease, menstruation, recent surgery/invasive procedures, severe liver/renal disease.

LIFESPAN CONSIDERATIONS: Pregnancy/lactation: Use with caution, particularly during last trimester, immediate postpartum period (increased risk of maternal hemorrhage). Does not cross placenta. Not distributed in breast milk. **Pregnancy Category C. Children:** No age-related precautions noted. Benzyl alcohol preservative may cause gasping syndrome in infants. **Elderly:** More susceptible to hemorrhage. Age-related decreased renal function may increase risk of bleeding.

INTERACTIONS

DRUG: Anticoagulants, platelet aggregation inhibitors, thrombolytics may increase risk of bleeding. **Antithyroid medications, cefoperazone, cefotetan, valproic acid** may cause hypoprothrombinemia. **Probenecid** may increase effect. **HERBAL: Feverfew, Ginkgo biloba** may have additive effect. **FOOD:** None known. **LAB VALUES:** May increase free fatty acids, SGOT (AST), SGPT (ALT). May decrease triglycerides, cholesterol.

AVAILABILITY (Rx)

INJECTION: 10 units/ml, 100 units/ml, 1,000 units/ml, 2,500 units/ml, 5,000 units/ml, 7,500 units/ml, 10,000 units/ml, 20,000 units/ml, 40,000 units/ml, 25,000 units/500 ml infusion.

ADMINISTRATION/HANDLING

Alert: Do **not** give by IM injection (pain, hematoma, ulceration, erythema).

SUBCUTANEOUS

Alert: Used in low-dose therapy.

• After withdrawal of heparin from vial, change needle before injection (prevents leakage along needle track). • Inject above iliac crest or in abdominal fat layer. Do not inject within 2 inches of umbilicus, or any scar tissue. • Withdraw needle rapidly, apply prolonged pressure at injection site. Do not massage. • Rotate injection sites.

IV

Alert: Used in full-dose therapy. Intermittent IV produces higher incidence of bleeding abnormalities. Continuous IV preferred.

Storage • Store at room temperature.

Reconstitution • Dilute IV infusion in isotonic sterile saline, D_5W, or lactated Ringer's. • Invert container at least 6 times (ensures mixing, prevents pooling of medication).

Rate of administration • Use constant-rate IV infusion pump.

∅ IV INCOMPATIBILITIES

Amiodarone (Cordarone), amphotericin B complex (Abelcet, AmBisome, Amphotec), ciprofloxacin (Cipro), dacarbazine (DTIC), diazepam (Valium), dobutamine (Dobutrex), doxorubicin (Adriamycin), droperidol (Inapsine), filgrastim (Neupogen), gentamicin (Garamycin), haloperidol (Haldol), idarubicin (Idamycin), labetalol (Trandate), nicardipine (Cardene), phenytoin (Dilantin), quinidine, tobramycin (Nebcin), vancomycin (Vancocin).

IV COMPATIBILITIES

Aminophylline, ampicillin/sulbactam (Unasyn), aztreonam (Azactam), calcium gluconate, cefazolin (Ancef), ceftazidime (Fortaz), ceftriaxone (Rocephin), digoxin (Lanoxin), diltiazem (Cardizem), dopamine (Intropin), enalapril (Vasotec), famotidine (Pepcid), fentanyl (Sublimaze), furosemide (Lasix), hydromorphone (Dilaudid), insulin, lidocaine, lorazepam (Ativan), magnesium sulfate, methylprednisolone (Solu-Medrol), midazolam (Versed), milrinone (Primacor), morphine, nitroglycerin, norepinephrine (Levophed), oxytocin (Pitocin), piperacillin/tazobactam (Zosyn), procainamide (Pronestyl), propofol (Diprivan).

INDICATIONS/ROUTES/DOSAGE

LINE FLUSHING

IV: ADULTS, ELDERLY, CHILDREN: 100 units q6–8h. INFANTS <10 KG: 10 units q6–8h.

USUAL ADULT, ELDERLY DOSAGE

PROPHYLAXIS: **Subcutaneous:** 5,000 units q8–12h.

TREATMENT: **Intermittent IV:** Initially, 10,000 units, then 50–70 units/kg (5,000–10,000 units) q4–6h.

IV infusion: Loading dose: 80 units/kg, then 18 units/kg/hr with adjustments according to aPTT. RANGE: 10–30 units/kg/hr.

USUAL DOSAGE FOR CHILDREN

Intermittent IV: >1 YR: Initially, 50–100 units/kg, then 50–100 units q4h.

IV infusion: >1 YR: Loading dose: 75 units/kg, then 20 units/kg/hr with adjustments according to aPTT.

IV infusion: <1 YR: Loading dose: 75 units/kg, then 28 units/kg/hr.

SIDE EFFECTS

OCCASIONAL: Itching, burning, particularly on soles of feet (due to vasospastic reaction). **RARE:** Pain, cyanosis of extremity 6–10 days after initial therapy, lasts 4–6 hrs; hypersensitivity reaction (chills, fever, pruritus, urticaria, asthma, rhinitis, lacrimation, headache).

ADVERSE REACTIONS/ TOXIC EFFECTS

Bleeding complications ranging from local ecchymoses to major hemorrhage occur more frequently in high-dose therapy, intermittent IV infusion, and in women >60 yrs. **ANTIDOTE:** Protamine sulfate 1–1.5 mg for every 100 units heparin subcutaneous if overdosage occurred before 30 min, 0.5–0.75 mg for every 100 units heparin subcutaneous if overdosage occurred within 30–60 min, 0.25–0.375 mg for every 100 units heparin subcutaneous if 2 hrs have elapsed since overdosage, 25–50 mg if heparin given by IV infusion.

NURSING IMPLICATIONS

BASELINE ASSESSMENT

Cross-check dose with co-worker. Determine aPTT prior to administration and 24 hrs following initiation of therapy, then 24–48 hrs for first week of therapy or until maintenance dose is established. Follow with aPTT determinations 1–2 times weekly for 3–4 wks. In long-term therapy, monitor 1–2 times/mo.

INTERVENTION/EVALUATION

Monitor aPTT (therapeutic dosage at 1.5–2.5 times normal) diligently. Assess Hct, platelet count, urine/stool culture for occult blood, SGOT (AST), SGPT (ALT), regardless of route of administration. Assess for decrease in B/P, increase in pulse rate, complaint of abdominal/back pain, severe headache (may be evidence of hemorrhage). Question for increase in amount of discharge during menses. Check peripheral pulses; skin for bruises, petechiae. Check for excessive bleeding from minor cuts, scratches. Assess gums for erythema, gingival bleeding. Assess urine output for hematuria. Avoid IM injections of other medications due to potential for hematomas. When converting to Coumadin therapy, monitor PT results (will be 10%–20% higher while heparin is given concurrently).

PATIENT/FAMILY TEACHING

Use electric razor, soft toothbrush to prevent bleeding. Report any sign of red/dark urine, black/red stool, coffee-ground vomitus, red-speckled mucus from cough. Do not use any OTC medication without physician approval (may interfere with platelet aggregation). Wear/carry identification that notes anticoagulant therapy. Inform dentist, other physicians of heparin therapy.

hepatitis A vaccine

(Havrix, Vaqta)

ACTION

Inactivated virus vaccine. **Therapeutic Effect:** Provides active immunization against hepatitis A virus infection.

USES

Active immunization of persons >2 yrs against disease caused by hepatitis A virus.

PRECAUTIONS

CONTRAINDICATIONS: None known. **CAUTIONS:** Serious active infection, cardiovascular disease, respiratory disorders. **Pregnancy Category C.**

INDICATIONS/ROUTES/DOSAGE

IM: ADULTS, ELDERLY: 1 ml with a booster dose at 6–12 mos. CHILDREN 2–18 YRS: 0.5 ml with a booster at 6–18 mos.

SIDE EFFECTS

OCCASIONAL (1%–10%): Injection site soreness, pain, tenderness, induration, redness, swelling, fatigue, fever, malaise, nausea, anorexia, headache.

hepatitis B immune globulin (human)

(Bayhep B✱, Nabi-HB)

◆ **CLASSIFICATION**

CLINICAL: Immunization agent.

ACTION

Immune globulin of inactivated hepatitis B virus. **Therapeutic Effect:** Provides passive immunization against hepatitis B virus.

USES

Passive immunity to hepatitis B infection to those exposed.

PRECAUTIONS

CONTRAINDICATIONS: Allergies to gamma globulin, thimerosal, IgA deficiency, IM injections in those with thrombocytopenia/coagulation disorders. **CAUTIONS:** None known.

AVAILABILITY (Rx)

INJECTION: 5-ml vial.

INDICATIONS/ROUTES/DOSAGE

ACUTE EXPOSURE

IM: ADULTS, ELDERLY: 0.06 ml/kg usual dose; 3–5 ml for postexposure prophylaxis.

SIDE EFFECTS

FREQUENT: Headache (26%), local pain (12%). **OCCASIONAL (5%):** Malaise, nausea, myalgia.

Hepsera

see adefovir

hetastarch

het-ah-starch

(Hespan, Hextend)

Do not confuse with heparin.

◆ **CLASSIFICATION**

CLINICAL: Plasma volume expander.

ACTION

Exerts osmotic pull on tissue fluids. **Therapeutic Effect:** Reduces hemoconcentration, blood viscosity; increases circulating blood volume.

PHARMACOKINETICS

Onset	Peak	Duration
IM		
30 min	—	24–36 hrs

Smaller molecules (<50,000 molecular weight) rapidly excreted by kidneys; larger molecules (>50,000 molecular weight) slowly degraded to smaller molecules, then excreted. **Half-life:** 17 days.

USES

Fluid replacement, plasma volume expansion in treatment of shock due to hemorrhage, burns, surgery, sepsis, trauma, leukapheresis.

H

PRECAUTIONS

CONTRAINDICATIONS: Severe bleeding disorders, severe CHF, oliguria, anuria. **CAUTIONS:** Thrombocytopenia, elderly or very young, pulmonary edema, CHF, impaired renal function, hepatic disease, those on sodium restriction.

LIFESPAN CONSIDERATIONS: Pregnancy/lactation: Do not use in pregnancy unless benefits outweigh risk to fetus. **Pregnancy Category C. Children:** Safety and efficacy not established. **Elderly:** No age-related precautions noted.

H

INTERACTIONS

DRUG: None known. **HERBAL:** None known. **FOOD:** None known. **LAB VALUES:** May prolong prothrombin time (PT), partial thromboplastin time (PTT), bleeding, clotting times; decreases Hct.

AVAILABILITY (Rx)

INJECTION: 6 g/100 ml 0.9% NaCl (500-ml infusion container).

ADMINISTRATION/HANDLING

IV

Storage • Store solutions at room temperature. • Solution should appear clear, pale yellow to amber. Do not use if discolored (deep turbid brown) or if precipitate forms.

Rate of administration • Administer only by IV infusion. • Do not add drugs or mix with other IV fluids. • In acute hemorrhagic shock, administer at rate approaching 1.2 g/kg (20 ml/kg) per hour. Use slower rates for burns, septic shock. • Monitor central venous pressure (CVP) when given by rapid infusion. If there is a precipitous rise in CVP, immediately discontinue drug (overexpansion of blood volume).

IV INCOMPATIBILITIES

Amikacin (Amikin), ampicillin (Polycillin), cefazolin (Ancef, Kefzol), cefotaxime (Claforan), cefoxitin (Mefoxin), gentamicin (Garamycin), ranitidine (Zantac), tobramycin (Nebcin).

IV COMPATIBILITIES

Cimetidine (Tagamet), digoxin (Lanoxin), diltiazem (Cardizem), dobutamine (Dobutrex), dopamine (Intropin), enalapril (Vasotec), fentanyl (Sublimaze), heparin, hydromorphone (Dilaudid), labetalol (Trandate), lidocaine, lorazepam (Ativan), magnesium sulfate, metoclopramide (Reglan), midazolam (Versed), milrinone (Primacor), morphine, nitroglycerin, potassium chloride.

INDICATIONS/ROUTES/DOSAGE

PLASMA VOLUME EXPANSION

IV: ADULTS, ELDERLY: 500–1,000 ml/day up to 1,500 ml/day (20 mg/kg) at a rate up to 20 ml/kg/hr in hemorrhagic shock (slower rates for burns or septic shock). CHILDREN: 10 ml/kg/dose. **Maximum total daily dose:** Not to exceed 20 ml/kg.

LEUKAPHERESIS

IV: ADULTS, ELDERLY: 250–700 ml infused at constant rate, usually 1:8 to venous whole blood.

SIDE EFFECTS

RARE: Allergic reaction resulting in vomiting, mild temperature elevation, chills, itching; submaxillary/parotid gland enlargement, peripheral edema of lower extremities, mild flulike symptoms: headache, muscle aches.

ADVERSE REACTIONS/TOXIC EFFECTS

Fluid overload (headache, weakness, blurred vision, behavioral changes, incoordination, isolated muscle twitching), pulmonary edema (rapid breathing, rales, wheezing, coughing, increased B/P, distended neck veins) may occur. Anaphylactoid reaction may be observed as periorbital edema, urticaria, wheezing.

NURSING IMPLICATIONS

INTERVENTION/EVALUATION

Monitor for fluid overload (peripheral and/or pulmonary edema, impending CHF symptoms). Assess lung sounds for wheezing, rales. During leukapheresis, monitor CBC, leukocyte/platelet counts, differential, Hgb, Hct, PT, PTT, I&O. Monitor central venous B/P (detects overexpansion of blood volume). Monitor urine output closely (increase in output generally occurs in oliguric pts following administration). Assess for periorbital edema, itching, wheezing, urticaria (allergic reaction). Monitor for oliguria, anuria, any change in output ratio. Monitor for bleeding from surgical/trauma sites.

Hivid

see zalcitabine

hydralazine hydrochloride

hy-**dral**-ah-zeen

(Apresoline, Novohylazin ✤)

Do not confuse with hydroxyzine.

FIXED-COMBINATION(S)

Apresazide: hydralazine/hydrochlorothiazide (a diuretic): 25 mg/25 mg; 50 mg/50 mg; 100 mg/50 mg.

◆ CLASSIFICATION

PHARMACOTHERAPEUTIC: Vasodilator. **CLINICAL:** Antihypertensive (see p. 53C).

ACTION

Direct vasodilation on arterioles. **Therapeutic Effect:** Decreases B/P, systemic resistance.

PHARMACOKINETICS

Onset	Peak	Duration
PO		
20–30 min	—	2–4 hrs
IV		
5–20 min	—	2–6 hrs

Well absorbed from GI tract. Widely distributed. Protein binding: 85%–90%. Metabolized in liver to active metabolite. Primarily excreted in urine. Not removed by hemodialysis. **Half-life:** 3–7 hrs (half-life increased with impaired renal function).

USES

Management of moderate/severe hypertension. **Unlabeled:** Treatment of CHF, hypertension secondary to preeclampsia, eclampsia, primary pulmonary hypertension.

PRECAUTIONS

CONTRAINDICATIONS: Coronary artery disease, rheumatic heart disease, lupus erythematosus. **CAUTIONS:** Impaired renal function, cerebrovascular disease.

LIFESPAN CONSIDERATIONS: Pregnancy/lactation: Drug crosses placenta. Unknown if drug is distributed in breast milk. Thrombocytopenia, leukopenia, petechial bleeding, hematomas have occurred in newborns (resolved within 1–3 wks). **Pregnancy Category C. Children:** No age-related precautions noted. **Elderly:** More sensitive to

H

hypotensive effects. Age-related renal impairment may require dosage adjustment.

INTERACTIONS

DRUG: Diuretics, other hypotensives may increase hypotensive effect. **HERBAL:** None known. **FOOD:** None known. **LAB VALUES:** May produce positive direct Coombs' test.

AVAILABILITY (Rx)

TABLETS: 10 mg, 25 mg, 50 mg, 100 mg. **INJECTION:** 20 mg/ml.

H

ADMINISTRATION/HANDLING

PO

• Best given with food or regularly spaced meals. • Tablets may be crushed.

IV

Storage • Store at room temperature.

Rate of administration • May give undiluted. • Give single dose over 1 min.

IV INCOMPATIBILITIES

Aminophylline, ampicillin (Polycillin), furosemide (Lasix).

IV COMPATIBILITIES

Dobutamine (Dobutrex), heparin, hydrocortisone (Solu-Cortef), nitroglycerin, potassium.

INDICATIONS/ROUTES/DOSAGE

HYPERTENSION

PO: ADULTS: Initially, 10 mg 4 times/day. May increase by 10–25 mg/dose q2–5days. **Maximum:** 300 mg/day. CHILDREN: Initially, 0.75–1 mg/kg/day in 2–4 divided doses, not to exceed 25 mg/dose. May increase over 3–4 wks. **Maximum:** 7.5 mg/kg/day (5 mg/kg/day in infants).

IM/IV: ADULTS, ELDERLY: Initially, 10–20 mg/dose q4–6h. May increase to 40 mg/dose. CHILDREN: Initially, 0.1–0.2 mg/kg/dose q4–6h as needed up to 1.7–3.5 mg/kg/day in divided doses q4–6h. **Maximum:** 20 mg.

DOSAGE IN RENAL IMPAIRMENT

Creatinine Clearance	Dosage Interval
10–50 ml/min	q8h
<10 ml/min	q8–24h

SIDE EFFECTS

FREQUENT: Headache, palpitations, tachycardia (generally disappears in 7–10 days). **OCCASIONAL:** GI disturbance (nausea, vomiting, diarrhea), paresthesia, fluid retention, peripheral edema, dizziness, flushed face, nasal congestion.

ADVERSE REACTIONS/ TOXIC EFFECTS

High dosage may produce lupus erythematosus–like reaction (fever, facial rash, muscle/joint aches, splenomegaly). Severe orthostatic hypotension, skin flushing, severe headache, myocardial ischemia, cardiac arrhythmias may develop. Profound shock may occur in cases of severe overdosage.

NURSING IMPLICATIONS

BASELINE ASSESSMENT

Obtain B/P, pulse immediately prior to each dose, in addition to regular monitoring (be alert to fluctuations).

INTERVENTION/EVALUATION

Monitor for headache, palpitations, tachycardia. Assess for peripheral edema of hands, feet (usually, first area of lower extremity swelling is behind medial malleolus in ambulatory, sacral area in bedridden). Monitor pattern of daily bowel activity, stool consistency.

PATIENT/FAMILY TEACHING

To reduce hypotensive effect, rise slowly from lying to sitting position, permit legs to dangle from bed momentarily before standing. Unsalted crackers, dry toast may relieve nausea. If taking high-dose therapy, report muscle/joint aches, fever (lupus-like reaction).

hydrochlorothiazide

high-drow-chlor-oh-**thigh**-ah-zide (Apo-Hydro ✤, Microzide)

FIXED-COMBINATION(S)

Accuretic: hydrochlorothiazide/quinapril (an ACE inhibitor): 12.5 mg/10 mg; 12.5 mg/20 mg; 25 mg/20 mg. **Aldactazide:** hydrochlorothiazide/spironolactone (a potassium-sparing diuretic): 25 mg/25 mg; 50 mg/50 mg. **Aldoril:** hydrochlorothiazide/methyldopa (an antihypertensive): 15 mg/250 mg; 25 mg/250 mg; 30 mg/500 mg; 50 mg/500 mg. **Apresazide**: hydrochlorothiazide/hydralazine (a vasodilator): 25 mg/25 mg; 50 mg/50 mg; 50 mg/100 mg. **Atacand HCT:** hydrochlorothiazide/candesartan (an angiotensin II receptor antagonist): 12.5 mg/16 mg; 12.5 mg/32 mg. **Avalide:** hydrochlorothiazide/irbesartan (an angiotensin II receptor antagonist): 12.5 mg/150 mg; 12.5 mg/300 mg. **Benicar HCT:** hydrochlorothiazide/olmesartan (an angiotensin II receptor antagonist): 12.5 mg/20 mg; 12.5 mg/40 mg; 25 mg/40 mg. **Capozide:** hydrochlorothiazide/captopril (an ACE inhibitor): 15 mg/25 mg; 15 mg/50 mg; 25 mg/25 mg; 25 mg/50 mg. **Diovan HCT:** hydrochlorothiazide/valsartan (an angiotensin II receptor antagonist): 12.5 mg/80 mg; 12.5 mg/160 mg. **Dyazide/Maxide:** hydrochlorothiazide/triamterene (a potassium-sparing diuretic): 25 mg/37.5 mg; 25mg/50 mg; 50 mg/75 mg. **Hyzaar:** hydrochlorothiazide/losartan (an angiotensin II receptor antagonist): 12.5 mg/50 mg; 25 mg/100 mg. **Inderide:** hydrochlorothiazide/propranolol (a beta-blocker): 25 mg/40 mg; 25 mg/80 mg; 50 mg/80 mg; 50 mg/120 mg; 50 mg/160 mg. **Lopressor HCT:** hydrochlorothiazide/metoprolol (a beta-blocker): 25 mg/50 mg; 25 mg/100 mg; 50 mg/100 mg. **Lotensin HCT:** hydrochlorothiazide/bepridil (a calcium channel blocker): 6.25 mg/5 mg; 12.5 mg/10 mg; 12.5 mg/20 mg; 25 mg/20 mg. **Micardis HCT:** hydrochlorothiazide/telmisartan (an angiotensin II receptor antagonist): 12.5 mg/40 mg; 12.5 mg/80 mg. **Moduretic:** hydrochlorothiazide/amiloride (a potassium-sparing diuretic): 50 mg/5 mg. **Normozide:** hydrochlorothiazide/labetalol (a beta-blocker): 25 mg/100 mg; 25 mg/300 mg. **Prinzide/Zestoretic:** hydrochlorothiazide/lisinopril (an ACE inhibitor): 12.5 mg/10 mg; 12.5 mg/20 mg; 25 mg/20 mg. **Teveten HCT:** hydrochlorothiazide/eprosartan (an angiotensin II receptor antagonist): 12.5 mg/600 mg; 25 mg/600 mg. **Timolide:** hydrochlorothiazide/timolol (a beta-blocker): 25 mg/10 mg. **Uniretic:** hydrochlorothiazide/moexipril (an ACE inhibitor): 12.5 mg/7.5 mg; 25 mg/15 mg. **Vaseretic:** hydrochlorothiazide/enalapril (an ACE inhibitor): 12.5 mg/5 mg; 25 mg/10 mg. **Ziac:** hydrochlorothiazide/bisoprolol (a beta-blocker): 6.25 mg/5 mg; 6.25 mg/10 mg.

CLASSIFICATION

PHARMACOTHERAPEUTIC: Sulfonamide derivative. **CLINICAL:** Thiazide diuretic, antihypertensive (see p. 86C).

H

ACTION

Diuretic: Blocks reabsorption of water, electrolytes (sodium, potassium) at cortical diluting segment of distal tubule. **Antihypertensive:** Reduces plasma, extracellular fluid volume, decreases peripheral vascular resistance (PVR) by direct effect on blood vessels. **Therapeutic Effect:** Promotes diuresis, reduces B/P.

PHARMACOKINETICS

Onset	Peak	Duration
PO (diuretic)		
2 hrs	4–6 hrs	6–12 hrs

Variably absorbed from GI tract. Primarily excreted unchanged in urine. Not removed by hemodialysis. **Half-life:** 5.6–14.8 hrs.

USES

Treatment of mild to moderate hypertension, edema in CHF, nephrotic syndrome. **Unlabeled:** Treatment of diabetes insipidus, prevention of calcium-containing renal stones.

PRECAUTIONS

CONTRAINDICATIONS: History of hypersensitivity to sulfonamides or thiazide diuretics, renal decompensation, anuria. **CAUTIONS:** Severe renal disease, impaired hepatic function, diabetes mellitus, elderly/debilitated, thyroid disorders.

LIFESPAN CONSIDERATIONS: Pregnancy/lactation: Crosses placenta. Small amount distributed in breast milk; nursing not advised. **Pregnancy Category B (D** if used in pregnancy-induced hypertension). **Children:** No age-related precautions noted, except jaundiced infants may be at risk for hyperbilirubinemia. **Elderly:** May be more sensitive to hypotensive, electrolyte effects. Age-related renal impairment may require caution.

INTERACTIONS

DRUG: Cholestyramine, colestipol may decrease absorption, effects. May increase **digoxin** toxicity (due to hypokalemia). May increase **lithium** toxicity. **HERBAL:** None known. **FOOD:** None known. **LAB VALUES:** May increase bilirubin, serum calcium, LDL, cholesterol, triglycerides, creatinine, glucose, uric acid. May decrease urinary calcium, magnesium, potassium, sodium.

AVAILABILITY (Rx)

CAPSULES: 12.5 mg. **TABLETS:** 25 mg, 50 mg, 100 mg. **ORAL SOLUTION:** 50 mg/5 ml.

ADMINISTRATION/HANDLING

PO

- May give with food or milk if GI upset occurs, preferably with breakfast (may prevent nocturia).

INDICATIONS/ROUTES/DOSAGE

EDEMA

PO: ADULTS: 12.5–100 mg/day. **Maximum:** 200 mg/day. CHILDREN 6 MOS–12 YRS: 2 mg/kg/day. **Maximum:** 200 mg/day. CHILDREN <6 MOS: 2–4 mg/kg/day. **Maximum:** 37.5 mg/day.

SIDE EFFECTS

EXPECTED: Increase in urine frequency/volume. **FREQUENT:** Potassium depletion. **OCCASIONAL:** Postural hypotension, headache, GI disturbances, photosensitivity reaction.

ADVERSE REACTIONS/ TOXIC EFFECTS

Vigorous diuresis may lead to profound water loss/electrolyte depletion, resulting in hypokalemia, hyponatremia, dehydration. Acute hypotensive episodes may occur. Hyperglycemia may be noted during prolonged therapy. GI upset, pancreatitis, dizziness, paresthesias, headache, blood dyscrasias, pulmonary edema, allergic pneumonitis, dermatologic reactions occur rarely. Overdosage can lead to lethargy, coma without changes in electrolytes or hydration.

NURSING IMPLICATIONS

BASELINE ASSESSMENT

Check vital signs, esp. B/P for hypotension prior to administration. Assess baseline electrolytes; particularly check for hypokalemia. Evaluate skin turgor, mucous membranes for hydration status. Evaluate for peripheral edema. Assess muscle strength, mental status. Note skin temperature, moisture. Obtain baseline weight. Initiate I&O.

INTERVENTION/EVALUATION

Continue to monitor B/P, vital signs, electrolytes, I&O, daily weight. Note extent of diuresis. Watch for changes from initial assessment (hypokalemia may result in weakness, tremor, muscle cramps, nausea, vomiting, change in mental status, tachycardia; hyponatremia may result in confusion, thirst, cold/clammy skin). Be esp. alert for potassium depletion in pts taking digoxin (cardiac arrhythmias). Potassium supplements are frequently ordered. Check for constipation (may occur with exercise diuresis).

PATIENT/FAMILY TEACHING

Expect increased frequency/volume of urination. To reduce hypotensive effect, rise slowly from lying to sitting position, permit legs to dangle momentarily before standing. Eat foods high in potassium, such as whole grains (cereals), legumes, meat, bananas, apricots, orange juice, potatoes (white, sweet), raisins. Protect skin from sun/ultraviolet rays (photosensitivity may occur).

hydrocodone bitartrate

high-drough-**koe**-doan
(Hycodan✤, Robidone✤)

FIXED-COMBINATION(S)

Anexsia: hydrocodone/acetaminophen (a non-narcotic analgesic): 5 mg/500 mg; 7.5 mg/650 mg; 10 mg/650 mg. **Duocet:** hydrocodone/acetaminophen: 5 mg/500 mg. **Lorcet:** hydrocodone/acetaminophen: 7.5 mg/650 mg; 10 mg/650 mg. **Lortab Elixer:** hydrocodone/acetaminophen: 2.5 mg/167 mg per 5 ml. **Lortab with ASA:** hydrocodone/aspirin: 5 mg/500 mg. **Lortab:** hydrocodone/acetaminophen: 2.5 mg/500 mg; 5 mg/500 mg; 7.5 mg/500 mg; 10 mg/500 mg. **Norco:** hydrocodone/acetaminophen: 10 mg/325 mg. **Vicodin ES:** hydrocodone/acetaminophen: 7.5 mg/750 mg. **Vicodin HP:** hydrocodone/acetaminophen: 10 mg/650 mg. **Vicodin:** hydrocodone/acetaminophen: 5 mg/500 mg. **Vicoprofen:** hydrocodone/ibuprofen (an NSAID): 7.5 mg/200 mg. **Zydone:** hydrocodone/acetaminophen: 5 mg/400 mg; 7.5 mg/400 mg; 10 mg/400 mg.

CLASSIFICATION

PHARMACOTHERAPEUTIC: Opioid agonist **(Schedule III). CLINICAL:** Narcotic analgesic, antitussive (see p. 120C).

ACTION

Binds at opiate receptor sites in CNS. **Therapeutic Effect:** Reduces intensity of pain stimuli incoming from sensory nerve endings, altering pain perception, emotional response to pain; suppresses cough reflex.

H

PHARMACOKINETICS

Onset	Peak	Duration
PO (analgesic)		
10–20 min	30–60 min	4–6 hrs
PO (antitussive)		
—	—	4–6 hrs

Well absorbed from GI tract. Metabolized in liver. Primarily excreted in urine. **Half-life:** 3.8 hrs (increased in elderly).

USES

Relief of moderate to moderately severe pain, nonproductive cough.

PRECAUTIONS

CONTRAINDICATIONS: None known. **EXTREME CAUTION:** CNS depression, anoxia, hypercapnia, respiratory depression, seizures, acute alcoholism, shock, untreated myxedema, respiratory dysfunction. **CAUTIONS:** Increased intracranial pressure, impaired hepatic function, acute abdominal conditions, hypothyroidism, prostatic hypertrophy, Addison's disease, urethral stricture, COPD.

LIFESPAN CONSIDERATIONS: Pregnancy/lactation: Readily crosses placenta. Distributed in breast milk. May prolong labor if administered in latent phase of first stage of labor, or prior to cervical dilation of 4–5 cm has occurred. Respiratory depression may occur in neonate if mother received opiates during labor. Regular use of opiates during pregnancy may produce withdrawal symptoms (irritability, excessive crying, tremors, hyperactive reflexes, fever, vomiting, diarrhea, yawning, sneezing, seizures) in the neonate. **Pregnancy Category C** (**D** if used for prolonged periods or at high dosages at term). **Children:** Those <2 yrs may be more susceptible to respiratory depression. **Elderly:** May be more susceptible to respiration depression, may cause paradoxical excitement. Age-related renal impairment, prostatic hypertrophy/obstruction may increase risk of urinary retention; dosage adjustment recommended.

INTERACTIONS

DRUG: Alcohol, CNS depressants may increase CNS or respiratory depression, hypotension. **MAOIs** may produce severe, fatal reaction (reduce dose to ¼ usual dose). **HERBAL:** None known. **FOOD:** None known. **LAB VALUES:** May increase amylase, lipase plasma concentrations.

ADMINISTRATION/HANDLING

PO

- Give without regard to meals.
- Tablets may be crushed.

INDICATIONS/ROUTES/DOSAGE

ANALGESIA

PO: ADULTS, CHILDREN >12 YRS: 5–10 mg q4–6h. ELDERLY: 2.5–5 mg q4–6h.

ANTITUSSIVE

PO: ADULTS: 5–10 mg q4–6h as needed. **Maximum:** 15 mg/dose. CHILDREN: 0.6 mg/kg/day in 3–4 divided doses at intervals of no less than 4 hrs. **Maximum single dose in children 2–12 yrs:** 5 mg. **Maximum single dose in children <2 yrs:** 1.25 mg.

EXTENDED-RELEASE

PO: ADULTS: 10 mg q12h. CHILDREN 6–12 YRS: 5 mg q12h.

SIDE EFFECTS

Alert: Effects depend on dosage amount but occur infrequently with oral antitussives. Ambulatory pts and those not in severe pain may experience dizziness, nausea, vomiting, hypotension more frequently than those who are in supine position or having severe pain.

FREQUENT: Sedation, decreased B/P, increased diaphoresis, flushed face, dizziness, drowsiness, hypotension. **OCCASIONAL:** Decreased urination, blurred vision, constipation, dry mouth, headache, nausea, vomiting, difficult/painful urination, euphoria, dysphoria.

ADVERSE REACTIONS/ TOXIC EFFECTS

Overdosage results in respiratory depression, skeletal muscle flaccidity, cold/ clammy skin, cyanosis, extreme somnolence progressing to convulsions, stupor, coma. Tolerance to analgesic effect, physical dependence may occur with repeated use. Prolonged duration of action, cumulative effect may occur in those with impaired hepatic, renal function.

NURSING IMPLICATIONS

BASELINE ASSESSMENT

Obtain vital signs prior to giving medication. If respirations are ≤12/min (≤20/min in children), withhold medication, contact physician. **Analgesic:** Assess onset, type, location, duration of pain. Effect of medication is reduced if full pain recurs before next dose. **Antitussive:** Assess type, severity, frequency of cough.

INTERVENTION/EVALUATION

Palpate bladder for urinary retention. Monitor pattern of daily bowel activity/ stool consistency. Initiate deep breathing/coughing exercises, particularly in pts with impaired pulmonary function. Assess for clinical improvement; record onset of relief of pain or cough.

PATIENT/FAMILY TEACHING

Change positions slowly to avoid orthostatic hypotension. Avoid tasks that require alertness, motor skills until response to drug is established. Tolerance/dependence may occur with prolonged use at high dosages. Avoid alcohol. Report nausea, vomiting, constipation, shortness of breath, difficulty breathing. May take with food.

hydrocortisone ⓔ

high-droe-**core**-tah-sewn
(Cort-Dome, Cortef ♣, Cortenema, Emcort, Hydrocortone, Hytone, Locoid, Pandel)

hydrocortisone acetate

(Cortaid, Cortamed ♣, Corticaine, Proctocort)

hydrocortisone sodium phosphate

(Hydrocortone Phosphate)

hydrocortisone sodium succinate

(A-HydroCort, Solu-Cortef)

hydrocortisone valerate

(WestCort)

FIXED-COMBINATION(S)

Cortisporin: hydrocortisone/neomycin/polymyxin (anti-infective): 5 mg/10,000 units/5 mg; 10 mg/ 10,000 units/5 mg.

◆ CLASSIFICATION

PHARMACOTHERAPEUTIC: Adrenal corticosteroid. **CLINICAL:** Glucocorticoid (see pp. 81C, 85C).

ACTION

Inhibits accumulation of inflammatory cells at inflammation sites, phagocytosis, lysosomal enzyme release and synthesis and/or release of mediators of inflammation. **Therapeutic Effect:** Prevents/ suppresses cell-mediated immune reactions. Decreases/prevents tissue response to inflammatory process.

PHARMACOKINETICS

Onset	Peak	Duration
IV		
—	4–6 hrs	8–12 hrs

Well absorbed following IM administration. Widely distributed. Metabolized in liver. **Half-life:** plasma: 1.5–2 hrs; biologic: 8–12 hrs.

USES

Management of adrenocortical insufficiency; relief of inflammation of corticosteroid-responsive dermatoses; adjunctive treatment of ulcerative colitis, status asthmaticus, shock.

PRECAUTIONS

CONTRAINDICATIONS: Serious infections; viral, fungal, tubercular skin lesions. **CAUTIONS:** Hyperthyroidism, cirrhosis, ulcerative colitis, hypertension, osteoporosis, thromboembolic tendencies, CHF, seizure disorders, thrombophlebitis, peptic ulcer, diabetes.

LIFESPAN CONSIDERATIONS: Pregnancy/lactation: Crosses placenta, distributed in breast milk. May produce cleft palate if used chronically during first trimester. Breast-feeding contraindicated. **Pregnancy Category C** (**D** if used in first trimester). **Children:** Prolonged treatment or high dosages may decrease short-term growth rate, cortisol secretion. **Elderly:** May be more susceptible to developing hypertension or osteoporosis.

INTERACTIONS

DRUG: **Amphotericin** may increase hypokalemia. May decrease effect of **oral hypoglycemics, insulin, diuretics, potassium supplements.** May increase **digoxin** toxicity (due to hypokalemia). **Hepatic enzyme inducers** may decrease effect. **Live virus vaccines** may potentiate virus replication, increase vaccine side effects, decrease pt's antibody response to vaccine. **HERBAL:** None known. **FOOD:** None known. **LAB VALUES:** May decrease calcium, potassium, thyroxine. May increase cholesterol, lipids, glucose, sodium, amylase.

AVAILABILITY (Rx)

HYDROCORTISONE: **GEL:** 0.5%, 1% (OTC). **LOTION:** 0.25%, 0.5%, 1%, 2%, 2.5%. **CREAM:** 0.5%, 1% (OTC), 2.5%. **OINTMENT:** 0.5%, 1% (OTC), 2.5%. **TOPICAL SOLUTION:** 1%. **ORAL SUSPENSION:** 10 mg/5 ml.

SODIUM PHOSPHATE: **INJECTION:** 50 mg/ml.

SODIUM SUCCINATE: **INJECTION:** 100 mg, 250 mg, 500 mg, 1,000 mg.

ACETATE: **INJECTION:** 25 mg/ml, 50 mg/ml. **SUPPOSITORY:** 10 mg, 25 mg, 30 mg. **CREAM:** 0.5%, 1%. **OINTMENT:** 0.5%, 1%.

VALERATE: **CREAM:** 0.2%.

ADMINISTRATION/HANDLING

IV

Storage • Store at room temperature.

HYDROCORTISONE SODIUM SUCCINATE

• After reconstitution, use solution within 72 hrs. Use immediately if further diluted with D_5W, 0.9% NaCl, or other compatible diluent. • Once reconstituted, solution is stable for 72 hrs at room temperature.

Reconstitution • May further dilute with D_5W or 0.9% NaCl. For IV push, dilute to 50 mg/ml; for intermittent infusion, dilute to 1 mg/ml.

Rate of administration • Administer IV push over 3–5 min. Give intermittent infusion over 20–30 min.

TOPICAL

• Gently cleanse area before application. • Use occlusive dressings only as ordered. • Apply sparingly and rub into area thoroughly.

RECTAL
• Shake homogeneous suspension well. • Instruct pt to lie on left side with left leg extended, right leg flexed. • Gently insert applicator tip into rectum, pointed slightly toward navel (umbilicus). Slowly instill medication.

⊘ IV INCOMPATIBILITIES
Ciprofloxacin (Cipro), diazepam (Valium), idarubicin (Idamycin), midazolam (Versed), phenytoin (Dilantin).

IV COMPATIBILITIES
Aminophylline, amphotericin, calcium gluconate, cefepime (Maxipime), digoxin (Lanoxin), diltiazem (Cardizem), diphenhydramine (Benadryl), dopamine (Intropin), insulin, lidocaine, lorazepam (Ativan), magnesium sulfate, morphine, norepinephrine (Levophed), procainamide (Pronestyl), potassium chloride, propofol (Diprivan).

INDICATIONS/ROUTES/DOSAGE

ACUTE ADRENAL INSUFFICIENCY
IV: ADULTS, ELDERLY: 100 mg IV bolus, then 300 mg/day in divided doses q8h. CHILDREN: 1–2 mg/kg IV bolus, then 150–250 mg/day in divided doses q6–8h. INFANTS: 1–2 mg/kg/dose IV bolus, then 25–150 mg/day in divided doses q6–8h.

ANTI-INFLAMMATORY/ IMMUNOSUPPRESSION
IM/IV: ADULTS, ELDERLY: 15–240 mg q12h. CHILDREN: 1–5 mg/kg/day in divided doses q12h.

PHYSIOLOGIC REPLACEMENT
IM: CHILDREN: 0.25–0.35 mg/kg/day as a single daily dose.

PO: CHILDREN: 0.5–0.75 mg/kg/day in divided doses q8h.

STATUS ASTHMATICUS
IV: ADULTS, ELDERLY: 100–500 mg q6h. CHILDREN: 2 mg/kg/dose q6h.

SHOCK
IV: ADULTS, ELDERLY, CHILDREN ≥12 YRS: 100–500 mg q6h. CHILDREN <12 YRS: 50 mg/kg. May repeat in 4 hrs, then q24h as needed.

USUAL RECTAL DOSAGE
Rectal: ADULTS, ELDERLY: 100 mg at bedtime for 21 nights or until clinical and proctologic remission occurs (may require 2–3 mos of therapy).

Cortifoam: ADULTS, ELDERLY: 1 applicator 1–2 times/day for 2–3 wks, then every second day thereafter.

USUAL TOPICAL DOSAGE
ADULTS, ELDERLY: Apply sparingly 2–4 times/day.

SIDE EFFECTS

FREQUENT: Insomnia, heartburn, nervousness, abdominal distention, diaphoresis, acne, mood swings, increased appetite, facial flushing, delayed wound healing, increased susceptibility to infection, diarrhea/constipation. **OCCASIONAL:** Headache, edema, change in skin color, frequent urination. **Topical:** Itching, redness, irritation. **RARE:** Tachycardia, allergic reaction (rash, hives), psychic changes, hallucinations, depression. **Topical:** Allergic contact dermatitis, purpura. Systemic absorption more likely with occlusive dressings or extensive application in young children.

ADVERSE REACTIONS/ TOXIC EFFECTS

LONG-TERM THERAPY: Hypocalcemia, hypokalemia, muscle wasting (esp. arms, legs), osteoporosis, spontaneous fractures, amenorrhea, cataracts, glaucoma, peptic ulcer, CHF. **ABRUPT WITHDRAWAL AFTER LONG-TERM THERAPY:** Anorexia, nausea, fever, headache, sudden severe joint pain, rebound inflammation, fatigue, weakness, lethargy, dizziness, orthostatic hypotension.

NURSING IMPLICATIONS

BASELINE ASSESSMENT

Obtain baseline values for weight, B/P, glucose, cholesterol, electrolytes. Check results of initial tests (e.g., TB skin test, x-rays, EKG).

INTERVENTION/EVALUATION

Assess for edema. Be alert to infection (reduced immune response): sore throat, fever, vague symptoms. Evaluate bowel activity. Monitor electrolytes. Watch for hypocalcemia (muscle twitching, cramps), hypokalemia (weakness, numbness/tingling [esp. lower extremities], nausea/vomiting, irritability, EKG changes). Assess emotional status, ability to sleep.

PATIENT/FAMILY TEACHING

Notify physician of fever, sore throat, muscle aches, sudden weight gain/swelling. Do not take aspirin or any other medication without consulting physician. Limit caffeine, avoid alcohol. Inform dentist, physicians of cortisone therapy now or within past 12 mos. Caution against overuse of joints injected for symptomatic relief. **Topical:** Apply after shower/bath for best absorption. Do not cover unless physician orders; do not use tight diapers, plastic pants, coverings. Avoid contact with eyes.

Hydrodiuril

see hydrochlorothiazide

hydromorphone hydrochloride

high-dro-**more**-phone
(Dilaudid, Dilaudid HP, Hydromorph Contin✱)

◆ CLASSIFICATION

PHARMACOTHERAPEUTIC: Opioid agonist **(Schedule II). CLINICAL:** Narcotic analgesic, antitussive (see p. 121C).

ACTION

Binds at opiate receptor sites in CNS. **Therapeutic Effect:** Reduces intensity of pain stimuli incoming from sensory nerve endings, altering pain perception, emotional response to pain; suppresses cough reflex.

PHARMACOKINETICS

Onset	Peak	Duration
PO		
30 min	90–120 min	4 hrs
Subcutaneous		
15 min	30–90 min	4 hrs
IM		
15 min	30–60 min	4–5 hrs
IV		
10–15 min	15–30 min	2–3 hrs
Rectal		
15–30 min	—	—

Well absorbed from GI tract after IM administration. Widely distributed. Metabolized in liver. Excreted in urine. **Half-life:** 1–3 hrs.

USES

Relief of moderate to severe pain, persistent nonproductive cough.

PRECAUTIONS

CONTRAINDICATIONS: None known. **EXTREME CAUTION:** CNS depression, anoxia, hypercapnia, respiratory depression, seizures, acute alcoholism, shock, untreated myxedema, respiratory dysfunction. **CAUTIONS:** Increased intracranial pressure, impaired hepatic function, acute abdominal conditions, hypothyroidism, prostatic hypertrophy, Addison's disease, urethral stricture, COPD.

LIFESPAN CONSIDERATIONS: Pregnancy/lactation: Readily crosses placenta. Unknown if distributed in breast milk. May prolong labor if administered in latent phase of first stage of labor or before cervical dilation of 4–5 cm has occurred. Respiratory depression may occur in neonate if mother receives opiates during labor. Regular use of opiates during pregnancy may produce withdrawal symptoms in the neonate (irritability, excessive crying, tremors, hyperactive reflexes, fever, vomiting, diarrhea, yawning, sneezing, seizures). **Pregnancy Category B** (**D** if used for prolonged periods or at high dosages at term). **Children:** Those <2 yrs may be more susceptible to respiratory depression. **Elderly:** May be more susceptible to respiratory depression, may cause paradoxical excitement. Age-related renal impairment, prostatic hypertrophy/obstruction may increase risk of urinary retention; dosage adjustment recommended.

INTERACTIONS

DRUG: Alcohol, CNS depressants may increase CNS or respiratory depression, hypotension. **MAOIs** may produce severe, fatal reaction (reduce dose to ¼ usual dose). **HERBAL:** None known. **FOOD:** None known. **LAB VALUES:** May increase amylase, lipase plasma concentrations.

AVAILABILITY (Rx)

TABLETS: 2 mg, 4 mg, 8 mg. **LIQUID:** 5 mg/5 ml. **INJECTION:** 1 mg/ml, 2 mg/ml, 4 mg/ml, 10 mg/ml. **SUPPOSITORY:** 3 mg.

ADMINISTRATION/HANDLING

PO

• Give without regard to meals. • Tablets may be crushed.

SUBCUTANEOUS/IM

• Use short 30-gauge needle for subcutaneous injection. • Administer slowly, rotating injection sites. • Pts with circulatory impairment experience higher risk of overdosage because of delayed absorption of repeated administration.

IV

Alert: High concentration injection (10 mg/ml) should be used only in those tolerant to opiate agonists, currently receiving high doses of another opiate agonist for severe, chronic pain due to cancer.

Storage • Store at room temperature; protect from light. • Slight yellow discoloration of parenteral form does not indicate loss of potency.

Reconstitution • May give undiluted. • May further dilute with 5 ml Sterile Water for Injection or 0.9% NaCl.

Rate of administration • Administer IV push very slowly (over 2–5 min). • Rapid IV increases risk of severe adverse reactions (chest wall rigidity, apnea, peripheral circulatory collapse, anaphylactoid effects, cardiac arrest).

RECTAL

• Refrigerate suppositories. • Moisten suppository with cold water before inserting well up into rectum.

IV INCOMPATIBILITIES

Amphotericin B complex (Abelcet, AmBisome, Amphotec), cefazolin (Ancef, Kefzol), diazepam (Valium), phenobarbital, phenytoin (Dilantin).

IV COMPATIBILITIES

Diltiazem (Cardizem), diphenhydramine (Benadryl), dobutamine (Dobutrex), dopamine (Intropin), fentanyl (Sublimaze), furosemide (Lasix), heparin, lorazepam (Ativan), magnesium sulfate, metoclopramide (Reglan), midazolam (Versed), milrinone (Primacor), morphine, propofol (Diprivan).

INDICATIONS/ROUTES/DOSAGE

ANALGESIC

IV: ADULTS, ELDERLY, CHILDREN >50 KG: 0.2–0.6 mg q2–3h.

PO: ADULTS, ELDERLY, CHILDREN >50 KG: 2–4 mg q3–4h. RANGE: 2–8 mg/dose. CHILDREN >6 MONTHS, <50 KG: 0.03–0.08 mg/kg/dose q3–4h.

H

USUAL RECTAL DOSAGE

ADULTS, ELDERLY: 3 mg q4–8h.

ANTITUSSIVE

PO: ADULTS, CHILDREN >12 YRS, ELDERLY: 1 mg q3–4h. CHILDREN 6–12 YRS: 0.5 mg q3–4h.

PATIENT CONTROLLED ANALGESIA (PCA)

ADULTS, ELDERLY: 0.05–0.5 mg at 5- to 15-min lockout. **4-hr maximum:** 4–6 mg.

USUAL EPIDURAL DOSAGE

ADULTS, ELDERLY: Bolus of 1–1.5 mg, rate of 0.04–0.4 mg/hr. Demand dose of 0.15 mg at 30-min lockout.

SIDE EFFECTS

Alert: Effects depend on dosage amount, route of administration but occur infrequently with oral antitussives. Ambulatory pts and those not in severe pain may experience dizziness, nausea, vomiting, hypotension more frequently than those in supine position or having severe pain.

FREQUENT: Drowsiness, dizziness, hypotension, decreased appetite. **OCCASIONAL:** Confusion, diaphoresis, facial flushing, urinary retention, constipation, dry mouth, nausea, vomiting, headache, pain at injection site. **RARE:** Allergic reaction, depression.

ADVERSE REACTIONS/ TOXIC EFFECTS

Overdosage results in respiratory depression, skeletal muscle flaccidity, cold/clammy skin, cyanosis, extreme somnolence progressing to seizures, stupor, coma. Tolerance to analgesic effect, physical dependence may occur with repeated use. Prolonged duration of action, cumulative effect may occur in those with impaired hepatic, renal function.

NURSING IMPLICATIONS

BASELINE ASSESSMENT

Obtain vital signs prior to giving medication. If respirations are ≤12/min (≤20/min in children), withhold medication, contact physician. **Analgesic:** Assess onset, type, location, duration of pain. Effect of medication is reduced if full pain recurs prior to next dose. **Antitussive:** Assess type, severity, frequency of cough.

INTERVENTION/EVALUATION

Monitor vital signs; assess for pain relief, cough. Assess breath sounds. Increase fluid intake, environmental humidity to decrease viscosity of lung secretions. To prevent pain cycles, instruct pt to request pain medication as soon as discomfort begins. Assess pattern of daily bowel activity/stool consistency. (esp. in long-term use). Initiate deep breathing/coughing exercises, particularly in pts with impaired pulmonary function. Assess for clinical improvement; record onset of relief of pain or cough.

PATIENT/FAMILY TEACHING

Avoid alcohol, tasks that require alertness/motor skills until response to drug is established. Tolerance/dependence may occur with prolonged use at high dosages. Change positions slowly to avoid orthostatic hypotension.

hydroxychloroquine sulfate

hi-drocks-ee-**klor**-oh-kwin
(Plaquenil)

Do not confuse with hydrocortisone, hydroxyzine.

◆CLASSIFICATION

CLINICAL: Antimalarial, antirheumatic.

ACTION

Concentrates in parasite acid vesicles, interfering with parasite protein synthesis, increasing pH. Antirheumatic action unknown but may involve suppressing formation of antigens responsible for hypersensitivity reactions. **Therapeutic Effect:** Inhibits parasite growth.

USES

Treatment of falciparum malaria (terminates acute attacks, cures nonresistant strains); suppression of acute attacks and prolongation of interval between treatment/relapse in vivax, ovale, malariae malaria. Treatment of discoid or systematic lupus erythematosus, acute and chronic rheumatoid arthritis. **Unlabeled:** Treatment of juvenile arthritis, sarcoid-associated hypercalcemia.

PRECAUTIONS

CONTRAINDICATIONS: Retinal/visual field changes, long-term therapy for children, psoriasis, porphyria. **CAUTIONS:** Alcoholism, hepatic disease, G6PD deficiency. Children are esp. susceptible to hydroxychloroquine fatalities. **Pregnancy Category C.**

INTERACTIONS

DRUG: May increase concentration of **penicillamine** (may increase risk of hematologic/renal or severe skin reaction). **HERBAL:** None known. **FOOD:** None known. **LAB VALUES:** None known.

AVAILABILITY (Rx)

TABLETS: 200 mg (155 mg base).

INDICATIONS/ROUTES/DOSAGE

Alert: 200 mg hydroxychloroquine = 155 mg base.

SUPPRESSION OF MALARIA

PO: ADULTS: 310 mg base weekly on same day each week. CHILDREN: 5 mg base/kg/wk. Begin 2 wks before exposure; continue 6–8 wks after leaving endemic area or if therapy is not begun before exposure.

PO: ADULTS: 620 mg base. CHILDREN: 10 mg base/kg given in 2 divided doses 6 hrs apart.

TREATMENT OF MALARIA (acute attack; dose [mg base])

Dose	Times	Adults	Children
Initial	Day 1	620 mg	10 mg/kg
Second	6 hrs later	310 mg	5 mg/kg
Third	Day 2	310 mg	5 mg/kg
Fourth	Day 3	310 mg	5 mg/kg

RHEUMATOID ARTHRITIS

PO: ADULTS: Initially, 400–600 mg (310–465 mg base) daily for 5–10 days; gradually increase dosage to optimum response level. MAINTENANCE (USUALLY WITHIN 4–12 WKS): Decrease dose by 50%, continue at level of 200–400 mg/day. Maximum effect may not be seen for several months.

LUPUS ERYTHEMATOSUS

PO: ADULTS: Initially, 400 mg 1–2 times/day for several weeks or months. MAINTENANCE: 200–400 mg/day.

SIDE EFFECTS

FREQUENT: Mild transient headache, anorexia, nausea, vomiting. **OCCASIONAL:** Visual disturbances, nervousness, fatigue, pruritus (esp. of palms, soles, scalp), irritability, personality changes, diarrhea. **RARE:** Stomatitis, dermatitis, impaired hearing.

ADVERSE REACTIONS/ TOXIC EFFECTS

Ocular toxicity (esp. retinopathy, which may progress even after drug is discontinued). **PROLONGED THERAPY:** Peripheral neuritis, neuromyopathy, hypotension, EKG changes, agranulocytosis, aplastic anemia, thrombocytopenia, seizure, psychosis. **OVERDOSAGE:** Headache, vomiting, visual disturbance, drowsiness, seizure, hypokalemia followed by cardiovascular collapse, death.

NURSING IMPLICATIONS

BASELINE ASSESSMENT

Evaluate CBC, hepatic function.

INTERVENTION/EVALUATION

Monitor, report any visual disturbances promptly. Evaluate for GI distress. Give dose with food (for malaria). Monitor hepatic function tests. Assess skin/buccal mucosa; inquire about pruritus. Report impaired hearing immediately.

PATIENT/FAMILY TEACHING

Continue drug for full length of treatment. In long-term therapy, therapeutic response may not be evident for up to 6 mos. Immediately notify physician of **any** new symptom of visual difficulties, muscular weakness, impaired hearing, tinnitus.

hydroxyurea

high-**drocks**-ee-your-e-ah
(Droxia, Hydrea, Mylocel)

CLASSIFICATION

PHARMACOTHERAPEUTIC: Synthetic urea analogue. **CLINICAL:** Antineoplastic (see p. 73C).

ACTION

Cell cycle–specific for S phase. Inhibits DNA synthesis without interfering with RNA synthesis or protein. **Therapeutic Effect:** Interferes with the normal repair process of cells damaged by irradiation.

USES

Treatment of melanoma; resistant chronic myelocytic leukemia; recurrent, metastatic, inoperable ovarian carcinoma. Also used in combination with radiation therapy for local control of primary squamous cell carcinoma of head/neck, excluding lip. Treatment of sickle cell anemia. **Unlabeled:** Treatment of cervical carcinoma, polycythemia vera. Long-term suppression of HIV.

PRECAUTIONS

CONTRAINDICATIONS: WBC $<2,500/mm^3$ or platelet count $<100,000/mm^3$. **CAUTIONS:** Previous irradiation therapy, other cytoxic drugs, impaired renal/hepatic function. **Pregnancy Category D.**

INTERACTIONS

DRUG: May decrease effect of **antigout medications. Bone marrow depressants** may increase bone marrow depression. **Live virus vaccines** may potentiate virus replication, increase vaccine side effects, decrease pt's antibody response to vaccine. **HERBAL:** None known. **FOOD:** None known. **LAB VALUES:** May increase BUN, creatinine, uric acid.

AVAILABILITY (Rx)

CAPSULES: 200 mg, 300 mg, 400 mg, 500 mg. **TABLETS:** 1,000 mg.

INDICATIONS/ROUTES/DOSAGE

Alert: Dosage individualized based on clinical response, tolerance to adverse effects. When used in combination therapy, consult specific protocols for optimum dosage, sequence of drug administration. Dosage based on actual or ideal body weight, whichever is less. Therapy interrupted when platelets fall below 100,000/mm^3 or leukocytes fall below 2,500/mm^3. Resume when counts rise toward normal.

SOLID TUMORS
PO: ADULTS, ELDERLY: 80 mg/kg q3days or 20–30 mg/kg/day as a single dose daily.

THERAPY WITH IRRADIATION
PO: ADULTS, ELDERLY: 80 mg/kg q3days beginning at least 7 days before starting irradiation.

RESISTANT CHRONIC MYELOCYTIC LEUKEMIA (CML)
PO: ADULTS, ELDERLY: 20–30 mg/kg once daily. CHILDREN: Initially, 10–20 mg/kg once daily.

HIV INFECTION
PO: ADULTS, ELDERLY: 500 mg 2 times/day (with didanosine).

SICKLE CELL ANEMIA
PO: ADULTS, ELDERLY, CHILDREN: Initially, 15 mg/kg once daily. May increase by 5 mg/kg/day. **Maximum:** 35 mg/kg/wk.

SIDE EFFECTS

FREQUENT: Nausea, vomiting, anorexia, constipation/diarrhea. **OCCASIONAL:** Mild reversible rash, facial flushing, pruritus, fever, chills, malaise. **RARE:** Alopecia, headache, drowsiness, dizziness, disorientation.

ADVERSE REACTIONS/ TOXIC EFFECTS

Bone marrow depression manifested as hematologic toxicity (leukopenia and, to lesser extent, thrombocytopenia, anemia).

NURSING IMPLICATIONS

BASELINE ASSESSMENT

Obtain bone marrow studies, hepatic/renal function tests before therapy begins, periodically thereafter. Obtain Hgb, WBC, platelet count, uric acid at baseline, and weekly during therapy. Those with marked renal impairment may develop visual/auditory hallucinations, marked hematologic toxicity.

INTERVENTION/EVALUATION

Assess pattern of daily bowel activity, stool consistency. Monitor for hematologic toxicity (fever, sore throat, signs of local infection, unusual bleeding/bruising from any site), symptoms of anemia (excessive tiredness, weakness). Assess skin for rash, erythema. Monitor CBC with differential, platelet count, Hgb, renal/liver function, uric acid.

PATIENT/FAMILY TEACHING

Promptly report fever, sore throat, signs of local infection, unusual bleeding/bruising from any site.

hydroxyzine

high-**drox**-ih-zeen
(Apo-Hydroxyzine ✤, Atarax, Novo-hydroxyzin ✤, Vistaril)

Do not confuse with hydralazine, hydroxyurea.

CLASSIFICATION

PHARMACOTHERAPEUTIC: Piperazine derivative. **CLINICAL:** Antihistamine, antianxiety, antispasmodic, antiemetic, antipruritic (see pp. 11C, 48C).

ACTION

Competes with histamine for receptor sites in GI tract, blood vessels, respiratory tract. Diminishes vestibular stimulation, depresses labyrinthine function. **Therapeutic Effect:** Produces anticholinergic, antihistaminic, analgesic effects; relaxes skeletal muscle. Controls nausea, vomiting.

PHARMACOKINETICS

Onset	Peak	Duration
PO		
15–30 min	—	4–6 hrs

Well absorbed from GI tract, parenteral administration. Metabolized in liver. Primarily excreted in urine. Not removed by hemodialysis. **Half-life:** 20–25 hrs (half-life increased in elderly).

USES

Relief of anxiety/tension; pruritus caused by allergic conditions, preop and postop sedation, control of muscle spasm, nausea/vomiting.

PRECAUTIONS

CONTRAINDICATIONS: None known. **CAUTIONS:** Narrow-angle glaucoma, prostatic hypertrophy, bladder neck obstruction, asthma, COPD.

LIFESPAN CONSIDERATIONS: Pregnancy/lactation: Unknown if drug crosses placenta or is distributed in breast milk. **Pregnancy Category C. Children:** Not recommended in newborns/premature infants (increased risk of anticholinergic effects). Paradoxical excitement may occur. **Elderly:** Increased risk of dizziness, sedation, confusion; hypotension, hyperexcitability may occur.

INTERACTIONS

DRUG: Alcohol, CNS depressants may increase CNS depressant effects. **MAOIs** may increase anticholinergic, CNS depressant effects. **HERBAL:** None known. **FOOD:** None known. **LAB VALUES:** May cause false positives with 17-hydroxy corticosteroid determinations.

AVAILABILITY (Rx)

TABLETS: 10 mg, 25 mg, 50 mg, 100 mg. **CAPSULES:** 25 mg, 50 mg, 100 mg. **ORAL SUSPENSION:** 25 mg/5 ml. **INJECTION:** 25 mg/ml, 50 mg/ml.

ADMINISTRATION/HANDLING

PO

• Shake oral suspension well. • Scored tablets may be crushed; do not crush or break capsule.

IM

Alert: Significant tissue damage, thrombosis, gangrene may occur if injection is given subcutaneous, intra-arterial, or by IV. • IM may be given undiluted. • Use Z-track technique of injection to prevent subcutaneous infiltration. • Inject deep IM into gluteus maximus or midlateral thigh in adults, midlateral thigh in children.

INDICATIONS/ROUTES/DOSAGE

ANTIEMETIC

IM: ADULTS, ELDERLY: 25–100 mg/dose q4–6h.

ANXIETY

PO: ADULTS, ELDERLY: 25–100 mg 4 times/day. **Maximum:** 600 mg/day.

PRURITUS

PO: ADULTS, ELDERLY: 25 mg 3–4 times/day.

USUAL CHILDREN'S DOSAGE

PO: 2 mg/kg/day in divided doses q6–8h.

IM: 0.5–1 mg/kg/dose q4–6h.

SIDE EFFECTS

Side effects are generally mild and transient. **FREQUENT:** Drowsiness, dry mouth, marked discomfort with IM injection. **OCCASIONAL:** Dizziness, ataxia (muscular incoordination), weakness, slurred speech, headache, agitation, increased anxiety. **RARE:** Paradoxical CNS hyperactivity/nervousness in children, excitement/restlessness in elderly/debilitated pts (generally noted during first 2 wks of therapy, particularly noted in presence of uncontrolled pain).

ADVERSE REACTIONS/ TOXIC EFFECTS

Hypersensitivity reaction (wheezing, dyspnea, chest tightness).

NURSING IMPLICATIONS

BASELINE ASSESSMENT

Anxiety: Offer emotional support to anxious pt. Assess motor responses (agitation, trembling, tension), autonomic responses (cold/clammy hands, sweating). **Antiemetic:** Assess for dehydration (poor skin turgor, dry mucous membranes, longitudinal furrows in tongue).

INTERVENTION/EVALUATION

For those on long-term therapy, liver/renal function tests, blood counts should be performed periodically. Monitor lung sounds for signs of hypersensitivity reaction. Monitor serum electrolytes in pts with severe vomiting. Assess for paradoxical reaction, particularly during early therapy. Assist with ambulation if drowsiness, lightheadedness occurs.

PATIENT/FAMILY TEACHING

Marked discomfort may occur with IM injection. Sugarless gum, sips of tepid water may relieve dry mouth. Drowsiness usually diminishes with continued therapy. Avoid tasks that require alertness, motor skills until response to drug is established.

hyoscyamine

high-oh-**sigh**-ah-meen
(Anaspaz, Buscopan✦, Cystospaz, Levsin, Levsinex, Nulev)

Do not confuse with Anaprox.

◆CLASSIFICATION

PHARMACOTHERAPEUTIC: Anticholinergic. **CLINICAL:** Antimuscarinic, antispasmodic.

H

ACTION

Inhibits action of acetylcholine at postganglionic (muscarinic) receptor sites. **Therapeutic Effect:** Decreases secretions (bronchial, salivary, sweat glands, gastric secretions). Reduces motility of GI and urinary tract.

USES

Treatment of GI tract disorders caused by spasm. Adjunct in treatment of peptic ulcer disease, GI hypermotility, infantile colic, hypermotility of lower urinary tract.

PRECAUTIONS

CONTRAINDICATIONS: Narrow-angle glaucoma, GI/GU obstruction, paralytic ileus, severe ulcerative colitis, myasthenia gravis. **CAUTIONS:** Hyperthyroidism, CHF, cardiac arrhythmias, prostatic hypertrophy, neuropathy, chronic lung disease. **Pregnancy Category C.**

INTERACTIONS

DRUG: **Antacids, antidiarrheals** may decrease absorption. **Anticholinergics** may increase effects. May decrease absorption of **ketoconazole.** May increase severity of GI lesions with **potassium chloride (wax matrix).** **HERBAL:** None known. **FOOD:** None known. **LAB VALUES:** None known.

AVAILABILITY (Rx)

TABLETS: 0.125 mg, 0.15 mg. **TABLETS (sublingual):** 0.125 mg. **CAPSULES (time-release):** 0.375 mg. **ELIXIR:** 0.125 mg/5 ml. **DROPS. INJECTION:** 0.5 mg/ml.

ADMINISTRATION/HANDLING

PO

• Give without regard to meals. • Tablets may be crushed, chewed. • Extended-release capsule should be swallowed whole.

H

PARENTERAL

• May give undiluted.

INDICATIONS/ROUTES/DOSAGE

GI TRACT DISORDERS

IM/subcutaneous: ADULTS, ELDERLY, CHILDREN >12 YRS: 0.25–0.5 mg q4h for 1–4 doses.

PO/sublingual: ADULTS, ELDERLY, CHILDREN >12 YRS: 0.125–0.25 mg q4h. **Maximum:** 1.5 or 0.375–0.75 mg q12h (time-release capsule). CHILDREN 2–12 YRS: 0.0625–0.125 mg q4h as needed. **Maximum:** 0.75 mg/day. CHILDREN <2 YRS: Drops dose q4h (using drop formulation).

HYPERMOTILITY OF LOWER URINARY TRACT

PO/sublingual: ADULTS, ELDERLY: 0.15–0.3 mg 4 times/day or 0.375 mg q12h (time-release capsule).

DUODENOGRAPHY

IV: ADULTS, ELDERLY: 0.25–0.5 mg 10 min before procedure.

PREOP

IM: ADULTS, ELDERLY: 0.5 mg (0.005 mg/kg) 30–60 min before induction of anesthesia or administration of preop medications.

SIDE EFFECTS

FREQUENT: Dry mouth (sometimes severe), decreased sweating, constipation. **OCCASIONAL:** Blurred vision, bloated feeling, urinary hesitancy, drowsiness (with high dosage), headache, intolerance to light, loss of taste, nervousness, flushing, insomnia, impotence, mental confusion/excitement (particularly in elderly, children). Parenteral form may produce temporary lightheadedness, local irritation. **RARE:** Dizziness, faintness.

ADVERSE REACTIONS/ TOXIC EFFECTS

Overdosage may produce temporary paralysis of ciliary muscle, pupillary dilation, tachycardia, palpitations, hot/dry/flushed skin, absence of bowel sounds, hyperthermia, increased respiratory rate, EKG abnormalities, nausea, vomiting, rash over face/upper trunk, CNS stimulation, psychosis (agitation, restlessness, rambling speech, visual hallucination, paranoid behavior, delusions), followed by depression.

NURSING IMPLICATIONS

BASELINE ASSESSMENT

Before giving medication, instruct pt to void (reduces risk of urinary retention).

INTERVENTION/EVALUATION

Monitor daily bowel activity/stool consistency. Palpate bladder for urinary retention. Monitor changes in B/P, temperature. Assess skin turgor, mucous membranes to evaluate hydration status (encourage adequate fluid intake), bowel sounds for peristalsis. Be alert for fever (increased risk of hyperthermia).

PATIENT/FAMILY TEACHING

May cause dry mouth; maintain good oral hygiene habits (lack of saliva may increase risk of cavities). Inform physician of rash, eye pain, difficulty in urinating, constipation. Avoid tasks that require alertness, motor skills until response to drug is established. Avoid hot baths, saunas.

ibandronate

eye-**band**-droh-nate
(Boniva)

CLASSIFICATION

PHARMACOTHERAPEUTIC: Bisphosphonate. **CLINICAL:** Calcium regulator.

ACTION

Binds to bone hydroxyapatite (part of the mineral matrix of bone), inhibits osteoclast activity. **Therapeutic Effect:** Reduces rate of bone turnover/resorption, resulting in net gain in bone mass.

PHARMACOKINETICS

Absorbed in upper GI tract. Extent of absorption impaired by food/beverages (other than plain water). Rapidly binds to bone. Unabsorbed portion is eliminated in the urine. Protein binding: 90%. **Half-life:** 10–60 hrs.

USES

Treatment/prevention of osteoporosis in postmenopausal women.

PRECAUTIONS

CONTRAINDICATIONS: Hypersensitivity to other bisphosphonates (etidronate, tiludronate, risedronate, alendronate, pamidronate), uncorrected hypocalcemia, inability to stand or sit upright for at least 60 min, severe renal impairment (creatinine clearance <30 ml/min). **CAUTIONS:** GI diseases (duodenitis, dysphagia, esophagitis, gastritis, ulcers [drug may exacerbate these conditions]), mild to moderate renal impairment.

LIFESPAN CONSIDERATIONS: Pregnancy/lactation: Potential for teratogenic effects. Unknown if excreted in breast milk. Do not breast-feed. **Pregnancy Category C. Children:** Safety and efficacy not established. **Elderly:** No age-related precautions noted.

INTERACTIONS

DRUG: Concurrent **dietary supplements,** food, beverages other than plain water interfere with ibandronate absorption. Antacids with **calcium, magnesium, aluminum, vitamin D** decrease absorption. **HERBAL:** None known. **FOOD:** Food, beverages (including mineral water) other than plain water likely reduce drug absorption. **LAB VALUES:** May decrease alkaline phosphatase. May increase cholesterol.

AVAILABILITY (Rx)

TABLETS: 2.5 mg

ADMINISTRATION/HANDLING

- Give 60 min prior to first food, beverage of the day, on an empty stomach with 6–8 oz plain water (not mineral water) while the pt is standing or sitting in an upright position. Pt cannot lie down for 60 min following drug administration. Pt should not chew or suck the tablet (potential for oropharangeal ulceration).

INDICATIONS/ROUTES/DOSAGE

OSTEOPOROSIS

PO: ADULTS, ELDERLY: 2.5 mg daily.

SIDE EFFECTS

FREQUENT (6%–13%): Back pain, dyspepsia (epigastric distress, heartburn), peripheral discomfort, diarrhea, headache, myalgia. **OCCASIONAL (3%–4%):** Dizziness, arthralgia, asthenia (lack of strength, energy). **RARE (≤2%):** Vomiting, hypersensitivity reaction.

ADVERSE REACTIONS/ TOXIC EFFECTS

Upper respiratory infection occurs occa-

I

sionally. Overdosage results in hypocalcemia, hypophosphatemia, significant GI disturbances.

NURSING IMPLICATIONS

BASELINE ASSESSMENT

Hypocalcemia, vitamin D deficiency must be corrected prior to beginning therapy. Obtain laboratory baselines, esp. electrolytes, renal function. Obtain results of bone density study.

INTERVENTION/EVALUATION

Monitor electrolytes, esp. calcium, alkaline phosphatase serum levels.

PATIENT/FAMILY TEACHING

Instruct pt that expected benefits occur only when medication is taken with full glass (6–8 oz) of plain water, first thing in the morning and at least 60 min prior to first food, beverage, medication of the day. Any other beverage (mineral water, orange juice, coffee) significantly reduces absorption of medication. Do not lie down for at least 60 min after taking medication (potentiates delivery to stomach, reduces risk of esophageal irritation). Consider weight-bearing exercises, modify behavioral factors (e.g., cigarette smoking, alcohol consumption).

ibritumomab tiuxetan

ih-brit-uh-**moe**-mab tea-**ux**-eh-tan
(Zevalin)

CLASSIFICATION

PHARMACOTHERAPEUTIC: Monoclonal antibody. **CLINICAL:** Antineoplastic (see p. 73C).

ACTION

Radioimmunotherapeutic agent that aims to combine the targeting power of monoclonal antibodies (MAbs) with the cancer-killing ability of radiation. Ibritumomab tiuxetan is an immunoconjugate resulting from a bond between the monoclonal antibody ibritumomab with the chelator tiuxetan. This conjugate tightly binds yttrium-90 (Y-90) for radioimmunotherapy of B-cell non-Hodgkin's lymphoma and indium-111 for imaging in this protocol. **Therapeutic Effect:** Targets the CD antigen (present on B cells in >90% of pts with B-cell non-Hodgkin's lymphoma), inducing cellular damage via formation of free radicals in the target and neighboring cells.

PHARMACOKINETICS

Tumor uptake is greater than normal tissue in non-Hodgkin's lymphoma. Most of dose is cleared by binding to tumor. Minimally excreted in urine. **Half-life:** 27–30 hrs.

USES

Treatment of non-Hodgkin's lymphoma in combination with rituxumab in pts with relapsed or refractory low-grade, follicular, or CD20-positive transformed B-cell non-Hodgkin's lymphoma.

PRECAUTIONS

CONTRAINDICATIONS: Platelet count <100,000 cells/mm^3, neutrophil count <1,500 cells/mm^3, history of failed stem cell collection. **CAUTIONS:** Prior radio/immunotherapy with the rituzimab/ibritumomab tiuxetan regimen, mild thrombocytopenia, prior external beam radiation to ≥25% of bone marrow, breast-feeding period, pregnancy, cardiovascular disease, hypertension/hypotension, history of hypersensitivity or anaphylaxis after use of other medications.

LIFESPAN CONSIDERATIONS: Pregnancy/lactation: Has potential to cause fetal harm. Substitute formula feedings for breast-feedings. Those with childbearing potential should use contraceptive methods during treatment and up to 12 mos after therapy. **Pregnancy Category D.** **Children:** Safety and efficacy not established. **Elderly:** No age-related precautions noted.

INTERACTIONS

DRUG: Any medication that interferes with platelet function or anticoagulants increases potential for prolonged/severe thrombocytopenia. **Bone marrow depressants** may increase bone marrow depression. **Live virus vaccines** may potentiate virus replication, increase vaccine side effects, decrease pt's antibody response to vaccine. **HERBAL:** None known. **FOOD:** None known. **LAB VALUES:** Severe reduction of Hgb, Hct, platelet count, WBC count.

AVAILABILITY (Rx)

INJECTION: 3.2-mg vial of ibritumomab tiuxetan.

ADMINISTRATION/HANDLING

Indium-111 ibritumomab tiuxetan and Y-90 ibritumomab tiuxetan are radiopharmaceuticals and should be used only by physicians and other professionals trained and experienced in the safe use/handling of radionuclides.

Rate of administration • Administer IV push over 10 min (see Indications/Routes/Dosage).

∅ **IV INCOMPATIBILITY**

Do not mix with any medications.

INDICATIONS/ROUTES/DOSAGE

NON-HODGKIN'S LYMPHOMA

IV: ADULTS, ELDERLY: Regimen consists of two steps: STEP 1: Single infusion of 250 mg/m^2 rituximab preceding (≤4 hrs) a fixed dose of 5 mCi (1.56 mg total antibody dose) of indium-111 ibritumomab administered IV push over 10 min. STEP 2: Follows step 1 by 7–9 days and consists of a second infusion of 250 mg/m^2 rituximab preceding (≤4 hrs) a fixed dose of 0.4 mCi/kg of Y-90 ibritumomab administered IV push over 10 min.

Alert: Reduce dosage of ibritumomab to 0.3 mCi/kg in pts whose platelet count is 100,000–149,000 cells/mm^3.

SIDE EFFECTS

FREQUENT (24%–43%): Asthenia (loss of strength, energy), nausea, chills. **OCCASIONAL (10%–17%):** Fever, abdominal pain, dyspnea, headache, vomiting, dizziness, cough, oral candidiasis. **RARE (5%–9%):** Pruritus, diarrhea, back pain, peripheral edema, anorexia, rash, flushing, arthralgia, myalgia, ecchymosis, rhinitis, constipation, insomnia.

ADVERSE REACTIONS/ TOXIC EFFECTS

Thrombocytopenia (95%), neutropenia (77%), anemia (61%) may be severe and prolonged; may be followed by infection (29%). Hypersensitivity reaction produces hypotension, bronchospasm, angioedema.

NURSING IMPLICATIONS

BASELINE ASSESSMENT

Pretreatment with acetaminophen and diphenhydramine prior to each infusion may prevent infusion-related effects. Give emotional support to pt/family. Use strict asepsis; protect pt from infection. CBC, platelet count, blood chemistries should be obtained as a baseline prior to beginning therapy. ANC nadir is 62 days before recovery begins.

INTERVENTION/EVALUATION

Diligently monitor lab values for possibly severe/prolonged thrombocytopenia, neutropenia, anemia. Monitor

I

for hematologic toxicity (fever, sore throat, signs of local infections, unusual bleeding/bruising), symptoms of anemia (excessive tiredness, weakness). Assess for GI symptoms (nausea, vomiting, abdominal pain, diarrhea).

PATIENT/FAMILY TEACHING

Do not have immunizations without physician's approval (drug lowers body's resistance). Avoid crowds, persons with known infections. Report signs of infection at once (fever, flulike symptoms). Contact physician if nausea/vomiting continues at home. Avoid pregnancy during therapy.

I

ibuprofen

eye-byew-**pro**-fen

(Advil, Apo-Ibuprofen✱ Motrin, Novoprofen✱, Nuprin)

FIXED-COMBINATION(S)

Vicoprofen: ibuprofen/hydrocodone (a narcotic analgesic): 200 mg/7.5 mg. **Children's Advil Cold:** ibuprofen/pseudoephedrine (a nasal decongestant): 100 mg/15 mg per 5 ml.

CLASSIFICATION

PHARMACOTHERAPEUTIC: Nonsteroidal anti-inflammatory. **CLINICAL:** Antirheumatic, analgesic, antipyretic, antidysmenorrheal, vascular headache suppressant (see p. 110C).

ACTION

Inhibits prostaglandin synthesis. Produces vasodilation in hypothalamus. **Therapeutic Effect:** Produces analgesic/anti-inflammatory effect, decreases elevated body temperature.

PHARMACOKINETICS

Onset	Peak	Duration
PO (analgesic)		
0.5 hr	—	4–6 hrs
PO (antirheumatic)		
2 days	1–2 wks	—

Rapidly absorbed from GI tract. Protein binding: >90%. Metabolized in liver. Primarily excreted in urine. Not removed by hemodialysis. **Half-life:** 2–4 hrs.

USES

Treatment of inflammatory diseases, rheumatoid disorders (e.g., juvenile rheumatoid arthritis), mild to moderate pain, migraine pain, fever, dysmenorrhea, gout. **Unlabeled:** Treatment of psoriatic arthritis, vascular headaches.

PRECAUTIONS

CONTRAINDICATIONS: Active peptic ulcer, GI ulceration, chronic inflammation of GI tract, GI bleeding disorders, history of hypersensitivity to aspirin, NSAIDs. **CAUTIONS:** CHF, hypertension, reduced renal/liver function, dehydration, GI disease (e.g., bleeding, ulcers), concurrent anticoagulant use.

LIFESPAN CONSIDERATIONS: Pregnancy/lactation: Unknown if drug crosses placenta or is distributed in breast milk. Avoid use during third trimester (may adversely affect fetal cardiovascular system: premature closure of ductus arteriosus). **Pregnancy Category B** (**D** if used in third trimester or near delivery). **Children:** Safety and efficacy not established in those <6 mos. **Elderly:** GI bleeding/ulceration more likely to cause serious adverse effects. Age-related renal impairment may increase risk of liver/renal toxicity; reduced dosage recommended.

INTERACTIONS

DRUG: May increase effects of **oral anticoagulants, heparin, thrombolytics.** May decrease effect of **antihy-**

pertensives, diuretics. **Salicylates, aspirin** may increase risk of GI side effects, bleeding. **Bone marrow depressants** may increase risk of hematologic reactions. May increase concentration, toxicity of **lithium.** May increase **methotrexate** toxicity. **Probenecid** may increase concentration. **HERBAL: Feverfew** effect may be decreased. **Ginkgo biloba** may increase risk of bleeding. **FOOD:** None known. **LAB VALUES:** May prolong bleeding time. May alter blood glucose. May increase BUN, creatinine, potassium, liver function tests. May decrease Hgb, Hct.

AVAILABILITY (Rx)

CAPSULE: 200 mg **TABLETS:** 20 mg, 100 mg, (OTC), 300 mg, 400 mg, 600 mg, 800 mg. **TABLETS (chewable):** 50 mg, 100 mg. **ORAL SUSPENSION:** 100 mg/5 ml (OTC). **ORAL DROPS:** 40 mg/ml.

ADMINISTRATION/HANDLING

PO

• Do not crush or break enteric-coated form. • Give with food, milk, antacids if GI distress occurs.

INDICATIONS/ROUTES/DOSAGE

ACUTE/CHRONIC RHEUMATOID ARTHRITIS, OSTEOARTHRITIS

PO: ADULTS, ELDERLY: 400–800 mg 3–4 times/day. **Maximum:** 3.2 g.

MILD TO MODERATE PAIN, PRIMARY DYSMENORRHEA

PO: ADULTS, ELDERLY: 200–400 mg q4–6h as needed. **Maximum:** 1.6 g.

FEVER, MINOR ACHES/PAIN

PO: ADULTS, ELDERLY: 200–400 mg q4–6h. **Maximum:** 1.6 g/day. CHILDREN: 5–10 mg/kg/dose q6–8h. **Maximum:** 40 mg/kg/day. **OTC:** 7.5 mg/kg/dose q6–8h. **Maximum:** 30 mg/kg/day.

JUVENILE ARTHRITIS

PO: CHILDREN: 30–70 mg/kg/24 hrs in 3–4 divided doses. **Maximum:** <20 KG: 400 mg/day. 20–30 KG: 600 mg/day. 30–40 KG: 800 mg/day.

SIDE EFFECTS

OCCASIONAL (3%–9%): Nausea (with or without vomiting), dyspepsia (heartburn, indigestion, epigastric pain), dizziness, rash. **RARE (<3%):** Diarrhea/constipation, flatulence, abdominal cramping/pain, itching.

ADVERSE REACTIONS/ TOXIC EFFECTS

Acute overdosage may result in metabolic acidosis. Peptic ulcer, GI bleeding, gastritis, severe hepatic reaction (cholestasis, jaundice) occur rarely. Nephrotoxicity (dysuria, hematuria, proteinuria, nephrotic syndrome), severe hypersensitivity reaction (particularly in pts with systemic lupus erythematosus, other collagen diseases) occur rarely.

NURSING IMPLICATIONS

BASELINE ASSESSMENT

Assess onset, type, location, duration of pain/inflammation. Inspect appearance of affected joints for immobility, deformities, skin condition. Assess temperature.

INTERVENTION/EVALUATION

Monitor for evidence of nausea, dyspepsia. Monitor CBC, liver/renal function tests. Monitor pattern of daily bowel activity/stool consistency. Assess skin for evidence of rash. Evaluate for therapeutic response: relief of pain, stiffness, swelling; increase in joint mobility; reduced joint tenderness; improved grip strength. Monitor temperature for evidence of fever.

PATIENT/FAMILY TEACHING

Avoid aspirin, alcohol during therapy (increases risk of GI bleeding). If GI upset occurs, take with food, milk, antacids. Do not crush/chew enteric-coated tablet. May cause dizziness.

I

ibutilide fumarate

eye-**byewt**-ih-lied
(Corvert)

◆**CLASSIFICATION**

CLINICAL: Antiarrhythmic (see p. 15C).

ACTION

Prolongs both atrial and ventricular action potential duration; increases atrial and ventricular refractory period. **Therapeutic Effect:** Activates slow, inward current (sodium), produces mild slowing of sinus rate and AV conduction, dose-related prolongation of QT interval. Converts arrhythmias to sinus rhythm.

PHARMACOKINETICS

After IV administration, highly distributed, rapidly cleared. Protein binding: 40%. Primarily excreted in urine as metabolite. **Half-life:** 2–12 hrs (avg: 6 hrs).

USES

Rapid conversion of atrial fibrillation/flutter of new or recent onset to sinus rhythm (arrhythmias of longer duration less likely to respond to therapy).

PRECAUTIONS

CONTRAINDICATIONS: None known. **CAUTIONS:** Abnormal liver function, heart block.

LIFESPAN CONSIDERATIONS: Pregnancy/lactation: Teratogenic, embryocidal in animals. Discourage breast-feeding during therapy. **Pregnancy Category C. Children:** Safety and efficacy not established. **Elderly:** No age-related precautions noted.

INTERACTIONS

DRUG: Do not give concurrently with **class Ia (disopyramide, quinidine, procainamide, moricizine)** or **class III (amiodarone, sotalol, bretylium) antiarrhythmics** or within 4 hrs postinfusion of ibutilide. **Phenothiazines, tricyclic** and **tetracyclic antidepressants, H_1 receptor antagonists** may prolong QT interval. **HERBAL:** None known. **FOOD:** None known. **LAB VALUES:** None known.

AVAILABILITY (Rx)

INJECTION: 0.1 mg/ml solution.

ADMINISTRATION/HANDLING

IV

Storage • Compatible with D_5W, 0.9% NaCl. Compatible with polyvinyl chloride plastic, polyolefin bag admixtures. • Admixtures with diluent are stable at room temperature for 24 hrs, 48 hrs if refrigerated.

Reconstitution • Give undiluted or may dilute in 50 ml diluent.

Rate of administration • Give over 10 min. • Monitor pt with continuous EKG reading for at least 4 hrs after infusion or until QT interval has returned to baseline.

IV INCOMPATIBILITY

No information available for Y-site administration.

INDICATIONS/ROUTES/DOSAGE

ATRIAL ARRHYTHMIAS

IV infusion: ADULTS, ELDERLY ≥60 KG (132 LBS): One vial (1 mg) given over 10 min. If arrhythmia does not stop within 10 min after end of initial infusion, a second 1 mg/10 min infusion may be given. ADULTS, ELDERLY <60 KG (132 LBS): 0.01 mg/kg given over 10 min. If arrhythmia does not stop within 10 min after end of initial infusion, a second 0.01 mg/kg, 10 min infusion may be given.

SIDE EFFECTS

Generally well tolerated. **OCCASIONAL:** Ventricular extrasystoles (5.1%); ventricular tachycardia (4.9%); headache (3.6%); hypotension, postural hypotension (2%). **RARE:** Bundle-branch block, AV block, bradycardia, hypertension.

ADVERSE REACTIONS/ TOXIC EFFECTS

Sustained polymorphic ventricular tachycardia, occasionally with QT prolongation (torsades de pointes) occurs rarely. Overdosage results in CNS toxicity (CNS depression, rapid gasping breathing, seizures). May exaggerate expected prolongation of repolarization. May worsen existing arrhythmias, produce new arrhythmias.

NURSING IMPLICATIONS

BASELINE ASSESSMENT

Those with atrial fibrillation of >2–3 days' duration must be treated with anticoagulants generally for at least 2 wks prior to ibutilide therapy. Advanced cardiac life support equipment, medications, and trained personnel must be available during and after administration. Anticipate proarrhythmic events.

INTERVENTION/EVALUATION

Observe pt with continuous EKG monitoring for at least 4 hrs following infusion or until QT interval has returned to baseline. If any arrhythmic activity is noted, continue EKG monitoring. Monitor for symptoms of electrolyte abnormalities, esp. magnesium and potassium, and for arrhythmias requiring overdrive cardiac pacing, electrical cardioversion, defibrillation.

idarubicin hydrochloride

eye-dah-**roo**-bi-sin
(Idamycin PFS)
Do not confuse with Adriamycin, doxorubicin.

CLASSIFICATION

PHARMACOTHERAPEUTIC: Anthracycline antibiotic. **CLINICAL:** Antineoplastic (see p. 73C).

ACTION

Inhibits nucleic acid synthesis by interacting with the enzyme topoisomerase II (an enzyme promoting DNA strand supercoiling). **Therapeutic Effect:** Produces death of rapidly dividing cells.

PHARMACOKINETICS

Widely distributed. Protein binding: 97%. Rapidly metabolized in liver to active metabolite. Primarily eliminated via biliary excretion. Not removed by hemodialysis. **Half-life:** 4–46 hrs; metabolite: 8–92 hrs.

USES

Treatment of acute myeloid leukemia (AML).

PRECAUTIONS

CONTRAINDICATIONS: Preexisting bone marrow suppression, severe CHF, cardiomyopathy, arrhythmias, pregnancy. **CAUTIONS:** Impaired renal/liver function, concurrent radiation therapy.

LIFESPAN CONSIDERATIONS: Pregnancy/lactation: If possible, avoid use during pregnancy (may be embryotoxic). Unknown if drug is distributed in breast milk (advise to discontinue breast-feeding before drug initiation). **Pregnancy Category D. Children:** Safety and efficacy not established. **Elderly:** Cardiotoxicity may be more frequent. Caution in those with inadequate bone marrow reserves. Age-related renal impairment may require dosage adjustment.

INTERACTIONS

DRUG: May decrease effect of **antigout medications. Bone marrow depressants** may increase bone marrow depression. **Live virus vaccines** may potentiate virus replication, increase vaccine side effects, decrease pt's antibody response to vaccine. **HERBAL:** None known. **FOOD:** None known. **LAB VALUES:** May increase uric acid, SGOT (AST), SGPT (ALT), alkaline phosphatase, bilirubin. May cause EKG changes.

I

AVAILABILITY (Rx)

INJECTION: 5 mg, 10 mg, 20 mg.

ADMINISTRATION/HANDLING

Alert: Give by free-flowing IV infusion (**never** subcutaneous or IM). Gloves, gowns, eye goggles recommended during preparation/administration of medication. If powder/solution comes in contact with skin, wash thoroughly. Avoid small veins, swollen/edematous extremities, areas overlying joints/tendons.

IV

Storage • Reconstituted solution is stable for 72 hrs (3 days) at room temperature or 168 hrs (7 days) if refrigerated. • Discard unused solution.

Alert: Idamycin Prefilled Syringe (PFS) does not require reconstitution and is stored refrigerated.

Reconstitution • Reconstitute each 10-mg vial with 10 ml 0.9% NaCl (5 ml/5 mg vial) to provide a concentration of 1 mg/ml.

Rate of administration • Administer into tubing of freely running IV infusion of D_5W or 0.9% NaCl, preferably via butterfly needle, **slowly** (>10–15 min). • Extravasation produces immediate pain, severe local tissue damage. Terminate infusion immediately. Apply cold compresses for ½ hr immediately, then ½ hr 4 times/day for 3 days. Keep extremity elevated.

IV INCOMPATIBILITIES

Acyclovir (Zovirax), allopurinol (Aloprim), ampicillin-sulbactam (Unasyn), cefazolin (Ancef, Kefzol), cefepime (Maxipime), ceftazidime (Fortaz), clindamycin (Cleocin), dexamethasone (Decadron), furosemide (Lasix), hydrocortisone (Solu-Cortef), lorazepam (Ativan), meperidine (Demerol), methotrexate, piperacillin/tazobactam (Zosyn), sodium bicarbonate, teniposide (Vumon), vancomycin (Vancocin), vincristine (Oncovin).

IV COMPATIBILITIES

Diphenhydramine (Benadryl), granisetron (Kytril), magnesium, potassium.

INDICATIONS/ROUTES/DOSAGE

Alert: Dosage individualized based on clinical response, tolerance to adverse effects. When used in combination therapy, consult specific protocols for optimum dosage, sequence of drug administration.

USUAL DOSE

IV: ADULTS: 8–12 mg/m^2/day for 3 days (combined with Ara-C). CHILDREN (solid tumor): 5 mg/m^2 once daily for 3 days. CHILDREN (leukemia): 10–12 mg/m^2 once daily for 3 days.

DOSAGE IN HEPATIC/RENAL IMPAIRMENT

	Dose Reduction
Serum creatinine ≥2	25%
Bilirubin >2.5	50%
Bilirubin >5	Do not give

SIDE EFFECTS

FREQUENT: Nausea, vomiting (82%); complete alopecia (scalp, axillary, pubic hair) (77%); abdominal cramping, diarrhea (73%); mucositis (50%). **OCCA-**

SIONAL: Hyperpigmentation of nailbeds, phalangeal/dermal creases (46%); fever (36%); headache (20%). **RARE:** Conjunctivitis, neuropathy.

ADVERSE REACTIONS/ TOXIC EFFECTS

Bone marrow depression manifested as hematologic toxicity (principally leukopenia and, to lesser extent, anemia, thrombocytopenia) generally occurs within 10–15 days, returns to normal levels by third week. Cardiotoxicity noted as either acute, transient abnormal EKG findings and/or cardiomyopathy manifested as CHF may occur.

NURSING IMPLICATIONS

BASELINE ASSESSMENT

Determine baseline renal/hepatic function, CBC results. Obtain EKG prior to therapy. Antiemetic prior to and during therapy may prevent/relieve nausea/vomiting. Inform pt of high potential for alopecia.

INTERVENTION/EVALUATION

Monitor CBC with differential, platelet count, EKG, renal/liver function tests. Monitor for hematologic toxicity (fever, sore throat, signs of local infection, unusual bleeding/bruising from any site), symptoms of anemia (excessive tiredness, weakness). Avoid IM injections, rectal temperatures, other trauma that may precipitate bleeding. Check infusion site frequently for extravasation (causes severe local necrosis). Assess for potentially fatal CHF (dyspnea, rales, pulmonary edema), life-threatening arrhythmias.

PATIENT/FAMILY TEACHING

Total body alopecia is frequent but reversible. Assist with ways to cope with hair loss. New hair growth resumes 2–3 mos after last therapy dose and may have different color, texture. Maintain fastidious oral hygiene. Avoid crowds, those with infections. Teach pt/family the early signs of bleeding/infection. Inform physician of fever, sore throat, bleeding, bruising. Urine may turn pink/red. Use contraceptive measures during therapy.

ifosfamide

eye-**fos**-fah-mid
(Ifex)

◆CLASSIFICATION

PHARMACOTHERAPEUTIC: Alkylating agent. **CLINICAL:** Antineoplastic (see p. 73C).

ACTION

Converted to active metabolite, binds with intracellular structures. Action primarily due to cross-linking strands of DNA, RNA. **Therapeutic Effect:** Inhibits protein synthesis.

PHARMACOKINETICS

Metabolized in liver to active metabolite. Crosses blood-brain barrier (limited). Primarily excreted in urine. Removed by hemodialysis. **Half-life:** 15 hrs.

USES

Chemotherapy of germ cell testicular carcinoma (used in combination with agents that protect against hemorrhagic cystitis). **Unlabeled:** Treatment of soft tissue sarcoma, Ewing's sarcoma, non-Hodgkin's lymphoma, lung/pancreatic carcinoma.

PRECAUTIONS

CONTRAINDICATIONS: Severely depressed bone marrow function, pregnancy. **CAUTIONS:** Impaired renal/liver function, compromised bone marrow function.

I

LIFESPAN CONSIDERATIONS: Pregnancy/lactation: If possible, avoid use during pregnancy, esp. first trimester. May cause fetal harm. Drug is distributed in breast milk. Breast-feeding not recommended. **Pregnancy Category D. Children:** Not intended for this pt population. **Elderly:** Age-related renal impairment may require dosage adjustment.

INTERACTIONS

DRUG: Bone marrow depressants may increase bone marrow depression. **Live virus vaccines** may potentiate virus replication, increase vaccine side effects, decrease pt's antibody response to vaccine. **HERBAL:** None known. **FOOD:** None known. **LAB VALUES:** May increase BUN, creatinine, uric acid, SGOT (AST), SGPT (ALT), LDH, bilirubin.

AVAILABILITY (Rx)

POWDER FOR INJECTION: 1 g, 3 g.

ADMINISTRATION/HANDLING

Alert: May be carcinogenic, mutagenic, or teratogenic. Handle with extreme care during preparation/administration.

IV

Storage • Store vial at room temperature. • After reconstitution with Bacteriostatic Water for Injection, solution is stable for 1 wk at room temperature, 3 wks if refrigerated (further diluted solution is stable for 6 wks if refrigerated). • Solution prepared with other diluents should be used within 6 hrs.

Reconstitution • Reconstitute 1-g vial with 20 ml Sterile Water for Injection or Bacteriostatic Water for Injection to provide a concentration of 50 mg/ml. Shake to dissolve. • Further dilute with D_5W or 0.9% NaCl to provide concentration of 0.6–20 mg/ml.

Rate of administration • Infuse over a minimum of 30 min. • Give with at least 2,000 ml PO or IV fluid (prevents bladder toxicity). • Give with a protectant against hemorrhagic cystitis (i.e., mesna).

⊘ IV INCOMPATIBILITIES

Cefepime (Maxipime), methotrexate.

IV COMPATIBILITIES

Granisetron (Kytril), ondansetron (Zofran).

INDICATIONS/ROUTES/DOSAGE

Alert: Dosage individualized based on clinical response, tolerance to adverse effects. When used in combination therapy, consult specific protocols for optimum dosage, sequence of drug administration.

GERM CELL TESTICULAR CARCINOMA

IV: ADULTS: 700–2,000 mg/m^2/day for 5 consecutive days. Repeat q3wks or after recovery from hematologic toxicity. Administer with mesna.

USUAL PEDIATRIC DOSAGE

IV: 1,200–1,800 mg/m^2/day for 5 days q21–28days.

SIDE EFFECTS

FREQUENT: Alopecia (83%); nausea, vomiting (58%). **OCCASIONAL (5%–15%):** Confusion, somnolence, hallucinations, infection. **RARE (<5%):** Dizziness, seizures, disorientation, fever, malaise, stomatitis (mucosal irritation, glossitis, gingivitis).

ADVERSE REACTIONS/ TOXIC EFFECTS

Hemorrhagic cystitis with hematuria, dysuria occurs frequently if a protective agent (mesna) is not used. Myelosuppression characterized as leukopenia, and, to a lesser extent, thrombocytopenia, occurs frequently. Pulmonary toxicity, hepatotoxicity, nephrotoxicity, cardiotoxicity, CNS toxicity (confusion, hallucinations, somnolence, coma) may require discontinuation of therapy.

NURSING IMPLICATIONS

BASELINE ASSESSMENT

Obtain urinalysis prior to each dose. If hematuria occurs (>10 RBCs per field), therapy should be withheld until resolution occurs. Obtain WBC, platelet count, Hgb prior to each dose.

INTERVENTION/EVALUATION

Monitor hematologic studies, urinalysis diligently. Assess for fever, sore throat, signs of local infection, unusual bleeding/easy bruising from any site, symptoms of anemia (excessive tiredness, weakness).

PATIENT/FAMILY TEACHING

Maintain copious daily fluid intake (protects against cystitis). Do not have immunizations without physician's approval (drug lowers body's resistance). Avoid contact with those who have recently received live virus vaccine. Avoid crowds, those with infections. Report unusual bleeding/bruising, fever, chills, sore throat, joint pain, sores in mouth or on lips, yellowing skin/eyes. Hemorrhagic cystitis occurs if mesna not given concurrently. Mesna should always be given with ifosfamide.

imatinib mesylate

ih-**mah**-tin-ib
(Gleevec)

◆CLASSIFICATION

PHARMACOTHERAPEUTIC: Protein-tyrosine kinase inhibitor. **CLINICAL:** Antineoplastic (see p. 73C).

ACTION

Inhibits the Bcr-Abl tyrosine kinase, a translocation-created enzyme, created by the Philadelphia chromosome abnormality noted in chronic myeloid leukemia (CML). **Therapeutic Effect:** Inhibits proliferation, tumor growth during the three stages of CML: CML in myeloid blast crisis, CML in accelerated phase, CML in chronic phase.

PHARMACOKINETICS

Well absorbed following PO administration. Binds to plasma proteins, particularly albumin. Metabolized in the liver. Eliminated mainly in the feces as metabolites. **Half-life:** 18 hrs.

USES

Treatment of pts with CML in blast crisis, accelerated phase, or chronic phase after failure of interferon-alfa therapy. First-line treatment for CML.

PRECAUTIONS

CONTRAINDICATIONS: Known hypersensitivity to imatinib. **CAUTIONS:** Hepatic/renal impairment.

LIFESPAN CONSIDERATIONS: Pregnancy/lactation: Has potential for severe teratogenic effects. Avoid breastfeeding. **Pregnancy Category D. Children:** Safety and efficacy not established. **Elderly:** Increased frequency of fluid retention noted.

INTERACTIONS

DRUG: Ketoconazole, itraconazole, erythromycin, clarithromycin increase imatinib plasma concentration. **Dexamethasone, phenytoin, carbamazepine, rifampicin, phenobarbital** decrease imatinib plasma concentration. Increases **simvastatin, triazolobenzodiazepines, dihydropyridine, calcium channel blockers** concentration. May alter **cyclosporine, pimozide** therapeutic effect. Reduces **warfarin** effect. **HERBAL: St. John's wort** decreases imatinib concentration. **FOOD:** None known. **LAB VALUES:** May decrease WBC, platelets, potassium. May increase transaminase, bilirubin.

AVAILABILITY (Rx)

TABLETS: 100 mg, 400 mg.

ADMINISTRATION/HANDLING

PO

- Give with a meal and a large glass of water.

INDICATIONS/ROUTES/DOSAGE

CHRONIC MYELOID LEUKEMIA (CML)

PO: ADULTS, ELDERLY: 400 mg/day for pts in chronic phase CML; 600 mg/day for pts in accelerated phase or blast crisis. May increase dose 400–600 mg/day for pts in chronic phase or 600–800 mg (given as 400 mg twice/day) for pts in accelerated phase/blast crisis in absence of severe drug reaction or severe neutropenia/thrombocytopenia in the following circumstances: progression of the disease, failure to achieve satisfactory hematologic response after ≥3 mos treatment, loss of previously achieved hematologic response. CHILDREN: 260 mg/m^2 daily as a single daily dose or 2 divided doses.

SIDE EFFECTS

FREQUENT (24%–68%): Nausea, diarrhea, vomiting, headache, fluid retention (periorbital, lower extremities), rash, musculoskeletal pain, muscle cramps, arthralgia. **OCCASIONAL (10%–23%):** Abdominal pain, cough, myalgia, fatigue, pyrexia, anorexia, dyspepsia (heartburn, gastric upset), constipation, night sweats, pruritus. **RARE (<10%):** Nasopharyngitis, petechiae, weakness, epistaxis.

ADVERSE REACTIONS/ TOXIC EFFECTS

Severe fluid retention (pleural effusion, pericardial effusion, pulmonary edema, ascites), hepatotoxicity occur rarely. Neutropenia, thrombocytopenia are expected responses to the drug. Respiratory toxicity is manifested as dyspnea, pneumonia.

NURSING IMPLICATIONS

BASELINE ASSESSMENT

Obtain CBC weekly for first month, biweekly for second month, and periodically thereafter. Monitor liver function tests (transaminase, bilirubin, alkaline phosphatase) prior to beginning treatment and monthly thereafter.

INTERVENTION/EVALUATION

Assess eye area, lower extremities for early evidence of fluid retention. Weigh and monitor for unexpected rapid weight gain. Offer antiemetics to control nausea, vomiting. Monitor stool frequency, consistency. Monitor CBC for evidence of neutropenia, thrombocytopenia; assess liver function tests for hepatotoxicity. Duration of neutropenia/thrombocytopenia ranges from 2–4 wks.

PATIENT/FAMILY TEACHING

Avoid crowds, those with known infection. Avoid contact with anyone who recently received live virus vaccine; do not receive vaccinations. Take with food and a full glass of water.

Imdur

see isosorbide

imiglucerase

im-ih-**gloo**-sir-ace
(Cerezyme)

Do not confuse with Cerebyx, Ceredase.

CLASSIFICATION

CLINICAL: Enzyme.

ACTION

Analogue of enzyme beta-glucocerebrosidase, which catalyzes hydrolysis of glycolipid glucocerebroside to glucose and ceramide. **Therapeutic Effect:** Minimizes conditions associated with Gaucher's disease (e.g., anemia, bone disease).

USES

Long-term treatment of Gaucher's disease.

PRECAUTIONS

CONTRAINDICATIONS: None known. **CAUTIONS:** None known. **Pregnancy Category C.**

INTERACTIONS

DRUG: None known. **HERBAL:** None known. **FOOD:** None known. **LAB VALUES:** None known.

AVAILABILITY (Rx)

POWDER FOR INJECTION: 214 units, 424 units.

ADMINISTRATION/HANDLING

IV

Storage • Refrigerate. • Once reconstituted, stable for 24 hrs if refrigerated.

Reconstitution • Reconstitute with 5.1 ml sterile water to provide concentration of 40 units/ml. • Further dilute with 100–200 ml 0.9% NaCl.

Rate of administration • Infuse over 1–2 hrs.

IV INCOMPATIBILITY

Do not mix with any other medication.

INDICATIONS/ROUTES/DOSAGE

GAUCHER'S DISEASE

IV infusion (over 1–2 hrs): ADULTS, ELDERLY, CHILDREN: Initially, 2.5 units/kg 3 times/wk up to 60 units/kg/wk. MAINTENANCE: Progressive reduction in dosage while monitoring pt response.

SIDE EFFECTS

FREQUENT (3%): Headache. **OCCASIONAL (1%–<3%):** Nausea, abdominal discomfort, dizziness, pruritus, rash, small decrease in B/P, urinary frequency.

NURSING IMPLICATIONS

INTERVENTION/EVALUATION

Monitor CBC, platelets, liver function.

imipenem/cilastatin sodium

im-ih-**peh**-nem/sill-as-**tah**-tin (Primaxin)

CLASSIFICATION

PHARMACOTHERAPEUTIC: Fixed-combination carbapenem. **CLINICAL:** Antibiotic.

ACTION

Imipenem: Binds to bacterial membrane. **Therapeutic Effect:** Inhibits cell wall synthesis. Bactericidal. **Cilastatin:** Competitively inhibits the enzyme, dehydropeptidase. **Therapeutic Effect:** Prevents renal metabolism of imipenem.

PHARMACOKINETICS

Readily absorbed after IM administration. Widely distributed. Protein binding: 13%–21%. Metabolized in kidney. Primarily excreted in urine. Removed by hemodialysis. **Half-life:** 1 hr (half-life increased with impaired renal function).

USES

Treatment of respiratory tract, skin/skin structure, gynecologic, bone/joint, intra-abdominal, complicated/uncomplicated urinary tract infections; endocarditis; polymicrobic infections; septicemia; serious nosocomial infections.

PRECAUTIONS

CONTRAINDICATIONS: None known. **CAUTIONS:** History of seizures, sensitivity to penicillins, impaired renal function.

LIFESPAN CONSIDERATIONS: Pregnancy/lactation: Crosses placenta. Distributed in cord blood, amniotic fluid, breast milk. **Pregnancy Category C. Children:** No precautions in those <12 yrs. **Elderly:** Age-related renal function impairment may require dosage adjustment.

INTERACTIONS

DRUG: None known. **HERBAL:** None known. **FOOD:** None known. **LAB VALUES:** May increase SGOT (AST), SGPT (ALT), alkaline phosphatase, LDH, bilirubin, BUN, creatinine. May decrease Hgb, Hct.

AVAILABILITY (Rx)

INJECTION FOR IM: 500 mg, 750 mg. **INJECTION FOR IV:** 250 mg, 500 mg.

ADMINISTRATION/HANDLING

IM

• Prepare with 1% lidocaine without epinephrine; 500-mg vial with 2 ml, 750-mg vial with 3 ml lidocaine HCl. • Administer suspension within 1 hr of preparation. • Do not mix with any other medications. • Inject deep in large muscle; aspirate to decrease risk of injection into a blood vessel.

IV

Storage • Solution appears colorless to yellow; discard if solution turns brown. • IV infusion (piggyback) is stable for 4 hrs at room temperature, 24 hrs if refrigerated. • Discard if precipitate forms.

Reconstitution • Dilute each 250- or 500-mg vial with 100 ml D_5W; 0.9% NaCl.

Rate of administration • Give by intermittent IV infusion (piggyback). Do not give IV push. • Infuse over 20–30 min (1-g dose >40–60 min). • Observe pt during first 30 min of infusion for possible hypersensitivity reaction.

IV INCOMPATIBILITIES

Allopurinol (Aloprim), amphotericin B complex (Abelcet, AmBisome, Amphotec), fluconazole (Diflucan).

IV COMPATIBILITIES

Diltiazem (Cardizem), insulin, propofol (Diprivan).

INDICATIONS/ROUTES/DOSAGE

SERIOUS INFECTIONS

IV: ADULTS, ELDERLY: 2–4 g/day in divided doses q6h.

MILD TO MODERATE INFECTIONS

IV: ADULTS, ELDERLY: 1–2 g/day in divided doses q6–8h.

USUAL PEDIATRIC DOSAGE

IV: ≥3 MOS–12 YRS: 60–100 mg/kg/day in divided doses q6h. **Maximum:** 4 g/day. 1–3 MOS: 100 mg/kg/day in divided doses q6h. <1 MO: 20–25 mg/kg/dose q8–24h.

USUAL IM DOSAGE

ADULTS, ELDERLY: 500–750 mg q12h.

DOSAGE IN RENAL IMPAIRMENT

Dose and/or frequency is modified based on creatinine clearance and/or severity of infection.

Creatinine Clearance	Dosage
31–70 ml/min	500 mg q8h
21–30 ml/min	500 mg q12h
0–20 ml/min	250 mg q12h

SIDE EFFECTS

OCCASIONAL (2%–3%): Diarrhea, nausea, vomiting. **RARE (1%–2%):** Rash.

ADVERSE REACTIONS/ TOXIC EFFECTS

Antibiotic-associated colitis, other superinfections may occur. Anaphylactic reactions in pts receiving beta-lactams have occurred.

NURSING IMPLICATIONS

BASELINE ASSESSMENT

Question for history of allergies, particularly to beta-lactams, penicillins, cephalosporins. Inquire about history of seizures.

INTERVENTION/EVALUATION

Monitor renal, liver, hematologic function tests. Evaluate for phlebitis (heat, pain, red streaking over vein), pain at IV injection site. Assess for GI discomfort, nausea, vomiting. Determine pattern of bowel activity/stool consistency. Assess skin for rash. Be alert to tremors, possible seizures.

imipramine

ih-**mih**-prah-meen
(Apo-Imipramine✤, Tofranil, Tofranil-PM)

Do not confuse with desipramine.

CLASSIFICATION

PHARMACOTHERAPEUTIC: Tricyclic. **CLINICAL:** Antidepressant, antineuritic, antipanic, antineuralgic, antinarcoleptic adjunct, anticataplectic, antibulimic (see p. 35C).

ACTION

Blocks reuptake of neurotransmitters (norepinephrine, serotonin) at presynaptic membranes, increasing concentration at postsynaptic receptor sites. **Therapeutic Effect:** Results in antidepressant effect. Anticholinergic effect controls nocturnal enuresis.

USES

Treatment of various forms of depression, often in conjunction with psychotherapy. Treatment of nocturnal enuresis in children >6 yrs. **Unlabeled:** Treatment of panic disorder, neurogenic pain, attention deficit hyperactivity disorder (ADHD), cataplexy associated with narcolepsy.

PRECAUTIONS

CONTRAINDICATIONS: Acute recovery period after MI, within 14 days of MAOI ingestion. **CAUTIONS:** Prostatic hypertrophy, history of urinary retention/obstruction, glaucoma, diabetes mellitus, history of seizures, hyperthyroidism, cardiac/hepatic/renal disease, schizophrenia, increased intraocular pressure, hiatal hernia. **Pregnancy Category D.**

INTERACTIONS

DRUG: **Alcohol, CNS depressants** may increase CNS, respiratory depression, hypotensive effects. **Antithyroid agents** may increase risk of agranulocytosis. **Phenothiazines** may increase sedative, anticholinergic effects. **Cimetidine** may increase concentration, toxicity. May decrease effects of **clonidine, guanadrel.** May increase cardiac effects with **sympathomimetics.** May increase risk of hypertensive crisis, hyperpyrexia, seizures with **MAOIs. Phenytoin** may decrease concentrations. **HERBAL:** **Ginkgo biloba** may decrease seizure threshold. **St. John's wort** may have additive effect. **FOOD:** None known. **LAB VALUES:** May alter EKG readings, glucose. Therapeutic blood serum level: 225–300 ng/ml; toxic blood serum level: >500 ng/ml.

AVAILABILITY (Rx)

TABLETS: 10 mg, 25 mg, 50 mg. **CAPSULES:** 75 mg, 100 mg, 125 mg, 150 mg.

ADMINISTRATION/HANDLING

PO

• Give with food or milk if GI distress occurs. • Do not crush or break film-coated tablets.

INDICATIONS/ROUTES/DOSAGE

DEPRESSION

PO: ADULTS: Initially, 75–100 mg daily. Dosage may be gradually increased to 300 mg daily for hospitalized pts, 200 mg for outpts, then reduce dosage to effective maintenance level (50–150 mg daily). ELDERLY: Initially, 10–25 mg/day at bedtime. May increase by 10–25 mg q3–7days. RANGE: 50–150 mg. CHILDREN: 1.5 mg/kg/day. May increase 1 mg/kg q3–4days. **Maximum:** 5 mg/kg/day.

CHILDHOOD ENURESIS

PO: CHILDREN >6 YRS: Initially, 10–25 mg at bedtime. May increase by 25 mg/day. **Maximum 6–12 yrs:** 50 mg. **Maximum >12 yrs:** 75 mg.

SIDE EFFECTS

FREQUENT: Drowsiness, fatigue, dry mouth, blurred vision, constipation, delayed micturition, postural hypotension, diaphoresis, disturbed concentration, increased appetite, urinary retention, photosensitivity. **OCCASIONAL:** GI disturbances (nausea, metallic taste sensation). **RARE:** Paradoxical reaction (agitation, restlessness, nightmares, insomnia), extrapyramidal symptoms (particularly fine hand tremor).

ADVERSE REACTIONS/ TOXIC EFFECTS

High dosage may produce cardiovascular effects (severe postural hypotension, dizziness, tachycardia, palpitations, arrhythmias), seizures. May result in altered temperature regulation (hyperpyrexia, hypothermia). Abrupt withdrawal from prolonged therapy may produce headache, malaise, nausea, vomiting, vivid dreams.

NURSING IMPLICATIONS

BASELINE ASSESSMENT

For pts on long-term therapy, liver/renal function tests, blood counts should be performed periodically.

INTERVENTION/EVALUATION

Supervise suicidal-risk pt closely during early therapy (as depression lessens, energy level improves, causing increased suicide potential). Assess appearance, behavior, speech pattern, level of interest, mood. Monitor pattern of daily bowel activity/stool consistency. Monitor B/P, pulse for hypotension, arrhythmias. Assess for urinary retention by bladder palpation. Therapeutic blood serum level: 225–300 ng/ml; toxic blood serum level: >500 ng/ml.

PATIENT/FAMILY TEACHING

Change positions slowly to avoid hypotensive effect. Tolerance to postural hypotension, sedative, anticholinergic effects usually develops during early therapy. Therapeutic effect may be noted within 2–5 days, maximum effect within 2–3 wks. Dry mouth may be relieved by sugarless gum, sips of tepid water. Do not abruptly discontinue medication. Avoid tasks that require alertness, motor skills until response to drug is established.

Imitrex

see sumatriptan

immune globulin IV (IGIV)

(Baygam ✤, Gamimune N, Gammagard, Gammar-IV, Gamunex, Polygam, Sandoglobulin, Venoglobulin-I)

Do not confuse with Sandimmune, Sandostatin.

CLASSIFICATION

CLINICAL: Immune serum.

ACTION

Increases antibody titer and antigen-antibody reaction. **Therapeutic Effect:** Provides passive immunity against infection. Induces rapid increase in platelet counts. Produces anti-inflammatory effect.

PHARMACOKINETICS

Evenly distributed between intravascular and extravascular space. **Half-life:** 21–23 days.

USES

Treatment of pts with primary immunodeficiency syndromes, idiopathic thrombocytopenia purpura (ITP), Kawasaki disease; prevention of recurrent bacterial infections in pts with hypogammaglobulinemia associated with B-cell chronic lymphocytic leukemia (CLL). Treatment adjunct in bone marrow transplantation. **Unlabeled:** Prevention of acute infections in immunosuppressed pts, control/prevention of infections in infants/children immunosuppressed in association with AIDS or ARC. Prophylaxis/treatment of infections in high-risk, preterm, low birth-weight neonates. Treatment of chronic inflammatory demyelinating polyneuropathies. Treatment of multiple sclerosis.

PRECAUTIONS

CONTRAINDICATIONS: History of allergic response to gamma globulin or anti-immunoglobulin A (IgA) antibodies, allergic response to thimerosal, pts with isolated immunoglobulin A (IgA) deficiency. IM also contraindicated in pts who have severe thrombocytopenia and any coagulation disorder. **CAUTIONS:** Cardiovascular disease, history of thrombosis, impaired renal function, diabetes, volume depletion, sepsis, concomitant nephrotoxic drugs.

LIFESPAN CONSIDERATIONS: Pregnancy/lactation: Unknown if drug crosses placenta or is distributed in breast milk. **Pregnancy Category C. Children/elderly:** No age-related precautions noted.

INTERACTIONS

DRUG: Live virus vaccines may potentiate virus replication, increase vaccine side effects, decrease pt's antibody response to vaccine. **HERBAL:** None known. **FOOD:** None known. **LAB VALUES:** None known.

AVAILABILITY (Rx)

INJECTION: 5%, 10%. **POWDER FOR INJECTION:** 0.5 g, 2.5 g, 6 g, 10 g, 20 g.

ADMINISTRATION/HANDLING

IV

Storage • Refer to individual IV preparations for storage requirements, stability after reconstitution.

Reconstitution • Reconstitute only with diluent provided by manufacturer. • Discard partially used or turbid preparations.

Rate of administration • Give by infusion only. • After reconstituted, administer via separate tubing. • Avoid mixing with other medication/IV infusion fluids. • Rate of infusion varies with product used. • Monitor vital signs, B/P diligently during and immediately after IV administration (precipitous fall in B/P may indicate anaphylactic reaction). Stop infusion immediately. Epinephrine should be readily available.

∅ **IV INCOMPATIBILITY**

Do not mix with any other medications.

INDICATIONS/ROUTES/DOSAGE

PRIMARY IMMUNODEFICIENCY SYNDROME

IV infusion: ADULTS, ELDERLY, CHILDREN: 200–400 mg/kg q1mo.

IDIOPATHIC THROMBOCYTOPENIA PURPURA (ITP)

IV infusion: ADULTS, ELDERLY, CHILDREN: 400–1,000 mg/kg/day for 2–5 days.

KAWASAKI DISEASE

IV infusion: ADULTS, ELDERLY, CHILDREN: 2 g/kg as a single dose.

CHRONIC LYMPHOCYTIC LEUKEMIA (CLL)

IV infusion: ADULTS, ELDERLY, CHILDREN: 400 mg/kg q3–4wks.

SIDE EFFECTS

FREQUENT: Tachycardia, backache, headache, joint/muscle pain. **OCCASIONAL:** Fatigue, wheezing, rash/pain at injection site, leg cramps, hives, bluish color of lips/nailbeds, lightheadedness.

ADVERSE REACTIONS/ TOXIC EFFECTS

Anaphylactic reactions occur rarely but there is increased incidence when repeated injections of immune globulin are given. Epinephrine should be readily available. Overdose may produce chest tightness, chills, diaphoresis, dizziness, flushed face, nausea, vomiting, fever, hypotension.

NURSING IMPLICATIONS

BASELINE ASSESSMENT

Inquire about history of exposure to disease for both pt and family as appropriate. Have epinephrine readily available. Well hydrate pt prior to use.

INTERVENTION/EVALUATION

Control rate of IV infusion carefully; too rapid infusion increases risk of precipitous fall in B/P, signs of anaphylaxis (facial flushing, chest tightness, chills, fever, nausea, vomiting, diaphoresis). Assess pt closely during infusion, esp. first hour; monitor vital signs continuously. Stop infusion temporarily if aforementioned signs noted. For treatment of ITP, monitor platelets.

PATIENT/FAMILY TEACHING

Explain rationale for therapy. Rapid response, lasts 1–3 mos. Inform physician if sudden weight gain, fluid retention, edema, decreased urine output, shortness of breath occur.

Imodium

see loperamide

indapamide

in-**dap**-ah-myd

(Lozide♣, Lozol)

Do not confuse with iodamide, iopamidol.

◆ CLASSIFICATION

PHARMACOTHERAPEUTIC: Thiazide. **CLINICAL:** Diuretic, antihypertensive (see p. 86C).

ACTION

Diuretic: Blocks reabsorption of water, electrolytes (sodium, potassium) at cortical diluting segment of distal tubule. **Therapeutic Effect:** Promotes renal excretion. **Antihypertensive:** Reduces plasma, extracellular fluid volume; decreases peripheral vascular resistance (PVR) by direct effect on blood vessels. **Therapeutic Effect:** Reduces B/P.

USES

Treatment of hypertension, edema associated with CHF. May be used alone or with antihypertensive agents.

PRECAUTIONS

CONTRAINDICATIONS: None known. **CAUTIONS:** History of hypersensitivity to sulfonamides or thiazide diuretics, renal decompensation, anuria. Severe renal disease, impaired hepatic function, diabetes mellitus, elderly/debilitated, thyroid disorders. **Pregnancy Category B** (**D** if used in pregnancy-induced hypertension).

INTERACTIONS

DRUG: May increase risk of **digoxin** toxicity (due to hypokalemia). May decrease clearance, increase toxicity of **lithium. HERBAL:** None known. **FOOD:** None known. **LAB VALUES:** May increase plasma renin activity. May decrease calcium, protein-bound iodine, potassium, sodium.

AVAILABILITY (Rx)

TABLETS: 1.25 mg, 2.5 mg.

ADMINISTRATION/HANDLING

PO

• Give with food, milk if GI upset occurs, preferably with breakfast (may prevent nocturia). • Do not crush or break tablets.

INDICATIONS/ROUTES/DOSAGE

EDEMA

PO: ADULTS: Initially, 2.5 mg/day, may increase to 5 mg/day after 1 wk.

HYPERTENSION

PO: ADULTS, ELDERLY: Initially, 1.25 mg, may increase to 2.5 mg/day after 4 wks or 5 mg/day after additional 4 wks.

SIDE EFFECTS

FREQUENT (>5%): Fatigue, numbness of extremities, tension, irritability, agitation, headache, dizziness, lightheadedness, insomnia, muscle cramping. **OCCASIONAL (<5%):** Tingling of extremities, frequent urination, polyuria, hives, rhinorrhea, flushing, weight loss, orthostatic hypotension, depression, blurred vision, nausea, vomiting, diarrhea/constipation, dry mouth, impotence, rash, pruritus.

ADVERSE REACTIONS/ TOXIC EFFECTS

Vigorous diuresis may lead to profound water loss/electrolyte depletion, resulting in hypokalemia, hyponatremia, dehydration. Acute hypotensive episodes may occur. Hyperglycemia may be noted during prolonged therapy. GI upset, pancreatitis, dizziness, paresthesias, headache, blood dyscrasias, pulmonary edema, allergic pneumonitis, dermatologic reactions occur rarely. Overdosage can lead to lethargy, coma without changes in electrolytes/hydration.

NURSING IMPLICATIONS

BASELINE ASSESSMENT

Check vital signs, esp. B/P for hypotension, prior to administration. Assess baseline electrolytes, particularly check for hypokalemia. Observe for edema; assess skin turgor, mucous membranes for hydration status. Assess muscle strength, mental status. Note skin temperature, moisture. Obtain baseline weight. Initiate I&O.

INTERVENTION/EVALUATION

Continue to monitor B/P, vital signs, electrolytes, I&O, weight. Note extent of diuresis. Watch for electrolyte disturbances (hypokalemia may result in weakness, tremor, muscle cramps, nausea, vomiting, change in mental status, tachycardia; hyponatremia may result in confusion, thirst, cold/clammy skin).

PATIENT/FAMILY TEACHING

Expect increased frequency/volume of urination. To reduce hypotensive effect, rise slowly from lying to sitting position, permit legs to dangle momentarily before standing. Eat foods high in potassium such as whole grains (cereals), legumes, meat, bananas, apricots, orange juice, potatoes (white, sweet), raisins. Take early in the day to avoid nocturia.

I

Inderal

see propranolol

indinavir

in-**din**-oh-vir
(Crixivan)
Do not confuse with Denavir.

CLASSIFICATION

PHARMACOTHERAPEUTIC: Protease inhibitor. **CLINICAL:** Antiviral (see pp. 59C, 100C).

ACTION

Suppresses HIV protease, an enzyme necessary for splitting viral polyprotein precursors into mature and infectious virus particles. **Therapeutic Effect:** Resultant effect interrupts HIV replication, forms immature noninfectious viral particles.

PHARMACOKINETICS

Rapidly absorbed following PO administration. Protein binding: 60%. Metabolized in liver. Primarily excreted in urine. Unknown if removed by hemodialysis. **Half-life:** 1.8 hrs (half-life increased with impaired liver function).

USES

Treatment of HIV when antiretroviral therapy is warranted. **Unlabeled:** Prophylaxis following occupational exposure to HIV.

PRECAUTIONS

CONTRAINDICATIONS: Hypersensitivity to indinavir; nephrolithiasis. **CAUTIONS:** Renal, hepatic function impairment.

LIFESPAN CONSIDERATIONS: Pregnancy/lactation: Unknown if excreted in breast milk. Breast-feeding not recommended in HIV-infected women. **Pregnancy Category C. Children:** Safety and efficacy not established. **Elderly:** Information not available.

INTERACTIONS

DRUG: Avoid concurrent administration of indinavir with **triazolam, midazolam** (potential for arrhythmias, prolonged sedation). **HERBAL: St. John's wort** may decrease concentration, effect. **FOOD:** Avoid meals high in fat, calories, and protein. **Grapefruit** may decrease concentration/effect. **LAB VALUES:** May increase bilirubin (occurs in 10% of pts), SGOT (AST), SGPT (ALT).

AVAILABILITY (Rx)

CAPSULES: 100 mg, 200 mg, 333 mg, 400 mg.

ADMINISTRATION/HANDLING

PO

• Store at room temperature. • Protect from moisture (capsules sensitive to moisture; keep in original bottle). • Best given without food but with water only (optimal absorption) 1 hr prior to or 2 hrs following a meal but may give with water, skim milk, juice, coffee, tea, light meal (e.g., dry toast with jelly). • Do not give with meal high in fat, calories, protein. • If indinavir and didanosine are given concurrently, give at least 1 hr apart on an empty stomach.

INDICATIONS/ROUTES/DOSAGE

HIV INFECTION

PO: ADULTS: 800 mg (two 400-mg capsules) q8h.

DOSAGE WITH HEPATIC INSUFFICIENCY

PO: ADULTS: 600 mg q8h.

SIDE EFFECTS

FREQUENT: Nausea (12%), abdominal pain (9%), headache (6%), diarrhea (5%). **OCCASIONAL:** Vomiting, asthenia, fatigue (4%); insomnia; accumulation of fat in waist, abdomen, back of neck. **RARE:** Abnormal taste sensation, heartburn, symptomatic urinary tract disease, transient kidney dysfunction.

ADVERSE REACTIONS/ TOXIC EFFECTS

Nephrolithiasis (flank pain with or without hematuria) occurs in 4% of pts.

NURSING IMPLICATIONS

BASELINE ASSESSMENT

Offer emotional support. Establish baseline lab values. Emphasize need for close monitoring of renal function (urinalysis, serum creatinine) during therapy.

INTERVENTION/EVALUATION

Encourage adequate hydration. Pt should drink 48 oz (1.5 L) of liquid for each 24 hrs during therapy. Monitor for evidence of nephrolithiasis (flank pain, hematuria), contact physician if symptoms occur (therapy should be interrupted for 1–3 days). Monitor stool frequency/consistency (watery, loose, soft). Assess for abdominal discomfort, headache. Monitor bilirubin, cholesterol, triglycerides, amylase, lipase, liver function tests, blood glucose, CD4 cell count, CBC.

PATIENT/FAMILY TEACHING

Advise that indinavir is not a cure for HIV; condition may progress despite treatment. If dose is missed, take next dose at regularly scheduled time (do **not** double the dose). Best taken without food but water only (optimal absorption) 1 hr prior to or 2 hrs following a meal but may take with water, skim milk, juice, coffee, tea, light meal. Avoid the herb St. John's wort and grapefruit/grapefruit juice.

indomethacin ⓔ

in-doe-**meth**-ah-sin

(Apo-Indomethacin ✤, Indocid ✤, Indocin, Indocin-SR, Novomethacin ✤)

◆CLASSIFICATION

PHARMACOTHERAPEUTIC: Nonsteroidal anti-inflammatory. **CLINICAL:** Anti-inflammatory, analgesic (see p. 110C).

ACTION

Produces analgesic, anti-inflammatory effect by inhibiting prostaglandin synthesis. **Therapeutic Effect:** Reduces inflammatory response, intensity of pain stimulus reaching sensory nerve endings. **Patent Ductus (in neonates):** Inhibits prostaglandin synthesis, increases sensitivity of premature ductus to dilating effects of prostaglandins. **Therapeutic Effect:** Causes closure of patent ductus arteriosus.

USES

Treatment of active stages of rheumatoid arthritis, osteoarthritis, ankylosing spondylitis, acute gouty arthritis. Relief of acute bursitis and/or tendonitis. For closure of hemodynamically significant patent ductus arteriosus of premature infants weighing 500–1,750 g. **Unlabeled:** Treatment of psoriatic arthritis, rheumatic complications associated with Paget's disease of bone, fever due to malignancy, vascular headache, pericarditis.

PRECAUTIONS

CONTRAINDICATIONS: Hypersensitivity to indomethacin, aspirin, other NSAIDs; active GI bleeding; ulcers; thrombocytopenia; impaired renal function. **CAUTIONS:** Cardiac dysfunction, hypertension, renal/liver impairment, epilepsy, concurrent anticoagulant therapy. **Pregnancy Category B** (**D** if used >48 hrs or after 34 wks' gestation or close to delivery).

INTERACTIONS

DRUG: May increase effects of **oral anticoagulants, heparin, thrombolytics.** May decrease effect of **antihypertensives, diuretics.** Do not give concurrently with **triamterene** (may potentiate acute renal failure). **Salicylates, aspirin** may increase risk of GI side effects, bleeding. **Bone marrow depressants** may increase risk of hematologic reactions. May increase concentration, toxicity of **lithium.** May increase **methotrexate** toxicity. **Probenecid** may increase concentration. May increase concentration of **aminoglycosides** in neonates. **HERBAL: Feverfew** effect may be decreased. **Ginkgo biloba** may increase risk of bleeding. **FOOD:** None known. **LAB VALUES:** May prolong bleeding time. May alter blood glucose. May increase BUN, creatinine, potassium, liver function tests. May decrease sodium, platelet count.

AVAILABILITY (Rx)

CAPSULES: 25 mg, 50 mg. **CAPSULES (sustained-release):** 75 mg. **ORAL SUSPENSION:** 25 mg/5 ml. **SUPPOSITORY:** 50 mg. **POWDER FOR INJECTION:** 1 mg.

ADMINISTRATION/HANDLING

PO

• Give after meals or with food or antacids. • Do not crush sustained-release capsules.

RECTAL

• If suppository is too soft, chill for 30 min in refrigerator or run cold water over foil wrapper. • Moisten suppository with cold water prior to inserting well into rectum.

Alert: IV injection preferred for patent ductus arteriosus in neonate (may give dose PO via NG tube or rectally).

IV

Storage • IV solutions made without preservatives should be used immediately. • Use IV immediately following reconstitution. IV solution appears clear; discard if cloudy or if precipitate forms. • Discard unused portion.

Reconstitution • To 1-mg vial, add 1–2 ml preservative-free Sterile Water for Injection or 0.9% NaCl to provide concentration of 1 mg or 0.5 mg/ml, respectively. • Do not further dilute.

Rate of administration • Administer over 5–10 sec. • Restrict fluid intake.

IV INCOMPATIBILITIES

Amino acid injection, calcium gluconate, cimetidine (Tagamet), dobutamine (Dobutrex), dopamine (Intropin), gentamicin (Garamycin), tobramycin (Nebcin).

IV COMPATIBILITIES

Insulin, potassium.

INDICATIONS/ROUTES/DOSAGE

MODERATE TO SEVERE RHEUMATOID ARTHRITIS, OSTEOARTHRITIS, ANKYLOSING SPONDYLITIS

PO: ADULTS, ELDERLY: Initially, 25 mg 2–3 times/day. Increase by 25–50 mg/wk up to 150–200 mg/day. CHILDREN: 1–2 mg/kg/day. **Maximum:** 150–200 mg/day. **Extended-release:**

ADULTS, ELDERLY: Initially, 75 mg/day up to 75 mg 2 times/day.

ACUTE GOUTY ARTHRITIS

PO: ADULTS, ELDERLY: Initially, 100 mg, then 50 mg 3 times/day.

ACUTE PAINFUL SHOULDER

PO: ADULTS, ELDERLY: 75–150 mg/day in 3–4 divided doses.

USUAL RECTAL DOSAGE

ADULTS, ELDERLY: 50 mg 4 times/day. CHILDREN: Initially, 1.5–2.5 mg/kg/day, up to 4 mg/kg/day. Do not exceed 150–200 mg/day.

PATENT DUCTUS ARTERIOSUS

Alert: May give up to 3 doses at 12- to 24-hr intervals.

IV: NEONATES: Initially, 0.2 mg/kg. >7 DAYS OLD: 0.25 mg/kg for 2nd and 3rd doses. 2–7 DAYS OLD: 0.2 mg/kg for 2nd and 3rd doses. <48 HRS OLD: 0.1 mg/kg for 2nd and 3rd doses.

SIDE EFFECTS

FREQUENT (3%–11%): Headache, nausea, vomiting, dyspepsia (heartburn, indigestion, epigastric pain), dizziness. **OCCASIONAL (<3%):** Depression, tinnitus, diaphoresis, drowsiness, constipation, diarrhea. **Patent ductus arteriosus:** Bleeding disturbances. **RARE:** Increased B/P, confusion, hives, itching, rash, blurred vision.

ADVERSE REACTIONS/ TOXIC EFFECTS

Paralytic ileus; ulceration of esophagus, stomach, duodenum, small intestine may occur. In pts with impaired renal function, hyperkalemia along with worsening of impairment may occur. May aggravate depression or psychiatric disturbances, epilepsy, parkinsonism. Nephrotoxicity (dysuria, hematuria, proteinuria, nephrotic syndrome) occurs rarely. **PATENT DUCTUS ARTERIOSUS:** Acidosis, apnea, bradycardia, alkalosis occur rarely.

NURSING IMPLICATIONS

BASELINE ASSESSMENT

May mask signs of infection. Assess onset, type, location, duration of pain, fever, inflammation. Inspect appearance of affected joints for immobility, deformities, skin condition.

INTERVENTION/EVALUATION

Monitor for evidence of nausea, dyspepsia. Assist with ambulation if dizziness occurs. Evaluate for therapeutic response: relief of pain, stiffness, swelling; increase in joint mobility; reduced joint tenderness; improved grip strength. Monitor BUN, creatinine, potassium, liver function tests. In neonates, also monitor heart rate, heart sounds for murmur, B/P, urine output, EKG, sodium, glucose, platelets.

PATIENT/FAMILY TEACHING

Avoid aspirin, alcohol during therapy (increases risk of GI bleeding). If GI upset occurs, take with food, milk. Avoid tasks that require alertness, motor skills until response to drug is established. Swallow capsule whole; do not crush or chew.

infliximab

in-**flicks**-ih-mab
(Remicade)
Do not confuse with Reminyl.

◆ CLASSIFICATION

PHARMACOTHERAPEUTIC: Monoclonal antibody. **CLINICAL:** GI anti-inflammatory.

ACTION

Binds to tumor necrosis factor (TNF), inhibits functional activity of TNF. **Therapeutic Effect:** Reduces infiltration of inflammatory cells, decreases inflamed areas of the intestine.

PHARMACOKINETICS

Onset	Peak	Duration
Crohn's		
1–2 wks	—	8–48 wks
RA		
3–7 days	—	6–12 wks

Absorbed into GI tissue; primarily distributed in the vascular compartment. **Half-life:** 9.5 days.

USES

Treatment of moderate to severe Crohn's disease, treatment of pts with fistulizing Crohn's disease for reduction in number of draining enterocutaneous fistula(s). Treatment of rheumatoid arthritis (with methotrexate). **Unlabeled:** Ankylosing spondylitis, sciatica.

PRECAUTIONS

CONTRAINDICATIONS: Sensitivity to infliximab, murine proteins, serious active infection, sepsis. **CAUTIONS:** History of recurrent infections.

LIFESPAN CONSIDERATIONS: Pregnancy/lactation: Unknown if distributed in breast milk. **Pregnancy Category C. Children:** Safety and efficacy not established. **Elderly:** Use cautiously due to a higher rate of infection.

INTERACTIONS

DRUG: Live vaccines may decrease immune response. **Immunosuppressants** may reduce frequency of infusion reactions and antibodies to infliximab. **HERBAL:** None known. **FOOD:** None known. **LAB VALUES:** None known.

AVAILABILITY (Rx)

POWDER FOR INJECTION: 100 mg.

ADMINISTRATION/HANDLING

IV

Storage • Refrigerate vials.

Reconstitution • Reconstitute each vial with 10 ml Sterile Water for Injection, using 21-gauge or smaller needle. Direct the stream of sterile water to the glass wall of the vial. • Swirl the vial gently to dissolve the contents. Do not shake. • Allow the solution to stand for 5 min. • Because infliximab is a protein, the solution may develop a few translucent particles; do not use if particles are opaque or foreign particles are present. • Solution should appear colorless to light yellow and opalescent; do not use if discolored. • Withdraw and waste a volume of 0.9% NaCl from a 250-ml bag to equal the volume of reconstituted solution to be injected into the 250-ml bag (approximately 10 ml). Total dose to be infused should equal 250 ml. • Slowly add the reconstituted infliximab solution to the 250-ml infusion bag. Gently mix. Infusion concentration should range between 0.4 and 4 mg/ml. • Begin infusion within 3 hrs after reconstitution.

Rate of administration • Administer IV infusion >2 hrs, using set with a low-protein-binding filter.

IV INCOMPATIBILITY

Do not infuse infliximab concurrently in the same IV line with other agents.

INDICATIONS/ROUTES/DOSAGE

MODERATE TO SEVERE CROHN'S DISEASE

IV infusion: ADULTS, ELDERLY: 5 mg/kg as a single IV infusion.

FISTULIZING CROHN'S DISEASE

IV infusion: ADULTS, ELDERLY: Initially, 5 mg/kg, followed by additional 5 mg/kg doses at 2 and 6 wks after the first infusion.

RHEUMATOID ARTHRITIS

IV infusion: ADULTS, ELDERLY: 3 mg/kg; follow with additional doses at 2 and 6 wks after the first infusion, then q8wks thereafter.

SIDE EFFECTS

FREQUENT (10%–22%): Headache, nausea, fatigue, fever. **OCCASIONAL (5%–9%):** Fever/chills during infusion, pharyngitis, vomiting, pain, dizziness, bronchitis, rash, rhinitis, coughing, pruritus, sinusitis, myalgia, back pain. **RARE (1%–4%):** Hypotension/hypertension, paresthesia, anxiety, depression, insomnia, diarrhea, urinary tract infection.

ADVERSE REACTIONS/ TOXIC EFFECTS

Potential for hypersensitivity reaction, lupus-like syndrome.

NURSING IMPLICATIONS

BASELINE ASSESSMENT

Determine pattern of bowel activity. Check baseline hydration status: skin turgor, mucous membranes for dryness, urinary status.

INTERVENTION/EVALUATION

Monitor urinalysis, ESR, B/P, signs of infection. **Crohn's Disease:** C-reactive protein, frequency of stools, abdominal pain. **Rheumatoid Arthritis:** C-reactive protein, decrease in pain, swollen joints, stiffness.

insulin

in-sull-in

Rapid acting:

INSULIN LISPRO:

(Humalog)

INSULIN ASPART:

(Novolog)

REGULAR INSULIN:

(Humulin R, Novolin R, Regular Iletin II)

Intermediate acting:

NPH:

(Humulin N, Novolin N, Pork)

LENTE:

(Humulin L, Lente Iletin II, Novolin L)

NPH/regular mixture (70%/30%):

HUMULIN 70/30, NOVOLIN 70/30

NPH/regular mixture (50%/50%):

HUMULIN 50/50

NPH/Lispro mixture (75%/25%):

HUMALOG MIX 75/25
NOVALOG MIX 70/30

Long acting:

INSULIN GLARGINE:

(Lantus)

◆CLASSIFICATION

PHARMACOTHERAPEUTIC: Exogenous insulin. **CLINICAL:** Antidiabetic (see p. 38C).

ACTION

Facilitates passage of glucose, potassium, magnesium across cellular membranes of skeletal/cardiac muscle, adipose tissue; controls storage/metabolism of carbohydrates, protein, fats. Promotes conversion of glucose to glycogen in liver. **Therapeutic Effect:** Controls glucose levels in diabetic patients.

PHARMACOKINETICS

	Onset (hrs)	Peak (hrs)	Duration (hrs)
Lispro	¼	½–1½	4–5
Insulin aspart	⅙	1–3	3–5
Regular	½–1	2–4	5–7
NPH	1–2	6–14	24+
Lente	1–3	6–14	24+
Insulin glargine	—	—	24

USES

Treatment of insulin-dependent type 1 diabetes mellitus; non–insulin-dependent type 2 diabetes mellitus when diet/weight control therapy has failed to maintain satisfactory blood glucose levels or in event of pregnancy, surgery, trauma, infection, fever, severe renal/hepatic/endocrine dysfunction. Regular insulin used in emergency treatment of ketoacidosis, to promote passage of glucose across cell membrane in hyperalimentation, to facilitate intracellular shift of potassium in hyperkalemia.

PRECAUTIONS

CONTRAINDICATIONS: Hypersensitivity or insulin resistance may require change of type, species source of insulin.

LIFESPAN CONSIDERATIONS: Pregnancy/lactation: Insulin is drug of choice for diabetes in pregnancy; close medical supervision is needed. Following delivery, insulin needs may drop for 24–72 hrs, then rise to prepregnancy levels. Not secreted in breast milk; lactation may decrease insulin requirements. **Pregnancy Category B. Children:** No age-related precautions noted. **Elderly:** Decreased vision, shakiness may lead to inaccurate dosage.

INTERACTIONS

DRUG: Glucocorticoids, thiazide diuretics may increase blood glucose. **Alcohol** may increase insulin effect. **Beta-adrenergic blockers** may increase risk of hypoglycemia/hyperglycemia, mask signs of hypoglycemia, prolong period of hypoglycemia. **HERBAL:** None known. **FOOD:** None known. **LAB VALUES:** May decrease potassium, magnesium, phosphate concentrations.

AVAILABILITY (OTC)

HUMALOG, NOVOLOG, REGULAR, NPH, 70/30, 50/50, LENTE: 100 units/ml.

ADMINISTRATION/HANDLING

SUBCUTANEOUS

• Store currently used insulin at room temperature (avoid extreme temperatures, direct sunlight). Store extra vials in refrigerator. • Discard unused vials if not used for several weeks. No insulin should have precipitate or discoloration. • Give subcutaneously only. (Regular insulin is the **only** insulin that may be given IV, IM for ketoacidosis or other specific situations.) • Do not give cold insulin; warm to room temperature. • Rotate vial gently between hands; do not shake. Regular insulin should be clear; no insulin should have precipitate or discoloration. • Usually administered approx 30 min before a meal (Insulin Lispro is given up to 15 min before meals). Check blood glucose concentration before administration; dosage highly individualized. • When insulin is mixed, regular insulin is always drawn up first. Mixtures must be administered at once (binding can occur within 5 min). Humalog may be mixed with Humulin N, Humulin L. • Subcutaneous injections may be given in thigh, abdomen, upper arm, buttocks, upper back if there is adequate adipose tissue. • Rotation of injection sites is essential; maintain careful record. • For home situations, prefilled syringes are stable for 1 wk under refrigeration (this includes mixtures once they have stabilized, e.g., 15 min for NPH/Regular, 24 hrs for Lente/Regular). Prefilled syringes should be stored in vertical or oblique position to avoid plugging; plunger should be pulled back slightly and the syringe rocked to remix the solution before injection.

IV (Regular):

• Use only if solution is clear. • May give undiluted.

IV INCOMPATIBILITIES

Digoxin (Lanoxin), diltiazem (Cardizem), dopamine (Intropin), nafcillin (Nafcil).

IV COMPATIBILITIES

Amiodarone (Cordarone), ampicillin-sulbactam (Unasyn), cefazolin (Ancef), cimetidine (Tagamet), digoxin (Lanoxin), dobutamine (Dobutrex), famotidine (Pepcid), gentamicin, heparin, magnesium sulfate, metoclopramide (Reglan), midazolam (Versed), milrinone (Primacor), morphine, nitroglycerin, potassium chloride, propofol (Diprivan).

INDICATIONS/ROUTES/DOSAGE

Dosage for insulin is individualized/monitored.

USUAL DOSAGE GUIDELINES

Alert: Adjust dosage to achieve premeal and bedtime glucose level of 80–140 mg/dl (children <5 yrs: 100–200 mg/dl).

Subcutaneous: ADULTS, ELDERLY, CHILDREN: 0.5–1 units/kg/day. ADOLESCENTS (during growth spurt): 0.8–1.2 units/kg/day.

SIDE EFFECTS

OCCASIONAL: Local redness, swelling, itching (due to improper injection technique, allergy to cleansing solution or insulin). **INFREQUENT:** Somogyi effect (rebound hyperglycemia) with chronically excessive insulin doses. Systemic allergic reaction (rash, angioedema, anaphylaxis), lipodystrophy (depression at injection site due to breakdown of adipose tissue), lipohypertrophy (accumulation of subcutaneous tissue at injection site due to lack of adequate site rotation). **RARE:** Insulin resistance.

ADVERSE REACTIONS/ TOXIC EFFECTS

Severe hypoglycemia (due to hyperinsulinism) may occur in overdose of insulin, decrease/delay of food intake, excessive exercise, or in pts with brittle diabetes. Diabetic ketoacidosis may result from stress, illness, omission of insulin dose, long-term poor insulin control.

I

NURSING IMPLICATIONS

BASELINE ASSESSMENT

Check blood glucose level. Discuss lifestyle to determine extent of learning, emotional needs.

INTERVENTION/EVALUATION

Assess for hypoglycemia (refer to pharmacokinetics table for peak times/duration): cool/wet skin, tremors, dizziness, headache, anxiety, tachycardia, numbness in mouth, hunger, diplopia. Check sleeping pt for restlessness, diaphoresis. Check for hyperglycemia: polyuria (excessive urine output), polyphagia (excessive food intake), polydipsia (excessive thirst), nausea/vomiting, dim vision, fatigue, deep/rapid breathing. Be alert to conditions altering glucose requirements: fever, increased activity/stress, surgical procedure.

PATIENT/FAMILY TEACHING

Prescribed diet is essential part of treatment; do not skip/delay meals. Carry candy, sugar packets, other sugar supplements for immediate response to hypoglycemia. Wear/carry medical alert identification. Check with physician when insulin demands are altered (e.g., fever, infection, trauma, stress, heavy physical activity). Do not take other medication without consulting physician. Weight control, exercise, hygiene (including foot care), and not smoking are integral parts of therapy. Protect skin, limit sun exposure. Inform dentist, physician, surgeon of medication before any treatment is given.

interferon alfa-2a

inn-ter-**fear**-on
(Roferon-A)

Do not confuse with interferon alfa-2b.

CLASSIFICATION

PHARMACOTHERAPEUTIC: Biologic response modifier. **CLINICAL:** Antineoplastic (see p. 73C).

ACTION

Inhibits viral replication in virus-infected cells. **Therapeutic Effect:** Suppresses cell proliferation; increases phagocytic action of macrophages; augments specific lymphocytic cell toxicity.

PHARMACOKINETICS

Well absorbed after IM, subcutaneous administration. Undergoes proteolytic degradation during reabsorption in kidney. **Half-life:** *IM:* 2 hrs; *subcutaneous:* 3 hrs.

USES

Treatment of hairy cell leukemia, AIDS-related Kaposi's sarcoma, chronic myelocytic leukemia (CML), chronic hepatitis C. **Unlabeled:** Treatment of active, chronic hepatitis; bladder, renal carcinoma; non-Hodgkin's lymphoma, malignant melanoma, multiple myeloma, mycosis fungoides.

PRECAUTIONS

CONTRAINDICATIONS: None known. **CAUTIONS:** Renal/hepatic impairment, seizure disorders, compromised CNS function, cardiac disease, history of cardiac abnormalities, myelosuppression.

LIFESPAN CONSIDERATIONS: Pregnancy/lactation: If possible, avoid use during pregnancy. Breast-feeding not recommended. **Pregnancy Category C. Children:** Safety and efficacy not established. **Elderly:** Neurotoxicity, cardiotoxicity may occur more frequently. Age-related renal impairment may require caution.

INTERACTIONS

DRUG: Bone marrow depressants may have additive effect. **HERBAL:** None known. **FOOD:** None known. **LAB VALUES:** May increase SGOT (AST), SGPT (ALT), alkaline phosphatase, LDH. May decrease Hgb, Hct, leukocyte, platelet counts.

AVAILABILITY (Rx)

INJECTION: 3 million units, 6 million units, 9 million units, 36 million units.

ADMINISTRATION/HANDLING

Alert: subcutaneous preferred for thrombocytopenic pts, those at risk for bleeding.

SUBCUTANEOUS/IM

• Refrigerate.• Do not shake vial. Solution appears colorless. Do not use if precipitate or discoloration occurs.

INDICATIONS/ROUTES/DOSAGE

Alert: Dosage individualized based on clinical response, tolerance to adverse effects. When used in combination therapy, consult specific protocols for optimum dosage, sequence of drug administration. If severe adverse reactions occur, modify dosage or temporarily discontinue medication.

HAIRY CELL LEUKEMIA
Subcutaneous/IM: ADULTS: Initially, 3 million units/day for 16–24 wks. MAINTENANCE: 3 million units 3 times/wk. Do not use 36-million-unit vial.

CHRONIC MYELOCYTIC LEUKEMIA (CML)
Subcutaneous/IM: ADULTS: 9 million units daily.

MELANOMA
Subcutaneous/IM: ADULTS, ELDERLY: 12 million units/m^2 3 times/wk for 3 mo.

AIDS-RELATED KAPOSI'S SARCOMA
Subcutaneous/IM: ADULTS: Initially, 36 million units/day for 10–12 wks (may give 3 million units on day 1; 9 million units on day 2; 18 million units on day 3; then begin 36 million units/day for remainder of 10–12 wks). MAINTENANCE: 36 million units/day 3 times/wk.

CHRONIC HEPATITIS C
Subcutaneous/IM: ADULTS: Initially, 6 million units once daily for 3 wks, then 3 million units 3 times/wk for 6 mos.

SIDE EFFECTS

FREQUENT (>20%): Flulike symptoms (fever, fatigue, headache, aches, pains, anorexia, chills), nausea, vomiting, coughing, dyspnea, hypotension, edema, chest pain, dizziness, diarrhea, weight loss, taste change, abdominal discomfort, confusion, paresthesia, depression, visual/sleep disturbances, diaphoresis, lethargy. **OCCASIONAL (5%–20%):** Partial alopecia, rash, dry throat/skin, pruritus, flatulence, constipation, hypertension, palpitations, sinusitis. **RARE (<5%):** Hot flashes, hypermotility, Raynaud's syndrome, bronchospasm, earache, ecchymosis.

ADVERSE REACTIONS/ TOXIC EFFECTS

Arrhythmias, stroke, transient ischemic attacks, CHF, pulmonary edema, MI occur rarely.

NURSING IMPLICATIONS

BASELINE ASSESSMENT

CBC, platelet counts, blood chemistries, urinalysis, renal/liver function tests should be performed prior to initial therapy and routinely thereafter.

INTERVENTION/EVALUATION

Offer emotional support. Monitor all levels of clinical function (numerous side effects). Encourage ample fluid intake, particularly during early therapy.

PATIENT/FAMILY TEACHING

Clinical response may take 1–3 mos. Flulike symptoms tend to diminish with continued therapy. Contact physician if nausea/vomiting continues at home. Avoid alcohol while taking medication. Use caution driving, performing tasks requiring mental alertness.

interferon alfa-2b

inn-ter-**fear**-on
(Intron-A)
Do not confuse with interferon alfa-2a.

FIXED-COMBINATION(S)

Rebetron: interferon alfa-2b/ribavirin (an antiviral): 3 million U/200 mg.

CLASSIFICATION

PHARMACOTHERAPEUTIC: Biologic response modifier. **CLINICAL:** Antineoplastic (see p. 73C).

ACTION

Inhibits viral replication in virus-infected cells, suppresses cell proliferation. **Therapeutic Effect:** Increases phagocytic action of macrophages, augments specific cytotoxicity of lymphocytes.

PHARMACOKINETICS

Well absorbed after IM, subcutaneous administration. Undergoes proteolytic degradation during reabsorption in kidney. **Half-life:** 2–3 hrs.

USES

Treatment of hairy cell leukemia, condylomata acuminata (genital, venereal warts), AIDS-related Kaposi's sarcoma, chronic hepatitis (non-A, non-B/C), chronic hepatitis B (including children ≥1 yr), non-Hodgkin's lymphoma. **Unlabeled:** Treatment of bladder, cervical, renal carcinoma; chronic myelocytic leukemia, laryngeal papillomatosis, multiple myeloma, mycosis fungoides.

PRECAUTIONS

CONTRAINDICATIONS: None known. **CAUTIONS:** Renal/hepatic impairment, seizure disorders, compromised CNS function, cardiac diseases, history of cardiac abnormalities, myelosuppression.

LIFESPAN CONSIDERATIONS: Pregnancy/lactation: If possible, avoid use during pregnancy. Breast-feeding not recommended. **Pregnancy Category C. Children:** Safety and efficacy not established. **Elderly:** Neurotoxicity, cardiotoxicity may occur more frequently. Age-related renal impairment may require caution.

INTERACTIONS

DRUG: Bone marrow depressants may have additive effect. **HERBAL:** None known. **FOOD:** None known. **LAB VALUES:** May increase SGOT (AST), SGPT (ALT), alkaline phosphatase, LDH, prothrombin time, partial thromboplastin time. May decrease Hgb, Hct; leukocyte, platelet counts.

AVAILABILITY (Rx)

INJECTION, POWDER FOR RECONSTITUTION: 3 million international units, 5 million international units, 6 million international units, 10 million international units, 18 million international units, 25 million international units, 50 million international units. **INJECTION, PREFILLED SYRINGES.**

ADMINISTRATION/HANDLING

SUBCUTANEOUS/IM

• Do not give IM if platelets <50,000/m^3; give subcutaneous. • For hairy cell leukemia, reconstitute each 3-million-international units vial with 1 ml Bacteriostatic Water for Injection to provide concentration of 3 million international units/ml (1-ml to 5-million-international units vial; 2-ml to 10-million-international units vial; 5-ml to 25-million-international units vial provides concentration of 5 million international units/ml). • For condylomata acuminata, reconstitute each 10-million-international units vial with 1 ml Bacteriostatic Water for Injection to provide concentration of 10 million international units/ml. • For AIDS-related Kaposi's sarcoma, reconstitute 50-million-international units vial with 1 ml Bacteriostatic Water for Injection to provide concentration of 50 million international units/ml. • Agitate vial gently, withdraw with sterile syringe.

IV

Storage • Refrigerate unopened vials (stable for 7 days at room temperature).

Reconstitution • Prepare immediately before use. • Reconstitute with diluent provided by manufacturer. • Withdraw desired dose and further dilute with 100 ml 0.9% NaCl to provide final concentration at least 10 million international units/100 ml.

Rate of administration • Administer over 20 min.

IV INCOMPATIBILITY
No information available. Do not mix with other medications via Y-site administration.

INDICATIONS/ROUTES/DOSAGE

Alert: Dosage individualized based on clinical response, tolerance to adverse effects. When used in combination therapy, consult specific protocols for optimum dosage, sequence of drug administration.

HAIRY CELL LEUKEMIA
IM/subcutaneous: ADULTS: 2 million international units/m^2 3 times/wk. If severe adverse reactions occur, modify dose or temporarily discontinue.

CONDYLOMATA ACUMINATA
Intralesional: ADULTS: 1 million international units/lesion 3 times/wk for 3 wks. Use only 10 million international units vial, reconstitute with no more than 1 ml diluent. Use TB syringe with 25- or 26-gauge needle. Give in evening with acetaminophen (alleviates side effects).

AIDS-RELATED KAPOSI'S SARCOMA
IM/subcutaneous: ADULTS: 30 million international units/m^2 3 times/wk. Use only 50 million international units vials. If severe adverse reactions occur, modify dose or temporarily discontinue.

CHRONIC HEPATITIS C
IM/subcutaneous: ADULTS: 3 million international units 3 times/wk for up to 6 mos (for up to 18–24 mos for chronic hepatitis C).

CHRONIC HEPATITIS B
IM/subcutaneous: ADULTS: 30–35 million international units/wk (5 million international units/day or 10 million international units 3 times/wk).

MALIGNANT MELANOMA
IV: ADULTS: Initially, 20 million international units/m^2 5 times/wk for 4 wks. MAINTENANCE: 10 million U IM/subcutaneous for 48 wks.

SIDE EFFECTS

Alert: Dose-related effects. **FREQUENT:** Flulike symptoms (fever, fatigue, headache, aches, pains, anorexia, chills), rash (hairy cell leukemia, Kaposi's sarcoma only). **Kaposi's sarcoma:** All previously mentioned side effects plus depression, dyspepsia, dry mouth/thirst, alopecia, rigors. **OCCASIONAL:** Dizziness, pruritus, dry skin, dermatitis, alteration in taste. **RARE:** Confusion, leg cramps, back pain, gingivitis, flushing, tremor, nervousness, eye pain.

ADVERSE REACTIONS/ TOXIC EFFECTS

Hypersensitivity reaction occurs rarely. Severe adverse reactions of flulike symptoms appear dose related.

NURSING IMPLICATIONS

BASELINE ASSESSMENT

CBC, platelet counts, blood chemistries, urinalysis, renal/liver function tests should be performed prior to initial therapy and routinely thereafter.

INTERVENTION/EVALUATION

Offer emotional support. Monitor all levels of clinical function (numerous side effects). Encourage ample fluid intake, particularly during early therapy.

PATIENT/FAMILY TEACHING

Clinical response occurs in 1–3 mos. Flulike symptoms tend to diminish with continued therapy. Some symptoms may be alleviated/minimized by bedtime doses. Do not have immunizations without physician's approval (drug lowers body's resistance). Avoid contact with those who have recently received live virus vaccine. Avoid tasks that require alertness, motor skills until response to drug is established. Sips of tepid water may relieve dry mouth.

interferon alfacon-1

inn-ter-**fear**-on
(Infergen)

◆CLASSIFICATION

PHARMACOTHERAPEUTIC: Biologic response modifier. **CLINICAL:** Antiviral

ACTION

Stimulates immune system. **Therapeutic Effect:** Inhibits hepatitis C virus.

USES

Treatment of chronic hepatitis C viral (HCV) infections in pts with compensated liver disease who have anti-HCV serum antibodies and/or presence of HCV RNA.

AVAILABILITY (Rx)

INJECTION: 15-mcg vials, 9-mcg vials.

INDICATIONS/ROUTES/DOSAGE

HEPATITIS C

Subcutaneous: ADULTS: 9 mcg 3 times/wk for 24 wks. May increase to 15 mcg in pts tolerating 9-mcg dose and not responding adequately.

Alert: At least 48 hrs should elapse between doses.

SIDE EFFECTS

FREQUENT (>50%): Headache, fatigue, fever, depression.

interferon alfa-n3

inn-ter-**fear**-on
(Alferon N)

◆CLASSIFICATION

PHARMACOTHERAPEUTIC: Biologic response modifier. **CLINICAL:** Antineoplastic.

ACTION

Inhibits viral replication in virus-infected cells. **Therapeutic Effect:** Suppresses cell proliferation, increases phagocytic action of macrophages, augments specific cytotoxicity of lymphocytes.

USES

Treatment of refractory/recurring condylomata acuminata (genital, venereal warts). **Unlabeled:** Treatment of active chronic hepatitis, bladder carcinoma, chronic myelocytic leukemia, laryngeal papillomatosis, non-Hodgkin's lymphoma, malignant melanoma, multiple myeloma, mycosis fungoides.

PRECAUTIONS

CONTRAINDICATIONS: Previous history of anaphylactic reaction to mouse immunoglobulin (IgG), egg protein, or neomycin. **CAUTIONS:** Unstable angina, uncontrolled CHF, severe pulmonary disease, diabetes mellitus with ketoacidosis, thrombophlebitis, pulmonary embolism, hemophilia, severe myelosuppression, seizure disorders.

LIFESPAN CONSIDERATIONS: Pregnancy Category C.

INTERACTIONS

DRUG: Bone marrow depressants may have additive effect. **HERBAL:** None known. **FOOD:** None known. **LAB VALUES:** May increase SGOT (AST), SGPT (ALT), alkaline phosphatase, LDH. May decrease Hgb, Hct; leukocyte, platelet counts.

AVAILABILITY (Rx)

INJECTION: 5 million units.

ADMINISTRATION/HANDLING

INTRALESIONAL

• Refrigerate vial. Do not freeze or shake. • Inject into base of each wart with 30-gauge needle.

INDICATIONS/ROUTES/DOSAGE

CONDYLOMATA ACUMINATA

Intralesional: ADULTS >18 YRS: 0.05 ml (250,000 international units) per wart 2 times/wk up to 8 wks. **Maximum dose/treatment session:** 0.5 ml (2.5 million international units). Do not repeat for 3 mos after initial 8 wks unless warts enlarge or new warts appear.

SIDE EFFECTS

FREQUENT: Flulike symptoms (fever, fatigue, headache, aches, pains, anorexia, chills). **OCCASIONAL:** Dizziness, pruritus, dry skin, dermatitis, alteration in taste. **RARE:** Confusion, leg cramps, back pain, gingivitis, flushing, tremor, nervousness, eye pain.

ADVERSE REACTIONS/TOXIC EFFECTS

Hypersensitivity reaction occurs rarely. Severe adverse reactions of flulike symptoms appear dose related.

NURSING IMPLICATIONS

INTERVENTION/EVALUATION

Monitor all levels of clinical function (numerous side effects). Encourage ample fluid intake, particularly during early therapy.

PATIENT/FAMILY TEACHING

Flulike symptoms tend to diminish with continued therapy. Some symptoms may be alleviated/minimized by bedtime doses.

interferon beta-1a

inn-ter-**fear**-on
(Avonex, Rebif)
Do not confuse with Avelox, interferon beta-1b.

◆ CLASSIFICATION

PHARMACOTHERAPEUTIC: Biologic response modifier. **CLINICAL:** Multiple sclerosis agent.

ACTION

Interacts with specific cell receptors found on surface of human cells. **Therapeutic Effect:** Possesses antiviral, immunoregulatory activities.

PHARMACOKINETICS

After IM administration, peak serum levels attained in 3–15 hrs. Biologic markers increase within 12 hrs and remain elevated for 4 days. **Half-life:** 10 hrs (IM).

USES

Treatment of relapsing multiple sclerosis to slow progression of physical disability, decrease frequency of clinical exacerbations. **Unlabeled:** Treatment of AIDS, AIDS-related Kaposi's sarcoma, renal cell carcinoma, malignant melanoma, acute non-A, non-B hepatitis.

PRECAUTIONS

CONTRAINDICATIONS: Hypersensitivity to interferon, albumin. **CAUTIONS:** Chronic progressive multiple sclerosis, children <18 yrs.

LIFESPAN CONSIDERATIONS: Pregnancy/lactation: Interferon beta-1a has abortifacient potential. Unknown if distributed in breast milk. **Pregnancy Category C. Children:** Safety and efficacy not established. **Elderly:** No information available.

INTERACTIONS

DRUG: None known. **HERBAL:** None known. **FOOD:** None known. **LAB VALUES:** May increase SGOT (AST), SGPT (ALT), bilirubin, alkaline phosphatase, BUN, calcium, glucose. May decrease Hgb, platelets, WBCs, neutrophils.

AVAILABILITY (Rx)

POWDER FOR INJECTION: 30 mcg. **REBIF:** 22 mg, 44 mcg. **PRE-FILLED SYRINGE (AVONEX).**

ADMINISTRATION/HANDLING

I

IM

• Refrigerate vials. • Following reconstitution, use within 6 hrs if refrigerated. Discard if discolored, contains a precipitate. • Reconstitute 33-mcg (6.6-million-international units) vial with 1.1 ml diluent (supplied by manufacturer). • Gently swirl to dissolve medication; do not shake. • Discard if discolored, contains particulate matter. • Discard unused portion (contains no preservative).

SUBCUTANEOUS ADMINISTRATION

Administer at same time of day 3 days each wk. Doses to be separated by at least 48 hrs.

INDICATIONS/ROUTES/DOSAGE

RELAPSING-REMITTING MULTIPLE SCLEROSIS

IM: ADULTS: (Avonex): 30 mcg once weekly.

Subcutaneous: ADULTS: (Rebif): Initially, 8.8 mcg 3 times/wk, may increase over 4–6 wks to 44 mcg 3 times/wk.

SIDE EFFECTS

FREQUENT: Headache (67%), flulike symptoms (61%), myalgia (34%), upper respiratory infection (31%), pain (24%), asthenia, chills (21%), sinusitis (18%), infection (11%). **OCCASIONAL:** Abdominal pain, arthralgia (9%), chest pain, dyspnea (6%), malaise, syncope (4%). **RARE:** Injection site reaction, hypersensitivity reaction (3%).

ADVERSE REACTIONS/ TOXIC EFFECTS

Anemia occurs in 8% of pts.

NURSING IMPLICATIONS

BASELINE ASSESSMENT

Obtain Hgb, CBC, platelet count, blood chemistries including liver function tests. Assess home situation for support of therapy.

INTERVENTION/EVALUATION

Assess for headache, flulike symptoms, muscle ache (see Side Effects). Periodically monitor lab results, reevaluate injection technique. Assess for depression, suicidal ideation.

PATIENT/FAMILY TEACHING

Do not change schedule/dosage without consultation with physician. Instruct on correct reconstitution of product and administration, including aseptic technique. Provide puncture-resistant container for used needles, syringes; explain proper disposal. Explain that injection site reactions may occur. These do not require discontinuation of therapy, but note type/extent carefully. Depression, suicidal ideation must be reported immediately.

interferon beta-1b

inn-ter-**fear**-on

(Betaferon, Betaseron)

Do not confuse with interferon beta-1a.

CLASSIFICATION

PHARMACOTHERAPEUTIC: Biologic response modifier. **CLINICAL:** Multiple sclerosis, cancer, AIDS agent.

ACTION

Interacts with specific cell receptors found on surface of human cells. **Therapeutic Effect:** Possesses antiviral, immunoregulatory activities.

PHARMACOKINETICS

Half-life: 8 min–4.3 hrs.

USES

Reduces frequency of clinical exacerbations in pts with relapsing-remitting multiple sclerosis (recurrent attacks of neurologic dysfunction). **Unlabeled:** Treatment of AIDS, AIDS-related Kaposi's sarcoma, renal cell carcinoma, malignant melanoma, acute non-A/non-B hepatitis.

PRECAUTIONS

CONTRAINDICATIONS: Hypersensitivity to interferon, albumin. **CAUTIONS:** Chronic progressive multiple sclerosis, children <18 yrs.

LIFESPAN CONSIDERATIONS: Pregnancy/lactation: Unknown if distributed in breast milk. **Pregnancy Category C. Children:** Safety and efficacy not established. **Elderly:** No information available.

INTERACTIONS

DRUG: None known. **HERBAL:** None known. **FOOD:** None known. **LAB VALUES:** May increase SGOT (AST), SGPT (ALT), bilirubin, alkaline phosphatase, BUN, calcium, glucose. May decrease Hgb, platelets, WBCs, neutrophils.

AVAILABILITY (Rx)

POWDER FOR INJECTION: 0.3 mg (9.6 million units).

ADMINISTRATION/HANDLING

SUBCUTANEOUS

• Store vials at room temperature. • After reconstitution, stable for 3 hrs if refrigerated. • Use within 3 hrs of reconstitution. • Discard if discolored, contains a precipitate. • Reconstitute 0.3-mg (9.6 million international units) vial with 1.2 ml diluent (supplied by manufacturer) to provide concentration of 0.25 mg/ml (8 million units/ml). • Gently swirl to dissolve medication; do not shake. • Discard if discolored, contains particulate matter. • Withdraw 1 ml solution and inject subcutaneous into arms, abdomen, hips, or thighs using 27-gauge needle. • Discard unused portion (contains no preservative).

INDICATIONS/ROUTES/DOSAGE

RELAPSING-REMITTING MULTIPLE SCLEROSIS

Subcutaneous: ADULTS: 0.25 mg (8 million international units) every other day.

SIDE EFFECTS

FREQUENT: Injection site reaction (85%), headache (84%), flulike symptoms (76%), fever (59%), pain (52%), asthenia (49%), myalgia (44%), sinusitis (36%), diarrhea, dizziness (35%), mental status changes (29%), constipation (24%), diaphoresis (23%), vomiting (21%). **OCCASIONAL:** Malaise (15%), somnolence (6%), alopecia (4%).

ADVERSE REACTIONS/ TOXIC EFFECTS

Seizures occur rarely.

NURSING IMPLICATIONS

BASELINE ASSESSMENT

Obtain Hgb, CBC, platelet count, blood chemistries (including liver function tests). Assess home situation for support of therapy.

INTERVENTION/EVALUATION

Periodically monitor lab results, reevaluate injection technique. Assess for nausea (high incidence). Monitor sleep pattern. Monitor stool frequency/ consistency (watery, loose, soft). Assist with ambulation if dizziness occurs.

Question for evidence of heartburn, epigastric discomfort. Monitor food intake. Assess for depression, suicidal ideation.

PATIENT/FAMILY TEACHING

Inform physician of flulike symptoms (occur commonly but decrease over time). Wear sunscreens, protective clothing if exposed to sunlight/ultraviolet light until tolerance known. Report depression, suicidal ideation immediately.

interferon gamma-1b

inn-ter-**fear**-on
(Actimmune)

CLASSIFICATION

PHARMACOTHERAPEUTIC: Biologic response modifier. **CLINICAL:** Immunologic agent.

ACTION

Induces activation of macrophages in blood monocytes to phagocytes (necessary in cellular immune response to intracellular, extracellular pathogens). **Therapeutic Effect:** Enhances phagocytic function, antimicrobial activity of monocytes.

PHARMACOKINETICS

Slowly absorbed after subcutaneous administration.

USES

Reduces frequency, severity of serious infections due to chronic granulomatous disease. Treatment of severe, malignant osteopetrosis.

PRECAUTIONS

CONTRAINDICATIONS: Hypersensitivity to *Escherichia coli* products. **CAUTIONS:** Seizure disorders, compromised CNS function, preexisting cardiac disease (including ischemia, CHF, arrhythmia), myelosuppression.

LIFESPAN CONSIDERATIONS: Pregnancy/lactation: Unknown if drug crosses placenta or is distributed in breast milk. **Pregnancy Category C. Children:** Safety and efficacy not established in those <1 yr. Flulike symptoms may occur more frequently. **Elderly:** No information available.

INTERACTIONS

DRUG: Bone marrow depressants may increase bone marrow depression. **HERBAL:** None known. **FOOD:** None known. **LAB VALUES:** None known.

AVAILABILITY (Rx)

INJECTION: 100 mcg (3 million units).

ADMINISTRATION/HANDLING

Alert: Avoid excessive agitation of vial; do not shake.

SUBCUTANEOUS

• Refrigerate vials. Do not freeze. • Do not keep at room temperature >12 hrs; discard after 12 hrs. • Vials are single dose; discard unused portion. • Clear, colorless solution. Do not use if discolored, precipitate formed. • When given 3 times/wk, give in left deltoid, right deltoid, anterior thigh.

INDICATIONS/ROUTES/DOSAGE

CHRONIC GRANULOMATOUS DISEASE, OSTEOPETROSIS

Subcutaneous: ADULTS, CHILDREN >1 YR: 50 mcg/m^2 (1.5 million units/m^2) in pts with body surface area (BSA) >0.5 m^2; 1.5 mcg/kg/dose in pts with BSA ≤0.5 m^2. Give 3 times/wk.

SIDE EFFECTS

FREQUENT: Fever (52%); headache (33%); rash (17%); chills, fatigue, diarrhea (14%). **OCCASIONAL (10%–13%):** Vomiting, nausea. **RARE (3%–6%):** Weight loss, myalgia, anorexia.

ADVERSE REACTIONS/ TOXIC EFFECTS

May exacerbate preexisting CNS dysfunction (demonstrated as decreased mental status, gait disturbance, dizziness), cardiac abnormalities.

NURSING IMPLICATIONS

BASELINE ASSESSMENT

CBC, platelet, blood chemistries, urinalysis, renal/liver function tests should be performed prior to initial therapy and at 3-mo intervals during course of treatment.

INTERVENTION/EVALUATION

Monitor for flulike symptoms (fever, chills, fatigue, muscle aches). Assess skin for evidence of rash.

PATIENT/FAMILY TEACHING

Flulike symptoms (fever, chills, fatigue, muscle aches) are generally mild and tend to disappear as treatment continues. Symptoms may be minimized with bedtime administration. Avoid tasks that require alertness, motor skills until response to drug is established. If home use prescribed, instruct in proper technique of administration; care in proper disposal of needles, syringes. Vials should remain refrigerated.

interleukin-2 (aldesleukin)

in-tur-**lew**-kin

(IL-2, Proleukin)

Do not confuse with interferon 2.

CLASSIFICATION

PHARMACOTHERAPEUTIC: Biologic response modifier. **CLINICAL:** Antineoplastic (see p. 68C).

ACTION

Modifies human recombinant interleukin-2. **Therapeutic Effect:** Promotes proliferation, differentiation, recruitment of T and B cells, natural killer cells, thymocytes. Causes cytolytic activity in lymphocytes.

PHARMACOKINETICS

Primarily distributed into plasma, lymphocytes, lungs, liver, kidney, spleen. Metabolized to amino acids in the cells lining the kidney. **Half-life:** 85 min.

USES

Treatment of metastatic renal cell carcinoma, metastatic melanoma. **Unlabeled:** Treatment of Kaposi's sarcoma, colorectal cancer, non-Hodgkin's lymphoma.

PRECAUTIONS

CONTRAINDICATIONS: Abnormal thallium stress test or pulmonary function tests, organ allografts, retreatment in those who experience the following toxicities: sustained ventricular tachycardia, cardiac rhythm disturbances (uncontrolled or unresponsive), recurrent chest pain with EKG changes, angina, MI, intubation >72 hrs, pericardial tamponade, renal dysfunction requiring dialysis >72 hrs, coma or toxic psychosis >48 hrs, repetitive or difficult-to-control seizures, bowel ischemia/perforation, GI bleeding requiring surgery. **EXTREME CAUTION:** Pts with normal thallium stress tests and pulmonary function tests who have history of prior cardiac or pulmonary disease. **CAUTIONS:** Pts with fixed requirements for large volumes of fluid (e.g., those with hypercalcemia), history of seizures.

LIFESPAN CONSIDERATIONS: Pregnancy/lactation: Avoid use in those of either sex not practicing effective contraception. **Pregnancy Category C. Children:** Safety and efficacy not established. **Elderly:** Age-related decreased renal function may require caution; will not tolerate toxicity.

I

INTERACTIONS

DRUG: **Antihypertensives** may increase hypotensive effect. **Glucocorticoids** may decrease effects. **Cardiotoxic-, hepatotoxic-, nephrotoxic-, myelotoxic**-producing medications may increase toxicity. **HERBAL:** None known. **FOOD:** None known. **LAB VALUES:** May increase bilirubin, BUN, serum creatinine, transaminase, alkaline phosphatase. May decrease magnesium, calcium, phosphorus, potassium, sodium.

AVAILABILITY (Rx)

POWDER FOR INJECTION: 22 million units (1.3 mg).

ADMINISTRATION/HANDLING

Alert: Hold administration in pts who develop moderate to severe lethargy or somnolence (continued administration may result in coma).

IV

Storage • Refrigerate vials, do not freeze. • Reconstituted solution is stable for 48 hrs refrigerated or at room temperature (refrigerated preferred).

Reconstitution • Reconstitute 22-million-units vial with 1.2 ml Sterile Water for Injection to provide concentration of 18 million units/ml. Bacteriostatic Water for Injection or NaCl should not be used to reconstitute because of increased aggregation. • During reconstitution, direct the Sterile Water for Injection at the side of vial. Swirl contents gently to avoid foaming. Do not shake.

Rate of administration • Further dilute dose in 50 ml D_5W and infuse over 15 min. Do not use an in-line filter. • Solution should be warmed to room temperature before infusion. • Monitor diligently for drop in mean arterial B/P (sign of capillary leak syndrome [CLS]). Continued treatment may result in significant hypotension (<90 mm Hg or a 20 mm Hg drop from baseline systolic pressure), edema, pleural effusion, mental status changes.

∅ IV INCOMPATIBILITIES

Ganciclovir (Cytovene), pentamidine (Pentam), prochlorperazine (Compazine), promethazine (Phenergan).

IV COMPATIBILITIES

Calcium gluconate, dopamine (Intropin), heparin, lorazepam (Ativan), magnesium, potassium.

INDICATIONS/ROUTES/DOSAGE

Alert: Restrict therapy to those with normal cardiac and pulmonary function as defined by thallium stress testing, pulmonary function testing. Dosage individualized based on clinical response, tolerance to adverse effects.

METASTATIC MELANOMA, METASTATIC RENAL CELL CARCINOMA

IV: ADULTS >18: 600,000 international units/kg q8h for 14 doses; rest 9 days, repeat 14 doses. Total: 28 doses. May repeat treatment no sooner than 7 wks from date of hospital discharge.

SIDE EFFECTS

Alert: Side effects generally self-limiting and reversible within 2–3 days after discontinuation of therapy.

FREQUENT (48%–89%): Fever, chills, nausea, vomiting, hypotension, diarrhea, oliguria/anuria, mental status changes, irritability, confusion, depression, sinus tachycardia, pain (abdomen, chest, back), fatigue, dyspnea, pruritus. **OCCASIONAL (17%–47%):** Edema, erythema, rash, stomatitis, anorexia, weight gain, infection (urinary tract, injection site, catheter tip), dizziness. **RARE (4%–15%):** Dry skin, sensory disorders (vision, speech, taste), dermatitis, headache, arthralgia, myalgia, weight loss, hematuria, conjunctivitis, proteinuria.

ADVERSE REACTIONS/ TOXIC EFFECTS

Anemia, thrombocytopenia, leukopenia occur commonly. GI bleeding, pulmonary edema occur occasionally. CLS results in hypotension (<90 mm Hg or a 20 mm Hg drop from baseline systolic pressure), extravasation of plasma proteins and fluid into extravascular space, loss of vascular tone. May result in cardiac arrhythmias, angina, MI, respiratory insufficiency. Fatal malignant hyperthermia, cardiac arrest or stroke, pulmonary emboli as well as bowel perforation/gangrene, severe depression leading to suicide have occurred in <1% of pts.

NURSING IMPLICATIONS

BASELINE ASSESSMENT

Pts with bacterial infection and with indwelling central lines should be treated with antibiotic therapy before treatment begins. All pts should be neurologically stable with a negative CT scan before treatment begins. CBC, blood chemistries (including electrolytes), renal/hepatic function tests, chest x-ray should be performed before therapy begins and daily thereafter.

INTERVENTION/EVALUATION

Monitor CBC with differential, platelets, electrolytes, renal/liver functions, weight, pulse oximetry. Determine serum amylase concentration frequently during therapy. Discontinue medication at first sign of hypotension and hold for moderate to severe lethargy (physician must decide whether therapy should continue). Assess mental status changes (irritability, confusion, depression), weight gain/loss. Maintain strict I&O. Assess for extravascular fluid accumulation (rales in lungs, edema in dependent areas).

PATIENT/FAMILY TEACHING

Nausea may decrease during therapy. At home, increase fluid intake (protects against renal impairment). Do not have immunizations without physician's approval (drug lowers body resistance); avoid contact with those who have recently taken live virus vaccine.

Invanz

see ertapenem

ipecac syrup

ip-eh-**kak**
(PMS Ipecac Syrup ✤)

CLASSIFICATION

PHARMACOTHERAPEUTIC: Antidote.
CLINICAL: Antidote.

ACTION

Acts centrally by stimulating medullary chemoreceptor trigger zone and locally by irritating gastric mucosa. **Therapeutic Effect:** Produces emesis.

USES

Induces vomiting in early treatment of unabsorbed oral poisons, drug overdosage.

PRECAUTIONS

CONTRAINDICATIONS: Do not use in unconscious pts, those with absent gag reflex, seizures. Do not use for ingestion of strong bases or acids, corrosive substances, volatile oils, hydrocarbons with high potential for aspiration. **CAUTIONS:** Cardiovascular disease, bulimia. **Pregnancy Category C.**

I

INTERACTIONS

DRUG: **Antiemetics** may decrease effect. **HERBAL:** None known. **FOOD:** Avoid **carbonated beverages** (causes stomach distention), **milk/milk products** (decreases effectiveness). **LAB VALUES:** None known.

AVAILABILITY (OTC)

ELIXIR; SYRUP.

INDICATIONS/ROUTES/DOSAGE

Alert: If vomiting has not occurred within 20 min after first dose, repeat with 15 ml. If vomiting has not occurred within 30 min after last dose, initiate gastric lavage, activated charcoal.

EMETIC

PO: ADULTS, ELDERLY, CHILDREN >12 YRS: 15–30 ml; give with 3–4 glasses of water immediately following administration. CHILDREN 1–12 YRS: 15 ml; follow with 1–2 glasses of water. CHILDREN 6 MOS–1 YR: 5–10 ml; follow with 1 glass of water. If vomiting has not occurred within 30 min, repeat initial dosage.

SIDE EFFECTS

EXPECTED RESPONSE: Nausea, vomiting. After vomiting, diarrhea and CNS symptoms (drowsiness, mild CNS depression) commonly occur.

ADVERSE REACTIONS/ TOXIC EFFECTS

Cardiotoxicity may occur if ipecac syrup is not vomited (noted as hypotension, tachycardia/precordial chest pain, pulmonary congestion, dyspnea, ventricular tachycardia/fibrillation, cardiac arrest). Overdose may produce diarrhea, fast/irregular heartbeat, nausea continuing >30 min, stomach pain, respiratory difficulty, aching/stiff muscles.

NURSING IMPLICATIONS

BASELINE ASSESSMENT

Do not administer to semiconscious, unconscious, convulsing pt. Gastric lavage, activated charcoal is necessary if vomiting does not occur within 30 min of second dose to avoid drug toxicity (bloody stools, vomiting, abdominal pain, hypotension, dyspnea, shock, cardiac disturbances, seizures, coma). Maintain pt in upright position to enhance emetic effect.

INTERVENTION/EVALUATION

Closely monitor vital signs, EKG during and following drug administration. Watch for changes from initial assessment. Check for reversal of poisoning or overdosage symptoms. Monitor daily bowel activity/stool consistency (watery, loose, soft, semisolid, solid); record time of evacuation. Assess for dehydration in excessive vomiting (poor skin turgor, dry mucous membranes, longitudinal furrows in tongue).

ipratropium bromide

ih-prah-**trow**-pea-um

(Atrovent)

Do not confuse with Alupent.

FIXED COMBINATION(S)

Combivent, Duoneb: ipratropime/albuterol (a bronchodilator): *Aerosol:* 18 mcg/103 mcg per actuation. *Solution:* 0.5 ml/2.5 ml per 3 ml.

◆CLASSIFICATION

PHARMACOTHERAPEUTIC: Anticholinergic. **CLINICAL:** Bronchodilator.

ACTION

Blocks action of acetylcholine at parasympathetic sites in bronchial smooth muscle. **Therapeutic Effect:** Causes bronchodilation, inhibits secretions from the glands lining the nasal mucosa.

PHARMACOKINETICS

Onset	Peak	Duration
Inhalation		
1–3 min	1–2 hrs	4–6 hrs

Minimal systemic absorption. Metabolized in liver (systemic absorption). Primarily eliminated in feces. **Half-life:** 1.5–4 hrs.

USES

Maintenance treatment of bronchospasm due to chronic obstructive airway disease, including bronchitis, emphysema. Adjunct to bronchodilators for maintenance treatment of bronchial asthma. Not to be used for immediate bronchospasm relief. **Nasal Spray:** Rhinorrhea (0.03% associated with perineal rhinitis, 0.06% associated with common cold).

PRECAUTIONS

CONTRAINDICATIONS: History of hypersensitivity to atropine. **CAUTIONS:** Narrow-angle glaucoma, prostatic hypertrophy, bladder neck obstruction.

LIFESPAN CONSIDERATIONS: Pregnancy/lactation: Unknown if distributed in breast milk. **Pregnancy Category B. Children/elderly:** No age-related precautions noted.

INTERACTIONS

DRUG: Avoid mixing with **cromolyn inhalation** solution (forms precipitate). **HERBAL:** None known. **FOOD:** None known. **LAB VALUES:** None known.

AVAILABILITY (Rx)

ORAL INHALATION: 18 mcg/actuation. **AEROSOL SOLUTION FOR INHALATION:** 0.02% (500-mcg vial). **NASAL SPRAY:** 0.03%, 0.06%.

ADMINISTRATION/HANDLING

INHALATION

• Shake container well, exhale completely through mouth; place mouthpiece into mouth, close lips, holding inhaler upright. • Inhale deeply through mouth while fully depressing the top of canister. Hold breath as long as possible before exhaling slowly. • Wait 2 min before inhaling second dose (allows for deeper bronchial penetration). • Rinse mouth with water immediately after inhalation (prevents mouth/throat dryness).

INDICATIONS/ROUTES/DOSAGE

BRONCHOSPASM

Inhalation: ADULTS, ELDERLY: 2 inhalations 4 times/day. Wait 1–10 min before administering second inhalation. **Maximum:** 12 inhalations/24 hrs. CHILDREN 3–12 YRS: 1–2 inhalations 3 times/day. **Maximum:** 6 inhalations/24 hrs.

Nebulization: ADULTS, ELDERLY: 500 mcg 3–4 times/day. CHILDREN: 125–250 mcg 3 times/day. NEONATES: 25 mcg/kg/dose 3 times/day.

RHINORRHEA

Intranasal: ADULTS, CHILDREN >6 YRS: 0.03%: 2 sprays 2–3 times/day. ADULTS, CHILDREN >12 YRS: 0.06%: 2 sprays 3–4 times/day.

SIDE EFFECTS

FREQUENT: Inhalation (3%–6%): Cough, dry mouth, headache, nausea. **Nasal:** Dry nose/mouth, headache, nasal irritation. **OCCASIONAL: Inhalation (2%):** Dizziness, transient increased bronchospasm. **RARE (<1%):** Hypotension, insomnia, metallic/unpleasant taste, palpitations, urinary retention. **Nasal:** Diarrhea/constipation, dry throat, stomach pain, stuffy nose.

ADVERSE REACTIONS/ TOXIC EFFECTS

Worsening of narrow-angle glaucoma, acute eye pain, hypotension occur rarely.

NURSING IMPLICATIONS

BASELINE ASSESSMENT

Offer emotional support (high incidence of anxiety due to difficulty in breathing, sympathomimetic response to drug).

INTERVENTION/EVALUATION

Monitor rate, depth, rhythm, type of respiration; quality, rate of pulse. Assess lung sounds for rhonchi, wheezing, rales. Monitor ABGs. Observe lips, fingernails for blue or dusky color in light-skinned pts; gray in dark-skinned pts. Observe for clavicular, sternal, intercostal retractions, hand tremor. Evaluate for clinical improvement (quieter, slower respirations, relaxed facial expression, cessation of retractions).

PATIENT/FAMILY TEACHING

Increase fluid intake (decreases lung secretion viscosity). Do not take >2 inhalations at any one time (excessive use may produce paradoxical bronchoconstriction or a decreased bronchodilating effect). Rinsing mouth with water immediately after inhalation may prevent mouth/throat dryness. Avoid excessive use of caffeine derivatives (chocolate, coffee, tea, cola, cocoa).

irbesartan

ir-beh-**sar**-tan
(Avapro)

FIXED-COMBINATION(S)

Avalide: irbesartan/hydrochlorothiazide (a diuretic): 150 mg/12.5 mg; 300 mg/12.5 mg.

◆CLASSIFICATION

PHARMACOTHERAPEUTIC: Angiotensin II receptor antagonist. **CLINICAL:** Antihypertensive (see p. 7C).

ACTION

Potent vasodilator. An angiotensin II receptor (type AT_1) antagonist; blocks vasoconstrictor and aldosterone-secreting effects of angiotensin II, inhibiting the binding of angiotensin II to the AT_1 receptors. **Therapeutic Effect:** Produces vasodilation, decreases peripheral resistance, decreases B/P.

PHARMACOKINETICS

Rapidly and completely absorbed after PO administration. Protein binding: 90%. Undergoes hepatic metabolism to inactive metabolite. Excreted primarily in feces and, to a lesser extent, in urine. Not removed by hemodialysis. **Half-life:** 11–15 hrs.

USES

Treatment of hypertension alone or in combination with other antihypertensives. Treatment of diabetic nephropathy. **Unlabeled:** Treatment of heart failure.

PRECAUTIONS

CONTRAINDICATIONS: Severe liver insufficiency, biliary cirrhosis/obstruction, primary hyperaldosteronism, bilateral renal artery stenosis. **CAUTIONS:** Mild to moderate liver dysfunction, sodium/water depletion, CHF, unilateral renal artery stenosis, coronary artery disease.

LIFESPAN CONSIDERATIONS: Unknown if distributed in breast milk. May cause fetal/neonatal morbidity/mortality. **Pregnancy/lactation:** Category C (D if used in second or third trimester). **Children:** Safety and efficacy not established. **Elderly:** No age-related precautions noted.

INTERACTIONS

DRUG: **Hydrochlorothiazide** produces further reduction in B/P. **HERBAL:** None known. **FOOD:** None known. **LAB VALUES:** Minor increase in BUN, serum creatinine. May decrease Hgb.

AVAILABILITY (Rx)

TABLETS: 75 mg, 150 mg, 300 mg.

ADMINISTRATION/HANDLING

PO

- Give without regard to meals.

INDICATIONS/ROUTES/DOSAGE

Alert: May be given concurrently with other antihypertensives. If B/P is not controlled by irbesartan alone, a diuretic may be added.

HYPERTENSION

PO: ADULTS, ELDERLY, CHILDREN ≥13 YRS: Initially, 75–150 mg/day. May increase to 300 mg/day. CHILDREN 6–12 YRS: Initially, 75 mg/day. May increase to 150 mg/day.

SIDE EFFECTS

OCCASIONAL (3%–9%): Upper respiratory infection, fatigue, diarrhea, cough. **RARE (1%–2%):** Heartburn, dizziness, headache, nausea, rash.

ADVERSE REACTIONS/ TOXIC EFFECTS

Overdosage may manifest as hypotension, tachycardia; bradycardia occurs less often. Institute supportive measures.

NURSING IMPLICATIONS

BASELINE ASSESSMENT

Obtain B/P, apical pulse immediately prior to each dose, in addition to regular monitoring (be alert to fluctuations). If excessive reduction in B/P occurs, place pt in supine position, feet slightly elevated. Question possibility of pregnancy (see Pregnancy Category). Assess medication history (esp. diuretic therapy).

INTERVENTION/EVALUATION

Maintain hydration (offer fluids frequently). Assess for evidence of upper respiratory infection. Assist with ambulation if dizziness occurs. Monitor electrolytes, renal/liver function tests, urinalysis, B/P, pulse. Assess for hypotension.

PATIENT/FAMILY TEACHING

Inform female pt regarding consequences of second- and third-trimester exposure to irbesartan. Avoid tasks that require alertness, motor skills (possible dizziness effect). Report any sign of infection (sore throat, fever). Caution against exercising during hot weather (risk of dehydration, hypotension).

irinotecan

eye-rin-**oh**-teh-can
(Camptosar)

CLASSIFICATION

PHARMACOTHERAPEUTIC: DNA topoisomerase inhibitor. **CLINICAL:** Antineoplastic (see p. 73C).

ACTION

Interacts with topoisomerase I, an enzyme, which relieves torsional strain in DNA by inducing reversible single-strand breaks. Binds to topoisomerase-DNA complex preventing relegation of these single-strand breaks. **Therapeutic Effect:** Produces cytotoxic effect due to double-strand DNA damage produced during DNA synthesis.

PHARMACOKINETICS

Following IV administration, metabolized to active metabolite in liver. Protein binding (metabolite): 95%. Excreted in urine and eliminated via biliary route. **Half-life:** 6 hrs; metabolite: 10 hrs.

USES

I

Treatment of metastatic carcinoma of colon/rectum in pts whose disease has recurred or progressed after 5-fluorouracil-based therapy.

PRECAUTIONS

CONTRAINDICATIONS: None known. **CAUTIONS:** Pt previously receiving pelvic/abdominal irradiation (increased risk of myelosuppression), elderly >65 yrs.

LIFESPAN CONSIDERATIONS: Pregnancy/lactation: May cause fetal harm. Unknown if distributed in breast milk; discontinue breast-feeding. **Pregnancy Category C (1st trimester), D (2nd and 3rd trimester). Children:** Safety and efficacy not established. **Elderly:** Risk of diarrhea significantly increased.

INTERACTIONS

DRUG: Other myelosuppressants may increase risk of myelosuppression. May increase akathisia with **prochlorperazine. Laxatives** may increase severity of diarrhea. **Diuretics** may increase risk of dehydration (due to vomiting/diarrhea with irinotecan therapy). **Live virus vaccines** may potentiate virus replication, increase vaccine side effects, decrease pt's antibody response to vaccine. **HERBAL:** None known. **FOOD:** None known. **LAB VALUES:** May increase SGOT (AST), alkaline phosphatase.

AVAILABILITY (Rx)

INJECTION: 20 mg/ml vial.

ADMINISTRATION/HANDLING

IV

Storage • Store vials at room temperature, protect from light. • Solution diluted in D_5W is stable for 48 hrs if refrigerated. • Use within 24 hrs if refrigerated or 6 hrs if kept at room temperature. • Do not refrigerate solution if diluted with 0.9% NaCl.

Reconstitution • Dilute in D_5W (preferred) or 0.9% NaCl to concentration of 0.12 to 1.1 mg/ml.

Rate of administration • Administer all doses as IV infusion over 90 min. • Assess for extravasation (flush site with sterile water, apply ice if extravasation occurs).

IV INCOMPATIBILITY

Gemcitabine (Gemzar).

INDICATIONS/ROUTES/DOSAGE

CARCINOMA OF COLON/RECTUM

IV infusion: ADULTS, ELDERLY: Initially, 125 mg/m² once weekly for 4 wks. Rest 2 wks. Additional courses may be repeated q6wks. Subsequent doses adjusted in 25–50 mg/m² increments as high as 150 mg/m², as low as 50 mg/m².

Alert: Do not begin a new course until granulocyte count recovered to >1,500/mm³, platelet count recovered to >100,000/mm³, and treatment-related diarrhea fully resolved.

SIDE EFFECTS

COMMON: Nausea (64%), alopecia (49%), vomiting (45%), diarrhea (32%). **FREQUENT:** Constipation, fatigue (29%), fever (28%), asthenia (loss of strength, energy) (25%), skeletal pain (23%), abdominal pain, dyspnea (22%). **OCCASIONAL:** Anorexia (19%), headache, stomatitis (18%), rash (16%).

ADVERSE REACTIONS/ TOXIC EFFECTS

Expect myelosuppression characterized as neutropenia in 97% of pts, neutrophil count <500/mm^3 in 78%. Thrombocytopenia, anemia sepsis occur frequently.

NURSING IMPLICATIONS

BASELINE ASSESSMENT

Offer emotional support to pt/family. Assess hydration status, electrolytes, CBC prior to each dose. Premedicate with antiemetics on day of treatment, starting at least 30 min prior to administration.

INTERVENTION/EVALUATION

Assess for early signs of diarrhea (preceded by complaints of diaphoresis, abdominal cramping). Monitor hydration status, I&O, electrolytes, CBC, Hgb, platelets. Monitor infusion site for signs of inflammation. Inform pt of possibility of alopecia. Assess skin for evidence of rash.

PATIENT/FAMILY TEACHING

Inform pt of possible late diarrhea causing dehydration, electrolyte depletion. Provide antiemetic/antidiarrheal regimen for subsequent use. Do not have immunizations without physician's approval (drug lowers body's resistance). Avoid contact with those who have recently received live virus vaccine. Avoid crowds, those with infections.

iron dextran

iron **dex**-tran
(Dexiron ✤, Infed, Infufer ✤)

◆CLASSIFICATION

PHARMACOTHERAPEUTIC: Trace element. **CLINICAL:** Hematinic iron preparation.

ACTION

Essential component of formation of Hgb. Necessary for effective erythropoiesis, O_2 transport capacity of blood. Serves as cofactor of several essential enzymes. **Therapeutic Effect:** Replenishes Hgb, depleted iron stores.

PHARMACOKINETICS

Readily absorbed after IM administration. Major portion of absorption occurs within 72 hrs; remainder within 3–4 wks. Iron is bound to protein to form hemosiderin, ferritin, or transferrin. No physiologic system of elimination. Small amounts lost daily in shedding of skin, hair, nails and in feces, urine, perspiration. **Half-life:** 5–20 hrs.

USES

Treatment of established iron deficiency anemia. Use only when PO administration is not feasible or when rapid replenishment of iron is warranted.

PRECAUTIONS

CONTRAINDICATIONS: All anemias except iron deficiency anemia (pernicious, aplastic, normocytic, refractory). **EXTREME CAUTION:** Serious liver impairment. **CAUTIONS:** History of allergies, bronchial asthma, rheumatoid arthritis.

LIFESPAN CONSIDERATIONS: Pregnancy/lactation: May cross placenta in some form (unknown). Trace distributed in breast milk. **Pregnancy Category C. Children/elderly:** No age-related precautions noted.

INTERACTIONS

DRUG: None known. **HERBAL:** None known. **FOOD:** None known. **LAB VALUES:** None known.

AVAILABILITY (Rx)

INJECTION: 50 mg/ml.

ADMINISTRATION/HANDLING

Alert: Test dose is generally given before the full dosage; stay with pt for several minutes after injection due to potential for anaphylactic reaction.

IM

• Draw up medication with one needle; use new needle for injection (minimizes skin staining). • Administer deep IM in upper outer quadrant of buttock only. • Use Z-tract technique (displacement of subcutaneous tissue lateral to injection site before inserting needle) to minimize skin staining.

IV

Storage • Store at room temperature.

Reconstitution • May give undiluted or dilute in 0.9% NaCl for infusion.

Rate of administration • Do not exceed IV administration rate of 50 mg/min (1 ml/min). A too rapid IV rate may produce flushing, chest pain, shock, hypotension, tachycardia. • Pt must remain recumbent 30–45 min after IV administration (avoid postural hypotension).

IV INCOMPATIBILITY

No information available via Y-site administration.

INDICATIONS/ROUTES/DOSAGE

Alert: Discontinue oral iron form before administering iron dextran. Dosage expressed in terms of milligrams of elemental iron. Dosage individualized based on degree of anemia, pt weight, presence of any bleeding. Use periodic hematologic determinations as guide to therapy.

IRON DEFICIENCY ANEMIA (no blood loss)

IM/IV: ADULTS, ELDERLY: Mg iron = 0.66 × weight (kg) × (100 − Hgb <g/dl>/14.8).

REPLACEMENT SECONDARY TO BLOOD LOSS

IM/IV: ADULTS, ELDERLY: Replacement iron (mg) = blood loss (ml) × Hct.

SIDE EFFECTS

FREQUENT: Allergic reaction (rash, itching), backache, muscle pain, chills, dizziness, headache, fever, nausea, vomiting, flushed skin, pain or redness at injection site, brown discoloration of skin, metallic taste.

ADVERSE REACTIONS/ TOXIC EFFECTS

Anaphylaxis has occurred during the first few minutes following injection, causing death on rare occasions. Leukocytosis, lymphadenopathy occur rarely.

NURSING IMPLICATIONS

BASELINE ASSESSMENT

Do not give concurrently with oral iron form (excessive iron may produce excessive iron storage [hemosiderosis]). Be alert to pts with rheumatoid arthritis or iron deficiency anemia (acute exacerbation of joint pain/swelling may occur). Inguinal lymphadenopathy may occur with IM injection. Assess for adequate muscle mass before injecting medication.

INTERVENTION/EVALUATION

Monitor IM site for abscess formation, necrosis, atrophy, swelling, brownish color to skin. Question pt regarding soreness, pain, inflammation at or near IM injection site. Check IV site for phlebitis. Monitor serum ferritin levels.

PATIENT/FAMILY TEACHING

Pain, brown staining may occur at injection site. Oral iron should not be taken when receiving iron injections. Stools often become black with iron therapy; this is harmless unless accompanied by red streaking, sticky consistency of stool, abdominal pain/cramping, which should be reported to physician. Oral hygiene, hard candy, gum may reduce metallic taste. Notify physician immediately if fever, back pain, headache occur.

iron sucrose

iron **sue**-crose
(Venofer)

CLASSIFICATION

PHARMACOTHERAPEUTIC: Trace element. **CLINICAL:** Hematinic iron preparation.

ACTION

Essential component of formation of Hgb. Necessary for effective erythropoiesis, O_2 transport capacity of blood. Serves as cofactor of several essential enzymes. **Therapeutic Effect:** Replenishes body iron stores in pts on chronic hemodialysis who have iron deficiency anemia and are receiving erythropoietin.

USES

Treatment of iron deficiency anemia in pts undergoing chronic hemodialysis who are receiving supplemental erythropoietin therapy. **Unlabeled:** Treatment of dystrophic epidermolysis bullosa.

PRECAUTIONS

CONTRAINDICATIONS: All anemias except iron deficiency anemia (pernicious, aplastic, normocytic, refractory anemia), evidence of iron overload. **CAUTIONS:** History of allergies, bronchial asthma; hepatic, renal, cardiac dysfunction. **Pregnancy Category B.**

INTERACTIONS

DRUG: None known. **HERBAL:** None known. **FOOD:** None known. **LAB VALUES:** Increases Hgb, Hct, serum ferritin, serum transferrin saturation.

AVAILABILITY (Rx)

INJECTION: 20 mg/ml (100 mg elemental iron) in 5-ml single-dose vial.

ADMINISTRATION/HANDLING

Alert: Administer directly into dialysis line during hemodialysis.

IV

Storage • Store at room temperature.

Reconstitution • May give undiluted as slow IV injection or IV infusion. For IV infusion, dilute each vial in maximum of 100 ml 0.9% NaCl immediately before infusion.

Rate of administration • For IV injection, administer into the dialysis line at a rate of 1 ml (20 mg iron) undiluted solution per min (5 min per vial). Do not exceed 1 vial per injection. • For IV infusion, administer into dialysis line (reduces risk of hypotensive episodes) at a rate of 100 mg iron over at least 15 min.

IV INCOMPATIBILITIES

Do not mix with other medication or add to parenteral nutrition solution for IV infusion.

INDICATIONS/ROUTES/DOSAGE

Alert: Dosage expressed in terms of milligrams of elemental iron.

IRON DEFICIENCY ANEMIA

IV: ADULTS, ELDERLY: 5 ml iron sucrose (100 mg elemental iron) delivered by IV during dialysis; administer 1–3 times/wk to total dose of 1,000 mg in 10 doses. Give no more than 3 times/wk.

SIDE EFFECTS

FREQUENT (23%–36%): Hypotension, leg cramps, diarrhea.

ADVERSE REACTIONS/TOXIC EFFECTS

A too rapid IV administration may produce severe hypotension, headache, vomiting, nausea, dizziness, paresthesia, abdominal/muscle pain, edema, cardiovascular collapse. Hypersensitivity reaction occurs rarely.

NURSING IMPLICATIONS

INTERVENTION/EVALUATION

Initially, monitor Hgb, Hct, serum ferritin, serum transferrin levels monthly then q2–3mos thereafter. Reliable serum iron values can be obtained 48 hrs following administration.

isoetharine

(Bronkosol)

See Classification section under: Bronchodilators

isoflurophate

(Floropryl)

See Classification section under: Antiglaucoma agents

isoniazid

eye-sew-**nye**-ah-zid

(INH, Isotamine✤, Nydrazid, PMS Isoniazid✤)

FIXED-COMBINATION(S)

Rifamate: isoniazid/rifampin (antitubercular): 150 mg/300 mg. **Rifater:** isoniazid/pyrazinamide/rifampin (antituberculars): 50 mg/300 mg/120 mg.

◆CLASSIFICATION

PHARMACOTHERAPEUTIC: Isonicotinic acid derivative. **CLINICAL:** Antitubercular

ACTION

Inhibits mycolic acid synthesis. Active only during cell division. **Therapeutic Effect:** Causes disruption of bacterial cell wall, loss of acid-fast properties in susceptible mycobacteria. Bactericidal.

PHARMACOKINETICS

Readily absorbed from GI tract. Protein binding: 10%–15%. Widely distributed (including CSF). Metabolized in liver. Primarily excreted in urine. Removed by hemodialysis. **Half-life:** 0.5–5 hrs.

USES

Drug of choice in tuberculosis prophylaxis. Used in combination with one or more other antitubercular agents for treatment of all forms of active tuberculosis.

PRECAUTIONS

CONTRAINDICATIONS: Acute liver disease, history of hypersensitivity reactions, hepatic injury with previous isoniazid therapy. **CAUTIONS:** Chronic liver disease, alcoholism, severe renal impairment. May be cross-sensitive with nicotinic acid, other chemically related medications.

LIFESPAN CONSIDERATIONS: Pregnancy/lactation: Prophylaxis usually postponed until after delivery. Crosses placenta. Distributed in breast milk. **Pregnancy Category C. Children:** No age-related precautions noted. **Elderly:** More susceptible to developing hepatitis.

INTERACTIONS

DRUG: Alcohol may increase hepatotoxicity, metabolism. May increase toxicity of **carbamazepine, phenytoin.** May decrease **ketoconazole** concentrations. **Disulfiram** may increase CNS effects. **Hepatotoxic medications** may increase hepatotoxicity. **HERBAL:** None known. **FOOD:** None known. **LAB VALUES:** May increase SGOT (AST), SGPT (ALT), bilirubin.

AVAILABILITY (Rx)

TABLETS: 100 mg, 300 mg. **SYRUP:** 50 mg/5 ml. **INJECTION:** 100 mg/ml.

ADMINISTRATION/HANDLING

PO

• Give 1 hr prior to or 2 hrs following meals (may give with food to decrease GI upset, but will delay absorption).
• Administer at least 1 hr before antacids, esp. those containing aluminum.

INDICATIONS/ROUTES/DOSAGE

TUBERCULOSIS (TREATMENT)

PO/IM: ADULTS, ELDERLY: 5 mg/kg/day as single dose. **Maximum:** 300 mg/day. CHILDREN: 10–15 mg/kg/day as single dose. **Maximum:** 300 mg/day.

TUBERCULOSIS (PREVENTION)

PO/IM: ADULTS, ELDERLY: 300 mg/day as single dose. CHILDREN: 10 mg/kg/day as single dose. **Maximum:** 300 mg/day.

SIDE EFFECTS

FREQUENT: Nausea, vomiting, diarrhea, abdominal pain. **RARE:** Pain at injection site, hypersensitivity reaction.

ADVERSE REACTIONS/ TOXIC EFFECTS

Neurotoxicity (clumsiness/unsteadiness, numbness, tingling, burning/pain in hands/feet), optic neuritis, hepatotoxicity occur rarely.

NURSING IMPLICATIONS

BASELINE ASSESSMENT

Question for history of hypersensitivity reactions, hepatic injury from isoniazid, sensitivity to nicotinic acid/chemically related medications. Ensure collection of specimens for culture, sensitivity. Evaluate initial hepatic function results.

INTERVENTION/EVALUATION

Monitor hepatic function test results and assess for hepatitis: anorexia, nausea, vomiting, weakness, fatigue, dark urine, jaundice (hold INH and inform physician promptly). Assess for tingling, numbness, burning of extremities (those esp. at risk for neuropathy may be given pyridoxine prophylactically: malnourished, elderly, diabetics, pts with chronic liver disease [including alcoholics]). Be alert for fever, skin eruptions (hypersensitivity reaction).

PATIENT/FAMILY TEACHING

Do not skip doses; continue taking isoniazid for full length of therapy (6–24 mos). Take preferably 1 hr prior to or 2 hrs following meals (with food if GI upset). Avoid alcohol during treatment. Do not take any other medications including antacids without consulting physician. Must take isoniazid at least 1 hr before antacid. Avoid tuna, sauerkraut, aged cheeses, smoked fish (provide list of tyramine-containing foods) that may cause reaction such as red/itching skin, pounding heartbeat, lightheadedness, hot/clammy feeling, headache; contact physician. Notify physician of any new symptom, immediately for vision difficulties, nausea/vomiting, dark urine, yellowing of skin/eyes, fatigue, numbness/tingling of hands/feet.

isoproterenol

(Isuprel)

See Classification section under: Sympathomimetics

isosorbide dinitrate

eye-sew-**sore**-bide
(Apo-ISDN✤, Cedocard✤, Dilatrate, Isordil)

isosorbide mononitrate

(Imdur, ISMO, Monoket)

Do not confuse with Inderal, Isuprel, K-Dur, Plendil.

◆ CLASSIFICATION

PHARMACOTHERAPEUTIC: Nitrate. **CLINICAL:** Antianginal (see p. 108C).

ACTION

Stimulates intracellular cyclic GMP. **Therapeutic Effect:** Relaxes vascular smooth muscle of both arterial and venous vasculature. Decreases preload, afterload.

PHARMACOKINETICS

Onset	Peak	Duration
Sublingual		
2–10 min	—	1–2 hrs
Chewable		
3 min	—	0.5–2 hrs
PO		
45–60 min	—	4–6 hrs
SR		
30 min	—	6–12 hrs

Mononitrate well absorbed after PO administration. Dinitrate poorly absorbed and metabolized in the liver to activate metabolite (mononitrate). Excreted in urine and feces. **Half-life:** Dinitrate: 1–4 hrs. Mononitrate: 4 hrs.

USES

Prophylaxis, treatment of angina pectoris. **Unlabeled:** CHF, pain relief, dysphagia, relief of esophageal spasm with GE reflux.

PRECAUTIONS

CONTRAINDICATIONS: Hypersensitivity to nitrates, severe anemia, closed-angle glaucoma, postural hypotension, head trauma, increased intracranial pressure. **Extended-release:** GI hypermotility/malabsorption, severe anemia. **CAUTIONS:** Acute MI, hepatic/renal disease, glaucoma (contraindicated in closed-angle glaucoma), blood volume depletion from diuretic therapy, systolic B/P <90 mm Hg.

LIFESPAN CONSIDERATIONS: Pregnancy/lactation: Unknown if drug crosses placenta or is distributed in breast milk. **Pregnancy Category C. Children:** Safety and efficacy not established. **Elderly:** May be more sensitive to hypotensive effects. Age-related decreased renal function may require cautious use.

INTERACTIONS

DRUG: Alcohol, antihypertensives, vasodilators may increase risk of orthostatic hypotension. **HERBAL:** None known. **FOOD:** None known. **LAB VALUES:** May increase urine catecholamines, urine VMA (vanillylmandelic acid).

AVAILABILITY (Rx)

DINITRATE: TABLETS: 5 mg, 10 mg, 20 mg, 30 mg, 40 mg. **TABLETS (sublingual):** 10 mg. **CAPSULES (sustained-release):** 40 mg.

MONONITRATE: TABLETS: 10 mg, 20 mg. **TABLETS (extended-release):** 30 mg, 60 mg, 120 mg.

ADMINISTRATION/HANDLING

PO

• Best if taken on an empty stomach. • Oral tablets may be crushed. • Do not crush or break sublingual or extended-release form. • Do not crush chewable form before administering.

SUBLINGUAL

• Do not crush/chew sublingual tablets. • Dissolve tablets under tongue; do not swallow.

INDICATIONS/ROUTES/DOSAGE

ACUTE ANGINA, PROPHYLACTIC MANAGEMENT IN SITUATIONS LIKELY TO PROVOKE ATTACK

Sublingual: ADULTS, ELDERLY: Initially, 2.5–5 mg. Repeat at 5- to 10-min intervals. No more than 3 doses in 15- to 30-min period.

ACUTE PROPHYLACTIC MANAGEMENT OF ANGINA

Sublingual: ADULTS, ELDERLY: 5–10 mg q2–3h.

LONG-TERM PROPHYLAXIS OF ANGINA

PO: ADULTS, ELDERLY: Initially, 5–20 mg 3–4 times/day. MAINTENANCE: 10–40 mg q6h. Consider 2–3 times/day, last dose no later than 7 PM to minimize intolerance.

Mononitrate: ADULTS, ELDERLY: 20 mg 2 times/day, 7 hrs apart. First dose upon awakening in morning.

Extended-release: ADULTS, ELDERLY: Initially, 40 mg. MAINTENANCE: 40–80 mg 2–3 times/day. Consider 1–2 times/day, last dose at 2 PM to minimize intolerance.

Imdur: 60–120 mg/day as single dose.

SIDE EFFECTS

FREQUENT: Headache (may be severe) occurs mostly in early therapy, diminishes rapidly in intensity, usually disappears during continued treatment; transient flushing of face/neck, dizziness (esp. if pt is standing immobile or is in a warm environment), weakness, postural hypotension, nausea, vomiting, restlessness. **Sublingual:** Burning, tingling sensation at oral point of dissolution. **OCCASIONAL:** GI upset, blurred vision, dry mouth.

ADVERSE REACTIONS/ TOXIC EFFECTS

Drug should be discontinued if blurred vision, dry mouth occurs. Severe postural hypotension manifested by fainting, pulselessness, cold/clammy skin, diaphoresis. Tolerance may occur with repeated, prolonged therapy (minor tolerance with intermittent use of sublingual tablets). Tolerance may not occur with extended-release form. High dose tends to produce severe headache.

NURSING IMPLICATIONS

BASELINE ASSESSMENT

Record onset, type (sharp, dull, squeezing), radiation, location, intensity, duration of anginal pain; precipitating factors (exertion, emotional stress). If headache occurs during management therapy, administer medication with meals.

INTERVENTION/EVALUATION

Assist with ambulation if lightheadedness, dizziness occurs. Assess for facial/neck flushing. Monitor number of anginal episodes, orthostatic B/P.

PATIENT/FAMILY TEACHING

Do not chew or crush sublingual or sustained-release forms. Take sublingual tablets while sitting down. Notify physician if angina persists for >20 min. Rise slowly from lying to sitting position, dangle legs momentarily before standing. Take oral form on empty stomach (however, if headache occurs during management therapy, take medication with meals). Dissolve sublingual tablet under tongue; do not swallow. Take at first signal of angina. If not relieved within 5 min, dissolve second tablet under tongue. Repeat if no relief in another 5 min. If pain continues, contact physician. Expel from mouth any remaining sublingual tablet after pain is completely relieved. Do not change from one brand of drug to another. Avoid alcohol (intensifies hypotensive effect). If alcohol is ingested soon after taking nitrates, possible acute hypotensive episode (marked drop in B/P, vertigo, pallor) may occur.

isotretinoin

eye-sew-**tret**-ih-noyn
(Accutane, Accutane Roche, Sotret)

Do not confuse with Accupril, Accurbron.

CLASSIFICATION

PHARMACOTHERAPEUTIC: Keratinization stabilizer. **CLINICAL:** Antiacne, antirosacea agent.

ACTION

Reduces sebaceous gland size, inhibiting its activity. **Therapeutic Effect:** Produces antikeratinizing, anti-inflammatory effects.

USES

Treatment of severe, recalcitrant cystic acne that is unresponsive to conventional acne therapies. **Unlabeled:** Treatment of gram-neg folliculitis, severe rosacea, correcting severe keratinization disorders.

PRECAUTIONS

CONTRAINDICATIONS: Hypersensitivity to isotretinoin, parabens (component of capsules). **CAUTIONS:** Renal, hepatic dysfunction. **Pregnancy Category X.**

INTERACTIONS

DRUG: Etretinate, tretinoin, vitamin A may increase toxic effects. **Tetracycline** may increase potential of pseudotumor cerebri. **HERBAL:** None known. **FOOD:** None known. **LAB VALUES:** May increase triglycerides, cholesterol, SGOT (AST), SGPT (ALT), alkaline phosphatase, LDH, sedimentation rate, fasting blood glucose, uric acid; may decrease HDL.

AVAILABILITY (Rx)

CAPSULES: 10 mg, 20 mg, 40 mg.

INDICATIONS/ROUTES/DOSAGE

RECALCITRANT CYSTIC ACNE

PO: ADULTS: Initially, 0.5–2 mg/kg/day divided in 2 doses for 15–20 wks. May repeat after at least 2 mos of therapy.

SIDE EFFECTS

FREQUENT: Cheilitis (inflammation of lips) (90%), skin/mucous membrane dryness (80%), skin fragility, pruritus, epistaxis, dry nose/mouth, conjunctivitis (40%), hypertriglyceridemia (25%), nausea, vomiting, abdominal pain (20%). **OCCASIONAL:** Musculoskeletal symptoms (16%) including bone or joint pain, arthralgia, generalized muscle aches; photosensitivity (5%–10%). **RARE:** Decreased night vision, depression.

ADVERSE REACTIONS/ TOXIC EFFECTS

Inflammatory bowel disease, pseudotumor cerebri (benign intracranial hypertension) have been associated with isotretinoin therapy.

NURSING IMPLICATIONS

BASELINE ASSESSMENT

Assess baselines for blood lipids, glucose.

INTERVENTION/EVALUATION

Assess acne for decreased cysts. Evaluate skin/mucous membranes for excessive dryness. Monitor blood glucose, lipids.

PATIENT/FAMILY TEACHING

A transient exacerbation of acne may occur during initial period. May have decreased tolerance to contact lenses during and following therapy. Do not take vitamin supplements with vitamin A due to additive effects. Notify physician immediately of onset of abdominal pain, severe diarrhea, rectal bleeding (possible inflammatory bowel disease), headache, nausea/vomiting, visual disturbances (possible pseudotumor cerebri). Decreased night vision may occur suddenly; take caution with night driving. Avoid prolonged exposure to sunlight; use sunscreens, protective clothing. Do not donate blood during or for 1 mo following treatment. **Women:** Explain the serious risk to fetus if pregnancy occurs (both oral and written warnings are given, with pt acknowledging in writing that she understands the warnings and consents to treatment). Must have a negative serum pregnancy test within 2 wks prior to starting therapy; therapy will begin on the second or third day of the next normal menstrual period. Effective contraception (using 2 reliable forms of contraception simultaneously) must be used for at least 1 mo before, during, and for at least 1 mo after therapy.

isradipine

iss-**rah**-dih-peen
(DynaCirc, DynaCirc CR)

Do not confuse with Dynabac, Dynacin.

◆CLASSIFICATION

PHARMACOTHERAPEUTIC: Calcium channel blocker. **CLINICAL:** Antihypertensive (see p. 67C).

ACTION

Inhibits calcium movement across cardiac, vascular smooth muscle. Potent peripheral vasodilator (does not depress SA, AV nodes). **Therapeutic Effect:** Produces relaxation of coronary vascular smooth muscle and coronary vasodilation. Increases myocardial oxygen delivery to those with vasospastic angina.

PHARMACOKINETICS

Onset	Peak	Duration
PO		
2–3 hrs	2–4 wks	—

Well absorbed from GI tract. Protein binding: 95%. Metabolized in liver (undergoes first-pass effect). Primarily excreted in urine. Not removed by hemodialysis. **Half-life:** 8 hrs.

USES

Management of hypertension. May be used alone or with thiazide-type diuretics. **Unlabeled:** Treatment of chronic angina pectoris, Raynaud's phenomena.

PRECAUTIONS

CONTRAINDICATIONS: Sinus bradycardia, heart block, ventricular tachycardia, cardiogenic shock, hypotension, CHF. **CAUTIONS:** Sick sinus syndrome; severe left ventricular dysfunction; liver disease; edema; concurrent therapy with beta-blockers, digoxin.

LIFESPAN CONSIDERATIONS: Pregnancy/lactation: Unknown if drug crosses placenta or is distributed in breast milk. **Pregnancy Category C. Children:** Safety and efficacy not established. **Elderly:** Age-related renal impairment may require cautious use.

INTERACTIONS

DRUG: Beta-blockers may have additive effect. **HERBAL:** None known. **FOOD: Grapefruit/grapefruit juice** may increase absorption. **LAB VALUES:** None known.

AVAILABILITY (Rx)

CAPSULES: 2.5 mg, 5 mg. **CAPSULES (extended-release):** 5 mg, 10 mg.

ADMINISTRATION/HANDLING

PO

- Do not crush or break capsule.

INDICATIONS/ROUTES/DOSAGE

HYPERTENSION

PO: ADULTS, ELDERLY: Initially, 2.5 mg 2 times/day. May increase by 2.5 mg at 2- to 4-wk intervals. RANGE: 5–20 mg/day.

SIDE EFFECTS

FREQUENT (4%–7%): Peripheral edema, palpitations (higher frequency in females). **OCCASIONAL (3%):** Facial flushing, cough. **RARE (1%–2%):** Angina, tachycardia, rash, pruritus.

ADVERSE REACTIONS/ TOXIC EFFECTS

CHF occurs rarely. Overdosage produces nausea, drowsiness, confusion, slurred speech.

NURSING IMPLICATIONS

BASELINE ASSESSMENT

Assess baseline renal/liver function tests. Assess B/P, apical pulse immediately before drug is administered (if pulse is ≤60/min or systolic B/P is <90 mm Hg, withhold medication, contact physician).

INTERVENTION/EVALUATION

Assess for peripheral edema behind medial malleolus (sacral area in bedridden pts). Monitor pulse rate for bradycardia. Monitor B/P; observe for signs, symptoms of CHF. Assess skin for flushing.

PATIENT/FAMILY TEACHING

Do not abruptly discontinue medication. Compliance with therapy regimen is essential to control hypertension. To avoid hypotensive effect, rise slowly from lying to sitting position, wait momentarily before standing. Contact physician/nurse if irregular heartbeat, shortness of breath, pronounced dizziness, nausea occurs. Avoid use of grapefruit/grapefruit juice.

itraconazole

eye-tra-**con**-ah-zoll
(Sporanox)
Do not confuse with Suprax.

CLASSIFICATION

CLINICAL: Antifungal.

ACTION

Inhibits synthesis of ergosterol (vital component of fungal cell formation), damaging fungal cell membrane. **Therapeutic Effect:** Fungistatic.

PHARMACOKINETICS

Moderately absorbed from GI tract (increased with food). Protein binding: 99%. Widely distributed (primarily in liver, kidney, fatty tissue). Metabolized in liver to active metabolite. Primarily excreted in urine. Not removed by hemodialysis. **Half-life:** 21 hrs; metabolite: 12 hrs.

USES

Treatment of blastomycosis (pulmonary, extrapulmonary), histoplasmosis, aspergillosis, onychomycosis, dermatophyte skin infections, tinea pedis in pts unable to take topical therapy. **Solution:** Oral, esophageal candidiasis. **Unlabeled:** Suppression of histoplasmosis; treatment of fungal pneumonia/septicemia, disseminated sporotrichosis, ringworm of hand.

PRECAUTIONS

CONTRAINDICATIONS: Hypersensitivity to itraconazole, fluconazole, ketoconazole, miconazole. **CAUTIONS:** Hepatitis, HIV-infected pts, pts with achlorhydria, hypochlorhydria (decreases absorption), impaired liver function.

LIFESPAN CONSIDERATIONS: Pregnancy/lactation: Distributed in breast milk. **Pregnancy Category C. Children:** Safety and efficacy not established. **Elderly:** Age-related renal impairment may require dosage adjustment.

INTERACTIONS

DRUG: May increase **buspirone, cyclosporine, digoxin, lovastatin, simvastatin** concentrations. May increase effect of **oral anticoagulants. Phenytoin, rifampin** may decrease concentrations. **Antacids, H_2 antagonists, didanosine** may decrease absorption. **HERBAL:** None known. **FOOD: Grapefruit juice** may alter absorption. **LAB VALUES:** May increase SGOT (AST), SGPT (ALT), alkaline phosphatase, LDH, bilirubin. May decrease potassium.

AVAILABILITY (Rx)

CAPSULES: 100 mg. **ORAL SOLUTION:** 10 mg/ml. **INJECTION:** 10 mg/ml, 25-ml amp.

ADMINISTRATION/HANDLING

PO

• Give capsules with food (increases absorption). • Give solution on an empty stomach.

IV

Storage • Store at room temperature. Do not freeze.

Reconstitution • Use only components provided by manufacturer. • Do not dilute with any other diluent. • Add full contents of amp (250 mg/10 ml) to infusion bag provided (50 ml 0.9% NaCl). • Mix gently.

Rate of administration • Infuse over 60 min using extension line and infusion set provided. • After administration, flush infusion set with 15–20 ml 0.9% NaCl over 30 sec to 15 min. • Discard entire infusion line.

IV INCOMPATIBILITIES

Alert: Dilution compatibility other than 0.9% NaCl unknown. Do not mix with D_5W or lactated Ringer's. Do not give any medication in same bag of itraconazole or through same IV line. Not for IV bolus administration. Do not mix with any other medication.

INDICATIONS/ROUTES/DOSAGE

Alert: Doses >200 mg given in 2 divided doses.

BLASTOMYCOSIS, HISTOPLASMOSIS

IV: ADULTS, ELDERLY: 200 mg 2 times/day for 4 doses then 200 mg once daily.

PO: Initially, 200 mg once daily. May increase to maximum of 400 mg/day in 2 divided doses.

ASPERGILLOSIS

IV: ADULTS, ELDERLY: 200 mg 2 times/day for 4 doses then 200 mg once daily.

PO: 600 mg/day in 3 divided doses for 3–4 days, then 200–400 mg/day in 2 divided doses.

ESOPHAGEAL CANDIDIASIS

PO: ADULTS, ELDERLY: Swish 10 ml in the mouth for several seconds then swallow. **Maximum dose:** 200 mg/day.

OROPHARYNGEAL CANDIDIASIS

PO: ADULTS, ELDERLY: Swish 10 ml in the mouth for several seconds.

SIDE EFFECTS

FREQUENT (9%–11%): Nausea, rash. **OCCASIONAL (3%–5%):** Vomiting, headache, diarrhea, hypertension, peripheral

I

edema, fatigue, fever. **RARE (≤2%):** Abdominal pain, dizziness, anorexia, pruritus.

ADVERSE REACTIONS/ TOXIC EFFECTS

Hepatitis (anorexia, abdominal pain, unusual tiredness/weakness, jaundice, dark urine) occurs rarely.

NURSING IMPLICATIONS

BASELINE ASSESSMENT

Determine baseline temperature, liver function tests. Assess allergies.

INTERVENTION/EVALUATION

Assess for signs, symptoms of liver dysfunction and monitor hepatic enzyme test results in pts with preexisting liver dysfunction.

PATIENT/FAMILY TEACHING

Take capsules with food, solution on empty stomach. Therapy will continue for at least 3 mos, until lab tests clinical presentation indicate infection is controlled. Report the following at once: unusual fatigue, yellow skin, dark urine, pale stool, anorexia/nausea/vomiting. Avoid grapefruit/grapefruit juice.

Kadian

see morphine

Kaletra

see lopinavir/ritonavir

kanamycin sulfate

can-ah-**my**-sin
(Kantrex)

CLASSIFICATION

PHARMACOTHERAPEUTIC: Aminoglycoside. **CLINICAL:** Antibiotic.

ACTION

Irreversibly binds to protein on bacterial ribosome. **Therapeutic Effect:** Interferes in protein synthesis of susceptible microorganisms.

USES

Treatment of wound, surgical site irrigation.

AVAILABILITY (Rx)

INJECTION: 1 g/3 ml.

INDICATIONS/ROUTES/DOSAGE

IRRIGATION ADULTS: 0.25% solution to irrigate pleural space, ventricular/abscess cavities, wounds, surgical sites.

SIDE EFFECTS

OCCASIONAL: Hypersensitivity reactions: rash, fever, urticaria, pruritus. **RARE:** Headache.

kaolin/pectin

kay-oh-lyn
(Kaopectate, Kapectolin)
Do not confuse with Kayexalate.

FIXED-COMBINATION(S)

Parepectolin: kaolin/pectin/opium: 5.5 g/162 mg/15 mg.

◆ **CLASSIFICATION**

PHARMACOTHERAPEUTIC: Magnesium/aluminum silicate. **CLINICAL:** Antidiarrheal (see p. 41C).

ACTION

Adsorbent, protectant. **Therapeutic Effect:** Adsorbs bacteria, toxins; reduces water loss.

PHARMACOKINETICS

Not absorbed orally. Up to 90% of pectin decomposed in GI tract.

USES

Symptomatic treatment of mild to moderate acute diarrhea.

PRECAUTIONS

CONTRAINDICATIONS: None known. **CAUTIONS:** None known.

LIFESPAN CONSIDERATIONS: Pregnancy/lactation: Unknown if drug crosses placenta or is distributed in breast milk. **Pregnancy Category C. Children:** Not recommended in those <3 yrs. **Elderly:** More sensitive to fluid and electrolyte loss; use caution.

INTERACTIONS

DRUG: May decrease absorption of **digoxin. HERBAL:** None known. **FOOD:** None known. **LAB VALUES:** None known.

AVAILABILITY (OTC)

ORAL SUSPENSION.

ADMINISTRATION/HANDLING

PO

- Shake suspension well before administration.

INDICATIONS/ROUTES/DOSAGE

ANTIDIARRHEAL

PO: ADULTS, ELDERLY: 60–120 ml after each loose bowel movement (LBM). CHILDREN >12 YRS: 60 ml after each LBM. CHILDREN 6–12 YRS: 30–60 ml after each LBM. CHILDREN 3–5 YRS: 15–30 ml after each LBM.

SIDE EFFECTS

RARE: Constipation.

ADVERSE REACTIONS/ TOXIC EFFECTS

None known.

NURSING IMPLICATIONS

INTERVENTION/EVALUATION

Encourage adequate fluid intake. Assess bowel sounds for peristalsis and stools for frequency, consistency (watery, loose, soft, semisolid, solid).

PATIENT/FAMILY TEACHING

Do not use >2 days or in presence of high fever.

K

kava kava

Also known as ava, kew, sakau, tonga, yagona

Alert: May be removed from market.

◆ **CLASSIFICATION**

HERBAL.

ACTION

Exact mechanism of action unknown, but possesses CNS effects. **Effect:** Anxiolytic, sedative, analgesic effects.

USES

Treatment of anxiety disorders, stress, restlessness. Also used for sedation, sleep enhancement.

PRECAUTIONS

CONTRAINDICATIONS: Pregnancy, lactation (may cause loss of uterine tone).

CAUTIONS: Depression, history of recurrent hepatitis.

LIFESPAN CONSIDERATIONS: Pregnancy/lactation: Contraindicated. **Children:** Safety and efficacy not established. **Elderly:** No age-related precautions noted.

INTERACTIONS

DRUG: **Alcohol, benzodiazepines** may increase risk of drowsiness. **HERBAL:** **Chamomile, goldenseal, melatonin, St. John's wort, ginseng, valerian** may increase risk of excessive drowsiness. **FOOD:** None known. **LAB VALUES:** May increase liver function tests.

K

AVAILABILITY (OTC)

CAPSULES: 140 mg, 150 mg, 250 mg, 300 mg, 425 mg, 500 mg. **LIQUID. EXTRACT. TINCTURE.**

INDICATIONS/ROUTES/DOSAGE

ANXIETY

PO: ADULTS, ELDERLY: 100 mg 3 times/day or 1 cup of the tea 3 times/day.

SIDE EFFECTS

GI upset, headache, dizziness, vision changes (blurred vision, red eyes), allergic skin reactions, dermopathy (dry, flaky skin, yellowing sclera of the eyes, skin, hair, nails), nausea, vomiting, weight loss, shortness of breath.

ADVERSE REACTIONS/ TOXIC EFFECTS

None known.

NURSING IMPLICATIONS

BASELINE ASSESSMENT

Assess if pregnant/breast-feeding (contraindicated). Determine baseline liver function tests. Assess for use of other CNS depressants.

INTERVENTION/EVALUATION

Monitor liver function tests. Assess for allergic skin reactions.

PATIENT/FAMILY TEACHING

Avoid use if pregnant, planning to become pregnant, or breast-feeding; not for use in children <12 yrs. Avoid tasks that require alertness, motor skills until response to herbal is established. Do not use for >3 mos (may be habit forming).

Keflex

see cephalexin

Kefzol

see cefazolin

Keppra

see levetiracetam

ketamine hydrochloride

key-tah-meen
(Ketalar)

CLASSIFICATION

CLINICAL: Rapid-acting general anesthetic (see p. 2C).

ACTION

Selectively blocks afferent impulses, interacts with CNS transmitter systems.

Therapeutic Effect: Produces an anesthetic state characterized by profound analgesia, normal pharyngeal-laryngeal reflexes.

PHARMACOKINETICS

Onset	Peak	Duration
IM (anesthetic)		
3–4 min	—	12–25 min
IM (analgesic)		
30 min	—	15–30 min
IV (anesthetic)		
30 sec	—	5–10 min
IV (analgesic)		
10–15 min	—	—

Rapidly distributed. Metabolized in liver. Primarily excreted in urine. **Half-life:** distribution: 10–15 min, elimination: 2–3 hrs.

USES

Sole anesthetic for short diagnostic and surgical procedures that do not require skeletal muscle relaxation. Induction of anesthesia before administering other general anesthetics. Used to supplement low-potency agents.

PRECAUTIONS

CONTRAINDICATIONS: Elevated intracranial pressure, hypertension, aneurysms, thyrotoxicosis, CHF, angina, psychotic disorders. **CAUTIONS:** GERD, impaired liver function, patients with a full stomach, chronic alcoholics, acutely intoxicated patients.

LIFESPAN CONSIDERATIONS: Pregnancy/lactation: Not recommended; safety not established. **Pregnancy Category B. Children/elderly:** No age-related precautions noted.

INTERACTIONS

DRUG: Antihypertensives, CNS depressants may increase risk of hypotension or respiratory depression. **HERBAL:** None known. **FOOD:** None known. **LAB VALUES:** May increase intraocular pressure.

AVAILABILITY (Rx)

INJECTION: 10 mg/ml, 50 mg/ml, 100 mg/ml.

ADMINISTRATION/HANDLING

IM

- Use 10 mg/ml vial.

IV

Reconstitution • For induction anesthesia using IV push, dilute 100 mg/ml with equal volume Sterile Water for Injection, D_5W, or 0.9% NaCl. • For maintenance IV infusion, dilute 50 mg/ml vial (10 ml) or 100 mg/ml vial (5 ml) to 250–500 ml D_5W or 0.9% NaCl to provide a concentration of 1–2 mg/ml.

Rate of administration • Administer IV push slowly over 60 sec (too rapid IV may produce severe hypotension, respiratory depression). • Administer IV infusion at rate of 0.5 mg/kg/min.

IV INCOMPATIBILITY

No information available via Y-site administration.

IV COMPATIBILITIES

Bupivacaine (Marcaine), clonidine (Duraclon), fentanyl (Sublimaze), lidocaine, morphine, propofol (Diprivan).

INDICATIONS/ROUTES/DOSAGE

USUAL DOSAGE

IM: ADULTS, ELDERLY: 3–8 mg/kg. CHILDREN: 3–7 mg/kg.

IV: ADULTS, ELDERLY: 1–4.5 mg/kg. CHILDREN: 0.5–2 mg/kg.

SIDE EFFECTS

FREQUENT: Increase in B/P, pulse. Emergence reaction occurs frequently (12%), resulting in dreamlike state, vivid imagery, hallucination, delirium; occasionally with confusion, excitement, irrational behavior. Lasts from few hours to 24 hrs after administration. **OCCASIONAL:** Pain at injection site. **RARE:** Rash.

K

ADVERSE REACTIONS/ TOXIC EFFECTS

Continuous or repeated intermittent infusion may result in extreme somnolence, respiratory/circulatory depression. A too rapid IV dose may produce marked severe hypotension, respiratory depression, irregular muscular movements.

NURSING IMPLICATIONS

BASELINE ASSESSMENT

Resuscitative equipment, endotracheal tube, suction, O_2 must be available. Obtain vital signs prior to induction.

INTERVENTION/EVALUATION

Monitor vital signs q3–5min during and after administration until recovery is achieved. Assess for emergence reaction (hypnotic/barbiturate may be needed). Keep verbal, tactile, visual stimulation at minimum during recovery.

PATIENT/FAMILY TEACHING

Avoid tasks that require alertness, motor skills for 24 hrs after anesthesia.

K

ketoconazole

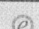

keet-oh-**con**-ah-zol

(Apo-Ketocomazole ✤, Nizoral, Nizoral AD)

Do not confuse with Nasarel.

◆CLASSIFICATION

PHARMACOTHERAPEUTIC: Imidazole derivative. **CLINICAL:** Antifungal (see p. 42C).

ACTION

Changes permeability of cell wall. **Therapeutic Effect:** Inhibits fungal biosynthesis of triglycerides, phospholipids. Fungistatic.

USES

Treatment of histoplasmosis, blastomycosis, candidiasis, chronic mucocutaneous candidiasis, coccidioidomycosis, paracoccidioidomycosis, chromomycosis, seborrheic dermatitis, tineas (ringworm): corporis, capitis, manus, cruris, pedis, unguium (onychomycosis), oral thrush, candiduria. **Shampoo:** Reduces scaling due to dandruff. Treatment of tinea versicolor. **Topical:** Treatment of tineas, pityriasis versicolor, cutaneous candidiasis, seborrhea dermatitis, dandruff. **Unlabeled: Systemic:** Treatment of fungal pneumonia, septicemia, prostate cancer.

PRECAUTIONS

CONTRAINDICATIONS: None known. **CAUTIONS:** Hepatic impairment. **Pregnancy Category C.**

INTERACTIONS

DRUG: **Alcohol, hepatotoxic medications** may increase hepatotoxicity. **Antacids, anticholinergics, H_2 antagonists, omeprazole** may decrease absorption (allow 2-hr interval). May increase concentration, toxicity of **cyclosporine, lovastatin, simvastatin. Isoniazid, rifampin** may decrease concentration. **HERBAL:** **Echinacea** may have additive hepatotoxic effects. **FOOD:** None known. **LAB VALUES:** May increase SGOT (AST), SGPT (ALT), alkaline phosphatase, bilirubin. May decrease corticosteroid, testosterone concentrations.

AVAILABILITY (Rx)

TABLETS: 200 mg. **CREAM:** 2%. **SHAMPOO:** 2%, 1% (OTC).

ADMINISTRATION/HANDLING

PO

• Give with food to minimize GI irritation. • Tablets may be crushed. • Ketoconazole requires acidity; give antacids, anticholinergics, H_2 blockers **at least** 2 hrs following dosing.

SHAMPOO

- Apply to wet hair, massage for 1 min, rinse thoroughly, reapply for 3 min, rinse.

TOPICAL

- Apply, rub gently into affected/surrounding area.

INDICATIONS/ROUTES/DOSAGE

USUAL ORAL DOSAGE

ADULTS, ELDERLY: 200–400 mg/day. CHILDREN: 3.3–6.6 mg/kg/day. **Maximum:** 800 mg/day in 2 divided doses.

USUAL TOPICAL DOSAGE

ADULTS, ELDERLY: Apply 1–2 times/day for 2–4 wks.

DANDRUFF

Shampoo: ADULTS, ELDERLY: 2 times/wk for 4 wks, allowing at least 3 days between shampooing. Intermittent use to maintain control.

SIDE EFFECTS

OCCASIONAL (3%–10%): Nausea, vomiting. **RARE (<2%):** Abdominal pain, diarrhea, headache, dizziness, photophobia, pruritus. Topical application may cause itching, burning, irritation.

ADVERSE REACTIONS/ TOXIC EFFECTS

Hematologic toxicity occurs occasionally (thrombocytopenia, hemolytic anemia, leukopenia). Hepatotoxicity may occur within first week to several months of therapy. Anaphylaxis occurs rarely.

NURSING IMPLICATIONS

BASELINE ASSESSMENT

Confirm that a culture or histologic test was done for accurate diagnosis; therapy may begin before results known.

INTERVENTION/EVALUATION

Monitor hepatic function tests; be alert for hepatotoxicity: dark urine, pale stools, fatigue, anorexia/nausea/vomiting (unrelieved by giving medication with food). Monitor CBC for evidence of hematologic toxicity. Determine pattern of bowel activity, stool consistency. Assess for dizziness, provide assistance as needed. Evaluate skin for rash, urticaria, itching. **Topical:** Check for local burning, itching, irritation.

PATIENT/FAMILY TEACHING

Prolonged therapy (weeks or months) is usually necessary. Do not miss a dose; continue therapy as long as directed. Avoid alcohol (potential for hepatotoxicity). May cause dizziness; avoid tasks that require alertness, motor skills until response to drug is established. Take antacids/antiulcer medications at least 2 hrs after ketoconazole. Notify physician of dark urine, pale stool, yellow skin/eyes, increased irritation in topical use, onset of other new symptoms. **Topical:** Rub well into affected areas. Avoid contact with eyes. Keep skin clean, dry; wear light clothing for ventilation. Separate personal items in direct contact with affected area. **Shampoo:** Initially, use twice weekly for 4 wks with at least 3 days between shampooing; frequency then determined by response to medication.

K

ketoprofen

key-toe-**pro**-fen

(Actron, Apo-Keto✤, Novo-Keto-EC✤, Orudis, Orudis KT, Oruvail, Rhodis✤)

◆ CLASSIFICATION

PHARMACOTHERAPEUTIC: Nonsteroidal anti-inflammatory. **CLINICAL:** Antirheumatic, analgesic, antidysmenorrheal, vascular headache suppressant (see p. 110C).

ACTION

Produces analgesic, anti-inflammatory effect by inhibiting prostaglandin synthesis. **Therapeutic Effect:** Reduces inflammatory response, intensity of pain stimulus reaching sensory nerve endings.

USES

Symptomatic treatment of acute and chronic rheumatoid arthritis, osteoarthritis. Relief of mild to moderate pain, primary dysmenorrhea. **Unlabeled:** Treatment of ankylosing spondylitis, psoriatic arthritis, acute gouty arthritis, vascular headache.

PRECAUTIONS

CONTRAINDICATIONS: Active peptic ulcer, GI ulceration, chronic inflammation of GI tract, GI bleeding disorders, history of hypersensitivity to aspirin, NSAIDs. **CAUTIONS:** Impaired renal/hepatic function, history of GI tract disease, predisposition to fluid retention. **Pregnancy Category B** (**D** if used in third trimester or near delivery).

K

INTERACTIONS

DRUG: May increase effects of **oral anticoagulants, heparin, thrombolytics.** May decrease effect of **antihypertensives, diuretics. Salicylates, aspirin** may increase risk of GI side effects, bleeding. **Bone marrow depressants** may increase risk of hematologic reactions. May increase concentration, toxicity of **lithium.** May increase **methotrexate** toxicity. **Probenecid** may increase concentration. **HERBAL: Feverfew** effects may be decreased. **Ginkgo biloba** may increase risk of bleeding. **FOOD:** None known. **LAB VALUES:** May prolong bleeding time. May increase alkaline phosphatase, LDH, liver function tests. May decrease sodium, Hgb, Hct.

AVAILABILITY (Rx)

TABLETS: (OTC): 12.5 mg. **CAPSULES:** 50 mg, 75 mg. **CAPSULES (extended-release):** 100 mg, 150 mg, 200 mg.

ADMINISTRATION/HANDLING

PO

• May give with food, milk, full glass (8 oz) of water (minimizes potential GI distress). • Do not break, chew extended-release capsules.

INDICATIONS/ROUTES/DOSAGE

Alert: Do not exceed 300 mg/day. Oruvail not recommended as initial therapy in pts who are small, >75 yrs, or with renal impairment.

ACUTE AND CHRONIC RHEUMATOID ARTHRITIS, OSTEOARTHRITIS

PO: ADULTS: Initially, 75 mg 3 times/day or 50 mg 4 times/day. ELDERLY: Initially, 25–50 mg 3–4 times/day. MAINTENANCE: 150–300 mg/day in 3–4 divided doses. **Extended-release:** 100–200 mg/day as single dose.

MILD TO MODERATE PAIN, DYSMENORRHEA

PO: ADULTS, ELDERLY: 25–50 mg q6–8h. **Maximum:** 300 mg/day.

SIDE EFFECTS

FREQUENT (11%): Dyspepsia (heartburn, indigestion, epigastric pain). **OCCASIONAL (>3%):** Nausea, diarrhea/constipation, flatulence, abdominal cramping, headache. **RARE (<2%):** Anorexia, vomiting, visual disturbances, fluid retention.

ADVERSE REACTIONS/ TOXIC EFFECTS

Peptic ulcer, GI bleeding, gastritis, severe hepatic reaction (cholestasis, jaundice) occur rarely. Nephrotoxicity (dysuria, hematuria, proteinuria, nephrotic syndrome), severe hypersensitivity reaction (bronchospasm, angioedema) occur rarely.

NURSING IMPLICATIONS

BASELINE ASSESSMENT

Assess onset, type, location, duration of pain/inflammation. Inspect appearance of affected joints for immobility, deformities, skin condition.

INTERVENTION/EVALUATION

Monitor for evidence of nausea, dyspepsia. Monitor for therapeutic response (pain, range of motion, grip strength, mobility). Monitor renal/liver function tests, mental function.

PATIENT/FAMILY TEACHING

Avoid aspirin, alcohol during therapy (increases risk of GI bleeding). If GI upset occurs, take with food, milk. Swallow capsule whole; do not crush or chew.

ketorolac tromethamine

key-**tore**-oh-lack
(Acular, Acular PF, Toradol)
Do not confuse with Acthar.

♦CLASSIFICATION

PHARMACOTHERAPEUTIC: Nonsteroidal anti-inflammatory. **CLINICAL:** Analgesic, intraocular anti-inflammatory (see p. 111C).

ACTION

Inhibits prostaglandin synthesis, reduces prostaglandin levels in aqueous humor. **Therapeutic Effect:** Reduces intensity of pain stimulus reaching sensory nerve endings, reduces intraocular inflammation.

PHARMACOKINETICS

Onset	Peak	Duration
PO		
30–60 min	1.5–4 hrs	4–6 hrs
IV/IM		
30 min	1–2 hrs	4–6 hrs

Readily absorbed from GI tract, after IM administration. Protein binding: >99%. Partially metabolized primarily in kidneys. Primarily excreted in urine. Not removed by hemodialysis. **Half-life:** 3.8–6.3 hrs (half-life increased with impaired renal function, in elderly).

USES

Short-term relief of mild to moderate pain. **Ophthalmic:** Relief of ocular itching due to seasonal allergic conjunctivitis. Treatment postop for inflammation following cataract extraction, pain following incisional refractive surgery. **Unlabeled: Ophthalmic:** Prophylaxis/treatment of ocular inflammation.

PRECAUTIONS

CONTRAINDICATIONS: Active peptic ulcer, GI ulceration, chronic inflammation of GI tract, GI bleeding disorders, history of hypersensitivity to aspirin, NSAIDs. **CAUTIONS:** Impaired renal/hepatic function, history of GI tract disease, predisposition to fluid retention.

LIFESPAN CONSIDERATIONS: Pregnancy/lactation: Unknown if drug is excreted in breast milk. Avoid use during third trimester (may adversely affect fetal cardiovascular system: premature closure of ductus arteriosus). **Pregnancy Category C** (**D** if used in third trimester). **Children:** Safety and efficacy not established, but doses of 0.5 mg/kg have been used. **Elderly:** GI bleeding or ulceration more likely to cause serious adverse effects. Age-related renal impair-

K

ment may increase risk of liver/renal toxicity; decreased dosage recommended.

INTERACTIONS

DRUG: May increase effects of **oral anticoagulants, heparin, thrombolytics.** May decrease effect of **antihypertensives, diuretics. Salicylates, aspirin** may increase risk of GI side effects, bleeding. **Bone marrow depressants** may increase risk of hematologic reactions. May increase concentration, toxicity of **lithium.** May increase **methotrexate** toxicity. **Probenecid** may increase concentration. **HERBAL: Feverfew** effects may be decreased. **Ginkgo biloba** may increase risk of bleeding. **FOOD:** None known. **LAB VALUES:** May prolong bleeding time. May increase liver function tests.

K

AVAILABILITY (Rx)

TABLETS: 10 mg. **INJECTION:** 15 mg/ml, 30 mg/ml. **OPHTHALMIC SOLUTION:** 0.4%, 0.5%.

ADMINISTRATION/HANDLING

PO

• Give with food, milk, antacids if GI distress occurs.

IM

• Give deep IM slowly into large muscle mass.

IV

• Give undiluted as IV push. • Give over at least 15 sec.

OPHTHALMIC

• Place finger on lower eyelid, pull out until pocket is formed between eye and lower lid. Hold dropper above pocket, place prescribed number of drops in pocket. • Close eye gently. Apply digital pressure to lacrimal sac for 1–2 min (minimized drainage into nose and throat, reducing risk of systemic effects). • Remove excess solution with tissue.

IV INCOMPATIBILITY

Promethazine (Phenergan).

IV COMPATIBILITIES

Fentanyl (Sublimaze), hydromorphone (Dilaudid), morphine, nalbuphine (Nubain).

INDICATIONS/ROUTES/DOSAGE

Alert: Combined duration of IM/IV and PO not to exceed 5 days. May give as single dose, routine, or as-needed schedule.

ANALGESIC (multiple dosing)

PO: ADULTS, ELDERLY: 10 mg q4–6h. **Maximum:** 40 mg/24 hrs.

IV/IM: ADULTS <65 YRS: 30 mg q6h. **Maximum:** 120 mg/24 hrs. ADULTS >65 YRS, RENAL IMPAIRMENT, <50 KG: 15 mg q6h. **Maximum:** 60 mg/24 hrs. CHILDREN 2–16 YRS: 0.5 mg/kg q6h.

ANALGESIC (single dose)

IM: ADULTS <65 YRS: 60 mg. ADULTS >65 YRS, RENAL IMPAIRMENT, <50 KG: 30 mg. CHILDREN 2–16 YRS: 0.4–1 mg/kg.

IV: ADULTS <65 YRS: 30 mg. ADULTS >65 YRS, RENAL IMPAIRMENT, <50 KG: 15 mg. CHILDREN: 0.4–1 mg/kg.

USUAL OPHTHALMIC DOSAGE

ADULTS, ELDERLY: 1 drop 4 times/day.

SIDE EFFECTS

FREQUENT (12%–17%): Headache, nausea, abdominal cramping/pain, dyspepsia (heartburn, indigestion, epigastric pain). **OCCASIONAL (3%–9%):** Diarrhea. **Ophthalmic:** Transient stinging, burning. **RARE (1%–3%):** Constipation, vomiting, flatulence, stomatitis. **Ophthalmic:** Ocular irritation, allergic reactions, superficial ocular infection, keratitis.

ADVERSE REACTIONS/ TOXIC EFFECTS

GI bleeding, peptic ulcer occur infrequently. Nephrotoxicity (glomerular nephritis, interstitial nephritis, nephrotic syndrome) may occur in pts with preexisting impaired renal function. Acute hypersensitivity reaction (fever, chills, joint pain) occurs rarely.

NURSING IMPLICATIONS

BASELINE ASSESSMENT

Assess onset, type, location, duration of pain.

INTERVENTION/EVALUATION

Monitor renal/liver function tests, occult blood loss, urine output. Evaluate for therapeutic response: relief of pain, stiffness, swelling; increase in joint mobility, reduced joint tenderness, improved grip strength. Be alert to signs of bleeding (may also occur with ophthalmic route due to systemic absorption).

PATIENT/FAMILY TEACHING

Avoid aspirin, alcohol during therapy with oral or ophthalmic ketorolac (increases tendency to bleed). If GI upset occurs, take with food, milk. Avoid tasks that require alertness, motor skills until response to drug is established. **Ophthalmic:** Transient stinging, burning may occur upon instillation. Do not administer while wearing soft contact lenses.

Klonopin

see clonazepam

Kytril

see granisetron

labetalol hydrochloride

lah-**bet**-ah-lol
(Normodyne, Trandate)
Do not confuse with Trental.

FIXED-COMBINATION(S)

Normozide: labetalol/hydrochlorothiazide (a diuretic): 100 mg/25 mg; 200 mg/25 mg; 300 mg/25 mg.

◆CLASSIFICATION

PHARMACOTHERAPEUTIC: Alpha-, beta-adrenergic blocker. **CLINICAL:** Antihypertensive.

ACTION

Blocks alpha$_1$-, beta$_1$-, beta$_2$- (large doses) adrenergic receptor sites. **Therapeutic Effect:** Slows sinus heart rate; decreases peripheral vascular resistance, cardiac output, B/P. Large doses increase airway resistance.

PHARMACOKINETICS

Onset	Peak	Duration
PO		
0.5–2 hrs	2–4 hrs	8–12 hrs
IV		
2–5 min	5–15 min	2–4 hrs

Completely absorbed from GI tract. Protein binding: 50%. Undergoes first-pass metabolism. Metabolized in liver. Primarily excreted in urine. Not removed by hemodialysis. **Half-life:** PO: 6–8 hrs; IV: 5.5 hrs.

USES

Management of mild, moderate, severe hypertension. May be used alone or in combination with other antihypertensives. **Unlabeled:** Treatment of chronic angina pectoris. Produces controlled hypotension during surgery.

PRECAUTIONS

CONTRAINDICATIONS: Bronchial asthma, uncontrolled CHF, second- or third-degree heart block, severe bradycardia, cardiogenic shock. **CAUTIONS:** Drug-controlled CHF, nonallergic bronchospastic disease (chronic bronchitis, emphysema), impaired hepatic, cardiac function, pheochromocytoma, diabetes mellitus.

LIFESPAN CONSIDERATIONS: Pregnancy/lactation: Drug crosses placenta. Small amount distributed in breast milk. **Pregnancy Category C** (**D** if used in second or third trimester). **Children:** Safety and efficacy not established. **Elderly:** Age-related peripheral vascular disease may increase susceptibility to decreased peripheral circulation.

INTERACTIONS

L

DRUG: **Diuretics, other hypotensives** may increase hypotensive effect; **sympathomimetics, xanthines** may mutually inhibit effects; may mask symptoms of hypoglycemia, prolong hypoglycemic effect of **insulin, oral hypoglycemics. MAOIs** may produce hypertension. **HERBAL:** None known. **FOOD:** None known. **LAB VALUES:** May increase ANA titer, SGOT (AST), SGPT (ALT), alkaline phosphatase, LDH, bilirubin, BUN, creatinine, potassium uric acid, lipoproteins, triglycerides.

AVAILABILITY (Rx)

TABLETS: 100 mg, 200 mg, 300 mg. **INJECTION:** 5 mg/ml.

ADMINISTRATION/HANDLING

PO

• Give without regard to food. • Tablets may be crushed.

IV

Alert: Pt must be in supine position for IV administration and for 3 hrs after receiving medication (substantial drop in B/P upon standing should be expected).

Storage • Store at room temperature. • After dilution, IV solution is stable for 24 hrs. • Solution appears clear, colorless to light yellow. • Discard if precipitate forms or discoloration occurs.

Reconstitution • For IV infusion, dilute 200 mg in 160 ml D_5W, 0.9% NaCl, lactated Ringer's, or any combination thereof to provide concentration of 1 mg/ml.

Rate of administration • For IV push, give over 2 min at 10-min intervals. • For IV infusion, administer at rate of 2 mg/min (2 ml/min) initially. Rate is adjusted according to B/P. • Monitor B/P immediately before and q5–10min during IV administration (maximum effect occurs within 5 min).

∅ IV INCOMPATIBILITIES

Amphotericin B complex (Abelcet, AmBisome, Amphotec), ceftriaxone (Rocephin), furosemide (Lasix), heparin, nafcillin (Nafcil), thiopental.

IV COMPATIBILITIES

Aminophylline, amiodarone (Cordarone), calcium gluconate, diltiazem (Cardizem), dobutamine (Dobutrex), dopamine (Intropin), enalapril (Vasotec), fentanyl (Sublimaze), hydromorphone (Dilaudid), lidocaine, lorazepam (Ativan), magnesium sulfate, midazolam (Versed), milrinone (Primacor), morphine, nitroglycerin, norepinephrine (Levophed), potassium chloride, potassium phosphate, propofol (Diprivan).

INDICATIONS/ROUTES/DOSAGE

HYPERTENSION

PO: ADULTS: Initially, 100 mg 2 times/day adjusted in increments of 100 mg 2 times/day q2–3days. MAINTENANCE: 200–400 mg 2 times/day. **Maximum:** 2.4 g/day.

USUAL ELDERLY DOSAGE

PO: Initially, 100 mg 1–2 times/day. May increase as needed.

SEVERE HYPERTENSION, HYPERTENSIVE EMERGENCY

IV: ADULTS: Initially, 20 mg. Additional doses of 20–80 mg may be given at 10-min intervals, up to total dose of 300 mg.

IV infusion: ADULTS: Initially, 2 mg/min up to total dose of 300 mg.

PO: ADULTS: (AFTER IV THERAPY): Initially, 200 mg; then, 200–400 mg in 6–12 hrs. Increase dose at 1-day intervals to desired level.

SIDE EFFECTS

FREQUENT: Drowsiness, excessive fatigue, weakness, trouble sleeping, decreased sexual function, transient scalp tingling. **OCCASIONAL:** Dizziness, difficulty breathing, swelling of hands/feet, depression, anxiety, constipation, diarrhea, nasal congestion, nausea, vomiting, stomach discomfort. **RARE:** Altered taste, dry eyes, increased urination, numbness/tingling in fingers/toes/scalp.

ADVERSE REACTIONS/ TOXIC EFFECTS

May precipitate, aggravate CHF (due to decreased myocardial stimulation). Abrupt withdrawal may precipitate myocardial ischemia, producing chest pain, diaphoresis, palpitations, headache, tremor. Beta-blockers may mask signs, symptoms of acute hypoglycemia (tachycardia, B/P changes) in diabetic pts.

NURSING IMPLICATIONS

BASELINE ASSESSMENT

Assess baseline renal/liver function tests. Assess B/P, apical pulse immediately prior to drug administration (if pulse is ≤60/min or systolic B/P is <90 mm Hg, withhold medication, contact physician).

INTERVENTION/EVALUATION

Monitor B/P for hypotension. Assess pulse for quality, irregular rate, bradycardia. Monitor EKG for cardiac arrhythmias. Monitor stool frequency/consistency. Assist with ambulation if dizziness occurs. Assess for evidence of CHF: dyspnea (particularly on exertion or lying down), night cough, peripheral edema, distended neck veins. Monitor I&O (increase in weight, decrease in urine output may indicate CHF).

PATIENT/FAMILY TEACHING

Do not discontinue drug except upon advice of physician (abrupt discontinuation may precipitate heart failure). Compliance with therapy regimen is essential to control hypertension, arrhythmias. Avoid tasks that require alertness, motor skills until response to drug is established. Report shortness of breath, excessive fatigue, weight gain, prolonged dizziness or headache. Do not use nasal decongestants, OTC cold preparations (stimulants) without physician approval.

L

lactulose

lack-tyoo-lows

(Acilac ✱, Constulose, Duphalac ✱, Enulose, Generlac, Kristalose, Laxilose ✱)

Do not confuse with lactose.

CLASSIFICATION

PHARMACOTHERAPEUTIC: Lactose derivative. **CLINICAL:** Hyperosmotic laxative, ammonia detoxicant (see p. 105C).

ACTION

Retains ammonia in colon (decreases serum ammonia concentration), producing osmotic effect. **Therapeutic Effect:** Promotes increased peristalsis, bowel evacuation (expelling ammonia from colon).

PHARMACOKINETICS

Onset	Peak	Duration
PO		
24–48 hrs	—	—
Rectal		
30–60 min	—	—

Poorly absorbed from GI tract. Acts in colon. Primarily excreted in feces.

USES

Prevention/treatment of portal systemic encephalopathy (including hepatic precoma, coma); treatment of constipation.

PRECAUTIONS

CONTRAINDICATIONS: Those on galactose-free diet, abdominal pain, nausea, vomiting, appendicitis. **CAUTIONS:** Diabetes mellitus.

L

LIFESPAN CONSIDERATIONS: Pregnancy/lactation: Unknown if drug crosses placenta or is distributed in breast milk. **Pregnancy Category B. Children:** Avoid use in children <6 yrs (usually unable to describe symptoms). **Elderly:** No age-related precautions noted.

INTERACTIONS

DRUG: May decrease transit time of concurrently administered **oral medication,** decreasing absorption. **HERBAL:** None known. **FOOD:** None known. **LAB VALUES:** May decrease potassium concentration.

AVAILABILITY (Rx)

SYRUP: 10 g/15 ml. **PACKETS:** 10 g, 20 g.

ADMINISTRATION/HANDLING

PO

• Store solution at room temperature. • Solution appears pale yellow to yellow, sweet, viscous liquid. Cloudiness, darkened solution does not indicate potency loss. • Drink water, juice, milk with each dose (aids stool softening, increases palatability).

RECTAL

• Lubricate anus with petroleum jelly before enema insertion. • Insert carefully (prevents damage to rectal wall) with nozzle toward navel. • Squeeze container until entire dose expelled. • Retain until definite lower abdominal cramping felt.

INDICATIONS/ROUTES/DOSAGE

CONSTIPATION

PO: ADULTS, ELDERLY: 15–30 ml/day up to 60 ml/day. CHILDREN: 7.5 ml/day after breakfast.

PORTAL-SYSTEMIC ENCEPHALOPATHY

PO: ADULTS, ELDERLY: Initially, 30–45 ml every hr. Then, 30–45 ml 3–4 times/day. Adjust dose q1–2days to produce 2–3 soft stools/day. CHILDREN: 40–90 ml/day in divided doses. INFANTS: 2.5–10 ml/day in divided doses.

USUAL RECTAL DOSAGE (AS RETENTION ENEMA)

ADULTS, ELDERLY: 300 ml with 700 ml water or saline; retain 30–60 min; repeat q4–6h. (If evacuation occurs too promptly, repeat immediately.)

SIDE EFFECTS

OCCASIONAL: Cramping, flatulence, increased thirst, abdominal discomfort. **RARE:** Nausea, vomiting.

ADVERSE REACTIONS/ TOXIC EFFECTS

Diarrhea indicates overdosage. Long-term use may result in laxative dependence, chronic constipation, loss of normal bowel function.

NURSING IMPLICATIONS

INTERVENTION/EVALUATION

Encourage adequate fluid intake. Assess bowel sounds for peristalsis. Monitor daily bowel activity, stool consistency (watery, loose, soft, semisolid, solid); record time of evacuation. Assess for abdominal disturbances. Monitor serum electrolytes in pts exposed to prolonged, frequent, or excessive use of medication.

PATIENT/FAMILY TEACHING

Evacuation occurs in 24–48 hrs of initial dose. Institute measures to promote defecation: increase fluid intake, exercise, high-fiber diet.

lamivudine

lah-**mih**-view-deen
(Epivir, Heptovir✤)

Do not confuse with lamotrigine.

FIXED-COMBINATION(S)

Combivir: lamivudine/zidovudine (an antiviral): 150 mg/300 mg. **Trizivir:** lamivudine/zidovudine/abacavir (an antiviral): 150 mg/300 mg/300 mg.

◆CLASSIFICATION

PHARMACOTHERAPEUTIC: Nucleoside reverse transcriptase inhibitor. **CLINICAL:** Antiviral (see pp. 59C, 98C).

ACTION

Inhibits HIV reverse transcriptase via viral DNA chain termination. Also inhibits RNA- and DNA-dependent DNA polymerase, an enzyme necessary for viral HIV replication. **Therapeutic Effect:** Slows HIV replication, reduces progression of HIV infection.

PHARMACOKINETICS

Rapidly, completely absorbed from GI tract. Protein binding: <36%. Widely distributed (crosses blood-brain barrier). Primarily excreted unchanged in urine. Not removed by hemodialysis/peritoneal dialysis. **Half-life:** 11–15 hrs (intracellular); serum (adults) 2–11 hrs, (children) 1.7–2 hrs. Half-life increased with impaired renal function.

USES

Treatment of HIV infection in combination with other antiretroviral agents. Treatment for chronic hepatitis B. **Unlabeled:** Prophylaxis in health care workers at risk of acquiring HIV after occupational exposure to virus.

PRECAUTIONS

CONTRAINDICATIONS: None known. **CAUTIONS:** Peripheral neuropathy, or history of peripheral neuropathy, history of pancreatitis in children, impaired renal function.

LIFESPAN CONSIDERATIONS: Pregnancy/lactation: Drug crosses placenta. Unknown if distributed in breast milk. Breast-feeding not recommended (possibility of HIV transmission). **Pregnancy Category C. Children:** Safety and efficacy not established in those <3 mos. **Elderly:** Age-related renal impairment may require dosage adjustment.

INTERACTIONS

DRUG: Trimethoprim-sulfamethoxazole increases lamivudine concentration. **HERBAL: St. John's wort** may decrease concentration, effect. **FOOD:** None known. **LAB VALUES:** May increase neutrophil count, SGOT (AST), SGPT (ALT), amylase serum level, Hgb.

AVAILABILITY (Rx)

TABLETS: 100 mg, 150 mg, 300 mg. **ORAL SOLUTION:** 5 mg/ml, 10 mg/ml.

ADMINISTRATION/HANDLING

PO

- Give without regard to meals.

INDICATIONS/ROUTES/DOSAGE

HIV INFECTION

PO: ADULTS, CHILDREN 12–16 YRS, >50 KG (>100 LBS): 150 mg twice daily or 300 mg once daily. ADULTS <50 KG: 2 mg/kg twice daily. CHILDREN 3 MOS–11 YRS: 4 mg/kg twice daily (up to 150 mg/dose).

CHRONIC HEPATITIS B

PO: ADULTS, CHILDREN ≥17 YRS: 100 mg daily. CHILDREN <17 YRS: 3 mg/kg/day. **Maximum:** 100 mg/day.

DOSAGE IN RENAL IMPAIRMENT

Dose and/or frequency is modified based on creatinine clearance.

Creatinine Clearance	Dosage
≥50	150 mg twice daily
30–49	150 mg once daily
15–29	150 mg first dose, then 100 mg once daily
5–14	150 mg first dose, then 50 mg once daily
<5	50 mg first dose, then 25 mg once daily

L

SIDE EFFECTS

FREQUENT: Headache (35%), nausea (33%), malaise/fatigue (27%), nasal disturbances (20%), diarrhea, cough (18%), musculoskeletal pain, neuropathy (12%), insomnia (11%), anorexia, dizziness, fever/chills (10%). **OCCASIONAL:** Depression, (9%), myalgia (8%), abdominal cramps (6%), dyspepsia, arthralgia (5%).

ADVERSE REACTIONS/ TOXIC EFFECTS

Pancreatitis occurs in 13% of pediatric pts. Anemia, neutropenia, thrombocytopenia occur rarely.

NURSING IMPLICATIONS

BASELINE ASSESSMENT

Establish baseline lab values, esp. renal function.

INTERVENTION/EVALUATION

Monitor amylase, lipase, BUN, serum creatinine. Assess for headache, nausea, cough. Determine pattern of bowel activity, stool consistency. Modify diet or administer laxative as needed. Assess for dizziness, sleep pattern. If pancreatitis in children occurs, movement aggravates abdominal pain; sitting up, flexing at the waist relieves the pain.

PATIENT/FAMILY TEACHING

Continue therapy for full length of treatment. Doses should be evenly spaced. Inform pt lamivudine is not a cure, pt may continue to experience illnesses, including opportunistic infections. Do not engage in activities that require mental acuity if experiencing dizziness. Advise parents to closely monitor pediatric pts for symptoms of pancreatitis (severe, steady abdominal pain often radiating to the back, clammy skin, hypotension; nausea/vomiting may accompany abdominal pain).

lamotrigine

lam-**oh**-trih-geen

(Lamictal)

Do not confuse with lamivudine.

CLASSIFICATION

CLINICAL: Anticonvulsant (see p. 33C).

ACTION

Exact mechanism unknown. May be due to inhibition of voltage-sensitive sodium channels, stabilizing neuronal membranes and regulating presynaptic transmitter release of excitatory amino acids. **Therapeutic Effect:** Produces anticonvulsant activity.

USES

Adjunctive therapy in adults and children with partial seizures, treatment of adults and children with generalized seizures of Lennox-Gastaut syndrome. Conversion to monotherapy in adults treated with another enzyme-inducing antiepileptic drug (EIAED). Long-term maintenance treatment of bipolar disorder.

PRECAUTIONS

CONTRAINDICATIONS: None known. **CAUTIONS:** Renal/hepatic/cardiac function impairment. **Pregnancy Category C.**

INTERACTIONS

DRUG: May increase **carbamazepine, valproic acid** serum levels. **Phenobarbital, primidone, phenytoin, carbamazepine, valproic acid** decreases lamotrigine concentration. **HERBAL:** None known. **FOOD:** None known. **LAB VALUES:** None known.

AVAILABILITY (Rx)

TABLETS: 25 mg, 100 mg, 150 mg, 200 mg. **TABLETS (chewable):** 5 mg, 25 mg.

ADMINISTRATION/HANDLING

PO

- Give without regard to food.

INDICATIONS/ROUTES/DOSAGE

Alert: If pt currently on valproic acid, reduce lamotrigine dosage to less than half the normal dosage.

SEIZURE CONTROL IN PTS RECEIVING EIAEDs, BUT NOT VALPROATE

PO: ADULTS, ELDERLY, CHILDREN >12 YRS: Recommended as add-on therapy: 50 mg once/day for 2 wks, followed by 100 mg/day in 2 divided doses for 2 wks. MAINTENANCE: Dosage may be increased by 100 mg/day every week, up to 300–500 mg/day in 2 divided doses. CHILDREN 2–12 YRS: 0.6 mg/kg/day in 2 divided doses for 2 wks, then 1.2 mg/kg/day in 2 divided doses for wks 3 and 4. MAINTENANCE: 5–15 mg/kg/day. **Maximum:** 400 mg/day.

SEIZURE CONTROL IN PTS RECEIVING COMBINATION THERAPY OF VALPROIC ACID AND EIAEDs

PO: ADULTS, ELDERLY, CHILDREN >12 YRS: 25 mg every other day for 2 wks, followed by 25 mg once/day for 2 wks. MAINTENANCE: Dosage may be increased by 25–50 mg/day q1–2wks, up to 150 mg/day in 2 divided doses. CHILDREN 2–12 YRS: 0.15 mg/kg/day in 2 divided doses for 2 wks, then 0.3 mg/kg/day in 2 divided doses for wks 3 and 4. MAINTENANCE: 1–5 mg/kg/day in 2 divided doses. **Maximum:** 200 mg/day.

CONVERSION TO MONOTHERAPY

PO: ADULTS, CHILDREN >12 YRS: Add lamotrigine 50 mg/day for 2 wks, then 100 mg/day during wks 3 and 4. Increase by 100 mg/day q1–2wks until maintenance dosage achieved (300–500 mg/day in 2 divided doses/day). Gradually discontinue other EIAEDs over 4 wks once maintenance dose achieved.

BIPOLAR DISORDER

PO: ADULTS, ELDERLY: Initially, 25 mg/day. May double dose after wks 2, 4, 5. Target dose: 200 mg/day.

RENAL FUNCTION IMPAIRMENT

Alert: Same dosage as combination therapy (see previous).

DISCONTINUATION THERAPY

Alert: A reduction in dosage over at least 2 wks (approx. 50% per week) is recommended.

SIDE EFFECTS

FREQUENT: Dizziness (38%), double vision (28%), headache (29%), ataxia

L

(muscular incoordination) (22%), nausea (19%), blurred vision (16%), somnolence, rhinitis (14%). **OCCASIONAL (5%–10%):** Rash, pharyngitis, vomiting, cough, flu syndrome, diarrhea, dysmenorrhea, fever, insomnia, dyspepsia. **RARE:** Constipation, tremor, anxiety, pruritus, vaginitis, sensitivity reaction.

ADVERSE REACTIONS/ TOXIC EFFECTS

Abrupt withdrawal may increase seizure frequency.

NURSING IMPLICATIONS

BASELINE ASSESSMENT

Review history of seizure disorder (type, onset, intensity, frequency, duration, LOC), drug history (esp. other anticonvulsants), other medical conditions (e.g., renal function impairment). Provide safety precautions, quiet, dark environment.

INTERVENTION/EVALUATION

Report to physician promptly if evidence of rash occurs (drug discontinuation may be necessary). Assist with ambulation if dizziness, ataxia occurs. Assess for clinical improvement (decrease in intensity/frequency of seizures). Assess for visual abnormalities, headache.

PATIENT/FAMILY TEACHING

Take medication only as prescribed; do not abruptly withdraw medication after long-term therapy. Avoid alcohol, tasks that require alertness, motor skills until response to drug is established. Carry identification card/bracelet to note anticonvulsant therapy. Strict maintenance of drug therapy is essential for seizure control. Report any rash, fever, swelling of glands to physician. May cause photosensitivity reaction; avoid exposure to sunlight, artificial light.

Lanoxin

see digoxin

lansoprazole

lan-sew-**prah**-zoll
(Prevacid)
Do not confuse with Pepcid, Pravachol, Prevpac.

CLASSIFICATION

CLINICAL: Proton pump inhibitor (see p. 128C).

ACTION

Selectively inhibits parietal cell membrane enzyme system (H^+, K^+, ATPase) or proton pump. **Therapeutic Effect:** Suppresses gastric acid secretion.

PHARMACOKINETICS

	Onset	Peak	Duration
15 mg	2–3 hrs	—	24 hrs
30 mg	1–2 hrs	—	>24 hrs

Once leaving stomach, rapid and complete absorption (food may decrease absorption). Protein binding: 97%. Distributed primarily to gastric parietal cells, converted to two active metabolites. Extensively metabolized in liver. Eliminated from body in bile and urine. Not removed by hemodialysis. **Half-life:** 1.5 hrs (half-life increased in elderly, those with liver impairment).

USES

Short-term treatment (≤4 wks) for healing, symptomatic relief of active duodenal ulcer, short-term treatment (≤8 wks) for healing, symptomatic relief of erosive esophagitis. Long-term treatment of pathologic hypersecretory conditions, including Zollinger-Ellison syndrome. Short-term treatment (≤8 wks) of active gastric ulcer, *H. pylori*–associated duodenal ulcer, maintenance treatment for healed duodenal ulcer. Treatment for gastroesophageal reflux disease (GERD), NSAID-associated gastric ulcer.

PRECAUTIONS

CONTRAINDICATIONS: None known. **CAUTIONS:** Impaired hepatic function.

LIFESPAN CONSIDERATIONS: Pregnancy/lactation: Unknown if distributed in breast milk. **Pregnancy Category B. Children:** Safety and efficacy not established. **Elderly:** No age-related precautions noted but doses >30 mg not recommended.

INTERACTIONS

DRUG: May interfere with **ketoconazole, ampicillin, iron salts, digoxin** absorption. **Sucralfate** may delay lansoprazole absorption (give lansoprazole 30 min before sucralfate). **HERBAL:** None known. **FOOD:** None known. **LAB VALUES:** May increase SGOT (AST), SGPT (ALT), serum creatinine, alkaline phosphatase, bilirubin, triglycerides, uric acid, LDH, cholesterol. May produce abnormal WBC, RBC, platelet counts; albumin/globulin ratio; electrolyte balance. May increase Hct, Hgb.

AVAILABILITY (Rx)

CAPSULES (extended-release): 15 mg, 30 mg. **GRANULES FOR ORAL SUSPENSION:** 15 mg/pack; 30 mg/pack.

ADMINISTRATION/HANDLING

PO

• Give while fasting or before meals (food diminishes absorption). • Do not chew or crush delayed-release capsules. • If pt has difficulty swallowing capsules, open capsules, sprinkle granules on 1 tbsp of applesauce, swallow immediately.

INDICATIONS/ROUTES/DOSAGE

DUODENAL ULCER

PO: ADULTS, ELDERLY: 15 mg/day, before eating, preferably in AM, for up to 4 wks.

EROSIVE ESOPHAGITIS

PO: ADULTS, ELDERLY: 30 mg/day, before eating, for up to 8 wks. If healing does not occur within 8 wks (5%–10%), may give for additional 8 wks. MAINTENANCE: 15 MG/DAY

GASTRIC ULCER

PO: ADULTS: 30 mg/day for up to 8 wks.

HEALED DUODENAL ULCER, GERD

PO: ADULTS: 15 mg/day.

H. PYLORI

PO: ADULTS: 30 mg 2 times/day for 10 days (with amoxicillin, clarithromycin).

PATHOLOGIC HYPERSECRETORY CONDITIONS (including Zollinger-Ellison syndrome)

PO: ADULTS, ELDERLY: 60 mg/day. Individualize dosage according to pt needs and for as long as clinically indicated. May increase to >120 mg/day in divided doses.

USUAL DOSAGE FOR CHILDREN

3 MOS–14 YRS, <10 KG: 7.5 mg; 10–20 KG: 15 mg; >20 KG: 30 mg.

SIDE EFFECTS

OCCASIONAL (2%–3%): Diarrhea, abdominal pain, rash, pruritus, altered appetite. **RARE (1%):** Nausea, headache.

ADVERSE REACTIONS/ TOXIC EFFECTS

Bilirubinemia, eosinophilia, hyperlipidemia occur rarely.

NURSING IMPLICATIONS

BASELINE ASSESSMENT

Obtain baseline lab values. Assess drug history, esp. use of sucralfate.

INTERVENTION/EVALUATION

Monitor ongoing laboratory results. Assess for therapeutic response (i.e., relief of GI symptoms). Question if diarrhea, abdominal pain, nausea occurs.

PATIENT/FAMILY TEACHING

Do not chew or crush delayed-release capsules. For pts who have difficulty swallowing capsules, open capsules, sprinkle granules on 1 tbsp of applesauce, swallow immediately.

laronidase

lar-**on**-ih-dase
(Aldurazyme)

◆CLASSIFICATION

PHARMACOTHERAPEUTIC: Enzyme. **CLINICAL:** Pulmonary agent.

ACTION

Increases catabolism of glycosaminoglycans in pts deficient in lysosomal enzymes required for glycosaminoglycans catabolism. **Therapeutic Effect:** Prevents glycosaminoglycans from causing widespread cellular, tissue, organ dysfunction.

USES

Treatment of pts with moderate to severe symptoms of Hurler, Hurler-Scheie form of mucopolysaccharidosis I.

PRECAUTIONS

CONTRAINDICATIONS: None known. **CAUTIONS:** None known. **Pregnancy Category B.**

INTERACTIONS

DRUG: None known. **HERBAL:** None known. **FOOD:** None known. **LAB VALUES:** None known.

AVAILABILITY (Rx)

INJECTION: 2.9 mg/5 ml vial.

ADMINISTRATION/HANDLING

Storage: • Refrigerate. Do not shake. • Once reconstituted, use immediately but may be stored in refrigerator no longer than 36 hrs from time of preparation to completion of administration. • Pretreat with antipyretics and/or antihistamines 60 min prior to start of IV infusion. • Total volume of infusion is determined by pt's body weight. Pts with body weight ≤20 kg should receive a total volume of 100 ml. Pts with a body weight >20 kg should receive a total volume of 250 ml.

Reconstitution • Dilute with 0.1% albumin (human) in 0.9% NaCl. • Administer using a 0.2-micrometer filter.

Rate of administration • Initial infusion rate should begin at 10 mcg/kg/hr; may be increased incrementally every 15 min to 20 mcg/kg/hr, then 50 mcg/kg/hr, and then 100 mcg/kg/hr during the first hour. • Remainder of the infusion may be infused at 200 mcg/kg/hr over 2–3 hrs. • Total infusion time: 3–4 hrs.

INDICATIONS/ROUTES/DOSAGE

MUCOPOLYSACCHARIDOSIS

IV infusion: ADULTS, ELDERLY: 0.58 mg/kg once weekly.

SIDE EFFECTS

FREQUENT (18%–36%): Infusion-related reactions (facial flushing, rash, fever, headache). **OCCASIONAL (9%):** Cough, bronchospasm, urticaria, pruritus, angioedema, dependent edema, hypotension, hyperreflexia.

ADVERSE REACTIONS/ TOXIC EFFECTS

Upper respiratory tract infection occurs commonly. Anaphylactic reaction (angioedema, severe bronchospasm, dyspnea) occurs rarely.

NURSING IMPLICATIONS

BASELINE ASSESSMENT

Pretreat with antipyretics, antihistamines 60 min prior to start of IV infusion.

INTERVENTION/EVALUATION

Assess skin for evidence of rash, facial flushing. Monitor carefully for infusion-related reactions. Slowing infusion rate, temporarily stopping infusion and/or administering additional antipyretics, antihistamines will reduce, impede infusion-related reactions.

PATIENT/FAMILY TEACHING

A registry for patients with mucopolysaccharidosis I has been established to monitor, evaluate treatments. Information regarding the registry program can be obtained by the physician.

Lasix

see furosemide

latanoprost

See Classification section under: Antiglaucoma agents (p. 45C)

leflunomide

lee-**flew**-no-mide
(Arava)

CLASSIFICATION

PHARMACOTHERAPEUTIC: Immunomodulatory agent. **CLINICAL:** Anti-inflammatory.

ACTION

Extends the immune response exhibited in rheumatoid synovium, hinders proliferation of lymphocytes, possesses anti-inflammatory action. **Therapeutic Effect:** Reduces signs/symptoms of rheumatoid arthritis, retards structural damage.

PHARMACOKINETICS

Well absorbed after PO administration. Protein binding: >99%. Metabolized to active metabolite in GI wall and liver. Mechanisms of excretion include both renal and biliary systems. Not removed by hemodialysis. **Half-life:** 16 days.

USES

Treatment of active rheumatoid arthritis. Improve physical function in pts with rheumatoid arthritis.

PRECAUTIONS

CONTRAINDICATIONS: Pregnancy or planning to become pregnant (Pregnancy Category X). **CAUTIONS:** Impaired hepatic/renal function, positive hepatitis B or C serology, those with immunodeficiency or bone marrow dysplasias, breast-feeding mothers.

LIFESPAN CONSIDERATIONS: Pregnancy/lactation: Can cause fetal harm. Unknown if excreted in breast milk. Avoid use in nursing mothers. **Pregnancy Category X. Children:** Safety and efficacy not established in those <18 yrs. **Elderly:** No age-related precautions noted.

INTERACTIONS

DRUG: Rifampin increases concentration of leflunomide. Leflunomide may increase effects of **warfarin.** **HERBAL:** None known. **FOOD:** None known. **LAB VALUES:** May increase liver enzymes (esp. SGOT [AST], SGPT [ALT]).

AVAILABILITY (Rx)

TABLETS: 10 mg, 20 mg.

ADMINISTRATION/HANDLING

PO

- Give without regard to food.

INDICATIONS/ROUTES/DOSAGE

RHEUMATOID ARTHRITIS

PO: ADULTS, ELDERLY: Initially, 100 mg daily for 3 days, then 10–20 mg daily.

SIDE EFFECTS

FREQUENT (10%–20%): Diarrhea, respiratory tract infection, hair loss, rash, nausea.

ADVERSE REACTIONS/ TOXIC EFFECTS

Transient thrombocytopenia, leukopenia occur rarely.

NURSING IMPLICATIONS

BASELINE ASSESSMENT

Question for possibility of pregnancy (Pregnancy Category X). Assess limitations in activities of daily living due to rheumatoid arthritis.

INTERVENTION/EVALUATION

Monitor tolerance to medication. Assess symptomatic relief of rheumatoid arthritis. Monitor liver function tests.

PATIENT/FAMILY TEACHING

May take without regard to food. Improvement may take >8 wks. Avoid pregnancy (Pregnancy Category X).

lepirudin

leh-**pier**-ruh-din
(Refludan)

CLASSIFICATION

PHARMACOTHERAPEUTIC: Thrombin inhibitor. **CLINICAL:** Anticoagulant.

ACTION

Inhibits thrombogenic action of thrombin (independent of antithrombin II, not inhibited by platelet factor 4). **Therapeutic Effect:** Produces increase in activated partial thromboplastin time (aPTT).

PHARMACOKINETICS

Distributed primarily in extracellular fluid. Primarily eliminated by kidneys. Removed by hemodialysis. **Half-life:** 1.3 hrs (half-life increased with impaired renal function).

USES

Anticoagulant in pts with heparin-induced thrombocytopenia, associated thromboembolic disease to prevent further thromboembolic complications.

PRECAUTIONS

CONTRAINDICATIONS: None known. **CAUTIONS:** Conditions associated with increased risk of bleeding (e.g., bacterial endocarditis, recent major bleeding, CVA, stroke, intracerebral surgery, hemorrhagic diathesis, severe hypertension, severe renal/liver function impairment, recent major surgery).

LIFESPAN CONSIDERATIONS: **Pregnancy/lactation:** Unknown if distributed in breast milk or crosses placenta. **Pregnancy Category B.** **Children:** Safety and efficacy not established. **Elderly:** Age-related renal function impairment may require dosage adjustment.

INTERACTIONS

DRUG: **Warfarin, platelet aggregation inhibitors, thrombolytics** may increase risk of bleeding complications. **HERBAL:** **Ginkgo biloba** may increase risk of bleeding. **FOOD:** None known. **LAB VALUES:** Increases aPTT, thrombin time.

AVAILABILITY (Rx)

POWDER FOR INJECTION: 50 mg.

ADMINISTRATION/HANDLING

IV

Storage • Store unreconstituted vials at room temperature. • Reconstituted solution to be used immediately. • IV infusion stable for up to 24 hrs at room temperature.

Reconstitution • Add 1 ml Sterile Water for Injection or 0.9% NaCl to 50-mg vial. • Shake gently. • Produces a clear, colorless solution (do not use if cloudy). • For IV push, further dilute by transferring to syringe and adding sufficient Sterile Water for Injection, 0.9% NaCl, or D_5W to produce concentration of 5 mg/ml. • For IV infusion, add contents of 2 vials (100 mg) to 250 ml or 500 ml 0.9% NaCl or D_5W, providing a concentration of 0.4 or 0.2 mg/ml, respectively.

Rate of administration • IV push given over 15–20 sec. • Adjust IV infusion based on aPTT or pt's body weight.

IV INCOMPATIBILITY
Do not mix with any other medication.

INDICATIONS/ROUTES/DOSAGE

Alert: Give initial dose as soon as possible after surgery but not more than 24 hrs after surgery.

ANTICOAGULANT

Alert: Dosage adjusted according to aPTT ratio with target range of 1.5–2.5 normal.

IV/IV infusion: ADULTS, ELDERLY: 0.2–0.4 mg/kg, IV slowly over 15–20 sec, followed by IV infusion of 0.1–0.15 mg/kg/hr for 2–10 days or longer.

Alert: For pts >110 kg, maximum initial dose is 44 mg, with maximum rate of 16.5 mg/hr.

DOSAGE IN RENAL IMPAIRMENT
Initial dose decreased to 0.2 mg/kg with infusion rate adjusted based on creatinine clearance (Ccr).

Ccr (ml/min)	% of Standard Infusion Rate	Infusion Rate (mg/kg/hr)
45–60	50	0.075
30–44	30	0.045
15–29	15	0.0225

SIDE EFFECTS

FREQUENT (5%–14%): Bleeding (from puncture sites/wound), hematuria, fever, GI/rectal bleeding. **OCCASIONAL (1%–3%):** Epistaxis, allergic reaction (rash, pruritus, vaginal bleeding).

ADVERSE REACTIONS/ TOXIC EFFECTS

Overdosage is characterized by excessively high aPTT values. Intracranial bleeding occurs rarely. Abnormal liver function occurs in 6% of pts.

NURSING IMPLICATIONS

BASELINE ASSESSMENT

Assess CBC, including platelet count. Determine initial B/P. Assess renal/liver function.

INTERVENTION/EVALUATION

Monitor aPTT diligently. Assess Hct, platelet count, urine/stool culture for occult blood, SGOT (AST), SGPT (ALT), renal function studies. Assess for decrease in B/P, increase in pulse rate, complaint of abdominal/back pain, severe headache (may be evidence of hemorrhage). Question for increase in amount of discharge during menses. Check peripheral pulses; skin for bruises, petechiae. Check for excessive bleeding from minor cuts, scratches. Assess gums for erythema, gingival bleeding. Assess urine output for hematuria.

PATIENT/FAMILY TEACHING

Report bleeding, bruising, dizziness/lightheadedness, rash, itching, fever, swelling, breathing difficulty.

Lescol

see fluvastatin

letrozole

leh-troe-zoll
(Femara)

CLASSIFICATION

PHARMACOTHERAPEUTIC: Aromatase inhibitor, hormone. **CLINICAL:** Antineoplastic (see p. 74C).

ACTION

Decreases circulating estrogen by inhibiting aromatase, an enzyme that catalyzes the final step in estrogen production. **Therapeutic Effect:** Suppresses estrogen biosynthesis in hormonally responsive breast cancers.

PHARMACOKINETICS

Rapidly and completely absorbed. Metabolized in liver. Primarily eliminated via the kidneys. Unknown if removed by hemodialysis. **Half-life:** Approx. 2 days.

USES

Treatment of advanced breast cancer in postmenopausal women whose disease progressed after antiestrogen therapy. First-line treatment of advanced breast cancer.

PRECAUTIONS

CONTRAINDICATIONS: None known. **CAUTIONS:** Renal/liver impairment.

LIFESPAN CONSIDERATIONS: Pregnancy/lactation: Unknown if distributed in breast milk. **Pregnancy Category D. Children:** Safety and efficacy not established. **Elderly:** No age-related precautions noted.

INTERACTIONS

DRUG: None known. **HERBAL:** None known. **FOOD:** None known. **LAB VALUES:** May increase serum calcium cholesterol, SGOT (AST), SGPT (ALT), GGT.

AVAILABILITY (Rx)

TABLETS: 2.5 mg.

ADMINISTRATION/HANDLING

PO

- Give without regard to food.

INDICATIONS/ROUTES/DOSAGE

BREAST CANCER

PO: ADULTS, ELDERLY: 2.5 mg daily. Continue until tumor progression is evident.

SIDE EFFECTS

FREQUENT (9%–21%): Musculoskeletal pain (back, arm, leg), nausea, headache. **OCCASIONAL (5%–8%):** Constipation, arthralgia, fatigue, vomiting, hot flashes, diarrhea, abdominal pain, cough, rash, anorexia, hypertension, peripheral edema. **RARE (1%–4%):** Asthenia (loss of strength, energy), somnolence, dyspepsia (heartburn, indigestion, epigastric pain), weight increase, pruritus.

ADVERSE REACTIONS/ TOXIC EFFECTS

None known.

NURSING IMPLICATIONS

INTERVENTION/EVALUATION

Monitor for, assist with ambulation if asthenia/dizziness occurs. Assess for headache. Offer antiemetic for nausea/vomiting. Monitor CBC, thyroid function, electrolytes, liver/renal function tests. Monitor for evidence of musculoskeletal pain; offer analgesics for pain relief.

PATIENT/FAMILY TEACHING

Notify physician if nausea, asthenia, hot flashes become unmanageable.

leucovorin calcium (folinic acid, citrovorum factor)

lou-**koe**-vor-in
(Lederle Leucovorin, Wellcovorin)
Do not confuse with Wellbutrin, Wellferon.

CLASSIFICATION

PHARMACOTHERAPEUTIC: Folic acid antagonist. **CLINICAL:** Antidote.

ACTION

Competes with methotrexate for same transport processes into cells (limits methotrexate action on normal cells). **Therapeutic Effect:** Allows purine, DNA, RNA, protein synthesis.

PHARMACOKINETICS

Readily absorbed from GI tract. Widely distributed. Primarily concentrated in liver. Metabolized in liver, intestinal mucosa to active metabolite. Primarily excreted in urine. **Half-life:** 15 min; metabolite: 30–35 min.

USES

Prophylaxis, treatment of methotrexate, pyrimethamine, trimethoprim toxicity. Treatment of folate-deficient megaloblastic anemia of infancy, sprue, pregnancy, colorectal carcinoma. **Unlabeled:** Treatment adjunct for head/neck carcinoma, Ewing's sarcoma, non-Hodgkin's lymphoma, gestational trophoblastic neoplasms.

PRECAUTIONS

CONTRAINDICATIONS: Pernicious anemia, other megaloblastic anemias secondary to vitamin B_{12} deficiency. **CAUTIONS:** History of allergies, bronchial asthma. **With 5-fluorouracil:** Those with GI toxicities (more common/severe).

LIFESPAN CONSIDERATIONS: Pregnancy/lactation: Unknown if drug crosses placenta or is distributed in breast milk. **Pregnancy Category C. Children:** May increase risk of seizures by counteracting anticonvulsant effects of barbiturate, hydantoins. **Elderly:** Age-related renal impairment may require dosage adjustment when used in rescue from effects of high-dose methotrexate therapy.

INTERACTIONS

DRUG: May decrease effect of **anticonvulsants.** May increase effect, toxicity of **5-fluorouracil. HERBAL:** None known. **FOOD:** None known. **LAB VALUES:** None known.

AVAILABILITY (Rx)

TABLETS: 5 mg, 10 mg, 15 mg, 25 mg. **INJECTION:** 10 mg/ml. **POWDER FOR**

INJECTION: 50 mg, 100 mg, 200 mg, 350 mg, 500 mg.

ADMINISTRATION/HANDLING

PO

- Scored tablets may be crushed.

IV

Storage • Store vials for parenteral use at room temperature. • Injection appears as clear, yellowish solution. • Use immediately if reconstituted with Sterile Water for Injection; is stable for 7 days if reconstituted with Bacteriostatic Water for Injection.

Reconstitution • Reconstitute each 50-mg vial with 5 ml Sterile Water for Injection or Bacteriostatic Water for Injection containing benzyl alcohol to provide concentration of 10 mg/ml. • Due to benzyl alcohol in 1-mg ampoule and in Bacteriostatic Water for Injection, reconstitute doses >10 mg/m^2 with Sterile Water for Injection. • Further dilute with D_5W or 0.9% NaCl.

Rate of administration • Do not exceed 160 mg/min if given by IV infusion (because of calcium content).

IV INCOMPATIBILITIES

Amphotericin B complex (Abelcet, AmBisome, Amphotec), droperidol (Inapsine), foscarnet (Foscavir).

IV COMPATIBILITIES

Cisplatin (Platinol AQ), cyclophosphamide (Cytoxan), doxorubicin (Adriamycin), etoposide (VePesid), filgrastim (Neupogen), fluorouracil, gemcitabine (Gemzar), granisetron (Kytril), heparin, methotrexate, metoclopramide (Reglan), mitomycin (Mutamycin), piperacillin-tazobactam (Zosyn), vinblastine (Velban), vincristine (Oncovin).

INDICATIONS/ROUTES/DOSAGE

ANTIDOTE, PREVENTION/TREATMENT OF HEMATOPOIETIC EFFECTS OF FOLIC ACID ANTAGONISTS

Alert: For rescue therapy in cancer chemotherapy, refer to specific protocol being used for optimal dosage and sequence of leucovorin administration.

CONVENTIONAL RESCUE DOSAGE

10 mg/m^2 parenterally one time then q6h orally until serum methotrexate $<10^{-8}$ M. If 24-hr serum creatinine increased by ≥50% or more over baseline or methotrexate $>5 \times 10^{-6}$ M or 48-hr level $>9 \times 10^{-7}$ M, increase to 100 mg/m^2 IV q3h until methotrexate level $<10^{-8}$ M.

FOLIC ACID ANTAGONIST OVERDOSAGE

PO: ADULTS, ELDERLY, CHILDREN: 2–15 mg/day for 3 days or 5 mg q3days.

FOLATE DEFICIENT MEGALOBLASTIC ANEMIA

IM: ADULTS, ELDERLY, CHILDREN: 1 mg/day.

MEGALOBLASTIC ANEMIA

IM: ADULTS, ELDERLY, CHILDREN: 3–6 mg/day.

PREVENTION OF HEMATOLOGIC TOXICITY (for toxoplasmosis):

IV/PO: ADULTS, ELDERLY, CHILDREN: 5–10 mg/day, repeat q3days.

PREVENTION OF HEMATOLOGIC TOXICITY

IV/PO: ADULTS, CHILDREN: 25 mg once weekly.

SIDE EFFECTS

FREQUENT: With 5-fluorouracil: Diarrhea, stomatitis, nausea, vomiting, lethargy/malaise/fatigue, alopecia, anorexia. **OCCASIONAL:** Urticaria, dermatitis.

ADVERSE REACTIONS/TOXIC EFFECTS

Excessive dosage may negate chemotherapeutic effect of folic acid antagonists.

Anaphylaxis occurs rarely. Diarrhea may cause rapid clinical deterioration and death.

NURSING IMPLICATIONS

BASELINE ASSESSMENT

Give as soon as possible, preferably within 1 hr, for treatment of accidental overdosage of folic acid antagonists.

INTERVENTION/EVALUATION

Monitor for vomiting—may need to change from oral to parenteral therapy. Observe elderly, debilitated closely because of risk of severe toxicities. Assess CBC, differential, platelet count (also electrolytes and liver function tests for combination with 5-fluorouracil).

PATIENT/FAMILY TEACHING

Explain purpose of medication in treatment of cancer. Report allergic reaction, vomiting.

leuprolide acetate

leu-pro-lied

(Eligard, Lupron, Lupron Depot-Ped, Viadur)

Do not confuse with Lopurin, Nuprin.

CLASSIFICATION

PHARMACOTHERAPEUTIC: Gonadotropin-releasing hormone analogue. **CLINICAL:** Antineoplastic (see pp. 74C, 90C).

ACTION

Initial or intermittent administration stimulates release of luteinizing hormone (LH), follicle-stimulating hormone (FSH) from anterior pituitary, increasing (within 1 wk) testosterone level in males, estradiol in premenopausal women. Continuous daily administration suppresses secretion of gonadotropin-releasing hormone. **Therapeutic Effect:** Produces fall (within 2–4 wks) in testosterone levels to castrate level in males, estrogen level in premenopausal women to postmenopausal levels. In central precocious puberty, gonadotropins reduced to prepubertal levels.

PHARMACOKINETICS

Rapidly, well absorbed after subcutaneous administration. Slow absorption after IM administration. Protein binding: 43%–49%. **Half-life:** 3–4 hrs.

USES

Treatment of advanced prostatic carcinoma, endometriosis, central precocious puberty, uterine fibroid tumors, anemia caused by uterine leiomyomata.

PRECAUTIONS

CONTRAINDICATIONS: Pernicious anemia, pregnancy. **CAUTIONS:** Long-term use in children.

LIFESPAN CONSIDERATIONS: Pregnancy/lactation: Depot: Contraindicated in pregnancy. May cause spontaneous abortion. **Pregnancy Category X. Children:** Long-term safety not established. **Elderly:** No age-related precautions noted.

INTERACTIONS

DRUG: None known. **HERBAL:** None known. **FOOD:** None known. **LAB VALUES:** May increase serum acid phosphatase. Initially increases testosterone, then decreases testosterone concentration.

AVAILABILITY (Rx)

IMPLANT: (Viadur): 65 mg. **INJECTION SOLUTION: (Lupron):** 5 mg/ml. **INJECTION DEPOT FORMULATION: (Eligard):** 7.5 mg, 22.5 mg, 30 mg. **(Lupron Depot):** 3.75 mg, 7.5 mg. **(Lupron Depot monthly):** 11.25 mg, 22.5 mg, 30 mg.

(Lupron Depot-Ped): 7.5 mg, 11.25 mg, 15 mg.

ADMINISTRATION/HANDLING

Alert: May be carcinogenic, mutagenic, teratogenic. Handle with extreme care during preparation/administration.

SUBCUTANEOUS

• Injection appears clear, colorless. • Refrigerate. • Store opened vial at room temperature. • Discard if precipitate forms or solution appears discolored. • Depot vials: Store at room temperature. Reconstitute only with diluent provided; use immediately. Do not use needles <22 gauge. • Use syringes provided by manufacturer (0.5-ml low-dose insulin syringe may be used as alternative).

L

INDICATIONS/ROUTES/DOSAGE

PROSTATIC CARCINOMA

Subcutaneous: ADULTS, ELDERLY: 1 mg daily.

IM: ADULTS, ELDERLY: DEPOT: 7.5 mg q28–33days or 22.5 mg q3mos or 30 mg q4mos.

ENDOMETRIOSIS, UTERINE LEIOMYOMATA

IM: ADULTS: DEPOT: 3.75 mg monthly or 11.25 mg as single injection.

CENTRAL PRECOCIOUS PUBERTY

Subcutaneous: CHILDREN: Initially, 35–50 mcg/kg/day; if down regulation not achieved, titrate upward by 10 mcg/kg/day.

IM: CHILDREN: Initially, 0.15–0.3 mg/kg/4 wks (minimum: 7.5 mg); if down regulation not achieved, titrate upward in 3.75-mg increments q4wks.

SIDE EFFECTS

FREQUENT: Hot flashes (ranging from mild flushing to diaphoresis). **Females:** Amenorrhea, spotting. **OCCASIONAL:** Arrhythmias, palpitations, blurred vision, dizziness, edema, headache, burning/itching/swelling at injection site, nausea, insomnia, increased weight. **Females:** Deepening voice, increased hair growth, decreased libido, increased breast tenderness, vaginitis, altered mood. **Males:** Constipation, decreased testicle size, gynecomastia, impotence, decreased appetite, angina. **RARE: Males:** Thrombophlebitis.

ADVERSE REACTIONS/ TOXIC EFFECTS

Occasionally, a worsening of signs/symptoms of prostatic carcinoma occurs 1–2 wks after initial dosing (subsides during continued therapy). Increased bone pain and less frequently dysuria or hematuria, weakness/paresthesia of lower extremities may be noted. MI, pulmonary embolism occur rarely.

NURSING IMPLICATIONS

BASELINE ASSESSMENT

Question for possibility of pregnancy prior to initiating therapy (Pregnancy Category X). Obtain serum testosterone, prostatic acid phosphatase (PAP) levels periodically during therapy. Serum testosterone, and PAP levels should increase during first week of therapy. Testosterone level then should decrease to baseline level or less within 2 wks, PAP level within 4 wks.

INTERVENTION/EVALUATION

Monitor for arrhythmias, palpitations. Assess for peripheral edema behind medial malleolus (sacral area in bedridden pts). Assess sleep pattern. Monitor for visual difficulties. Assist with ambulation if dizziness occurs. Offer antiemetics if nausea occurs.

PATIENT/FAMILY TEACHING

Hot flashes tend to decrease during continued therapy. A temporary exacerbation of signs/symptoms of disease may occur during first few wks of therapy. Use contraceptive measures during therapy. Inform physician if regular menstruation persists, pregancy occurs.

levalbuterol

lee-val-**bwet**-err-all
(Xopenex)
Do not confuse with Xanax.

◆ CLASSIFICATION

PHARMACOTHERAPEUTIC: Sympathomimetic. **CLINICAL:** Bronchodilator (see p. 64C).

ACTION

Stimulates beta$_2$-adrenergic receptors in the lungs resulting in relaxation of bronchial smooth muscle. **Therapeutic Effect:** Relieves bronchospasm, reduces airway resistance.

PHARMACOKINETICS

Onset	Peak	Duration
Inhalation		
10–17 min	1.5 hrs	5–6 hrs

Metabolized in the liver to inactive metabolite. **Half-life:** 3.3–4 hrs.

USES

Treatment, prevention of bronchospasm due to reversible obstructive airway disease.

PRECAUTIONS

CONTRAINDICATIONS: History of hypersensitivity to sympathomimetics. **CAUTIONS:** Cardiovascular disorders (e.g., cardiac arrhythmias), seizures, hypertension, diabetes mellitus.

LIFESPAN CONSIDERATIONS: Pregnancy/lactation: Crosses placenta. Unknown if distributed in breast milk. **Pregnancy Category C. Children:** Safety and efficacy not established in those <12 yrs. **Elderly:** Lower initial dosages recommended.

INTERACTIONS

DRUG: **Beta-adrenergic blocking agents (beta-blockers)** antagonize effects. May increase risk of arrhythmias with **digoxin. MAOIs, tricyclic antidepressants** may potentiate cardiovascular effects. **HERBAL:** **Ma huang (ephedra)** may increase CNS stimulation. **FOOD:** None known. **LAB VALUES:** May increase potassium.

AVAILABILITY (Rx)

SOLUTION FOR NEBULIZATION: 0.31 mg in 3-ml vials; 0.63 mg in 3-ml vials; 1.25 mg in 3-ml vials.

ADMINISTRATION/HANDLING

NEBULIZATION

• No diluent necessary. • Protect from light/excessive heat. Store at room temperature. • Once foil is opened, use within 2 wks. • Discard if solution is not colorless. • Do not mix with other medications. • Give over 5–15 min.

INDICATIONS/ROUTES/DOSAGE

BRONCHOSPASM

Nebulization: ADULTS, CHILDREN >12 YRS: Initially, 0.63 mg 3 times/day 6–8 hrs apart. May increase to 1.25 mg 3 times/day with dose monitoring. CHILDREN 6–11 YRS: Initially, 0.31 mg 3 times/day. **Maximum:** 0.63 mg 3 times/day.

SIDE EFFECTS

FREQUENT: Tremor, nervousness, headache, throat dryness/irritation. **OCCASIONAL:** Dry, irritated mouth/throat, coughing, bronchial irritation. **RARE:** Drowsiness, diarrhea, dry mouth, flushing, diaphoresis, anorexia.

ADVERSE REACTIONS/ TOXIC EFFECTS

Excessive sympathomimetic stimulation may produce palpitations, extrasystoles, tachycardia, chest pain, slight increase in B/P followed by substantial decrease, chills, diaphoresis, blanching of skin. Too frequent or excessive use may lead to loss of bronchodilating effectiveness and/or severe paradoxical bronchoconstriction.

NURSING IMPLICATIONS

BASELINE ASSESSMENT

Offer emotional support (high incidence of anxiety due to difficulty in breathing, sympathomimetic response to drug).

INTERVENTION/EVALUATION

Monitor rate, depth, rhythm, type of respiration; quality/rate of pulse, EKG, serum potassium, ABG determinations. Assess lung sounds for wheezing (bronchoconstriction), rales.

PATIENT/FAMILY TEACHING

Increase fluid intake (decreases lung secretion viscosity). Rinsing mouth with water immediately after inhalation may prevent mouth/throat dryness. Avoid excessive use of caffeine derivatives (chocolate, coffee, tea, cola, cocoa). Notify physician if palpitations, tachycardia, chest pain, tremors, dizziness, headache occurs.

Levaquin

see levofloxacin

levetiracetam

leave-ty-rah-**see**-tam

(Keppra)

Do not confuse with Kaletra.

CLASSIFICATION

CLINICAL: Anticonvulsant (see p. 33c).

ACTION

Inhibits burst firing without affecting normal neuronal excitability. **Therapeutic Effect:** Prevents seizure activity.

USES

Adjunctive therapy in treatment of partial-onset seizures in adults and children with epilepsy.

PRECAUTIONS

CONTRAINDICATIONS: Hypersensitivity reaction. **CAUTIONS:** Renal function impairment. **Pregnancy Category C.**

INTERACTIONS

DRUG: None known. **HERBAL:** None known. **FOOD:** None significant. **LAB VALUES:** May increase Hgb, Hct, RBC, WBC.

AVAILABILITY (Rx)

TABLETS: 250 mg, 500 mg, 750 mg. **LIQUID:** 100 mg/ml.

INDICATIONS/ROUTES/DOSAGE

PARTIAL-ONSET SEIZURES

PO: ADULTS, ELDERLY: Initially, 500 mg q12h. May increase by 1,000 mg/day q2wks. **Maximum:** 3,000 mg/day.

DOSAGE IN RENAL IMPAIRMENT

Creatinine Clearance (ml/min)	Dosage
>80	500–1,500 mg q12h
50–80	500–1,000 mg q12h
30–49	250–750 mg q12h
<30	250–500 mg q12h
ESRD using dialysis	500–1,000 mg q12h (following dialysis, a 250- to 500-mg supplemental dose is recommended)

SIDE EFFECTS

FREQUENT (10%–15%): Somnolence, asthenia (loss of strength, energy), headache, infection. **OCCASIONAL (3%–9%):** Dizziness, pharyngitis, pain, depression, nervousness, vertigo, rhinitis, anorexia. **RARE (<3%):** Amnesia, anxiety, emotional lability, cough, sinusitis, anorexia, diplopia.

ADVERSE REACTIONS/ TOXIC EFFECTS

None known.

NURSING IMPLICATIONS

BASELINE ASSESSMENT

Review history of seizure disorder (intensity, frequency, duration, LOC). Initiate seizure precautions. Assess for hypersensitivity to levetiracetam, renal function tests.

INTERVENTION/EVALUATION

Observe for recurrence of seizure activity. Assess for clinical improvement (decrease in intensity/frequency of seizures). Monitor renal function tests. Assist with ambulation if dizziness occurs.

PATIENT/FAMILY TEACHING

Somnolence, drowsiness usually diminishes with continued therapy. Do not abruptly discontinue medication (may precipitate seizures). Strict maintenance of drug therapy is essential for seizure control. Avoid tasks that require alertness, motor skills until response to drug is established.

levobunolol hydrochloride

(Betagan Liquifilm)

See Classification section under: Antiglaucoma agents (p. 46C)

levobupivacaine

(Chirocaine)

See Classification section under: Anesthetics: local (p. 5C)

levofloxacin

leave-oh-**flocks**-ah-sin

(Levaquin, Quixin)

◆ CLASSIFICATION

PHARMACOTHERAPEUTIC: Fluoroquinolone. **CLINICAL:** Antibiotic (see p. 23C).

ACTION

Inhibits the DNA enzyme gyrase in susceptible microorganisms, interfering with bacterial DNA replication and repair. **Therapeutic Effect:** Produces bactericidal activity.

PHARMACOKINETICS

Well absorbed after both PO and IV administration. Protein binding: 24%–38%. Penetrates rapidly, extensively into leukocytes, epithelial cells, macrophages. Lung concentrations are 2–5 times higher than those of plasma. Eliminated unchanged in the urine. Partially removed by hemodialysis. **Half-life:** 8 hrs.

USES

Treatment of acute bacterial exacerbation of chronic bronchitis, community-acquired pneumonia, nosocomial pneumonia, acute maxillary sinusitis, complicated urinary tract infections, acute pyelonephritis, uncomplicated mild to moderate skin/skin structure infections prostatitis. **Ophthalmic:** Treatment of superficial infections to conjunctiva, cornea.

PRECAUTIONS

CONTRAINDICATIONS: History of hypersensitivity to fluoroquinolones, cinoxacin, nalidixic acid. **CAUTIONS:** Suspected CNS disorders, seizure disorder, impaired renal function, bradycardia, cardiomyopathy, hypokalemia, or hypomagnesemia.

LIFESPAN CONSIDERATIONS: Pregnancy/lactation: Excreted in breast milk. Avoid use in pregnancy. **Pregnancy Category C. Children:** Safety and efficacy not established in those <18 yrs. **Elderly:** Age-related renal impairment may require dosage adjustment.

L

INTERACTIONS

DRUG: Antacids, sucralfate, iron preparations decrease levofloxacin absorption. **NSAIDs** may increase risk of CNS stimulation/seizures. **HERBAL:** None known. **FOOD:** None known. **LAB VALUES:** May alter blood glucose concentrations.

AVAILABILITY (Rx)

TABLETS: 250 mg, 500 mg, 750 mg. **INJECTION:** 500 mg/20 ml vials. **PREMIX:** 250 mg/50 ml, 500 mg/100 ml, 750 mg/150 ml. **OPHTHALMIC SOLUTION:** 0.5%.

ADMINISTRATION/HANDLING

PO

• Do not administer antacids (aluminum, magnesium), sucralfate, iron/multivitamin preparations with zinc within 2 hrs of levofloxacin administration (significantly reduces levofloxacin absorption). • Encourage use of cranberry juice, citrus fruits (acidifies urine). • Give without regard to food.

IV

Storage • Available in single-dose 20-ml (500-mg) vials and premixed with D_5W, ready to infuse.

Reconstitution • For infusion using single-dose vial, withdraw desired amount (10 ml for 250 mg, 20 ml for 500 mg). Dilute each 10 ml (250 mg) with minimum 40 ml 0.9% NaCl, D_5W.

Rate of administration • Administer slowly, over not less than 60 min.

OPHTHALMIC

• Place finger on lower eyelid, pull out until a pocket is formed between eye and lower lid. Hold dropper above pocket, place correct number of drops into pocket. • Close eye gently. Apply digital pressure to lacrimal sac for 1–2 min (minimizes drainage into nose/throat, reducing risk of systemic effects).

∅ IV INCOMPATIBILITIES

Furosemide (Lasix), heparin, insulin, nitroglycerin, propofol (Diprivan).

IV COMPATIBILITIES

Aminophylline, dobutamine (Dobutrex), dopamine (Intropin), fentanyl (Sublimaze), lidocaine, lorazepam (Ativan), morphine.

INDICATIONS/ROUTES/DOSAGE

BRONCHITIS

PO/IV: ADULTS, ELDERLY: 500 mg q24h for 7 days.

PNEUMONIA

PO/IV: ADULTS, ELDERLY: 500 mg q24h for 7–14 days.

ACUTE MAXILLARY SINUSITIS

PO/IV: ADULTS, ELDERLY: 500 mg q24h for 10–14 days.

SKIN, SKIN STRUCTURE
PO/IV: ADULTS, ELDERLY: 500 mg q24h for 7–10 days.

URINARY TRACT INFECTION, ACUTE PYELONEPHRITIS
PO/IV: ADULTS, ELDERLY: 250 mg q24h for 10 days.

DOSAGE IN RENAL IMPAIRMENT
BRONCHITIS, PNEUMONIA, SINUSITIS, SKIN/SKIN STRUCTURE INFECTIONS

Creatinine Clearance	Dosage
50–80 ml/min	No change
20–49 ml/min	500 mg initially, then 250 mg q24h
10–19 ml/min	500 mg initially, dialysis then 250 mg q48h

URINARY TRACT INFECTION, PYELONEPHRITIS

Creatinine Clearance	Dosage
20 ml/min	No change
10–19 ml/min	250 mg initially, then 250 mg q48h

BACTERIAL CONJUNCTIVITIS
Ophthalmic: ADULTS, ELDERLY, CHILDREN <1 YR: 1–2 drops q2h for 2 days (up to 8 times/day), then 1–2 drops q4h for 5 days.

SIDE EFFECTS

OCCASIONAL (1%–3%): Diarrhea, nausea, stomach pain, dizziness, drowsiness, headache, lightheadedness. **Ophthalmic:** Local burning/discomfort, margin crusting, crystals/scales, foreign body sensation, itching, bad taste. **RARE (<1%):** Flatulence, taste perversion, pain, inflammation/swelling in calves, hands, shoulder. **Ophthalmic:** Corneal staining, keratitis, allergic reaction, eyelid edema, tearing, reduced vision.

ADVERSE REACTIONS/ TOXIC EFFECTS

Pseudomembranous colitis (severe abdominal pain/cramps, severe watery diarrhea, fever) may occur. Superinfection (genital-anal pruritus, ulceration/changes in oral mucosa, moderate to severe diarrhea) may occur. Hypersensitivity reactions, including photosensitivity (rash, pruritus, blistering, swelling, sensation of skin burning), have occurred in those receiving fluoroquinolone therapy.

NURSING IMPLICATIONS

BASELINE ASSESSMENT

Question for hypersensitivity to levofloxacin, other fluoroquinolones.

INTERVENTION/EVALUATION

Monitor blood glucose, renal/liver function tests. Report hypersensitivity reaction: skin rash, urticaria, pruritus, photosensitivity promptly. Be alert for superinfection (e.g., genital-anal pruritus, ulceration/changes in oral mucosa, moderate to severe diarrhea, new/increased fever). Provide symptomatic relief for nausea. Evaluate food tolerance, change in taste sensation.

PATIENT/FAMILY TEACHING

Drink 6–8 glasses of fluid/day (citrus, cranberry juice acidifies urine). Avoid tasks that require alertness, motor skills until response to drug is established (may cause dizziness, drowsiness). Notify physician if tendon pain/swelling, palpitations, chest pain, difficulty breathing, persistent diarrhea occurs.

levorphanol tartrate

leh-**vor**-phan-ole
(Levo-Dromoran)
See Classification section under: Opioid analgesics (p. 121C)

levothyroxine

lee-voe-thye-**rox**-een
(Eltroxin, Levothroid, Levoxyl, Novothyrox, Synthroid, Unithroid)
Do not confuse with liothyronine.

FIXED-COMBINATION(S)

With liothyronine, T_3 **(Thyrolar).**

CLASSIFICATION

PHARMACOTHERAPEUTIC: Synthetic isomer of thyroxine. **CLINICAL:** Thyroid hormone (T_4) (see p. 135C).

ACTION

Involved in normal metabolism, growth, development (esp. CNS of infants). Possesses catabolic and anabolic effects. **Therapeutic Effect:** Increases basal metabolic rate, enhances gluconeogenesis, stimulates protein synthesis.

PHARMACOKINETICS

Variable, incomplete absorption from GI tract. Protein binding: >99%. Widely distributed. Deiodinated in peripheral tissues, minimal metabolism in liver. Eliminated by biliary excretion. **Half-life:** 6–7 days.

USES

Replacement in decreased, absent thyroid function (partial/complete absence of gland, primary atrophy, functional deficiency, effects of surgery/radiation/antithyroid agents, pituitary/hypothalamic hypothyroidism). Management of simple (nontoxic) goiter, chronic lymphocytic thyroiditis. Treatment of thyrotoxicosis (with antithyroid drugs) to prevent goitrogenesis, hypothyroidism. Management of thyroid cancer. Diagnostic aid in thyroid suppression tests.

PRECAUTIONS

CONTRAINDICATIONS: Thyrotoxicosis and MI uncomplicated by hypothyroidism, hypersensitivity to any component (with tablets: tartrazine, allergy to aspirin, lactose intolerance), treatment of obesity. **CAUTIONS:** Elderly, angina pectoris, hypertension, other cardiovascular disease.

LIFESPAN CONSIDERATIONS: Pregnancy/lactation: Drug does not cross placenta. Minimal excretion in breast milk. **Pregnancy Category A. Children:** No age-related precautions noted. Caution in neonates in interpreting thyroid function tests. **Elderly:** May be more sensitive to thyroid effects; individualized dosage recommended.

INTERACTIONS

DRUG: May alter effect of **oral anticoagulants. Cholestyramine, colestipol** may decrease absorption. **Sympathomimetics** may increase effects, coronary insufficiency. **HERBAL:** None known. **FOOD:** None known. **LAB VALUES:** None known.

AVAILABILITY (Rx)

TABLETS: 0.025 mg, 0.05 mg, 0.075 mg, 0.088 mg, 0.1 mg, 0.112 mg, 0.125 mg, 0.137 mg, 0.15 mg, 0.175 mg, 0.2 mg, 0.3 mg. **INJECTION:** 200 mcg, 500 mcg.

ADMINISTRATION/HANDLING

Alert: Do not interchange brands (problems with bioequivalence between manufacturers).

PO

• Give at same time each day to maintain hormone levels. • Administer before breakfast to prevent insomnia. • Tablets may be crushed.

IV

Storage • Store vials at room temperature.

Reconstitution • Reconstitute 200-mcg or 500-mcg vial with 5 ml 0.9% NaCl to provide a concentration of 40 or 100 mcg/ml, respectively; shake until clear.

Rate of administration • Use immediately and discard unused portions. • Give each 100 mcg or less over 1 min.

⊘ **IV INCOMPATIBILITIES**

Do not use or mix with other IV solutions.

INDICATIONS/ROUTES/DOSAGE

Alert: Begin therapy with small doses, increase gradually.

HYPOTHYROIDISM

PO: ADULTS, ELDERLY: Initially, 12.5–50 mcg. May increase by 25–50 mcg/day q2–4wks.

MYXEDEMA COMA OR STUPOR

IV: ADULTS, ELDERLY: 200–500 mcg once, then 75–300 mcg/day.

THYROID SUPPRESSION TEST

PO: ADULTS, ELDERLY: 2–6 mcg/kg/day for 7–10 days.

TSH SUPPRESSION IN THYROID CANCER, NODULES, EUTHYROID GOITERS

PO: ADULTS, ELDERLY: Use larger doses than those used for replacement therapy.

USUAL PEDIATRIC DOSAGE

PO: >12 YRS: 150 mcg/day. 6–12 YRS: 100–125 mcg/day. >1–5 YRS: 75–100 mcg/day. 7–12 MOS: 50–75 mcg/day. 3–6 MOS: 25–50 mcg/day. <3 MOS: 10–15 mcg/kg.

USUAL PARENTERAL DOSAGE

IV: ADULTS, ELDERLY, CHILDREN: Initial dosage approximately half the previously established oral dosage.

SIDE EFFECTS

OCCASIONAL: Children may have reversible hair loss upon initiation. **RARE:** Dry skin, GI intolerance, skin rash, hives, pseudotumor cerebri (severe headache in children).

ADVERSE REACTIONS/ TOXIC EFFECTS

Excessive dosage produces signs/symptoms of hyperthyroidism: weight loss, palpitations, increased appetite, tremors, nervousness, tachycardia, hypertension, headache, insomnia, menstrual irregularities. Cardiac arrhythmias occur rarely.

NURSING IMPLICATIONS

BASELINE ASSESSMENT

Question for hypersensitivity to tartrazine, aspirin, lactose. Obtain baseline weight, vital signs. Signs/symptoms of diabetes mellitus, diabetes insipidus, adrenal insufficiency, hypopituitarism may become intensified. Treat with adrenocortical steroids prior to thyroid therapy in coexisting hypothyroidism and hypoadrenalism.

INTERVENTION/EVALUATION

Monitor pulse for rate, rhythm (report pulse of 100 or marked increase). Assess for tremors, nervousness. Check appetite, sleep pattern.

PATIENT/FAMILY TEACHING

Do not discontinue drug therapy; replacement for hypothyroidism is lifelong. Follow-up office visits, thyroid function tests are essential. Take medication at the same time each day, preferably in the morning. Monitor pulse, report marked increase, pulse of ≥100, change of rhythm. Do not change brands. Notify physician promptly of chest pain, weight loss, nervousness/tremors, insomnia. Children may have reversible hair loss, increased aggressiveness during the first few months of therapy. Full therapeutic effect may take 1–3 wks.

Levoxyl

see levothyroxine

Lexapro

see escitalopram

lidocaine hydrochloride

lie-doe-cane
(Lidoderm, Xylocaine, Xylocard❖, Zilactin-L❖)

FIXED-COMBINATION(S)

Lidocaine with epinephrine: lidocaine/epinephrine (a sympathomimetic): 2%/1:50,000; 1%/1:100,000; 1%/1:200,000; 0.5%/1:200,000. **EMLA:** lidocaine/prilocaine (an anesthetic): 2.5%/2.5%.

CLASSIFICATION

PHARMACOTHERAPEUTIC: Amide anesthetic. **CLINICAL:** Antiarrhythmic, anesthetic (see pp. 5C, 13C).

ACTION

Anesthetic: Inhibits conduction of nerve impulses. **Therapeutic Effect:** Causes temporary loss of feeling/sensation. **Antiarrhythmic:** Decreases depolarization, automaticity, excitability of ventricle during diastole by direct action. **Therapeutic Effect:** Reverses ventricular arrhythmias.

PHARMACOKINETICS

Onset	Peak	Duration
IV		
30–90 sec	—	10–20 min
Local anesthetic		
2.5 min	—	30–60 min

Completely absorbed after IM administration. Protein binding: 60%–80%. Widely distributed. Metabolized in liver. Primarily excreted in urine. Minimally removed by hemodialysis. **Half-life:** 1–2 hrs.

USES

Antiarrhythmic: Rapid control of acute ventricular arrhythmias following MI, cardiac catheterization, cardiac surgery, digitalis-induced ventricular arrhythmias. **Local Anesthetic:** Infiltration/nerve block for dental/surgical procedures, childbirth. **Topical Anesthetic:** Local skin disorders (minor burns, insect bites, prickly heat, skin manifestations of chickenpox, abrasions). Mucous membranes (local anesthesia of oral, nasal, laryngeal mucous membranes; local anesthesia of respiratory, urinary tracts; relief of discomfort of pruritus ani, hemorrhoids, pruritus vulvae). **Dermal Patch:** Treatment of shingles-related skin pain.

PRECAUTIONS

CONTRAINDICATIONS: Hypersensitivity to amide-type local anesthetics, Adams-Stokes syndrome, supraventricular arrhythmias, Wolff-Parkinson-White syndrome. Spinal anesthesia contraindicated in septicemia. **CAUTIONS:** Liver disease, marked hypoxia, severe respiratory depression, hypovolemia, heart block, bradycardia, atrial fibrillation.

LIFESPAN CONSIDERATIONS: Pregnancy/lactation: Crosses placenta. Distributed in breast milk. **Pregnancy Category B. Children:** No age-related precautions noted. **Elderly:** More sensitive to adverse effects. Dose, rate of infusion should be reduced. Age-related renal impairment may require dosage adjustment.

INTERACTIONS

DRUG: May increase cardiac effects with **other antiarrhythmics. Anticonvulsants** may increase cardiac depressant effects. **Beta-adrenergic blockers** may increase risk of toxicity. **HERBAL:** None known. **FOOD:** None known. **LAB VALUES:** IM lidocaine may increase CPK level (used in diagnostic test for presence of acute MI). Therapeutic blood serum level: 1.5–6 mcg/ml; toxic blood serum level: >6 mcg/ml.

AVAILABILITY (Rx)

INJECTION: **IM:** 300 mg/3 ml. **DIRECT IV:** 10 mg/ml, 20 mg/ml. **IV ADMIXTURE:** 40 mg/ml, 100 mg/ml, 200 mg/ml. **IV INFUSION:** 2 mg/ml, 4 mg/ml, 8 mg/ml. **INJECTION (anesthesia):** 0.5%, 1%, 1.5%, 2%, 4%.

TOPICAL: **LIQUID:** 2.5%, 5%. **OINTMENT:** 2.5%, 5%. **CREAM:** 0.5%. **GEL:** 0.5%, 2.5%. **SPRAY:** 0.5%. **SOLUTION:** 2%, 4%. **JELLY:** 2%. **DERMAL PATCH:** 5%.

ADMINISTRATION/HANDLING

Alert: Resuscitative equipment, drugs (including O_2) must always be readily available when administering lidocaine by any route.

IM

• Use 10% (100 mg/ml); clearly identify lidocaine that is **for IM use.** • Give in deltoid muscle (blood level is significantly higher than if injection is given in gluteus muscle or lateral thigh).

IV

Alert: Use only lidocaine without preservative, clearly marked **for IV use.**

Storage • Store at room temperature.

Reconstitution • For IV infusion, prepare solution by adding 1 g to 1 L D_5W to provide concentration of 1 mg/ml (0.1%). • Commercially available preparations of 0.2%, 0.4%, and 0.8% may be used for IV infusion. Maximum concentration: 4 g/250 ml.

Rate of administration • For IV push, use 1% (10 mg/ml) or 2% (20 mg/ml). • Administer IV push at rate of 25–50 mg/min. • Administer for IV infusion at rate of 1–4 mg/min (1–4 ml); use volume control IV set.

TOPICAL

• Not for ophthalmic use. • For skin disorders, apply directly to affected area or put on gauze or bandage, which is then applied to the skin. • For mucous membrane use, apply to desired area using manufacturer's insert. • Administer the lowest dosage possible that still provides anesthesia.

IV INCOMPATIBILITIES

Amphotericin B complex (Abelcet, AmBisome, Amphotec), thiopental.

IV COMPATIBILITIES

Aminophylline, amiodarone (Cordarone), calcium gluconate, digoxin (Lanoxin), diltiazem (Cardizem), dobutamine (Dobutrex), dopamine (Intropin), enalapril (Vasotec), furosemide (Lasix), heparin, insulin, nitroglycerin, potassium chloride.

INDICATIONS/ROUTES/DOSAGE

VENTRICULAR ARRHYTHMIAS

IM: ADULTS, ELDERLY: 300 mg (or 4.3 mg/kg). May repeat in 60–90 min.

IV: ADULTS, ELDERLY: Initially, 50–100 mg (1 mg/kg) IV bolus at rate of 25–50 mg/min. May repeat in 5 min. Give no more than 200–300 mg in 1 hr. MAINTENANCE: 20–50 mcg/kg/min (1–4 mg/min) as IV infusion. CHILDREN, INFANTS: Initially, 0.5–1 mg/kg IV bolus; may repeat but total dose not to exceed 3–5 mg/kg. MAINTENANCE: 10–50 mcg/kg/min as IV infusion.

USUAL LOCAL ANESTHETIC DOSAGE

Dose varies with procedure, degree of anesthesia, vascularity, duration. **Maximum dose:** 4.5 mg/kg. Do not repeat within 2 hrs.

USUAL TOPICAL DOSAGE

Topical: ADULTS, ELDERLY: Apply to affected areas as needed. **Dermal patch:** Apply to intact skin over most painful area (up to 3 patches/application once for up to 12 hrs in a 24-hr period).

SIDE EFFECTS

CNS effects generally dose related and of short duration. **OCCASIONAL: IM:** Pain at injection site. **Topical:** Burning, stinging, tenderness. **RARE:** Generally with high dose: Drowsiness, dizziness, disorientation, lightheadedness, tremors, apprehension, euphoria, sensation of heat/cold/numbness, blurred/double vision, ringing/roaring in ears (tinnitus), nausea.

ADVERSE REACTIONS/ TOXIC EFFECTS

Although serious adverse reactions to lidocaine are uncommon, high dosage by any route may produce cardiovascular depression: bradycardia, somnolence, hypotension, arrhythmias, heart block, cardiovascular collapse, cardiac arrest. Potential for malignant hyperthermia. CNS toxicity may occur, esp. with regional anesthesia use, progressing rapidly from mild side effects to tremors, convulsions, vomiting, respiratory depression. Methemoglobinemia (evidenced by cyanosis) has occurred following topical application of lidocaine for teething discomfort and laryngeal anesthetic spray. Overuse of oral lidocaine has caused seizures in children. Allergic reactions are rare.

NURSING IMPLICATIONS

BASELINE ASSESSMENT

Question for hypersensitivity to lidocaine, amide anesthetics. Obtain baseline B/P, pulse, respirations, EKG, electrolytes.

INTERVENTION/EVALUATION

Monitor EKG, vital signs closely during and following drug administration for cardiac performance. If EKG shows arrhythmias, prolongation of PR interval or QRS complex, inform physician immediately. Assess pulse for irregularity, quality, bradycardia. Assess B/P for evidence of hypotension. Monitor for therapeutic serum level (1.5–6 mcg/ml). For lidocaine given by all routes, monitor vital signs, pt's state of consciousness. Drowsiness should be considered a warning sign of high blood levels of lidocaine. Therapeutic blood serum level: 1.5–6 mcg/ml; toxic blood serum level: >6 mcg/ml.

PATIENT/FAMILY TEACHING

Local Anesthesia: Ensure that pt understands loss of feeling/sensation, need for protection until anesthetic wears off (e.g., no ambulation, including special positions for some regional anesthesia; no chewing gum, eating, drinking after administration to oral area, etc.). **Oral Mucous Membrane Anesthesia:** Do not eat, drink, chew gum for 1 hr after application (swallowing reflex may be impaired, increasing risk of aspiration; numbness of tongue/buccal mucosa may lead to biting trauma).

linezolid

lyn-eh-**zoe**-lid
(Zyvox)
Do not confuse with Vioxx.

◆ **CLASSIFICATION**

PHARMACOTHERAPEUTIC: Oxalodinone. **CLINICAL:** Antibiotic.

ACTION

Binds to a site on bacterial 23S ribosomal RNA, preventing formation of complex that is an essential component of bacterial translation process. **Therapeutic Effect:** Bacteriostatic against enterococci, staphylococci; bactericidal against streptococci.

PHARMACOKINETICS

Rapidly, extensively absorbed following PO administration. Protein binding: 31%. Metabolized in liver by oxidation. Excreted in urine. **Half-life:** 4–5.4 hrs.

USES

Treatment of vancomycin-resistant *Enterococcus faecium* (VRE) infections, nosocomial pneumonia, uncomplicated/complicated skin/skin structure infections, community-acquired pneumonia (CAP), diabetic foot infections.

PRECAUTIONS

CONTRAINDICATIONS: None known. **CAUTIONS:** Uncontrolled hypertension, pheochromocytoma, carcinoid syndrome, severe renal/liver impairment, untreated hyperthyroidism.

LIFESPAN CONSIDERATIONS: Pregnancy/lactation: Unknown if distributed in breast milk. **Pregnancy Category C. Children:** Safety and efficacy not established. **Elderly:** No age-related precautions noted.

INTERACTIONS

DRUG: Decreases effect of **MAOIs. Adrenergic agents (sympathomimetics)** increase effect. **HERBAL:** None known. **FOOD:** None known. **LAB VALUES:** May decrease platelets, Hgb, WBC, SGPT (ALT).

AVAILABILITY (Rx)

TABLETS: 400 mg, 600 mg. **POWDER FOR RECONSTITUTION (PO):** 100 mg/5 ml. **INJECTION:** 2 mg/ml in 100-ml, 300-ml bags.

ADMINISTRATION/HANDLING

PO

• Give without regard to meals. • Use suspension within 21 days after reconstitution.

IV

Storage • Store at room temperature • Protect from light. • Yellow color does not affect potency.

Rate of administration • Infuse over 30–120 min.

IV INCOMPATIBILITIES

Alert: Do not mix with other medications. If same line is used, flush with compatible fluid (D_5W, 0.9% NaCl, lactated Ringer's).

Amphotericin B complex (Abelcet, AmBisome, Amphotec), chlorpromazine (Thorazine), diazepam (Valium), erythromycin (Erythrocin), pentamidine (Pentam IV), phenytoin (Dilantin), sulfamethoxazole-trimethoprim (Bactrim).

INDICATIONS/ROUTES/DOSAGE

VRE

PO/IV: ADULTS, ELDERLY, CHILDREN >12 YRS: 600 mg q12h for 14–28 days.

NOSOCOMIAL PNEUMONIA, CAP, COMPLICATED SKIN INFECTIONS

PO/IV: ADULTS, ELDERLY: 600 mg q12h for 10–14 days.

UNCOMPLICATED SKIN INFECTIONS

PO/IV: ADULTS, ELDERLY: 400 mg q12h for 10–14 days. CHILDREN ≥12 YRS: 600

mg q12. CHILDERN 5–11 YRS: 10 mg/kg/dose q12h.

SIDE EFFECTS

OCCASIONAL (2%–5%): Diarrhea, nausea, headache. **RARE (<2%):** Taste alteration, vaginal candidiasis (itching, discharge), fungal infection, dizziness, tongue discoloration.

ADVERSE REACTIONS/ TOXIC EFFECTS

Thrombocytopenia occurs rarely. Myelosuppression. Antibiotic-associated colitis (severe abdominal pain/tenderness, fever, watery/severe diarrhea) may result from altered bacterial balance.

NURSING IMPLICATIONS

INTERVENTION/EVALUATION

Monitor bowel activity/stool consistency carefully; mild GI effects may be tolerable, but increasing severity may indicate onset of antibiotic-associated colitis. Be alert for superinfection: severe genital/anal pruritus, abdominal pain, severe mouth soreness, moderate to severe diarrhea. Monitor CBC weekly.

PATIENT/FAMILY TEACHING

Continue therapy for full length of treatment. Doses should be evenly spaced. May cause GI upset (may take with food, milk). Avoid excessive amounts of tyramine-containing foods (e.g., red wine, aged cheese). Notify physician of persistent, worsening of symptoms of infection.

liothyronine

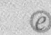

lye-oh-**thigh**-roe-neen
(Cytomel, Triostat)
Do not confuse with levothyroxine.

FIXED-COMBINATION(S)

With levothyroxine, T_4 **(Thyrolar).**

CLASSIFICATION

PHARMACOTHERAPEUTIC: Synthetic form thyroid hormone T_3. **CLINICAL:** Thyroid hormone (see p. 135C).

ACTION

Involved in normal metabolism, growth, development (esp. CNS of infants). Possesses catabolic, anabolic effects. **Therapeutic Effect:** Increases basal metabolic rate, enhances gluconeogenesis, stimulates protein synthesis.

USES

PO: Replacement in decreased, absent thyroid function (partial, complete absence of gland; primary atrophy; functional deficiency; effects of surgery, radiation, antithyroid agents; pituitary, hypothalamic hypothyroidism). Management of simple (nontoxic) goiter; diagnostically in T_3 suppression test (differentiates hyperthyroidism from euthyroidism). **IV:** Myxedema coma, precoma.

PRECAUTIONS

CONTRAINDICATIONS: Thyrotoxicosis and MI uncomplicated by hypothyroidism, treatment of obesity. **CAUTIONS:** Cardiovascular disease, adrenal insufficiency, coronary artery disease, diabetes mellitus, diabetes insipidus. **Pregnancy Category A.**

INTERACTIONS

DRUG: May alter effect of **oral anticoagulants. Cholestyramine, colestipol** may decrease absorption. **Sympathomimetics** may increase effects, coronary insufficiency. **HERBAL:** None known. **FOOD:** None known. **LAB VALUES:** None known.

AVAILABILITY (Rx)

TABLETS: 5 mcg, 25 mcg, 50 mcg. **INJECTION:** 10 mcg/ml.

INDICATIONS/ROUTES/DOSAGE

HYPOTHYROIDISM

PO: ADULTS, ELDERLY: Initially, 25 mcg/day. May increase in 12.5–25 mcg/day increments q1–2wks. **Maximum:** 100 mcg/day. CHILDREN: Initially 5 mcg/day. May increase by 5 mcg/day q3–4days. MAINTENANCE: INFANTS: 20 mcg/day. CHILDREN 1–3 YRS: 50 mcg/day. CHILDREN >3 YRS: 100 mcg/day.

MYXEDEMA

PO: ADULTS, ELDERLY: Initially, 5 mcg/day. Increase by 5–10 mcg q1–2wks (after 25 mcg/day reached, may increase by 12.5-mcg increments). MAINTENANCE: 50–100 mcg/day.

NONTOXIC GOITER

PO: ADULTS, ELDERLY: Initially, 5 mcg/day. Increase by 5–10 mcg/day q1–2wks. When 25 mcg/day obtained, may increase by 12.5–25 mcg/day q1–2wks. MAINTENANCE: 75 mcg/day. CHILDREN: 5 mcg/day. May increase by 5 mcg q1–2wks. MAINTENANCE: 15–20 mcg/day.

CONGENITAL HYPOTHYROIDISM

PO: CHILDREN: Initially, 5 mcg/day. Increase by 5 mcg/day q3–4days. MAINTENANCE: (INFANTS): 20 mcg/day. (1 YR): 50 mcg/day. (>3 YRS): Full adult dosage.

T_3 SUPPRESSION TEST

PO: ADULTS, ELDERLY: 75–100 mcg/day for 7 days, then repeat ^{131}I thyroid uptake test.

MYXEDEMA COMA, PRECOMA

Alert: Initial and subsequent dosage based on pt's clinical status, response. Administer IV dose at least 4 hrs but no longer than 12 hrs apart.

IV: ADULTS, ELDERLY: Initially, 25–50 mcg (10–20 mcg in pts with cardiovascular disease). Total dose at least 65 mcg/day.

SIDE EFFECTS

OCCASIONAL: Children may have reversible hair loss upon initiation. **RARE:** Dry skin, GI intolerance, skin rash, hives, pseudotumor cerebri (severe headache in children).

ADVERSE REACTIONS/ TOXIC EFFECTS

Excessive dosage produces signs/symptoms of hyperthyroidism: weight loss, palpitations, increased appetite, tremors, nervousness, tachycardia, increased B/P, headache, insomnia, menstrual irregularities. Cardiac arrhythmias occur rarely.

L

NURSING IMPLICATIONS

BASELINE ASSESSMENT

Question for hypersensitivity to tartrazine, aspirin. Obtain baseline weight, vital signs. Signs, symptoms of diabetes mellitus, diabetes insipidus, adrenal insufficiency, hypopituitarism may become intensified. Treat with adrenocortical steroids prior to thyroid therapy in coexisting hypothyroidism and hypoadrenalism.

INTERVENTION/EVALUATION

Monitor pulse for rate, rhythm (report pulse ≥100 or marked increase). Assess for tremors, nervousness. Assess appetite, sleep pattern.

PATIENT/FAMILY TEACHING

Do not discontinue drug therapy; replacement for hypothyroidism is lifelong. Follow-up office visits, thyroid function tests are essential. Take medication at the same time each day, preferably in morning. Teach pt/family to take pulse correctly, report marked increase, pulse of ≥100, change of rhythm. Notify physician promptly of chest pain, weight loss, nervousness/tremors, insomnia. Children may have reversible hair loss, increased aggressiveness during first few months of therapy.

Lipitor

see atorvastatin

lisinopril

lih-**sin**-oh-prill
(Prinivil, Zestril)

Do not confuse with Desyrel, fosinopril, Lioresal, Plendil, Prilosec, Proventil, Restoril, Zostrix.

FIXED-COMBINATION(S)

Prinzide/Zestoretic: lisinopril/hydrochlorothiazide (a diuretic): 10 mg/12.5 mg; 20 mg/12.5 mg; 20 mg/25 mg.

CLASSIFICATION

PHARMACOTHERAPEUTIC: Angiotensin-converting enzyme (ACE) inhibitor. **CLINICAL:** Antihypertensive (see p. 6C).

ACTION

Suppresses renin-angiotensin-aldosterone system (prevents conversion of angiotensin I to angiotensin II, a potent vasoconstrictor; may also inhibit angiotensin II at local vascular, renal sites). Decreases plasma angiotensin II, increases plasma renin activity, decreases aldosterone secretion. **Therapeutic Effect:** Reduces peripheral arterial resistance, B/P (afterload), pulmonary capillary wedge pressure (preload), pulmonary vascular resistance. In those with heart failure, also decreases heart size, increases cardiac output, exercise tolerance time.

PHARMACOKINETICS

Onset	Peak	Duration
PO		
1 hr	6 hrs	24 hrs

Incompletely absorbed from GI tract. Protein binding: 25%. Primarily excreted unchanged in urine. Removed by hemodialysis. **Half-life:** 12 hrs (half-life prolonged with impaired renal function).

USES

Treatment of hypertension. Used alone or in combination with other antihypertensives. Adjunctive therapy in management of heart failure. Improves survival in pts who had an MI. **Unlabeled:** Treatment of hypertension/renal crises with scleroderma.

PRECAUTIONS

CONTRAINDICATIONS: History of angioedema with previous treatment with ACE inhibitors. **CAUTIONS:** Renal impairment, those with sodium depletion or on diuretic therapy, dialysis, hypovolemia, coronary/cerebrovascular insufficiency, severe CHF.

LIFESPAN CONSIDERATIONS: Pregnancy/lactation: Crosses placenta. Unknown if distributed in breast milk. **Pregnancy Category C** (**D** if used in second or third trimester). Has caused fetal/neonatal mortality, morbidity. **Children:** Safety and efficacy not established. **Elderly:** May be more sensitive to hypotensive effects.

INTERACTIONS

DRUG: **Alcohol, diuretics, hypotensive agents** may increase effects. **NSAIDs** may decrease effect. **Potassium-sparing diuretics, potassium supplements** may cause hyperkalemia. May increase **lithium** concentration, toxicity. **HERBAL:** None known. **FOOD:** None known. **LAB VALUES:** May increase potassium, SGOT (AST), SGPT (ALT), alkaline phosphatase, bilirubin, BUN, creatinine. May decrease sodium. May cause positive ANA titer.

AVAILABILITY (Rx)

TABLETS: 2.5 mg, 5 mg, 10 mg, 20 mg, 30 mg, 40 mg.

ADMINISTRATION/HANDLING

PO

• Give without regard to food. • Tablets may be crushed.

INDICATIONS/ROUTES/DOSAGE

HYPERTENSION (used alone)

PO: ADULTS: Initially, 10 mg/day. May increase by 5–10 mg/day at 1- to 2-wk intervals. **Maximum:** 40 mg/day. ELDERLY: Initially, 2.5–5 mg/day. May increase by 2.5–5 mg/day at 1- to 2-wk intervals. **Maximum:** 40 mg/day.

HYPERTENSION (combination therapy)

Alert: Discontinue diuretic 2–3 days before initiating lisinopril therapy.

PO: ADULTS: Initially, 2.5–5 mg/day titrated to pt's needs.

CHF

PO: ADULTS, ELDERLY: Initially, 2.5–5 mg/day. May increase by no more than 10 mg/day at intervals of at least 2 wks. MAINTENANCE: 5–40 mg/day.

MI

PO: ADULTS, ELDERLY: Initially, 5 mg, then 5 mg after 24 hrs, 10 mg after 48 hrs, then 10 mg/day for 6 wks. (Pts with low systolic B/P: 2.5 mg/day for 3 days, then 2.5–5 mg/day.)

USUAL ELDERLY DOSAGE

PO: Initially, 2.5–5 mg/day. May increase by 2.5–5 mg/day at 1- to 2-wk intervals. **Maximum:** 40 mg/day.

DOSAGE IN RENAL IMPAIRMENT

Titrate to pt's needs after giving the following initial dose:

Creatinine Clearance	% Normal Dose
10–50 ml/min	50–75
<10 ml/min	25–50

SIDE EFFECTS

FREQUENT (5%–12%): Headache, dizziness, postural hypotension. **OCCASIONAL (2%–4%):** Chest discomfort, fatigue, rash, abdominal pain, nausea, diarrhea, upper respiratory infection. **RARE (≤1%):** Palpitations, tachycardia, peripheral edema, insomnia, paresthesia, confusion, constipation, dry mouth, muscle cramps.

ADVERSE REACTIONS/ TOXIC EFFECTS

Excessive hypotension ("first-dose syncope") may occur in pts with CHF, severe salt/volume depletion. Angioedema (swelling of face/lips), hyperkalemia occurs rarely. Agranulocytosis, neutropenia may be noted in pts with impaired renal function, collagen vascular disease (systemic lupus erythematosus, scleroderma). Nephrotic syndrome may be noted in pts with history of renal disease.

NURSING IMPLICATIONS

BASELINE ASSESSMENT

Obtain B/P, apical pulse immediately prior to each dose, in addition to regular monitoring (be alert to fluctuations). If excessive reduction in B/P occurs, place pt in supine position, feet slightly elevated. In pts with renal impairment, autoimmune disease, taking drugs that affect leukocytes or immune response, CBC and differential count should be performed prior to beginning therapy and q2wks for 3 mos, then periodically thereafter.

L

INTERVENTION/EVALUATION

Assess for edema. Check lungs for rales. Monitor I&O, weigh daily. Assess stools for frequency, consistency. Assist with ambulation if dizziness occurs. Monitor B/P, renal function tests, WBC, potassium.

PATIENT/FAMILY TEACHING

To reduce hypotensive effect, rise slowly from lying to sitting position, permit legs to dangle from bed momentarily before standing. Limit alcohol. Inform physician if vomiting, diarrhea, diaphoresis, swelling of face/lips/tongue, difficulty in breathing occur.

L

lithium carbonate

lith-ee-um
(Duralith✱, Eskalith, Lithobid)

lithium citrate

(Cibalith-S)

Do not confuse with Levbid, Lithostat, Lithotabs.

CLASSIFICATION

PHARMACOTHERAPEUTIC: Psychotherapeutic. **CLINICAL:** Antimanic, antidepressant, vascular headache prophylactic.

ACTION

Affects storage, release, reuptake of neurotransmitters. Antimanic effect may be result of increase in norepinephrine reuptake and increase in serotonin receptor sensitivity. **Therapeutic Effect:** Produces antimanic, antidepressant effects.

PHARMACOKINETICS

Rapid, complete absorption from GI tract. Primarily excreted unchanged in urine. Removed by hemodialysis. **Half-life:** 18–24 hrs (half-life increased in elderly).

USES

Prophylaxis, treatment of acute mania, manic phase of bipolar disorder (manic-depressive illness). **Unlabeled:** Treatment of mental depression, neutropenia; prophylaxis of vascular headache.

PRECAUTIONS

CONTRAINDICATIONS: Severe cardiovascular disease, severe renal disease, severe dehydration/sodium depletion, debilitated pts. **CAUTIONS:** Cardiovascular disease, thyroid disease, elderly.

LIFESPAN CONSIDERATIONS: Pregnancy/lactation: Freely crosses placenta. Distributed in breast milk. **Pregnancy Category D. Children:** May increase bone formation/density (alter parathyroid hormone concentrations). **Elderly:** More susceptible to develop lithium-induced goiter/clinical hypothyroidism, CNS toxicity. Increased thirst, urination more frequent; lower dosage recommended.

INTERACTIONS

DRUG: May increase effects of **antithyroid medication, iodinated glycerol, potassium iodide. NSAIDs** may increase concentration, toxicity. May decrease absorption of **phenothiazines. Phenothiazines** may increase intracellular concentration, increase renal excretion, extrapyramidal symptoms (EPS), delirium, mask early signs of lithium toxicity. **Diuretics** may increase concentration, toxicity. **Haloperidol** may increase EPS, neurologic toxicity. **Molindone** may increase risk of neurotoxic symptoms. **HERBAL:** None known. **FOOD:** None known. **LAB VALUES:** May increase blood glucose, calcium, immunoreactive parathyroid hormone. Therapeutic blood serum level: 0.6–1.2 mEq/L; toxic blood serum level: >1.5 mEq/L.

AVAILABILITY (Rx)

CAPSULES: 150 mg, 300 mg, 600 mg. **TABLETS:** 300 mg. **TABLETS (slow-release):** 300 mg, 450 mg. **SYRUP:** 300 mg/5 ml.

ADMINISTRATION/HANDLING

PO

• Preferable to administer with meals or milk. • Do not crush, chew, or break extended-release or film-coated tablets.

INDICATIONS/ROUTES/DOSAGE

Alert: During acute phase, therapeutic serum lithium concentration of 1–1.4 mEq/L is required. Desired level during long-term control: 0.5–1.3 mEq/L. Monitor serum concentrations, clinical response to determine proper dosage.

USUAL DOSAGE

PO: ADULTS: 300 mg 3–4 times/day. **Maximum:** 2.4 g/day or 450–900 mg slow-release form 2 times/day. ELDERLY: 300 mg 2 times/day. May increase by 300 mg/day q1wk. MAINTENANCE: 900–1,200 mg/day. CHILDREN ≥12 YRS: 600–1,800 mg/day in 3–4 divided doses (2 doses/day for slow release). CHILDREN <12 YRS: 15–60 mg/kg/day in 3–4 divided doses.

SIDE EFFECTS

Alert: Effects are dose related and seldom occur at serum lithium levels <1.5 mEq/L.

OCCASIONAL: Fine hand tremor, polydipsia (excessive thirst), polyuria (increased urination), mild nausea. **RARE:** Weight gain, fast/slow heartbeat, acne, rash, muscle twitching, blue hue in fingers/toes, coldness in arms/legs, pseudotumor cerebri (eye pain, headache, vision problems, tinnitus).

ADVERSE REACTIONS/ TOXIC EFFECTS

Serum lithium concentration of 1.5–2.0 mEq/L may produce vomiting, diarrhea, drowsiness, incoordination, coarse hand tremor, muscle twitching, EKG T-wave depression, mental confusion. Serum lithium concentration of 2.0–2.5 mEq/L may result in ataxia, giddiness, tinnitus, blurred vision, clonic movements, severe hypotension. Acute toxicity characterized by seizures, oliguria, circulatory failure, coma, death.

NURSING IMPLICATIONS

BASELINE ASSESSMENT

Serum lithium levels should be tested q3–4days during initial phase of therapy, q1–2mos thereafter, and weekly if there is no improvement of disorder or adverse effects occur.

INTERVENTION/EVALUATION

Serum lithium testing should be performed as close as possible to 12th hr following last dose. Besides serum lithium concentration levels, clinical assessment of therapeutic effect, tolerance to drug effect is necessary for correct dosing-level management. Assess behavior, appearance, emotional status, response to environment, speech pattern, thought content. Monitor serum lithium concentrations, differential count, urinalysis, creatinine clearance. Assess for increased urine output, persistent thirst. Report polyuria, prolonged vomiting, diarrhea, fever to physician (may need to temporarily reduce or discontinue dosage). Monitor for signs of lithium toxicity. Assess for therapeutic response (interest in surroundings, improvement in self-care, increased ability to concentrate, relaxed facial

L

expression). Monitor lithium levels q3–4days at initiation of therapy (then q1–2mos). Levels obtained 8–12 hrs postdose. Monitor renal, liver, thyroid, cardiovascular function; CBC with differential; electrolytes. Therapeutic blood serum level: 0.6–1.2 mEq/L; toxic blood serum level: >1.5 mEq/L.

PATIENT/FAMILY TEACHING

Limit alcohol, caffeine. Avoid tasks requiring coordination until CNS effects of drug are known. May cause dry mouth. Maintain steady salt/fluid intake (avoid dehydration). Inform physician if vomiting, diarrhea, muscle weakness, tremor, drowsiness, ataxia occurs. Blood level monitoring is necessary to determine proper dose.

lomefloxacin hydrochloride

low-meh-**flocks**-ah-sin
(Maxaquin)

CLASSIFICATION

PHARMACOTHERAPEUTIC: Quinolone. **CLINICAL:** Antibiotic (see p. 23C).

ACTION

Inhibits the enzyme DNA-gyrase in susceptible microorganisms. **Therapeutic Effect:** Interferes with bacterial DNA replication and repair. Bactericidal.

PHARMACOKINETICS

Well absorbed from GI tract. Protein binding: 10%. Widely distributed. Metabolized in liver. Primarily excreted in urine. Not removed by hemodialysis. **Half-life:** 4–6 hrs (half-life increased with impaired renal function, elderly).

USES

Treatment of infections of urinary tract, lower respiratory tract; postop prophylaxis in pts undergoing transurethral procedures.

PRECAUTIONS

CONTRAINDICATIONS: Hypersensitivity to quinolones. **CAUTIONS:** Renal impairment, CNS disorders, seizures, those taking theophylline, caffeine.

LIFESPAN CONSIDERATIONS: Pregnancy/lactation: Unknown if distributed in breast milk. If possible, do not use during pregnancy/lactation (risk of arthropathy to fetus/infant). **Pregnancy Category C. Children:** Safety and efficacy not established. **Elderly:** Age-related renal impairment may require dosage adjustment.

INTERACTIONS

DRUG: Antacids, iron prep, sucralfate may decrease absorption. Decreases clearance, may increase concentration, toxicity of **theophylline.** May increase effects of **oral anticoagulants. HERBAL:** None known. **FOOD:** None known. **LAB VALUES:** May increase SGOT (AST), SGPT (ALT), alkaline phosphatase, LDH, serum bilirubin, BUN, serum creatinine concentration.

AVAILABILITY (Rx)

TABLETS: 400 mg.

ADMINISTRATION/HANDLING

PO

• May be given without regard to meals (preferred dosing time: 2 hrs after meals). • Do not administer antacids (aluminum, magnesium) within 2 hrs of lomefloxacin. • Encourage cranberry juice, citrus fruits (acidify urine).

INDICATIONS/ROUTES/DOSAGE

UTI

PO: ADULTS, ELDERLY: 400 mg/day for 10–14 days.

UNCOMPLICATED UTI
PO: ADULTS (FEMALES): 400 mg/day for 3 days.

LOWER RESPIRATORY TRACT INFECTIONS
PO: ADULTS, ELDERLY: 400 mg/day for 10 days.

SURGICAL PROPHYLAXIS
PO: ADULTS, ELDERLY: 400 mg 2–6 hrs before surgery.

DOSAGE IN RENAL IMPAIRMENT
Dose and/or frequency is modified in pts based on severity of renal impairment:

Creatinine Clearance	Dosage
>40 ml/min	No change
10–40 ml/min	400 mg initially, then 200 mg/day for 10–14 days

SIDE EFFECTS

OCCASIONAL (2%–3%): Nausea, headache, photosensitivity, dizziness. **RARE (1%):** Diarrhea.

ADVERSE REACTIONS/ TOXIC EFFECTS

Antibiotic-associated colitis (severe abdominal pain/tenderness, fever, watery/ severe diarrhea), fungal superinfection may result from altered bacterial balance.

NURSING IMPLICATIONS

BASELINE ASSESSMENT

Question for history of hypersensitivity to lomefloxacin, quinolones.

INTERVENTION/EVALUATION

Monitor signs, symptoms of infection, WBC count, mental status. Check for dizziness, headache. Be alert for superinfection (e.g., genital pruritus, vaginitis, fever, oral candidiasis).

PATIENT/FAMILY TEACHING

Do not skip doses; take full course of therapy. Do not take antacids (reduces/destroys effectiveness). Avoid sunlight/ultraviolet exposure; wear sunscreen, protective clothing if photosensitivity develops.

Lomotil

see diphenoxylate with atropine

lomustine

low-**meuw**-steen
(CeeNU)

CLASSIFICATION

PHARMACOTHERAPEUTIC: Alkylating agent (nitrosourea). **CLINICAL:** Antineoplastic (see p. 74C).

ACTION

Inhibits DNA, RNA synthesis by cross-linking with DNA, RNA strands, preventing cellular division. Cell cycle–phase nonspecific. **Therapeutic Effect:** Interferes with DNA/RNA function.

USES

Treatment of primary and metastatic brain tumors, disseminated Hodgkin's disease. **Unlabeled:** Treatment of GI, lung, renal, breast carcinoma; multiple myeloma, malignant melanoma.

PRECAUTIONS

CONTRAINDICATIONS: Pregnancy. **CAUTIONS:** Depressed platelet, leukocyte, erythrocyte counts. **Pregnancy Category D.**

INTERACTIONS

DRUG: Bone marrow depressants may increase bone marrow depression. **Live virus vaccines** may potentiate virus replication, increase vaccine side effects, decrease pt's antibody response to vaccine. **HERBAL:** None known. **FOOD:** None known. **LAB VALUES:** May increase liver function tests.

AVAILABILITY (Rx)

CAPSULES: 10 mg, 40 mg, 100 mg, 300 mg.

INDICATIONS/ROUTES/DOSAGE

Alert: Dosage is individualized based on clinical response, tolerance to adverse effects. When used in combination therapy, consult specific protocols for optimum dosage, sequence of drug administration.

USUAL DOSAGE

PO: ADULTS, ELDERLY: 100–130 mg/m^2 as single dose. Repeat dose at intervals of at least 6 wks but not until circulating blood elements have returned to acceptable levels. Adjust dose based on hematologic response to previous dose. CHILDREN: 75–150 mg/m^2 as single dose q6wks.

SIDE EFFECTS

FREQUENT: Nausea, vomiting occur 45 min–6 hrs after dosing, lasts 12–24 hrs. Anorexia often follows for 2–3 days. **OCCASIONAL:** Neurotoxicity (confusion, slurred speech), stomatitis, darkening of skin, diarrhea, skin rash, itching, hair loss.

ADVERSE REACTIONS/ TOXIC EFFECTS

Bone marrow depression manifested as hematologic toxicity (principally leukopenia, mild anemia, thrombocytopenia). Leukopenia occurs at about 6 wks, thrombocytopenia at about 4 wks, and persists for 1–2 wks. Refractory anemia, thrombocytopenia occur commonly if therapy continued for >1 yr. Hepatotoxicity occurs infrequently. Large cumulative doses may result in renal damage.

NURSING IMPLICATIONS

BASELINE ASSESSMENT

Manufacturer recommends weekly blood counts; experts recommend first blood count obtained 2–3 wks following initial therapy, subsequent blood counts indicated by prior toxicity. Antiemetics can reduce duration, frequency of nausea, vomiting.

INTERVENTION/EVALUATION

Monitor CBC with differential; platelet count; liver, renal, pulmonary function tests. Monitor for stomatitis (burning/erythema of oral mucosa at inner margin of lips, sore throat, difficulty swallowing). Monitor for hematologic toxicity (fever, sore throat, signs of local infection, unusual bruising/bleeding from any site), symptoms of anemia (excessive tiredness, weakness).

PATIENT/FAMILY TEACHING

Nausea, vomiting generally abates in <1 day. Fasting before therapy can reduce frequency/duration of GI effects. Maintain fastidious oral hygiene. Do not have immunizations without physician's approval (drug lowers body's resistance). Avoid crowds, those with known illness. Promptly report fever, sore throat, signs of local infection, unusual bruising/bleeding from any site, swelling of legs/feet, jaundice.

loperamide hydrochloride

low-**pear**-ah-myd
(Apo-Loperamide✤, Imodium A-D, Loperacap✤, Novo-Loperamide✤)
Do not confuse with Ionamin.

FIXED-COMBINATION(S)

Imodium Advanced: loperamide/simethicone (an antiflatulant): 2 mg/125 mg.

CLASSIFICATION

CLINICAL: Antidiarrheal (see p. 41C).

ACTION

Direct effect on intestinal wall muscles. **Therapeutic Effect:** Slows intestinal motility, prolongs transit time of intestinal contents (reduces fecal volume, diminishes loss of fluid/electrolytes, increases viscosity, bulk).

PHARMACOKINETICS

Poorly absorbed from GI tract. Protein binding: 97%. Metabolized in liver. Eliminated in feces, excreted in urine. Not removed by hemodialysis. **Half-life:** 9.1–14.4 hrs.

USES

Controls, provides symptomatic relief of acute nonspecific diarrhea, chronic diarrhea associated with inflammatory bowel disease, traveler's diarrhea. Reduces volume of discharge from ileostomy.

PRECAUTIONS

CONTRAINDICATIONS: Those who must avoid constipation, diarrhea associated with pseudomembranous enterocolitis due to broad-spectrum antibiotics or with organisms that invade intestinal mucosa (*Escherichia coli,* shigella, salmonella), acute ulcerative colitis (may produce toxic megacolon). **CAUTIONS:** Those with fluid/electrolyte depletion, hepatic impairment.

LIFESPAN CONSIDERATIONS: Pregnancy/lactation: Unknown if drug crosses placenta or is distributed in breast milk. **Pregnancy Category B. Children:** Not recommended in those <6 yrs (infants <3 mos more susceptible to CNS effects). **Elderly:** May mask dehydration, electrolyte depletion.

INTERACTIONS

DRUG: Opioid (narcotic) analgesics may increase risk of constipation. **HERBAL:** None known. **FOOD:** None known. **LAB VALUES:** None known.

AVAILABILITY (OTC)

TABLETS: 2 mg. **CAPSULES (Rx):** 2 mg. **LIQUID:** 1 mg/5 ml.

INDICATIONS/ROUTES/DOSAGE

ACUTE DIARRHEA (capsules)

PO: ADULTS, ELDERLY: Initially, 4 mg, then 2 mg after each unformed stool. **Maximum:** 16 mg/day. CHILDREN 9–12 YRS, >30 KG: Initially, 2 mg 3 times/day for 24 hrs; CHILDREN 6–8 YRS, 20–30 KG: Initially, 2 mg 2 times/day for 24 hrs. CHILDREN 2–5 YRS, 13–20 KG: Initially, 1 mg 3 times/day for 24 hrs. MAINTENANCE: 1 mg/10 kg only after loose stool.

CHRONIC DIARRHEA

PO: ADULTS, ELDERLY: Initially, 4 mg, then 2 mg after each unformed stool until diarrhea is controlled. CHILDREN: 0.08–0.24 mg/kg/day in 2–3 divided doses. **Maximum:** 2 mg/dose.

TRAVELER'S DIARRHEA

PO: ADULTS, ELDERLY: Initially, 4 mg, then 2 mg after each loose bowel movement (LBM). **Maximum:** 8 mg/day for 2 days. CHILDREN 9–11 YRS: Initially, 2 mg, then 1 mg after each LBM. **Maximum:** 6 mg/day for 2 days. CHILDREN 6–8 YRS: Initially, 1 mg, then 1 mg after each LBM. **Maximum:** 4 mg/day for 2 days.

SIDE EFFECTS

RARE: Dry mouth, drowsiness, abdominal discomfort, allergic reaction (rash, itching).

L

ADVERSE REACTIONS/ TOXIC EFFECTS

Toxicity results in constipation, GI irritation (including nausea, vomiting); CNS depression. **TREATMENT:** Activated charcoal.

NURSING IMPLICATIONS

BASELINE ASSESSMENT

Do not administer in presence of bloody diarrhea, temperature >101°F.

INTERVENTION/EVALUATION

Encourage adequate fluid intake. Assess bowel sounds for peristalsis. Monitor stool frequency, consistency (watery, loose, soft, semisolid, solid). Withhold drug, notify physician promptly in event of abdominal pain, distention, fever.

PATIENT/FAMILY TEACHING

Do not exceed prescribed dose. May cause dry mouth. Avoid alcohol. Avoid tasks that require alertness, motor skills until response to drug is established. Notify physician if diarrhea does not stop within 3 days, abdominal distention/pain occurs, fever develops.

L

lopinavir/ritonavir

low-**pin**-ah-veer/rih-**ton**-ah-veer (Kaletra)

Do not confuse with Keppra.

CLASSIFICATION

PHARMACOTHERAPEUTIC: Protease inhibitor combination. **CLINICAL:** Antiretroviral (see pp. 59C, 100C).

ACTION

Lopinavir: Acts on protease enzyme late in the HIV replication process, inhibits its activity. **Therapeutic Effect:** Formation of immature, noninfectious viral particles. **Ritonavir:** Inhibits the metabolism of lopinavir. **Therapeutic Effect:** Increases plasma concentrations of lopinavir.

PHARMACOKINETICS

Readily absorbed following PO administration (increased when taken with food). Protein binding: 98%–99%. Metabolized in liver. Primarily eliminated in feces. Not removed by hemodialysis. **Half-life:** 5–6 hrs. (See ritonavir for pharmacokinetics.)

USES

In combination with other antiretroviral agents for the treatment of HIV infection.

PRECAUTIONS

CONTRAINDICATIONS: Hypersensitivity to lopinavir, ritonavir. Concomitant use of flecainide, pimozide, propafenone (increased risk of serous cardiac arrhythmias), midazolam, triazolam (increases sedation or respiratory depression), ergot derivatives (peripheral vasospasm, ischemia of extremities). **CAUTIONS:** Impaired liver function, hepatitis B or C. High-dose itraconazole, ketoconazole not recommended. Metronidazole may cause disulfiram-type reaction with oral solution (contains alcohol).

LIFESPAN CONSIDERATIONS: Pregnancy/lactation: Unknown if excreted in breast milk. Not recommended that HIV-infected mothers breast-feed. **Pregnancy Category C. Children:** Safety and efficacy not established in those <6 mos. **Elderly:** Age-related renal/hepatic impairment, cardiac function impairment requires caution.

INTERACTIONS

DRUG: Carbamazepine, corticosteroids, efavirenz, nevirapine, phenobarbital, phenytoin, rifampin may decrease concentration, effect. May increase concentration, effect of **cla-**

rithromycin, felodipine, immunosuppressants, nicardipine, nifedipine, rifabutin. May decrease concentration, effect of **atovaquone, methadone, oral contraceptives.** May increase concentration, risk of myopathy with **atorvastatin.** **HERBAL:** **St. John's wort** may decrease concentrations, effect. **FOOD:** None known. **LAB VALUES:** May increase glucose, uric acid, SGOT (AST), SGPT (ALT), GGT, total cholesterol, triglycerides.

AVAILABILITY (Rx)

CAPSULES: 133.3 mg lopinavir/33.3 mg ritonavir. **ORAL SOLUTION:** 80 mg lopinavir/20 mg ritonavir per ml.

ADMINISTRATION/HANDLING

PO

• Refrigerate until dispensed. • Avoid exposure to excessive heat. • If stored at room temperature, use within 2 mos. • Give with food.

INDICATIONS/ROUTES/DOSAGE

HIV

PO: ADULTS: 400/100 mg of lopinavir/ritonavir (3 capsules or 5 ml) twice daily. Increase to 533/133 mg (4 capsules or 6.5 ml) when taken with efavirenz or nevirapine. CHILDREN 7 TO <15 KG WITHOUT EFAVIRENZ OR NEVIRAPINE: 12 mg/kg 2 times/day. CHILDREN 15–40 KG: 10 mg/kg 2 times/day. CHILDREN 7 TO <15 KG WITH EFAVIRENZ OR NEVIRAPINE: 13 mg/kg 2 times/day. CHILDREN 15–50 KG: 11 mg/kg 2 times/day.

SIDE EFFECTS

FREQUENT (14%): Diarrhea (mild to moderate). **OCCASIONAL (2%–6%):** Nausea, asthenia (loss of strength, energy), abdominal pain, headache, vomiting. **RARE (<2%):** Insomnia, rash.

ADVERSE REACTIONS/ TOXIC EFFECTS

Anemia, leukopenia, lymphadenopathy, deep vein thrombosis, Cushing's syndrome, pancreatitis, hemorrhagic colitis occur rarely.

NURSING IMPLICATIONS

BASELINE ASSESSMENT

Obtain baseline CBC, renal/hepatic function tests, weight.

INTERVENTION/EVALUATION

Monitor consistency, frequency of stools. Assess for opportunistic infections: onset of fever, oral mucosa changes, cough, other respiratory symptoms. Check weight at least twice a week. Assess for nausea, vomiting. Monitor for signs/symptoms of pancreatitis (nausea, vomiting, abdominal pain), electrolytes, blood glucose, cholesterol, liver function, CBC with differential, platelets, CD4 cell count, viral load.

PATIENT/FAMILY TEACHING

Explain correct administration of medication. Eat small, frequent meals to offset nausea, vomiting. Medication is not a cure for HIV infection, nor does it reduce risk of transmission to others.

Lopressor

see metoprolol

loracarbef

laur-ah-**car**-bef
(Lorabid)
Do not confuse with Lortab.

♣CLASSIFICATION

PHARMACOTHERAPEUTIC: Cephalosporin. **CLINICAL:** Antibiotic (see p. 21C).

L

ACTION

Bactericidal. Binds to bacterial membranes. **Therapeutic Effect:** Inhibits bacterial cell wall synthesis.

USES

Treatment of bronchitis, otitis media, pharyngitis, pneumonia, sinusitis, skin/soft tissue infections, urinary tract infections (uncomplicated cystitis, pyelonephritis).

PRECAUTIONS

CONTRAINDICATIONS: History of hypersensitivity to cephalosporins, anaphylactic reaction to penicillins. **CAUTIONS:** Renal impairment, history of colitis. **Pregnancy Category B.**

INTERACTIONS

DRUG: **Probenecid** increases serum concentrations, half-life of loracarbef. **HERBAL:** None known. **FOOD:** None known. **LAB VALUES:** May increase SGOT (AST), SGPT (ALT), alkaline phosphatase, BUN, creatinine. May decrease leukocytes, platelets.

AVAILABILITY (Rx)

CAPSULES: 200 mg, 400 mg. **POWDER FOR PO SUSPENSION:** 100 mg/5 ml, 200 mg/5 ml.

ADMINISTRATION/HANDLING

PO

• Give 1 hr before or 2 hrs after meal. • After reconstitution, powder for suspension may be kept at room temperature for 14 days. Discard unused portion after 14 days. • Shake oral suspension well before using.

INDICATIONS/ROUTES/DOSAGE

BRONCHITIS

PO: ADULTS, ELDERLY, CHILDREN >12 YRS: 200–400 mg q12h for 7 days.

PHARYNGITIS

PO: ADULTS, ELDERLY, CHILDREN >12 YRS: 200 mg q12h for 10 days. CHILDREN 6 MOS–12 YRS: 7.5 mg/kg q12h for 10 days.

PNEUMONIA

PO: ADULTS, ELDERLY, CHILDREN >12 YRS: 400 mg q12h for 14 days.

SINUSITIS

PO: ADULTS, ELDERLY, CHILDREN >12 YRS: 400 mg q12h for 10 days. CHILDREN 6 MOS–12 YRS: 15 mg/kg q12h for 10 days.

SKIN, SOFT TISSUE INFECTIONS

PO: ADULTS, ELDERLY, CHILDREN >12 YRS: 200 mg q12h for 7 days. CHILDREN 6 MOS–12 YRS: 7.5 mg/kg q12h for 7 days.

URINARY TRACT INFECTIONS

PO: ADULTS, ELDERLY, CHILDREN 6 MOS–12 YRS: 200–400 mg q12h for 7–14 days.

OTITIS MEDIA

PO: CHILDREN 6 MOS–12 YRS: 15 mg/kg q12h for 10 days.

SIDE EFFECTS

FREQUENT: Abdominal pain, anorexia, nausea, vomiting, diarrhea. **OCCASIONAL:** Skin rash, itching. **RARE:** Dizziness, headache, vaginitis.

ADVERSE REACTIONS/ TOXIC EFFECTS

Antibiotic-associated colitis, other superinfections may result from altered bacterial balance. Hypersensitivity reactions (ranging from rash, urticaria, fever to anaphylaxis) occur in <5%, generally those with history of allergies, esp. penicillin.

NURSING IMPLICATIONS

BASELINE ASSESSMENT

Question for history of allergies, particularly cephalosporins, penicillins.

INTERVENTION/EVALUATION

Assess for nausea, vomiting. Check stool frequency, consistency. Assess skin for rash (diaper area in children). Monitor I&O, urinalysis, renal function reports for nephrotoxicity. Be alert for superinfection: genital/anal pruritus, moniliasis, abdominal pain, sore mouth/tongue, moderate to severe diarrhea.

PATIENT/FAMILY TEACHING

Continue antibiotic therapy for full length of treatment. Doses should be evenly spaced, given at least 1 hr before or 2 hrs after a meal.

loratadine

low-**rah**-tah-deen
(Claritin, Claritin Reditabs)

FIXED-COMBINATION(S)

Claritin-D: loratadine/pseudoephedrine (a sympathomimetic): 5 mg/120 mg; 10 mg/240 mg.

◆ CLASSIFICATION

PHARMACOTHERAPEUTIC: H_1 antagonist. **CLINICAL:** Antihistamine (see p. 49C).

ACTION

Long acting with selective peripheral histamine H_1 receptor antagonist action. Competes with histamine for receptor site. **Therapeutic Effect:** Prevents allergic responses mediated by histamine (urticaria, pruritus).

PHARMACOKINETICS

Onset	Peak	Duration
PO		
1–3 hrs	8–12 hrs	>24 hrs

Rapidly, almost completely absorbed from GI tract. Protein binding: 97% (metabolite: 73%–77%). Distributed mainly in liver, lungs, GI tract, bile. Metabolized in liver to active metabolite (undergoes extensive first-pass metabolism). Excreted in urine, eliminated in feces. Not removed by hemodialysis. **Half-life:** 8.4 hrs; metabolite: 28 hrs (half-life increased in elderly, liver disease).

USES

Relief of nasal/non-nasal symptoms of seasonal allergic rhinitis (hayfever). Treatment of idiopathic chronic urticaria (hives). **Unlabeled:** Adjunct treatment of bronchial asthma.

PRECAUTIONS

CONTRAINDICATIONS: Hypersensitivity to loratadine or any ingredient. **CAUTIONS:** Liver impairment, breast-feeding women. Safety in children unknown.

LIFESPAN CONSIDERATIONS: Pregnancy/lactation: Excreted in breast milk. **Pregnancy Category B. Children/elderly:** More sensitive to anticholinergic effects (e.g., dry mouth, nose, throat).

INTERACTIONS

DRUG: Ketoconazole, erythromycin, fluconazole, clarithromycin may increase concentrations. **HERBAL:** None known. **FOOD:** None known. **LAB VALUES:** May suppress wheal, flare reactions to antigen skin testing, unless antihistamines are discontinued 4 days prior to testing.

AVAILABILITY (Rx)

TABLETS: 10 mg. **RAPID DISSOLUTION TABLET:** 10 mg. **SYRUP:** 10 mg/10 ml.

ADMINISTRATION/HANDLING

PO

- Preferably give on an empty stomach (food delays absorption).

INDICATIONS/ROUTES/DOSAGE

ALLERGIC RHINITIS, HIVES

PO: ADULTS, ELDERLY, CHILDREN ≥6 YRS: 10 mg once daily. CHILDREN 2–5 YRS: 5 mg once daily. HEPATIC FUNCTION IMPAIRMENT: 10 mg every other day.

L

SIDE EFFECTS

FREQUENT (8%–12%): Headache, fatigue, drowsiness. **OCCASIONAL (3%):** Dry mouth, nose, throat. **RARE:** Photosensitivity.

ADVERSE REACTIONS/ TOXIC EFFECTS

None known.

NURSING IMPLICATIONS

BASELINE ASSESSMENT

Assess lung sounds, skin for urticaria, other allergy symptoms.

INTERVENTION/EVALUATION

For upper respiratory allergies, increase fluids to maintain thin secretions and offset thirst, loss of fluids from increased sweating. Monitor symptoms for therapeutic response.

PATIENT/FAMILY TEACHING

Drink plenty of water (may cause dry mouth). Avoid alcohol. May cause drowsiness, impair ability to perform hazardous tasks requiring mental alertness. May cause photosensitivity reactions (avoid direct exposure to sunlight.)

L

lorazepam

low-**raz**-ah-pam
(Apo-Lorazepam, Ativan, Novo-lorazepam)

Do not confuse with Alprazolam.

CLASSIFICATION

PHARMACOTHERAPEUTIC: Benzodiazepine **(Schedule IV). CLINICAL:** Antianxiety, sedative-hypnotic, antiemetic, skeletal muscle relaxant, amnesiac, anticonvulsant, antitremor (see p. 11C).

ACTION

Enhances inhibitory neurotransmitter gamma-aminobutyric acid (GABA) neurotransmission at CNS, affecting memory, motor, sensory, cognitive functions. **Therapeutic Effect:** Produces anxiolytic, muscle relaxation, anticonvulsant, sedative, antiemetic effect.

PHARMACOKINETICS

Onset	Peak	Duration
PO		
60 min	—	8–12 hrs
IM		
30–60 min	—	8–12 hrs
IV		
15–30 min	—	8–12 hrs

Well absorbed after PO, IM administration. Protein binding: 85%. Widely distributed. Metabolized in liver. Primarily excreted in urine. Not removed by hemodialysis. **Half-life:** 10–20 hrs.

USES

Management of anxiety, status epilepticus, preop sedation, amnesia. **Unlabeled:** Treatment of alcohol withdrawal, adjunct to endoscopic procedures (diminishes pt recall), panic disorders, skeletal muscle spasms, chemotherapy–induced nausea/vomiting, tension headache, tremors.

PRECAUTIONS

CONTRAINDICATIONS: Preexisting CNS depression, narrow-angle glaucoma, severe uncontrolled pain, severe hypotension. **CAUTIONS:** Neonates, renal/liver impairment, compromised pulmonary function, concomitant CNS depressant use.

LIFESPAN CONSIDERATIONS: Pregnancy/lactation: May cross placenta. May be distributed in breast milk. May increase risk of fetal abnormalities if administered during first trimester of pregnancy. Chronic ingestion during pregnancy may produce fetal toxicity, withdrawal symptoms, CNS depression in neonates. **Pregnancy Category D.** **Children:** Safety and efficacy not established in those <12 yrs. **Elderly:** Use small initial doses with gradual increases to avoid ataxia or excessive sedation.

INTERACTIONS

DRUG: **Alcohol, CNS depressants** may increase CNS depressant effect. **HERBAL:** **Kava kava, valerian** may increase CNS depression. **FOOD:** None known. **LAB VALUES:** None known. Therapeutic blood serum level: 50–240 ng/ml; toxic blood serum level: N/A.

AVAILABILITY (Rx)

TABLETS: 0.5 mg, 1 mg, 2 mg. **INJECTION:** 2 mg/ml, 4 mg/ml.

ADMINISTRATION/HANDLING

PO

• Give with food. • Tablets may be crushed.

IM

• Give deep IM into large muscle mass.

IV

Storage • Refrigerate parenteral form. • Do not use if precipitate forms or solution appears discolored. • Avoid freezing.

Reconstitution • Dilute with equal volume of Sterile Water for Injection, 0.9% NaCl, or D_5W. • To dilute prefilled syringe, remove air from half-filled syringe, aspirate equal volume of diluent, pull plunger back slightly to allow for mixing, gently invert syringe several times (do not shake vigorously).

Rate of administration • Give by IV push into tubing of free-flowing IV infusion (0.9% NaCl, D_5W) at rate not to exceed 2 mg/min.

IV INCOMPATIBILITIES

Aldesleukin (Proleukin), aztreonam (Azactam), idarubicin (Idamycin), ondansetron (Zofran), sufentanil (Sufenta).

IV COMPATIBILITIES

Bumetanide (Bumex), cefepime (Maxipime), diltiazem (Cardizem), dobutamine (Dobutrex), dopamine (Intropin), heparin, labetalol (Normodyne, Trandate), milrinone (Primacor), norepinephrine (Levophed), piperacillin/tazobactam (Zosyn), potassium, propofol (Diprivan).

INDICATIONS/ROUTES/DOSAGE

ANXIETY

PO: ADULTS: 1–10 mg/day in 2–3 divided doses. AVERAGE: 2–6 mg/day. ELDERLY: Initially, 0.5–1 mg/day. May increase gradually.

IV: ADULTS, ELDERLY: Titrate to desired effect.

PO/IV: CHILDREN: 0.05 mg/kg/dose q4–8h. RANGE: 0.02–0.1 mg/kg. **Maximum:** 2 mg/dose.

INSOMNIA DUE TO ANXIETY

PO: ADULTS: 2–4 mg at bedtime. ELDERLY: 0.5–1 mg at bedtime.

PREOP

IM: ADULTS, ELDERLY: 0.05 mg/kg given 2 hrs before procedure. Do not exceed 4 mg.

IV: ADULTS, ELDERLY: 0.044 mg/kg (up to 2 mg total) 15–20 min before surgery.

STATUS EPILEPTICUS

IV: ADULTS, ELDERLY: 4 mg/dose over 2–5 min. May repeat in 10–15 min (8 mg maximum in 12-hr period). CHILDREN: 0.1 mg/kg over 2–5 min. **Maximum:** 4 mg. May repeat second dose of 0.05 mg/kg in 15–20 min. NEONATE: 0.05 mg/kg. May repeat in 10–15 min.

SIDE EFFECTS

FREQUENT: Drowsiness, ataxia (incoordination), confusion. Morning drowsiness may occur initially. **OCCASIONAL:** Blurred vision, slurred speech, hypoten-

L

sion, headache. **RARE:** Paradoxical CNS restlessness, excitement in elderly/debilitated.

ADVERSE REACTIONS/ TOXIC EFFECTS

Abrupt or too rapid withdrawal may result in pronounced restlessness, irritability, insomnia, hand tremors, abdominal/muscle cramps, diaphoresis, vomiting, seizures. Overdosage results in somnolence, confusion, diminished reflexes, coma.

NURSING IMPLICATIONS

BASELINE ASSESSMENT

Offer emotional support to anxious pt. Pt must remain recumbent for up to 8 hrs (individualized) following parenteral administration to reduce hypotensive effect. Assess motor responses (agitation, trembling, tension), autonomic responses (cold/clammy hands, diaphoresis).

INTERVENTION/EVALUATION

Monitor B/P, respiratory rate, heart rate, CBC with differential, liver function tests. For those on long-term therapy, liver/renal function tests, blood counts should be performed periodically. Assess for paradoxical reaction, particularly during early therapy. Evaluate for therapeutic response: calm facial expression, decreased restlessness, insomnia. Therapeutic blood serum level: 50–240 ng/ml; toxic blood serum level: N/A.

PATIENT/FAMILY TEACHING

Drowsiness usually disappears during continued therapy. Avoid tasks that require alertness, motor skills until response to drug is established. Smoking reduces drug effectiveness. Do not abruptly withdraw medication after long-term therapy. Do not use alcohol, CNS depressants. Contraception recommended for long-term therapy. Notify physician at once if pregnancy is suspected.

losartan

loh-**sar**-tan
(Cozaar)
Do not confuse with Zocor.

FIXED-COMBINATION(S)

Hyzaar: losartan/hydrochlorothiazide (a diuretic): 50 mg/12.5 mg; 100 mg/25 mg.

CLASSIFICATION

PHARMACOTHERAPEUTIC: Angiotensin II receptor antagonist. **CLINICAL:** Antihypertensive (see p. 7C).

ACTION

Potent vasodilator. An angiotensin II receptor (type AT_1) antagonist, blocks vasoconstrictor, aldosterone-secreting effects of angiotensin II, inhibiting the binding of angiotensin II to the AT_1 receptors. **Therapeutic Effect:** Causes vasodilation, decreased peripheral resistance, decrease in B/P.

PHARMACOKINETICS

Onset	Peak	Duration
PO		
—	6 hrs	24 hrs

Well absorbed after PO administration. Protein binding: >98%. Undergoes first-pass metabolism in liver to active metabolites. Excreted in urine and via biliary system. Not removed by hemodialysis. **Half-life:** 2 hrs (metabolite: 6–9 hrs).

USES

Treatment of hypertension. Used alone or in combination with other antihypertensives. Treatment of diabetic nephropathy, prevention of stroke.

PRECAUTIONS

CONTRAINDICATIONS: None known. **CAUTIONS:** Renal/hepatic function impairment, renal arterial stenosis.

LIFESPAN CONSIDERATIONS: Pregnancy/lactation: Has caused fetal/neonatal morbidity, mortality. Potential for adverse effects on nursing infant. Do not breast-feed. **Pregnancy Category C** (**D** if used in second or third trimesters [fetal/neonatal morbidity/mortality]). **Children:** Safety and efficacy not established. **Elderly:** No age-related precautions noted.

INTERACTIONS

DRUG: **Cimetidine** may increase effects. **Phenobarbital, rifampin** may decrease effects. May inhibit effects of **ketoconazole, troleandomycin.** May increase concentration, toxicity of **lithium. HERBAL:** None known. **FOOD: Grapefruit juice** may alter absorption. **LAB VALUES:** May increase BUN, serum creatinine, SGOT (AST), SGPT (ALT), alkaline phosphatase, bilirubin. May decrease Hgb/Hct.

AVAILABILITY (Rx)

TABLETS: 25 mg, 50 mg, 100 mg.

ADMINISTRATION/HANDLING

PO

• May give without regard to food. • Do not crush or break tablets.

INDICATIONS/ROUTES/DOSAGE

HYPERTENSION

PO: ADULTS, ELDERLY: Initially, 50 mg once daily. **Maximum:** May be given once or twice daily with total daily doses ranging from 25–100 mg.

NEPHROPATHY

PO: ADULTS, ELDERLY: Initially, 50 mg/day. May increase to 100 mg/day based on B/P response.

HEPATIC FUNCTION IMPAIRMENT

PO: Initially, 25 mg daily.

SIDE EFFECTS

FREQUENT (8%): Upper respiratory infection. **OCCASIONAL (2%–4%):** Dizziness, diarrhea, cough. **RARE (≤1%):** Insomnia, dyspepsia, heartburn, back/leg pain, muscle cramps/ache, nasal congestion, sinusitis.

ADVERSE REACTIONS/ TOXIC EFFECTS

Overdosage may manifest as hypotension, tachycardia; bradycardia occurs less often. Institute supportive measurement.

NURSING IMPLICATIONS

BASELINE ASSESSMENT

Obtain B/P, apical pulse immediately before each dose, in addition to regular monitoring (be alert to fluctuations). If excessive reduction in B/P occurs, place pt in supine position, feet slightly elevated. Question for possibility of pregnancy (see Pregnancy/Lactation). Assess medication history (esp. diuretic).

INTERVENTION/EVALUATION

Maintain hydration (offer fluids frequently). Assess for evidence of upper respiratory infection, cough. Assist with ambulation if dizziness occurs. Monitor stool frequency, consistency (watery, loose, soft). Monitor B/P, pulse.

PATIENT/FAMILY TEACHING

Inform female pt regarding consequences of second- and third-trimester exposure to losartan. Report pregnancy to physician as soon as possible. Avoid tasks that require alertness, motor skills (possible dizziness effect).

Report any sign of infection (sore throat, fever), chest pain. Do not take cold preparations, nasal decongestants. Do not stop taking medication.

Lotensin

see benazepril

lovastatin

low-vah-**stah**-tin
(Altocor, Mevacor)

Do not confuse with Leustatin, Livostin, Mivacron.

CLASSIFICATION

PHARMACOTHERAPEUTIC: HMG-CoA reductase inhibitor. **CLINICAL:** Antihyperlipidemic (see p. 50C).

ACTION

Inhibits HMG-CoA reductase, the enzyme that catalyzes the early step in cholesterol synthesis. **Therapeutic Effect:** Decreases LDL cholesterol, VLDL cholesterol, plasma triglycerides; increases HDL cholesterol.

PHARMACOKINETICS

Onset	Peak	Duration
PO		
3 days	4–6 wks	—

Incompletely absorbed from GI tract (increased on empty stomach). Protein binding: >95%. Hydrolyzed in liver to active metabolite. Primarily eliminated in feces. Not removed by hemodialysis. **Half-life:** 1.1–1.7 hrs.

USES

Decreases elevated total and LDL cholesterol in primary hypercholesterolemia; primary prevention of coronary artery disease.

PRECAUTIONS

CONTRAINDICATIONS: Active liver disease, unexplained elevated liver function tests, pregnancy. **CAUTIONS:** History of heavy alcohol use; renal impairment; concomitant use of cyclosporine, fibrates, niacin. (See Interactions.)

LIFESPAN CONSIDERATIONS: Pregnancy/lactation: Contraindicated in pregnancy (suppression of cholesterol biosynthesis may cause fetal toxicity) and lactation. Unknown if drug is distributed in breast milk. **Pregnancy Category X. Children:** Safety and efficacy not established. **Elderly:** No age-related precautions noted.

INTERACTIONS

DRUG: Increased risk of rhabdomyolysis, acute renal failure with **cyclosporine, erythromycin, gemfibrozil, niacin, other immunosuppressants. Erythromycin, itraconazole, ketoconazole** may increase concentration causing severe muscle pain, inflammation, weakness. **HERBAL:** None known. **FOOD:** Large amounts of **grapefruit juice** may increase risk of side effects (e.g., muscle pain, weakness). **LAB VALUES:** May increase creatinine kinase, serum transaminase concentrations.

AVAILABILITY (Rx)

TABLETS: 10 mg, 20 mg, 40 mg. **TABLETS (extended-release):** 20 mg, 40 mg, 60 mg.

ADMINISTRATION/HANDLING

PO

- Give with meals.

INDICATIONS/ROUTES/DOSAGE

HYPERLIPOPROTEINEMIA

PO: ADULTS, ELDERLY: Initially, 20–40 mg/day with evening meal. Increase at

4-wk intervals up to maximum of 80 mg/day. MAINTENANCE: 20–80 mg/day in single or divided doses. **Extended-release:** Initially, 20 mg/day. May increase at 4-wk intervals up to 60 mg/day. CHILDREN 10–17 YRS: 10–40 mg/day with evening meal.

SIDE EFFECTS

Generally well tolerated. Side effects usually mild and transient. **FREQUENT (5%–9%):** Headache, flatulence, diarrhea, abdominal pain/cramps, rash/pruritus. **OCCASIONAL (3%–4%):** Nausea, vomiting, constipation, dyspepsia. **RARE (1%–2%):** Dizziness, heartburn, myalgia, blurred vision, eye irritation.

ADVERSE REACTIONS/ TOXIC EFFECTS

Potential for cataracts.

NURSING IMPLICATIONS

BASELINE ASSESSMENT

Question for possibility of pregnancy before initiating therapy (Pregnancy Category X). Assess baseline lab results: cholesterol, triglycerides, liver function tests.

INTERVENTION/EVALUATION

Determine pattern of bowel activity. Check for headache, dizziness, blurred vision. Assess for rash, pruritus. Monitor cholesterol, triglyceride levels for therapeutic response. Be alert for malaise, muscle cramping/weakness.

PATIENT/FAMILY TEACHING

Take with meals. Follow special diet (important part of treatment). Periodic lab tests are essential part of therapy. Avoid grapefruit juice. Inform physician of severe gastric upset, vision changes, muscle pain/weakness, changes in color of urine/stool, yellowing of eyes/skin, unusual bruising.

Lovenox

see enoxaparin

loxapine hydrochloride

lox-ah-peen
(Apo-Loxapine ♣, Loxapac ♣, Loxitane)

loxapine succinate

(Loxitane)
See classification section under: Antipsychotics (p. 56C)

L

lymphocyte immune globulin N

lym-phow-site
(Atgam)
Do not confuse with Ativan.

◆CLASSIFICATION

PHARMACOTHERAPEUTIC: Biologic response modifier. **CLINICAL:** Immunosuppressant.

ACTION

Lymphocyte selective immunosuppressant; reduces number of circulating thymus-dependent lymphocytes (T lymphocytes), altering function of T lymphocytes, which are responsible for cell-mediated and humoral immunity. Stimulates release of hematopoietic growth factors. **Therapeutic Effect:** Prevents allograft rejection, treats aplastic anemia.

USES

Prevention and/or treatment of allograft rejection, treatment of moderate to severe aplastic anemia in those not suitable for bone marrow transplant, prevention of graft-vs-host disease after bone marrow transplant. **Unlabeled:** Immunosuppressant in liver, bone marrow, heart transplants; treatment of multiple sclerosis, myasthenia gravis, pure red cell aplasia, scleroderma.

PRECAUTIONS

CONTRAINDICATIONS: Systemic hypersensitivity reaction to previous injection of antithymocyte globulin. **CAUTIONS:** Concurrent immunosuppressive therapy. **Pregnancy Category C.**

L

INTERACTIONS

DRUG: None known. **HERBAL:** None known. **FOOD:** None known. **LAB VALUES:** May alter renal function tests.

AVAILABILITY

INJECTION: 250 mg/5 ml.

ADMINISTRATION/HANDLING

IV

Storage • Keep refrigerated before and after dilution. • Discard diluted solution after 24 hrs.

Reconstitution • Total daily dose must be further diluted with 0.9% NaCl (do not use D_5W). • Gently rotate diluted solution. Do not shake. • Final concentration must not exceed 4 mg/ml.

Rate of administration • Use 0.2- to 1-micron filter. • Give total daily dose over minimum of 4 hrs.

IV INCOMPATIBILITY

No information available via Y-site administration.

INDICATIONS/ROUTES/DOSAGE

RENAL ALLOGRAFT RECIPIENTS

IV infusion: ADULTS: 10–30 mg/kg/day. CHILDREN: 5–25 mg/kg/day. DELAY OF ONSET OF REJECTION: 15 mg/kg/day for 14 days, then 15 mg/kg/day every other day for 14 days. Give first dose within 24 hrs before or after transplant. TREATMENT OF REJECTION: 10–15 mg/kg/day for 14 days. May continue with alternate-day therapy up to 21 doses.

APLASTIC ANEMIA

IV infusion: ADULTS: 10–20 mg/kg/day for 8–14 days. May continue alternate-day therapy up to 21 doses.

SIDE EFFECTS

FREQUENT: Fever (51%), thrombocytopenia (30%), rash (2%), chills (16%), leukopenia (14%), systemic infection (13%). **OCCASIONAL (5%–10%):** Serum sickness–like symptoms, dyspnea, apnea, arthralgia, chest/back/flank pain, nausea, vomiting, diarrhea, phlebitis.

ADVERSE REACTIONS/ TOXIC EFFECTS

Thrombocytopenia occurs but is generally transient. Severe hypersensitivity reaction, including anaphylaxis, occurs rarely.

NURSING IMPLICATIONS

BASELINE ASSESSMENT

Use of high-flow vein (CVL, PICC, Groshong catheter) may prevent chemical phlebitis that may occur if peripheral vein is used.

INTERVENTION/EVALUATION

Monitor frequently for chills, fever, erythema, itching. Obtain order for prophylactic antihistamines or corticosteroids.

magnesium

magnesium chloride

(Citro-Mag♣, Phillips' Magnesia Tablets♣, Slow-Mag)

magnesium citrate

(Citrate of Magnesia, Citroma)

magnesium hydroxide

(MOM)

magnesium oxide

(Mag-Ox 400, Maox 420)

magnesium protein complex

(Mg-PLUS)

magnesium sulfate

(Epsom salt, magnesium sulfate injection)

Do not confuse with manganese sulfate.

FIXED-COMBINATION(S)

With aluminum, an antacid **(Aludrox, Delcid, Gaviscon, Maalox);** with aluminum and simethicone, an antiflatulent **(Di-Gel, Gelusil, Maalox Plus, Mylanta, Silain-Gel);** with aluminum and calcium, an antacid **(Camalox);** with mineral oil, a lubricant laxative **(Haley's MO);** with magnesium oxide and aluminum oxide, antacids **(Riopan).**

◆ CLASSIFICATION

CLINICAL: Antacid, anticonvulsant, electrolyte, laxative (see pp. 9C, 104C, 105C).

ACTION

Antacid: Acts in stomach to neutralize gastric acid. **Therapeutic Effect:** Increases pH. **Laxative:** Osmotic effect primarily in small intestine. Draws water into intestinal lumen. **Therapeutic Effect:** Produces distention; promotes peristalsis, bowel evacuation. **Systemic (dietary supplement, replacement):** Found primarily in intracellular fluids. Essential for enzyme activity, nerve conduction, muscle contraction. **Anticonvulsant:** Blocks neuromuscular transmission, amount of acetylcholine released at motor end plate. **Therapeutic Effect:** Produces seizure control.

PHARMACOKINETICS

Antacid, Laxative: Minimal absorption through intestine. Absorbed dose primarily excreted in urine. **Systemic:** Widely distributed. Primarily excreted in urine.

USES

Treatment/prevention of hypomagnesemia. Treatment of hypertension, torsades de pointes, encephalopathy, seizures associated with acute nephritis, constipation, hyperacidity.

PRECAUTIONS

CONTRAINDICATIONS: Antacids: Severe renal impairment, appendicitis/symptoms of appendicitis, ileostomy, intestinal obstruction. **Laxative:** Appendicitis, undiagnosed rectal bleeding, CHF, intestinal obstruction, hypersensitivity, colostomy, ileostomy. **Systemic:** Heart block, myocardial damage, renal failure. **CAUTIONS:** Safety in children <6 yrs not known. **Antacids:** Undiagnosed GI/rectal bleeding, ulcerative colitis, colostomy, diverticulitis, chronic diarrhea. **Laxative:** Diabetes mellitus or pts on low-salt diet (some products contain sugar, sodium). **Systemic:** Severe renal impairment.

LIFESPAN CONSIDERATIONS: Pregnancy/lactation: ANTACID: Unknown if distributed in breast milk. **Pregnancy**

M

Category B. PARENTERAL: Readily crosses placenta. Distributed in breast milk for 24 hrs after magnesium therapy is discontinued. Continuous IV infusion increases risk of magnesium toxicity in neonate. IV administration should not be used 2 hrs preceding delivery. **Pregnancy Category B (anticonvulsant/laxative). Children:** No age-related precautions noted. **Elderly:** Increased risk of developing magnesium deficiency (e.g., poor diet, decreased absorption, medications).

INTERACTIONS

DRUG: Antacids: May decrease absorption of **ketoconazole, tetracyclines.** May decrease effect of **methenamine. Antacids, laxatives:** May decrease effects of **oral anticoagulants, digoxin, phenothiazines.** May form nonabsorbable complex with **tetracyclines. Systemic: Calcium** may neutralize effects. **CNS depression-producing medications** may increase CNS depression. May cause changes in cardiac conduction/heart block with **digoxin. HERBAL:** None known. **FOOD:** None known. **LAB VALUES:** Antacid: May increase gastrin, pH. **Laxative:** May decrease potassium. **Systemic:** None known.

AVAILABILITY

MAGNESIUM CHLORIDE (Slow-Mag): 64 mg. **MAGNESIUM CITRATE: Solution:** 300 ml. **MAGNESIUM HYDROXIDE: Liquid:** 400 mg/5 ml, 800 mg/5 ml; **Chewable tablets:** 311 mg. **MAGNESIUM OXIDE (Mag-Ox):** 400 mg. **MAGNESIUM SULFATE: (Premix solution):** 10 mg/ml, 20 mg/ml, 40 mg/ml, 80 mg/ml. **(Injection solution):** 125 mg/ml, 500 mg/ml.

ADMINISTRATION/HANDLING

PO (ANTACID)

• Shake suspension well before use. • Chewable tablets should be chewed thoroughly before swallowing, followed with full glass of water.

PO (LAXATIVE)

• Drink full glass of liquid (8 oz) with each dose (prevents dehydration). • Flavor may be improved by following with fruit juice, citrus carbonated beverage. • Refrigerate citrate of magnesia (retains potency, palatability).

IM

• For adults, elderly, use 250 mg/ml (25%) or 500 mg/ml (50%) magnesium sulfate concentration. • For infants, children, do not exceed 200 mg/ml (20%).

IV

Storage • Store at room temperature.

Reconstitution • Must dilute (do not exceed 20 mg/ml concentration).

Rate of administration • For IV infusion, do not exceed magnesium sulfate concentration 200 mg/ml (20%). • Do not exceed IV infusion rate of 150 mg/min.

IV INCOMPATIBILITIES

Amphotericin B complex (Abelcet, AmBisome, Amphotec), cefepime (Maxipime).

IV COMPATIBILITIES

Amikacin (Amikin), cefazolin (Ancef), cefepime (Maxipime), ciprofloxacin (Cipro), dobutamine (Dobutrex), enalapril (Vasotec), gentamicin, heparin, hydromorphone (Dilaudid), insulin, milrinone (Primacor), morphine, piperacillin-tazobactam (Zosyn), potassium chloride, propofol (Diprivan), tobramycin (Nebcin), vancomycin (Vancocin).

INDICATIONS/ROUTES/DOSAGE

HYPOMAGNESEMIA (magnesium sulfate)

IM/IV: ADULTS, ELDERLY: 1 g q6h for 4 doses. CHILDREN: 25–50 mg/kg/dose q4–6h for 3–4 doses.

PO: ADULTS, ELDERLY: 3 g q6h for 4 doses. CHILDREN: 10–20 mg/kg (elemental magnesium)/dose 4 times/day.

HYPERTENSION, SEIZURES (magnesium sulfate)
IM/IV: ADULTS, ELDERLY: 1 g q6h for 4 doses as needed. CHILDREN: 20–100 mg/kg/dose q4–6h as needed.

TORSADES DE POINTES (magnesium sulfate)
IV: ADULTS, ELDERLY: 1–2 g >60–90 sec followed by 1–2 g/hr diluted in 100 ml 0.9% NaCl or D_5W.

LAXATIVE (magnesium citrate)
PO: ADULTS, ELDERLY, CHILDREN >12 YRS: 150–300 ml. CHILDREN 6–12 YRS: 100–150 ml. CHILDREN <6 YRS: 2–4 ml/kg.

LAXATIVE (magnesium hydroxide)
PO: ADULTS, ELDERLY, CHILDREN ≥12 YRS: 30–60 ml/day. CHILDREN 6–11 YRS: 15–30 ml/day. CHILDREN 2–5 YRS: 5–15 ml/day. CHILDREN <2 YRS: 0.5 ml/kg/dose.

ANTACID (magnesium hydroxide)

Alert: Up to 4 times/day.

PO: ADULTS, ELDERLY: (TABLET): 622–1,244 mg/dose. (LIQUID CONCENTRATE): 2.5–7.5 ml/dose. (LIQUID): 5–15 ml/dose. CHILDREN: (LIQUID): 2.5–5 ml/dose.

SIDE EFFECTS

FREQUENT: Antacid: Chalky taste, diarrhea, laxative effect. **OCCASIONAL: Antacid:** Nausea, vomiting, stomach cramps. **Antacid, laxative:** Prolonged use or large dose with renal impairment may cause increased magnesium (dizziness, irregular heartbeat, mental changes, tiredness, weakness). **Laxative:** Cramping, diarrhea, increased thirst, gas. **Systemic:** Reduced respiratory rate, decreased reflexes, flushing, hypotension, decreased heart rate.

ADVERSE REACTIONS/ TOXIC EFFECTS

ANTACID, LAXATIVE: None known. **SYSTEMIC:** May produce prolonged PQ interval, widening of QRS intervals. May cause loss of deep tendon reflexes, heart block, respiratory paralysis, cardiac arrest. **ANTIDOTE:** 10–20 ml 10% calcium gluconate (5–10 mEq of calcium).

NURSING IMPLICATIONS

BASELINE ASSESSMENT

Assess if pt is sensitive to magnesium. **Antacid:** Assess GI pain (duration, location, time of occurrence, relief with food, caused by food/alcohol, constant/sporadic, worsened when lying down/bending over). **Laxative:** Assess color, amount, consistency of stool. Assess bowel habits (usual pattern), bowel sound for peristalsis. Assess pt for weight loss, nausea, vomiting, history of recent abdominal surgery. **Systemic:** Assess renal function, magnesium level.

INTERVENTION/EVALUATION

Antacid: Assess for relief of gastric distress. Monitor renal function (esp. if dosing is long term or frequent). **Laxative:** Monitor stools for diarrhea, constipation. Maintain adequate fluid intake. **Systemic:** Monitor renal function, magnesium levels, EKG for cardiac function. Test patellar reflex or knee jerk reflexes prior to giving repeat parenteral doses (used as indication of CNS depression; suppressed reflex may be sign of impending respiratory arrest). Patellar reflex must be present, respiratory rate should be >16/min prior to each parenteral dose. Provide seizure precautions.

PATIENT/FAMILY TEACHING

Antacid: Give at least 2 hrs apart from other medication. Do not take >2 wks unless directed by physician. For peptic ulcer, take 1 and 3 hrs after meals and at bedtime for 4–6 wks. Chew tablets thoroughly, followed with glass of water; shake suspensions well. Repeat dosing/large doses may have laxative effect. **Laxative:** Drink full glass (8 oz) liquid to aid stool softening. Use only for short term. Do not use if abdominal pain, vomiting, nausea is present. **Systemic:** Inform physician of any signs of hypermagnesemia (confusion, irregular heartbeat, cramping, unusual tirednes weakness, lightheadedness, dizziness).

mannitol

man-ih-toll
(Osmitrol)

CLASSIFICATION

CLINICAL: Osmotic diuretic, antiglaucoma, antihemolytic.

ACTION

Elevates osmotic pressure of glomerular filtrate; increases flow of water into interstitial fluid/plasma, inhibiting renal tubular reabsorption of sodium, chloride. Enhances flow of water from eye into plasma. **Therapeutic Effect:** Produces diuresis, reduces intraocular pressure (IOP).

PHARMACOKINETICS

Onset	Peak	Duration
Diuresis		
1–3 hrs	—	—
Reduced IOP		
15 min	—	3–6 hrs

Remains in extracellular fluid. Primarily excreted in urine. Removed by hemodialysis. **Half-life:** 100 min. Onset diuresis occurs in 1–3 hrs, decreases IOP in 0.5–1 hr, duration 4–6 hrs. Decreases CSF pressure in 15 min, duration 3–8 hrs.

USES

Prevention, treatment of oliguric phase of acute renal failure (before evidence of permanent renal failure). Reduces increased intracranial pressure due to cerebral edema, edema of injured spinal cord, IOP due to acute glaucoma. Promotes urinary excretion of toxic substances (aspirin, bromides, imipramine, barbiturates).

PRECAUTIONS

CONTRAINDICATIONS: Severe renal disease, dehydration, intracranial bleeding, severe pulmonary edema/congestion. **CAUTIONS:** None known.

LIFESPAN CONSIDERATIONS: Pregnancy/lactation: Unknown if drug crosses placenta or is distributed in breast milk. **Pregnancy Category C. Children:** Safety and efficacy not established in those <12 yrs. **Elderly:** Age-related renal impairment may require caution.

INTERACTIONS

DRUG: May increase **digoxin** toxicity (due to hypokalemia). **HERBAL:** None known. **FOOD:** None known. **LAB VALUES:** May decrease phosphate, potassium, sodium.

AVAILABILITY (Rx)

INJECTION: 5%, 10%, 15%, 20%, 25%.

ADMINISTRATION/HANDLING

Alert: Assess IV site for patency before each dose. Pain, thrombosis noted with extravasation.

IV

Storage • Store at room temperature. • If crystals are noted in solution, warm bottle in hot water, shake vigorously at intervals. Cool to body temperature before administration. Do not use if crystals remain after warming procedure.

Rate of administration In-line filter (<5 micron) used for concentrations >20%. Test dose for oliguria. IV push over 3–5 min; over 20–30 min for cerebral edema, elevated intracranial pressure. Maximum concentration: 25%.

• Do not add KCl or NaCl to mannitol 20% or greater. Do not add to whole blood for transfusion.

⊘ IV INCOMPATIBILITIES

Cefepime (Maxipime), doxorubicin liposome (Doxil), filgrastim (Neupogen).

IV COMPATIBILITIES

Cisplatin (Platinol), ondansetron (Zofran), propofol (Diprivan).

INDICATIONS/ROUTES/DOSAGE

USUAL IV DOSAGE

Alert: Test dose of 12.5 g for adults (200 mg/kg for children) over 3–5 min to produce a urine flow of at least 30–50 ml/hr over 2–3 hrs (1 ml/kg/hr for children).

ADULTS, ELDERLY, CHILDREN: Initially, 0.5–1 g/kg, then 0.25–0.5 g/kg q4–6h.

SIDE EFFECTS

FREQUENT: Dry mouth, thirst. **OCCASIONAL:** Blurred vision, increased urination, headache, arm pain, backache, nausea, vomiting, urticaria (hives), dizziness, hypotension/hypertension, tachycardia, fever, angina-like chest pain.

ADVERSE REACTIONS/ TOXIC EFFECTS

Fluid, electrolyte imbalance may occur because of rapid administration of large doses or inadequate urinary output resulting in overexpansion of extracellular fluid. Circulatory overload may produce pulmonary edema, CHF. Excessive diuresis may produce hypokalemia, hyponatremia. Fluid loss in excess of electrolyte excretion may produce hypernatremia, hyperkalemia.

NURSING IMPLICATIONS

BASELINE ASSESSMENT

Check B/P, pulse prior to giving medication. Assess skin turgor, mucous membranes, mental status, muscle strength. Obtain baseline weight. Monitor I&O.

INTERVENTION/EVALUATION

Monitor urinary output to ascertain therapeutic response. Monitor electrolytes, BUN, renal/hepatic reports. Assess vital signs, skin turgor, mucous membranes. Weigh daily. Signs of hyponatremia include confusion, drowsiness, thirst/dry mouth, cold/clammy skin. Signs of hypokalemia include changes in muscle strength, tremors, muscle cramps, changes in mental status, cardiac arrhythmias. Signs of hyperkalemia include colic, diarrhea, muscle twitching followed by weakness/paralysis, arrhythmias.

PATIENT/FAMILY TEACHING

Expect increased frequency, volume of urination. May cause dry mouth.

maprotiline hydrochloride

(Ludiomil)

See Classification section under: Antidepressants

Mavik

see trandolapril

Maxalt

see rizatriptan

Maxipime

see cefepime

mechlorethamine hydrochloride

(Mustargen)

See Classification section under: Cancer chemotherapeutic agents (p. 74C)

meclizine

mek-lih-zeen

(Antivert, Bonamine, Bonine)

CLASSIFICATION

PHARMACOTHERAPEUTIC: Anticholinergic. **CLINICAL:** Antiemetic, antivertigo.

ACTION

Reduces labyrinth excitability, diminishes vestibular stimulation of labyrinth, affecting chemoreceptor trigger zone (CTZ). Possesses anticholinergic activity. **Therapeutic Effect:** Reduces nausea, vomiting, vertigo.

PHARMACOKINETICS

Onset	Peak	Duration
PO		
30–60 min	—	12–24 hrs

Well absorbed from GI tract. Widely distributed. Metabolized in liver. Primarily excreted in urine. **Half-life:** 6 hrs.

USES

Prevention, treatment of nausea, vomiting, vertigo due to motion sickness. Treatment of vertigo associated with diseases affecting vestibular system.

PRECAUTIONS

CONTRAINDICATIONS: None known. **CAUTIONS:** Narrow-angle glaucoma, obstructive diseases of the GI/GU tract.

LIFESPAN CONSIDERATIONS: Pregnancy/lactation: Unknown if drug crosses placenta or is distributed in breast milk (may produce irritability in nursing infants). **Pregnancy Category B. Children/elderly:** May be more sensitive to anticholinergic effects (e.g., dry mouth).

INTERACTIONS

DRUG: Alcohol, CNS depression-producing medications may increase CNS depressant effect. **HERBAL:** None known. **FOOD:** None known. **LAB VALUES:** May suppress wheal, flare reactions to antigen skin testing, unless meclizine discontinued 4 days before testing.

AVAILABILITY (Rx)

TABLETS: 12.5 mg, 25 mg, 50 mg. **TABLETS (chewable):** 25 mg.

ADMINISTRATION/HANDLING

PO

- Give without regard to meals.
- Scored tablets may be crushed.
- Do not crush or break capsule form.

INDICATIONS/ROUTES/DOSAGE

MOTION SICKNESS

PO: ADULTS, ELDERLY, CHILDREN ≥12 YRS: 12.5–25 mg 1 hr before travel. May repeat q12–24h. May require dose of 50 mg q12–24h.

VERTIGO

PO: ADULTS, ELDERLY, CHILDREN ≥12 YRS: 25–100 mg/day in divided doses as needed.

SIDE EFFECTS

Alert: Elderly (>60 yrs) tend to develop sedation, dizziness, hypotension, mental confusion, disorientation, agitation, psychotic-like symptoms.

FREQUENT: Drowsiness. **OCCASIONAL:** Blurred vision; dry mouth, nose, throat.

ADVERSE REACTIONS/ TOXIC EFFECTS

Children may experience dominant paradoxical reaction (restlessness, insomnia, euphoria, nervousness, tremors). Overdosage in children may result in hallucinations, convulsions, death. Hypersensitivity reaction (eczema, pruritus, rash, cardiac disturbances, photosensitivity) may occur. Overdosage may vary from CNS depression (sedation, apnea, cardiovascular collapse, death) to severe paradoxical reaction (hallucinations, tremor, seizures).

NURSING IMPLICATIONS

INTERVENTION/EVALUATION

Monitor B/P, esp. in elderly (increased risk of hypotension). Monitor children closely for paradoxical reaction. Monitor serum electrolytes in those with severe vomiting. Assess skin turgor, mucous membranes to evaluate hydration status.

PATIENT/FAMILY TEACHING

Tolerance to sedative effect may occur. Avoid tasks that require alertness, motor skills until response to drug is established. Dry mouth, drowsiness, dizziness may be an expected response of drug. Avoid alcoholic beverages during therapy. Sugarless gum, sips of tepid water may relieve dry mouth. Coffee, tea may help reduce drowsiness.

meclofenamate sodium

(Meclodium, Meclomen)

See Classification section under: Nonsteroidal Anti-Inflammatory Drugs (NSAIDs)

medroxyprogesterone acetate

meh-drocks-ee-pro-**jes**-ter-own

(Depo-Provera, Novo-Medrone ✤, Provera)

Do not confuse with hydroxyprogesterone, methylprednisolone, methyltestosterone.

FIXED-COMBINATION(S)

Prempro, Premphase: medroxyprogesterone/conjugated estrogens: 1.5 mg/0.3 mg; 1.5 mg/0.45 mg; 2.5 mg/0.625 mg; 5 mg/0.625 mg.

◆CLASSIFICATION

PHARMACOTHERAPEUTIC: Hormone. **CLINICAL:** Progestin, antineoplastic.

ACTION

Transforms endometrium from proliferative to secretory (in an estrogen-primed endometrium); inhibits secretion of pituitary gonadotropins. **Therapeutic Effect:** Prevents follicular maturation, ovulation. Stimulates growth of mammary alveolar tissue; relaxes uterine smooth muscle. Restores hormonal imbalance.

PHARMACOKINETICS

Slow absorption after IM administration. Protein binding: 90%. Metabolized in

M

liver. Primarily excreted in urine. **Half-life:** 30 days.

USES

PO: Prevention of endometrial hyperplasia (concurrently given with estrogen to women with intact uterus), treatment of secondary amenorrhea, abnormal uterine bleeding. **IM:** Adjunctive therapy, palliative treatment of inoperable, recurrent, metastatic endometrial carcinoma, renal carcinoma; prevention of pregnancy. **Unlabeled:** Treatment of endometriosis, hormonal replacement therapy in estrogen-treated menopausal women.

PRECAUTIONS

CONTRAINDICATIONS: History of or active thrombotic disorders (cerebral apoplexy, thrombophlebitis, thromboembolic disorders), hypersensitivity to progestins, severe liver dysfunction, estrogen-dependent neoplasia, undiagnosed abnormal genital bleeding, missed abortion, use as pregnancy test, undiagnosed vaginal bleeding, carcinoma of breast, known/suspected pregnancy. **CAUTIONS:** Those with conditions aggravated by fluid retention (asthma, seizures, migraine, cardiac/renal dysfunction), diabetes, history of mental depression.

LIFESPAN CONSIDERATIONS: Pregnancy/lactation: Avoid use during pregnancy, esp. first 4 mos (congenital heart, limb reduction defects may occur). Distributed in breast milk. **Pregnancy Category X. Children:** Safety and efficacy not established. **Elderly:** No age-related precautions noted.

INTERACTIONS

DRUG: May interfere with effects of **bromocriptine. HERBAL:** None known. **FOOD:** None known. **LAB VALUES:** Altered thyroid, liver function tests, prothrombin time, metyrapone test.

AVAILABILITY (Rx)

TABLETS: 2.5 mg, 5 mg, 10 mg. **INJECTION:** 150 mg/ml, 400 mg/ml.

ADMINISTRATION/HANDLING

PO

- Give without regard to meals.

IM

- Shake vial immediately before administering (ensures complete suspension).
- Rarely, a residual lump, change in skin color, sterile abscess occurs at injection site. Inject IM only in upper arm, upper outer aspect of buttock.

INDICATIONS/ROUTES/DOSAGE

ENDOMETRIAL HYPERPLASIA

PO: ADULTS: 2–10 mg/day for 14 days.

SECONDARY AMENORRHEA

PO: ADULTS: 5–10 mg/day for 5–10 days (begin at any time during menstrual cycle) or 2.5 mg/day.

ABNORMAL UTERINE BLEEDING

PO: ADULTS: 5–10 mg/day for 5–10 days (begin on calculated day 16 or day 21 of menstrual cycle).

ENDOMETRIAL, RENAL CARCINOMA

IM: ADULTS, ELDERLY: Initially, 400–1,000 mg, repeat at 1-wk intervals. If improvement occurs and disease stabilized, begin maintenance with as little as 400 mg/mo.

PREGNANCY PREVENTION

IM: ADULTS: 150 mg q3mos.

SIDE EFFECTS

FREQUENT: Transient menstrual abnormalities (spotting, change in menstrual flow/cervical secretions, amenorrhea) at initiation of therapy. **OCCASIONAL:** Edema, weight change, breast tenderness, nervousness, insomnia, fatigue, dizziness. **RARE:** Alopecia, mental depression, dermatologic changes, headache, fever, nausea.

ADVERSE REACTIONS/ TOXIC EFFECTS

Thrombophlebitis, pulmonary/cerebral embolism, retinal thrombosis occurs rarely.

NURSING IMPLICATIONS

BASELINE ASSESSMENT

Question for hypersensitivity to progestins, possibility of pregnancy before initiating therapy (Pregnancy Category X). Obtain baseline weight, blood glucose, B/P.

INTERVENTION/EVALUATION

Check weight daily; report weekly gain of ≥5 lbs. Check B/P periodically. Assess skin for rash, hives. Report immediately the development of chest pain, sudden shortness of breath, sudden decrease in vision, migraine headache, pain (esp. with swelling, warmth, redness) in calves, numbness of an arm/leg (thrombotic disorders).

PATIENT/FAMILY TEACHING

Inform physician of sudden loss of vision, severe headache, chest pain, coughing up of blood (hemoptysis), numbness in arm/leg, severe pain/swelling in calf, unusual heavy vaginal bleeding, severe pain/tenderness in abdominal area.

megestrol acetate

meh-**geh**-stroll
(Apo-Megestrol✱, Megace, Megace OS✱)

CLASSIFICATION

PHARMACOTHERAPEUTIC: Hormone. **CLINICAL:** Antineoplastic (see p. 74C).

ACTION

Suppresses release of luteinizing hormone from anterior pituitary by inhibiting pituitary function. **Therapeutic Effect:** Regresses tumor size. Increases appetite (mechanism unknown).

PHARMACOKINETICS

Well absorbed from GI tract. Metabolized in liver; excreted in urine.

USES

Palliative management of recurrent, inoperable, metastatic endometrial/breast carcinoma. Treatment of anorexia, cachexia, unexplained significant weight loss in pts with AIDS. **Unlabeled:** Treatment of hormonally dependent/advanced prostate carcinoma.

PRECAUTIONS

CONTRAINDICATIONS: None known. **CAUTIONS:** History of thrombophlebitis.

LIFESPAN CONSIDERATIONS: Pregnancy/lactation: If possible, avoid use during pregnancy, esp. first 4 mos. Breast-feeding not recommended. **Pregnancy Category X** (suspension), **D** (tablets). **Children:** Safety and efficacy not established. **Elderly:** No age-related precautions noted.

INTERACTIONS

DRUG: None known. **HERBAL:** None known. **FOOD:** None known. **LAB VALUES:** May increase serum glucose levels.

AVAILABILITY (Rx)

TABLETS: 20 mg, 40 mg. **SUSPENSION:** 40 mg/ml.

M

melatonin

Also known as pineal hormone

CLASSIFICATION

HERBAL.

ACTION

Hormone synthesized endogenously by the pineal gland. Interacts with melatonin receptors in the brain. **Effect:** Regulates the body's circadian rhythm, sleep patterns. Acts as an antioxidant, protecting cells from oxidative damage by free radicals.

USES

Treatment for insomnia, jet lag. Also used as an antioxidant.

PRECAUTIONS

CONTRAINDICATIONS: Pregnancy/breastfeeding. **CAUTIONS:** Depression (may worsen dysphoria), seizures (may increase incidence), cardiovascular/hepatic disease.

LIFESPAN CONSIDERATIONS: Pregnancy/lactation: Contraindicated. **Children:** Safety and efficacy not established. **Elderly:** No age-related precautions noted.

INTERACTIONS

DRUG: May be additive with **alcohol, benzodiazepines.** May interfere with **immunosuppressants.** May enhance effects of **isoniazid. HERBAL: Chamomile, ginseng, goldenseal, kava kava, valerian** may increase sedative effects. **FOOD:** None known. **LAB VALUES:** May increase human growth hormone levels. May decrease LH levels.

AVAILABILITY (OTC)

LOZENGES: 3 mg. **POWDER. TABLETS:** 0.5 mg, 3 mg.

INDICATIONS/ROUTES/DOSAGE

PALLIATIVE TREATMENT OF ADVANCED BREAST CANCER

PO: ADULTS, ELDERLY: 160 mg/day in 4 equally divided doses.

PALLIATIVE TREATMENT OF ADVANCED ENDOMETRIAL CARCINOMA

PO: ADULTS, ELDERLY: 40–320 mg/day in divided doses. **Maximum:** 800 mg/day in 1–4 divided doses.

ANOREXIA, CACHEXIA, WEIGHT LOSS

PO: ADULTS, ELDERLY: 800 mg (20 ml)/day.

SIDE EFFECTS

FREQUENT: Weight gain secondary to increased appetite. **OCCASIONAL:** Nausea, breakthrough bleeding, backache, headache, breast tenderness, carpal tunnel syndrome. **RARE:** Feeling of coldness.

ADVERSE REACTIONS/ TOXIC EFFECTS

Thrombophlebitis, pulmonary embolism occur rarely.

NURSING IMPLICATIONS

BASELINE ASSESSMENT

Question for possibility of pregnancy before initiating therapy (Pregnancy Category X [suspension], D [tablets]). Provide support to pt, family, recognizing this drug is palliative, not curative.

EVALUATION/INTERVENTION

Monitor for tumor response.

PATIENT/FAMILY TEACHING

Contraception is imperative. Report any calf pain, difficulty breathing, vaginal bleeding. May cause headache, nausea, vomiting, breast tenderness, backache.

INDICATIONS/ROUTES/DOSAGE

INSOMNIA

PO: ADULTS, ELDERLY: 0.5–5 mg at bedtime.

JET LAG

PO: ADULTS, ELDERLY: 5 mg/day beginning 3 days before flight and 3 days after flight.

SIDE EFFECTS

Headache, transient depression, fatigue, drowsiness, dizziness, abdominal cramps/irritability, decreased alertness, hypersensitivity reaction, tachycardia, nausea, vomiting, anorexia, changes in sleep patterns, confusion.

ADVERSE REACTIONS/ TOXIC EFFECTS

None known.

NURSING IMPLICATIONS

BASELINE ASSESSMENT

Assess whether pregnant/breast-feeding (avoid use). Determine whether pt has history of seizures, depression. Assess sleep patterns if used for insomnia. Determine medication usage (esp. CNS depressants).

INTERVENTION/EVALUATION

Monitor effectiveness in improving insomnia. Assess for hypersensitivity reactions, CNS effects.

PATIENT/FAMILY TEACHING

Do not use if pregnant, planning to become pregnant, breast-feeding. Avoid tasks that require mental alertness or motor skills (e.g., driving).

meloxicam

meh-**locks**-ih-cam
(Mobic)

◆CLASSIFICATION

PHARMACOTHERAPEUTIC: Nonsteroidal anti-inflammatory. **CLINICAL:** Anti-inflammatory, analgesic (see p. 111C).

ACTION

Produces analgesic, anti-inflammatory effect by inhibiting prostaglandin synthesis. **Therapeutic Effect:** Reduces inflammatory response, intensity of pain stimulus reaching sensory nerve endings.

PHARMACOKINETICS

Onset	Peak	Duration
PO analgesic		
30 min	4–5 hrs	—

Well absorbed after PO administration. Protein binding: 99%. Metabolized in liver. Eliminated via the kidney/feces. Not removed by hemodialysis. **Half-life:** 15–20 hrs.

USES

Relief of signs/symptoms of osteoarthritis.

PRECAUTIONS

CONTRAINDICATIONS: Aspirin-induced nasal polyps associated with bronchospasm. **CAUTIONS:** History of GI disease (e.g., ulcers), impaired renal/liver function, CHF, dehydration, hypertension, asthma, hemostatic disease. Concurrent use of anticoagulants.

LIFESPAN CONSIDERATIONS: Pregnancy/lactation: Excreted in breast milk. **Pregnancy Category C** (**D** if used in third trimester or near term). **Children:** Safety and efficacy not established. **Elderly:** Age-related renal impairment may require dosage adjustment. More susceptible to GI toxicity; lower dosage recommended.

M

INTERACTIONS

DRUG: None known. **HERBAL: Ginkgo biloba** may increase risk of bleeding. **FOOD:** None known. **LAB VALUES:** May increase serum creatinine, SGOT (AST), SGPT (ALT).

AVAILABILITY (Rx)

TABLETS: 7.5 mg, 15 mg.

ADMINISTRATION/HANDLING

PO

- Give without regard to meals.

INDICATIONS/ROUTES/DOSAGE

OSTEOARTHRITIS

PO: ADULTS: Initially, 7.5 mg/day. **Maximum:** 15 mg/day.

SIDE EFFECTS

FREQUENT (7%–9%): Dyspepsia (heartburn, indigestion, epigastric pain), headache, diarrhea, nausea. **OCCASIONAL (3%–4%):** Dizziness, insomnia, rash, pruritus, flatulence, constipation, vomiting. **RARE (<2%):** Somnolence/drowsiness, urticaria, photosensitivity.

M

ADVERSE REACTIONS/ TOXIC EFFECTS

In those treated chronically, peptic ulcer, GI bleeding, gastritis, severe hepatic reaction (jaundice), nephrotoxicity (hematuria, dysuria, proteinuria), severe hypersensitivity reaction (bronchospasm, angioedema) occur rarely.

NURSING IMPLICATIONS

BASELINE ASSESSMENT

Assess onset, type, location, duration of pain/inflammation. Inspect appearance of affected joints for immobility, deformities, skin condition.

INTERVENTION/EVALUATION

Monitor CBC, liver/renal function tests. Evaluate for therapeutic response: relief of pain/stiffness/swelling, increase in joint mobility, reduced joint tenderness, improved grip strength.

PATIENT/FAMILY TEACHING

Take with food, milk to reduce GI upset. Inform physician of ringing in ears, persistent cramping/pain in stomach, severe nausea/vomiting, difficulty breathing, unusual bruising/bleeding, rash, swelling of extremities, chest pain, palpitations.

melphalan

mel-fah-lan

(Alkeran)

Do not confuse with Leukeran, Mephyton, Myleran.

CLASSIFICATION

PHARMACOTHERAPEUTIC: Alkylating agent. **CLINICAL:** Antineoplastic (see p. 74C).

ACTION

Primarily cross-links strands of DNA, RNA. Cell cycle–phase nonspecific. **Therapeutic Effect:** Inhibits protein synthesis, producing cell death.

USES

Treatment of multiple myeloma, nonresectable epithelial carcinoma of ovary. **Unlabeled:** Treatment of breast, testicular carcinoma; neuroblastoma; rhabdomyosarcoma.

PRECAUTIONS

CONTRAINDICATIONS: Severe bone marrow suppression, pregnancy. **CAUTIONS:** Leukocyte count <3,000/mm^3 or platelet count <100,000/mm^3, bone marrow suppression, impaired renal function. **Pregnancy Category D.**

INTERACTIONS

DRUG: May decrease effect of **antigout** medications. **Bone marrow depressants** may increase bone marrow depression. **Live virus vaccines** may potentiate virus replication, increase vaccine side effects, decrease pt's antibody response to vaccine. **HERBAL:** None known. **FOOD:** None known. **LAB VALUES:** May increase uric acid, positive Coombs' (direct).

AVAILABILITY (Rx)

TABLETS: 2 mg. **POWDER FOR INJECTION:** 50 mg.

ADMINISTRATION/HANDLING:

IV

Storage • Store at room temperature; protect from light. • Once reconstituted, stable for 90 min at room temperature (do not refrigerate).

Reconstitution • Reconstitute 50-mg vial with diluent supplied by manufacturer to yield a 5 mg/ml solution. • Further dilute with 0.9% NaCl to final concentration, not to exceed 2 mg/ml (central line) or 0.45 mg/ml (peripheral line).

Rate of administration • Infuse over 15–30 min at a rate not to exceed 10 mg/min.

∅ **IV INCOMPATIBILITY**

Do not mix with any other medications.

INDICATIONS/ROUTES/DOSAGE

Alert: May be carcinogenic, mutagenic, or teratogenic. Handle with extreme care during preparation/administration. Dosage individualized on the basis of clinical response, tolerance to adverse effects. When used in combination therapy, consult specific protocols for optimum dosage, sequence of drug administration. Leukocyte count usually maintained between 3,000–4,000/mm^3.

OVARIAN CARCINOMA

PO: ADULTS, ELDERLY: 0.2 mg/kg/day for 5 successive days. Repeat at 4- to 6-wk intervals.

MULTIPLE MYELOMA

PO: ADULTS: 6 mg once daily, initially adjusted as indicated or 0.15 mg/kg/day for 7 days or 0.25 mg/kg/day for 4 days. Repeat at 4- to 6-wk intervals.

IV: ADULTS: 16 mg/m^2/dose q2wks for 4 doses; then repeat monthly as per protocol.

Alert: Decrease dosage by 50% in pts with BUN >30 mg/dl or serum creatinine >1.5 mg/dl.

SIDE EFFECTS

FREQUENT: Nausea, vomiting (may be severe with large dose). **OCCASIONAL:** Diarrhea, stomatitis (burning/erythema of oral mucosa, sore throat, difficulty swallowing, oral ulceration), rash, pruritus, alopecia.

ADVERSE REACTIONS/ TOXIC EFFECTS

Bone marrow depression manifested as hematologic toxicity (principally leukopenia, thrombocytopenia, and, to lesser extent, anemia, pancytopenia, agranulocytosis). Leukopenia may occur as early as 5 days. WBC, platelet counts return to normal levels during fifth wk, but leukopenia, thrombocytopenia may last >6 wks after discontinuing drug. Hyperuricemia noted by hematuria, crystalluria, flank pain.

NURSING IMPLICATIONS

BASELINE ASSESSMENT

Obtain blood counts weekly. Dosage may be decreased or discontinued if WBC falls below 3,000/mm^3 or platelet

M

count falls below 100,000/mm^3. Antiemetics may be effective in preventing, treating nausea, vomiting.

INTERVENTION/EVALUATION

Monitor CBC with diffferential, platelet count, electrolytes, Hgb. Monitor for stomatitis. Monitor for hematologic toxicity (fever, sore throat, signs of local infection, unusual bruising/bleeding from any site), symptoms of anemia (excessive tiredness, weakness), signs of hyperuricemia (hematuria, flank pain). Avoid IM injections, rectal temperatures, other traumas that may induce bleeding.

PATIENT/FAMILY TEACHING

Increase fluid intake (may protect against hyperuricemia). Maintain fastidious oral hygiene. Alopecia is reversible, but new hair growth may have different color, texture. Avoid crowds, those with infections. Inform physician if fever, shortness of breath, cough, sore throat, bleeding, bruising occurs.

M

memantine hydrochloride

meh-**man**-teen
(Namenda)

CLASSIFICATION

PHARMACOTHERAPEUTIC: Neurotransmitter inhibitor. **CLINICAL:** Anti-Alzheimer's agent.

ACTION

Decreases the effects of glutamate, the principal excitatory neurotransmitter in the brain (Alzheimer's disease involves degeneration of cholinergic neuronal pathways). **Therapeutic Effect:** May reduce clinical deterioration in moderate to severe Alzheimer's disease.

PHARMACOKINETICS

Rapidly and completely absorbed following PO administration. Undergoes little metabolism with the majority of the dose excreted unchanged in the urine. Protein binding: 45%. **Half-life:** 60–80 hrs.

USES

Treatment of moderate to severe Alzheimer's disease.

PRECAUTIONS

CONTRAINDICATIONS: Not recommended in pts with severe renal impairment. **CAUTIONS:** Moderately impaired renal function.

LIFESPAN CONSIDERATIONS: Pregnancy/lactation: Unknown if drug crosses placenta or is distributed in breast milk. **Pregnancy Category B. Children:** Not prescribed for this pt population. **Elderly:** No age-related precautions noted, but use is not recommended in those with severe renal impairment (creatinine clearance <9 ml/min).

INTERACTIONS

DRUG: Carbonic anhydrase inhibitors, sodium bicarbonate may reduce memantine renal elimination. **HERBAL:** None known. **FOOD:** None known. **LAB VALUES:** None known.

AVAILABILITY (Rx)

TABLETS: 5 mg, 10 mg.

ADMINISTRATION/HANDLING

PO

- Give without regard to food.

INDICATIONS/ROUTES/DOSAGE

ALZHEIMER'S DISEASE

PO: ADULTS, ELDERLY: 5 mg once daily, with target dose of 20 mg/day. Increase in 5-mg increments to 10 mg/day (5 mg twice daily), 15 mg/day (5 mg and 10 mg as separate doses), 20 mg/day (10 mg twice daily). Recommended minimum interval between dose increases is 1 wk.

SIDE EFFECTS

OCCASIONAL (4%–7%): Dizziness, headache, confusion, constipation, hypertension, cough. **RARE (2%–3%):** Back pain, nausea, fatigue, anxiety, peripheral edema, arthralgia, insomnia.

ADVERSE REACTIONS/ TOXIC EFFECTS

None known.

NURSING IMPLICATIONS

BASELINE ASSESSMENT

Assess cognitive, behavioral, functional deficits of pt. Assess renal function.

INTERVENTION/EVALUATION

Monitor cognitive, behavioral, functional status of pt. Monitor urine pH (alterations of urine pH toward the alkaline condition may lead to accumulation of the drug with possible increase in side effects)

PATIENT/FAMILY TEACHING

Do not reduce or stop medication; do not increase dosage without physician direction. Ensure adequate fluid intake. If therapy is interrupted for several days, restart at lowest dose, titrate to current dose at minimum of 1-wk intervals. Inform family of local chapter of Alzheimer's Disease Association (provides a guide to services for these pts).

menotropins

(Humegon, Pergonal, Repronex)

See Classification section under: Fertility agents (p. 90C)

meperidine hydrochloride

meh-**pear**-ih-deen
(Demerol)

CLASSIFICATION

PHARMACOTHERAPEUTIC: Narcotic agonist. **CLINICAL:** Opiate analgesic **(Schedule II)** (see p. 121C).

ACTION

Binds with opioid receptors within CNS. **Therapeutic Effect:** Alters processes, affecting pain perception, emotional response to pain.

PHARMACOKINETICS

Onset	Peak	Duration
PO		
15 min	60 min	2–4 hrs
Subcutaneous		
10–15 min	30–50 min	2–4 hrs
IM		
10–15 min	30–50 min	2–4 hrs
IV		
<5 min	5–7 min	2–3 hrs

Variably absorbed from GI tract, well absorbed after IM administration. Protein binding: 60%–80%. Widely distributed. Metabolized in liver to active metabolite. Primarily excreted in urine. Not removed by hemodialysis. **Half-life:** 2.4–4 hrs (half-life increased in elderly); metabolite: 8–16 hrs.

USES

Relief of moderate to severe pain, preop sedation, obstetric support, anesthesia adjunct.

PRECAUTIONS

CONTRAINDICATIONS: Those receiving MAOIs in past 14 days, diarrhea due to poisoning, delivery of premature infant. **CAUTION:** Impaired renal/hepatic function, elderly/debilitated, supraventricular

M

tachycardia, cor pulmonale, history of seizures, acute abdominal conditions, increased intracranial pressure, respiratory abnormalities.

LIFESPAN CONSIDERATIONS: Pregnancy/lactation: Crosses placenta. Distributed in breast milk. Respiratory depression may occur in neonate if mother received opiates during labor. Regular use of opiates during pregnancy may produce withdrawal symptoms in neonate (irritability, excessive crying, tremors, hyperactive reflexes, fever, vomiting, diarrhea, yawning, sneezing, seizures). **Pregnancy Category B** (**D** if used for prolonged periods or at high dosages at term). **Children:** Paradoxical excitement may occur. Those <2 yrs more susceptible to respiratory depressant effects. **Elderly:** More susceptible to respiratory depressant effects. Age-related renal impairment may increase risk of urinary retention.

M

INTERACTIONS

DRUG: **Alcohol, CNS depressants** may increase CNS or respiratory depression, hypotension. **MAOIs** may produce severe, fatal reaction (reduce dose to ¼ usual dose). **HERBAL:** **Valerian** may increase CNS depression. **FOOD:** None known. **LAB VALUES:** May increase amylase, lipase. Therapeutic blood serum level: 100–550 ng/ml; toxic blood serum level: >1,000 ng/ml.

AVAILABILITY (Rx)

TABLETS: 50 mg, 100 mg. **SYRUP:** 50 mg/5 ml. **INJECTION:** 25 mg/ml, 50 mg/ml, 75 mg/ml, 100 mg/ml.

ADMINISTRATION/HANDLING

PO

• Give without regard to meals. • Dilute syrup in glass of water (prevents anesthetic effect on mucous membranes).

SUBCUTANEOUS/IM

Alert: IM preferred over subcutaneous route (subcutaneous produces pain, local irritation, induration).

• Administer slowly. • Those with circulatory impairment experience higher risk of overdosage due to delayed absorption of repeated administration.

IV

Alert: Give by slow IV push or IV infusion.

Storage • Store at room temperature.

Reconstitution • May give undiluted or may dilute in D_5W, lactated Ringer's, dextrose-saline combination (2.5%, 5%, or 10% dextrose in water—0.45% or 0.9% NaCl), Ringer's, lactated Ringer's, or molar sodium lactate diluent for IV injection or infusion.

Rate of administration • IV dosage must always be administered very slowly, over 2–3 min. • Rapid IV increases risk of severe adverse reactions (chest wall rigidity, apnea, peripheral circulatory collapse, anaphylactoid effects, cardiac arrest).

IV INCOMPATIBILITIES

Allopurinol (Aloprim), amphotericin B complex (Abelcet, AmBisome, Amphotec), cefepime (Maxipime), cefoperazone (Cefobid), doxorubicin liposome (Doxil), furosemide (Lasix), idarubicin (Idamycin), nafcillin (Nafcil).

IV COMPATIBILITIES

Bumetanide (Bumex), diltiazem (Cardizem), dobutamine (Dobutrex), dopamine (Intropin), heparin, insulin, lidocaine, magnesium, oxytocin (Pitocin), potassium.

INDICATIONS/ROUTES/DOSAGE

PAIN

PO/IM/subcutaneous: ADULTS, ELDERLY: 50–150 mg q3–4h. CHILDREN:

1.1–1.5 mg/kg q3–4h. Do not exceed single pediatric dose 100 mg.

USUAL PCA DOSAGE FOR ADULTS
Loading dose: 50–100 mg. **Intermittent bolus:** 5–30 mg. **Lockout interval:** 10–20 min. **Continuous infusion:** 5–40 mg/hr. **4-hr limit:** 200–300 mg.

DOSAGE IN RENAL IMPAIRMENT

Creatinine Clearance	% Normal Dose
10–50 ml/min	75
<10 ml/min	50

SIDE EFFECTS

Alert: Effects are dependent on dosage amount, route of administration. Ambulatory pts and those not in severe pain may experience dizziness, nausea, vomiting more frequently than those in supine position or having severe pain.

FREQUENT: Sedation, decreased B/P, diaphoresis, flushed face, dizziness, nausea, vomiting, constipation. **OCCASIONAL:** Confusion, irregular heartbeat, tremors, decreased urination, abdominal pain, dry mouth, headache, irritation at injection site, euphoria, dysphoria. **RARE:** Allergic reaction (rash, itching), insomnia.

ADVERSE REACTIONS/ TOXIC EFFECTS

Overdosage results in respiratory depression, skeletal muscle flaccidity, cold/clammy skin, cyanosis, extreme somnolence progressing to convulsions, stupor, coma. **ANTIDOTE:** 0.4 mg naloxone (Narcan). Tolerance to analgesic effect, physical dependence may occur with repeated use.

NURSING IMPLICATIONS

BASELINE ASSESSMENT

Pt should be in recumbent position before drug is administered by parenteral route. Assess onset, type, location, duration of pain. Obtain vital signs before giving medication. If respirations are ≤12/min (≤20/min in children), withhold medication, contact physician. Effect of medication is reduced if full pain recurs before next dose.

INTERVENTION/EVALUATION

Monitor vital signs 15–30 min after subcutaneous/IM dose, 5–10 min after IV dose (monitor for decreased B/P, change in rate/quality of pulse). Monitor pain level, sedation. Monitor stools; avoid constipation. Check for adequate voiding. Initiate deep breathing, coughing exercises, particularly in pts with impaired pulmonary function. Therapeutic blood serum level: 100–550 ng/ml; toxic blood serum level: >1,000 ng/ml.

PATIENT/FAMILY TEACHING

Medication should be taken before pain fully returns, within ordered intervals. Discomfort may occur with injection. Change positions slowly to avoid orthostatic hypotension. Increase fluids, bulk to prevent constipation. Tolerance/dependence may occur with prolonged use of high doses. Avoid alcohol and other CNS depressants. Avoid tasks requiring mental alertness, motor control until response to drug is established.

M

mepivacaine hydrochloride

(Carbocaine, Polocaine)

FIXED-COMBINATION(S)

With levonordefrin, a vasoconstrictor **(Isocaine).**
See Classification section under: Anesthetics: local (p. 5C)

mercaptopurine

(Purinethol)

See Classification section under: Cancer chemotherapeutic agents (p. 74C)

meropenem

murr-**oh**-pen-em

(Merrem IV)

CLASSIFICATION

PHARMACOTHERAPEUTIC: Carbapenem. **CLINICAL:** Antibiotic.

ACTION

Binds to penicillin-binding proteins. **Therapeutic Effect:** Inhibits bacterial cell wall synthesis. Bactericidal.

PHARMACOKINETICS

After IV administration, widely distributed into tissues/fluid, including CSF. Protein binding: 2%. Primarily excreted unchanged in urine. Removed by hemodialysis. **Half-life:** 1 hr.

USES

Treatment of intra-abdominal infections, bacterial meningitis (pediatric pts ≥3 mos only), cystic fibrosis. **Unlabeled:** Lower respiratory tract infections, febrile neutropenia, obstetric/gynecologic infections, sepsis.

PRECAUTIONS

CONTRAINDICATIONS: None known. **CAUTIONS:** Hypersensitivity to penicillins, cephalosporins, other allergens; renal function impairment; CNS disorders, particularly with history of seizures.

LIFESPAN CONSIDERATIONS: Pregnancy/lactation: Unknown if distributed in breast milk. **Pregnancy Category B. Children:** Safety and efficacy not established in those <3 mos. **Elderly:** Age-related renal impairment may require dosage adjustment.

INTERACTIONS

DRUG: **Probenecid** inhibits renal excretion of meropenem (do not use concurrently). **HERBAL:** None known. **FOOD:** None known. **LAB VALUES:** May increase SGOT (AST), SGPT (ALT), alkaline phosphatase, LDH, bilirubin, BUN, creatinine. May decrease Hgb, Hct, potassium.

AVAILABILITY (Rx)

POWDER FOR INJECTION: 500 mg, 1 g.

ADMINISTRATION/HANDLING

IV

Storage • Store vials at room temperature. • After reconstitution with 0.9% NaCl, stable for 2 hrs at room temperature, 18 hrs if refrigerated (with D_5W, stable for 1 hr at room temperature, 8 hrs if refrigerated).

Reconstitution • Reconstitute each 500 mg with 10 ml Sterile Water for Injection to provide a concentration of 50 mg/ml. • Shake to dissolve until clear. • May further dilute with 100 ml 0.9% NaCl or D_5W.

Rate of administration • May give by IV push or IV intermittent infusion (piggyback). • If administering as IV intermittent infusion (piggyback), give over 15–30 min; if administered by IV push (5–20 ml), give over 3–5 min.

IV INCOMPATIBILITIES

Acyclovir (Zovirax), amphotericin B (Fungizone), diazepam (Valium), doxycycline (Vibramycin), metronidazole (Flagyl), ondansetron (Zofran).

M

IV COMPATIBILITIES

Dobutamine (Dobutrex), dopamine (Intropin), heparin, magnesium.

INDICATIONS/ROUTES/DOSAGE

Alert: Space doses evenly around the clock.

MILD-MODERATE INFECTIONS

IV: ADULTS, ELDERLY: 0.5–1 g q8h.

MENINGITIS

IV: ADULTS, ELDERLY, CHILDREN ≥50 KG: 2g q8h. CHILDREN: >3 MOS, <50 KG: 40 mg/kg q8h. **Maximum:** 2 g/dose.

USUAL PEDIATRIC DOSE

IV: CHILDREN ≥3 MOS: 20 mg/kg/dose q8h. CHILDREN <3 MOS: 20 mg/kg/dose q8–12h.

DOSAGE IN RENAL IMPAIRMENT

Reduce dosage in pts with creatinine clearance <50 ml/min.

Creatinine Clearance	Dosage	Interval
26–49 ml/min	Recommended dose (1,000 mg)	q12h
10–25 ml/min	½ recommended dose	q12h
<10 ml/min	½ recommended dose	q24h

SIDE EFFECTS

FREQUENT (3%–5%): Diarrhea, nausea, vomiting, headache, inflammation at injection site. **OCCASIONAL (2%):** Oral moniliasis, rash, pruritus. **RARE (<2%):** Constipation, glossitis.

ADVERSE REACTIONS/ TOXIC EFFECTS

Antibiotic-associated colitis, other superinfections may occur. Anaphylactic reactions in pts receiving beta lactams have occurred. Seizures may occur in those with CNS disorders (brain lesions, history of seizures), bacterial meningitis, impaired renal function.

NURSING IMPLICATIONS

BASELINE ASSESSMENT

Inquire about history of seizures.

INTERVENTION/EVALUATION

Monitor daily bowel activity/stool consistency (watery, loose, soft). Monitor for nausea, vomiting. Evaluate hydration status. Evaluate for inflammation at IV injection site. Assess skin for rash. Monitor I&O, renal function tests. Check mental status; be alert to tremors, possible seizures. Assess temperature, B/P twice daily, more often if necessary. Monitor electrolytes, esp. potassium.

mesalamine (5-aminosalicylic acid, 5-ASA)

mess-**al**-ah-meen

(Asacol, Fiv-ASA, Mesasal ♣, Pentasa, Rowasa, Salofalk ♣)

Do not confuse with Os-Cal.

CLASSIFICATION

PHARMACOTHERAPEUTIC: Salicylic acid derivative. **CLINICAL:** Anti-inflammatory agent.

ACTION

Produces local inhibitory effect on arachidonic acid metabolite production (increased in pts with chronic inflammatory bowel disease). **Therapeutic Effect:** Blocks prostaglandin production, diminishes inflammation in colon.

PHARMACOKINETICS

Poorly absorbed from colon. Moderately absorbed from GI tract. Metabolized in liver to active metabolite. Unabsorbed portion eliminated in feces; absorbed

M

portion excreted in urine. Unknown if removed by hemodialysis. **Half-life:** 0.5–1.5 hrs; metabolite: 5–10 hrs.

USES

Treatment of active mild to moderate distal ulcerative colitis, proctosigmoiditis, or proctitis. **Asacol:** Maintenance of remission of ulcerative colitis.

PRECAUTIONS

CONTRAINDICATIONS: None known. **CAUTIONS:** Preexisting renal disease, sulfasalazine sensitivity.

LIFESPAN CONSIDERATIONS: Pregnancy/lactation: Unknown if drug crosses placenta or is distributed in breast milk. **Pregnancy Category B. Children:** Safety and efficacy not established. **Elderly:** Age-related renal impairment may require cautious use.

INTERACTIONS

DRUG: None known. **HERBAL:** None known. **FOOD:** None known. **LAB VALUES:** May increase SGOT (AST), SGPT (ALT), alkaline phosphatase, BUN, serum creatinine.

AVAILABILITY (Rx)

TABLETS (delayed-release): 400 mg. **CAPSULES (controlled-release):** 250 mg. **SUPPOSITORY:** 500 mg. **RECTAL SUSPENSION:** 4 g/60 ml.

ADMINISTRATION/HANDLING

Alert: Store rectal suspension, suppository, oral forms at room temperature.

PO

• Have pt swallow whole; do not break outer coating of tablet. • Give without regard to food.

RECTAL

• Shake bottle well. • Instruct pt to lie on left side with lower leg extended, upper leg flexed forward. • Knee-chest position may also be used. • Insert applicator tip into rectum, pointing toward umbilicus. • Squeeze bottle steadily until contents are emptied.

INDICATIONS/ROUTES/DOSAGE

ULCERATIVE COLITIS, PROCTOSIGMOIDITIS, PROCTITIS

PO: (Asacol): ADULTS, ELDERLY: 800 mg 3 times/day for 6 wks. CHILDREN: 50 mg/kg/day q8–12h. **(Pentasa):** 1 g 4 times/day for 8 wks. CHILDREN: 50 mg/kg/day q6–12h.

Rectal: (Retention enema): ADULTS, ELDERLY: 60 ml (4 g) at bedtime; retain overnight, about 8 hrs, for 3–6 wks. **(Suppository):** ADULTS, ELDERLY: 1 suppository (500 mg) 2 times/day, retain 1–3 hrs for 3–6 wks.

MAINTENANCE OF REMISSION, ULCERATIVE COLITIS

PO: ADULTS, ELDERLY: **(Asacol):** 1.6 g/day in divided doses. **(Pentasa):** 1 g 4 times/day.

SIDE EFFECTS

Alert: Generally well tolerated, with only mild and transient effects.

FREQUENT (>6%): PO: Abdominal cramps/pain, diarrhea, dizziness, headache, nausea, vomiting, rhinitis, unusual tiredness. **Rectal:** Abdominal/stomach cramps, flatulence, headache, nausea. **OCCASIONAL (2%–6%): PO:** Hair loss, decreased appetite, back/joint pain, flatulence, acne. **Rectal:** Hair loss. **RARE (<2%): Rectal:** Anal irritation.

ADVERSE REACTIONS/ TOXIC EFFECTS

Sulfite sensitivity in susceptible pts noted as cramping, headache, diarrhea, fever, rash, hives, itching, wheezing. Discontinue drug immediately. Hepatitis, pancreatitis, pericarditis occur rarely with oral dosage.

NURSING IMPLICATIONS

INTERVENTION/EVALUATION

Encourage adequate fluid intake. Assess bowel sounds for peristalsis. Monitor daily bowel activity, stool consistency (watery, loose, soft, semisolid, solid); record time of evacuation. Assess for abdominal disturbances. Assess skin for rash, hives. Discontinue medication if rash, fever, cramping, diarrhea occurs.

PATIENT/FAMILY TEACHING

Avoid tasks that require alertness, motor skills until response to drug is established. May discolor urine yellow-brown. Suppositories stain fabrics.

mesna

mess-nah
(Mesnex, Uromitexan ✤)

CLASSIFICATION

PHARMACOTHERAPEUTIC: Cytoprotective agent. **CLINICAL:** Antineoplastic adjunct, antidote.

ACTION

Binds with and detoxifies urotoxic metabolites of ifosfamide/cyclophosphamide. **Therapeutic Effect:** Inhibits ifosfamide/cyclophosphamide-induced hemorrhagic cystitis.

PHARMACOKINETICS

Rapidly metabolized after IV administration to mesna disulfide, which is reduced to mesna in kidney. Excreted in urine. **Half-life:** 24 min.

USES

Detoxifying agent used as a protectant against hemorrhagic cystitis induced by ifosamide, cyclophosphamide.

PRECAUTIONS

CONTRAINDICATIONS: None known. **CAUTIONS:** None known.

LIFESPAN CONSIDERATIONS: Pregnancy/lactation: Unknown if drug crosses placenta or is distributed in breast milk. **Pregnancy Category B. Children:** Safety and efficacy not established. **Elderly:** Information not available.

INTERACTIONS

DRUG: None known. **HERBAL:** None known. **FOOD:** None known. **LAB VALUES:** May produce false-positive test for urinary ketones.

AVAILABILITY (Rx)

INJECTION: 100 mg/ml. **TABLETS:** 400 mg.

ADMINISTRATION/HANDLING

PO

• Dilute mesna solution before oral administration to decrease sulfur odor. Can be diluted in carbonated cola drinks, fruit juices, milk.

IV

Storage • Store parenteral form at room temperature. • After dilution, is stable for 24 hrs at room temperature (recommended use within 6 hrs). Discard unused medication.

Reconstitution • May dilute with D_5W or 0.9% NaCl to concentration of 1–20 mg/ml. • May add to solutions containing ifosfamide or cyclophosphamide.

Rate of administration • Administer by IV infusion over 15–30 min or by continuous infusion.

IV INCOMPATIBILITIES

Amphotericin B complex (Abelcet, AmBisome, Amphotec).

IV COMPATIBILITIES

Allopurinol (Aloprim), docetaxel (Taxotere), doxorubicin (Adriamycim), etopo-

M

side (VePesid), gemcitabine (Gemczar), granisetron (Kytril), methotrexate, ondansetron (Zofran), paclitaxel (Taxol), vinorelbine (Navelbine).

INDICATIONS/ROUTES/DOSAGE

HEMORRHAGIC CYSTITIS (ifosfamide)
IV: ADULTS, ELDERLY: 20% of ifosfamide dose at time of ifosfamide administration and 4 and 8 hrs after each dose of ifosfamide. Total dose: 60% of ifosfamide dosage.

HEMORRHAGIC CYSTITIS (cyclophosphamide)
IV: ADULTS, ELDERLY: 20% of cyclophosphamide dose at time of cyclophosphamide administration and q3h for 3–4 doses.

PO: 40% of antineoplastic agent dose in 3 doses at 4-hr intervals.

SIDE EFFECTS

FREQUENT (>17%): Bad taste in mouth, soft stools. **Large doses:** Diarrhea, limb pain, headache, fatigue, nausea, hypotension, allergic reaction.

ADVERSE REACTIONS/ TOXIC EFFECTS

Hematuria occurs rarely.

NURSING IMPLICATIONS

BASELINE ASSESSMENT
Each dose must be administered with ifosfamide.

INTERVENTION/EVALUATION
Assess morning urine specimen for hematuria. If such occurs, dosage reduction or discontinuation may be necessary. Monitor daily bowel activity/stool consistency (watery, loose, soft, semisolid, solid); record time of evacuation. Monitor B/P for hypotension.

PATIENT/FAMILY TEACHING
Inform physician/nurse if headache, limb pain, nausea occurs.

mesoridazine besylate

mess-oh-**rid**-ah-zeen
(Serentil)
Do not confuse with Proventil, Serevent.

CLASSIFICATION

PHARMACOTHERAPEUTIC: Phenothiazine. **CLINICAL:** Antipsychotic (see p. 56C).

ACTION

Blocks dopamine at postsynaptic receptor sites in brain. Possesses anticholinergic, sedative effects. **Therapeutic Effect:** Suppresses behavioral response in psychosis.

USES

Treatment of schizophrenia in pts who fail to respond to other antipsychotic medication. Treatment of alcoholism.

PRECAUTIONS

CONTRAINDICATIONS: Severe CNS depression, comatose states, severe cardiovascular disease, bone marrow depression, subcortical brain damage. **CAUTIONS:** Impaired respiratory/hepatic/renal/cardiac function, alcohol withdrawal, history of seizures, urinary retention, glaucoma, prostatic hypertrophy. **Pregnancy Category C.**

INTERACTIONS

DRUG: **Alcohol, CNS depressants** may increase CNS, respiratory depression, hypotensive effects. **Tricyclic antidepressants, MAOIs** may increase sedative, anticholinergic effects. **Antithyroid** agents may increase risk of agranulocytosis. Extrapyramidal symptoms (EPS) may increase with **EPS-producing medications. Hypotensives** may increase hypotension. May decrease **levo-**

dopa effects. **Lithium** may decrease absorption, produce adverse neurologic effects. **HERBAL:** None known. **FOOD:** None known. **LAB VALUES:** May produce false-positive pregnancy, PKU tests. EKG changes may occur, including Q- and T-wave disturbances.

AVAILABILITY (Rx)

TABLETS: 10 mg, 25 mg, 50 mg, 100 mg. **ORAL SOLUTIONS:** 25 mg/ml. **INJECTION:** 25 mg/ml.

INDICATIONS/ROUTES/DOSAGE

SCHIZOPHRENIA

PO: ADULTS, ELDERLY: 25–50 mg 3 times/day. **Maximum:** 400 mg/day.

IM: ADULTS, ELDERLY: Initially, 25 mg. May repeat in 30–60 min. RANGE: 25–200 mg.

BEHAVIORAL SYMPTOMS

PO: ELDERLY: Initially, 10 mg 1–2 times/day. May increase at 4- to 7-day intervals. **Maximum:** 250 mg.

IM: ADULTS; ELDERLY: Initially, 25 mg. May repeat in 30–60 min. RANGE: 25-200 mg.

SIDE EFFECTS

FREQUENT: Orthostatic hypotension, dizziness, syncope occur frequently after first injection, occasionally after subsequent injections, rarely with oral dosage. **OCCASIONAL:** Drowsiness during early therapy, dry mouth, blurred vision, lethargy, constipation/diarrhea, nasal congestion, peripheral edema, urinary retention. **RARE:** Ocular changes, skin pigmentation (those taking high dosages for prolonged periods).

ADVERSE REACTIONS/ TOXIC EFFECTS

Abrupt withdrawal following long-term therapy may precipitate nausea, vomiting, gastritis, dizziness, tremors. Blood dyscrasias, particularly agranulocytosis, mild leukopenia may occur. May lower seizure threshold.

NURSING IMPLICATIONS

BASELINE ASSESSMENT

Avoid skin contact with solution (contact dermatitis). Assess behavior, appearance, emotional status, response to environment, speech pattern, thought content.

INTERVENTION/EVALUATION

Assess for orthostatic hypotension. Monitor stool frequency, consistency (watery, loose, soft, semisolid, solid). Supervise suicidal-risk pt closely during early therapy (as depression lessens, energy level improves, increasing suicide potential). Assess for therapeutic response (interest in surroundings, improvement in self-care, increased ability to concentrate, relaxed facial expression).

PATIENT/FAMILY TEACHING

Full therapeutic effect may take up to 6 wks. Urine may become pink, reddish brown. Do not abruptly withdraw from long-term drug therapy. Report visual disturbances. Drowsiness generally subsides during continued therapy. Do not use alcohol, other CNS depressants.

M

metaproterenol sulfate

met-ah-pro-**tair**-in-all
(Alupent)

Do not confuse with Atrovent, metipranolol, metoprolol.

CLASSIFICATION

PHARMACOTHERAPEUTIC: Sympathomimetic (an adrenergic agonist). **CLINICAL:** Bronchodilator (see p. 64C).

ACTION

Stimulates beta$_2$-adrenergic receptors, resulting in relaxation of bronchial smooth muscle. **Therapeutic Effect:** Relieves bronchospasm; reduces airway resistance.

USES

Relief of reversible bronchospasm due to bronchial asthma, bronchitis, emphysema.

PRECAUTIONS

CONTRAINDICATIONS: Preexisting cardiac arrhythmias associated with tachycardia, narrow-angle glaucoma. **CAUTIONS:** Ischemic heart disease, hypertension, hyperthyroidism, seizure disorder, CHF, diabetes, arrhythmias. **Pregnancy Category C.**

M

INTERACTIONS

DRUG: **Tricyclic antidepressants** may increase cardiovascular effects. **MAOIs** may increase risk of hypertensive crises. May decrease effects of **beta-blockers. Digoxin, other sympathomimetics** may increase risk of arrhythmias. **HERBAL: Ma huang (ephedra)** may increase CNS effects. **FOOD:** None known. **LAB VALUES:** May decrease serum potassium levels.

AVAILABILITY (Rx)

SOLUTION FOR ORAL INHALATION: 0.4%, 0.6%, 5%. **SYRUP:** 10 mg/5 ml. **TABLETS:** 10 mg, 20 mg.

INDICATIONS/ROUTES/DOSAGE

BRONCHOSPASM

PO: ADULTS, CHILDREN >9 YRS: 20 mg 3–4 times/day. ELDERLY: 10 mg 3–4 times/day. May increase to 20 mg/dose. CHILDREN 6–9 YRS: 10 mg 3–4 times/day. CHILDREN 2–5 YRS: 1.3–2.6 mg/kg/day in 3–4 divided doses. CHILDREN <2 YRS: 0.4 mg/kg 3–4 times/day.

Inhalation: ADULTS, ELDERLY, CHILDREN >12 YRS: 2–3 inhalations q3–4h. **Maximum:** 12 inhalations/24 hrs.

Nebulization: ADULTS, ELDERLY, CHILDREN >12 YRS: 10–15 mg (0.2–0.3 ml) of 5% q4–6h. CHILDREN <12 YRS, INFANTS: 0.5–1 mg/kg (0.01–0.02 ml/kg) of 5% q4–6h.

SIDE EFFECTS

FREQUENT (>10%): Shakiness, nervousness, nausea, dry mouth. **OCCASIONAL (1%–9%):** Dizziness, vertigo, weakness, headache, GI distress, vomiting, cough, dry throat. **RARE (<1%):** Drowsiness, diarrhea, unusual taste.

ADVERSE REACTIONS/ TOXIC EFFECTS

Excessive sympathomimetic stimulation may cause palpitations, extrasystoles, tachycardia, chest pain, slight increase in B/P followed by a substantial decrease, chills, diaphoresis, blanching of skin. Too frequent or excessive use may lead to loss of bronchodilating effectiveness and/or severe, paradoxical bronchoconstriction.

NURSING IMPLICATIONS

BASELINE ASSESSMENT

Offer emotional support (high incidence of anxiety because of difficulty in breathing, sympathomimetic response to drug).

INTERVENTION/EVALUATION

Monitor rate, depth, rhythm, type of respiration; quality/rate of pulse. Assess lung sounds for rhonchi, wheezing, rales. Monitor ABGs, pulmonary function tests. Observe lips, fingernails for blue/dusky color in light-skinned pts; gray in dark-skinned pts. Evaluate for clinical improvement (quieter, slower respirations; relaxed facial expression; cessation of clavicular, sternal, intercostal retractions).

PATIENT/FAMILY TEACHING

Increase fluid intake (decreases lung secretion viscosity). Do not exceed recommended dosage. May cause nervousness, restlessness, inability to sleep. Inform physician if palpitations, tachycardia, chest pain, tremors, dizziness, headache, flushing, difficulty in breathing persists. Avoid excessive use of caffeine derivatives (chocolate, coffee, tea, cola, cocoa).

metformin hydrochloride

met-**for**-min

(Glucophage, Glucophage XL, Glycon ✤, Novo-Metformin ✤, Riomet)

FIXED-COMBINATION(S)

Glucovance: metformin/glyburide (an antidiabetic): 250 mg/1.25 mg; 500 mg/2.5 mg; 500 mg/5 mg. **Metaglip:** metformin/glipizide (an antidiabetic): 250 mg/2.5 mg; 500 mg/2.5 mg; 500 mg/5 mg. **Avandamet:** metformin/rosiglitazone (an antidiabetic): 500 mg/1 mg; 500 mg/2 mg; 500 mg/4 mg; 1,000 mg/2 mg; 1,000 mg/4 mg.

CLASSIFICATION

PHARMACOTHERAPEUTIC: Antihyperglycemic. **CLINICAL:** Antidiabetic (see p. 40C).

ACTION

Decreases liver production of glucose, decreases absorption of glucose, improves insulin sensitivity. **Therapeutic Effect:** Provides improvement in glycemic control, stabilizes/decreases body weight, improves lipid profile.

PHARMACOKINETICS

Slowly, incompletely absorbed after PO administration (food delays/decreases extent of absorption). Protein binding: Negligible. Primarily distributed to intestinal mucosa, salivary glands. Primarily excreted unchanged in urine. Removed by hemodialysis. **Half-life:** 3–6 hrs.

USES

Management of type 2 diabetes mellitus as monotherapy or concomitantly with an oral sulfonylurea or insulin. **Unlabeled:** Treatment of metabolic complications of AIDS, weight reduction, prediabetes.

PRECAUTIONS

CONTRAINDICATIONS: Renal disease/dysfunction, cardiovascular collapse, respiratory failure, acute MI, acute CHF, septicemia.

Alert: Lactic acidosis, a rare but potentially severe consequence of metformin therapy. Withhold in pts with conditions that may predispose to lactic acidosis (e.g., hypoxemia, dehydration, hypoperfusion, sepsis).

CAUTIONS: Conditions delaying food absorption (e.g., diarrhea, high fever, malnutrition, gastroparesis, vomiting), causing hyperglycemia or hypoglycemia, uncontrolled hypothyroidism/hyperthyroidism, cardiovascular pts, concurrent drugs that affect renal function, hepatic impairment, elderly, malnourished/debilitated pts with decreased renal function, CHF, excessive alcohol intake, chronic respiratory difficulty.

LIFESPAN CONSIDERATIONS: Pregnancy/lactation: Insulin is drug of

M

choice during pregnancy. Distributed in breast milk in animals. **Pregnancy Category B.** **Children:** Safety and efficacy not established. **Elderly:** Age-related renal impairment or peripheral vascular disease may require dosage adjustment or discontinuation.

INTERACTIONS

DRUG: **Alcohol, amiloride, digoxin, morphine, procainamide, quinidine, quinine, ranitidine, triamterene, trimethoprim, vancomycin, cimetidine, furosemide, nifedipine** increase metformin concentration. **Furosemide, hypoglycemia-causing medication** may decrease dosage of metformin needed. **Iodinated contrast studies** may produce acute renal failure (increases risk of lactic acidosis). **HERBAL:** None known. **FOOD:** None known. **LAB VALUES:** None known.

M

AVAILABILITY (Rx)

TABLETS: 500 mg, 850 mg, 1,000 mg. **TABLETS (extended-release):** 500 mg, 750 mg. **ORAL SOLUTION:** 100 mg/ml.

ADMINISTRATION/HANDLING

PO

- Do not crush film-coated tablets.
- Give with meals.

INDICATIONS/ROUTES/DOSAGE

DIABETES MELLITUS (500-mg, 1,000-mg tablet)

PO: ADULTS, ELDERLY: Initially, 500 mg twice daily (with morning and evening meals). May increase dosage in 500-mg increments every week, in divided doses. Can be given twice daily up to 2,000 mg/day (e.g., 1,000 mg twice daily with morning and evening meals). If 2,500 mg/day dose is required, give 3 times/day with meals. **Maximum dose/day:** 2,500 mg/day. CHILDREN 10–16 YRS: Initially, 500 mg 2 times/day. May increase by 500 mg/day at weekly intervals. **Maximum:** 2,000 mg/day.

DIABETES MELLITUS (850-mg tablet)

PO: ADULTS, ELDERLY: Initially, 850-mg/day, with morning meal. May increase dosage in 850-mg increments every **other** week, in divided doses. MAINTENANCE: 850 mg twice daily (with morning and evening meals). **Maximum dose/day:** 2,550 mg (850 mg 3 times/day).

DIABETES MELLITUS (extended-release tablets)

PO: ADULTS, ELDERLY: Initially, 500 mg once daily. May increase by 500 mg/day at weekly intervals. **Maximum:** 2,000 mg/day once daily.

ADJUNCT TO INSULIN THERAPY

PO: ADULTS, ELDERLY: Initially, 500 mg/day. May increase by 500 mg at 7-day intervals. **Maximum:** 2,500 mg (2,000 mg for extended release).

Alert: Decreased insulin dosage may be needed if blood sugar falls below 120 mg/dl.

SIDE EFFECTS

OCCASIONAL (>3%): GI disturbances are transient and resolve spontaneously during therapy (diarrhea, nausea, vomiting, abdominal bloating, flatulence, anorexia). **RARE (1%–3%):** Unpleasant/metallic taste (resolves spontaneously during therapy).

ADVERSE REACTIONS/ TOXIC EFFECTS

Lactic acidosis occurs rarely (0.03 cases/1,000 pts) but is a serious, often fatal (50%) complication. Characterized by increase in blood lactate levels (>5 mmol/L), decrease in blood pH, electrolyte disturbances. Symptoms include unexplained hyperventilation, myalgia, malaise, somnolence. May advance to cardiovascular collapse (shock), acute CHF, acute MI, prerenal azotemia.

NURSING IMPLICATIONS

BASELINE ASSESSMENT

Inform pt of potential risks/advantages of therapy (see Adverse Reactions/Toxic Effects) and of alternative modes of therapy. Prior to initiation of therapy and annually thereafter, assess Hgb, Hct, RBC, serum creatinine.

INTERVENTION/EVALUATION

Monitor fasting blood glucose, Hgb A, renal function. Monitor folic acid, renal function tests for evidence of early lactic acidosis. If pt is on concurrent oral sulfonylureas, assess for hypoglycemia (cool/wet skin, tremors, dizziness, anxiety, headache, tachycardia, numbness in mouth, hunger, diplopia). Be alert to conditions that alter glucose requirements: fever, increased activity/stress, surgical procedure.

PATIENT/FAMILY TEACHING

Discontinue metformin, contact physician immediately if evidence of lactic acidosis appears (unexplained hyperventilation, muscle aches, extreme tiredness, unusual sleepiness). Prescribed diet is principal part of treatment; do not skip/delay meals. Diabetes mellitus requires lifelong control. Avoid alcohol. Inform physician if headache, nausea, vomiting, diarrhea persist or skin rash, unusual bruising/bleeding, change in color of urine/stool occurs.

methadone hydrochloride

meth-ah-doan
(Dolophine, Metadol✤, Methadose)

CLASSIFICATION

PHARMACOTHERAPEUTIC: Narcotic agonist. **CLINICAL:** Opioid analgesic **(Schedule II)** (see p. 121C).

ACTION

Binds with opioid receptors within CNS. **Therapeutic Effect:** Alters processes affecting analgesia, emotional response to acute withdrawal syndrome.

PHARMACOKINETICS

Onset	Peak	Duration
PO		
30–60 min	0.5–1 hr	6–8 hrs
Subcutaneous		
10–15 min	1–2 hrs	4–6 hrs
IM		
10–15 min	1–2 hrs	4–6 hrs

Well absorbed after IM injection. Protein binding: 80%–85%. Metabolized in liver. Primarily excreted in urine. Not removed by hemodialysis. **Half-life:** 15–25 hrs.

M

USES

Relief of severe pain, detoxification, temporary maintenance treatment of narcotic abstinence syndrome.

PRECAUTIONS

CONTRAINDICATIONS: Hypersensitivity to narcotics, diarrhea due to poisoning, delivery of premature infant, during labor. **EXTREME CAUTION:** Impaired renal/hepatic function, elderly/debilitated, supraventricular tachycardia, cor pulmonale, history of seizures, acute abdominal conditions, increased intracranial pressure, respiratory abnormalities.

LIFESPAN CONSIDERATIONS: Pregnancy/lactation: Crosses placenta. Distributed in breast milk. Respiratory depression may occur in neonate if mother received opiates during labor. Regular use of opiates during pregnancy may produce withdrawal symptoms in neonate (irritability, excessive crying, tremors, hyperactive reflexes, fever, vomiting, diarrhea, yawning, sneezing, seizures). **Pregnancy Category B** (**D** if used for prolonged periods or at high dosages at term). **Children:** Paradoxical excitement may occur. Those <2 yrs more susceptible to respiratory depressant effects. **Elderly:** More susceptible to respiratory depressant effects. Age-related renal impairment may increase risk of urinary retention.

INTERACTIONS

DRUG: Alcohol, CNS depressants may increase CNS or respiratory depression, hypotension. **MAOIs** may produce severe, fatal reaction (reduce dose to ¼ usual dose). **HERBAL: Valerian** may increase CNS depression. **FOOD:** None known. **LAB VALUES:** May increase amylase, lipase.

M

AVAILABILITY (Rx)

TABLETS: 5 mg, 10 mg. **TABLETS (dispersible):** 40 mg. **ORAL SOLUTION:** 5 mg/5 ml, 10 mg/5 ml. **ORAL CONCENTRATE:** 10 mg/ml. **INJECTION:** 10 mg/ml.

ADMINISTRATION/HANDLING

PO

• Give without regard to meals. • Dilute syrup in glass of H_2O (prevents anesthetic effect on mucous membranes).

SUBCUTANEOUS/IM

Alert: IM preferred over subcutaneous route (subcutaneous produces pain, local irritation, induration).

• Do not use if solution appears cloudy or contains a precipitate. • Administer slowly. • Those with circulating impairment experience higher risk of overdosage due to delayed absorption of repeated administration.

INDICATIONS/ROUTES/DOSAGE

ANALGESIA

PO/IM/IV/subcutaneous: ADULTS: 2.5–10 mg q3–8h as needed up to 5–20 mg q6–8h. ELDERLY: 2.5 mg q8–12h. CHILDREN: Initially, 0.1 mg/kg/dose q4h for 2–3 doses, then q6–12h. **Maximum:** 10 mg/dose.

DETOXIFICATION

PO: ADULTS, ELDERLY: 15–40 mg/day.

MAINTENANCE OF OPIATE DEPENDENCE

PO: ADULTS, ELDERLY: 20–120 mg/day.

SIDE EFFECTS

FREQUENT: Sedation, decreased B/P, diaphoresis, flushed face, constipation, dizziness, nausea, vomiting. **OCCASIONAL:** Confusion, decreased urination, pounding heartbeat, stomach cramps, visual changes, dry mouth, headache, decreased appetite, nervousness, inability to sleep. **RARE:** Allergic reaction (rash, itching).

ADVERSE REACTIONS/ TOXIC EFFECTS

Overdosage results in respiratory depression, skeletal muscle flaccidity, cold/clammy skin, cyanosis, extreme somnolence progressing to convulsions, stupor, coma. **ANTIDOTE:** 0.4 mg naloxone (Narcan). Tolerance to analgesic effect, physical dependence may occur with repeated use.

NURSING IMPLICATIONS

BASELINE ASSESSMENT

Pt should be in recumbent position prior to drug administration by parenteral route. Obtain vital signs before giving medication. If respirations are ≤12/min (≤20/min in children), withhold medication, contact physician.

INTERVENTION/EVALUATION

Monitor vital signs 15–30 min after subcutaneous/IM dose, 5–10 min following IV dose. Oral medication is one-half as potent as parenteral. Assess for adequate voiding. Assess for clinical improvement, record onset of relief of pain. Provide support to pt in detoxification program; monitor for withdrawal symptoms.

PATIENT/FAMILY TEACHING

Avoid alcohol. Do not stop taking abruptly after prolonged use. May cause dry mouth, drowsiness; impair ability to perform activities requiring mental alertness (e.g., driving).

methimazole

meth-**im**-ah-zole
(Tapazole)

CLASSIFICATION

PHARMACOTHERAPEUTIC: Thiomidazole derivative. **CLINICAL:** Antithyroid.

ACTION

Inhibits synthesis of thyroid hormone by interfering with incorporation of iodine into tyrosyl residues. **Therapeutic Effect:** Effective in the treatment of hyperthyroidism.

USES

Treatment of hyperthyroidism. Used to attain a normal metabolic state before thyroidectomy, to control thyrotoxic crisis that may accompany thyroidectomy.

PRECAUTIONS

CONTRAINDICATIONS: None known. **CAUTIONS:** Pts >40 yrs or in combination with other agranulocytosis-inducing drugs, impaired liver function. **Pregnancy Category D.**

INTERACTIONS

DRUG: Amiodarone, iodinated glycerol, iodine, potassium iodide may decrease response. May decrease effect of **oral anticoagulants.** May increase concentration of **digoxin** (as pt becomes euthyroid). May decrease thyroid uptake of ^{131}**I. HERBAL:** None known. **FOOD:** None known. **LAB VALUES:** May increase SGOT (AST), SGPT (ALT), alkaline phosphatase, LDH, bilirubin, prothrombin time. May decrease prothrombin level, WBC count.

AVAILABILITY (Rx)

TABLETS: 5 mg, 10 mg.

INDICATIONS/ROUTES/DOSAGE

HYPERTHYROIDISM

PO: ADULTS, ELDERLY: Initially, 15–60 mg/day in 3 divided doses. MAINTENANCE: 5–15 mg/day. CHILDREN: Initially, 0.4 mg/kg/day in 3 divided doses. MAINTENANCE: One-half the initial dose.

M

SIDE EFFECTS

FREQUENT (3%–5%): Fever, rash, pruritus. **OCCASIONAL (1%–3%):** Dizziness, loss of taste, nausea, vomiting, stomach pain, peripheral neuropathy (numbness in fingers, toes, face). **RARE (<1%):** Swollen lymph nodes/salivary glands.

ADVERSE REACTIONS/ TOXIC EFFECTS

Agranulocytosis (which may occur as long as 4 mos after therapy); pancytopenia, hepatitis have occurred.

NURSING IMPLICATIONS

BASELINE ASSESSMENT

Obtain baseline weight, pulse.

INTERVENTION/EVALUATION

Monitor pulse, weight daily. Assess skin for rash, pruritus, swollen lymph glands. Monitor CBC with differential, hepatic function, prothrombin time. Assess for signs of infection, bleeding.

PATIENT/FAMILY TEACHING

Do not exceed ordered dose. Space doses evenly around the clock. Take resting pulse daily to monitor therapeutic results. Seafood, iodine products may be restricted. Report illness, unusual bleeding/bruising immediately.

methocarbamol

(Robaxin)

FIXED-COMBINATION(S)

With aspirin, a salicylate **(Robaxisal).**
See Classification section under: Skeletal muscle relaxants

methohexital sodium

(Brevital)

See Classification section under: Anesthetics: general (p. 2C)

methotrexate sodium

meth-oh-**trex**-ate
(Rheumatrex)

CLASSIFICATION

PHARMACOTHERAPEUTIC: Antimetabolite. **CLINICAL:** Antineoplastic, antiarthritic, antipsoriatic (see p. 74C).

ACTION

Competes with enzymes necessary to reduce folic acid to tetrahydrofolic acid, a component essential to DNA, RNA, protein synthesis. **Therapeutic Effect:** Inhibits DNA, RNA, protein synthesis.

PHARMACOKINETICS

Variably absorbed from GI tract. Completely absorbed after IM administration. Protein binding: 50%–60%. Widely distributed. Metabolized in liver, intracellularly. Primarily excreted in urine. Removed by hemodialysis; not removed by peritoneal dialysis. **Half-life:** 8–12 hrs (large doses: 8–15 hrs).

USES

Treatment of trophoblastic neoplasms (gestational choriocarcinoma, chorioadenoma destruens, hydatidiform mole), acute leukemias, breast cancer, epidermoid cancers of head/neck, lung cancer, advanced stages of lymphosarcoma, mycosis fungoides, meningeal leukemia, severe psoriasis, rheumatoid arthritis. **Unlabeled:** Treatment of cervical, ovarian, bladder, renal, prostatic, testicular carcinoma; acute myelocytic leukemia; psoriatic arthritis; systemic dermatomyositis.

PRECAUTIONS

CONTRAINDICATIONS: Severe renal/liver impairment, preexisting bone marrow suppression. **CAUTIONS:** Peptic ulcer, ulcerative colitis, bone marrow suppression, ascites, pleural effusion.

LIFESPAN CONSIDERATIONS: Pregnancy/lactation: Avoid pregnancy during methotrexate therapy and minimum 3 mos after therapy in males or at least one ovulatory cycle after therapy in females. May cause fetal death, congenital anomalies. Drug is distributed in breast milk. Breast-feeding not recommended. **Pregnancy Category D** (**X** for psoriasis or rheumatoid arthritis pts). **Children/**

elderly: Decreased renal/liver function requires caution; may require dosage adjustment.

INTERACTIONS

DRUG: **Parenteral acyclovir** may increase neurotoxicity. **Alcohol, hepatotoxic medications** may increase hepatotoxicity. **NSAIDs** may increase toxicity. **Asparaginase** may decrease effects of methotrexate. **Bone marrow depressants** may increase bone marrow depression. **Probenecid, salicylates** may increase concentration, toxicity. **Live virus vaccines** may potentiate virus replication, increase vaccine side effects, decrease pt's antibody response to vaccine. **HERBAL:** None known. **FOOD:** None known. **LAB VALUES:** May increase uric acid, SGOT (AST).

AVAILABILITY (Rx)

TABLETS: 2.5 mg, 5 mg, 7.5 mg, 10 mg, 15 mg. **POWDER FOR INJECTION:** 20 mg, 1 g. **INJECTION:** 25 mg/ml. **INJECTION (preservative-free):** 25 mg/ml.

ADMINISTRATION/HANDLING

Alert: May be carcinogenic, mutagenic, or teratogenic. Handle with extreme care during preparation/administration. Wear gloves when preparing solution. If powder or solution comes in contact with skin, wash immediately, thoroughly with soap, water. May give IM, IV, intra-arterially, intrathecally.

IV

Storage • Store vials at room temperature.

Reconstitution • Reconstitute each 5 mg with 2 ml Sterile Water for Injection or 0.9% NaCl to provide a concentration of 2.5 mg/ml. Maximum concentration 25 mg/ml. • May further dilute with D_5W or 0.9% NaCl. • For intrathecal use, dilute with preservative-free 0.9% NaCl to provide a 1 mg/ml concentration.

Rate of administration • Give IV push at rate of 10 mg/min. • Give IV infusion over 30 min–4 hrs.

IV INCOMPATIBILITIES

Chlorpromazine (Thorazine), droperidol (Inapsine), gemcitabine (Gemzar), idarubicin (Idamycin), midazolam (Versed), nalbuphine (Nubain).

IV COMPATIBILITIES

Cisplatin (Platinol AQ), cyclophosphamide (Cytoxan), daunorubicin (DaunoXome), doxorubicin (Adriamycin), etoposide (VePesid), fluorouracil, granisetron (Kytril), leucovorin, mitomycin (Mutamycin), ondansetron (Zofran), paclitaxel (Taxol), vinblastine (Velban), vincristine (Oncovin), vinorelbine (Navelbine).

INDICATIONS/ROUTES/DOSAGE

Alert: Refer to individual protocols.

TROPHOBLASTIC NEOPLASMS
PO/IM: ADULTS, ELDERLY: 15–30 mg/day for 5 days; repeat in 7 days for 3–5 courses.

HEAD/NECK CANCER
PO/IM/IV: ADULTS, ELDERLY: 25–50 mg/m² once weekly.

RHEUMATOID ARTHRITIS
PO: ADULTS, ELDERLY: 7.5 mg once weekly or 2.5 mg q12h for 3 doses/wk. **Maximum:** 20 mg/wk.

PSORIASIS
PO: ADULTS, ELDERLY: 2.5–5 mg/dose q12h for 3 doses/wk given once weekly.

PO/IM: 10–25 mg once weekly.

CHORIOCARCINOMA, CHORIOADENOMA DESTRUENS, HYDATIDIFORM MOLE
IM/PO: ADULTS, ELDERLY: 15–30 mg/day for 5 days; repeat 3–5 times with 1–2 wks between courses.

ACUTE LYMPHOCYTIC LEUKEMIA
IM/IV/PO: ADULTS, ELDERLY: INDUCTION: 3.3 mg/m²/day (in combination).

IM/PO: MAINTENANCE: 30 $mg/m^2/wk$ in divided doses.

IV: 2.5 mg/kg q14days.

BURKITT'S LYMPHOMA

PO: ADULTS: 10–25 mg/day for 4–8 days; repeat with 7- to 10-day rest between courses.

LYMPHOSARCOMA

PO: ADULTS, ELDERLY: 0.625–2.5 mg/kg/day.

MYCOSIS FUNGOIDES

PO: ADULTS, ELDERLY: 2.5–10 mg/day.

IM: 50 mg/wk or 25 mg 2 times/wk.

JUVENILE RHEUMATOID ARTHRITIS

PO/IM/subcutaneous: CHILDREN: 5–15 $mg/m^2/wk$ as a single dose or in 3 divided doses given 12 hrs apart.

USUAL ANTINEOPLASTIC DOSAGE FOR CHILDREN

M

Alert: Refer to individual protocols.

PO/IM: 7.5–30 $mg/m^2/wk$ or q2wks.

IV: 10–33,000 mg/m^2 bolus or continuous infusion over 6–42 hrs.

SIDE EFFECTS

FREQUENT (3%–10%): Nausea, vomiting, stomatitis. In psoriatic pts, burning, erythema at psoriatic site. **OCCASIONAL (1%–3%):** Diarrhea, rash, dermatitis, pruritus, alopecia, dizziness, anorexia, malaise, headache, drowsiness, blurred vision.

ADVERSE REACTIONS/ TOXIC EFFECTS

High potential for various, severe toxicity. GI toxicity may produce oral ulcers of mouth, gingivitis, glossitis, pharyngitis, stomatitis, enteritis, hematemesis. Hepatotoxicity occurs more frequently with frequent, small doses than with large, intermittent doses. Pulmonary toxicity characterized as interstitial pneumonitis. Hematologic toxicity resulting from marked bone marrow depression may be manifested as leukopenia, thrombocytopenia, anemia, hemorrhage (may develop rapidly). Skin toxicity produces rash, pruritus, urticaria, pigmentation, photosensitivity, petechiae, ecchymosis, pustules. Severe nephropathy produces azotemia, hematuria, renal failure.

NURSING IMPLICATIONS

BASELINE ASSESSMENT

Question for possibility of pregnancy before initiating therapy (Pregnancy Category X) in pts with psoriasis, rheumatoid arthritis. Obtain all functional tests prior to therapy, repeat throughout therapy. Antiemetics may prevent nausea, vomiting.

INTERVENTION/EVALUATION

Monitor hepatic/renal function tests, Hgb, Hct, WBC, differential, platelet count, urinalysis, chest x-rays, serum uric acid level. Monitor for hematologic toxicity (fever, sore throat, signs of local infection, unusual bruising/bleeding from any site), symptoms of anemia (excessive tiredness, weakness). Assess skin for evidence of dermatologic toxicity. Keep pt well hydrated, urine alkaline. Avoid IM injections, rectal temperatures, traumas that induce bleeding. Apply 5 full min of pressure to IV sites.

PATIENT/FAMILY TEACHING

Maintain fastidious oral hygiene. Do not have immunizations without physician's approval (drug lowers body's resistance). Avoid crowds, those with infection. Avoid alcohol, salicylates. Avoid sunlamp/sunlight exposure. Use contraceptive measures during therapy and for 3 mos (males) or one ovulatory cycle (females) after therapy. Promptly report fever, sore throat, signs of local infection, unusual bruising/bleeding from any site. Alopecia is reversible, but new hair growth may have different color, texture. Contact physician if nausea/vomiting continues at home.

methylcellulose

meth-ill-**cell**-you-los
(Citrucel, Cologel)
Do not confuse with Citracal.

CLASSIFICATION

CLINICAL: Bulk-forming laxative (see p. 104C).

ACTION

Dissolves and expands in water. **Therapeutic Effect:** Provides increased bulk, moisture content in stool, increasing peristalsis, bowel motility.

PHARMACOKINETICS

Onset	Peak	Duration
PO		
12–24 hrs	—	—

Full effect may not be evident for 2–3 days. Acts in small/large intestine.

USES

Prophylaxis in those who should not strain during defecation. Facilitates defecation in those with diminished colonic motor response.

PRECAUTIONS

CONTRAINDICATIONS: Abdominal pain, nausea, vomiting, symptoms of appendicitis, partial bowel obstruction, dysphagia. **CAUTIONS:** None known.

LIFESPAN CONSIDERATIONS: Pregnancy/lactation: Safe for use in pregnancy. **Pregnancy Category C. Children:** Safety and efficacy not established in those <6 yrs. Not recommended in this age group. **Elderly:** No age-related precautions noted.

INTERACTIONS

DRUG: May interfere with effects of **potassium-sparing diuretics, potassium supplements.** May decrease effect of **oral anticoagulants, digoxin, salicylates** by decreasing absorption. **HERBAL:** None known. **FOOD:** None known. **LAB VALUES:** May increase glucose. May decrease potassium.

AVAILABILITY (OTC)

POWDER.

ADMINISTRATION/HANDLING

PO

- Instruct pt to drink 6–8 glasses of water/day (aids stool softening).
- Not to be swallowed in dry form; mix with at least 1 full glass (8 oz) of liquid.

INDICATIONS/ROUTES/DOSAGE

LAXATIVE

PO: ADULTS, ELDERLY: 1 tbsp (15 ml) in 8 oz water 1–3 times/day. CHILDREN 6–12 YRS: 1 tsp (5 ml) in 4 oz water 3–4 times/day.

SIDE EFFECTS

RARE: Some degree of abdominal discomfort, nausea, mild cramps, griping, faintness.

ADVERSE REACTIONS/ TOXIC EFFECTS

Esophageal/bowel obstruction may occur if administered with insufficient liquid (<250 ml or 1 full glass).

NURSING IMPLICATIONS

INTERVENTION/EVALUATION

Encourage adequate fluid intake. Assess bowel sounds for peristalsis. Monitor daily bowel activity/stool consistency (watery, loose, soft, semisolid, solid); record time of evacuation.

M

Monitor serum electrolytes in those exposed to prolonged, frequent, excessive use of medication.

PATIENT/FAMILY TEACHING

Institute measures to promote defecation: increase fluid intake, exercise, high-fiber diet.

methyldopa

meth-ill-**doe**-pah

(Aldomet, Apo-Methyldopa ♣, Novo-medopa ♣)

Do not confuse with Anzemet.

FIXED-COMBINATION(S)

Aldoril: methyldopa/hydrochlorothiazide (a diuretic): 250 mg/15 mg; 250 mg/25 mg; 500 mg/30 mg; 500 mg/50 mg.

◆CLASSIFICATION

PHARMACOTHERAPEUTIC: Alpha-adrenergic agonist. **CLINICAL:** Antihypertensive (see p. 52C).

ACTION

Stimulates central inhibitory alpha-adrenergic receptors (lowers arterial pressure, reduces plasma renin activity). **Therapeutic Effect:** Reduces standing, supine B/P.

USES

Management of moderate to severe hypertension.

PRECAUTIONS

CONTRAINDICATIONS: Liver disease, pheochromocytoma. **CAUTIONS:** Renal impairment. **Pregnancy Category B.**

INTERACTIONS

DRUG: **Tricyclic antidepressants, NSAIDs** may decrease effect. **Hypotensive-producing medications** may increase effect. May increase risk of toxicity of **lithium.** May cause hyperexcitability with **MAOIs. Sympathomimetics** may decrease effects. **HERBAL:** None known. **FOOD:** None known. **LAB VALUES:** May increase SGOT (AST), SGPT (ALT), alkaline phosphatase, bilirubin, BUN, creatinine, potassium, sodium, prolactin, uric acid. May produce false-positive Coombs' test, prolong prothrombin time.

AVAILABILITY (Rx)

TABLETS: 125 mg, 250 mg, 500 mg. **ORAL SUSPENSION:** 250 mg/5 ml. **INJECTION:** 250 mg/5 ml.

INDICATIONS/ROUTES/DOSAGE

HYPERTENSION

PO: ADULTS: Initially, 250 mg 2–3 times/day for 2 days. Adjust dosage at intervals of 2 days (minimum). ELDERLY: Initially, 125 mg 1–2 times/day. May increase by 125 mg q2–3days. MAINTENANCE: 500 mg to 2 g/day in 2–4 divided doses. CHILDREN: Initially, 10 mg/kg/day in 2–4 divided doses. Adjust dosage at intervals of 2 days (minimum). **Maximum:** 65 mg/kg/day or 3 g/day, whichever is less.

IV: ADULTS: 250–1,000 mg q6–8h. **Maximum:** 4 g/day. CHILDREN: Initially, 2–4 mg/kg/dose. May increase to 5–10 mg/kg/dose in 4–6 hrs if no response. **Maximum:** 65 mg/kg/day or 3 g/day, whichever is less.

SIDE EFFECTS

FREQUENT: Peripheral edema, drowsiness, headache, dry mouth. **OCCASIONAL:** Mental changes (e.g., anxiety, depression), decreased sexual function/interest, diarrhea, swelling of breasts, nausea, vomiting, lightheadedness, numbness in hands/feet, rhinitis.

ADVERSE REACTIONS/ TOXIC EFFECTS

Hepatotoxicity (abnormal liver function tests, jaundice, hepatitis), hemolytic anemia, unexplained fever/flulike symptoms: discontinue medication, contact physician.

NURSING IMPLICATIONS

BASELINE ASSESSMENT

Obtain baseline B/P, pulse, weight.

INTERVENTION/EVALUATION

Monitor B/P, pulse closely q30min until stabilized. Monitor weight daily during initial therapy. Monitor liver function tests. Assess for peripheral edema of hands, feet (usually, first area of low extremity swelling is behind medial malleolus in ambulatory, sacral area in bedridden).

PATIENT/FAMILY TEACHING

Avoid alcohol; may cause drowsiness. Avoid tasks requiring mental alertness, motor skills until response to drug is established.

methylergonovine

meth-ill-er-go-**noe**-veen
(Methergine)

CLASSIFICATION

PHARMACOTHERAPEUTIC: Ergot alkaloid. **CLINICAL:** Uterine stimulant.

ACTION

Stimulates alpha-adrenergic, serotonin receptors, producing arterial vasoconstriction. Causes vasospasm of coronary arteries. Directly stimulates uterine muscle. **Therapeutic Effect:** Increases strength, frequency of contractions, decreases uterine bleeding.

PHARMACOKINETICS

Onset	Peak	Duration
PO		
5–10 min	—	—
IM		
2–5 min	—	—
IV		
Immediate	—	3 hrs

Rapidly absorbed from GI tract, after IM administration. Distributed rapidly to plasma, extracellular fluid, tissues. Metabolized in liver (undergoes first-pass effect). Primarily excreted in urine.

USES

Prevents/treats postpartum, postabortion hemorrhage due to atony/involution (not for induction, augmentation of labor). **Unlabeled:** Treatment of incomplete abortion.

PRECAUTIONS

CONTRAINDICATIONS: Hypertension, pregnancy, toxemia, untreated hypocalcemia. **CAUTIONS:** Renal/hepatic impairment, coronary artery disease, occlusive peripheral vascular disease, sepsis.

LIFESPAN CONSIDERATIONS: Pregnancy/lactation: Contraindicated during pregnancy. Small amounts in breast milk. **Pregnancy Category C. Children/elderly:** No information available.

INTERACTIONS

DRUG: Vasoconstrictors, vasopressors may increase effect. **HERBAL:** None known. **FOOD:** None known. **LAB VALUES:** May decrease prolactin concentration.

AVAILABILITY (Rx)

TABLETS: 0.2 mg. **INJECTION:** 0.2 mg/ml.

M

ADMINISTRATION/HANDLING

Alert: May give PO, IM, or IV.

Storage • Refrigerate ampoules. • Initial dose may be given parenterally, followed by oral regimen. • IV use in life-threatening emergencies only.

Reconstitution • Dilute to volume of 5 ml with 0.9% NaCl.

Rate of administration • Give over at least 1 min, carefully monitoring B/P.

∅ IV INCOMPATIBILITY
No information available for Y-site administration.

IV COMPATIBILITIES
Heparin, potassium.

INDICATIONS/ROUTES/DOSAGE

USUAL ORAL DOSAGE
PO: ADULTS: 0.2 mg 3–4 times/day. Continue for up to 7 days.

USUAL PARENTERAL DOSAGE
IM/IV: ADULTS: Initially, 0.2 mg. May repeat no more often than q2–4h for no more than 5 doses total.

SIDE EFFECTS

FREQUENT: Nausea, uterine cramping, vomiting. **OCCASIONAL:** Abdominal/stomach pain, diarrhea, dizziness, diaphoresis, tinnitus, bradycardia, chest pain. **RARE:** Allergic reaction (rash, itching), dyspnea, sudden/severe hypertension.

ADVERSE REACTIONS/ TOXIC EFFECTS

Severe hypertensive episodes may result in cerebrovascular accident, serious arrhythmias, seizures; hypertensive effects more frequent with pt susceptibility, rapid IV administration, concurrent regional anesthesia, vasoconstrictors. Peripheral ischemia may lead to gangrene.

NURSING IMPLICATIONS

BASELINE ASSESSMENT
Determine calcium level, B/P, pulse baselines. Assess bleeding prior to administration.

INTERVENTION/EVALUATION
Monitor uterine tone, bleeding, B/P, pulse q15min until stable (about 1–2 hrs). Assess extremities for color, warmth, movement, pain. Report chest pain promptly. Provide support with ambulation if dizziness occurs.

PATIENT/FAMILY TEACHING
Avoid smoking because of added vasoconstriction. Report increased cramping, bleeding, foul-smelling lochia. Pale, cold hands/feet should be reported (possibility of decreased circulation).

methylphenidate hydrochloride

meh-thyl-**fen**-ih-date
(Concerta, Metadate, Ritalin, Ritalin LA, Ritalin SR)
Do not confuse with Rifadin.

CLASSIFICATION

PHARMACOTHERAPEUTIC: Piperidine derivative B **(Schedule II).** **CLINICAL:** CNS stimulant.

ACTION

Blocks reuptake mechanisms of dopaminergic neurons. **Therapeutic Effect:** Decreases motor restlessness, enhances ability to pay attention. Increases motor activity, mental alertness; diminishes sense of fatigue; enhances spirit; produces mild euphoria.

PHARMACOKINETICS

Onset	Peak	Duration
Immediate-release	2 hrs	3–5 hrs
SR	4–7 hrs	3–8 hrs
Extended-release	—	8–12 hrs

Slowly, incompletely absorbed from GI tract. Protein binding: 15%. Metabolized in liver. Excreted in urine, eliminated in feces via biliary system. Unknown if removed by hemodialysis. **Half-life:** 2–4 hrs.

USES

Adjunct to treatment of attention deficit hyperactivity disorder (ADHD) with moderate to severe distractibility, short attention spans, hyperactivity, emotional impulsivity in children >6 yrs. Management of narcolepsy in adults. **Unlabeled:** Treatment of secondary mental depression.

PRECAUTIONS

CONTRAINDICATIONS: Use of MAOIs within 14 days. **CAUTIONS:** Hypertension, seizures, acute stress reaction, emotional instability, history of drug dependence.

LIFESPAN CONSIDERATIONS: Pregnancy/lactation: Unknown if drug crosses placenta or is distributed in breast milk. **Pregnancy Category C. Children:** May be more susceptible to develop anorexia, insomnia, stomach pain, decreased weight. Chronic use may inhibit growth. **Elderly:** No age-related precautions noted.

INTERACTIONS

DRUG: CNS stimulants may have additive effect. **MAOIs** may increase effects. **HERBAL: Ma huang (ephedra)** may increase CNS stimulation. **FOOD:** None known. **LAB VALUES:** None known.

AVAILABILITY (Rx)

CAPSULES (extended-release): Metadate CD: 10 mg, 20 mg, 30 mg. **Ritalin LA:** 20 mg, 30 mg, 40 mg. **TABLETS: Ritalin:** 5 mg, 10 mg, 20 mg. **TABLETS (extended-release): Concerta:** 18 mg, 27 mg, 36 mg, 54 mg. **Metadate ER:** 10 mg, 20 mg. **TABLETS (sustained-release): Ritalin SR:** 20 mg.

ADMINISTRATION/HANDLING

PO

• Do not give drug in afternoon or evening (drug causes insomnia). • Do not crush, break sustained-release capsules. • Tablets may be crushed. • Give dose 30–45 min before meals. • **Metadate CD:** May be opened, sprinkled on applesauce.

INDICATIONS/ROUTES/DOSAGE

ADHD

PO: CHILDREN >6 YRS: Initially, 2.5–5 mg before breakfast and lunch. May increase by 5–10 mg/day at weekly intervals. **Maximum:** 60 mg/day.

Alert: Sustained-release forms **(Metadate SR, Ritalin SR)** may be given once the daily dose is titrated; the regular tablets and the titrated 8-hr dosage correspond to sustained-release size.

Concerta: Initially, 18 mg once daily; may increase by 18 mg/day at weekly intervals. **Maximum:** 54 mg/day.

Metadate CD: Initially, 20 mg/day. May increase by 20 mg/day at 7-day intervals. **Maximum:** 60 mg/day.

Ritalin LA: Initially, 20 mg/day. May increase by 10 mg/day at 7-day intervals. **Maximum:** 60 mg/day.

NARCOLEPSY

PO: ADULTS, ELDERLY: 10 mg 2–3 times/day. RANGE: 10–60 mg/day.

SIDE EFFECTS

FREQUENT: Nervousness, insomnia, anorexia. **OCCASIONAL:** Dizziness, drowsiness, headache, nausea, stomach pain, fever, rash, joint pain. **RARE:** Blurred vision, Tourette's syndrome (uncontrolled vocal outbursts, repetitive body movements, tics).

ADVERSE REACTIONS/ TOXIC EFFECTS

Prolonged administration to children with attention deficit disorder may produce a temporary suppression of normal weight gain pattern. Overdose may produce tachycardia, palpitations, cardiac irregularities, chest pain, psychotic episode, seizures, coma. Hypersensitivity reactions, blood dyscrasias occur rarely.

NURSING IMPLICATIONS

INTERVENTION/EVALUATION

CBC with differential, platelet count should be performed routinely during therapy. If paradoxical return of attention deficit occurs, dosage should be reduced or discontinued.

PATIENT/FAMILY TEACHING

Avoid tasks that require alertness, motor skills until response to drug is established. Dry mouth may be relieved by sugarless gum, sips of tepid water. Report any increase in seizures. Take last dose early in morning to avoid insomnia. Report nervousness, palpitations, fever, vomiting, skin rash. Avoid caffeine. Do not abruptly stop taking after prolonged use.

methylprednisolone

meth-ill-pred-**niss**-oh-lone
(Medrol)

methylprednisolone sodium succinate

(A-Methapred, Solu-Medrol)

methylprednisolone acetate

(Depo-Medrol)

Do not confuse with Mebaral, medroxyprogesterone.

CLASSIFICATION

PHARMACOTHERAPEUTIC: Adrenal corticosteroid. **CLINICAL:** Glucocorticoid (see p. 81C).

ACTION

Suppresses migration of polymorphonuclear leukocytes, reverses increased capillary permeability. **Therapeutic Effects:** Decreases inflammation.

PHARMACOKINETICS

Onset	Peak	Duration
PO		
—	1–2 hrs	30–36 hrs
IM		
—	4–8 days	1–4 wks

Well absorbed from GI tract following IM administration. Widely distributed. Metabolized in liver. Excreted in urine. Removed by hemodialysis. **Half-life:** >3.5 hrs.

USES

Substitution therapy of deficiency states: acute/chronic adrenal insufficiency, congenital adrenal hyperplasia, adrenal insufficiency secondary to pituitary insufficiency. **Nonendocrine Disorders:** Arthritis; rheumatic carditis; allergic, collagen, intestinal tract, liver, ocular, renal, skin diseases; bronchial asthma; cerebral edema; malignancies.

PRECAUTIONS

CONTRAINDICATIONS: Administration of live virus vaccines, systemic fungal infection. **CAUTIONS:** Hypothyroidism, cirrhosis, hypertension, diabetes, CHF, ulcerative colitis, thromboembolic disorders.

LIFESPAN CONSIDERATIONS: Pregnancy/lactation: Crosses placenta. Distributed in breast milk. May cause cleft palate (chronic use first trimester). Nursing contraindicated. **Pregnancy Category C. Children:** Prolonged treatment or high dosages may decrease short-term growth rate, cortisol secretion. **Elderly:** No age-related precaution noted.

INTERACTIONS

DRUG: **Amphotericin** may increase hypokalemia. May decrease effect of **oral hypoglycemics, insulin, diuretics, potassium supplements.** May increase **digoxin** toxicity (due to hypokalemia). **Hepatic enzyme inducers** may decrease effect. **Live virus vaccines** may potentiate virus replication, increase vaccine side effects, decrease pt's antibody response to vaccine. **HERBAL:** None known. **FOOD:** None known. **LAB VALUES:** May decrease calcium, potassium, thyroxine. May increase cholesterol, lipids, glucose, sodium, amylase.

AVAILABILITY (Rx)

TABLETS: 2 mg, 4 mg, 8 mg, 16 mg, 24 mg, 32 mg. **SUCCINATE: POWDER FOR INJECTION:** 40 mg, 125 mg, 500 mg, 1 g, 2 g. **ACETATE: INJECTION:** 20 mg/ml, 40 mg/ml, 80 mg/ml.

ADMINISTRATION/HANDLING

PO

• Give with food, milk. • Give single doses before 9 AM; give multiple doses at evenly spaced intervals.

IM

• Methylprednisolone acetate should not be further diluted. • Methylprednisolone sodium succinate should be reconstituted with Bacteriostatic Water for Injection. • Give deep IM in gluteus maximus.

IV

Storage • Store vials at room temperature.

Reconstitution • Follow directions with Mix-o-vial. • For infusion, add to D_5W, 0.9% NaCl.

Rate of administration • Give IV push over 2–3 min. • Give IV piggyback over 10–20 min. • Do **not** give methylprednisolone acetate IV.

IV INCOMPATIBILITIES

Ciprofloxacin (Cipro), diltiazem (Cardizem), docetaxel (Taxotere), etoposide (VePesid), filgrastim (Neupogen), gemcitabine (Gemzar), paclitaxel (Taxol), potassium chloride, propofol (Diprivan), vinorelbine (Navelbine).

IV COMPATIBILITIES

Dopamine (Intropin), heparin, midazolam (Versed), theophylline.

INDICATIONS/ROUTES/DOSAGE

Alert: Individualize dose based on disease, pt response.

ORAL METHYLPREDNISOLONE

PO: ADULTS, ELDERLY: Initially, 4–48 mg/day.

METHYLPREDNISOLONE SODIUM SUCCINATE

IV: ADULTS, ELDERLY: (HIGH DOSE): 30 mg/kg over at least 30 min. Repeat q4–6h for 48–72 hrs.

IV: ADULTS, ELDERLY: 40–250 mg q4–6h.

METHYLPREDNISOLONE ACETATE

IM: ADULTS, ELDERLY: 10–80 mg/day.

Intra-articular, intralesional: 4–40 mg, up to 80 mg q1–5wks.

SIDE EFFECTS

FREQUENT: Insomnia, heartburn, nervousness, abdominal distention, diaphoresis, acne, mood swings, increased appetite, facial flushing, GI distress, delayed wound healing, increased susceptibility to infection, diarrhea/constipation. **OCCASIONAL:** Headache, edema, tachycardia, change in skin color, frequent urination, depression. **RARE:** Psychosis, increased blood coagulability, hallucinations.

ADVERSE REACTIONS/ TOXIC EFFECTS

LONG-TERM THERAPY: Muscle wasting (esp. arms, legs), osteoporosis, spontaneous fractures, amenorrhea, cataracts, glaucoma, peptic ulcer, CHF. **ABRUPT WITHDRAWAL AFTER LONG-TERM THERAPY:** Anorexia, nausea, fever, headache, severe joint pain, rebound inflammation, fatigue, weakness, lethargy, dizziness, orthostatic hypotension.

NURSING IMPLICATIONS

BASELINE ASSESSMENT

Question for hypersensitivity to any of the corticosteroids, components. Obtain baselines for height, weight, B/P, glucose, electrolytes. Check results of initial tests (e.g., TB skin test, x-rays, EKG).

INTERVENTION/EVALUATION

Monitor I&O, weight; assess for edema. Evaluate bowel activity. Check vital signs at least 2 times/day. Be alert for infection: sore throat, fever, vague symptoms. Monitor electrolytes. Watch for hypocalcemia (muscle twitching, cramps, positive Trousseau's or Chvostek's signs), hypokalemia (weakness/muscle cramps, numbness/tingling [esp. lower extremities], nausea/vomiting, irritability, EKG changes). Assess emotional status, ability to sleep. Check lab results for blood coagulability, clinical evidence of thromboembolism.

PATIENT/FAMILY TEACHING

Take oral dose with food, milk. Do not change dose/schedule or stop taking drug; must taper off gradually under medical supervision. Notify physician of fever, sore throat, muscle aches, sudden weight gain/swelling. Maintain fastidious personal hygiene, avoid exposure to disease, trauma. Severe stress (serious infection, surgery, trauma) may require increased dosage. Follow-up visits, lab tests are necessary. Children must be assessed for growth retardation. Inform dentist, other physicians of methylprednisolone therapy now or within past 12 mos.

methysergide maleate

(Sansert)

See Classification section under: Antimigraine

metipranolol

(OptiPranolol)

See Classification section under: Antiglaucoma agents (p. 46C)

metoclopramide

meh-tah-**klo**-prah-myd
(Apo-Metoclop✱, Reglan)
Do not confuse with Renagel.

CLASSIFICATION

PHARMACOTHERAPEUTIC: Dopamine receptor antagonist. **CLINICAL:** GI emptying adjunct, peristaltic stimulant, antiemetic.

ACTION

Stimulates motility of upper GI tract. Decreases reflux into esophagus. Raises threshold activity of chemoreceptor trigger zone. **Therapeutic Effect:** Accelerates intestinal transit, gastric emptying. Produces antiemetic activity.

PHARMACOKINETICS

Onset	Peak	Duration
PO		
30–60 min	—	—
IM		
10–15 min	—	—
IV		
1–3 min	—	—

Well absorbed from GI tract. Metabolized in liver. Protein binding: 30%. Primarily excreted in urine. Not removed by hemodialysis. **Half-life:** 4–6 hrs.

USES

Relieves symptoms of acute, recurrent gastroparesis (nausea, vomiting, persistent fullness after meals). Prevents nausea, vomiting associated with cancer chemotherapy. Treatment of heartburn, delayed gastric emptying secondary to reflux esophagitis. **Unlabeled:** Treatment of slow gastric emptying, vascular headaches, persistent hiccups, drug-related postop nausea/vomiting. Prophylaxis of aspiration pneumonia.

PRECAUTIONS

CONTRAINDICATIONS: Pheochromocytoma, history of seizure disorders, concurrent use of medications likely to produce extrapyramidal reactions, GI obstruction/perforation/hemorrhage. **CAUTIONS:** Impaired renal function, CHF, cirrhosis.

LIFESPAN CONSIDERATIONS: Pregnancy/lactation: Crosses placenta. Distributed in breast milk. **Pregnancy Category B. Children:** More susceptible to having dystonia reactions. **Elderly:** More likely to have parkinsonism, tardive dyskinesias after long-term therapy.

INTERACTIONS

DRUG: Alcohol may increase CNS depressant effect. **CNS depressants** may increase sedative effect. **HERBAL:** None known. **FOOD:** None known. **LAB VALUES:** May increase aldosterone, prolactin concentrations.

AVAILABILITY (Rx)

TABLETS: 5 mg, 10 mg. **SYRUP:** 5 mg/5 ml. **INJECTION:** 5 mg/ml.

ADMINISTRATION/HANDLING

PO

• Give 30 min before meals and at bedtime. • Tablets may be crushed.

IV

Storage • Store vials at room temperature. • After dilution, IV infusion (piggyback) is stable for 48 hrs.

Reconstitution • Dilute doses >10 mg in 50 ml D_5W, 0.9% NaCl, or lactated Ringer's.

Rate of administration • Infuse >15 min. • May give slow IV push at rate of 10 mg over 1–2 min. • A too rapid IV injection may produce intense feeling of anxiety or restlessness, followed by drowsiness.

M

∅ IV INCOMPATIBILITIES

Allopurinol (Aloprim), cefepime (Maxipime), doxorubicin liposome (Doxil), furosemide (Lasix), propofol (Diprivan).

IV COMPATIBILITIES

Dexamethasone, diltiazem (Cardizem), diphenhydramine (Benadryl), fentanyl (Sublimaze), heparin, hydromorphone (Dilaudid), morphine, potassium chloride.

INDICATIONS/ROUTES/DOSAGE

Alert: May give PO, IM, direct IV, IV infusion.

DIABETIC GASTROPARESIS

PO/IV: ADULTS: 10 mg before meals and at bedtime for 2–8 wks.

PO: ELDERLY: Initially, 5 mg before meals and at bedtime. May increase to 10 mg.

IV: ELDERLY: 5 mg over 1–2 min. May increase to 10 mg.

SYMPTOMATIC GASTROESOPHAGEAL REFLUX

PO: ADULTS: 10–15 mg up to 4 times/day; single doses up to 20 mg as needed. ELDERLY: Initially, 5 mg 4 times/day. May increase to 10 mg. CHILDREN: 0.4–0.8 mg/kg/day in 4 divided doses.

PREVENTION OF CANCER CHEMOTHERAPY–INDUCED NAUSEA AND VOMITING

IV: ADULTS, ELDERLY, CHILDREN: 1–2 mg/kg 30 min prior to chemotherapy; repeat q2h for 2 doses, then q3h as needed.

TO FACILITATE SMALL BOWEL INTUBATION (single dose)

IV: ADULTS, ELDERLY: 10 mg. CHILDREN 6–14 YRS: 2.5–5 mg. CHILDREN <6 YRS: 0.1 mg/kg.

POSTOP NAUSEA/VOMITING

IV: ADULTS, ELDERLY, CHILDREN >14 YRS: 10 mg; repeat q6–8h as needed. CHILDREN ≤14 YRS: 0.1–0.2 mg/kg/dose; repeat q6–8h as needed.

DOSAGE IN RENAL IMPAIRMENT

Creatinine Clearance	% Normal Dose
40–50 ml/min	75%
10–40 ml/min	50%
<10 ml/min	25%–50%

SIDE EFFECTS

Alert: Doses of ≥2 mg/kg or increase in length of therapy may result in a greater incidence of side effects.

FREQUENT (10%): Drowsiness, restlessness, fatigue, lassitude. **OCCASIONAL (3%):** Dizziness, anxiety, headache, insomnia, breast tenderness, altered menstruation, constipation, rash, dry mouth, galactorrhea, gynecomastia. **RARE (<3%):** Hypotension/hypertension, tachycardia.

ADVERSE REACTIONS/ TOXIC EFFECTS

Extrapyramidal reactions occur most frequently in children, young adults (18–30 yrs) receiving large doses (2 mg/kg) during cancer chemotherapy and is usually limited to akathisia (motor restlessness), involuntary limb movement, facial grimacing.

NURSING IMPLICATIONS

BASELINE ASSESSMENT

Antiemetic: Assess for dehydration (poor skin turgor, dry mucous membranes, longitudinal furrows in tongue).

INTERVENTION/EVALUATION

Monitor for anxiety, restlessness, extrapyramidal symptoms during IV administration. Monitor pattern of daily bowel activity/stool consistency. Assess for periorbital edema. Assess skin for rash, hives. Evaluate for therapeutic response from gastroparesis (nausea, vomiting, persistent fullness after meals). Monitor renal function, B/P, heart rate.

PATIENT/FAMILY TEACHING

Avoid tasks that require alertness, motor skills until drug response is established. Report involuntary eye, facial, limb movement (extrapyramidal reaction). Avoid alcohol.

metolazone

me-**toh**-lah-zone
(Mykrox, Zaroxolyn)

Do not confuse with methazolamide, metoprolol, Zarontin.

CLASSIFICATION

PHARMACOTHERAPEUTIC: Thiazide-like. **CLINICAL:** Diuretic, antihypertensive (see p. 87C).

ACTION

Diuretic: Blocks reabsorption of sodium, potassium, chloride at distal convoluted tubule, promoting delivery of sodium to potassium side, increasing potassium excretion (Na-K) exchange. **Therapeutic Effect:** Produces renal excretion. **Antihypertensive:** Reduces plasma, extracellular fluid volume. **Therapeutic Effect:** Decreases peripheral vascular resistance, reduced B/P by direct effect on blood vessels.

PHARMACOKINETICS

Onset	Peak	Duration
PO (diuretic)		
1 hr	2 hrs	12–24 hrs

Incompletely absorbed from GI tract. Protein binding: 95%. Primarily excreted unchanged in urine. Not removed by hemodialysis. **Half-life:** 14 hrs.

USES

Zaroxolyn: Treatment of mild to moderate essential hypertension, edema of renal disease, edema due to CHF. **Mykrox:** Treatment of mild to moderate hypertension.

PRECAUTIONS

CONTRAINDICATIONS: History of hypersensitivity to sulfonamides or thiazide diuretics, renal decompensation, anuria, hepatic coma, precoma. **CAUTIONS:** Severe renal disease, impaired liver function, gout, lupus erythematosus, diabetes, elevated cholesterol/triglycerides.

LIFESPAN CONSIDERATIONS: Pregnancy/lactation: Crosses placenta. Small amount distributed in breast milk; breast-feeding not advised. **Pregnancy Category B** (**D** if used in pregnancy-induced hypertension). **Children:** No age-related precautions noted. **Elderly:** May be more sensitive to hypotensive/electrolyte effects. Age-related renal impairment may require caution.

INTERACTIONS

DRUG: **Cholestyramine, colestipol** may decrease absorption, effects. May increase **digoxin** toxicity (due to hypokalemia). May increase **lithium** toxicity. **HERBAL:** None known. **FOOD:** None known. **LAB VALUES:** May increase bilirubin, serum calcium, LDL, cholesterol, triglycerides, creatinine, glucose, uric acid. May decrease urinary calcium, magnesium, potassium, sodium.

AVAILABILITY (Rx)

TABLETS: 2.5 mg, 5 mg, 10 mg. **TABLETS (Mykrox):** 0.5 mg.

ADMINISTRATION/HANDLING

PO

- May give with food, milk if GI upset occurs, preferably with breakfast (may prevent nocturia).

M

INDICATIONS/ROUTES/DOSAGE

EDEMA (Zaroxolyn)

PO: ADULTS: 5–10 mg once daily in morning. Reduce dosage to lowest maintenance level when dry weight is achieved (nonedematous state).

EDEMA DUE TO RENAL DISEASE (Zaroxolyn)

PO: ADULTS: 5–20 mg once daily in morning. Reduce dosage to lowest maintenance level when dry weight is achieved (nonedematous state).

HYPERTENSION (Zaroxolyn)

PO: ADULTS: 2.5–5 mg once daily in morning.

USUAL ELDERLY DOSAGE (Zaroxolyn)

PO: Initially, 2.5 mg/day or every other day.

HYPERTENSION (Mykrox)

PO: ADULTS: 0.5 mg once daily in morning. Dosage may be increased to 1 mg once daily if B/P response is insufficient.

USUAL DOSAGE FOR CHILDREN (Mykrox)

PO: 0.2–0.4 mg/kg/day in divided doses q12–24h.

SIDE EFFECTS

EXPECTED: Increase in urine frequency/volume. **FREQUENT (9%–10%):** Dizziness, lightheadedness, headache. **OCCASIONAL (4%–6%):** Muscle cramps/spasm, fatigue, lethargy. **RARE (<2%):** Weakness, palpitations, depression, nausea, vomiting, abdominal bloating, constipation, diarrhea, urticaria.

ADVERSE REACTIONS/TOXIC EFFECTS

Vigorous diuresis may lead to profound water loss and electrolyte depletion, resulting in hypokalemia, hyponatremia, dehydration. Acute hypotensive episodes may occur. Hyperglycemia may be noted during prolonged therapy. GI upset, pancreatitis, dizziness, paresthesias, headache, blood dyscrasias, pulmonary edema, allergic pneumonitis, dermatologic reactions occur rarely. Overdosage can lead to lethargy, coma without changes in electrolytes or hydration.

NURSING IMPLICATIONS

BASELINE ASSESSMENT

Check vital signs, esp. B/P for hypotension, prior to administration. Assess baseline electrolytes, particularly check for hypokalemia. Assess edema, skin turgor, mucous membranes for hydration status. Assess muscle strength, mental status. Note skin temperature, moisture. Obtain baseline weight. Monitor I&O.

INTERVENTION/EVALUATION

Continue to monitor B/P, vital signs, electrolytes, I&O, weight. Note extent of diuresis. Watch for electrolyte disturbances (hypokalemia may result in weakness, tremor, muscle cramps, nausea, vomiting, change in mental status, tachycardia; hyponatremia may result in confusion, thirst, cold/clammy skin).

PATIENT/FAMILY TEACHING

Expect increased frequency/volume of urination. To reduce hypotensive effect, rise slowly from lying to sitting position, permit legs to dangle momentarily before standing. Eat foods high in potassium, such as whole grains (cereals), legumes, meat, bananas, apricots, orange juice, potatoes (white, sweet), raisins.

metoprolol tartrate

meh-**toe**-pro-lol

(Apo-Metoprolol✤, Betaloc✤, Lopressor, Nu-Metop✤, PMS-Metoprolol✤, Toprol XL)

Do not confuse with metaproterenol, metolazone.

FIXED-COMBINATION(S)

Lopressor HCT: metoprolol/hydrochlorothiazide (a diuretic): 50 mg/25 mg; 100 mg/25 mg; 100 mg/50 mg.

◆CLASSIFICATION

PHARMACOTHERAPEUTIC: Beta$_1$-adrenergic blocker. **CLINICAL:** Antianginal, antihypertensive, MI adjunct (see p. 62C).

ACTION

Selectively blocks beta$_1$-adrenergic receptors, high dosages may block beta$_2$-adrenergic receptors. Decreases O_2 requirements. **Therapeutic Effect:** Slows sinus heart rate, decreases cardiac output, reduces B/P. Decreases myocardial ischemia severity. Increases airway resistance at high dosages.

PHARMACOKINETICS

Onset	Peak	Duration
PO		
10–15 min	—	6 hrs
PO (extended-release)		
—	6–12 hrs	24 hrs
IV		
Immediate	20 min	5–8 hrs

Well absorbed from GI tract. Protein binding: 12%. Widely distributed. Metabolized in liver (undergoes significant first-pass metabolism). Primarily excreted in urine. Removed by hemodialysis. **Half-life:** 3–7 hrs.

USES

Management of mild to moderate hypertension. Used alone or in combination with diuretics, esp. thiazide type. Management of chronic stable angina pectoris. Reduces cardiovascular mortality in those with definite or suspected acute MI. **Extended-Release:** Management of hypertension, long-term treatment of angina pectoris. Treatment of heart failure. **Unlabeled:** Treatment/prophylaxis of cardiac arrhythmias, hypertrophic cardiomyopathy, pheochromocytoma, vascular headache, tremors, anxiety, thyrotoxicosis, mitral valve prolapse syndrome. Increases survival rate in diabetic pts with heart disease.

PRECAUTIONS

CONTRAINDICATIONS: Overt cardiac failure, cardiogenic shock, heart block greater than first degree, sinus bradycardia. **MI:** Heart rate <45 beats/min, systolic B/P <100 mm Hg. **CAUTIONS:** Bronchospastic disease, impaired renal function, peripheral vascular disease, hyperthyroidism, diabetes, inadequate cardiac function.

LIFESPAN CONSIDERATIONS: Pregnancy/lactation: Crosses placenta. Distributed in breast milk. Avoid use during first trimester. May produce bradycardia, apnea, hypoglycemia, hypothermia during delivery, low birth-weight infants. **Pregnancy Category C (D** if used in second or third trimester). **Children:** Safety and efficacy not established. **Elderly:** Age-related peripheral vascular disease may increase susceptibility to decreased peripheral circulation.

INTERACTIONS

DRUG: Diuretics, other hypotensives may increase hypotensive effect; **sympathomimetics, xanthines** may mutually inhibit effects; may mask symptoms of hypoglycemia, prolong hypoglycemic effect of **insulin, oral hypoglycemics; NSAIDs** may decrease antihypertensive effect; **cimetidine** may increase concentration. **HERBAL:** None known. **FOOD:** None known. **LAB VALUES:** May increase ANA titer, SGOT (AST), SGPT (ALT), alkaline phosphatase, LDH, bilirubin, BUN, creatinine, potassium, uric acid, lipoproteins, triglycerides.

AVAILABILITY (Rx)

TABLETS: 50 mg, 100 mg. **TABLETS (extended-release):** 25 mg, 50 mg, 100 mg, 200 mg. **INJECTION:** 1 mg/ml.

M

ADMINISTRATION/HANDLING

PO

• Tablets may be crushed; do not crush or break extended-release tablets. • Give at same time each day. • May be given with or immediately after meals (enhances absorption).

IV

Storage • Store at room temperature.

Rate of administration • May give undiluted. • Administer IV injection over 1 min. • Monitor EKG during administration.

IV INCOMPATIBILITIES

Amphotericin B complex (Abelcet, AmBisome, Amphotec).

IV COMPATIBILITY

Alteplase (Activase).

INDICATIONS/ROUTES/DOSAGE

HYPERTENSION, ANGINA PECTORIS

PO: ADULTS: Initially, 100 mg/day as single or divided dose. Increase at weekly (or longer) intervals. MAINTENANCE: 100–450 mg/day.

USUAL ELDERLY DOSAGE

PO: Initially, 25 mg/day. RANGE: 25–300 mg/day.

USUAL DOSAGE FOR EXTENDED-RELEASE TABLETS

PO: ADULTS: HYPERTENSION: 50–100 mg/day as single dose. May increase at least at weekly intervals until optimum B/P attained. ANGINA: Initially, 100 mg/day as single dose. May increase at least at weekly intervals until optimum clinical response achieved. HEART FAILURE: Initially, 25 mg/day. May double dose q2wks. **Maximum:** 200 mg/day.

MI (early treatment)

IV: ADULTS: 5 mg q2min for 3 doses, followed by 50 mg orally q6h for 48 hrs. Begin oral dose 15 min after last IV dose. Alternatively, in those who do not tolerate full IV dose, give 25–50 mg orally q6h, 15 min after last IV dose.

MI (late treatment, maintenance)

PO: ADULTS: 100 mg 2 times/day for at least 3 mos.

SIDE EFFECTS

Generally well tolerated, with transient and mild side effects. **FREQUENT:** Decreased sexual function, drowsiness, insomnia, unusual tiredness/weakness. **OCCASIONAL:** Anxiety, nervousness, diarrhea, constipation, nausea, vomiting, nasal congestion, stomach discomfort, dizziness, difficulty breathing, cold hands/feet. **RARE:** Altered taste, dry eyes, nightmares, numbness in fingers/feet, allergic reaction (rash, pruritus).

ADVERSE REACTIONS/ TOXIC EFFECTS

Excessive dosage may produce profound bradycardia, hypotension, bronchospasm. Abrupt withdrawal may result in diaphoresis, palpitations, headache, tremulousness, exacerbation of angina, MI, ventricular arrhythmias. May precipitate CHF, MI in pts with cardiac disease; thyroid storm in those with thyrotoxicosis; peripheral ischemia in pts with existing peripheral vascular disease. Hypoglycemia may occur in pts with previously controlled diabetes.

NURSING IMPLICATIONS

BASELINE ASSESSMENT

Assess baseline renal/liver function tests. Assess B/P, apical pulse immediately prior to drug administration (if pulse is ≤60/min or systolic B/P is <90 mm Hg, withhold medication, contact physician). **Antianginal:** Record onset, type (sharp, dull, squeezing), radiation, location, intensity, duration of anginal pain, precipitating factors (exertion, emotional stress).

INTERVENTION/EVALUATION

Measure B/P near end of dosing interval (determines whether B/P is controlled throughout day). Monitor B/P for hypotension, respiration for shortness of breath. Assess pulse for quality, irregular rate, bradycardia. Assess for evidence of CHF: dyspnea (particularly on exertion, lying down), night cough, peripheral edema, distended neck veins. Monitor I&O (increase in weight, decrease in urine output may indicate CHF). Therapeutic response to hypertension noted in 1–2 wks.

PATIENT/FAMILY TEACHING

Do not abruptly discontinue medication. Compliance with therapy regimen is essential to control hypertension, arrhythmias. If a dose is missed, take next scheduled dose (do not double dose). To avoid hypotensive effect, rise slowly from lying to sitting position, wait momentarily before standing. Report excessive fatigue, dizziness. Do not use nasal decongestants, OTC cold preparations (stimulants) without physician approval. Outpts should monitor B/P, pulse before taking medication. Restrict salt, alcohol intake.

metronidazole hydrochloride

meh-trow-**nye**-dah-zoll

(Apo-Metronidazole✤, Flagyl, MetroCream, MetroGel, MetroLotion, NidaGel✤, Noritate, Novonidazol✤, Satric-500)

FIXED-COMBINATION(S)

Helidac: metronidazole/bismuth/tetracycline (an anti-infective): 250 mg/262 mg/500 mg.

◆ CLASSIFICATION

PHARMACOTHERAPEUTIC: Nitroimidazole derivative. **CLINICAL:** Antibacterial, antiprotozoal.

ACTION

Disrupts DNA, inhibits nucleic acid synthesis. **Therapeutic Effect:** Produces bactericidal, amebicidal, trichomonacidal effects. Produces anti-inflammatory, immunosuppressive effects when applied topically.

PHARMACOKINETICS

Well absorbed from GI tract, minimal absorption after topical application. Protein binding: <20%. Widely distributed, crosses blood-brain barrier. Metabolized in liver to active metabolite. Primarily excreted in urine; partially eliminated in feces. Removed by hemodialysis. **Half-life:** 8 hrs (half-life increased in those with alcoholic liver disease, neonates).

USES

Treatment of anaerobic infections (skin/skin structure, CNS, lower respiratory tract, bone/joints, intra-abdominal, gynecologic infections, endocarditis, septicemia). Treatment of trichomoniasis, amebiasis, perioperatively for contaminated/potentially contaminated intra-abdominal surgery, antibiotic-associated pseudomembranous colitis (AAPC). **Unlabeled:** Treatment of *H. pylori*–associated gastritis/duodenal ulcer. Topical application in treatment of acne rosacea. Also used in treatment of grade III, IV decubitus ulcers with anaerobic infection. Treatment of bacterial vaginosis. Treatment of inflammatory bowel disease.

PRECAUTIONS

CONTRAINDICATIONS: Hypersensitivity to metronidazole or other nitroimidazole derivatives (also parabens with topical application). **CAUTIONS:** Blood dyscrasias, severe hepatic dysfunction, CNS dis-

M

ease, predisposition to edema, concurrent corticosteroid therapy. Safety and efficacy of topical administration in those <21 yrs not established.

LIFESPAN CONSIDERATIONS: Pregnancy/lactation: Readily crosses placenta. Distributed in breast milk. Contraindicated during first trimester in those with trichomoniasis. Topical use during pregnancy or lactation discouraged. **Pregnancy Category B. Children:** No age-related precautions noted. **Elderly:** Age-related liver impairment may require dosage adjustment.

INTERACTIONS

DRUG: Alcohol may cause disulfiram-type reaction. May increase effect of **oral anticoagulants.** May increase toxicity with **disulfiram. HERBAL:** None known. **FOOD:** None known. **LAB VALUES:** May increase SGOT (AST), SGPT (ALT), LDH.

M

AVAILABILITY (Rx)

TABLETS: 250 mg, 500 mg. **TABLETS (extended-release):** 750 mg. **CAPSULES:** 375 mg. **POWDER FOR INJECTION:** 500 mg. **INJECTION (infusion):** 500 mg/100 ml. **LOTION:** 0.75%. **VAGINAL GEL:** 0.75%. **TOPICAL GEL:** 0.75%. **TOPICAL CREAM:** 0.75%, 1%.

ADMINISTRATION/HANDLING

PO

• Give without regard to meals. Give with food to decrease GI irritation.

IV

Storage • Store at room temperature (ready-to-use infusion bags).

Rate of administration • Infuse >30–60 min. Do not give bolus. • Avoid prolonged use of indwelling catheters.

IV INCOMPATIBILITIES

Amphotericin B complex (Abelcet, AmBisome, Amphotec), filgrastim (Neupogen).

IV COMPATIBILITIES

Diltiazem (Cardizem), dopamine (Intropin), heparin, hydromorphone (Dilaudid), lorazepam (Ativan), magnesium sulfate, midazolam (Versed), morphine.

INDICATIONS/ROUTES/DOSAGE

AMEBIASIS

PO: ADULTS, ELDERLY: 500–750 mg q8h. CHILDREN: 35–50 mg/kg/day in divided doses q8h.

PARASITIC INFECTIONS

PO: ADULTS, ELDERLY: 250 mg q8h or 2 g as a single dose. CHILDREN: 15–30 mg/kg/day in divided doses q8h.

ANAEROBIC INFECTIONS

PO/IV: ADULTS, ELDERLY, CHILDREN: 30 mg/kg/day in divided doses q6h. **Maximum:** 4 g/day.

AAPC

PO: ADULTS, ELDERLY: 250–500 mg 3–4 times/day for 10–14 days. CHILDREN: 30 mg/kg/day in divided doses q6h for 7–10 days.

H. PYLORI

PO: ADULTS, ELDERLY: 250–500 mg 3 times/day (in combination). CHILDREN: 15–20 mg/kg/day in 2 divided doses.

BACTERIAL VAGINOSIS

Intravaginal: ADULTS: One applicatorful 2 times/day or once daily at bedtime for 5 days.

PO: ADULTS: 750 mg at bedtime for 7 days.

ROSACEA

Topical: ADULTS: Thin application 2 times/day to affected area. **Cream:** Once daily. **Lotion:** Apply twice daily.

SIDE EFFECTS

FREQUENT: Anorexia, nausea, dry mouth, metallic taste. **Vaginal:** Symptomatic cervicitis/vaginitis, abdominal cramps, uterine pain. **OCCASIONAL:** Diarrhea/constipation, vomiting, dizziness, erythematous rash, urticaria, reddish brown/

dark urine. **Topical:** Transient redness, mild dryness, burning, irritation, stinging (also tearing when applied too close to eyes). **Vaginal:** Vaginal, perineal, vulvar itching; vulvar swelling. **RARE:** Mild, transient leukopenia, thrombophlebitis with IV therapy.

ADVERSE REACTIONS/ TOXIC EFFECTS

Oral therapy may result in furry tongue, glossitis, cystitis, dysuria, pancreatitis, flattening of T waves with EKG readings. Peripheral neuropathy (numbness, tingling, paresthesia) is usually reversible if treatment is stopped immediately upon appearance of neurologic symptoms. Seizures occur occasionally.

NURSING IMPLICATIONS

BASELINE ASSESSMENT

Question for history of hypersensitivity to metronidazole or other nitroimidazole derivatives (and parabens with topical). Obtain specimens for diagnostic tests prior to giving first dose (therapy may begin before results are known).

INTERVENTION/EVALUATION

Determine pattern of bowel activity. Monitor I&O, assess for urinary problems. Be alert to neurologic symptoms: dizziness; numbness, tingling, paresthesia of extremities. Assess for rash, urticaria. Watch for onset of superinfection: ulceration/change of oral mucosa, furry tongue, vaginal discharge, genital/anal pruritus.

PATIENT/FAMILY TEACHING

Urine may be red-brown/dark. Avoid alcohol, alcohol-containing preparations (e.g., cough syrups, elixirs). Avoid tasks that require alertness, motor skills until response to drug established (may cause dizziness). If taking metronidazole for trichomoniasis, refrain from sexual intercourse until physician advises. For amebiasis, frequent stool specimen checks will be necessary. **Topical:** Avoid contact with eyes. May apply cosmetics after application. Metronidazole acts on redness, papules, pustules but has no effect on rhinophyma (hypertrophy of nose), telangiectasia, ocular problems (conjunctivitis, keratitis, blepharitis). Other recommendations for rosacea include avoidance of hot/spicy foods, alcohol, extremes of hot/cold temperatures, excessive sunlight.

Mevacor

see lovastatin

mexiletine hydrochloride

(Mexitil)

See Classification section under: Antiarrhythmics (p. 13C)

Miacalcin

see calcitonin

Micardis

see telmisartan

M

miconazole nitrate

mih-**kon**-nah-zoll
(Micatin, Micozole, Monistat, Monistat 3, Monistat 7, Monistat-Derm)

Do not confuse with Micronase, Micronor.

CLASSIFICATION

PHARMACOTHERAPEUTIC: Imidazole derivative. **CLINICAL:** Antifungal (see p. 42C).

ACTION

Inhibits synthesis of ergosterol (vital component of fungal cell formation), damaging fungal cell membrane. **Therapeutic Effect:** Fungistatic; may be fungicidal, depending on concentration.

M

PHARMACOKINETICS

Small amounts absorbed systemically after vaginal administration. Protein binding: 91%–93%. Primarily excreted in feces. **Half-life:** 24 hrs.

USES

Vaginal: Vulvovaginal candidiasis. **Topical:** Cutaneous candidiasis, tinea cruris, t. corporis, t. pedis, t. versicolor.

PRECAUTIONS

CONTRAINDICATIONS: Avoid vaginal preparations during first trimester. **CAUTIONS:** Pts allergic to other antifungals (e.g., clotrimazole, ketoconazole).

LIFESPAN CONSIDERATIONS: Pregnancy/lactation: Unknown if drug crosses placenta or is distributed in breast milk. **Pregnancy Category C. Children:** Safety in those <1 yr not established. **Elderly:** No age-related precautions noted.

INTERACTIONS

DRUG: May increase effects of **oral anticoagulants, oral hypoglycemics. Isoniazid, rifampin** may decrease concentrations. **HERBAL:** None known. **FOOD:** None known. **LAB VALUES:** None known.

AVAILABILITY (Rx)

VAGINAL SUPPOSITORY: 100 mg, 200 mg. **TOPICAL CREAM:** 2%. **VAGINAL CREAM:** 2%. **TOPICAL POWDER:** 2%. **TOPICAL SPRAY:** 2%.

INDICATIONS/ROUTES/DOSAGE

VULVOVAGINAL CANDIDIASIS

Intravaginal: ADULTS, ELDERLY: One 200-mg suppository at bedtime for 3 days; one 100-mg suppository or one applicatorful at bedtime for 7 days.

TOPICAL FUNGAL INFECTIONS, CUTANEOUS CANDIDIASIS

Topical: ADULTS, ELDERLY: Apply liberally 2 times/day, morning and evening.

SIDE EFFECTS

TOPICAL: Itching, burning, stinging, erythema, urticaria. **VAGINAL (2%):** Vulvovaginal burning, itching, irritation, headache, skin rash.

ADVERSE REACTIONS/ TOXIC EFFECTS

None known.

NURSING IMPLICATIONS

BASELINE ASSESSMENT

Topical: Avoid occlusive dressing. Apply only a small amount to cover area completely. **Spray:** Shake well before using.

INTERVENTION/EVALUATION

Topical/Vaginal: Assess for burning, itching, irritation.

PATIENT/FAMILY TEACHING

Vaginal Preparation: Base interacts with certain latex products such as contraceptive diaphragm. Ask physician about douching, sexual intercourse. **Topical:** Rub well into affected areas. Avoid getting in eyes. Keep areas clean, dry; wear light clothing for ventilation. Separate personal items in contact with affected areas.

midazolam hydrochloride

my-**day**-zoe-lam
(Versed)

Do not confuse with VePesid.

CLASSIFICATION

PHARMACOTHERAPEUTIC: Benzodiazepine **(Schedule IV). CLINICAL:** Sedative (see p. 3C).

ACTION

Enhances action of inhibitory neurotransmitter gamma-aminobutyric acid (GABA), one of the major inhibitory transmitters in the brain. **Therapeutic Effect:** Produces anxiolytic, hypnotic, anticonvulsant, muscle relaxant, amnestic effects.

PHARMACOKINETICS

Onset	Peak	Duration
PO		
10–20 min	—	—
IM		
5–15 min	15–60 min	2–6 hrs
IV		
1–5 min	5–7 min	20–30 min

Well absorbed after IM administration. Protein binding: 97%. Metabolized in liver to active metabolite. Primarily excreted in urine. Not removed by hemodialysis. **Half-life:** 1–5 hrs.

USES

Sedation, anxiolytic, amnesia prior to procedure or induction of anesthesia, conscious sedation prior to diagnostic/radiographic procedure, continuous IV sedation of intubated/mechanically ventilated pts, status epilepticus.

PRECAUTIONS

CONTRAINDICATIONS: Shock, coma, acute alcohol intoxication, acute narrow-angle glaucoma. **CAUTIONS:** Acute illness, severe fluid/electrolyte imbalance, impaired renal/liver/pulmonary function, CHF, treated open-angle glaucoma.

LIFESPAN CONSIDERATIONS: Pregnancy/lactation: Crosses placenta. Unknown if drug is distributed in breast milk. **Pregnancy Category D. Children:** Neonates more likely to have respiratory depression. **Elderly:** Age-related renal impairment may require dosage adjustment.

INTERACTIONS

DRUG: Alcohol, CNS depressants may increase CNS, respiratory depression, hypotensive effects. **Hypotension-producing medications** may increase hypotensive effects. **HERBAL: Kava kava, valerian** may increase CNS depression. **FOOD: Grapefruit juice** increases oral absorption. **LAB VALUES:** None known.

AVAILABILITY (Rx)

INJECTION: 1 mg/ml, 5 mg/ml. **SYRUP:** 2 mg/ml.

ADMINISTRATION/HANDLING

IM

- Give deep IM into large muscle mass.

IV

Storage • Store vials at room temperature.

Rate of administration • May give undiluted or as infusion. • Resuscitative equipment, O_2 must be readily available prior to IV administration. • Administer by slow IV injection, in incremental dosages: Give each incremental dose over ≥2 min at intervals of at least 2 min. • Reduce IV rate in those >60 yrs, and/or debilitated, pts with chronic disease states, and/or impaired pulmonary function. • A too rapid IV rate, excessive doses, or a single large dose increases risk of respiratory depression/arrest.

⊘ IV INCOMPATIBILITIES

Albumin, ampicillin/sulbactam (Unasyn), amphotericin B complex (Abelcet, AmBisome, Amphotec), ampicillin (Polycillin), bumetanide (Bumex), dexamethasone (Decadron), fosphenytoin (Cerebyx), furosemide (Lasix), hydrocortisone (Solu-Cortef), methotrexate, nafcillin (Nafcil), sodium bicarbonate, sodium pentothal (Thiopental), sulfamethoxazole-trimethoprim (Bactrim).

IV COMPATIBILITIES

Amiodarone (Cordarone), calcium gluconate, diltiazem (Cardizem), dobutamine (Dobutrex), dopamine (Intropin), etomidate (Amidate), fentanyl (Sublimaze), heparin, hydromorphone (Dilaudid), insulin, lorazepam (Ativan), milrinone (Primacor), morphine, nitroglycerin, norepinephrine (Levophed), potassium chloride, propofol (Diprivan).

INDICATIONS/ROUTES/DOSAGE

Alert: Dosage must be individualized based on age, underlying disease, medications, desired effect.

PREOP SEDATION

IM: ADULTS, ELDERLY: 0.07–0.08 mg/kg 30–60 min prior to surgery. CHILDREN: 0.1–0.15 mg/kg 30–60 min prior to surgery. **Maximum total dose:** 10 mg.

IV: CHILDREN 6–12 YRS: 0.025–0.05 mg/kg. CHILDREN 6 MOS–5 YRS: 0.05–0.1 mg/kg.

PO: CHILDREN: 0.25–0.5 mg/kg. **Maximum:** 20 mg.

CONSCIOUS SEDATION FOR PROCEDURES

IV: ADULTS, ELDERLY: 1–2.5 mg over 2 min. Titrate as needed. **Total dose:** 2.5–5 mg.

CONSCIOUS SEDATION DURING MECHANICAL VENTILATION

IV: ADULTS, ELDERLY: 0.01–0.05 mg/kg; may repeat at 10- to 15-min intervals until adequately sedated, then continuous infusion: initially, 0.02–0.1 mg/kg/hr (1–7 mg/hr). CHILDREN >32 WKS: Initially, 1 mcg/kg/min as continuous infusion. CHILDREN ≤32 WKS: Initially, 0.5 mcg/kg/min as continuous infusion.

STATUS EPILEPTICUS

IV: CHILDREN >2 MOS: Loading dose of 0.15 mg/kg followed by continuous infusion of 1 mcg/kg/min. Titrate. RANGE: 1–18 mcg/kg/min.

SIDE EFFECTS

FREQUENT (4%–10%): Decreased respiratory rate, tenderness at IM/IV injection site, pain during injection, desaturation, hiccups. **OCCASIONAL (2%–3%):** Pain at IM injection site, hypotension, paradoxical reaction. **RARE (<2%):** Nausea, vomiting, headache, coughing, hypotensive episodes.

ADVERSE REACTIONS/ TOXIC EFFECTS

Too much or too little dosage, improper administration may result in cerebral hypoxia: agitation, involuntary movements, hyperactivity, combativeness. Underventilation/apnea may produce hypoxia, cardiac arrest. A too rapid IV rate, excessive doses, or a single large dose increases risk of respiratory depression/arrest.

NURSING IMPLICATIONS

BASELINE ASSESSMENT

Resuscitative equipment, endotracheal tube, suction, O_2 must be available. Obtain vital signs before administration.

INTERVENTION/EVALUATION

Monitor respiratory rate and oxygen saturation continuously during parenteral administration for underventilation, apnea. Monitor vital signs, level of sedation q3–5min during recovery period.

midodrine

my-doe-dreen
(Amatine✤, ProAmatine)

Do not confuse with protamine.

◆CLASSIFICATION

PHARMACOTHERAPEUTIC: Vasopressor. **CLINICAL:** Orthostatic hypotension adjunct.

ACTION

Forms active metabolite desglymidodrine, which is an alpha$_1$-agonist, activating alpha receptors of arteriolar, venous vasculature. **Therapeutic Effect:** Increases vascular tone, B/P.

PRECAUTIONS

CONTRAINDICATIONS: Severe cardiac disease, persistent hypertension, pheochromocytoma, thyrotoxicosis, acute renal function impairment, urinary retention. **CAUTIONS:** Renal/liver impairment, history of visual problems. **Pregnancy Category C.**

INTERACTIONS

DRUG: Digoxin may have additive bradycardiac effects. **Sodium-retaining steroids (e.g., fludrocortisone)** may increase sodium retention. **Vasoconstrictors** may be additive. **HERBAL:** None known. **FOOD:** None known. **LAB VALUES:** None known.

USES

Treatment of symptomatic orthostatic hypotension.

AVAILABILITY (Rx)

TABLETS: 2.5 mg, 5 mg, 10 mg.

INDICATIONS/ROUTES/DOSAGE

ORTHOSTATIC HYPOTENSION

PO: ADULTS, ELDERLY: 10 mg 3 times/day. Give during day when pt is upright (upon arising, midday, late afternoon not later than 6 PM).

DOSAGE IN RENAL IMPAIRMENT

2.5 mg 3 times/day increase gradually as tolerated.

SIDE EFFECTS

FREQUENT (7%–20%): Paresthesia, piloerection, pruritus, dysuria, supine hypertension. **OCCASIONAL (1%–7%):** Pain, rash, chills, headache, facial flushing, confusion, dry mouth, anxiety.

ADVERSE REACTIONS/ TOXIC EFFECTS

None known.

NURSING IMPLICATIONS

BASELINE ASSESSMENT

Assess sensitivity to midodrine, taking of other medications (esp. digoxin sodium-retaining vasoconstrictors). Assess medical history, esp. for renal impairment, severe hypertension, cardiac disease.

INTERVENTION/EVALUATION

Monitor B/P, renal/liver/cardiac function.

M

PATIENT/FAMILY TEACHING

Do not take last dose of the day after evening meal or <4 hrs prior to bedtime. Do not give if pt will be supine. Use caution with OTC medications that may affect B/P: cough/cold, diet medications.

mifepristone

my-fih-**priss**-tone
(Mifeprex)
Do not confuse with Mirapex.

CLASSIFICATION

CLINICAL: Abortifacient.

ACTION

Has antiprogestational activity resulting from competitive interaction with progesterone; inhibits the activity of endogenous or exogenous progesterone. Also has antiglucocorticoid and weak antiandrogenic activity. **Therapeutic Effect:** Terminates pregnancy.

USES

Termination of intrauterine pregnancy. **Unlabeled:** Postcoital contraception/contragestation, intrauterine fetal death/nonviable early pregnancy, unresectable meningioma, endometriosis, Cushing's syndrome.

PRECAUTIONS

CONTRAINDICATIONS: Confirmed/suspected ectopic pregnancy, IUD in place, chronic adrenal failure, concurrent long-term steroid/anticoagulant therapy, hemorrhagic disorders, inherited porphyrias. **CAUTIONS:** Treatment of women >35 yrs or smoke >10 cigarettes/day, cardiovascular disease, hypertension, liver/renal impairment, diabetes, severe anemia. **Pregnancy Category X.**

INTERACTIONS

DRUG: Ketoconazole, itraconazole, erythromycin may inhibit metabolism. **Rifampin, phenytoin, phenobarbital, carbamazepine** may increase metabolism. **HERBAL: St. John's wort** may increase metabolism. **FOOD: Grapefruit** may inhibit metabolism. **LAB VALUES:** May decrease Hgb/Hct and RBC count.

AVAILABILITY (Rx)

TABLETS: 200 mg.

INDICATIONS/ROUTES/DOSAGE

Alert: Treatment with mifepristone and misoprostol requires three office visits.

TERMINATION OF PREGNANCY

PO: ADULTS: Day 1: 600 mg as single dose. Day 3: 400 mcg misoprostol. Day 14: Posttreatment examination.

SIDE EFFECTS

FREQUENT (>10%): Headache, dizziness, abdominal pain, nausea, vomiting, diarrhea, fatigue. **OCCASIONAL (3%–10%):** Uterine hemorrhage, back pain, insomnia, vaginitis, dyspepsia, back pain, fever, viral infections, rigors (chills/shaking). **RARE: (1%–2%):** Anxiety, syncope, anemia, asthenia, leg pain, sinusitis, leukorrhea.

ADVERSE REACTIONS/ TOXIC EFFECTS

None known.

NURSING IMPLICATIONS

BASELINE ASSESSMENT

Assess for use of ketoconazole, itraconazole, erythromycin, rifampin, anticonvulsants (inhibits metabolism).

INTERVENTION/EVALUATION

Monitor Hgb/Hct.

PATIENT/FAMILY TEACHING

Advise pts of treatment procedure/effects, need for follow-up visit. Vaginal bleeding/uterine cramping may occur.

miglitol

mig-lih-toll
(Glyset)

CLASSIFICATION

PHARMACOTHERAPEUTIC: Alpha-glucosidase inhibitor. **CLINICAL:** Antidiabetic (see p. 39C).

ACTION

An oral alpha-glucosidase inhibitor that delays the digestion of ingested carbohydrates into simple sugars such as glucose. **Therapeutic Effect:** Produces smaller rise in blood glucose concentration after meals.

USES

Treatment of type 2 non–insulin-dependent diabetes mellitus.

PRECAUTIONS

CONTRAINDICATIONS: Diabetic ketoacidosis, inflammatory bowel disease, colonic ulceration, partial intestinal obstruction, hypersensitivity to miglitol. **CAUTIONS:** Renal function impairment. **Pregnancy Category B.**

INTERACTIONS

DRUG: May decrease concentration/effect of **digoxin, propranolol, ranitidine. HERBAL:** None known. **FOOD:** None known. **LAB VALUES:** None known.

AVAILABILITY (Rx)

TABLETS: 25 mg, 50 mg, 100 mg.

INDICATIONS/ROUTES/DOSAGE

ANTIDIABETIC

PO: ADULTS, ELDERLY: Initially, 25 mg 3 times/day (with first bite of each main meal). MAINTENANCE: 50 mg 3 times/day. **Maximum:** 100 mg 3 times/day.

SIDE EFFECTS

FREQUENT (10%–40%): Flatulence, soft stools, diarrhea, abdominal pain. **OCCASIONAL (5%):** Rash.

NURSING IMPLICATIONS

BASELINE ASSESSMENT

Check blood glucose levels. Determine use of medications, esp. digoxin, propranolol, ranitidine. Discuss lifestyle to determine extent of learning needs.

INTERVENTION/EVALUATION

Monitor blood glucose levels, food intake. Assess for hypoglycemia (cool/wet skin, tremors, dizziness, anxiety, headache, tachycardia, hunger, circumoral numbness, diplopia) or hyperglycemia (polyuria, polydipsia, polyphagia, nausea, vomiting, dim vision, fatigue, deep/rapid breathing). Be alert for conditions altering glucose requirements (fever, stress, surgical procedures).

PATIENT/FAMILY TEACHING

Discuss diet (prescribed diet is a principal part of treatment). Wear medical alert identification. Check with physician when glucose demands are altered (e.g., fever, infection, trauma, heavy physical activity, stress).

miglustat

mig-**lew**-stat
(Zavesca)

M

◆CLASSIFICATION

PHARMACOTHERAPEUTIC: Enzyme inhibitor. **CLINICAL:** Gaucher's disease agent.

ACTION

Inhibits the enzyme glucosylceramide synthase, reducing the rate of synthesis of most glycosphingolipids. **Therapeutic Effect:** Allows the residual activity of the deficient enzyme glucocerebrosidase to be more effective in degrading lysosomal storage within tissue, minimizing conditions (e.g., anemia, bone disease) associated with Gaucher's disease.

USES

Treatment of adult pts with mild to moderate type 1 Gaucher's disease (anemia, thrombocytopenia, progressive hepatosplenomegaly, skeletal complications) for whom enzyme replacement is not feasible (allergy, hypersensitivity, poor venous access).

M

PRECAUTIONS

CONTRAINDICATIONS: Women who are or may become pregnant. **CAUTIONS:** Renal function impairment, fertility impairment. **Pregnancy Category X.**

INTERACTIONS

DRUG: May decrease effects of **imiglucerase. HERBAL:** None known. **FOOD:** None known. **LAB VALUES:** None known.

AVAILABILITY (Rx)

CAPSULES: 100 mg.

ADMINISTRATION/HANDLING

- Give without regard to food. Do not open, crush, or break capsule.

INDICATIONS/ROUTES/DOSAGE

GAUCHER'S DISEASE

PO: ADULTS, ELDERLY: One 100-mg capsule three times/day at regular intervals. MILD RENAL IMPAIRMENT, CREATININE CLEARANCE 50–70 ML/MIN: 100 mg twice daily. MODERATE RENAL IMPAIRMENT, CREATININE CLEARANCE 30–49 ML/MIN: 100 mg daily.

SIDE EFFECTS

COMMON (65%–89%): Diarrhea, weight loss. **FREQUENT (11%–39%):** Hand tremor, flatulence, headache, abdominal pain, nausea. **OCCASIONAL (4%–7%):** Paresthesia, anorexia, dyspepsia (heartburn, epigastric distress), leg cramps, vomiting.

ADVERSE REACTIONS/ TOXIC EFFECTS

Thrombocytopenia occurs in 7% of pts. Overdose produces dizziness, neutropenia.

NURSING IMPLICATIONS

BASELINE ASSESSMENT

Baseline neurological evaluation initially and at 6-mo intervals throughout treatment.

INTERVENTION/EVALUATION

Encourage adequate fluid intake. Assess bowel sounds for peristalsis. Monitor stool frequency/consistency (watery, loose, soft, semisolid, solid). Weigh weekly. Assess for evidence of hand tremor.

PATIENT/FAMILY TEACHING

Avoid high-carbohydrate foods during treatment if diarrhea occurs. Pt should maintain reliable contraceptive methods during treatment and, if seeking to conceive, stop miglustat therapy and maintain contraceptive methods for 3 mos thereafter.

milrinone lactate

mill-rih-known
(Primacor)

CLASSIFICATION

PHARMACOTHERAPEUTIC: Cardiac inotropic agent. **CLINICAL:** Vasodilator (see p. 78C).

ACTION

Inhibits phosphodiesterase, which increases cAMP, potentiating delivery of calcium to myocardial contractile systems. **Therapeutic Effect:** Relaxes vascular muscle, causes vasodilation. Increases cardiac output, decreases pulmonary capillary wedge pressure, vascular resistance.

PHARMACOKINETICS

Onset	Peak	Duration
IV		
5–15 min	—	—

Protein binding: 70%. Primarily excreted unchanged in urine. **Half-life:** 2.4 hrs.

USES

Short-term management of CHF.

PRECAUTIONS

CONTRAINDICATIONS: None known. **CAUTIONS:** Severe obstructive aortic/pulmonic valvular disease, history of ventricular arrhythmias, atrial fibrillation/flutter, impaired renal function.

LIFESPAN CONSIDERATIONS: Pregnancy/lactation: Unknown if drug crosses placenta or is distributed in breast milk. **Pregnancy Category C. Children:** Safety and efficacy not established. **Elderly:** Age-related renal impairment may require dosage adjustment.

INTERACTIONS

DRUG: Produces additive inotropic effects with **cardiac glycosides. HERBAL:** None known. **FOOD:** None known. **LAB VALUES:** None known.

AVAILABILITY (Rx)

INJECTION: 1 mg/ml. **INJECTION (premix):** 200 mcg/ml.

ADMINISTRATION/HANDLING

IV

Storage • Store at room temperature.

Reconstitution • For IV infusion, dilute 20-mg (20-ml) vial with 80 or 180 ml diluent (0.9% NaCl, D_5W) to provide concentration of 200 or 100 mcg/ml, respectively. Maximum concentration: 100 mg/250 ml.

Rate of administration • For IV injection (loading dose), administer undiluted slowly over 10 min. • Monitor for arrhythmias, hypotension during IV therapy; reduce or temporarily discontinue infusion until condition stabilizes.

IV INCOMPATIBILITY

Furosemide (Lasix).

IV COMPATIBILITIES

Calcium gluconate, digoxin (Lanoxin), diltiazem (Cardizem), dobutamine (Dobutrex), dopamine (Intropin), heparin, lidocaine, magnesium, midazolam (Versed), nitroglycerin, potassium, propofol (Diprivan).

INDICATIONS/ROUTES/DOSAGE

CHF

IV: ADULTS: Initially, 50 mcg/kg over 10 min. Continue with maintenance infusion rate of 0.375–0.75 mcg/kg/min based on hemodynamic, clinical response (total

M

daily dose: 0.59–1.13 mg/kg). Reduce dose to 0.2–0.43 mcg/kg/min in pts with severe renal impairment.

SIDE EFFECTS

OCCASIONAL (1%–3%): Headache, hypotension. **RARE (<1%):** Angina, chest pain.

ADVERSE REACTIONS/ TOXIC EFFECTS

Supraventricular/ventricular arrhythmias (12%), nonsustained ventricular tachycardia (2%), sustained ventricular tachycardia (1%).

NURSING IMPLICATIONS

BASELINE ASSESSMENT

Offer emotional support (difficulty breathing may produce anxiety). Assess B/P, apical pulse rate prior to treatment begins and during IV therapy. Assess lung sounds, check edema.

INTERVENTION/EVALUATION

Monitor B/P, heart rate, cardiac output, EKG, potassium, renal function, signs/symptoms of CHF.

M

minocycline hydrochloride

min-know-**sigh**-clean

(Dynacin, Minocin, Novo Minocycline)

Do not confuse with Dynabac, Mithracin.

CLASSIFICATION

PHARMACOTHERAPEUTIC: Tetracycline. **CLINICAL:** Antibiotic.

ACTION

Binds to ribosomes. **Therapeutic Effects:** Inhibits protein synthesis. Bacteriostatic.

USES

Treatment of prostate, urinary tract, CNS infections (not meningitis), uncomplicated gonorrhea, inflammatory acne, brucellosis, skin granulomas, cholera, trachoma, nocardiasis, yaws, syphilis when penicillins are contraindicated. **Unlabeled:** Treatment of atypical mycobacterial infections, rheumatoid arthritis, scleroderma.

PRECAUTIONS

CONTRAINDICATIONS: Hypersensitivity to tetracyclines, last half of pregnancy, children <8 yrs. **CAUTIONS:** Renal impairment, sun/ultraviolet exposure (severe photosensitivity reaction). **Pregnancy Category D.**

INTERACTIONS

DRUG: **Cholestyramine, colestipol** may decrease absorption. May decrease effect of **oral contraceptives. Carbamazepine, phenytoin** may decrease concentration. **HERBAL:** **St. John's wort** may increase risk of photosensitivity. **FOOD:** None known. **LAB VALUES:** May increase SGOT (AST), SGPT (ALT), alkaline phosphatase, amylase, bilirubin concentrations.

AVAILABILITY (Rx)

CAPSULES: 50 mg, 75 mg, 100 mg. **TABLETS:** 50 mg, 75 mg, 100 mg. **POWDER FOR INJECTION:** 100 mg.

ADMINISTRATION/HANDLING

PO

• Store at room temperature. • Give capsules, tablets with full glass of water.

IV

Storage • IV solution is stable for 24 hrs at room temperature. • Use IV infusion (piggyback) immediately after reconstitution. • Discard if precipitate forms.

Reconstitution • For intermittent IV infusion (piggyback), reconstitute each 100-mg vial with 5–10 ml Sterile Water for Injection to provide concentration of 20 or 10 mg/ml, respectively. • Further dilute with 500–1,000 ml D_5W or 0.9% NaCl.

Rate of administration • Infuse over 6 hrs.

⊘ IV INCOMPATIBILITY
Piperacillin/tazobactam (Zosyn).

IV COMPATIBILITIES
Heparin, magnesium, potassium.

INDICATIONS/ROUTES/DOSAGE

Alert: Space doses evenly around the clock.

MILD TO SEVERE INFECTIONS
PO: ADULTS, ELDERLY: Initially, 100–200 mg, then 100 mg q12h or 50 mg q6h.

IV: ADULTS, ELDERLY: Initially, 200 mg, then 100 mg q12h up to 400 mg/day.

PO/IV: CHILDREN >8 YRS: Initially, 4 mg/kg, then 2 mg/kg q12h.

SIDE EFFECTS

FREQUENT: Dizziness, lightheadedness, diarrhea, nausea, vomiting, stomach cramps, photosensitivity (may be severe). **OCCASIONAL:** Pigmentation of skin or mucous membranes, itching in rectal/genital area, sore mouth/tongue.

ADVERSE REACTIONS/ TOXIC EFFECTS

Superinfection (esp. fungal), anaphylaxis, increased intracranial pressure, bulging fontanelles occur rarely in infants.

NURSING IMPLICATIONS

BASELINE ASSESSMENT

Question for history of allergies, esp. tetracyclines, sulfite.

INTERVENTION/EVALUATION

Assess ability to ambulate (may cause vertigo, dizziness). Determine pattern of bowel activity/stool consistency. Assess skin for rash. Check B/P, LOC for increased intracranial pressure. Be alert for superinfection: diarrhea, ulceration/changes of oral mucosa, anal/genital pruritus.

PATIENT/FAMILY TEACHING

Continue antibiotic for full length of treatment. Space doses evenly. Drink full glass of water with capsules/tablets, avoid bedtime doses. Avoid tasks that require alertness, motor skills until response to drug is established. Notify physician if diarrhea, rash, other new symptom occurs. Protect skin from sun exposure.

minoxidil

min-**ox**-ih-dill
(Apo-Gain, Loniten, Milnox, Rogaine, Rogaine Extra Strength)
Do not confuse with Lotensin.

CLASSIFICATION

CLINICAL: Antihypertensive, hair growth stimulant (see p. 53C).

ACTION

Direct action of vascular smooth muscle, producing vasodilation of arterioles. **Therapeutic Effect:** Decreases peripheral vascular resistance, B/P; increases cutaneous blood flow; stimulates hair follicle epithelium, hair follicle growth.

PHARMACOKINETICS

Onset	Peak	Duration
PO		
0.5 hr	2–8 hrs	2–5 days

Well absorbed from GI tract, minimal absorption after topical application. Protein binding: None. Widely distributed. Metabolized in liver to active metabolite. Primarily excreted in urine. Removed by hemodialysis. **Half-life:** 4.2 hrs.

USES

Treatment of severe symptomatic hypertension/hypertension associated with organ damage. Used for pts who fail to respond to maximal therapeutic dosages of diuretic and two other antihypertensive agents. Treatment of alopecia androgenetica (males: baldness of vertex of scalp; females: diffuse hair loss/thinning of frontoparietal areas).

M

PRECAUTIONS

CONTRAINDICATIONS: Pheochromocytoma. **CAUTIONS:** Severe renal impairment, chronic CHF, coronary artery disease, recent MI (1 mo).

LIFESPAN CONSIDERATIONS: Pregnancy/lactation: Crosses placenta. Distributed in breast milk. **Pregnancy Category C. Children:** No age-related precautions noted. **Elderly:** More sensitive to hypotensive effects. Age-related renal impairment may require dosage adjustment.

INTERACTIONS

DRUG: Parenteral antihypertensives may increase hypotensive effect. **NSAIDs** may decrease effect. **HERBAL:** None known. **FOOD:** None known. **LAB VALUES:** May increase BUN, creatinine, plasma renin activity, alkaline phosphatase, sodium. May decrease Hgb, Hct, erythrocyte count.

AVAILABILITY (Rx)

TABLETS: 2.5 mg, 10 mg. **TOPICAL SOLUTION (OTC):** 2% (20 mg/ml), 5% (50 mg/ml).

ADMINISTRATION/HANDLING

PO

• Give without regard to food (with food if GI upset occurs). • Tablets may be crushed.

TOPICAL

• Shampoo, dry hair before applying medication. • Wash hands immediately after application. • Do not use hair dryer after application (reduces effectiveness).

INDICATIONS/ROUTES/DOSAGE

HYPERTENSION

PO: ADULTS: Initially, 5 mg/day. Increase with at least 3-day intervals to 10 mg, 20 mg, up to 40 mg/day in 1–2 doses. ELDERLY: Initially, 2.5 mg/day. May increase gradually. MAINTENANCE: 10–40 mg/day. **Maximum:** 100 mg/day. CHILDREN: Initially, 0.1–0.2 mg/kg (5 mg maximum) daily. Gradually increase at minimum 3-day intervals of 0.1–2 mg/kg. MAINTENANCE: 0.25–1 mg/kg/day in 1–2 doses. **Maximum:** 50 mg/day.

HAIR REGROWTH

Topical: ADULTS: 1 ml to total affected areas of scalp 2 times/day. Total daily dose not to exceed 2 ml.

SIDE EFFECTS

FREQUENT: PO: Edema with concurrent weight gain, hypertrichosis (elongation, thickening, increased pigmentation of fine body hair) develops in 80% of pts within 3–6 wks after beginning therapy. **OCCASIONAL:** EKG T-wave changes (usually revert to pretreatment state with continued therapy or drug withdrawal). **Topical:** Itching, skin rash, dry/flaking skin, erythema. **RARE:** Rash, pruritus, breast tenderness in male and female, headache, photosensitivity reaction.

Topical: Allergic reaction, alopecia, burning scalp, soreness at hair root, headache, visual disturbances.

ADVERSE REACTIONS/ TOXIC EFFECTS

Tachycardia, angina pectoris may occur because of increased O_2 demands associated with increased heart rate, cardiac output. Fluid/electrolyte imbalance, CHF may be observed (esp. if diuretic is not given concurrently). Too rapid reduction in B/P may result in syncope, cerebrovascular accident, MI, ischemia of sense organs (vision, hearing). Pericardial effusion, tamponade may be seen in pts with impaired renal function not on dialysis.

NURSING IMPLICATIONS

BASELINE ASSESSMENT

Assess B/P on both arms and take pulse for 1 full min immediately prior to giving medication. If pulse increases ≥20 beats/min over baseline or systolic or diastolic B/P decreases >20 mm Hg, withhold drug, contact physician.

INTERVENTION/EVALUATION

Monitor fluids/electrolytes, body weight, B/P. Assess for peripheral edema of hands, feet (usually, first area of low extremity swelling is behind medial malleolus in ambulatory, sacral area in bedridden). Assess for signs of CHF (cough, rales at base of lungs, cool extremities, dyspnea on exertion). Monitor fluid, electrolyte serum levels. Assess for distant/muffled heart sounds by auscultation (pericardial effusion, tamponade).

PATIENT/FAMILY TEACHING

Maximum B/P response occurs in 3–7 days. Reversible growth of fine body hair may begin 3–6 wks following initiation of treatment. When used topically for stimulation of hair growth, treatment must continue on a permanent basis—cessation of treatment will begin reversal of new hair growth. Avoid exposure to sunlight, artificial light sources.

mirtazapine

murr-**taz**-ah-peen
(Remeron, Remeron Soltab)
Do not confuse with Premarin.

◆ CLASSIFICATION

PHARMACOTHERAPEUTIC: Tetracyclic compound. **CLINICAL:** Antidepressant (see p. 36C).

ACTION

Acts as antagonist at presynaptic $alpha_2$-adrenergic receptors, increasing norepinephrine, serotonin neurotransmission. **Therapeutic Effect:** Produces antidepressant effect. Prominent sedative effects, low anticholinergic activity.

PHARMACOKINETICS

Rapidly, completely absorbed after PO administration (not affected by food). Protein binding: 85%. Metabolized in liver. Primarily excreted in urine. Unknown if removed by hemodialysis. **Half-life:** 20–40 hrs (longer in males than females [37 hrs vs. 26 hrs]).

USES

Treatment of depression.

PRECAUTIONS

CONTRAINDICATIONS: Within 14 days of MAOI ingestion. **CAUTIONS:** Cardiovascular or GI disorders, prostatic hyperplasia, urinary retention, narrow-angle glaucoma, renal/liver impairment.

LIFESPAN CONSIDERATIONS: Pregnancy/lactation: Unknown if distributed in breast milk. **Pregnancy Cate-**

M

gory C. **Children:** Safety and efficacy not established. **Elderly:** Age-related renal impairment may require cautious use.

INTERACTIONS

DRUG: **Alcohol, diazepam** may increase impairment of cognition, motor skills. **MAOIs** may increase risk of hypertensive crisis, severe convulsions. **HERBAL:** None known. **FOOD:** None known. **LAB VALUES:** May increase cholesterol, triglycerides, SGOT (ALT), SGPT (AST).

AVAILABILITY (Rx)

TABLETS: 15 mg, 30 mg, 45 mg. **ORAL DISINTEGRATING TABLETS:** 15 mg, 30 mg, 45 mg.

ADMINISTRATION/HANDLING

PO

• Give without regard to food. • May crush or break scored tablets.

M

INDICATIONS/ROUTES/DOSAGE

Alert: At least 14 days should elapse between discontinuing MAOIs and instituting mirtazapine therapy. Also, allow at least 14 days after discontinuing mirtazapine and instituting MAOI therapy.

DEPRESSION

PO: ADULTS: Initially, 15 mg at bedtime. May increase by 15 mg/day q1–2wks. **Maximum:** 45 mg/day. ELDERLY: Initially, 7.5 mg at bedtime. May increase by 7.5–15 mg/day q1–2wks. **Maximum:** 45 mg/day.

SIDE EFFECTS

FREQUENT: Somnolence (54%), dry mouth (25%), increase in appetite (17%), constipation (13%), weight gain (12%). **OCCASIONAL:** Asthenia (8%), dizziness (7%), flu syndrome (5%), abnormal dreams (4%). **RARE:** Abdominal discomfort, vasodilation, paresthesia, acne, dry skin, thirst, arthralgia.

ADVERSE REACTIONS/ TOXIC EFFECTS

Higher incidence of seizures than with tricyclic antidepressants (esp. in those with no previous history of seizures). High dosage may produce cardiovascular effects (severe postural hypotension, dizziness, tachycardia, palpitations, arrhythmias). Abrupt withdrawal from prolonged therapy may produce headache, malaise, nausea, vomiting, vivid dreams. Agranulocytosis occurs rarely.

NURSING IMPLICATIONS

BASELINE ASSESSMENT

For pts on long-term therapy, liver/renal function tests, blood counts should be performed periodically.

INTERVENTION/EVALUATION

Supervise suicidal-risk pt closely during early therapy (as depression lessens, energy level improves, increasing suicide potential). Assess appearance, behavior, speech pattern, level of interest, mood. Monitor B/P, pulse for hypotension, arrhythmias.

PATIENT/FAMILY TEACHING

Take as a single bedtime dose. Avoid alcohol, other sedating medications. Avoid tasks requiring mental alertness, motor skills until response to drug established.

misoprostol

mis-oh-**pros**-toll
(Cytotec)
Do not confuse with Cytoxan.

FIXED-COMBINATION(S)

Arthrotec: misoprostol/diclofenac (an NSAID): 200 mcg/50 mg; 200 mcg/75 mg.

◆CLASSIFICATION

PHARMACOTHERAPEUTIC: Prostaglandin. **CLINICAL:** Antisecretory, gastric protectant.

ACTION

Misoprostol, a gastric antisecretory agent, replaces the protective prostaglandins consumed with prostaglandin-inhibiting therapies (e.g., NSAIDs). **Therapeutic Effect:** Reduces acid secretion from the gastric parietal cell, stimulates bicarbonate production from gastric/duodenal mucosa.

PHARMACOKINETICS

Onset	Peak	Duration
PO		
30 min	1–1.5 hrs	3–6 hrs

Rapidly absorbed from GI tract. Protein binding: 80%–90%. Rapidly converted to active metabolite. Primarily excreted in urine. Unknown if removed by hemodialysis. **Half-life:** 20–40 min.

USES

Prevention of NSAID-induced gastric ulcers and in those at high risk of developing gastric ulcer/gastric ulcer complication. **Unlabeled:** Induction of labor. Treatment of duodenal/gastric ulcer, improvement of fat absorption in cystic fibrosis pts.

PRECAUTIONS

CONTRAINDICATIONS: Pregnancy (produces uterine contractions). **CAUTIONS:** Impaired renal function.

LIFESPAN CONSIDERATIONS: Pregnancy/lactation: Unknown if distributed in breast milk. Produces uterine contractions, uterine bleeding, expulsion of products of conception (abortifacient property). **Pregnancy Category X. Children:** Safety and efficacy not established. **Elderly:** No age-related precautions noted.

INTERACTIONS

DRUG: Magnesium antacids enhance diarrhea associated with misoprostol. **HERBAL:** None known. **FOOD:** None known. **LAB VALUES:** None known.

AVAILABILITY (Rx)

TABLETS: 100 mcg, 200 mcg.

ADMINISTRATION/HANDLING

PO

- Give with or after meals (minimizes diarrhea).

INDICATIONS/ROUTES/DOSAGE

PREVENTION OF NSAID-INDUCED GASTRIC ULCER

PO: ADULTS: 200 mcg 4 times/day with food (last dose at bedtime). Continue for duration of NSAID therapy. May reduce dosage to 100 mcg if 200-mcg dose is not tolerated. ELDERLY: 100–200 mcg 4 times/day with food.

M

SIDE EFFECTS

FREQUENT (20%–40%): Abdominal pain, diarrhea. **OCCASIONAL (2%–3%):** Nausea, flatulence, dyspepsia, headache. **RARE (1%):** Vomiting, constipation.

ADVERSE REACTIONS/ TOXIC EFFECTS

Overdosage may produce sedation, tremor, convulsions, dyspnea, palpitations, hypotension, bradycardia.

NURSING IMPLICATIONS

BASELINE ASSESSMENT

Question for possibility of pregnancy prior to initiating therapy (Pregnancy Category X).

PATIENT/FAMILY TEACHING

Avoid magnesium-containing antacids (minimizes potential for diarrhea). Women of childbearing potential must not be pregnant prior to or during medication therapy (may result in hospitalization, surgery, infertility, fetal death). Incidence of diarrhea may be lessened by taking right after meals.

mitomycin

my-toe-**my**-sin
(Mutamycin)

CLASSIFICATION

PHARMACOTHERAPEUTIC: Antibiotic. **CLINICAL:** Antineoplastic (see p. 74C).

ACTION

Alkylating agent, cross-links the strands of DNA. **Therapeutic Effect:** Inhibits DNA, RNA synthesis.

PHARMACOKINETICS

Widely distributed. Does not cross blood-brain barrier. Primarily metabolized in liver and excreted in urine. **Half-life:** 50 min.

USES

Treatment of disseminated adenocarcinoma of stomach, pancreas. **Unlabeled:** Treatment of colorectal, breast, head/neck, bladder, lung, biliary, cervical carcinoma; chronic myelocytic leukemia.

PRECAUTIONS

CONTRAINDICATIONS: Platelet count <75,000/mm^3, WBC <3,000/mm^3, serum creatinine >1.7 mg/dl, coagulation disorders/bleeding tendencies, serious infection. **CAUTIONS:** Myelosuppression, impaired renal/liver function.

LIFESPAN CONSIDERATIONS: Pregnancy/lactation: If possible, avoid use during pregnancy, esp. first trimester. Breast-feeding not recommended. Safety in pregnancy not established. **Children:** No age-related precautions noted. **Elderly:** Age-related renal impairment may require cautious use.

INTERACTIONS

DRUG: Bone marrow depressants may increase bone marrow depression. **Live virus vaccines** may potentiate virus replication, increase vaccine side effects, decrease pt's antibody response to vaccine. **HERBAL:** None known. **FOOD:** None known. **LAB VALUES:** May increase BUN, creatinine.

AVAILABILITY (Rx)

POWDER FOR INJECTION: 5 mg, 20 mg, 40 mg.

ADMINISTRATION/HANDLING

Alert: May be carcinogenic, mutagenic, or teratogenic. Handle with extreme care during preparation/administration. Give via IV push, IV infusion. Extremely irritating to vein. May produce pain on injection, with induration, thrombophlebitis, paresthesia.

IV

Storage • Use only clear, blue-gray solutions. • Concentration of 0.5 mg/ml is stable for 7 days at room temperature or 2 wks if refrigerated. Further diluted solution with D_5W is stable for 3 hrs, 24 hrs if diluted with 0.9% NaCl.

Reconstitution • Reconstitute 5-mg vial with 10 ml Sterile Water for Injection (40 ml for 20-mg vial) to provide solution containing 0.5 mg/ml. • Do not shake vial to dissolve. Allow vial to stand at room temperature until complete dissolution occurs. • For IV infusion, further dilute with 50–100 ml D_5W or 0.9% NaCl.

Rate of administration • Give IV push over 5–10 min. • Give IV through tubing of functional IV catheter or running IV infusion. • Extravasation may produce cellulitis, ulceration, tissue sloughing. Terminate administration immediately, inject ordered antidote. Apply ice intermittently for up to 72 hrs; keep area elevated.

∅ IV INCOMPATIBILITY
Do not mix with any other medications.

IV COMPATIBILITIES
Cisplatin (Platinol AQ), cyclophosphamide (Cytoxan), doxorubicin (Adriamycin), fluorouracil, granisetron (Kytril), leucovorin, methotrexate, ondansetron (Zofran), vinblastine (Velban), vincristine (Oncovin).

INDICATIONS/ROUTES/DOSAGE

Alert: Dosage individualized based on clinical response, tolerance to adverse effects. When used in combination therapy, consult specific protocols for optimum dosage, sequence of drug administration.

INITIAL DOSAGE

IV: ADULTS, ELDERLY, CHILDREN: 10–20 mg/m^2 as single dose. Repeat q6–8wks. Give additional courses only after circulating blood elements (platelets, WBC) are within acceptable levels.

DOSAGE IN RENAL IMPAIRMENT

Creatinine Clearance	% Normal Dose
<10 ml/min	75%

Leukocytes	Platelets	% of Prior Dose to Give
4,000	>100,000	100
3,000–3,999	75,000 99,000	100
2,000–2,999	25,000 74,999	70
<2,000	<25,000	50

SIDE EFFECTS

FREQUENT (>10%): Fever, anorexia, nausea, vomiting. **OCCASIONAL (2%–10%):** Stomatitis, numbness of fingers/toes, purple color bands on nails, skin rash, alopecia, unusual tiredness. **RARE (<1%):** Thrombophlebitis, cellulitis, extravasation.

ADVERSE REACTIONS/ TOXIC EFFECTS

Marked bone marrow depression results in hematologic toxicity manifested as leukopenia, thrombocytopenia, and, to a lesser extent, anemia (generally occurs within 2–4 wks after initial therapy). Renal toxicity may be evidenced by rise in BUN and/or serum creatinine. Pulmonary toxicity manifested as dyspnea, cough, hemoptysis, pneumonia. Long-term therapy may produce hemolytic uremic syndrome (HUS), characterized by hemolytic anemia, thrombocytopenia, renal failure, hypertension.

NURSING IMPLICATIONS

BASELINE ASSESSMENT

Obtain CBC with differential, prothrombin, bleeding time, prior to and periodically during therapy. Antiemetics prior to and during therapy may alleviate nausea/vomiting.

INTERVENTION/EVALUATION

Monitor hematologic status, BUN, serum creatinine, renal function studies. Assess IV site for phlebitis, extravasation. Monitor for hematologic toxicity (fever, sore throat, signs of local infection, unusual bruising/bleeding from any site), symptoms of anemia (excessive tiredness, weakness). Assess for renal toxicity (foul odor from urine, rise in BUN, serum creatinine).

PATIENT/FAMILY TEACHING

Maintain fastidious oral hygiene. Immediately report any stinging, burning, pain at injection site. Do not have immunizations without physician's approval (drug lowers body's resistance). Avoid contact with those who have recently received live virus vaccine. Promptly report fever, sore throat, signs of local infection, unusual

M

bruising/bleeding from any site, increased urinary frequency, dysuria. Alopecia is reversible, but new hair growth may have different color, texture. Contact physician if nausea/vomiting, fever, sore throat, bruising, bleeding, shortness of breath, painful urination occur.

mitotane

(Lysodren)

See Classification section under: Cancer chemotherapeutic agents (p. 74C)

mitoxantrone

my-toe-**zan**-trone
(Novantrone)

CLASSIFICATION

PHARMACOTHERAPEUTIC: Anthracenedione. **CLINICAL:** Nonvesicant, antineoplastic (see p. 75C).

ACTION

Inhibits DNA, RNA synthesis. Active throughout entire cell cycle. **Therapeutic Effect:** Inhibits B-cell, T-cell, macrophage proliferation. Causes cell death.

PHARMACOKINETICS

Protein binding: 78%. Widely distributed. Metabolized in liver. Primarily eliminated in feces via biliary system. Not removed by hemodialysis. **Half-life:** 2.3–13 days.

USES

Treatment of acute, nonlymphocytic leukemia (monocytic, myelogenous, promyelocytic), late-stage hormone-resistant prostate cancer, multiple sclerosis. **Unlabeled:** Treatment of breast, liver carcinoma; non-Hodgkin's lymphoma.

PRECAUTIONS

CONTRAINDICATIONS: Pts with multiple sclerosis with hepatic impairment, baseline left ventricular ejection fraction <50%, cumulative lifetime mitoxantrone dose ≥140 mg/m². **CAUTIONS:** Preexisting bone marrow suppression, previous treatment with cardiotoxic medications, impaired hepatobiliary function.

LIFESPAN CONSIDERATIONS: Pregnancy/lactation: If possible, avoid use during pregnancy, esp. first trimester. May cause fetal harm. Breast-feeding not recommended. **Pregnancy Category D. Children:** Safety and efficacy not established. **Elderly:** No age-related precautions noted.

INTERACTIONS

DRUG: May decrease effect of **antigout medications. Bone marrow depressants** may increase bone marrow depression. **Live virus vaccines** may potentiate virus replication, increase vaccine side effects, decrease pt's antibody response to vaccine. **HERBAL:** None known. **FOOD:** None known. **LAB VALUES:** May increase SGOT (AST), SGPT (ALT), bilirubin, uric acid.

AVAILABILITY (Rx)

INJECTION: 2 mg/ml.

ADMINISTRATION/HANDLING

Alert: May be carcinogenic, mutagenic, or teratogenic. Handle with extreme care during preparation/administration. Give by IV injection, IV infusion. Must dilute before administration.

IV

Storage • Store vials at room temperature.

Reconstitution • Dilute with at least 50 ml D_5W or 0.9% NaCl.

Rate of administration Do not administer by subcutaneous, IM, intrathecal, or intra-arterial injection. Do not give IV push over <3 min. May give IV bolus over >3 min, IV intermittent infusion over 15–60 min, or IV continuous infusion (0.02–0.5 mg/ml) in D_5W or 0.9% NaCl.

∅ IV INCOMPATIBILITIES
Heparin, paclitaxel (Taxol), piperacillin/tazobactam (Zosyn).

IV COMPATIBILITIES
Allopurinol (Aloprim), etoposide (VePesid), gemcitabine (Gemczar), granisetron (Kytril), ondansetron (Zofran), potassium chloride.

INDICATIONS/ROUTES/DOSAGE

LEUKEMIAS

IV: ADULTS, ELDERLY, CHILDREN >2 YRS: 12 mg/m^2/day once daily for 2–3 days. ACUTE LEUKEMIA IN RELAPSE: 8–12 mg/m^2/day once daily for 4–5 days. ACUTE NONLYMPHOCYTIC LEUKEMIA: 10 mg/m^2/day once daily for 3–5 days. CHILDREN <2 YRS: 0.4 mg/kg/day once daily for 3–5 days.

SOLID TUMORS

IV: ADULTS, ELDERLY: 12–14 mg/m^2 once q3–4wks. CHILDREN: 18–20 mg/m^2 once q3–4wks.

MULTIPLE SCLEROSIS

IV: ADULTS, ELDERLY: 12 mg/m^2/dose q3mos.

SIDE EFFECTS

FREQUENT (>10%): Nausea, vomiting, diarrhea, cough, headache, stomatitis, abdominal discomfort, fever, alopecia. **OCCASIONAL (4%–9%):** Easy bruising, fungal infection, conjunctivitis, urinary tract infection. **RARE (3%):** Arrhythmias.

ADVERSE REACTIONS/TOXIC EFFECTS

Bone marrow suppression may be severe, resulting in GI bleeding, sepsis, pneumonia. Renal failure, seizures, jaundice, CHF may occur.

NURSING IMPLICATIONS

BASELINE ASSESSMENT

Offer emotional support. Establish baseline for CBC with differential, temperature, pulse rate/quality, respiratory status.

INTERVENTION/EVALUATION

Monitor hematologic status, pulmonary function studies, hepatic/renal function tests. Monitor for stomatitis (burning/erythema of oral mucosa, ulceration, sore throat, difficulty swallowing), fever, signs of local infection, unusual bruising/bleeding from any site. Extravasation produces swelling, pain, burning, blue discoloration of skin.

PATIENT/FAMILY TEACHING

Urine will appear blue/green 24 hrs after administration. Blue tint to sclera may also appear. Maintain adequate daily fluid intake (may protect against renal impairment). Do not have immunizations without physician's approval (drug lowers body's resistance). Avoid crowds, those with infection. Contraceptive measures recommended during therapy.

mivacurium chloride

(Mivacron)

See Classification section under: Neuromuscular blockers (p. 106C)

M

modafinil

mode-ah-**feen**-awl
(Alertec, Provigil)

CLASSIFICATION

PHARMACOTHERAPEUTIC: Alpha$_1$-agonist. **CLINICAL:** Wakefulness-promoting agent.

ACTION

Binds to dopamine reuptake carrier site, increasing alpha activity, decreasing delta, theta, and beta activity. **Therapeutic Effect:** Reduces the number of sleep episodes and duration of total daytime sleep.

PHARMACOKINETICS

Well absorbed. Protein binding: 60%. Widely distributed. Metabolized in lever. Excreted in the kidney. Unknown if removed by hemodialysis. **Half-life:** 8–10 hrs.

M

USES

Treatment of excessive daytime sleepiness associated with narcolepsy, other sleep disorders. **Unlabeled:** Depression.

PRECAUTIONS

CONTRAINDICATIONS: None known. **CAUTIONS:** History of clinically significant manifestation of mitral valve prolapse, left ventricular hypertrophy, liver impairment, history of seizures.

LIFESPAN CONSIDERATIONS: Pregnancy/lactation: Unknown if excreted in breast milk. Use caution if given to pregnant women. **Pregnancy Category C. Children:** Safety and efficacy not established in those <16 yrs. **Elderly:** Age-related renal/liver impairment in the elderly may require decreased dosage.

INTERACTIONS

DRUG: May increase concentrations of **tricyclic antidepressants, phenytoin, warfarin, diazepam, propranolol.** May decrease concentrations of **cyclosporine, oral contraceptives, theophylline. CNS stimulants** may increase CNS stimulation. **HERBAL:** None known. **FOOD:** None known. **LAB VALUES:** None known.

AVAILABILITY (Rx)

TABLETS: 100 mg, 200 mg.

ADMINISTRATION/HANDLING

- Give without regard to meals.

INDICATIONS/ROUTES/DOSAGE

NARCOLEPSY, SLEEP DISORDERS

PO: ADULTS, ELDERLY: 200–400 mg/day.

SIDE EFFECTS

FREQUENT: Anxiety, headache, insomnia, nausea, nervousness. **OCCASIONAL:** Anorexia, diarrhea, dizziness, dry mouth/skin, muscle stiffness, increased thirst, rhinitis, tingling of skin, tremor, headache, vomiting.

ADVERSE REACTIONS/ TOXIC EFFECTS

Agitation, excitation, increased B/P, insomnia.

NURSING IMPLICATIONS

BASELINE ASSESSMENT

Obtain baseline evidence of narcolepsy or other sleep disorders, including pattern, environmental situations, lengths of sleep episodes. Question for sudden loss of muscle tone (cataplexy) precipitated by strong emotional responses prior to sleep episode. Assess frequency/severity of sleep episodes prior to drug therapy.

INTERVENTION/EVALUATION

Monitor sleep pattern, evidence of restlessness during sleep, length of insomnia episodes during night. Assess for dizziness, anxiety; initiate fall precautions. Sugarless gum, sips of tepid water may relieve dry mouth.

PATIENT/FAMILY TEACHING

Avoid tasks that require alertness, motor skills until response to drug is established. Do not increase dose without checking with physician. Use alternative steroidal contraceptives during and 1 mo after discontinuing modafinil.

moexipril hydrochloride

mow-**ex**-ih-prill
(Univasc)

FIXED-COMBINATION(S)

Uniretic: moexipril/hydrochlorothiazide (a diuretic): 7.5 mg/12.5 mg, 15 mg/12.5 mg, 15 mg/25 mg.

◆ CLASSIFICATION

PHARMACOTHERAPEUTIC: Angiotensin-converting enzyme (ACE) inhibitor. **CLINICAL:** Antihypertensive (see p. 6C).

ACTION

Suppresses renin-angiotensin-aldosterone system (prevents conversion of angiotensin I to angiotensin II, a potent vasoconstrictor; may also inhibit angiotensin II at local vascular and renal sites). **Therapeutic Effect:** Reduces peripheral arterial resistance, B/P.

PHARMACOKINETICS

Onset	Peak	Duration
PO		
1 hr	3–6 hrs	24 hrs

Incompletely absorbed from GI tract (food decreases absorption). Rapidly converted to active metabolite. Protein binding: 50%. Primarily recovered in feces, partially excreted in urine. Unknown if removed by dialysis. **Half-life:** 1 hr (metabolite 2–9 hrs).

USES

Treatment of hypertension. Used alone or in combination with thiazide diuretics.

PRECAUTIONS

CONTRAINDICATIONS: History of angioedema with previous treatment with ACE inhibitors. **CAUTIONS:** Renal impairment, those with sodium depletion or on diuretic therapy, dialysis, hypovolemia, coronary/cerebrovascular insufficiency, hyperkalemia, aortic stenosis, ischemic heart disease, angina, severe CHF cerebrovascular disease.

LIFESPAN CONSIDERATIONS: Pregnancy/lactation: Crosses placenta. Unknown if distributed in breast milk. **Pregnancy Category C** (**D** if used during second and third trimesters). Has caused fetal/neonatal mortality, morbidity. **Children:** Safety and efficacy not established. **Elderly:** Age-related renal impairment may require cautious use.

INTERACTIONS

DRUG: **Alcohol, diuretics, hypotensive agents** may increase effects. **NSAIDs** may decrease effect. **Potassium-sparing diuretics, potassium supplements** may cause hyperkalemia. May increase **lithium** concentration, toxicity. **HERBAL:** None known. **FOOD:** None known. **LAB VALUES:** May increase potassium, SGOT (AST), SGPT (ALT), alkaline phosphatase, bilirubin,

M

BUN, creatinine. May decrease sodium. May cause positive ANA titer.

AVAILABILITY (Rx)

TABLETS: 7.5 mg, 15 mg.

ADMINISTRATION/HANDLING

PO

• Give 1 hr before meals. • Tablets may be crushed.

INDICATIONS/ROUTES/DOSAGE

HYPERTENSION (used alone)

PO: ADULTS, ELDERLY: Initially, 7.5 mg once daily 1 hr before meals. Adjust according to B/P effect. MAINTENANCE: 7.5–30 mg daily in 1–2 divided doses 1 hr before meals.

HYPERTENSION (concurrent diuretic therapy)

Alert: To reduce risk of hypotension, discontinue diuretic 2–3 days before initiating moexipril therapy. If B/P not controlled, resume diuretic. If diuretic cannot be discontinued, give initial dose of 3.75 mg moexipril.

RENAL FUNCTION IMPAIRMENT

PO: ADULTS, ELDERLY: 3.75 mg once daily in pts with creatinine clearance of 40 ml/min/1.73 m^2. **Maximum:** May titrate up to 15 mg/day.

SIDE EFFECTS

OCCASIONAL: Cough, headache (6%); dizziness (4%); nausea, fatigue (3%). **RARE:** Flushing, rash, myalgia, nausea, vomiting.

ADVERSE REACTIONS/ TOXIC EFFECTS

Excessive hypotension ("first-dose syncope") may occur in those with CHF, severely salt/volume depleted. Angioedema (swelling of face/lips), hyperkalemia occur rarely. Agranulocytosis, neutropenia may be noted in pts with impaired renal function, collagen vascular disease (systemic lupus erythematosus, scleroderma). Nephrotic syndrome may be noted in pts with history of renal disease.

NURSING IMPLICATIONS

BASELINE ASSESSMENT

Obtain B/P, apical pulse immediately prior to each dose, in addition to regular monitoring (be alert to fluctuations). If excessive reduction in B/P occurs, place pt in supine position, feet slightly elevated. Renal function tests should be performed before therapy begins. In pts with renal impairment, autoimmune disease, taking drugs that affect leukocytes or immune response, CBC with differential count should be performed prior to when therapy begins and q2wks for 3 mos, then periodically thereafter.

INTERVENTION/EVALUATION

Monitor B/P, serum potassium, renal function, WBC count. Watch for hypotensive effect within 1–3 hrs of first dose or increase in dose. Assist with ambulation if dizziness occurs.

PATIENT/FAMILY TEACHING

Do not abruptly stop medication. Inform physician of sore throat, fever, difficulty breathing, chest pain, cough. Notify physician of signs of angioedema (swelling of hands, feet, face, eyes, lips, tongue). Irregular heartbeats may occur. To reduce hypotensive effect, rise slowly from lying to sitting position, permit legs to dangle momentarily before standing. May alter taste.

molindone hydrochloride

(Moban)

See Classification section under: Antipsychotics

mometasone

(Elocon)

See Classification section under: Corticosteroids: topical (p. 85C)

mometasone furoate monohydrate

(Nasonex)

◆CLASSIFICATION

PHARMACOTHERAPEUTIC: Adrenocorticosteroid. **CLINICAL:** Anti-inflammatory.

ACTION

Inhibits early activation of allergic reaction, release of inflammatory cells into nasal tissue. **Therapeutic Effect:** Decreases response to seasonal and perennial rhinitis.

PHARMACOKINETICS

Undetectable in plasma. Protein binding: 98%–99%. The portion of the dose that is swallowed undergoes extensive metabolism. Excreted via bile and, to a lesser extent, into the urine.

USES

Treatment of nasal symptoms of seasonal allergic/perennial allergic rhinitis in adults, children >2 yrs. Prophylaxis of nasal symptoms of seasonal allergic rhinitis in adults, adolescents >12 yrs.

PRECAUTIONS

CONTRAINDICATIONS: Hypersensitivity to any corticosteroid, systemic fungal infections, persistently positive sputum cultures for *Candida albicans,* untreated localized infection involving nasal mucosa. **CAUTIONS:** Adrenal insufficiency, cirrhosis, glaucoma, hypothyroidism, untreated infection, osteoporosis, tuberculosis.

LIFESPAN CONSIDERATIONS: Pregnancy/lactation: Unknown if drug crosses placenta or is distributed in breast milk. **Pregnancy Category C. Children:** Prolonged treatment/high doses may decrease short-term growth rate, cortisol secretion. **Elderly:** No age-related precautions noted.

INTERACTIONS

DRUG: None known. **HERBAL:** None known. **FOOD:** None known. **LAB VALUES:** None known.

AVAILABILITY (Rx)

NASAL SPRAY.

ADMINISTRATION/HANDLING

INTRANASAL

• Shake well before each use. • Clear nasal passages as much as possible. • Insert spray tip into nostril, pointing toward nasal passages, away from nasal septum. • Spray into nostril while holding other nostril closed, concurrently inspire through nose to permit medication as high into nasal passages as possible.

INDICATIONS/ROUTES/DOSAGE

ALLERGIC RHINITIS

Nasal spray: ADULTS, ELDERLY, CHILDREN ≥12 YRS: 2 sprays in each nostril once daily. CHILDREN 2–11 YRS: 1 spray in each nostril once daily. Improvement occurs within 11 hrs–2 days following first dose. Maximum benefit achieved within 1–2 wks.

SIDE EFFECTS

OCCASIONAL: Nasal irritation, stinging. **RARE:** Nasal/pharyngeal candidiasis.

ADVERSE REACTIONS/ TOXIC EFFECTS

Acute hypersensitivity reaction (urticaria, angioedema, severe bronchospasm) oc-

M

curs rarely. Transfer from systemic to local steroid therapy may unmask previously suppressed bronchial asthma condition.

NURSING IMPLICATIONS

BASELINE ASSESSMENT

Question for hypersensitivity to any corticosteroids.

INTERVENTION/EVALUATION

Teach proper use of nasal spray. Clear nasal passages prior to use. Contact physician if no improvement in symptoms, sneezing, nasal irritation occur.

PATIENT/FAMILY TEACHING

Do not change dose schedule or stop taking drug; must taper off gradually under medical supervision. Contact physician if no improvement in symptoms, sneezing, nasal irritation occur. Clear nasal passages prior to use.

M

Monopril

see fosinopril

montelukast

mon-**tee**-leu-cast
(Singulair)

CLASSIFICATION

PHARMACOTHERAPEUTIC: Leukotriene receptor inhibitor. **CLINICAL:** Antiasthmatic (see p. 66C).

ACTION

Inhibits the cysteinyl leukotriene receptor producing inhibition of the effects on bronchial smooth muscle. **Therapeutic Effect:** Attenuates bronchoconstriction, decreases vascular permeability, mucosal edema, mucus production.

PHARMACOKINETICS

Onset	Peak	Duration
PO		
—	—	24 hrs
PO, chewable		
—	—	24 hrs

Rapidly absorbed from GI tract. Protein binding: 99%. Extensively metabolized in the liver. Excreted almost exclusively in the feces. **Half-life:** 2.7–5.5 hrs (half-life slightly longer in the elderly).

USES

Prophylaxis, chronic treatment of asthma. Not for use in reversal of bronchospasm in acute asthma attacks, status asthmaticus, exercise-induced bronchospasm. Treatment of seasonal allergic rhinitis (hay fever).

PRECAUTIONS

CONTRAINDICATIONS: None known. **CAUTIONS:** Systemic corticosteroid treatment reduction during montelukast therapy, impaired liver function.

LIFESPAN CONSIDERATIONS: Pregnancy/lactation: Unknown if excreted in breast milk. Use during pregnancy only if necessary. **Pregnancy Category B. Children/elderly:** No age-related precautions noted in those >6 yrs or the elderly.

INTERACTIONS

DRUG: Phenobarbital, rifampin may reduce duration of action of montelukast. **HERBAL:** None known. **FOOD:** None known. **LAB VALUES:** May increase SGOT (AST), SGPT (ALT).

AVAILABILITY (Rx)

TABLETS: 10 mg. **TABLETS (chewable):** 4 mg, 5 mg. **ORAL GRANULES:** 4 mg.

ADMINISTRATION/HANDLING

PO

- Administer in the evening without regard to food ingestion.

INDICATIONS/ROUTES/DOSAGE

BRONCHIAL ASTHMA

PO: ADULTS, ELDERLY, ADOLESCENTS >14 YRS: One 10-mg tablet daily, taken in the evening. CHILDREN 6–14 YRS: One 5-mg chewable tablet daily, taken in the evening. CHILDREN 1–5 YRS: One 4-mg chewable tablet daily, taken in the evening.

SEASONAL ALLERGIC RHINITIS

PO: ADULTS, ELDERLY, CHILDREN ≥15 YRS: 10 mg once daily.

SIDE EFFECTS

ADULTS, ADOLESCENTS >14 YRS: **FREQUENT (18%):** Headache. **OCCASIONAL (4%):** Influenza. **RARE (2%–3%):** Abdominal pain, cough, dyspepsia, dizziness, fatigue, dental pain.

CHILDREN 6–14 YRS: **RARE (<2%):** Diarrhea, laryngitis, pharyngitis, nausea, otitis media, sinusitis, viral infection.

ADVERSE REACTIONS/ TOXIC EFFECTS

None known.

NURSING IMPLICATIONS

BASELINE ASSESSMENT

Chewable tablet contains phenylalanine (a component of aspartame); parents of phenylketonuric pts should be informed. Montelukast should not be abruptly substituted for inhaled or oral corticosteroids.

INTERVENTION/EVALUATION

Monitor rate, depth, rhythm, type of respirations; quality/rate of pulse. Assess lung sounds for rhonchi, wheezing, rales. Observe lips, fingernails for blue/dusky color in light-skinned pts, gray in dark-skinned pts.

PATIENT/FAMILY TEACHING

Increase fluid intake (decreases lung secretion viscosity). Take as prescribed, even during symptom-free periods as well as during excacerbations of asthma. Do not alter/stop other asthma medications. Drug is not for the treatment of acute asthma attacks. Pts with aspirin sensitivity should avoid aspirin, NSAIDs while taking montelukast.

moricizine hydrochloride

(Ethmozine)

See Classification section under: Antiarrhythmics (p. 14C)

morphine sulfate

(Astramorph, Avinza, Duramorph, Infumorph, Kadian, M-Eslon ✤, MS Contin, MSIR, Oramorph SR, RMS, Roxanol, Statex ✤)

Do not confuse with hydromorphone, Roxicet.

CLASSIFICATION

PHARMACOTHERAPEUTIC: Narcotic agonist. **CLINICAL:** Opiate analgesic **(Schedule II)** (see p. 121C).

ACTION

Binds with opioid receptors within CNS. **Therapeutic Effect:** Alters processes affecting pain perception, emotional response to pain; produces generalized CNS depression.

PHARMACOKINETICS

	Onset	Peak	Duration
Tablets	—	1 hr	3–5 hrs
Oral solution	—	1 hr	3–5 hrs
Epidural	—	1 hr	12–20 hrs
ER Tabs	—	3–4 hrs	8–12 hrs
Rectal	—	0.5–1 hr	3–7 hrs
Subcutaneous	—	1.1–5 hrs	3–5 hrs
IM	5–30 min	0.5–1 hr	3–5 hrs
IV	Rapid	0.3 hr	3–5 hrs

Variably absorbed from GI tract. Readily absorbed following subcutaneous, IM administration. Protein binding: 20%–35%. Widely distributed. Metabolized in liver. Primarily excreted in urine. Removed by hemodialysis. **Half-life:** 2–3 hrs.

USES

Relief of severe/acute/chronic pain, preop sedation, anesthesia supplement, analgesia during labor. Drug of choice for pain due to MI, dyspnea from pulmonary edema not resulting from chemical respiratory irritant.

PRECAUTIONS

CONTRAINDICATIONS: Severe respiratory depression, acute/severe asthma, severe liver/renal impairment, GI obstruction. **EXTREME CAUTION:** COPD, cor pulmonale, hypoxia, hypercapnia, preexisting respiratory depression, head injury, increased intracranial pressure, severe hypotension. **CAUTIONS:** Biliary tract disease, pancreatitis, Addison's disease, hypothyroidism, urethral stricture, prostatic hypertrophy, debilitated patients, those with CNS depression, toxic psychosis, seizure disorders, alcoholism.

LIFESPAN CONSIDERATIONS: Pregnancy/lactation: Crosses placenta. Distributed in breast milk. May prolong labor if administered in latent phase of first stage of labor or before cervical dilation of 4–5 cm has occurred. Respiratory depression may occur in neonate if mother received opiates during labor. Regular use of opiates during pregnancy may produce withdrawal symptoms in neonate (irritability, excessive crying, tremors, hyperactive reflexes, fever, vomiting, diarrhea, yawning, sneezing, seizures). **Pregnancy Category C (D** if used for prolonged periods or at high dosages at term). **Children:** Paradoxical excitement may occur; those <2 yrs more susceptible to respiratory depressant effects. **Elderly:** Paradoxical excitement may occur; age-related renal impairment may increase risk of urinary retention.

INTERACTIONS

DRUG: Alcohol, CNS depressants may increase CNS or respiratory depression, hypotension. **MAOIs** may produce severe, fatal reaction (reduce dose ¼ usual dose). **HERBAL:** None known. **FOOD:** None known. **LAB VALUES:** May increase amylase, lipase.

AVAILABILITY (Rx)

CAPSULES (sustained-release): (Kadian): 20 mg, 30 mg, 50 mg, 60 mg, 100 mg. **(extended release): (Avinza):** 30 mg, 60 mg, 90 mg, 120 mg. **SOLUTION FOR INJECTIONS:** 0.5 mg/ml, 1 mg/ml, 2 mg/ml, 4 mg/ml, 5 mg/ml, 8 mg/ml, 10 mg/ml, 15 mg/ml, 25 mg/ml, 50 mg/ml. **(Preservative-free):** 0.5 mg/ml, 1 mg/ml, 10 mg/ml, 25 mg/ml, 50 mg/ml. **EPIDURAL/INTRATHECAL VIA INFUSION DEVICE: (Infumorph):** 10 mg/ml, 25 mg/ml. **EPIDURAL, INTRATHECAL, IV INFUSION: (Astramorph, Duramorph):** 0.5 mg/ml, 1 mg/ml, 4 mg/ml. **IV INFUSION (via PCA):** 1 mg/ml, 5 mg/ml. **ORAL SOLUTION (Roxanol):** 10 mg/5 ml, 20 mg/5 ml, 20 mg/ml, 100 mg/5 mg. **SUPPOSITORY (RMS):** 5 mg, 10 mg, 20 mg, 30 mg. **TABLETS (MSIR):** 15 mg/30 mg. **TABLETS (extended-release): (MS Contin, Oramorph SR):** 15 mg, 30 mg, 60 mg, 100 mg, 200 mg.

ADMINISTRATION/HANDLING

PO

• Mix liquid form with fruit juice to improve taste. • Do not crush, break extended-release capsule. • **Kadian:** May mix with applesauce immediately prior to administration.

SUBCUTANEOUS/IM

• Administer slowly, rotating injection sites. • Pts with circulatory impairment experience higher risk of overdosage due to delayed absorption of repeated administration.

IV

Storage • Store at room temperature.

Reconstitution • May give undiluted. • For IV injection, may dilute 2.5–15 mg morphine in 4–5 ml Sterile Water for Injection. • For continuous IV infusion, dilute to concentration of 0.1–1 mg/ml in D_5W and give through controlled infusion device.

Rate of administration • Always administer very slowly. Rapid IV increases risk of severe adverse reactions (apnea, chest wall rigidity, peripheral circulatory collapse, cardiac arrest, anaphylactoid effects).

RECTAL

• If suppository is too soft, chill for 30 min in refrigerator or run cold water over foil wrapper. • Moisten suppository with cold water before inserting well into rectum.

IV INCOMPATIBILITIES

Amphotericin B complex (Abelcet, AmBisome, Amphotec), cefepime (Maxipime), doxorubicin liposome (Doxil), thiopental.

IV COMPATIBILITIES

Amiodarone (Cordarone), bumetanide (Bumex), bupivacaine (Marcaine, Sensorcaine), diltiazem (Cardizem), dobutamine (Dobutrex), dopamine (Intropin), heparin, lidocaine, lorazepam (Ativan), magnesium, midazolam (Versed), milrinone (Primacor), nitroglycerin, potassium, propofol (Diprivan).

INDICATIONS/ROUTES/DOSAGE

Alert: Reduce dosage in elderly/debilitated, those on concurrent CNS depressants. Doses to be titrated to desired effect.

PAIN

PO: ADULTS, ELDERLY: (Prompt-release): 10–30 mg q4h as needed. CHILDREN: 0.2–0.5 mg/kg/dose q4–6h. (Sustained-release): 15–30 mg q8–12h. CHILDREN: 0.3–0.6 mg/kg/dose q12h.

IV/IM/subcutaneous: ADULTS, ELDERLY: 2.5–20 mg/dose q2–6h. CHILDREN: 0.1–0.2 mg/kg/dose q2–4h. **Maximum:** 15 mg/dose.

IV continuous infusion: ADULTS, ELDERLY: 0.8–10 mg/hr. RANGE: Up to 80 mg/hr. CHILDREN: 0.025–2.6 mg/kg/hr.

Epidural: ADULTS, ELDERLY: Initially, 5 mg. May give 1–2 mg in 1 hr if no relief. **Maximum:** 10 mg/24 hrs.

Intrathecal: ADULTS, ELDERLY: 1/10 epidural dose: 0.2–1 mg/dose.

PCA: LOADING DOSE: 5–10 mg. INTERMITTENT BOLUS: 0.5–3 mg. LOCKOUT INTERVAL: 5–12 min. CONTINUOUS INFUSION: 1–10 mg/hr. 4-HR LIMIT: 20–30 mg.

SIDE EFFECTS

Alert: Effects depend on dosage amount, route of administration. Ambulatory pts, those not in severe pain may experience dizziness, nausea, vomiting, hypotension more frequently than those in supine position or who have severe pain.

FREQUENT: Sedation, decreased B/P, diaphoresis, flushed face, constipation, dizziness, drowsiness, nausea, vomiting. **OCCASIONAL:** Allergic reaction (rash, itching), difficulty breathing, confusion, pounding heartbeat, tremors, decreased urination, stomach cramps, vision changes, dry mouth, headache, decreased appetite, pain/burning at injection site. **RARE:** Paralytic ileus.

ADVERSE REACTIONS/ TOXIC EFFECTS

Overdosage results in respiratory depression, skeletal muscle flaccidity, cold/clammy skin, cyanosis, extreme somnolence progressing to convulsions, stupor, coma. Tolerance to analgesic effect, physical dependence may occur with repeated use. Prolonged duration of action, cumulative effect may occur in those with impaired hepatic, renal function.

NURSING IMPLICATIONS

BASELINE ASSESSMENT

Pt should be in a recumbent position before drug is given by parenteral route. Assess onset, type, location, duration of pain. Obtain vital signs before giving medication. If respirations are ≤12/min (≤20/min in children), withhold medication, contact physician. Effect of medication is reduced if full pain recurs before next dose.

INTERVENTION/EVALUATION

Monitor vital signs 5–10 min after IV administration, 15–30 min after subcutaneous, IM. Be alert for decreased respirations, B/P. Check for adequate voiding. Monitor stools; avoid constipation. Initiate deep breathing, coughing exercises, particularly in those with impaired pulmonary function. Assess for clinical improvement, record onset of pain relief. Consult physician if pain relief is not adequate.

PATIENT/FAMILY TEACHING

Discomfort may occur with injection. Change positions slowly to avoid orthostatic hypotension. Avoid tasks that require alertness, motor skills until response to drug is established. Avoid alcohol, CNS depressants. Tolerance/dependence may occur with prolonged use of high doses.

Motrin

see ibuprofen

moxifloxacin hydrochloride

mox-ih-**flocks**-ah-sin
(Avelox, Avelox IV, Vigamox)
Do not confuse with Avonex.

CLASSIFICATION

PHARMACOTHERAPEUTIC: Fluoroquinolone. **CLINICAL:** Antibacterial (see p. 23C).

ACTION

Inhibits two enzymes, topoisomerase II and IV, in susceptible microorganisms. **Therapeutic Effect:** Interferes with bacterial DNA replication. Prevents/delays resistance emergence. Bactericidal.

PHARMACOKINETICS

Well absorbed from GI tract after PO administration. Protein binding: 50%. Widely distributed throughout body with tissue concentration often exceeding plasma concentration. Metabolized in liver. Primarily excreted in urine with a lesser amount in feces. **Half-life:** 10.7–13.3 hrs.

USES

Treatment of acute bacterial exacerbation of chronic bronchitis, acute bacterial sinusitis, community-acquired pneumonia, uncomplicated skin/skin structure infections. **Ophthalmic:** Topical treatment of bacterial conjunctivitis due to susceptible strains of bacteria.

PRECAUTIONS

CONTRAINDICATIONS: Hypersensitivity to quinolones. **CAUTIONS:** Renal/hepatic impairment, CNS disorders, cerebral arthrosclerosis, seizures, those with prolonged QT interval, uncorrected hypokalemia, those receiving quinidine, procainamide, amiodarone, sotalol.

LIFESPAN CONSIDERATIONS: Pregnancy/lactation: May be distributed in breast milk. May produce teratogenic effects. **Pregnancy Category C. Children:** Safety and efficacy not established. **Elderly:** No age-related precautions noted.

INTERACTIONS

DRUG: Antacids, iron preparations, sucralfate, didanosine chewable/buffered tablets, pediatric powder for oral solution may decrease moxifloxacin absorption. **HERBAL:** None known. **FOOD:** None known. **LAB VALUES:** None known.

AVAILABILITY (Rx)

TABLETS: 400 mg. **INJECTION:** 400 mg. **OPHTHALMIC SOLUTION:** 0.5%.

ADMINISTRATION/HANDLING

PO

• Give without regard to meals. • Oral moxifloxacin should be administered 4 hrs before or 8 hrs after antacids, multivitamins, iron preparations, sucralfate, didanosine chewable/buffered tablets, pediatric powder for oral solution.

OPHTHALMIC

• Tilt head backward, have pt look up. Gently pull lower eyelid down until pocket formed. Hold dropper above pocket. Without touching eyelid or conjunctival sac place drops into center of pocket. Close eyes gently, apply gentle finger pressure to lacrimal sac at inner canthus. Remove excess solution around eye with a tissue.

IV

Storage • Store at room temperature. • Do not refrigerate.

Reconstitution • N/A. Available in ready-to-use containers.

Rate of administration • Give by IV infusion only. • Avoid rapid or bolus IV infusion. • Infuse over ≥60 min.

IV INCOMPATIBILITY

Do not add or infuse other drugs simultaneously through the same IV line. Flush line prior to and following use if same IV line is used with other medications.

INDICATIONS/ROUTES/DOSAGE

Alert: Infuse IV over 60 min.

ACUTE BACTERIAL SINUSITIS, COMMUNITY-ACQUIRED PNEUMONIA

IV/PO: ADULTS >18 YRS, ELDERLY: 400 mg q24h for 10 days.

ACUTE BACTERIAL EXACERBATION OF CHRONIC BRONCHITIS

IV/PO: ADULTS >18 YRS, ELDERLY: 400 mg q24h for 5 days.

SKIN/SKIN STRUCTURE INFECTIONS

IV/PO: ADULTS, ELDERLY: 400 mg once daily for 7 days.

USUAL OPHTHALMIC DOSAGE

Ophthalmic: ADULTS, ELDERLY, CHILDREN >1 YR: 1 drop 3 times/day for 7 days.

SIDE EFFECTS

FREQUENT (6%–8%): Nausea, diarrhea. **OCCASIONAL (2%–3%):** Dizziness, headache, abdominal pain, vomiting. **OPHTHALMIC (1%–6%):** Conjunctival irritation, reduced visual acuity, dry eye, keratitis, eye pain, ocular itching, swelling of tissue around cornea, eye discharge, fever, cough, pharyngitis, rash, rhinitis. **RARE (1%):** Change in sense of taste, dyspepsia (heartburn, indigestion), photosensitivity.

ADVERSE REACTIONS/ TOXIC EFFECTS

Pseudomembranous colitis (severe abdominal pain/cramps, severe watery diarrhea, fever) may occur. Superinfection (genital-anal pruritus, ulceration/changes in oral mucosa, moderate to severe diarrhea) may occur.

NURSING IMPLICATIONS

BASELINE ASSESSMENT

Question for history of hypersensitivity to moxifloxacin, quinolones.

INTERVENTION/EVALUATION

Determine pattern of bowel activity. Assist with ambulation if dizziness occurs. Assess for headache, abdominal pain, vomiting, change in sense of taste, dyspepsia (heartburn, indigestion). Monitor WBC, signs of infection.

PATIENT/FAMILY TEACHING

May be taken without regard to food. Drink plenty of fluids. Avoid exposure to direct sunlight; may cause photosensitivity reaction. Do not take antacids 4 hrs before or 8 hrs after dosing. Take full course of therapy.

mupirocin

mew-pie-ro-sin

(Bactroban, Bactroban Nasal)

Do not confuse with bacitracin, baclofen.

CLASSIFICATION

PHARMACOTHERAPEUTIC: Anti-infective. **CLINICAL:** Topical antibacterial.

ACTION

Inhibits bacterial protein, RNA synthesis. Less effective on DNA synthesis. **Nasal:** Eradicates nasal colonization of methicillin-resistant *staphylococcus aureus* (MRSA). **Therapeutic Effect:** Prevents bacterial growth, replication. Bacteriostatic.

PHARMACOKINETICS

Following topical administration, penetrates outer layer of skin (minimal through intact skin). Protein binding: 95%. Metabolized in liver; excreted in urine. **Half-life:** 17–36 min.

USES

Ointment: Topical treatment of impetigo caused by *S. aureus*, *S. pyogenes;* treatment of folliculitis, furunculosis, minor wounds, burns, ulcers caused by susceptible organisms. **Cream:** Treatment of traumatic skin lesions due to *S. aureus*, *S. pyogenes,* prophylactic agent applied to IV catheter exit sites. **Intranasal Ointment:** Eradication of *S. aureus* from nasal, perineal carriage sites. **Unlabeled:** Treatment of infected eczema, folliculitis, minor bacterial skin infections.

PRECAUTIONS

CONTRAINDICATIONS: None known. **CAUTIONS:** Impaired renal function, burn pts.

LIFESPAN CONSIDERATIONS: Pregnancy/lactation: Unknown if present in breast milk. Temporarily discontinue breast-feeding while using mupirocin. **Pregnancy Category B. Children:** Safety and efficacy not established. **Elderly:** No age-related precautions noted.

INTERACTIONS

DRUG: None known. **HERBAL:** None known. **FOOD:** None known. **LAB VALUES:** None known.

AVAILABILITY (Rx)

CREAM: 2%. **OINTMENT:** 2%. **NASAL OINTMENT:** 2%.

ADMINISTRATION/HANDLING

TOPICAL

• **Cream/ointment:** For topical use only. Do not apply into the eyes. May cover with gauze dressing. • **Intranasal:** Avoid contact with eyes. Apply ½ ointment from single-use tube into each nostril.

INDICATIONS/ROUTES/DOSAGE

USUAL TOPICAL DOSAGE

Topical: ADULTS, ELDERLY, CHILDREN: **Cream:** Apply small amount 3 times/day for 10 days. **Ointment:** Apply small amount 3–5 times/day for 5–14 days.

USUAL NASAL DOSAGE

Intranasal: ADULTS, ELDERLY, CHILDREN: Apply small amount 2–4 times/day for 5–14 days.

SIDE EFFECTS

FREQUENT: Nasal (3%–9%): Headache, rhinitis, upper respiratory congestion, pharyngitis, altered taste. **OCCASIONAL: Nasal (2%):** Burning, stinging, cough. **Topical (1%–2%):** Pain, burning, stinging, itching. **RARE: Nasal (<1%):** Pruritus, diarrhea, dry mouth, epistaxis, nausea, rash. **Topical (<1%):** Rash, nausea, dry skin, contact dermatitis.

ADVERSE REACTIONS/ TOXIC EFFECTS

Superinfection may result in bacterial, fungal infections, esp. with prolonged, repeated therapy.

NURSING IMPLICATIONS

BASELINE ASSESSMENT

Assess skin for type, extent of lesions.

INTERVENTION/EVALUATION

Keep neonates or pts with poor hygiene isolated. Wear gloves, gown if necessary when contact with discharges is likely; continue until 24 hrs after therapy is effective. Cleanse/dispose of articles soiled with discharge according to institutional guidelines. In event of skin reaction, stop applications, cleanse area gently, notify physician.

PATIENT/FAMILY TEACHING

For external use only. Avoid contact with eyes. Explain precautions to avoid spread of infection; teach how to apply medication. If skin reaction, irritation develops, notify physician. If there is no improvement in 3–5 days, pt should be reevaluated.

muromonab-CD3

meur-oh-**mon**-ab
(Orthoclone, OKT3)

◆ CLASSIFICATION

PHARMACOTHERAPEUTIC: Murine monoclonal antibody. **CLINICAL:** Immunosuppressant.

ACTION

Antibody (purified IgG_2 immune globulin) that reacts with T3 (CD3) antigen of human T-cell membranes. Blocks function of T cells (has major role in acute renal rejection). **Therapeutic Effect:** Reverses graft rejection.

USES

Treatment of acute allograft rejection in renal transplant pts; steroid-resistant acute allograft rejection in cardiac, hepatic transplant pts.

PRECAUTIONS

CONTRAINDICATIONS: History of hypersensitivity to muromonab-CD3 or any murine origin product, those in fluid overload evidenced by chest x-ray or >3% weight gain within the week before

M

initial treatment. **CAUTIONS:** Impaired hepatic, renal, cardiac function. **Pregnancy Category C.**

AVAILABILITY (Rx)

INJECTION: 1 mg/ml.

ADMINISTRATION/HANDLING

IV

Storage • Refrigerate ampoule. If left out of refrigerator for >4 hrs, do not use. • Do not shake ampoule before using. • Fine translucent particles may develop; does not affect potency.

Reconstitution • Draw solution into syringe through 0.22-micron filter. Discard filter; use needle for IV administration.

Rate of administration • Administer IV push over <1 min. • Give methylprednisolone 1 mg/kg before and 100 mg hydrocortisone 30 min after dose (decreases adverse reaction to first dose).

IV INCOMPATIBILITY

Do not mix with any other medications.

INDICATIONS/ROUTES/DOSAGE

PREVENTION OF ALLOGRAFT REJECTION

IV: ADULTS, ELDERLY, CHILDREN >30 KG: 5 mg/day for 10–14 days. Begin when acute renal rejection is diagnosed. CHILDREN <12 YRS: 0.1 mg/kg/day for 10–14 days.

INTERACTIONS

DRUG: Other immunosuppressants may increase risk of infection or development of lymphoproliferative disorders. **Live virus vaccines** may potentiate virus replication, increase vaccine side effects, decrease pt's antibody response to vaccine. **HERBAL: Echinacea** may decrease effect. **FOOD:** None known. **LAB VALUES:** None known.

SIDE EFFECTS

FREQUENT: First-dose reaction: Fever, chills, dyspnea, malaise occurs 30 min–6 hrs after first dose (reaction markedly reduced with subsequent dosing after first 2 days of treatment). **OCCASIONAL:** Chest pain, nausea, vomiting, diarrhea, tremors.

ADVERSE REACTIONS/ TOXIC EFFECTS

Cytokine release syndrome (CRS) may range from flulike illness to life-threatening shocklike reaction. Occasional fatal hypersensitivity reactions may occur. Severe pulmonary edema occurs in <2% of those treated with muromonab-CD3. Infection (due to immunosuppression) generally occurs within 45 days after initial treatment; cytomegalovirus occurs in 19%, herpes simplex in 27%. Severe, life-threatening infection occurs in <4.8%.

NURSING IMPLICATIONS

BASELINE ASSESSMENT

Chest x-ray must be taken within 24 hrs of initiation of therapy and be clear of fluid. Weight should be ≤3% above minimum weight the week prior to beginning treatment (pulmonary edema occurs when fluid overload is present before treatment). Have resuscitative drugs, equipment immediately available.

INTERVENTION/EVALUATION

Monitor WBC, differential, platelet count, renal/hepatic function tests, immunologic tests (plasma levels, quantitative T lymphocyte surface phenotyping) prior to and during therapy. If fever exceeds 100°F, antipyretics should be instituted. Monitor for fluid overload by chest x-ray and weight gain of >3% over weight prior to treatment. Assess lung sounds for evidence of fluid overload. Monitor I&O. Assess stool frequency/consistency.

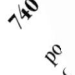

PATIENT/FAMILY TEACHING

Inform pt of first-dose reaction (fever, chills, chest tightness, wheezing, nausea, vomiting, diarrhea). Avoid crowds, those with infections. Do not receive immunizations.

mycophenolate mofetil

my-koe-**phen**-oh-late
(CellCept)

CLASSIFICATION

PHARMACOTHERAPEUTIC: Immunologic agent. **CLINICAL:** Immunosuppressant (see p. 102C).

ACTION

Inhibits inosine monophosphate dehydrogenase, an enzyme that deprives lymphocytes of nucleotides necessary for DNA and RNA synthesis. Inhibits proliferation of T and B lymphocytes. Suppresses immunologically mediated inflammatory response. **Therapeutic Effect:** Prevents transplant rejection.

PHARMACOKINETICS

Rapidly, extensively absorbed after PO administration (food does not alter the extent of absorption, but plasma concentration decreased in presence of food). Protein binding: 97%. Completely hydrolyzed to active metabolite mycophenolic acid (MPA). Primarily excreted in urine. Not removed by hemodialysis. **Half-life:** 17.9 hrs.

USES

Prophylaxis of organ rejection in pts receiving allogeneic liver/renal/cardiac transplants. Should be used concurrently with cyclosporine and corticosteroids. **Unlabeled:** Prevent… pts undergoing heart t…

PRECAUTIONS

CONTRAINDICATIONS: Mycop… acid. **CAUTIONS:** Active serious di… tive disease, renal impairment, neutropenia, women of childbearing potential.

LIFESPAN CONSIDERATIONS: Pregnancy/lactation: Unknown if drug crosses placenta or is distributed in breast milk. Avoid breast-feeding. **Pregnancy Category C. Children:** Safety and efficacy not established. **Elderly:** Age-related renal impairment may require dosage adjustments.

INTERACTIONS

DRUG: Acyclovir, ganciclovir competes with MPA (active metabolite for renal excretion); may increase plasma concentration of each in presence of renal impairment. **Antacids (magnesium, aluminum-containing), cholestyramine** may decrease absorption. **Other immunosuppressants** may increase risk of infection or development of lymphomas. **Live virus vaccines** may potentiate virus replication, increase vaccine side effects, decrease pt's antibody response to vaccine. **Probenecid** may increase concentration. **HERBAL: Echinacea** may decrease effect. **FOOD:** None known. **LAB VALUES:** May increase alkaline phosphatase, creatinine, SGOT (AST), SGPT (ALT), cholesterol, phosphate. Alters calcium, glucose, potassium, uric acid, lipid levels.

AVAILABILITY (Rx)

CAPSULES: 250 mg. **TABLETS:** 500 mg. **ORAL SUSPENSION:** 200 mg/ml. **INJECTION:** 500 mg.

ADMINISTRATION/HANDLING

PO

• Give on an empty stomach. • Do not open or crush capsules. Avoid inhalation of powder in capsules, direct contact of

M

powder on skin/mucous membranes. If contact occurs, wash thoroughly with soap/water. Rinse eyes profusely with plain water. • Store reconstituted suspension in refrigerator or at room temperature. • Suspension is stable for 60 days after reconstitution. • Suspension can be administered orally or via a nasogastric tube (minimum size 8 French).

IV

Storage • Store at room temperature.

Reconstitution • Reconstitute each 500-mg vial with 14 ml D_5W. Gently agitate. • For 1-g dose, further dilute with 140 ml D_5W; for 1.5-g dose further dilute with 210 ml D_5W, providing a concentration of 6 mg/ml.

Rate of administration • Infuse over at least 2 hrs.

IV INCOMPATIBILITIES

Compatible only with D_5W. Do not infuse concurrently with other drugs or IV solutions.

INDICATIONS/ROUTES/DOSAGE

RENAL TRANSPLANT

IV/PO: ADULTS, ELDERLY: 1 g 2 times/day.

CARDIAC TRANSPLANT

IV/PO: ADULTS, ELDERLY: 1.5 g 2 times/day.

LIVER TRANSPLANT

IV: ADULTS, ELDERLY: 1 g 2 times/day.

PO: ADULTS, ELDERLY: 1.5 g 2 times/day.

USUAL DOSAGE FOR CHILDREN

PO: 600 mg/m^2/dose 2 times/day. **Maximum:** 2 g/dose.

SIDE EFFECTS

FREQUENT (20%–37%): UTI, hypertension, peripheral edema, diarrhea, constipation, fever, headache, nausea. **OCCASIONAL (10%–18%):** Dyspepsia (heartburn, indigestion, epigastric pain), dyspnea, cough, hematuria, asthenia (loss of strength, energy), vomiting, edema, tremors, abdominal/chest/back pain, oral moniliasis, acne. **RARE (6%–9%):** Insomnia, respiratory infection, rash, dizziness.

ADVERSE REACTIONS/ TOXIC EFFECTS

Significant anemia, leukopenia, thrombocytopenia, neutropenia, leukocytosis may occur, particularly in pts undergoing kidney rejection. Sepsis, infection occur occasionally, GI tract hemorrhage rarely. There is an increased risk of neoplasia (new, abnormal growth tumor).

NURSING IMPLICATIONS

BASELINE ASSESSMENT

Women of childbearing potential should have a negative serum or urine pregnancy test within 1 wk prior to initiation of drug therapy. Assess medical history, esp. renal function, existence of active digestive system disease, drug history, esp. other immunosuppressants.

INTERVENTION/EVALUATION

CBC should be performed weekly during first month of therapy, twice monthly during second and third months of treatment, then monthly throughout the first year. If rapid fall in WBC occurs, dosage should be reduced or discontinued. Assess particularly for delayed bone marrow suppression. Report any major change in assessment of pt. Routinely watch for any change from normal.

PATIENT/FAMILY TEACHING

Effective contraception should be used before, during, and for 6 wks after discontinuing therapy, even if there has been a history of infertility, other than hysterectomy. Two forms of contraception must be used concurrently unless abstinence is absolute. Contact physician if unusual bleeding/bruising, sore throat, mouth sores, abdominal pain, fever occurs. Inform pts of need for laboratory tests while taking medication. Inform pts of risk of malignancies that may occur.

nabumetone

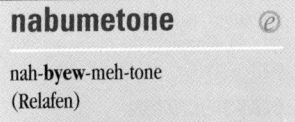

nah-**byew**-meh-tone
(Relafen)

CLASSIFICATION

PHARMACOTHERAPEUTIC: Nonsteroidal anti-inflammatory. **CLINICAL:** Analgesic, anti-inflammatory (see p. 111C).

ACTION

Produces analgesic, anti-inflammatory effect by inhibiting prostaglandin synthesis. **Therapeutic Effect:** Reduces inflammatory response, intensity of pain stimulus reaching sensory nerve endings.

PHARMACOKINETICS

Readily absorbed from GI tract. Protein binding: >99%. Widely distributed. Metabolized in liver to active metabolite. Primarily excreted in urine. Not removed by hemodialysis. **Half-life:** 22–30 hrs.

USES

Acute, chronic treatment of osteoarthritis, rheumatoid arthritis.

PRECAUTIONS

CONTRAINDICATIONS: Active peptic ulcer, GI ulceration, chronic inflammation of GI tract, GI bleeding disorders, history of hypersensitivity to aspirin or NSAIDs, history of significantly impaired renal function. **CAUTIONS:** CHF, hypertension, decreased liver/renal function, concurrent use of anticoagulants.

LIFESPAN CONSIDERATIONS: Pregnancy/lactation: Distributed in low concentration in breast milk. Avoid use during last trimester (may adversely affect fetal cardiovascular system: premature closing of ductus arteriosus). **Pregnancy Category C** (**D** if used in third trimester or near delivery). **Children:** Safety and efficacy not established. **Elderly:** Age-related renal impairment may increase risk of liver/renal toxicity; reduced dosage recommended. More likely to have serious adverse effects with GI bleeding/ulceration.

INTERACTIONS

DRUG: May increase effects of **oral anticoagulants, heparin, thrombolytics.** May decrease effect of **antihypertensives, diuretics. Salicylates, aspirin** may increase risk of GI side effects, bleeding. **Bone marrow depressants** may increase risk of hematologic reactions. May increase concentration, toxicity of **lithium.** May increase **methotrexate** toxicity. **Probenecid** may increase concentration. **HERBAL: Feverfew** effects may be decreased. **Ginkgo biloba** may increase risk of bleeding. **FOOD:** None known. **LAB VALUES:** May increase alkaline phosphatase, LDH, serum transaminase, potassium, urine protein, BUN, serum creatinine. May decrease uric acid.

AVAILABILITY (Rx)

TABLETS: 500 mg, 750 mg.

ADMINISTRATION/HANDLING

PO

• Give with food, milk, antacids if GI distress occurs. • Do not crush; swallow whole.

INDICATIONS/ROUTES/DOSAGE

RHEUMATOID ARTHRITIS, OSTEOARTHRITIS

PO: ADULTS, ELDERLY: Initially, 1,000 mg as single dose or in 2 divided doses.

M

May increase up to 2,000 mg/day as single or in 2 divided doses.

SIDE EFFECTS

FREQUENT (12%–14%): Diarrhea, abdominal cramping/pain, dyspepsia (heartburn, indigestion, epigastric pain). **OCCASIONAL (3%–9%):** Nausea, constipation, flatulence, dizziness, headache. **RARE (1%–3%):** Vomiting, stomatitis.

ADVERSE REACTIONS/ TOXIC EFFECTS

Overdose may result in acute hypotension, tachycardia. Peptic ulcer, GI bleeding, nephrotoxicity (dysuria, cystitis, hematuria, proteinuria, nephrotic syndrome), gastritis, severe hepatic reaction (cholestasis, jaundice), severe hypersensitivity reaction (bronchospasm, angiofacial edema) occur rarely.

NURSING IMPLICATIONS

BASELINE ASSESSMENT

Assess onset, type, location, duration of pain/inflammation. Inspect appearance of affected joints for immobility, deformities, skin condition.

INTERVENTION/EVALUATION

Assist with ambulation if somnolence/drowsiness/dizziness occurs. Monitor for evidence of dyspepsia, pattern of daily bowel activity/stool consistency. Evaluate for therapeutic response: relief of pain, stiffness, swelling. Assess for increase in joint mobility, reduced joint tenderness; improved grip strength.

PATIENT/FAMILY TEACHING

May cause serious GI bleeding with or without pain. Avoid aspirin. May take with food if GI upset occurs. May cause dizziness, confusion (use caution performing tasks requiring mental alertness, physical coordination).

nadolol

nay-**doe**-lol
(Apo-Nadol✤, Corgard, Novo-Nadolol✤)

FIXED-COMBINATION(S)

Corzide: nadolol/bendroflumethiazide (a diuretic): 40 mg/5 mg, 80 mg/5 mg.

◆CLASSIFICATION

PHARMACOTHERAPEUTIC: Beta-adrenergic blocker. **CLINICAL:** Antianginal, antihypertensive (see p. 62C).

ACTION

Nonselective beta-blocker. Blocks $beta_1$-, $beta_2$-adrenergic receptors. **Therapeutic Effect:** Slows sinus heart rate; decreases cardiac output, B/P; increases airway resistance. Decreases myocardial ischemia severity by decreasing O_2 requirements.

USES

Management of mild to moderate hypertension. Used alone or in combination with diuretics, esp. thiazide type. Management of chronic stable angina pectoris. **Unlabeled:** Treatment of cardiac arrhythmias, hypertrophic cardiomyopathy, MI, pheochromocytoma, vascular headaches, tremors, thyrotoxicosis, mitral valve prolapse syndrome, neuroleptic-induced akathisia.

PRECAUTIONS

CONTRAINDICATIONS: Bronchial asthma, COPD, uncontrolled cardiac failure, sinus bradycardia, heart block greater than first degree, cardiogenic shock, CHF unless secondary to tachyarrhythmias, those on MAOIs. **CAUTIONS:** Inadequate cardiac function, impaired renal/hepatic function, diabetes mellitus, hyperthyroidism. **Pregnancy Category C** (**D** if used in second or third trimester).

INTERACTIONS

DRUG: Diuretics, other hypotensives may increase hypotensive effect; **sympathomimetics, xanthines** may mutually inhibit effects; may mask symptoms of hypoglycemia, prolong hypoglycemic effect of **insulin, oral hypoglycemics; NSAIDs** may decrease antihypertensive effect; **cimetidine** may increase concentration. **HERBAL:** None known. **FOOD:** None known. **LAB VALUES:** May increase ANA titer, SGOT (AST), SGPT (ALT), alkaline phosphatase, LDH, bilirubin, BUN, creatinine, potassium, uric acid, lipoproteins, triglycerides.

AVAILABILITY (Rx)

TABLETS: 20 mg, 40 mg, 80 mg, 120 mg, 160 mg.

ADMINISTRATION/HANDLING

PO

• Give without regard to meals. • Tablets may be crushed.

INDICATIONS/ROUTES/DOSAGE

HYPERTENSION, ANGINA

PO: ADULTS: Initially, 40 mg/day. May increase by 40–80 mg at 3- to 7-day intervals. **Maximum:** 240–360 mg/day. ELDERLY: Initially, 20 mg/day. May increase gradually. RANGE: 20–240 mg/day.

DOSAGE IN RENAL IMPAIRMENT

Dosage is modified based on creatinine clearance.

Creatinine Clearance	% Normal Dosage
10–50 ml/min	50
<10 ml/min	25

SIDE EFFECTS

Generally well tolerated, with transient and mild side effects. **FREQUENT:** Decreased sexual function, drowsiness, unusual tiredness/weakness. **RARE:** Bradycardia, difficulty breathing, depression, cold hands/feet, diarrhea, constipation, anxiety, nasal congestion, nausea, vomiting. **RARE:** Altered taste, dry eyes, itching.

ADVERSE REACTIONS/ TOXIC EFFECTS

Excessive dosage may produce profound bradycardia, hypotension. Abrupt withdrawal may result in diaphoresis, palpitations, headache, tremulousness, exacerbation of angina, MI, ventricular arrhythmias. May precipitate CHF, MI in those with cardiac disease; thyroid storm in those with thyrotoxicosis; peripheral ischemia in those with existing peripheral vascular disease. Hypoglycemia may occur in pts with previously controlled diabetes.

NURSING IMPLICATIONS

BASELINE ASSESSMENT

Assess baseline renal/liver function tests. Assess B/P, apical pulse immediately prior to drug administration (if pulse is ≤60/min or systolic B/P is <90 mm Hg, withhold medication, contact physician). **Antianginal:** Record onset, type (sharp, dull, squeezing), radiation, location, intensity, duration of anginal pain; precipitating factors (exertion, emotional stress).

INTERVENTION/EVALUATION

Monitor B/P for hypotension, respiration for shortness of breath. Assess pulse for quality, irregular rate, bradycardia. Assess fingers for color, numbness (Raynaud's). Assess for evidence of CHF: dyspnea (particularly on exertion, lying down), night cough, peripheral edema, distended neck veins. Monitor I&O (increase in weight, decrease in urine output may indicate CHF).

PATIENT/FAMILY TEACHING

Do not discontinue abruptly (may precipitate angina). Inform physician if difficulty breathing, night cough, swelling of arms and legs, slow pulse, dizziness, confusion, depression, rash, fe-

N

ver, sore throat, unusual bleeding/bruising occurs. Use caution performing tasks requiring mental alertness, physical coordination.

nafarelin acetate

naf-ah-**rell**-in
(Synarel)

CLASSIFICATION

PHARMACOTHERAPEUTIC: Gonadotropin inhibitor. **CLINICAL:** Hormone agonist (see p. 90C).

ACTION

Initially stimulates the release of the pituitary gonadotropins, luteinizing hormone and follicle-stimulating hormone. **Therapeutic Effect:** Results in temporary increase of ovarian steroidogenesis. Continued dosing abolishes the stimulatory effect on the pituitary gland and, after about 4 wks, leads to decreased secretion of gonadal steroids.

N

USES

Management of endometriosis, including dysmenorrhea, dyspareunia, pelvic pain. Treatment of central precocious puberty.

PRECAUTIONS

CONTRAINDICATIONS: Hypersensitivity to nafarelin, other agonist analogues; undiagnosed abnormal vaginal bleeding. **CAUTIONS:** History of osteoporosis, chronic alcohol/tobacco use, intercurrent rhinitis. **Pregnancy Category X.**

AVAILABILITY (Rx)

NASAL SOLUTION: 2 mg/ml (each spray delivers 200 mcg).

INTERACTIONS

DRUG: None known. **HERBAL:** None known. **FOOD:** None known. **LAB VALUES:** None known.

INDICATIONS/ROUTES/DOSAGE

ENDOMETRIOSIS

Alert: Initiate treatment between days 2 and 4 of menstrual cycle. Duration of therapy is 6 mos.

Intranasal: ADULTS: 400 mcg/day: 200 mcg (1 spray) into 1 nostril in morning, 1 spray into other nostril in evening. For pts with persistent regular menstruation after months of treatment, increase dosage to 800 mcg/day (1 spray into each nostril in morning and evening).

CENTRAL PRECOCIOUS PUBERTY

Intranasal: CHILDREN: 1,600 mcg/day: 400 mcg (2 sprays into each nostril in morning and evening; total 8 sprays). May increase dose to 600 mcg (3 sprays) into alternating nostrils 3 times/day.

SIDE EFFECTS

FREQUENT (90%): Hot flashes, muscle pain, decreased breast size, myalgia, nasal irritation (10%). **OCCASIONAL (13%–22%):** Decreased libido, vaginal dryness, headache, emotional lability, acne. **RARE (2%–8%):** Insomnia, edema, weight gain, seborrhea, depression.

ADVERSE REACTIONS/TOXIC EFFECTS

None known.

NURSING IMPLICATIONS

BASELINE ASSESSMENT

Inquire about menstrual cycle; therapy should begin between days 2 and 4 of cycle.

INTERVENTION/EVALUATION

Check for pain relief as result of therapy. Inquire about menstrual cessation, other decreased estrogen effects.

PATIENT/FAMILY TEACHING

Pt should use nonhormonal contraceptive during therapy. Do not take drug if pregnancy is suspected (risk to fetus). Importance of full length of therapy, regular visits to physician's office. Notify physician if regular menstruation continues (menstruation should stop with therapy).

nafcillin sodium

naph-**sill**-in
(Nafcil, Nallpen, Unipen)
Do not confuse with Unicap.

CLASSIFICATION

PHARMACOTHERAPEUTIC: Penicillinase-resistant penicillin. **CLINICAL:** Antibiotic (see p. 26C).

ACTION

Binds to bacterial membranes. **Therapeutic Effect:** Inhibits cell wall synthesis. Bactericidal.

USES

Treatment of respiratory tract, skin/skin structure infections, osteomyelitis, endocarditis, meningitis; perioperatively, esp. in cardiovascular, orthopedic procedures. Predominantly treatment of infections caused by penicillinase-producing staphylococci.

PRECAUTIONS

CONTRAINDICATIONS: Hypersensitivity to any penicillin. **CAUTIONS:** History of allergies, particularly cephalosporins, severe renal/liver dysfunction. **Pregnancy Category B.**

INTERACTIONS

DRUG: **Probenecid** may increase concentration, toxicity risk. **HERBAL:** None known. **FOOD:** None known. **LAB VALUES:** May cause positive Coombs' test.

AVAILABILITY (Rx)

POWDER FOR INJECTION: 500 mg, 1 g, 2 g.

ADMINISTRATION/HANDLING

Alert: Space doses evenly around the clock.

IM

- Reconstitute each 500 mg with 1.7 ml Sterile Water for Injection or 0.9% NaCl to provide concentration of 250 mg/ml.
- Inject IM into large muscle mass.

IV

Storage

IV INFUSION (piggyback)

- Stable for 24 hrs at room temperature, 96 hrs if refrigerated. Discard if precipitate forms.

Reconstitution • For IV push, reconstitute each vial with 15–30 ml Sterile Water for Injection or 0.9% NaCl. Administer over 5–10 min. • For intermittent IV infusion (piggyback), further dilute with 50–100 ml D_5W, $D_{10}W$, 0.9% NaCl, 0.45% NaCl, 0.2% NaCl, Ringer's, lactated Ringer's, or any combination thereof.

Rate of administration • Infuse over 30–60 min. • Because of potential for hypersensitivity/anaphylaxis, start initial dose at few drops per min, increase slowly to ordered rate; stay with pt first 10–15 min, then check q10min. • Limit IV therapy to <48 hrs, if possible. Stop infusion if pt complains of pain.

IV INCOMPATIBILITIES

Diltiazem (Cardizem), droperidol (Inapsine), fentanyl, insulin, labetalol (Normodyne, Trandate), midazolam (Versed), nalbuphine (Nubain), vancomycin (Vancocin), verapamil (Isoptin).

IV COMPATIBILITIES

Heparin, lidocaine, magnesium, potassium chloride, propofol (Diprivan).

INDICATIONS/ROUTES/DOSAGE

USUAL DOSAGE

IV: ADULTS, ELDERLY: 0.5–2 g q4–6h. CHILDREN: 50–200 mg/kg/day in divided doses q4–6h. **Maximum:** 12 g/day. NEONATES: 50–100 mg/kg/day in divided doses q6–12h.

IM: ADULTS, ELDERLY: 500 mg q4–6h. CHILDREN: 50–200 mg/kg/day in divided doses q4–6h. **Maximum:** 12 g/day.

SIDE EFFECTS

FREQUENT: Mild hypersensitivity reaction (fever, rash, pruritus), GI effects (nausea, vomiting, diarrhea). **OCCASIONAL:** Hypokalemia with high IV dosages, phlebitis, thrombophlebitis (common in elderly). **RARE:** Extravasation with IV administration.

N

ADVERSE REACTIONS/ TOXIC EFFECTS

Superinfections, potentially fatal antibiotic-associated colitis may result from altered bacterial balance. Hematologic effects (esp. involving platelets, WBCs), severe hypersensitivity reactions, anaphylaxis occur rarely.

NURSING IMPLICATIONS

BASELINE ASSESSMENT

Question for history of allergies, esp. penicillins, cephalosporins.

INTERVENTION/EVALUATION

Hold medication, promptly report rash (possible hypersensitivity), diarrhea (fever, abdominal pain, mucus/blood in stool may indicate antibiotic-associated colitis). Evaluate IV site frequently for phlebitis (heat, pain, red streaking over vein), infiltration (potential extravasation). Monitor potassium, periodic CBC, urinalysis, renal/liver function. Be alert for superinfection: increased fever, onset of sore throat, vomiting, diarrhea, ulceration/changes of oral mucosa, anal/genital pruritus. Check hematology reports (esp. WBCs), periodic renal/hepatic reports in prolonged therapy.

PATIENT/FAMILY TEACHING

Continue antibiotic for full length of treatment. Doses should be evenly spaced. Discomfort may occur with IM injection. Report IV discomfort immediately. Notify physician in event of diarrhea, rash, other new symptoms.

naftifine hydrochloride

(Naftin)

See Classification section under: Antifungals: topical

nalbuphine hydrochloride

nail-**byew**-phin

(Nubain)

Do not confuse with Navane.

CLASSIFICATION

PHARMACOTHERAPEUTIC: Narcotic agonist, antagonist. **CLINICAL:** Opioid analgesic (see p. 121C).

ACTION

Binds with opioid receptors within the CNS. May displace opioid agonists and competitively inhibit their action (may precipitate withdrawal symptoms). **Therapeutic Effect:** Alters pain perception, emotional response to pain.

PHARMACOKINETICS

Onset	Peak	Duration
Subcutaneous		
<15 min	—	3–6 hrs
IM		
<15 min	60 min	3–6 hrs
IV		
2–3 min	30 min	3–6 hrs

Well absorbed following subcutaneous, IM administration. Protein binding: 50%. Metabolized in liver. Primarily eliminated in feces via biliary secretion. **Half-life:** 3.5–5 hrs.

USES

Relief of moderate to severe pain, preop sedation, obstetric analgesia, adjunct to anesthesia.

PRECAUTIONS

CONTRAINDICATIONS: Respirations <12/min. **CAUTIONS:** Liver/renal impairment, respiratory depression, recent MI, recent biliary tract surgery, head trauma, increased intracranial pressure, pregnancy, those suspected to be opioid dependent.

LIFESPAN CONSIDERATIONS: Pregnancy/lactation: Readily crosses placenta. Distributed in breast milk (breastfeeding not recommended). **Pregnancy Category B** (**D** if used for prolonged periods or at high dosages at term). **Children:** Paradoxical excitement may occur. Those <2 yrs more susceptible to respiratory depression. **Elderly:** More susceptible to respiratory depression. Age-related impaired renal function may increase risk of urinary retention.

INTERACTIONS

DRUG: Alcohol, CNS depressants may increase CNS or respiratory depression, hypotension. **MAOIs** may produce severe reaction (reduce dose to ¼ usual dose). Effects may be decreased with **buprenorphine. HERBAL:** None known. **FOOD:** None known. **LAB VALUES:** May increase amylase, lipase, serum levels.

AVAILABILITY (Rx)

INJECTION: 10 mg/ml, 20 mg/ml.

ADMINISTRATION/HANDLING

Alert: Store parenteral form at room temperature.

IM

- Rotate IM injection sites.

IV

Storage • Store at room temperature.

Reconstitution • May give undiluted.

Rate of administration • For IV push, administer each 10 mg >3–5 min.

IV INCOMPATIBILITIES

Amphotericin B complex (Abelcet, AmBisome, Amphotec), cefepime (Maxipime), docetaxel (Doxil), methotrexate, nafcillin (Nafcil), piperacillin/tazobactam (Zosyn), sargramostim (Leukine, Prokine), sodium bicarbonate.

IV COMPATIBILITIES

Diphenhydramine (Benadryl), droperidol (Inapsine), glycopyrrolate (Robinul), hydroxyzine (Vistaril), ketorolac (Toradol), lidocaine, midazolam (Versed), propofol (Diprivan).

INDICATIONS/ROUTES/DOSAGE

Alert: Dosage based on severity of pain, physical condition of pt, concurrent use of other medications.

ANALGESIA

Subcutaneous/IM/IV: ADULTS, ELDERLY: 10 mg q3–6h as needed. Do not exceed maximum single dose of 20 mg, maximum daily dose of 160 mg. In pts chronically receiving narcotic analgesics of similar duration of action, give 25%

N

of usual dosage. CHILDREN: 0.1–0.15 mg/kg q3–6h as needed.

SUPPLEMENT TO ANESTHESIA

IV: ADULTS, ELDERLY: Induction: 0.3–3 mg/kg over 10–15 min. MAINTENANCE: 0.25–0.5 mg/kg as needed.

SIDE EFFECTS

FREQUENT (35%): Sedation. **OCCASIONAL (3%–9%):** Sweaty/clammy feeling, nausea, vomiting, dizziness, vertigo, dry mouth, headache. **RARE (≤1%):** Restlessness, crying, euphoria, hostility, confusion, numbness, tingling, flushing, paradoxical reaction.

ADVERSE REACTIONS/ TOXIC EFFECTS

Abrupt withdrawal after prolonged use may produce symptoms of narcotic withdrawal (abdominal cramping, rhinorrhea, lacrimation, anxiety, increased temperature, piloerection [goose bumps]). Overdose results in severe respiratory depression, skeletal muscle flaccidity, cyanosis, extreme somnolence progressing to convulsions, stupor, coma. Tolerance to analgesic effect, physical dependence may occur with chronic use.

N

NURSING IMPLICATIONS

BASELINE ASSESSMENT

Raise bed rails. Obtain vital signs before giving medication. If respirations are ≤12/min (≤20/min in children), withhold medication, contact physician. Assess onset, type, location, duration of pain. Effect of medication is reduced if full pain recurs before next dose. Low abuse potential.

INTERVENTION/EVALUATION

Monitor for change in respirations, B/P/rate/quality of pulse. Monitor pattern of daily bowel activity, stool consistency. Initiate deep breathing, coughing exercises, particularly in pts with impaired pulmonary function. Assess for clinical improvement, record onset of relief of pain. Consult physician if pain relief is not adequate.

PATIENT/FAMILY TEACHING

Avoid alcohol. May cause drowsiness/ impair ability to perform activities requiring mental alertness, physical coordination (e.g., driving). May cause dry mouth. May be habit forming.

naloxone hydrochloride

nay-**lox**-own

(Narcan)

Do not confuse with Norcuron.

CLASSIFICATION

PHARMACOTHERAPEUTIC: Narcotic antagonist. **CLINICAL:** Antidote (see p. 122C).

ACTION

Displaces opiates at opiate-occupied receptor sites in CNS. **Therapeutic Effect:** Blocks narcotic effects. Reverses opiate-induced sleep/sedation. Increases respiratory rate, returns depressed B/P to normal rate.

PHARMACOKINETICS

	Onset	Peak	Duration
Subcutaneous	2–5 min	—	20–60 min
IM	2–5 min	—	20–60 min
IV	1–2 min	—	20–60 min

Well absorbed after subcutaneous, IM administration. Metabolized in liver. Primarily excreted in urine. **Half-life:** 60–100 min.

USES

Diagnosis, treatment of opioid toxicity, treatment of opioid-induced respiratory depression, other effects (e.g., sedation, coma, convulsions). Used in neonates to reverse respiratory depression caused by opioids given to mother during labor/delivery. Adjunctive therapy to treat hypotension in management of septic shock.

PRECAUTIONS

CONTRAINDICATIONS: Respiratory depression due to nonopiate drugs. **CAUTIONS:** Chronic cardiac/pulmonary disease, coronary artery disease. Those suspected of being opioid dependent, postop pts (to avoid cardiovascular changes).

LIFESPAN CONSIDERATIONS: Pregnancy/lactation: Unknown if drug crosses placenta or is distributed in breast milk. **Pregnancy Category B. Children/elderly:** No age-related precautions noted.

INTERACTIONS

DRUG: Reverses analgesic/side effects, may precipitate withdrawal symptoms of **butorphanol, nalbuphine, pentazocine, opioid agonist analgesics. HERBAL:** None known. **FOOD:** None known. **LAB VALUES:** None known.

AVAILABILITY (Rx)

INJECTION: 0.02 mg/ml, 0.4 mg/ml, 1 mg/ml.

ADMINISTRATION/HANDLING

IM

• Give in upper, outer quadrant of buttock.

IV

Storage • Store parenteral form at room temperature. • Use mixture within 24 hrs; discard unused solution. • Protect from light. Stable in D_5W or 0.9% NaCl at 4 mcg/ml for 24 hrs.

Reconstitution • May dilute 1 mg/ml with 50 ml Sterile Water for Injection to provide a concentration of 0.02 mg/ml. • For continuous IV infusion, dilute each 2 mg of naloxone with 500 ml of D_5W in water or 0.9% NaCl, producing solution containing 0.004 mg/ml.

Rate of administration • May administer undiluted. • Give each 0.4 mg as IV push over 15 sec. • Use the 0.4 mg/ml and 1 mg/ml for injection for adults, the 0.02 mg/ml concentration for neonates.

IV INCOMPATIBILITIES

Amphotericin B complex (Abelcet, AmBisome, Amphotec).

IV COMPATIBILITIES

Heparin, ondansetron (Zofran), propofol (Diprivan).

INDICATIONS/ROUTES/DOSAGE

OPIOID TOXICITY

Subcutaneous/IM/IV: ADULTS, ELDERLY: 0.4–2 mg q2–3 min as need. May repeat q20–60 min. CHILDREN ≥5 YRS OR ≥22 KG: 2 mg/dose; if no response may repeat q2–3 min. May need to repeat q20–60min. CHILDREN <5 YRS OR <22 KG: 0.1 mg/kg, repeat q2–3min. May need to repeat q20–60min.

POSTANESTHESIA NARCOTIC REVERSAL

IV: CHILDREN: 0.01 mg/kg. May repeat q2–3 min.

NEONATAL OPIOID-INDUCED DEPRESSION

IV: 0.01 mg/kg. May repeat q2–3min as needed. May need to repeat q1–2h.

SIDE EFFECTS

None known (little or no pharmacologic effect in absence of narcotics).

ADVERSE REACTIONS/TOXIC EFFECTS

Too rapid reversal of narcotic depression may result in nausea, vomiting, tremulousness, diaphoresis, increased B/P, tachycardia. Excessive dosage in postop pts may produce significant reversal of analgesia, excitement, tremulousness. Hypotension/hypertension, ventric-

N

ular tachycardia/fibrillation, pulmonary edema may occur in those with cardiovascular disease.

NURSING IMPLICATIONS

BASELINE ASSESSMENT

Maintain clear airway. Obtain weight of children to calculate drug dosage.

INTERVENTION/EVALUATION

Monitor vital signs, esp. rate, depth, rhythm of respiration, during and frequently following administration. Carefully observe pt after satisfactory response (duration of opiate may exceed duration of naloxone, resulting in recurrence of respiratory depression). Assess for increased pain with reversal of opiate.

naphazoline

na-**faz**-oh-leen

(Albalon, AK-Con, Clear Eyes, Naphcon, Privine, Vasocon)

FIXED-COMBINATION(S)

Naphcon-A: naphazoline/pheniramine (an antihistamine): 0.25%/0.3%.

CLASSIFICATION

PHARMACOTHERAPEUTIC: Sympathomimetic. **CLINICAL:** Decongestant.

ACTION

Directly acts on alpha-adrenergic receptors in arterioles of conjunctiva. **Therapeutic Effect:** Causes vasoconstriction, with subsequent decreased congestion to area.

USES

Ophthalmic: Relief of itching, congestion, minor irritation; control of hyperemia in pts with superficial corneal vascularity. Occasionally may be used during some ocular diagnostic procedures. **Intranasal:** Relief of nasal congestion due to common cold, acute/chronic rhinitis, hay fever, other allergies.

PRECAUTIONS

CONTRAINDICATIONS: Narrow-angle glaucoma or those with a narrow angle who do not have glaucoma; before peripheral iridectomy; eyes capable of angle closure. **CAUTIONS:** Hypertension, diabetes, hyperthyroidism, heart disease, hypertensive cardiovascular disease, coronary artery disease, cerebral arteriosclerosis, long-standing bronchial asthma.

INTERACTIONS

DRUG: **Tricyclic antidepressants, maprotiline** may increase effect. **HERBAL:** **Ma huang (ephedra)** may increase CNS effects. **FOOD:** None known. **LAB VALUES:** None known.

AVAILABILITY (Rx)

OPHTHALMIC SOLUTION: 0.012%, 0.1%. **NASAL DROPS:** 0.05%. **NASAL SPRAY:** 0.05%.

INDICATIONS/ROUTES/DOSAGE

USUAL NASAL DOSAGE

Intranasal: ADULTS, ELDERLY, CHILDREN >12 YRS: 1–2 drops/sprays (0.05%) in each nostril q3–6h. CHILDREN 6–12 YRS: 1 spray/drop q6h as needed.

USUAL OPHTHALMIC DOSAGE

Ophthalmic: ADULTS, ELDERLY, CHILDREN >6 YRS: 1–2 drops q3–4h for 3–4 days.

SIDE EFFECTS

OCCASIONAL: **Nasal:** Burning, stinging, drying nasal mucosa, sneezing, rebound congestion. **Ophthalmic:** Blurred vision, large pupils, increased eye irritation.

Alert: **Systemic absorption:** Fast/irregular/pounding heartbeat, headache, lightheadedness, nervousness, trembling, insomnia, nausea.

ADVERSE REACTIONS/ TOXIC EFFECTS

Large doses may produce tachycardia, palpitations, lightheadedness, nausea, vomiting. Overdosage in pts >60 yrs: hallucinations, CNS depression, seizures.

NURSING IMPLICATIONS

PATIENT/FAMILY TEACHING

Do not use for >72 hrs without consulting a physician. Use caution with activities that require visual acuity. Discontinue, consult physician if the following occur: vision changes, headache, eye pain, floating spots, pain with light exposure, acute eye redness, insomnia, dizziness, weakness, tremor, irregular heartbeat. Too frequent use may result in rebound effect.

Naprosyn

see naproxen

naproxen

nah-**prox**-en
(EC-Naprosyn, Naprelan, Naprosyn, Naxem ✤)

naproxen sodium

(Aleve, Anaprox, Apo-Napro ✤, Novonaprox ✤)

◆CLASSIFICATION

PHARMACOTHERAPEUTIC: Nonsteroidal anti-inflammatory. **CLINICAL:** Analgesic, anti-inflammatory (see p. 111C).

ACTION

Produces analgesic, anti-inflammatory effect by inhibiting prostaglandin synthesis. **Therapeutic Effect:** Reduces inflammatory response, intensity of pain stimulus reaching sensory nerve endings.

PHARMACOKINETICS

Onset	Peak	Duration
PO (analgesic)		
<1 hr	—	≤7 hrs
PO (antirheumatic)		
≤14 days	2–4 wks	—

Completely absorbed from GI tract. Protein binding: 99%. Metabolized in liver. Primarily excreted in urine. Not removed by hemodialysis. **Half-life:** 13 hrs.

USES

Treatment of acute or long-term mild to moderate pain, primary dysmenorrhea, mild to moderately severe pain, rheumatoid arthritis, juvenile rheumatoid arthritis, osteoarthritis, ankylosing spondylitis, acute gouty arthritis, bursitis, tendinitis. **Unlabeled:** Treatment of vascular headaches.

PRECAUTIONS

CONTRAINDICATIONS: Hypersensitivity to naproxen, aspirin, other NSAIDs. **CAUTIONS:** GI/cardiac disease, impaired renal/liver function. Concurrent use of anticoagulants.

LIFESPAN CONSIDERATIONS: Pregnancy/lactation: Crosses placenta. Distributed in breast milk. Avoid use during third trimester (may adversely affect fetal cardiovascular system: premature closing of ductus arteriosus). **Pregnancy Category B** (**D** if used in third trimester or near delivery). **Children:** Safety and efficacy not established in those <2 yrs. Children >2 yrs at increased risk of skin rash. **Elderly:** Age-related renal impairment may increase risk of liver and renal toxicity; reduced dosage recommended. More likely to have serious adverse effects with GI bleeding/ulceration.

INTERACTIONS

DRUG: May increase effects of **oral anticoagulants, heparin, thrombolytics.** May decrease effect of **antihypertensives, diuretics. Salicylates, aspirin** may increase risk of GI side effects, bleeding. **Bone marrow depressants** may increase risk of hematologic reactions. May increase concentration, toxicity of **lithium.** May increase **methotrexate** toxicity. **Probenecid** may increase concentration. **HERBAL: Feverfew** effects may be decreased. **Ginkgo biloba** may increase risk of bleeding. **FOOD:** None known. **LAB VALUES:** May prolong bleeding time, alter blood glucose levels. May increase liver function tests. May decrease sodium, uric acid.

AVAILABILITY (Rx)

N

GELCAP (OTC): 220 mg. **TABLETS (OTC):** 200 mg. **TABLETS (Rx):** 250 mg, 375 mg, 500 mg. **TABLETS (delayed-release):** 375 mg, 500 mg. **ORAL SUSPENSION:** 125 mg/5 ml.

ADMINISTRATION/HANDLING

PO

• Swallow enteric-coated form whole; scored tablets may be broken or crushed. • May give with food, milk, antacids if GI distress occurs.

INDICATIONS/ROUTES/DOSAGE

Alert: Each 275- or 550-mg tablet of naproxen sodium equals 250 or 500 mg naproxen, respectively.

RHEUMATOID ARTHRITIS, OSTEOARTHRITIS, ANKYLOSING SPONDYLITIS

PO: ADULTS, ELDERLY: 250–500 mg (275–550 mg) 2 times/day or 250 mg (275 mg) in morning and 500 mg (550 mg) in evening. **Naprelan:** 750–1,000 mg daily as single dose.

JUVENILE RHEUMATOID ARTHRITIS (naproxen only)

PO: CHILDREN: 10–15 mg/kg/day in 2 divided doses. **Maximum:** 1,000 mg/day.

ACUTE GOUTY ARTHRITIS

PO: ADULTS, ELDERLY: Initially, 750 (825) mg, then 250 (275) mg q8h until attack subsides. **Naprelan:** Initially, 1,000–1,500 mg, then 1,000 mg/day as single dose until attack subsides.

MILD TO MODERATE PAIN, DYSMENORRHEA, BURSITIS, TENDINITIS

PO: ADULTS, ELDERLY: Initially, 500 (550) mg, then 250 (275) mg q6–8h as needed. Total daily dose not to exceed 1.25 (1.375) g. **Naprelan:** 1,000 mg/day as single dose.

SIDE EFFECTS

FREQUENT (3%–9%): Nausea, constipation, abdominal cramps/pain, heartburn, dizziness, headache, drowsiness. **OCCASIONAL (1%–3%):** Stomatitis, diarrhea, indigestion. **RARE (<1%):** Vomiting, confusion.

ADVERSE REACTIONS/ TOXIC EFFECTS

Peptic ulcer, GI bleeding, gastritis, severe hepatic reaction (cholestasis, jaundice) occur rarely. Nephrotoxicity (dysuria, hematuria, proteinuria, nephrotic syndrome), severe hypersensitivity reaction (fever, chills, bronchospasm) occur rarely.

NURSING IMPLICATIONS

BASELINE ASSESSMENT

Assess onset, type, location, duration of pain/inflammation. Inspect appearance of affected joints for immobility, deformities, skin condition.

INTERVENTION/EVALUATION

Assist with ambulation if dizziness occurs. Monitor CBC, platelet count, renal/liver function tests, Hgb, pattern of daily bowel activity/stool consistency. Evaluate for therapeutic response: relief of pain, stiffness, swelling; increase in joint mobility; reduced joint tenderness; improved grip strength.

PATIENT/FAMILY TEACHING

Avoid tasks that require alertness, motor skills until response to drug is established. If GI upset occurs, take with food, milk. Avoid aspirin, alcohol during therapy (increases risk of GI bleeding). Report headache, rash, visual disturbances, weight gain, black stools, persistent headache.

naratriptan

nar-ah-**trip**-tan
(Amerge)
Do not confuse with Amaryl.

CLASSIFICATION

PHARMACOTHERAPEUTIC: Serotonin receptor agonist. **CLINICAL:** Antimigraine (see p. 54C).

ACTION

Binds selectively to vascular receptors producing a vasoconstrictive effect on cranial blood vessels. **Therapeutic Effect:** Produces relief of migraine headache.

PHARMACOKINETICS

Well absorbed following PO administration. Protein binding: 28%–31%. Metabolized by the liver to inactive metabolite. Eliminated primarily in the urine with lesser amount excreted in the feces. **Half-life:** 6 hrs (half-life increased in renal/hepatic impairment).

USES

Treatment of acute migraine attack with or without aura in adults.

PRECAUTIONS

CONTRAINDICATIONS: Coronary artery disease, uncontrolled hypertension, severe renal impairment (Ccr <15 ml/min), severe hepatic impairment (Child-Pugh grade C), cerebrovascular/peripheral vascular syndromes, ischemic heart disease (angina pectoris, history of MI, silent ischemia), Prinzmetal's angina, concurrent use (or within 24 hrs) of ergotamine-containing preparations, concurrent (or within 2 wks) of MAOI therapy, hemiplegic or basilar migraine, within 24 hrs of another serotonin receptor agonist. **CAUTIONS:** Mild to moderate renal/hepatic impairment, pt profile suggesting cardiovascular risks.

LIFESPAN CONSIDERATIONS: Pregnancy/lactation: Unknown if excreted in human breast milk. **Pregnancy Category C. Children:** Safety and efficacy not established. **Elderly:** Not recommended in the elderly.

INTERACTIONS

DRUG: Ergotamine-containing drugs may produce vasospastic reaction. **Oral contraceptives** reduce naratriptan's clearance, volume of distribution. Combined use of **fluoxetine, fluvoxamine, paroxetine, sertraline** may produce weakness, hyperreflexia, incoordination. **HERBAL:** None known. **FOOD:** None known. **LAB VALUES:** None known.

AVAILABILITY (Rx)

TABLETS: 1 mg, 2.5 mg.

ADMINISTRATION/HANDLING

PO

- Give without regard to food.

N

INDICATIONS/ROUTES/DOSAGE

MIGRAINE

PO: ADULTS: Give 1 mg or 2.5 mg. If headache returns or pt received only a partial response to initial dose, may repeat dose once after 4 hrs. **Maximum:** 5 mg per 24-hr period.

MILD TO MODERATE RENAL/HEPATIC IMPAIRMENT

PO: ADULTS: Consider low starting dosage. Do not exceed 2.5 mg over a 24-hr period.

SIDE EFFECTS

OCCASIONAL (5%): Nausea. **RARE (2%):** Paresthesia, dizziness, fatigue, drowsiness, neck/throat/jaw pressure.

ADVERSE REACTIONS/ TOXIC EFFECTS

May produce corneal opacities, defects. Cardiac events (ischemia, coronary artery vasospasm, MI), noncardiac vasospasm-related reactions (hemorrhage, stroke) occur rarely but particularly in those with hypertension, obesity, smokers, diabetics, strong family history of coronary artery disease, male >40 yrs, postmenopausal women.

NURSING IMPLICATIONS

BASELINE ASSESSMENT

Question for history of peripheral vascular disease, renal/hepatic impairment, possibility of pregnancy. Question pt regarding onset, location, duration of migraine; possible precipitating symptoms.

INTERVENTION/EVALUATION

Assess for relief of migraine headache; potential for photophobia, phonophobia (sound sensitivity), nausea, vomiting.

PATIENT/FAMILY TEACHING

Do not crush, chew tablet; swallow whole with water. May repeat dose after 4 hrs (maximum of 5 mg/24 hrs). May cause dizziness, fatigue, drowsiness. Use caution driving, engaging in tasks requiring mental alertness, physical coordination. Inform physician of any chest pain, heart throbbing, tightness in throat, rash, hallucinations, anxiety, panic.

natamycin

(Natacyn)

See Classification section under: Antifungals: topical

nateglinide

nah-**teg**-glih-nide

(Starlix)

◆ CLASSIFICATION

PHARMACOTHERAPEUTIC: Antihyperglycemic. **CLINICAL:** Antidiabetic (see p. 40C).

ACTION

Stimulates release of insulin from beta cells of the pancreas by depolarizing beta cells, leading to an opening of calcium channels. Resulting calcium influx induces insulin secretion. **Therapeutic Effect:** Lowers glucose concentration.

USES

Treatment of type 2 diabetes mellitus in pts whose disease cannot be adequately controlled with diet and exercise and in pts who have not been chronically treated with other antidiabetic agents. Used as monotherapy or in combination form.

PRECAUTIONS

CONTRAINDICATIONS: Diabetic ketoacidosis, type 1 diabetes mellitus. **CAUTIONS:** Hepatic/renal function impairment. **Pregnancy Category C.**

INTERACTIONS

DRUG: **NSAIDs, salicylates, MAOIs, beta-blockers** may increase hypoglycemic effect. **Thiazide diuretics, corticosteroids, thyroid medication, sympathomimetics** may decrease hypoglycemic effect. **HERBAL:** None known. **FOOD:** Peak plasma levels may be significantly reduced if administered 10 min before a liquid meal. **LAB VALUES:** None known.

AVAILABILITY (Rx)

TABLETS: 60 mg, 120 mg.

ADMINISTRATION/HANDLING

PO

- Ideally, give within 15 min of a meal, but may be given immediately before a meal to as long as 30 min before a meal.

INDICATIONS/ROUTES/DOSAGE

DIABETES MELLITUS

PO: ADULTS, ELDERLY: 120 mg 3 times/day before meals. Initially, 60 mg may be given.

SIDE EFFECTS

FREQUENT (10%): Upper respiratory tract infection. **OCCASIONAL (3%–4%):** Back pain, flu symptoms, dizziness, arthropathy, diarrhea. **RARE (≤2%):** Bronchitis, cough.

ADVERSE REACTIONS/ TOXIC EFFECTS

Hypoglycemia occurs in <2%.

NURSING IMPLICATIONS

BASELINE ASSESSMENT

Check fasting blood glucose, glycosylated Hgb (HbA_{1C}) periodically to determine minimum effective dose. Discuss lifestyle to determine extent of learning, emotional needs. Ensure follow-up instruction if pt/family do not thoroughly understand diabetes management or glucose-testing technique. At least 1 wk should elapse to assess response to drug before new dose adjustment is made.

INTERVENTION/EVALUATION

Monitor blood glucose, food intake. Assess for hypoglycemia (cool/wet skin, tremors, dizziness, anxiety, headache, tachycardia, numbness in mouth, hunger, diplopia), hyperglycemia (polyuria, polyphagia, polydipsia, nausea, vomiting, dim vision, fatigue, deep rapid breathing). Be alert to conditions that alter glucose requirements: fever, increased activity/stress, surgical procedures.

PATIENT/FAMILY TEACHING

Diabetes mellitus requires lifelong control. Prescribed diet, exercise are principal parts of treatment; do not skip or delay meals. Continue to adhere to dietary instructions, a regular exercise program, regular testing of blood glucose.

Natrecor

see nesiritide

Nebcin

see tobramycin

nedocromil sodium

ned-oh-**crow**-mul
(Alocril, Mireze, Tilade)

CLASSIFICATION

PHARMACOTHERAPEUTIC: Mast cell stabilizer. **CLINICAL:** Respiratory inhalant anti-inflammatory (see p. 65C).

ACTION

Prevents activation, release of mediators of inflammation (e.g., histamine, leukotrienes, mast cells, eosinophils, monocytes). **Therapeutic Effect:** Prevents both early and late asthmatic responses.

USES

Maintenance therapy for preventing airway inflammation, bronchoconstriction in pts with mild to moderate bronchial asthma. **Ophthalmic:** Treatment of itching associated with allergic conjunctivitis. **Unlabeled:** Prevention of bronchospasm in pts with reversible obstructive airway disease.

N

PRECAUTIONS

CONTRAINDICATIONS: None known. **CAUTIONS:** Not used for reversing acute bronchospasm. **Pregnancy Category B.**

INTERACTIONS

DRUG: None known. **HERBAL:** None known. **FOOD:** None known. **LAB VALUES:** None known.

AVAILABILITY (Rx)

AEROSOL FOR INHALATION: 1.75 mg/activation. **OPHTHALMIC SOLUTION:** 2%.

INDICATIONS/ROUTES/DOSAGE

ASTHMA

Oral inhalation: ADULTS, ELDERLY, CHILDREN ≥6 YRS: 2 inhalations 4 times/day. May decrease to 3 times/day then 2 times/day as control of asthma occurs.

ALLERGIC CONJUNCTIVITIS

Ophthalmic: ADULTS, ELDERLY, CHILDREN: ≥3 yrs 1–2 drops in each eye 2 times/day.

SIDE EFFECTS

FREQUENT (5%–10%): Cough, pharyngitis, bronchospasm, headache, unpleasant taste. **OCCASIONAL (1%–5%):** Rhinitis, upper respiratory tract infection, abdominal pain, fatigue. **RARE (<1%):** Diarrhea, dizziness.

ADVERSE REACTIONS/ TOXIC EFFECTS

None known.

NURSING IMPLICATIONS

INTERVENTION/EVALUATION

Evaluate therapeutic response: reduced dependence on antihistamine, less frequent/less severe asthmatic attacks.

PATIENT/FAMILY TEACHING

Increase fluid intake (decreases lung secretion viscosity). Must be administered at regular intervals (even when symptom free) to achieve optimal results of therapy. Unpleasant taste after inhalation may be relieved by rinsing mouth with water immediately.

nefazodone hydrochloride

nef-**ah**-zoh-doan
(Serzone)

CLASSIFICATION

CLINICAL: Antidepressant (see p. 36C).

ACTION

Exact mechanism unknown. Appears to inhibit neuronal uptake of serotonin and norepinephrine, antagonize alpha$_1$-adrenergic receptors. **Therapeutic Effect:** Produces antidepressant effect.

PHARMACOKINETICS

Rapidly, completely absorbed from GI tract. Protein binding: >99%. Food delays absorption. Widely distributed in body tissues, including CNS. Extensively metabolized to active metabolites. Excreted in urine and eliminated in feces. Unknown if removed by hemodialysis. **Half-life:** 2–4 hrs.

USES

Treatment of depression. Maintenance treatment for prevention of relapse of acute depressive episode.

PRECAUTIONS

CONTRAINDICATIONS: Within 14 days of MAOI ingestion. **CAUTIONS:** Recent MI, unstable heart disease, hepatic cirrhosis, dehydration, hypovolemia, cerebrovascular disease, history of mania/hypomania, history of seizures.

LIFESPAN CONSIDERATIONS: Pregnancy/lactation: Unknown if drug crosses placenta or is distributed in breast milk. **Pregnancy Category C. Children:** Safety and efficacy not established. **Elderly:** No age-related precautions noted; lower dosage recommended.

INTERACTIONS

DRUG: May increase concentration, toxicity of **alprazolam, triazolam** (dosage reduction advised). **MAOIs** may produce severe reactions (see Adverse Reactions/Toxic Effects). At least 14 days should elapse between discontinuing MAOIs and initiating of nefazodone therapy. At least 7 days should elapse after discontinuing nefazodone and initiating MAOI therapy. **HERBAL: St. John's wort** may increase risk of adverse effects. **FOOD:** None known. **LAB VALUES:** None known.

AVAILABILITY (Rx)

TABLETS: 50 mg, 100 mg, 150 mg, 200 mg, 250 mg.

ADMINISTRATION/HANDLING

PO

- Give without regard to meals.

INDICATIONS/ROUTES/DOSAGE

Alert: At least 14 days should elapse between discontinuing MAOIs and initiating nefazodone therapy. At least 7 days should elapse after discontinuing nefazodone and initiating MAOI therapy.

DEPRESSION, PREVENTION OF RELAPSE OF ACUTE EPISODE

PO: ADULTS: Initially, 200 mg/day, given in 2 divided doses. Gradually increase dose in increments of 100–200 mg/day on a twice-daily schedule, at intervals of at least 1 wk. RANGE: 300–600 mg/day. ELDERLY: Initially, 100 mg/day on a twice daily schedule. Adjust the rate of subsequent dose titration based on clinical response. RANGE: 200–400 mg/day. CHILDREN: 300–400 mg/day.

SIDE EFFECTS

Elderly/debilitated experience increased susceptibility to side effects. **FREQUENT:** Headache (36%); dry mouth, somnolence (25%); nausea (22%); dizziness (17%); constipation (14%); insomnia, asthenia (loss of strength, energy), lightheadedness (10%). **OCCASIONAL:** Dyspepsia, blurred vision (9%); diarrhea, infection (8%); confusion, abnormal vision (7%); pharyngitis (6%); increased appetite (5%); postural hypotension, vasodilation (flushing, feeling of warmth)

(4%); peripheral edema, cough, flu syndrome (3%).

ADVERSE REACTIONS/ TOXIC EFFECTS

Concurrent MAOI administration or if time frame between discontinuation and initiation of drug therapy (see Indications/Routes/Dosage) is not followed, serious reactions (hyperthermia, rigidity, myoclonus, extreme agitation, delirium, coma) occur.

NURSING IMPLICATIONS

BASELINE ASSESSMENT

Question for history of sensitivity to nefazodone, trazodone, other medication (esp. alprazolam, triazolam, MAOIs, terfenadine). Obtain history of cardiovascular/cerebrovascular disease, mania/hypomania, seizures.

INTERVENTION/EVALUATION

Monitor B/P, pulse. Supervise suicidal-risk pt closely during early therapy (as energy level improves, suicide potential increases). Assess appearance, behavior, speech pattern, level of interest, mood. Assist with ambulation if dizziness, lightheadedness occurs. Monitor stool frequency/consistency.

PATIENT/FAMILY TEACHING

Maximum therapeutic response may require several weeks of therapy. Dry mouth may be relieved by sugarless gum, sips of tepid water. Report headache, nausea, visual disturbances. May cause dizziness. Avoid tasks that require alertness, motor skills until response to drug is established. Avoid alcohol.

nelfinavir

nell-**fine**-ah-veer
(Viracept)

CLASSIFICATION

PHARMACOTHERAPEUTIC: Protease inhibitor. **CLINICAL:** Antiviral (see pp. 59C, 100C).

ACTION

Inhibits activity of HIV-1 protease, the enzyme necessary for the formation of infectious HIV. **Therapeutic Effect:** Formation of immature noninfectious viral particles rather than HIV replication.

PHARMACOKINETICS

Well absorbed after PO administration. Protein binding: >98%. Absorption increased with food. Metabolized by the liver. Highly bound to plasma proteins. Eliminated primarily in feces. Unknown if removed by hemodialysis. **Half-life:** 3.5–5 hrs.

USES

Treatment of HIV infection when antiretroviral therapy is warranted.

PRECAUTIONS

CONTRAINDICATIONS: Concurrent administration with midazolam, triazolam, rifampin. **CAUTIONS:** Hepatic function impairment.

LIFESPAN CONSIDERATIONS: Pregnancy/lactation: Unknown if distributed in breast milk. **Pregnancy Category B. Children:** No age-related precautions noted in those >2 yrs. **Elderly:** No information available.

INTERACTIONS

DRUG: Alcohol, psychoactive drugs may produce additive CNS effects. **Anticonvulsants, rifampin, rifabutin** lower nelfinavir plasma concentration.

Increases **indinavir, saquinavir** plasma concentration. **Ritonavir** increases nelfinavir plasma concentration. Decreases effects of **oral contraceptives.** **HERBAL:** **St. John's wort** may decrease concentrations, effect. **FOOD:** **Food** increases plasma concentration. **LAB VALUES:** May decrease Hgb, WBCs, neutrophils; increase SGOT (AST), SGPT (ALT), creatine kinase.

AVAILABILITY (Rx)

TABLETS: 250 mg, 625 mg. **POWDER:** 50 mg/g.

ADMINISTRATION/HANDLING

PO

• Give with food (light meal, snack). • Mix oral powder with small amount of water, milk, formula, soy formula, soy milk, dietary supplement. • Entire contents must be consumed in order to ingest full dose. • Do not mix with acidic food, orange juice, apple juice, applesauce (bitter taste), or with water in its original container.

INDICATIONS/ROUTES/DOSAGE

HIV INFECTION

PO: ADULTS: 750 mg (three 250-mg tablets) 3 times/day, or 1,250 mg 2 times/day in combination with nucleoside analogues (enhances antiviral activity). CHILDREN 2–13 YRS: 20–30 mg/kg/dose, 3 times daily. **Maximum:** 750 mg q8h.

SIDE EFFECTS

FREQUENT (20%): Diarrhea. **OCCASIONAL (3%–7%):** Nausea, rash. **RARE (1%–2%):** Flatulence, asthenia.

ADVERSE REACTIONS/ TOXIC EFFECTS

None known.

NURSING IMPLICATIONS

BASELINE ASSESSMENT

Check hematology, liver function tests for accurate baseline.

INTERVENTION/EVALUATION

Determine pattern of bowel activity, stool consistency. Monitor liver enzyme studies for abnormalities. Be alert to development of opportunistic infections, (e.g., fever, chills, cough, myalgia).

PATIENT/FAMILY TEACHING

Take with food (optimizes absorption). Take medication every day as prescribed. Doses should be evenly spaced around the clock. Do not alter dose or discontinue medication without informing physician. Medication is not a cure for HIV infection, pt may continue to experience illnesses, including opportunistic infections. Medication does not reduce risk of transmission to others.

N

neomycin sulfate

nee-oh-**my**-sin
(Mycifradin, Myciguent)

FIXED-COMBINATION(S)

Neosporin GU Irrigant: neomycin/polymyxin B: 40 mg/200,000 units/ml. **Neosporin Ointment, TripleAntibiotic:** neomycin/polymyxin B/bacitracin: 3.5 mg/5,000 units/400 units/g; 3.5 mg/10,000 units/400 units/g.

◆CLASSIFICATION

PHARMACOTHERAPEUTIC: Aminoglycoside. **CLINICAL:** Antibiotic (see p. 18C).

ACTION

Binds to bacterial microorganisms. **Therapeutic Effect:** Interferes with bactererial protein synthesis.

USES

Preparation of GI tract for surgery. Treatment of minor skin infections, diarrhea caused by *E. coli*. Adjunct in treatment of hepatic encephalopathy.

PRECAUTIONS

CONTRAINDICATIONS: Hypersensitivity to aminoglycosides. **CAUTIONS:** Elderly, infants with renal insufficiency/immaturity; neuromuscular disorders, prior hearing loss, vertigo, renal impairment. **Pregnancy Category C.**

INTERACTIONS

DRUG: If significant systemic absorption occurs, may increase nephrotoxicity, ototoxicity with **aminoglycosides, other nephrotoxic, ototoxic medications.** **HERBAL:** None known. **FOOD:** None known. **LAB VALUES:** None known.

N

AVAILABILITY

TOPICAL OINTMENT (OTC): 0.5%. **TABLETS (Rx):** 500 mg.

INDICATIONS/ROUTES/DOSAGE

PREOP BOWEL ANTISEPSIS

PO: ADULTS, ELDERLY: 1 g each hr for 4 doses; then 1 g q4h for 5 doses or 1 g at 1 PM, 2 PM, 10 PM (with erythromycin) on day prior to surgery. CHILDREN: 90 mg/kg/day in divided doses q4h for 2 days or 25 mg/kg at 1 PM, 2 PM, 10 PM on day prior to surgery.

HEPATIC ENCEPHALOPATHY

PO: ADULTS, ELDERLY: 4–12 g/day in divided doses q4–6h. CHILDREN: 2.5–7 g/m^2/day in divided doses q4–6h.

DIARRHEA CAUSED BY *E. COLI*

PO: ADULTS, ELDERLY: 3 g/day in divided doses q6h. CHILDREN: 50 mg/kg/day in divided doses q6h.

USUAL TOPICAL DOSAGE

ADULTS, ELDERLY, CHILDREN: Apply 1–3 times/day.

SIDE EFFECTS

FREQUENT: Systemic: Nausea, vomiting, diarrhea, irritation of mouth/rectal area. **Topical:** Itching, redness, swelling, rash. **RARE: Systemic:** Malabsorption syndrome, neuromuscular blockade (drowsiness, weakness, difficulty breathing).

ADVERSE REACTIONS/ TOXIC EFFECTS

Nephrotoxicity (evidenced by increased BUN, serum creatinine, decreased creatinine clearance) may be reversible if drug stopped at first sign of symptoms; irreversible ototoxicity (tinnitus, dizziness, ringing/roaring in ears, reduced hearing), neurotoxicity (headache, dizziness, lethargy, tremors, visual disturbances) occur occasionally. Severe respiratory depression, anaphylaxis occur rarely. Superinfections, particularly with fungi, may occur.

NURSING IMPLICATIONS

BASELINE ASSESSMENT

Dehydration must be treated before aminoglycoside therapy. Establish pt's baseline hearing acuity before beginning therapy.

INTERVENTION/EVALUATION

Be alert to ototoxic, neurotoxic symptoms (see Adverse Reactions/Toxic Effects). Assess for hypersensitivity reaction (**topical:** assess for rash, redness, itching). Be alert for superinfection, particularly genital/anal pruritus, changes of oral mucosa, diarrhea.

PATIENT/FAMILY TEACHING

Continue antibiotic for full length of treatment. Space doses evenly. **Topical:** Cleanse area gently before application; report redness, itching. Inform physician if ringing in the ears, impaired hearing, dizziness occurs.

neostigmine

nee-oh-**stig**-meen
(Prostigmin)

Do not confuse with physostigmine.

CLASSIFICATION

PHARMACOTHERAPEUTIC: Cholinergic. **CLINICAL:** Antimyasthenic, antidote (see p. 80C).

ACTION

Prevents destruction of acetylcholine by attaching to enzyme, anticholinesterase. **Therapeutic Effect:** Improves intestinal/skeletal muscle tone; increases secretions, salivation.

USES

Improvement of muscle strength in control of myasthenia gravis, diagnosis of myasthenia gravis, prevention/treatment of postop distention and urinary retention, antidote for reversal of effects of nondepolarizing neuromuscular blocking agents after surgery.

PRECAUTIONS

CONTRAINDICATIONS: GI/GU obstruction, peritonitis. **CAUTIONS:** Epilepsy, asthma, bradycardia, hyperthyroidism, arrhythmias, peptic ulcer, recent coronary occlusion. **Pregnancy Category C.**

INTERACTIONS

DRUG: Anticholinergics reverse/prevent effects. **Cholinesterase inhibitors** may increase toxicity. Antagonizes **neuromuscular blocking agents. Quinidine, procainamide** may antagonize action. **HERBAL:** None known. **FOOD:** None known. **LAB VALUES:** None known.

∅ IV INCOMPATIBILITY

None known.

IV COMPATIBILITIES

Glycopyrrolate (Robinul), heparin, ondansetron (Zofran), potassium chloride, thiopental (Pentothal).

AVAILABILITY (Rx)

INJECTION: 0.5 mg/ml, 1 mg/ml. **TABLETS:** 15 mg.

INDICATIONS/ROUTES/DOSAGE

MYASTHENIA GRAVIS

PO: ADULTS, ELDERLY: Initially, 15–30 mg 3–4 times/day. Increase as necessary. USUAL MAINTENANCE DOSE: 150 mg/day (range of 15–375 mg). CHILDREN: 2 mg/kg/day or 60 mg/m^2/day divided q3–4h.

Subcutaneous/IM/IV: ADULTS: 0.5–2.5 mg as needed. CHILDREN: 0.01–0.04 mg/kg q2–4h.

N

DIAGNOSIS OF MYASTHENIA GRAVIS

Alert: Discontinue all anticholinesterase therapy at least 8 hrs before testing. Give 0.011 mg/kg atropine sulfate IV simultaneously with neostigmine or IM 30 min prior to administering neostigmine (prevents adverse effects).

IM: ADULTS, ELDERLY: 0.022 mg/kg. If cholinergic reaction occurs, discontinue tests and administer 0.4–0.6 mg or more atropine sulfate IV. CHILDREN: 0.025–0.04 mg/kg IM preceded by atropine sulfate 0.011 mg/kg subcutaneously.

PREVENTION OF POSTOP URINARY RETENTION

Subcutaneous/IM: ADULTS, ELDERLY: 0.25 mg q4–6h for 2–3 days.

POSTOP DISTENTION, URINARY RETENTION

Subcutaneous/IM: ADULTS, ELDERLY: 0.5–1 mg. Catheterize if voiding does not occur within 1 hr. After voiding, continue 0.5 mg q3h for 5 injections.

REVERSAL OF NEUROMUSCULAR BLOCKADE

IV: ADULTS, ELDERLY: 0.5–2.5 mg given slowly. CHILDREN: 0.025–0.08 mg/kg/dose. INFANTS: 0.025–0.1 mg/kg/dose.

SIDE EFFECTS

FREQUENT: Muscarinic effects (diarrhea, increased sweating/watering of mouth, nausea, vomiting, stomach cramps/pain). **OCCASIONAL:** Muscarinic effects (increased frequency/urge to urinate, increased bronchial secretions, unusually small pupils/watering of eyes).

ADVERSE REACTIONS/ TOXIC EFFECTS

Overdose produces a cholinergic reaction manifested as abdominal discomfort/cramping, nausea, vomiting, diarrhea, flushing, feeling of warmth/heat about face, excessive salivation, diaphoresis, lacrimation, pallor, bradycardia/tachycardia, hypotension, urinary urgency, blurred vision, bronchospasm, pupillary contraction, involuntary muscular contraction visible under the skin (fasciculation).

NURSING IMPLICATIONS

BASELINE ASSESSMENT

Larger doses should be given at time of greatest fatigue. Avoid large doses in those with megacolon, reduced GI motility.

INTERVENTION/EVALUATION

Monitor muscle strength, vital signs. Monitor for therapeutic response to medication (increased muscle strength, decreased fatigue, improved chewing, swallowing functions).

PATIENT/FAMILY TEACHING

Report nausea, vomiting, diarrhea, diaphoresis, increased salivary secretions, irregular heartbeat, muscle weakness, severe abdominal pain, difficulty in breathing.

Neo-Synephrine

see phenylephrine

nesiritide

ness-**ear**-ih-tide
(Natrecor)

CLASSIFICATION

PHARMACOTHERAPEUTIC: Brain natriuretic peptide. **CLINICAL:** Endogenous hormone.

ACTION

Facilitates cardiovascular homeostasis, fluid status through counterregulation of the renin-angiotensin-aldosterone system, stimulating cyclic guanosine monophosphate, leading to smooth muscle cell relaxation. **Therapeutic Effect:** Promotes vasodilation, natriuresis, diuresis, correcting CHF.

PHARMACOKINETICS

	Onset	Peak	Duration
IV	15–30 min	1–2 hrs	4 hrs

Excreted primarily in the heart by the left ventricle. Metabolized by the natriuretic neutral endopeptidase enzymes on the vascular luminal surface. **Half-life:** 18–23 min.

USES

Treatment of acutely decompensated CHF in pts who have dyspnea at rest or with minimal activity.

PRECAUTIONS

CONTRAINDICATIONS: Systolic B/P <90 mm Hg, cardiogenic shock. **CAUTIONS:** Significant valvular stenosis, restrictive/obstructive cardiomyopathy, constrictive pericarditis, pericardial tamponade, suspected low cardiac filling pressures, atrial/ventricular arrhythmias/conduction defects, hypotension, hepatic/renal insufficiency.

LIFESPAN CONSIDERATIONS: Pregnancy/lactation: Unknown if drug crosses placenta or is distributed in breast milk. **Pregnancy Category C. Children:** Safety and efficacy not established. **Elderly:** No age-related precautions noted.

INTERACTIONS

DRUG: IV nitroglycerin, angiotensin-converting enzyme (ACE) inhibitors, milrinone, nitroprusside may increase risk of hypotension. **HERBAL:** None known. **FOOD:** None known. **LAB VALUES:** None known.

AVAILABILITY (Rx)

INJECTION: 1.5 mg/5 ml vial.

ADMINISTRATION/HANDLING

Alert: Do not mix with other injections or infusions. Do not give IM.

IV

Storage • Store vial at room temperature. Once reconstituted, use within 24 hrs at room temperature or refrigerated.

Reconstitution • Reconstitute one 1.5-mg vial with 5 ml D_5W or 0.9% NaCl, 0.2% NaCl or any combination thereof. Swirl or rock gently, add to 250-ml bag D_5W or 0.9% NaCl, 0.2% NaCl, or any combination thereof yielding a solution of 6 mcg/ml.

Rate of administration • Give as an IV bolus over approx. 60 sec initially followed by continuous IV infusion.

IV INCOMPATIBILITIES

Bumetanide (Bumex), enalapril (Vasotec), ethacrynic acid (Edecrin), furosemide (Lasix), heparin, hydralazine (Apresoline), insulin, sodium metabisulfite.

INDICATIONS/ROUTES/DOSAGE

CHF

IV bolus: ADULTS, ELDERLY: 2 mcg/kg followed by a continuous IV infusion of 0.01 mcg/kg/min. May be incrementally increased q3h to a maximum of 0.03 mcg/kg/min.

SIDE EFFECTS

FREQUENT (11%): Hypotension. **OCCASIONAL (2%–8%):** Headache, nausea, bradycardia. **RARE (≤1%):** Confusion, paresthesia, somnolence, tremor.

ADVERSE REACTIONS/ TOXIC EFFECTS

Ventricular arrhythmias (ventricular tachycardia, atrial fibrillation, atrioventricular node conduction abnormalities), angina pectoris occur rarely.

NURSING IMPLICATIONS

BASELINE ASSESSMENT

Obtain B/P immediately prior to each dose, in addition to regular monitoring (be alert to fluctuations). If excessive reduction in B/P occurs, place pt in supine position with legs elevated.

INTERVENTION/EVALUATION

B/P readings, pulse rate should be frequently monitored for hypotension during therapy. With physician, establish parameters for adjusting rate or stopping infusion. Maintain accurate I&O; measure urine output frequently. Immediately notify physician of decreased urine output, cardiac arrhythmias, significant decrease in B/P or heart rate.

netilmicin sulfate

(Netromycin)

See Classification section under: Antibiotic: aminoglycosides (p. 18C)

Neupogen

see filgrastim

Neurontin

see gabapentin

nevirapine

neh-**vear**-ah-peen

(Viramune)

CLASSIFICATION

PHARMACOTHERAPEUTIC: Nonnucleoside reverse transcriptase inhibitor. **CLINICAL:** Antiviral (see p. 99C).

ACTION

Binds directly to virus type 1 (HIV-1) reverse transcriptase (RT), blocking RNA-dependent and DNA-dependent DNA polymerase activity (changes the shape of RT enzyme). **Therapeutic Effect:** Slows HIV replication, reducing progression of HIV infection.

PHARMACOKINETICS

Readily absorbed following PO administration. Protein binding: 60%. Widely distributed. Extensively metabolized in liver; primarily excreted in urine. **Half-life:** 45 hrs (single dose); 25–30 hrs (multiple doses).

USES

Used in combination with nucleoside analogues or protease inhibitors for treatment of HIV-1–infected adults who have experienced clinical and immunologic deterioration. **Unlabeled:** Reduces risk of transmitting HIV from infected mother to newborn.

PRECAUTIONS

CONTRAINDICATIONS: None known. **CAUTIONS:** Renal/liver dysfunction, elevated SGOT (AST) or SGPT (ALT), history of chronic hepatitis (B or C).

LIFESPAN CONSIDERATIONS: Pregnancy/lactation: Crosses placenta. Distributed in breast milk. Breast-feeding not recommended (possibility of HIV transmission). **Pregnancy Category C. Children:** Granulocytopenia occurs more frequently. **Elderly:** No information available.

INTERACTIONS

DRUG: May decrease **ketoconazole, protease inhibitors, oral contraceptives** plasma concentration. **Rifabutin, rifampin** may decrease concentration. **HERBAL: St. John's wort** may decrease concentrations, effects. **FOOD:** None known. **LAB VALUES:** May significantly increase SGOT (AST), SGPT (ALT), bilirubin, GGT. May significantly decrease Hgb, platelets, neutrophil count.

AVAILABILITY (Rx)

TABLETS: 200 mg. **ORAL SUSPENSION:** 50 mg/5 ml.

ADMINISTRATION/HANDLING

PO

- Give without regard to meals.

INDICATIONS/ROUTES/DOSAGE

Alert: Always administer nevirapine in combination with at least one additional antiretroviral agent (resistant HIV virus appears rapidly when nevirapine is given as monotherapy).

HIV-1 INFECTION

PO: ADULTS: 200 mg daily for 14 days (reduces risk of rash). MAINTENANCE: 200 mg twice daily in combination with nucleoside analogue antiretroviral agents. CHILDREN 2 MOS–8 YRS: 4 mg/kg once daily for 14 days; then 7 mg/kg 2 times/day. CHILDREN >8 YRS: 4 mg/kg once daily for 14 days; then 4 mg/kg 2 times/day. **Maximum:** 400 mg/day.

SIDE EFFECTS

FREQUENT (3%–8%): Rash, fever, headache, nausea. **OCCASIONAL (1%–3%):** Stomatitis (burning/erythema of oral mucosa, mucosal ulceration, dysphagia). **RARE (<1%):** Paresthesia, myalgia, abdominal pain.

ADVERSE REACTIONS/ TOXIC EFFECTS

Rash may become severe, life threatening. Hepatitis occurs rarely.

NURSING IMPLICATIONS

BASELINE ASSESSMENT

Establish baseline lab values, esp. liver function tests, prior to initiating therapy and at intervals during therapy. Obtain medication history (esp. use of oral contraceptives).

INTERVENTION/EVALUATION

Closely monitor for evidence of rash (usually appears on trunk, face, extremities; occurs within first 6 wks of drug initiation). Observe for rash accompanied by fever, blistering, oral lesions, conjunctivitis, swelling, muscle/joint aches, general malaise.

PATIENT/FAMILY TEACHING

If nevirapine therapy is missed for >7 days, restart by using one 200-mg tablet daily for first 14 days, followed by one 200-mg tablet twice daily. Continue therapy for full length of treatment. Doses should be evenly spaced. Nevirapine is not a cure for HIV infection, nor does it reduce risk of transmission to others. If rash appears, contact physician before continuing therapy.

Nexium

see esomeprazole

niacin, nicotinic acid

(Niacor, Niaspan, Nico-400, Nicotinex)

Do not confuse with Nitro-Bid.

✦CLASSIFICATION

CLINICAL: Antihyperlipidemic, water-soluble vitamin (see pp. 51C, 137C).

ACTION

Component of 2 coenzymes needed for tissue respiration, lipid metabolism, glycogenolysis. Inhibits synthesis of very-low-density lipoproteins (VLDLs). **Therapeutic Effect:** Reduces total and LDL cholesterol, triglycerides, increases HDL cholesterol. Necessary for lipid metabolism, tissue respiration, glycogenolysis. Lowers serum cholesterol, triglycerides (decreases LDL, VLDL, increases HDL).

PHARMACOKINETICS

Readily absorbed from GI tract. Widely distributed. Metabolized in liver. Primarily excreted in urine. **Half-life:** 45 min.

N

USES

Adjunct in treatment of hyperlipidemias, peripheral vascular disease; treatment of pellagra; dietary supplement.

PRECAUTIONS

CONTRAINDICATIONS: Hypersensitivity to niacin, tartrazine (frequently seen in pts sensitive to aspirin), active peptic ulcer, severe hypotension, hepatic dysfunction, arterial hemorrhaging. **CAUTIONS:** Diabetes mellitus, gallbladder disease, gout, history of jaundice/liver disease.

LIFESPAN CONSIDERATIONS: Pregnancy/lactation: Not recommended for use during pregnancy/lactation. Distributed in breast milk. **Pregnancy Category A** (**C** if used at dosages above RDA). **Children:** No age-related precautions noted. Not recommended in those <2 yrs. **Elderly:** No age-related precautions noted.

INTERACTIONS

DRUG: Lovastatin, pravastatin, simvastatin may increase risk of rhabdomyolysis and acute renal failure. **HERBAL:** None known. **FOOD:** None known. **LAB VALUES:** May increase uric acid.

AVAILABILITY (OTC)

TABLETS: 50 mg, 100 mg, 250 mg, 500 mg. **TABLETS (time-release):** 500 mg, 750 mg, 1,000 mg. **CAPSULES (time-release):** 125 mg, 250 mg, 400 mg, 500 mg. **ELIXIR:** 50 mg/5 ml.

ADMINISTRATION/HANDLING

PO

• Give without regard to meals. • Take at bedtime, avoid alcohol.

INDICATIONS/ROUTES/DOSAGE

HYPERLIPIDEMIA

PO: Immediate-release: ADULTS, ELDERLY: Initially, 50–100 mg 2 times/day for 7 days. Increase gradually by doubling dose qwk up to 1–1.5 g/day in 2–3 doses. **Maximum:** 3 g/day. CHILDREN: Initially, 100–250 mg/day (**Maximum:** 10 mg/kg/day) in 3 divided doses. May increase by 100 mg/wk or 250 mg q2–3wks. **Maximum:** 2,250 mg/day. **Extended-release:** Initially, 500 mg/day in divided doses 2 times/day for 1 wk; then increase to 500 mg 2 times/day. MAINTENANCE: 2 g/day.

NUTRITIONAL SUPPLEMENT

PO: ADULTS, ELDERLY: 10–20 mg/day.

SIDE EFFECTS

FREQUENT: Flushing (esp. of face, neck) occurring within 20 min of administration and lasting for 30–60 min, GI upset, pruritus. **OCCASIONAL:** Dizziness, hypotension, headache, blurred vision, burning/tingling of skin, flatulence, nausea, vomiting, diarrhea. **RARE:** Hyperglycemia, glycosuria, rash, hyperpigmentation, dry skin.

ADVERSE REACTIONS/ TOXIC EFFECTS

Cardiac arrhythmias occur rarely.

NURSING IMPLICATIONS

BASELINE ASSESSMENT

Question for history of hypersensitivity to niacin, tartrazine, aspirin. Assess baselines: cholesterol, triglyceride, blood glucose, liver function tests.

INTERVENTION/EVALUATION

Evaluate flushing, degree of discomfort. Check for headache, dizziness, blurred vision. Determine pattern of bowel activity. Monitor liver function, cholesterol, triglycerides. Check blood glucose levels carefully in those on insulin, oral antihyperglycemics. Assess skin for rash, dryness. Monitor blood glucose, uric acid.

PATIENT/FAMILY TEACHING

Transient flushing of the skin, sensation of warmth, itching, tingling may occur. Notify physician if dizziness occurs (avoid sudden changes in posture). Inform physician if nausea, vomiting, loss of appetite, yellowing of skin, dark urine, feeling of weakness occurs.

nicardipine hydrochloride

nigh-**car**-dih-peen
(Cardene, Cardene IV, Cardene SR)
Do not confuse with Cardizem SR, codeine, nifedipine.

CLASSIFICATION

PHARMACOTHERAPEUTIC: Calcium channel blocker. **CLINICAL:** Antianginal, antihypertensive (see p. 67C).

ACTION

Inhibits calcium ion movement across cell membrane, depressing contraction of cardiac and vascular smooth muscle. **Therapeutic Effect:** Increases heart rate, cardiac output. Decreases systemic vascular resistance, B/P.

PHARMACOKINETICS

	Onset	Peak	Duration
PO	—	1–2 hrs	8 hrs

Rapidly, completely absorbed from GI tract. Protein binding: >95%. Undergoes first-pass metabolism in liver. Primarily excreted in urine. Not removed by hemodialysis. **Half-life:** 2–4 hrs.

USES

PO: Treatment of chronic stable (effort-associated) angina, essential hypertension. **Sustained-Release:** Treatment of essential hypertension. **Parenteral:** Short-term treatment of hypertension when oral therapy not feasible or desirable. **Unlabeled:** Treatment of vasospastic angina, Raynaud's phenomena, subarachnoid hemorrhage, associated neurologic deficits.

PRECAUTIONS

CONTRAINDICATIONS: Severe hypotension, second- or third-degree heart block, sinus bradycardia, ventricular tachycardia, cardiogenic shock, CHF, atrial fibrillation/flutter associated with accessory conduction pathways. Within several hours of IV beta-blocker therapy. **CAUTIONS:** Sick sinus syndrome, severe left ventricular dysfunction, renal/liver impairment, cardiomyopathy, edema, concomitant beta-blocker or digoxin therapy.

LIFESPAN CONSIDERATIONS: Pregnancy/lactation: Unknown if distributed in breast milk. **Pregnancy Category C. Children:** Safety and efficacy not established. **Elderly:** Age-related renal impairment may require cautious use.

INTERACTIONS

DRUG: Beta-blockers may have additive effect. May increase **digoxin** concentration. **Procainamide, quinidine** may increase risk of QT interval prolongation. **Hypokalemia-producing agents** may increase risk of arrhythmias. **HERBAL:** None known. **FOOD: Grapefruit/grapefruit juice** may alter absorption. **LAB VALUES:** None known.

AVAILABILITY (Rx)

CAPSULES: 20 mg, 30 mg. **CAPSULES (sustained-release):** 30 mg, 45 mg, 60 mg. **INJECTION:** 2.5 mg/ml.

ADMINISTRATION/HANDLING

PO

• Do not crush or break oral, sustained-release capsules. • Give without regard to food.

N

IV

Storage • Store at room temperature. • Diluted IV solution is stable for 24 hrs at room temperature.

Reconstitution • Dilute each 25-mg ampoule with 250 ml D_5W, 0.9% NaCl, 0.45% NaCl, or any combination thereof to provide a concentration of 1 mg/10 ml.

Rate of administration • Give by slow IV infusion. • Change IV site q12h if administered peripherally.

IV INCOMPATIBILITIES

Furosemide (Lasix), heparin, thiopental (Pentothal).

IV COMPATIBILITIES

Diltiazem (Cardizem), dobutamine (Dobutrex), dopamine (Intropin), epinephrine, hydromorphone (Dilaudid), labetalol (Trandate), lorazepam (Ativan), midazolam (Versed), milrinone (Primacor), morphine, nitroglycerin, norepinephrine (Levophed).

N

INDICATIONS/ROUTES/DOSAGE

CHRONIC STABLE ANGINA

PO: ADULTS, ELDERLY: Initially, 20 mg 3 times/day. RANGE: 20–40 mg 3 times/day.

ESSENTIAL HYPERTENSION

PO: ADULTS, ELDERLY: Initially, 20 mg 3 times/day. RANGE: 20–40 mg 3 times/day.

Sustained-release: ADULTS, ELDERLY: Initially, 30 mg 2 times/day. RANGE: 30–60 mg 2 times/day.

DOSAGE IN LIVER IMPAIRMENT

Initially, 20 mg 2 times/day, then titrate.

DOSAGE IN RENAL IMPAIRMENT

Initially, 20 mg q8h (30 mg 2 times/day sustained-release), then titrate.

USUAL PARENTERAL DOSAGE: SUBSTITUTE FOR ORAL NICARDIPINE

IV: ADULTS, ELDERLY: 0.5 mg/hr (20 mg q8h), 1.2 mg/hr (30 mg q8h), 2.2 mg/hr (40 mg q8h).

DRUG-FREE PT

IV: ADULTS, ELDERLY: (GRADUAL B/P DECREASE): Initially, 5 mg/hr. May increase by 2.5 mg/hr q15min. (RAPID B/P DECREASE): Initially, 5 mg/hr. May increase by 2.5 mg/hr q5min. **Maximum:** 15 mg/hr until desired B/P attained.

Alert: After B/P goal achieved, decrease rate to 3 mg/hr.

CHANGING TO ORAL ANTIHYPERTENSIVE THERAPY

Begin 1 hr after IV discontinued; for nicardipine, give first dose 1 hr before discontinuing IV.

SIDE EFFECTS

FREQUENT (7%–10%): Headache, facial flushing, peripheral edema, lightheadedness, dizziness. **OCCASIONAL (3%–6%):** Asthenia (loss of strength, energy), palpitations, angina, tachycardia. **RARE (<2%):** Nausea, abdominal cramps, dyspepsia, dry mouth, rash.

ADVERSE REACTIONS/ TOXIC EFFECTS

Overdosage manifested as confusion, slurred speech, drowsiness, marked hypotension, bradycardia.

NURSING IMPLICATIONS

BASELINE ASSESSMENT

Concurrent therapy of sublingual nitroglycerin may be used for relief of anginal pain. Record onset, type (sharp, dull, squeezing), radiation, location, intensity, duration of anginal pain, precipitating factors (exertion, emotional stress).

INTERVENTION/EVALUATION

Monitor B/P during and following IV infusion. Assess for peripheral edema behind medial malleolus (sacral area in bedridden pts). Assess skin for facial flushing, dermatitis, rash. Question for asthenia, headache. Monitor liver enzyme results. Assess EKG, pulse for tachycardia, palpitations.

PATIENT/FAMILY TEACHING

Take sustained-release with food; do not crush. Avoid alcohol, limit caffeine. Inform physician if angina pains not relieved or irregular heartbeat, shortness of breath, swelling, dizziness, constipation, nausea, hypotension occurs.

nicotine

nick-oh-teen

(Commit, Habitrol Patch, Nicoderm CQ Patch✤, Nicorette DS Gum, Nicorette Plus✤, Nicorette Gum, Nicotrol NS, Nicotrol Patch)

Do not confuse with Nitroderm.

◆ CLASSIFICATION

PHARMACOTHERAPEUTIC: Cholinergic-receptor agonist. **CLINICAL:** Smoking deterrent.

ACTION

Produces autonomic effects by binding to acetylcholine receptors. Produces both stimulating and depressant effects on peripheral and central nervous systems; respiratory stimulant. **Therapeutic Effect:** Low amounts increase heart rate, B/P; high dosages may decrease B/P; may increase motor activity of GI smooth muscle. Nicotine produces psychological and physical dependence.

PHARMACOKINETICS

Absorption is slow following transdermal administration. Protein binding: 5%. Metabolized in the liver. Excreted primarily in urine. **Half-life:** 4 hrs.

USES

An alternative, less potent form of nicotine (without tar, carbon monoxide, carcinogenic substances of tobacco) used as part of a smoking cessation program.

PRECAUTIONS

CONTRAINDICATIONS: During immediate post-MI period, life-threatening arrhythmias, severe/worsening angina. **CAUTIONS:** Hyperthyroidism, pheochromocytoma, insulin-dependent diabetes mellitus, severe renal impairment, eczematous dermatitis, oral/pharyngeal inflammation, esophagitis, peptic ulcer (delays healing in peptic ulcer disease).

LIFESPAN CONSIDERATIONS: Pregnancy/lactation: Passes freely into breast milk. Use of cigarettes, nicotine gum associated with decrease in fetal breathing movements. **Pregnancy Category C** (chewing gum), **D** (transdermal nicotine). **Children:** Not recommended. **Elderly:** Age-related decrease in cardiac function may require cautious use.

INTERACTIONS

DRUG: Smoking cessation may increase effects of **beta-adrenergic blockers, bronchodilators (e.g., theophylline), insulin, propoxyphene. HERBAL:** None known. **FOOD:** None known. **LAB VALUES:** None known.

AVAILABILITY (OTC)

TRANSDERMAL: Nicoderm (OTC): 7 mg/day, 14 mg/day, 21 mg/day. **Nicotrol (Rx):** 5 mg/day, 10 mg/day; **(OTC):** 15 mg/day. **CHEWING GUM: Nicorette (OTC):** 2-mg, 4-mg squares. **NASAL SPRAY (Rx). INHALER: Nicotrol (Rx). LOZENGES: Commit:** 2 mg, 4 mg.

ADMINISTRATION/HANDLING

TRANSDERMAL

• Apply promptly upon removal from protective pouch (prevents evaporation, loss of nicotine). Use only intact pouch. Do not cut patch. • Apply only once/day

N

to hairless, clean, dry skin on upper body or outer arm. • Replace daily at different sites; do not use same site within 7 days; do not use same patch >24 hrs. • Wash hands with water alone after applying patch (soap may increase nicotine absorption). • Discard used patch by folding patch in half (sticky side together), placing in pouch of new patch, and throwing away in such a way as to prevent child/pet accessibility.

GUM

• Do not swallow. • Chew 1 piece when urge to smoke present. • Chew slowly/intermittently for 30 min. • Chew until distinctive nicotine taste (peppery) or slight tingling in mouth perceived, then stop; when tingling almost gone (about 1 min) repeat chewing procedure (this allows constant slow buccal absorption).• Too rapid chewing may cause excessive release of nicotine, resulting in adverse effects similar to oversmoking (e.g., nausea, throat irritation).

N

INHALER

• Insert cartridge into mouthpiece.
• Vigorously puff for 20 min.

INDICATIONS/ROUTES/DOSAGE

SMOKING DETERRENT

Alert: Individualize dose; stop smoking immediately.

Usual lozenge (Commit) dosage

Alert: Those who smoke first cigarette within 30 min of waking use 4 mg, otherwise use 2 mg. Do not use more than 1 lozenge at a time. **Maximum:** 5 lozenges/6 hrs, 20/day.

Week 1–6	one q1–2h
Week 7–9	one q2–4h
Week 10–12	one q4–8h

Usual transdermal dosage

≥10 cigarettes/day

Step One	21 mg/day for 4–6 wks
Step Two	14 mg/day for 2 wks
Step Three	7 mg/day for 2 wks

<10 cigarettes/day

Step One	14 mg/day for 6 wks
Step Two	7 mg/day for 2 wks

Alert: Initial starting dose for pts <100 lbs, history of cardiovascular disease: 14 mg/day for 4–6 wks, then 7 mg/day for 2–4 wks. Decrease dose in pts taking >600 mg cimetidine (Tagamet) daily.

Nicotrol: One patch daily for 6 wks.

Gum: ADULTS, ELDERLY: Usually, 10–12 pieces/day. **Maximum:** 30 pieces/day.

Nasal spray: ADULTS, ELDERLY: (1 dose = 2 sprays = 1 mg) 1–2 doses/hr up to 40 doses/day no more than 5 doses (10 sprays) per hour.

Inhaler: ADULTS, ELDERLY: Puff on nicotine cartridge mouthpiece for about 20 min as needed.

SIDE EFFECTS

FREQUENT: Hiccups, nausea. **Gum:** Mouth/throat soreness, nausea, hiccups. **Transdermal:** Erythema, pruritus, burning at application site. **OCCASIONAL:** Eructation, GI upset, dry mouth, insomnia, diaphoresis, irritability. **Gum:** Hiccups, hoarseness. **Inhaler:** Mouth/throat irritation, cough. **RARE:** Dizziness, muscle/joint pain.

ADVERSE REACTIONS/ TOXIC EFFECTS

Overdose produces palpitations, tachyarrhythmias, convulsions, depression, confusion, profuse diaphoresis, hypotension, rapid/weak pulse, difficulty breathing. Lethal dose, adults: 40–60 mg. Death results from respiratory paralysis.

NURSING IMPLICATIONS

BASELINE ASSESSMENT

Screen, evaluate those with coronary heart disease (history of MI, angina pectoris), serious cardiac arrhythmias, Buerger's disease, Prinzmetal's variant angina.

INTERVENTION/EVALUATION

Monitor smoking habit, B/P, pulse, sleep pattern, skin for erythema, pruritus, burning at application site if transdermal system used.

PATIENT/FAMILY TEACHING

Instruct pt on proper application of transdermal system. Inform patient to chew gum slowly to avoid jaw ache and maximize benefit. Inform physician if persistent rash, itching occurs with patch. Do not smoke while wearing patches.

nifedipine

nye-**fed**-ih-peen

(Adalat CC, Adalat FT ♣, Adalat PA ♣, Apo-Nifed ♣, Nifedicol XL, Novonifedin ♣, Procardia)

Do not confuse with nicardipine.

CLASSIFICATION

PHARMACOTHERAPEUTIC: Calcium channel blocker. **CLINICAL:** Antianginal, antihypertensive (see p. 67C).

ACTION

Inhibits calcium ion movement across cell membrane, depressing contraction of cardiac/vascular smooth muscle. **Therapeutic Effect:** Increases heart rate, cardiac output. Decreases systemic vascular resistance, B/P.

PHARMACOKINETICS

	Onset	Peak	Duration
SL	1–5 min	—	—
PO	20–30 min	—	4–8 hrs
ER	2 hrs	—	24 hrs

Rapidly, completely absorbed from GI tract. Protein binding: 92%–98%. Undergoes first-pass metabolism in liver. Primarily excreted in urine. Not removed by hemodialysis. **Half-life:** 2–5 hrs.

USES

Treatment of angina due to coronary artery spasm (Prinzmetal's variant angina), chronic stable angina (effort-associated angina). **Extended-Release:** Treatment of essential hypertension. **Unlabeled:** Treatment of Raynaud's phenomena.

PRECAUTIONS

CONTRAINDICATIONS: Severe hypotension, advanced aortic stenosis. **CAUTIONS:** Impaired renal/hepatic function.

LIFESPAN CONSIDERATIONS: Pregnancy/lactation: Insignificant amount distributed in breast milk. **Pregnancy Category C. Children:** Safety and efficacy not established. **Elderly:** Age-related renal impairment may require cautious use.

INTERACTIONS

DRUG: Beta-blockers may have additive effect. May increase **digoxin** concentration. **Hypokalemia-producing agents** may increase risk of arrhythmias. **HERBAL:** None known. **FOOD: Grapefruit/grapefruit juice** may increase plasma concentration. **LAB VALUES:** May cause positive ANA, direct Coombs' test.

AVAILABILITY (Rx)

CAPSULES: 10 mg, 20 mg. **TABLETS (extended-release):** 30 mg, 60 mg, 90 mg.

ADMINISTRATION/HANDLING

PO

• Do not crush/break film-coated tablet, sustained-release capsule. • Give with-

N

out regard to meals. • Grapefruit juice may alter absorption.

SUBLINGUAL

• Capsule must be punctured, chewed, and/or squeezed to express liquid into mouth.

INDICATIONS/ROUTES/DOSAGE

Alert: May give 10–20 mg sublingual as needed for acute attacks of angina.

PRINZMETAL'S VARIANT ANGINA, CHRONIC STABLE ANGINA

PO: ADULTS, ELDERLY: Initially, 10 mg 3 times/day. Increase at 7- to 14-day intervals. MAINTENANCE: 10 mg 3 times/day up to 30 mg 4 times/day.

Extended-release: ADULTS, ELDERLY: Initially, 30–60 mg/day. MAINTENANCE: Up to 120 mg/day.

HYPERTENSION

Extended-release: ADULTS, ELDERLY: Initially, 30–60 mg/day. MAINTENANCE: Up to 120 mg/day.

N

SIDE EFFECTS

FREQUENT (11%–30%): Peripheral edema, headache, flushed skin, dizziness. **OCCASIONAL (6%–12%):** Nausea, shakiness, muscle cramps/pain, drowsiness, palpitations, nasal congestion, cough, dyspnea, wheezing. **RARE (3%–5%):** Hypotension, rash, pruritus, urticaria, constipation, abdominal discomfort, flatulence, sexual dysfunction.

ADVERSE REACTIONS/ TOXIC EFFECTS

May precipitate CHF, MI in pts with cardiac disease, peripheral ischemia. Overdose produces nausea, drowsiness, confusion, slurred speech.

NURSING IMPLICATIONS

BASELINE ASSESSMENT

Concurrent therapy of sublingual nitroglycerin may be used for relief of anginal pain. Record onset, type (sharp, dull, squeezing), radiation, location, intensity, duration of anginal pain; precipitating factors (exertion, emotional stress). Check B/P for hypotension immediately prior to giving medication.

INTERVENTION/EVALUATION

Assist with ambulation if lightheadedness, dizziness occurs. Assess for peripheral edema behind medial malleolus (sacral area in bedridden pts). Assess skin for flushing. Monitor liver enzyme tests.

PATIENT/FAMILY TEACHING

Rise slowly from lying to sitting position, permit legs to dangle from bed momentarily before standing to reduce hypotensive effect. Contact physician/nurse if irregular heartbeat, shortness of breath, pronounced dizziness, nausea occurs. Avoid alcohol, concomitant grapefruit/juice use.

nilutamide

nih-**lute**-ah-myd

(Anandron, Nilandron)

CLASSIFICATION

PHARMACOTHERAPEUTIC: Hormone. **CLINICAL:** Antineoplastic (see p. 75C).

ACTION

Competitively inhibits androgen action by binding to androgen receptors in target tissue. **Therapeutic Effect:** Decreases growth of prostatic carcinoma.

USES

Treatment of metastatic prostatic carcinoma (stage D_2) in combination with surgical castration. For maximum benefit, begin on same day or day after surgical castration.

PRECAUTIONS

CONTRAINDICATIONS: Severe hepatic impairment, severe respiratory insufficiency. **CAUTIONS:** Hepatitis, marked increase in liver enzymes. **Pregnancy Category C.**

INTERACTIONS

DRUG: None known. **HERBAL:** None known. **FOOD:** None known. **LAB VALUES:** May increase SGOT (AST), SGPT (ALT), bilirubin, creatinine.

AVAILABILITY (Rx)

TABLETS: 150 mg.

INDICATIONS/ROUTES/DOSAGE

PROSTATIC CARCINOMA

PO: ADULTS, ELDERLY: 300 mg once a day for 30 days, then 150 mg once a day. Begin on same day or day after surgical castration.

SIDE EFFECTS

FREQUENT (>10%): Hot flashes, delay in recovering vision after bright illumination (sun, television, bright lights), loss of libido/sexual function, mild nausea, gynecomastia, alcohol intolerance. **OCCASIONAL (<10%):** Constipation, hypertension, dizziness, dyspnea, urinary tract infections.

ADVERSE REACTIONS/ TOXIC EFFECTS

Interstitial pneumonitis occurs rarely.

NURSING IMPLICATIONS

BASELINE ASSESSMENT

Baseline chest x-ray, hepatic enzyme levels should be obtained prior to beginning therapy.

INTERVENTION/EVALUATION

Monitor B/P periodically and hepatic function tests in long-term therapy.

PATIENT/FAMILY TEACHING

Contact physician if any side effects occur at home, esp. signs of liver toxicity (jaundice, dark urine, fatigue, abdominal pain). Caution about driving at night (tinted glasses may help).

nimodipine

nih-**moad**-ih-peen
(Nimotop)

CLASSIFICATION

PHARMACOTHERAPEUTIC: Calcium channel blocker. **CLINICAL:** Cerebral vasospasm agent (see p. 67C).

ACTION

Inhibits movement of calcium ions across cellular membranes in vascular smooth muscle. **Therapeutic Effect:** Produces favorable effect on severity of neurologic deficits due to cerebral vasospasm. Greatest effect on cerebral arteries; may prevent cerebral spasm.

PHARMACOKINETICS

Rapidly absorbed from GI tract. Protein binding: >95%. Metabolized in liver. Excreted in urine, eliminated in feces. Not removed by hemodialysis. **Half-life:** (terminal): 3 hrs.

USES

Improvement of neurologic deficits due to spasm following subarachnoid hemorrhage from ruptured congenital intracranial aneurysms in pts in good neurologic condition. **Unlabeled:** Treatment of chronic and classic migraine, chronic cluster headaches.

PRECAUTIONS

CONTRAINDICATIONS: Sinus bradycardia, heart block, ventricular tachycardia, cardiogenic shock, CHF, atrial fibrillation/flutter, within several hours of IV beta-blocker therapy. **CAUTIONS:** Impaired renal/hepatic function.

N

LIFESPAN CONSIDERATIONS: Pregnancy/lactation: Unknown if drug crosses placenta or is distributed in breast milk. **Pregnancy Category C. Children:** Safety and efficacy not established. **Elderly:** Age-related renal impairment may require cautious use. May experience greater hypotensive response, constipation.

INTERACTIONS

DRUG: Beta-blockers may increase cardiac and AV conduction depression. **Erythromycin, ketoconazole, itraconazole, protease inhibitors** may inhibit metabolism. Metabolism may be increased with **rifampin, rifabutin. HERBAL: Garlic** may increase antihypertensive effect. **Ephedra, yohimbe, ginseng** may worsen hypertension. **FOOD: Grapefruit juice** may increase concentration/toxicity. **LAB VALUES:** None known.

AVAILABILITY (Rx)

CAPSULES: 30 mg.

ADMINISTRATION/HANDLING

PO

- If pt unable to swallow, place hole in both ends of capsule with 18-gauge needle to extract contents into syringe.
- Empty into NG tube; flush tube with 30 ml normal saline.

INDICATIONS/ROUTES/DOSAGE

SUBARACHNOID HEMORRHAGE

PO: ADULTS, ELDERLY: 60 mg q4h for 21 days. Begin within 96 hrs of subarachnoid hemorrhage.

SIDE EFFECTS

OCCASIONAL (2%–6%): Hypotension, peripheral edema, diarrhea, headache. **RARE (<2%):** Allergic reaction (rash, hives), tachycardia, flushing of skin.

ADVERSE REACTIONS/ TOXIC EFFECTS

Overdosage produces nausea, weakness, dizziness, drowsiness, confusion, slurred speech.

NURSING IMPLICATIONS

BASELINE ASSESSMENT

Assess LOC, neurologic response, initially and throughout therapy. Monitor baseline liver function tests. Assess B/P, apical pulse immediately prior to drug administration (if pulse is ≤60/min or systolic B/P is <90 mm Hg, withhold medication, contact physician).

INTERVENTION/EVALUATION

Monitor CNS response, heart rate, B/P for evidence of hypotension, signs/ symptoms of CHF.

PATIENT/FAMILY TEACHING

Do not crush/chew capsules. Inform physician if irregular heartbeat, shortness of breath, swelling, constipation, nausea, dizziness occurs.

nisoldipine

(Sular)

See Classification section under: Calcium channel blockers

nitazoxanide

nye-tay-**zocks**-ah-nide
(Alinia)

CLASSIFICATION

PHARMACOTHERAPEUTIC: Antiparasitic. **CLINICAL:** Antiprotozoal.

ACTION

Interferes with body's reaction to pyruvate ferredoxin oxidoreductase, an enzyme, essential for anaerobic energy metabolism. **Therapeutic Effect:** Produces antiprotozoal activity, reducing or terminating diarrheal episodes.

PHARMACOKINETICS

Rapidly hydrolyzed to an active metabolite. Protein binding: 99%. Excreted in the urine, bile, feces. **Half-life:** 2–4 hrs.

USES

Treatment of diarrhea caused by *Cryptosporidium parvum* and *Giardia lamblia* in children 12 mos–11 yrs of age.

PRECAUTIONS

CONTRAINDICATIONS: History of sensitivity to aspirin/salicylates. **CAUTIONS:** GI disorders, hepatic/biliary disease, renal impairment.

LIFESPAN CONSIDERATIONS: Pregnancy/lactation: Unknown if distributed in breast milk. **Pregnancy Category B. Children:** Safety and efficacy in children >11 yrs has not been established. **Elderly:** Not for this age group.

INTERACTIONS

DRUG: None known. **HERBAL:** None known. **FOOD:** None known. **LAB VALUES:** May increase creatinine, ALT (SGPT).

AVAILABILITY (Rx)

POWDER FOR ORAL SUSPENSION: 100 mg/5ml.

ADMINISTRATION/HANDLING

PO

• Store unreconstituted powder at room temperature. • Reconstitute oral suspension with 48 ml water to provide a concentration of 100 mg/5 ml. • Shake vigorously to suspend powder. • Reconstituted solution is stable for 7 days at room temperature. • Give with food.

INDICATIONS/ROUTES/DOSAGE

DIARRHEA

PO: CHILDREN 5–11 YRS: 200 mg (10 ml) q12h for 3 days. CHILDREN 1–4 YRS: 100 mg (5 ml) q12h for 3 days.

SIDE EFFECTS

OCCASIONAL (8%): Abdominal pain. **RARE (1%–2%):** Diarrhea, vomiting, headache.

ADVERSE REACTIONS/TOXIC EFFECTS

None known.

NURSING IMPLICATIONS

BASELINE ASSESSMENT

Establish baseline B/P, weight, blood glucose, electrolytes. Assess for dehydration.

INTERVENTION/EVALUATION

Evaluate blood glucose levels in diabetics, electrolytes (therapy generally reduces abnormalities). Weigh pt daily. Encourage adequate fluid intake. Assess bowel sounds for peristalsis. Monitor stool frequency/consistency (watery, loose, soft, semisolid, solid).

PATIENT/FAMILY TEACHING

Older children with diabetes should be aware that the oral suspension contains 1.48 g of sucrose per 5 ml. Therapy should provide significant improvement of symptoms.

nitrofurantoin sodium

ny-tro-feur-**an**-twon
(Apo-Nitrofurantoin✤, Furadantin, Macrobid, Macrodantin, Novo-Furan✤)

◆ **CLASSIFICATION**

PHARMACOTHERAPEUTIC: Antibacterial. **CLINICAL:** Urinary tract infection prophylaxis.

ACTION

Inhibits bacterial enzyme systems that may alter ribosomal proteins. **Therapeutic Effect:** Inhibits protein, DNA, RNA, cell wall synthesis. Bacteriostatic (bactericidal at high concentration).

PHARMACOKINETICS

Microcrystalline: rapidly, completely absorbed; macrocrystalline: more slowly absorbed. Food increases absorption. Protein binding: 40%. Primarily concentrated in urine, kidneys. Metabolized in most body tissues. Primarily excreted in urine. Removed by hemodialysis. **Half-life:** 20–60 min.

USES

Treatment of urinary tract infections (UTIs), initial and chronic. **Unlabeled:** Prophylaxis of bacterial UTIs.

PRECAUTIONS

CONTRAINDICATIONS: Infants <1 mo because of hemolytic anemia, anuria, oliguria, substantial renal impairment (creatinine clearance <40 ml/min). **CAUTIONS:** Renal impairment, diabetes mellitus, electrolyte imbalance, anemia, vitamin B deficiency, debilitated (greater risk of peripheral neuropathy), G6PD deficiency (greater risk of hemolytic anemia).

LIFESPAN CONSIDERATIONS: Pregnancy/lactation: Readily crosses placenta. Distributed in breast milk. Contraindicated at term and during lactation when infant suspected of having G6PD deficiency. **Pregnancy Category B. Children:** No age-related precautions noted in those >1 mo. **Elderly:** More likely to develop acute pneumonitis and peripheral neuropathy. Age-related renal impairment may require dosage adjustment.

INTERACTIONS

DRUG: Hemolytics may increase risk of toxicity. **Neurotoxic medications** may increase risk of neurotoxicity. **Probenecid** may increase concentration, toxicity. **HERBAL:** None known. **FOOD:** None known. **LAB VALUES:** None known.

AVAILABILITY (Rx)

CAPSULES: (Macrodantin): 25 mg, 50 mg, 100 mg. **(Macrobid):** 100 mg. **PO SUSPENSION: (Furadantin):** 25 mg/5 ml.

ADMINISTRATION/HANDLING

PO

- Give with food, milk to enhance absorption, reduce GI upset.

INDICATIONS/ROUTES/DOSAGE

INITIAL OR RECURRENT UTI

PO: ADULTS, ELDERLY: 50–100 mg 4 times/day. **Maximum:** 400 mg/day. CHILDREN >1 MO: 5–7 mg/kg in 4 divided doses. **Maximum:** 400 mg/day.

LONG-TERM PROPHYLACTIC THERAPY OF UTI

PO: ADULTS, ELDERLY: 50–100 mg as single evening dose. CHILDREN: 1–2 mg/kg in 1–2 divided doses.

SIDE EFFECTS

FREQUENT: Anorexia, nausea, vomiting, dark yellow/brown urine. **OCCASIONAL:** Abdominal pain, diarrhea, rash, pruritus, urticaria, hypertension, headache, dizziness, drowsiness. **RARE:** Photosensitivity, transient alopecia, asthmatic attack in those with history of asthma.

ADVERSE REACTIONS/ TOXIC EFFECTS

Superinfection, hepatotoxicity, peripheral neuropathy (may be irreversible), Stevens-Johnson syndrome, permanent pulmonary function impairment, anaphylaxis occur rarely.

NURSING IMPLICATIONS

BASELINE ASSESSMENT

Question for history of asthma. Evaluate lab test results for renal/hepatic baseline values.

INTERVENTION/EVALUATION

Monitor I&O, renal function results. Determine pattern of bowel activity. Assess skin for rash, urticaria. Be alert for numbness/tingling, esp. of lower extremities (may signal onset of peripheral neuropathy). Watch for signs of hepatotoxicity: fever, rash, arthralgia, hepatomegaly. Perform respiratory assessment: Auscultate lungs, check for cough, chest pain, difficulty breathing.

PATIENT/FAMILY TEACHING

Urine may become dark yellow/brown. Take with food, milk for best results and to reduce GI upset. Complete full course of therapy. Avoid sun/ultraviolet light; use sunscreens, wear protective clothing. Notify physician if cough, fever, chest pain, difficult breathing, numbness/tingling of fingers/toes occurs. Rare occurrence of alopecia is transient.

nitroglycerin

nigh-trow-**glih**-sir-in

(Minitran, Nitrek, Nitro-Bid, Nitro-Dur, Nitrogard, Nitroject♣, Nitrolingual, Nitrong-SR♣, NitroQuick, Nitrostat, Nitro-Tab, Trinipatch♣)

Do not confuse with Hyperstat, Nicobid, Nicoderm, Nilstat, nitroprusside, Nizoral, Nystatin.

◆ CLASSIFICATION

PHARMACOTHERAPEUTIC: Nitrate. **CLINICAL:** Antianginal, antihypertensive, coronary vasodilator (see p. 108C).

ACTION

Decreases myocardial O_2 demand. Reduces left ventricular preload and afterload. **Therapeutic Effect:** Dilates coronary arteries, improves collateral blood flow to ischemic areas within myocardium. **IV:** Produces peripheral vasodilation.

PHARMACOKINETICS

Onset	Peak	Duration
Sublingual		
2–5 min	4–8 min	30–60 min
Transmucosal tablet		
2–5 min	4–10 min	3–5 hrs
Extended-release		
20–45 min	—	3–8 hrs
Topical		
15–60 min	0.5–2 hrs	3–8 hrs
Patch		
30–60 min	1–3 hrs	8–12 hrs
IV		
1–2 min	—	3–5 min

Well absorbed after PO, sublingual, topical administration. Undergoes extensive first-pass metabolism. Metabolized in liver, enzymes in bloodstream. Primarily excreted in urine. Not removed by hemodialysis. **Half-life:** 1–4 min.

USES

Lingual/sublingual/buccal dose used for acute relief of angina pectoris. Extended-release, topical forms used for prophylaxis, long-term angina management. IV form used in treatment of CHF associated with acute MI.

PRECAUTIONS

CONTRAINDICATIONS: Hypersensitivity to nitrates, severe anemia, closed-angle glaucoma, postural hypotension, head trauma, increased intracranial pressure. **Sublingual:** Early MI. **Transdermal:** Allergy to adhesives. **Extended-release:** GI hypermotility/malabsorption, severe anemia. **IV:** Uncorrected hypovolemia, hypotension, inadequate cerebral circulation, constrictive pericarditis, pericardial tamponade. **CAUTIONS:** Acute MI, hepatic/renal disease, glaucoma (contraindicated in closed-angle glaucoma), blood volume depletion from diuretic therapy, systolic B/P <90 mm Hg.

N

LIFESPAN CONSIDERATIONS: Pregnancy/lactation: Unknown if drug crosses placenta or is distributed in breast milk. **Pregnancy Category B. Children:** Safety and efficacy not established. **Elderly:** More susceptible to hypotensive effects. Age-related renal impairment may require cautious use.

INTERACTIONS

DRUG: **Alcohol, antihypertensives, vasodilators** may increase risk of orthostatic hypotension. **HERBAL:** None known. **FOOD:** None known. **LAB VALUES:** May increase methemoglobin, urine catecholamines, urine VMA.

AVAILABILITY (Rx)

TABLETS (sublingual): 0.3 mg, 0.4 mg, 0.6 mg. **SPRAY:** 0.4 mg/dose. **TABLETS (buccal, controlled-release):** 3 mg. **CAPSULES (sustained-release):** 2.5 mg, 6.5 mg, 9 mg. **TRANSDERMAL:** 0.1 mg/hr, 0.2 mg/hr, 0.3 mg/hr, 0.4 mg/hr, 0.6 mg/hr. **TOPICAL OINTMENT:** 2%. **INJECTION:** 5 mg/ml. **INJECTION SOLUTION:** 100 mcg/ml, 200 mcg/ml.

ADMINISTRATION/HANDLING

PO

• Do not chew extended-release form. • Do not shake oral aerosol canister before lingual spraying.

SUBLINGUAL

• Do not swallow; dissolve under the tongue. • Administer while seated. • Slight burning sensation under tongue may be lessened by placing tablet in buccal pouch. • Keep sublingual tablets in original container.

TOPICAL

• Spread thin layer on clean/dry/hairless skin of upper arm or body (not below knee or elbow), using applicator or dose-measuring papers. Do not use fingers; do not rub/massage into skin.

TRANSDERMAL

• Apply patch on clean/dry/hairless skin of upper arm or body (not below knee or elbow).

IV

Storage • Store at room temperature.

Reconstitution • Available in ready-to-use injectable containers. • Dilute vials in 250 or 500 ml D_5W or 0.9% NaCl. Maximum concentration: 250 mg/250 ml.

Rate of administration • Use microdrop or infusion pump.

IV INCOMPATIBILITY

Alteplase (Activase).

IV COMPATIBILITIES

Amiodarone (Cordarone), diltiazem (Cardizem), dobutamine (Dobutrex), dopamine (Intopin), epinephrine, famotidine (Pepcid), fentanyl (Sublimaze), furosemide (Lasix), heparin, hydromorphone (Dilaudid), insulin, labetalol (Trandate), lidocaine, lorazepam (Ativan), midazolam (Versed), milrinone (Primacor), morphine, nicardipine (Cardene), nitroprusside (Nipride), norepinephrine (Levophed), propofol (Diprivan).

INDICATIONS/ROUTES/DOSAGE

ACUTE ANGINA, ACUTE PROPHYLAXIS

Lingual spray: ADULTS, ELDERLY: 1 spray onto or under tongue q3–5min until relief is noted (no more than 3 sprays in 15-min period).

Sublingual: ADULTS, ELDERLY: 0.4 mg q5min until relief is noted (no more than 3 doses in 15-min period). Use prophylactically 5–10 min before activities that may cause an acute attack.

LONG-TERM PROPHYLAXIS OF ANGINA

PO (extended-release): ADULTS, ELDERLY: 2.5–9 mg q8–12h.

Topical: ADULTS, ELDERLY: Initially, ½ inch q8h. Increase by ½ inch with each application. RANGE: 1–2 inches q8h up to 4–5 inches q4h.

Transdermal patch: ADULTS, ELDERLY: Initially, 0.2–0.4 mg/hr. MAINTENANCE: 0.4–0.8 mg/hr. Consider patch on 12–14 hrs, patch off 10–12 hrs (prevents tolerance).

USUAL PARENTERAL DOSAGE

IV: ADULTS, ELDERLY: Initially, 5 mcg/min via infusion pump. Increase in 5 mcg/min increments at 3- to 5-min intervals until B/P response is noted or until dosage reaches 20 mcg/min; then increase as needed by 10 mcg/min. Dosage may be further titrated according to pt, therapeutic response up to 200 mcg/min. CHILDREN: Initially, 0.25–0.5 mcg/kg/min; titrate by 0.5–1 mcg/kg/min up to 20 mcg/kg/min.

SIDE EFFECTS

FREQUENT: Headache (may be severe) occurs mostly in early therapy, diminishes rapidly in intensity, usually disappears during continued treatment; transient flushing of face/neck; dizziness (esp. if pt is standing immobile or is in a warm environment); weakness; postural hypotension. **Sublingual:** Burning, tingling sensation at oral point of dissolution. **Ointment:** Erythema, pruritus. **OCCASIONAL:** GI upset. **Transdermal:** Contact dermatitis.

ADVERSE REACTIONS/ TOXIC EFFECTS

Drug should be discontinued if blurred vision, dry mouth occurs. Severe postural hypotension manifested by fainting, pulselessness, cold/clammy skin, profuse sweating. Tolerance may occur with repeated, prolonged therapy (minor tolerance with intermittent use of sublingual tablets). High dose tends to produce severe headache.

NURSING IMPLICATIONS

BASELINE ASSESSMENT

Record onset, type (sharp, dull, squeezing), radiation, location, intensity, duration of anginal pain; and precipitating factors (exertion, emotional stress). Assess B/P, apical pulse prior to administration and periodically following dose. Pt must have continuous EKG monitoring for IV administration.

INTERVENTION/EVALUATION

Monitor B/P, heart rate. Assess for facial/neck flushing. Cardioverter/defibrillator must not be discharged through paddle electrode overlying nitroglycerin system (may cause burns to pt or damage to paddle via arcing).

PATIENT/FAMILY TEACHING

Rise slowly from lying to sitting position, dangle legs momentarily before standing. Take oral form on empty stomach (however, if headache occurs during therapy, take medication with meals). Use inhalants only when lying down. Dissolve sublingual tablet under tongue; do not swallow. Take at first sign of angina. If not relieved within 5 min, dissolve second tablet under tongue. Repeat if no relief in another 5 min. If pain continues, contact physician or immediately go to emergency room. Do not change brands. Keep container away from heat, moisture. Do not inhale lingual aerosol but spray onto or under tongue (avoid swallowing after spray is administered). Expel from mouth any remaining lingual/sublingual/intrabuccal tablet after pain is completely relieved. Place transmucosal tablets under upper lip or buccal pouch (between cheek and gum); do not chew/swallow tablet. Avoid alcohol (intensifies hypotensive effect). If alcohol is ingested soon after taking nitroglycerin, possible acute hypotensive episode (marked drop in B/P, vertigo, pallor) may occur.

nitroprusside sodium

nigh-troe-**pruss**-eyd
(Nipride, Nitropress)
Do not confuse with nitroglycerin.

CLASSIFICATION

PHARMACOTHERAPEUTIC: Hypertensive emergency agent. **CLINICAL:** Antihypertensive, vasodilator, CHF/MI adjunct, antidote.

ACTION

Direct vasodilating action on arterial, venous smooth muscle. Decreases peripheral vascular resistance, preload, afterload; improves cardiac output. **Therapeutic Effect:** Dilates coronary arteries, decreases O_2 consumption, relieves persistent chest pain.

PHARMACOKINETICS

Onset	Peak	Duration
IV		
1–10 min	Dependent on infusion rate	Dissipates rapidly after stopping IV

Reacts with Hgb in erythrocytes, producing cyanmethemoglobin, cyanide ions. Primarily excreted in urine. **Half-life:** <10 min.

USES

Immediate reduction of B/P in hypertensive crisis. Produces controlled hypotension in surgical procedures to reduce bleeding. Treatment of acute CHF. **Unlabeled:** Controls paroxysmal hypertension prior to/during surgery for pheochromocytoma; treatment adjunct for MI, valvular regurgitation, peripheral vasospasm caused by ergot alkaloid overdose.

PRECAUTIONS

CONTRAINDICATIONS: Compensatory hypertension (AV shunt or coarctation of aorta), inadequate cerebral circulation, moribund pts. **CAUTIONS:** Severe hepatic/renal impairment, hypothyroidism, hyponatremia, elderly.

LIFESPAN CONSIDERATIONS: Pregnancy/lactation: Unknown if drug crosses placenta or is distributed in breast milk. **Pregnancy Category C. Children:** Safety and efficacy not established. **Elderly:** More sensitive to hypotensive effect. Age-related renal impairment may require cautious use.

INTERACTIONS

DRUG: **Dobutamine** may increase cardiac output, decrease pulmonary wedge pressure. **Hypotensive-producing medications** may increase hypotensive effect. **HERBAL:** None known. **FOOD:** None known. **LAB VALUES:** None known.

AVAILABILITY (Rx)

POWDER FOR INJECTION: 50 mg. **INJECTION:** 25 mg/ml.

ADMINISTRATION/HANDLING

IV

Storage • Protect solution from light. • Solution should appear very faint brown. • Use only freshly prepared solution. Once prepared, do not keep or use longer than 24 hrs. • Deterioration evidenced by color change from brown to blue, green, dark red. • Discard unused portion.

Reconstitution • Reconstitute 50-mg vial with 2–3 ml D_5W or Sterile Water for Injection without preservative. • Further dilute with 250–1,000 ml D_5W to provide concentration of 200 mcg, 50 mcg/ml, respectively. Maximum concentration: 200 mg/250 ml. • Wrap infusion bottle in aluminum foil immediately after mixing.

Rate of administration • Give by IV infusion only using infusion rate chart provided by manufacturer or protocol. • Administer using IV infusion pump or microdrip (60 gtt/ml). • Be alert for extravasation (produces severe pain, sloughing).

IV INCOMPATIBILITY

Cisatracurium (Nimbex).

IV COMPATIBILITIES

Diltiazem (Cardizem), dobutamine (Dobutrex), dopamine (Intropin), enalapril (Vasotec), heparin, insulin, labetalol (Normodyne, Trandate), lidocaine, midazolam (Versed), milrinone (Primacor), nitroglycerin, propofol (Diprivan).

INDICATIONS/ROUTES/DOSAGE

USUAL PARENTERAL DOSAGE

IV: ADULTS, ELDERLY, CHILDREN: Initially, 0.3 mcg/kg/min. RANGE: 0.5–10 mcg/kg/min. Do not exceed 10 mcg/kg/min (risk of precipitous drop in B/P).

SIDE EFFECTS

OCCASIONAL: Flushing of skin, increased intracranial pressure, rash, pain/redness at injection site.

ADVERSE REACTIONS/TOXIC EFFECTS

A too rapid IV rate reduces B/P too quickly. Nausea, retching, diaphoresis (sweating), apprehension, headache, restlessness, muscle twitching, dizziness, palpitations, retrosternal pain, abdominal pain may occur. Symptoms disappear rapidly if rate of administration is slowed or temporarily discontinued. Overdosage produces metabolic acidosis, tolerance to therapeutic effect.

NURSING IMPLICATIONS

N

BASELINE ASSESSMENT

Pt must have continuous monitoring of EKG, B/P. Check with physician for desired B/P level (B/P is normally maintained about 30%–40% below pretreatment levels). Medication should be discontinued if therapeutic response is not achieved within 10 min after IV infusion at 10 mcg/kg/min.

INTERVENTION/EVALUATION

Monitor rate of infusion frequently. Monitor blood acid-base balance, electrolytes, laboratory results, I&O. Assess for metabolic acidosis (weakness, disorientation, headache, nausea, hyperventilation, vomiting). Assess for therapeutic response to medication. Monitor B/P for potential rebound hypertension after infusion is discontinued.

nizatidine

nye-**zah**-tih-deen
(Axid, Axid AR)

◆CLASSIFICATION

PHARMACOTHERAPEUTIC: H_2 receptor antagonist. **CLINICAL:** Antiulcer, gastric acid secretion inhibitor (see p. 92C).

ACTION

Inhibits histamine action at H_2 receptors of parietal cells. **Therapeutic Effect:** Inhibits basal/nocturnal gastric acid secretion.

PHARMACOKINETICS

Rapidly, well absorbed from GI tract. Protein binding: 35%. Metabolized in liver. Primarily excreted in urine. Not removed by hemodialysis. **Half-life:** 1–2 hrs (half-life increased with renal function).

N

USES

Short-term treatment of active duodenal ulcer, active benign gastric ulcer. Prevention of duodenal ulcer recurrence. Treatment of gastroesophageal reflux disease (GERD), including erosive esophagitis. **Unlabeled:** Treatment of gastric hypersecretory conditions, Zollinger-Ellison syndrome, multiple endocrine adenoma; to decrease weight gain in pts taking Zyprexa.

PRECAUTIONS

CONTRAINDICATIONS: None known. **CAUTIONS:** Impaired renal/hepatic function.

LIFESPAN CONSIDERATIONS: Pregnancy/lactation: Unknown if drug crosses placenta or is distributed in breast milk. **Pregnancy Category B. Children:** Safety and efficacy not established in those <16 yrs. **Elderly:** No age-related precautions noted.

INTERACTIONS

DRUG: Antacids may decrease absorption (do not give within 1 hr). May decrease absorption of **ketoconazole** (give at least 2 hrs after). **HERBAL:** None known. **FOOD:** None known. **LAB VALUES:** Interferes with skin tests using allergen extracts. May increase SGOT (AST), SGPT (ALT), alkaline phosphatase.

AVAILABILITY (Rx)

CAPSULES: 75 mg (OTC), 150 mg, 300 mg.

ADMINISTRATION/HANDLING

PO

• Give without regard to meals. Best given after meals or at bedtime. • Do not administer within 1 hr of magnesium- or aluminum-containing antacids (decreases absorption). • May give right before eating for heartburn prevention.

INDICATIONS/ROUTES/DOSAGE

ACTIVE DUODENAL ULCER

PO: ADULTS, ELDERLY: 300 mg at bedtime or 150 mg 2 times/day.

MAINTENANCE OF HEALED ULCER

PO: ADULTS, ELDERLY: 150 mg at bedtime.

GERD

PO: ADULTS, ELDERLY: 150 mg 2 times/day.

ACTIVE BENIGN GASTRIC ULCER

PO: ADULTS, ELDERLY: 150 mg 2 times/day or 300 mg at bedtime.

USUAL OTC DOSAGE

PO: ADULTS, ELDERLY: 75 mg 30–60 min before meals; no more than 2 tablets/day.

DOSAGE IN RENAL IMPAIRMENT

Creatinine Clearance	Active Ulcer	Maintenance Therapy
20–50 ml/min	150 mg at bedtime	150 mg every other day
<20 ml/min	150 mg every other day	150 mg q3days

SIDE EFFECTS

OCCASIONAL (2%): Somnolence, fatigue. **RARE (<1%):** Sweating, rash.

ADVERSE REACTIONS/ TOXIC EFFECTS

Asymptomatic ventricular tachycardia, hyperuricemia (not associated with gout), nephrolithiasis occur rarely.

NURSING IMPLICATIONS

INTERVENTION/EVALUATION

Assess for abdominal pain, GI bleeding (overt blood in emesis/stool, tarry stools). Monitor blood tests for elevated SGOT (AST), SGPT (ALT), alkaline phosphatase (hepatocellular injury).

PATIENT/FAMILY TEACHING

Avoid tasks that require alertness, motor skills until drug response is established. Avoid alcohol, aspirin, smoking. Inform physician if symptoms of heartburn, acid indigestion, sour stomach persist after 2 wks of continuous use of nizatidine.

Nolvadex

see tamoxifen

norepinephrine bitartrate

nor-eh-pih-**nef**-rin
(Levophed)

◆CLASSIFICATION

PHARMACOTHERAPEUTIC: Sympathomimetic. **CLINICAL:** Vasopressor (see p. 134C).

ACTION

Stimulates $beta_1$-adrenergic receptors, alpha-adrenergic receptors, increasing peripheral resistance. **Therapeutic Effect:** Enhances contractile myocardial force, increases cardiac output. Constricts resistance and capacitance vessels. Increases systemic B/P, coronary blood flow.

PHARMACOKINETICS

Onset	Peak	Duration
IV		
Rapid	1–2 min	—

Localized in sympathetic tissue. Metabolized in liver. Primarily excreted in urine.

USES

Corrects hypotension unresponsive to adequate fluid volume replacement, as part of shock syndrome, caused by MI, bacteremia, open heart surgery, renal failure.

PRECAUTIONS

CONTRAINDICATIONS: Hypovolemic states (unless an emergency measure), mesenteric/peripheral vascular thrombosis, profound hypoxia. **CAUTIONS:** Severe cardiac disease, hypertensive/hypothyroid pts, those on MAOIs.

LIFESPAN CONSIDERATIONS: Pregnancy/lactation: Readily crosses placenta. May produce fetal anoxia due to uterine contraction, constriction of uter-

N

ine blood vessels. **Pregnancy Category C. Children/elderly:** No age-related precautions noted.

INTERACTIONS

DRUG: **Tricyclic antidepressants, maprotiline** may increase cardiovascular effects. May decrease effect of **methyldopa.** May have mutually inhibitory effects with **beta-blockers.** May increase risk of arrhythmias with **digoxin. Ergonovine, oxytocin** may increase vasoconstriction. **HERBAL:** None known. **FOOD:** None known. **LAB VALUES:** None known.

AVAILABILITY (Rx)

INJECTION: 1 mg/ml ampoules.

ADMINISTRATION/HANDLING

Alert: Blood, fluid volume depletion should be corrected before drug is administered.

IV

Storage • Do not use if brown or contains precipitate. • Store ampoules at room temperature.

Reconstitution • Add 4 ml (4 mg) to 250 ml (16 mcg/ml). Maximum concentration: 32 ml (32 mg) to 250 ml (128 mcg/ml).

Rate of administration • Avoid catheter tie-in technique (encourages stasis, increases local drug concentration). • Closely monitor IV infusion flow rate (use microdrip or infusion pump). • Monitor B/P q2min during IV infusion until desired therapeutic response is achieved, then q5min during remaining IV infusion. • Never leave pt unattended. • Maintain B/P at 80–100 mm Hg in previously normotensive pts, and 30–40 mm Hg below preexisting B/P in previously hypertensive pts. • Reduce IV infusion gradually. Avoid abrupt withdrawal. • If using peripherally inserted catheter, it is imperative to check the IV site frequently for free flow and infused vein for blanching, hardness to vein, coldness, pallor to extremity. • If extravasation occurs, area should be infiltrated with 10–15 ml sterile saline containing 5–10 mg phentolamine (does not alter pressor effects of norepinephrine).

∅ IV INCOMPATIBILITY

Insulin (Regular).

IV COMPATIBILITIES

Amiodarone (Cordarone), calcium gluconate, diltiazem (Cardizem), dobutamine (Dobutrex), dopamine (Intropin), epinephrine, esmolol (Brevibloc), fentanyl (Sublimaze), furosemide (Lasix), haloperidol (Haldol), heparin, hydromorphone (Dilaudid), labetalol (Trandate), lorazepam (Ativan), magnesium, midazolam (Versed), milrinone (Primacor), morphine, nicardipine (Cardene), nitroglycerin, potassium chloride, propofol (Diprivan).

INDICATIONS/ROUTES/DOSAGE

ACUTE HYPOTENSION

IV: ADULTS, ELDERLY: Initially, administer at 0.5–1 mcg/min. Adjust rate of flow to establish, maintain desired B/P (40 mm Hg below preexisting systolic pressure). AVERAGE MAINTENANCE DOSE: 8–12 mcg/min. CHILDREN: Initially, 0.05–0.1 mcg/kg/min, titrate to desired effect **Maximum:** 1–2 mcg/kg/min. RANGE: 0.5–30 mcg/min.

SIDE EFFECTS

Norepinephrine produces less pronounced, less frequent side effects than epinephrine. **OCCASIONAL (3%–5%):** Anxiety; bradycardia; awareness of slow, forceful heartbeat. **RARE (1%–2%):** Nausea, anginal pain, shortness of breath, fever.

ADVERSE REACTIONS/ TOXIC EFFECTS

Extravasation may produce tissue necrosis, sloughing. Overdosage manifested as severe hypertension with violent headache (may be first clinical sign of overdosage), arrhythmias, photophobia, retrosternal/pharyngeal pain, pallor, diaphoresis, vomiting. Prolonged therapy may result in plasma volume depletion. Hypotension may recur if plasma volume is not maintained.

NURSING IMPLICATIONS

BASELINE ASSESSMENT

Assess EKG, B/P continuously (be alert to precipitous B/P drop). Never leave pt alone during IV infusion. Be alert to pt complaint of headache.

INTERVENTION/EVALUATION

Monitor IV flow rate diligently. Assess for extravasation characterized by blanching of skin over vein, coolness (results from local vasoconstriction); color and temperature of IV site extremity (pallor, cyanosis, mottling). Assess nailbed capillary refill. Monitor I&O; measure output hourly, and report <30 ml IV should not be reinstated unless systolic B/P falls below 70–80 mm Hg.

norfloxacin

nor-**flocks**-ah-sin
(Noroxin, Noroxin Ophthalmic ✤)

CLASSIFICATION

PHARMACOTHERAPEUTIC: Quinolone. **CLINICAL:** Anti-infective (see p. 23C).

ACTION

Inhibits DNA replication, repair by interfering with DNA-gyrase in susceptible microorganisms. **Therapeutic Effect:** Produces bactericidal activity.

USES

Treatment of complicated and uncomplicated urinary tract infections, uncomplicated gonococcal infections, acute/chronic prostatitis. **Ophthalmic:** Conjunctival keratitis, keratoconjunctivitis, corneal ulcers, blepharitis, blepharoconjunctivitis, acute meibomianitis, dacryocystitis.

PRECAUTIONS

CONTRAINDICATIONS: Hypersensitivity to norfloxacin, quinolones, any component of preparation. Do not use in children <18 yrs (may produce arthropathy). **Ophthalmic:** Epithelial herpes simplex, keratitis, vaccinia, varicella, mycobacterial infection, fungal disease of ocular structure. Do not use after uncomplicated removal of foreign body. **CAUTIONS:** Impaired renal function; any predisposition to seizures. **Pregnancy Category C.**

N

INTERACTIONS

DRUG: **Antacids, sucralfate** may decrease absorption. Decrease clearance, may increase concentration, toxicity of **theophylline.** May increase effects of **oral anticoagulants.** **HERBAL:** None known. **FOOD:** None known. **LAB VALUES:** May increase SGOT (AST), SGPT (ALT), alkaline phosphatase, LDH, bilirubin, BUN, creatinine.

AVAILABILITY (Rx)

TABLETS: 400 mg. **OPHTHALMIC SOLUTION 0.3%:** 3 mg/ml.

ADMINISTRATION/HANDLING

PO

• Give 1 hr before or 2 hrs after meals, with 8 oz of water. • Encourage additional glasses of water between meals. • Do not administer antacids with or within 2 hrs of norfloxacin dose. • Encourage cranberry juice, citrus fruits (to acidify urine).

OPHTHALMIC

• Place finger on lower eyelid, pull out until a pocket is formed between eye and lower lid. • Hold dropper above pocket, place correct number of drops into pocket. Close eye gently. • Apply digital pressure to lacrimal sac for 1–2 min (minimizes drainage into nose/throat, reducing risk of systemic effects).

INDICATIONS/ROUTES/DOSAGE

COMPLICATED OR UNCOMPLICATED URINARY TRACT INFECTIONS

PO: ADULTS, ELDERLY: 400 mg 2 times/day for 7–21 days.

PROSTATITIS

PO: ADULTS: 400 mg 2 times/day for 28 days.

UNCOMPLICATED GONOCOCCAL INFECTIONS

PO: ADULTS: 800 mg as single dose.

DOSAGE IN RENAL IMPAIRMENT

Dose and/or frequency is modified based on degree of renal impairment.

Creatinine Clearance	Dosage
≥30 ml/min	400 mg twice daily
<30 ml/min	400 mg once daily

USUAL OPHTHALMIC DOSAGE

Ophthalmic: ADULTS, ELDERLY: 1–2 drops 4 times/day up to 7 days. For severe infections, may give 1–2 drops q2h while awake the first day.

SIDE EFFECTS

FREQUENT: Nausea, headache, dizziness. **Ophthalmic:** Bad taste in mouth. **OCCASIONAL:** **Ophthalmic:** Temporary blurring of vision, irritation, burning, stinging, itching. **RARE:** Vomiting, diarrhea, dry mouth, bitter taste, nervousness, drowsiness, insomnia, photosensitivity, tinnitus, crystalluria, rash, fever, seizures. **Ophthalmic:** Conjunctival hyperemia, photophobia, decreased vision, pain.

ADVERSE REACTIONS/ TOXIC EFFECTS

Superinfection, anaphylaxis, Stevens-Johnson syndrome, arthropathy (joint disease) occurs rarely.

NURSING IMPLICATIONS

BASELINE ASSESSMENT

Question for history of hypersensitivity to norfloxacin, quinolones.

INTERVENTION/EVALUATION

Assess for nausea, headache, dizziness. Evaluate food tolerance. Assess for chest, joint pain. **Ophthalmic:** Check for therapeutic response.

PATIENT/FAMILY TEACHING

Take 1 hr before or 2 hrs after meals. Complete full course of therapy. Take with 8 oz of water; drink several glasses of water between meals. May cause dizziness, drowsiness. Do not take antacids with or within 2 hrs of norfloxacin dose (reduces/destroys effectiveness).

Normodyne

see labetalol

nortriptyline hydrochloride

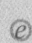

nor-**trip**-teh-leen

(Aventyl, Norventyl, Pamelor)

Do not confuse with Ambenyl, amitriptyline, Bentyl.

◆ CLASSIFICATION

PHARMACOTHERAPEUTIC: Tricyclic compound. **CLINICAL:** Antidepressant (see p.35C).

ACTION

Blocks reuptake of neurotransmitters (norepinephrine, serotonic) at neuronal presynaptic membranes, increasing availability at postsynaptic receptor sites. **Therapeutic Effect:** Resulting enhancements of synaptic activity produces antidepressant effect.

USES

Treatment of various forms of depression, often in conjunction with psychotherapy. **Unlabeled:** Treatment of panic disorder, neurogenic pain; prophylaxis of migraine headache.

PRECAUTIONS

CONTRAINDICATIONS: Acute recovery period following MI, within 14 days of MAOI ingestion. **CAUTIONS:** Prostatic hypertrophy, history of urinary retention/obstruction, glaucoma, diabetes mellitus, history of seizures, hyperthyroidism, cardiac/hepatic/renal disease, schizophrenia, increased intraocular pressure, hiatal hernia. **Pregnancy Category D.**

INTERACTIONS

DRUG: **Alcohol, CNS depressants** may increase CNS, respiratory depression; hypotensive effects. **Antithyroid agents** may increase risk of agranulocytosis. **Phenothiazines** may increase sedative, anticholinergic effects. **Cimetidine** may increase concentration, toxicity. May decrease effects of **clonidine, guanadrel.** May increase cardiac effects with **sympathomimetics.** May increase risk of hypertensive crisis, hyperpyretic convulsions with **MAOIs.** **HERBAL:** None known. **FOOD:** None known. **LAB VALUES:** May alter EKG readings, glucose. Therapeutic blood serum level: Peak: 6–10 mcg/ml; trough: 0.5–2 mcg/ml. Toxic blood serum level: Peak: >12 mcg/ml; trough: >2 mcg/ml.

AVAILABILITY (Rx)

CAPSULES: 10 mg, 25 mg, 50 mg, 75 mg. **ORAL SOLUTION:** 10 mg/5 ml.

ADMINISTRATION/HANDLING

PO

- Give with food or milk if GI distress occurs.

INDICATIONS/ROUTES/DOSAGE

PO: ADULTS: 75–100 mg/day in 1–4 divided doses until therapeutic response achieved. Reduce dosage gradually to effective maintenance level. ELDERLY: Initially, 10–25 mg at bedtime. May increase by 25 mg q3–7days. **Maximum:** 150 mg/day. CHILDREN >12 YRS: 30–50 mg/day in 3–4 divided doses. CHILDREN 6–12 YRS: 10–20 mg/day in 3–4 divided doses.

ENURESIS

PO: CHILDREN >11 YRS: 25–35 mg/day. CHILDREN 8–11 YRS: 10–20 mg/day; CHILDREN 6–7 YRS: 10 mg/day.

SIDE EFFECTS

FREQUENT: Drowsiness, fatigue, dry mouth, blurred vision, constipation, delayed micturition, postural hypotension, diaphoresis, disturbed concentration, increased appetite, urinary retention. **OCCASIONAL:** GI disturbances (nausea, GI distress, metallic taste sensation), photosensitivity. **RARE:** Paradoxical reaction (agitation, restlessness, nightmares, insomnia), extrapyramidal symptoms (particularly fine hand tremor).

ADVERSE REACTIONS/ TOXIC EFFECTS

High dosage may produce cardiovascular effects (severe postural hypotension, dizziness, tachycardia, palpitations,

N

arrhythmias), seizures. May also result in altered temperature regulation (hyperpyrexia, hypothermia). Abrupt withdrawal from prolonged therapy may produce headache, malaise, nausea, vomiting, vivid dreams.

NURSING IMPLICATIONS

BASELINE ASSESSMENT

For pts on long-term therapy, liver/renal function tests, blood counts should be performed periodically.

INTERVENTION/EVALUATION

Supervise suicidal-risk pt closely during early therapy (as depression lessens, energy level improves, increasing suicide potential). Assess appearance, behavior, speech pattern, level of interest, mood. Monitor stool consistency; avoid constipation with increased fluids, bulky foods. Monitor B/P, pulse for hypotension, arrhythmias. Assess for urinary retention, including output estimate and bladder palpation if indicated. Therapeutic blood serum level: Peak: 6–10 mcg/ml; trough: 0.5–2 mcg/ml. Toxic blood serum level: Peak: >12 mcg/ml; trough: >2 mcg/ml.

PATIENT/FAMILY TEACHING

Change positions slowly to avoid hypotensive effect. Tolerance to postural hypotension, sedative, anticholinergic effects usually develops during early therapy. Therapeutic effect may be noted in ≥2 wks. Photosensitivity to sun may occur. Use sunscreens, protective clothing. Dry mouth may be relieved by sugarless gum, sips of tepid water. Report visual disturbances. Do not abruptly discontinue medication. Avoid tasks that require alertness, motor skills until response to drug is established.

Norvasc

see amlodipine

Norvantrone

see mitoxantrone

nystatin

nigh-**stat**-in
(Mycostatin, Nilstat, Nyaderm ✦, Nystop)

Do not confuse with Nitrostat.

FIXED-COMBINATION(S)

Mycolog, Myco-Triacet: nystatin/triamcinolone (a steroid): 100,000 units/0.1%.

◆CLASSIFICATION

CLINICAL: Antifungal (see p. 43C).

ACTION

Binds to sterols in cell membrane, increasing permeability, permitting loss of potassium, other cell components. **Therapeutic Effect:** Fungistatic.

PHARMACOKINETICS

PO: Poorly absorbed from GI tract. Eliminated unchanged in feces. **Topical:** Not absorbed systemically from intact skin.

USES

Treatment of intestinal and oral candidiasis, cutaneous/mucocutaneous mycotic infections caused by *Candida albicans* (oral thrush, paronychia, vulvovaginal candidiasis, diaper rash, perlèche). Un-

labeled: Prophylaxis/treatment of oropharyngeal candidiasis, tinea barbae, capitis.

PRECAUTIONS

CONTRAINDICATIONS: None known. **CAUTIONS:** None known.

LIFESPAN CONSIDERATIONS: Pregnancy/lactation: Unknown if distributed in breast milk. Vaginal applicators may be contraindicated, requiring manual insertion of tablets during pregnancy. **Pregnancy Category C. Children:** No age-related precautions noted for suspension or topical use. Lozenges not recommended in those <5 yrs. **Elderly:** No age-related precautions noted.

INTERACTIONS

DRUG: None known. **HERBAL:** None known. **FOOD:** None known. **LAB VALUES:** None known.

AVAILABILITY (Rx)

TABLETS: 500,000 units. **ORAL SUSPENSION:** 100,000 units/ml. **TROCHES:** 200,000 units. **VAGINAL TABLETS:** 100,000 units. **CREAM. OINTMENT. POWDER.**

ADMINISTRATION/HANDLING

PO

• Dissolve lozenges (troches) slowly/completely in mouth (optimal therapeutic effect). Do not chew/swallow lozenges whole. • Shake suspension well before administration. • Place and hold suspension in mouth or swish throughout mouth as long as possible before swallowing.

INDICATIONS/ROUTES/DOSAGE

INTESTINAL CANDIDIASIS

PO: ADULTS, ELDERLY: 500,000–1,000,000 units 3 times/day. CHILDREN: 500,000 units 4 times/day.

ORAL CANDIDIASIS

PO: ADULTS, ELDERLY, CHILDREN: Oral suspension: 400,000–600,000 units 4 times/day. INFANTS: 100,000–200,000 units 4 times/day.

PO: ADULTS, ELDERLY, CHILDREN: Troches: 200,000–400,000 units 4–5 times/day up to 14 days.

VULVOVAGINAL CANDIDIASIS

Intravaginal: ADULTS, ELDERLY: 1 tablet high in vagina 1–2 times/day for 14 days.

TOPICAL FUNGAL INFECTIONS

Topical: ADULTS, ELDERLY: Apply 2–4 times/day.

SIDE EFFECTS

OCCASIONAL: PO: None known. **Topical:** Skin irritation. **Vaginal:** Vaginal irritation.

ADVERSE REACTIONS/TOXIC EFFECTS

High dosage with oral form may produce nausea, vomiting, diarrhea, GI distress.

NURSING IMPLICATIONS

BASELINE ASSESSMENT

Confirm that cultures or histologic tests were done for accurate diagnosis.

INTERVENTION/EVALUATION

Assess for increased irritation with topical, increased vaginal discharge with vaginal application.

PATIENT/FAMILY TEACHING

Do not miss dose; complete full length of treatment (continue vaginal use during menses). Notify physician if nausea, vomiting, diarrhea, stomach pain develops. **Vaginal:** Insert high in vagina. Check with physician regarding douching, sexual intercourse. **Topical:** Rub well into affected areas. Must not contact eyes. Use cream (sparingly)/powder on erythematous areas. Keep areas clean, dry; wear light clothing for ventilation. Separate personal items in contact with affected areas.

octreotide acetate

ock-**tree**-oh-tide
(Sandostatin, Sandostatin LAR)
Do not confuse with OctreoScan, Sandimmune, Sandoglobulin.

CLASSIFICATION

CLINICAL: Secretory inhibitory, growth hormone suppressant.

ACTION

Suppresses secretion of serotonin, gastroenteropancreatic peptides. Enhances fluid/electrolyte absorption from GI tract. **Therapeutic Effect:** Prolongs intestinal transit time.

PHARMACOKINETICS

	Onset	Peak	Duration
Subcutaneous	—	—	Up to 12 hrs

Rapidly, completely absorbed from injection site. Excreted in urine. Removed by hemodialysis. **Half-life:** 1.5 hrs.

USES

Controls symptoms in pts with metastatic carcinoid tumors, vasoactive intestinal peptic-secreting tumors (VIPomas), secretory diarrhea, acromegaly. **Unlabeled:** AIDS-associated secretory diarrhea, control of bleeding of esophageal varices, insulinomas, small bowel fistulas, chemotherapy-induced diarrhea.

PRECAUTIONS

CONTRAINDICATIONS: None known. **CAUTIONS:** Insulin-dependent diabetes, renal failure.

LIFESPAN CONSIDERATIONS: Pregnancy/lactation: Unknown if excreted in breast milk. **Pregnancy Category B. Children:** Dosage not established in children. **Elderly:** No age-related precautions noted.

INTERACTIONS

DRUG: May alter glucose concentrations with **insulin, oral hypoglycemics, glucagon, growth hormone. HERBAL:** None known. **FOOD:** None known. **LAB VALUES:** May decrease T_4 concentration.

AVAILABILITY (Rx)

INJECTION: 0.05 mg/ml, 0.1 mg/ml, 0.2 mg/ml, 0.5 mg/ml, 1 mg/ml. **SUSPENSION FOR INJECTION:** 10-mg, 20-mg, 30-mg vials.

ADMINISTRATION/HANDLING

Alert: Sandostatin may be given IV, IM, subcutaneous. Sandostatin LAR may be given only IM.

SUBCUTANEOUS

• Do not use if particulates or discoloration is noted. • Avoid multiple injections at the same site within short periods.

IM

• Give immediately after mixing. • Administer intragluteally at 4-wk intervals. • Avoid deltoid injections.

INDICATIONS/ROUTES/DOSAGE

DIARRHEA (Sandostatin)

Subcutaneous: ADULTS, ELDERLY: 50 mcg 1–2 times/day.

IV: ADULTS, ELDERLY: Initially, 50–100 mcg q8h. May increase by 100 mcg/dose q48h. **Maximum:** 500 mcg q8h.

Subcutaneous/IV: CHILDREN: 1–10 mcg/kg q12h.

CARCINOID TUMORS (Sandostatin)

Subcutaneous/IV: ADULTS, ELDERLY: 100–600 mcg/day in 2–4 divided doses.

VIPOMAS (Sandostatin)

Subcutaneous/IV: ADULTS, ELDERLY: 200–300 mcg/day in 2–4 divided doses.

ESOPHAGEAL VARICES (Sandostatin)
IV: ADULTS, ELDERLY: Bolus of 25–50 mcg followed by IV infusion of 25–50 mcg/hr.

ACROMEGALY (Sandostatin)
Subcutaneous/IV: ADULTS, ELDERLY: 50 mcg 3 times/day. Increase as needed. **Maximum:** 500 mcg 3 times/day.

ACROMEGALY (Sandostatin LAR)
IM: ADULTS, ELDERLY: 20 mg q4wks for 3 mos. **Maximum:** 40 mg q4wks.

VIPOMAS, CARCINOID TUMORS (Sandostatin LAR)
IM: ADULTS, ELDERLY: 20 mg q4wks.

SIDE EFFECTS

FREQUENT (6%–10%; 30–58% in acromegalics): Diarrhea, nausea, abdominal discomfort, headache, pain at injection site. **OCCASIONAL (1%–5%):** Vomiting, flatulence, constipation, alopecia, flushing, itching, dizziness, fatigue, arrhythmias, bruising, blurred vision. **RARE (<1%):** Depression, decreased libido, vertigo, palpitations, shortness of breath.

ADVERSE REACTIONS/ TOXIC EFFECTS

Increased risk of cholelithiasis. Potential for hypothyroidism with prolonged high therapy. Hepatitis, GI bleeding, seizures occur rarely.

NURSING IMPLICATIONS

BASELINE ASSESSMENT

Establish baseline B/P, weight, blood glucose, electrolytes.

INTERVENTION/EVALUATION

Monitor blood glucose, thyroid function tests, fluid/electrolyte balance, fecal fat. In acromegaly, monitor growth hormone levels. Weigh every 2–3 days, report >5 lbs gain/wk. Monitor B/P, pulse, respirations periodically during treatment. Be alert for decreased urinary output, swelling of ankles, fingers. Monitor stools for frequency, consistency.

PATIENT/FAMILY TEACHING

Therapy should provide significant improvement of symptoms.

ocular lubricant

ock-you-lar **lube**-rih-cant
(Hypotears, Lacrilube, Tears Naturale)

CLASSIFICATION

PHARMACOTHERAPEUTIC: Topical ophthalmic. **CLINICAL:** Lubricant, toner, buffer, viscosity agent.

ACTION

Forms an occlusive film on eye surface. **Therapeutic Effect:** Lubricates/protects eye from drying.

USES

Protection/lubrication of the eye in exposure keratitis, decreased corneal sensitivity, recurrent corneal erosions, keratitis sicca (particularly for nighttime use), after removal of a foreign body, during and following surgery.

PRECAUTIONS

CONTRAINDICATIONS: None known. **CAUTIONS:** None known.

LIFESPAN CONSIDERATIONS: Pregnancy/lactation: Pregnancy Category unknown. **Children/elderly:** No age-related precautions noted.

INTERACTIONS

DRUG: None known. **HERBAL:** None known. **FOOD:** None known. **LAB VALUES:** None known.

O

AVAILABILITY (OTC)

OPHTHALMIC OINTMENT. SOLUTION.

ADMINISTRATION/HANDLING

OPHTHALMIC

• Do not use with contact lenses. • **Ointment:** Hold tube in hand for a few minutes to warm ointment. • Avoid touching tip of tube or dropper to any surface. • Gently pull lower lid down to form pouch between eye and lower lid (conjunctival sac). • Place ordered amount of ointment into pouch with a sweeping motion. Instruct pt to close the eye for 1–2 min and roll the eyeball around in all directions. • Inform pt of temporary blurred vision. If possible, apply just before bedtime. • **Drops:** Instruct pt to lie down or tilt head backward and look up. • Gently pull lower lid down to form pouch between eye and lower lid (conjunctival sac). • Hold dropper above pouch. Instill drop(s); have pt close eye gently for 1–2 min (placing drops directly onto eye may cause a sudden squeezing of eyelid, with subsequent loss of solution). • Apply gentle pressure with fingers to bridge of nose (inside corner of eye) for 1–2 min (promotes absorption, minimizes drainage into nose/throat)

INDICATIONS/ROUTES/DOSAGE

USUAL OPHTHALMIC DOSAGE

Ophthalmic: ADULTS, ELDERLY: Small amount in conjunctival cul-de-sac as needed.

SIDE EFFECTS

FREQUENT: Temporary blurring after administration, esp. with ointment.

ADVERSE REACTIONS/ TOXIC EFFECTS

None known.

NURSING IMPLICATIONS

PATIENT/FAMILY TEACHING

Teach proper application. Do not use with contact lenses. Temporary blurring will occur, esp. with administration of ointment. Avoid activities requiring visual acuity until blurring clears. If eye pain, change of vision, worsening of condition occurs, or if condition is unchanged after 72 hrs, notify physician. Do not touch to any surface (may contaminate).

ofloxacin

oh-**flocks**-ah-sin

(Apo-Oflox ✦, Floxin, Floxin Otic, Ocuflox)

Do not confuse with Flexeril, Flexon, Ocufen.

CLASSIFICATION

PHARMACOTHERAPEUTIC: Fluoroquinolone. **CLINICAL:** Anti-infective (see p. 23C).

ACTION

Inhibits DNA-gyrase in susceptible microorganisms. **Therapeutic Effect:** Interferes with bacterial DNA replication/ repair. Bactericidal.

PHARMACOKINETICS

Rapidly, well absorbed from GI tract. Protein binding: 20%–25%. Widely distributed (penetrates CSF). Metabolized in liver. Primarily excreted in urine. Removed by hemodialysis. **Half-life:** 4.7–7 hrs (half-life increased with impaired renal function, elderly, cirrhosis).

USES

Treatment of infections of urinary tract, lower respiratory tract, skin/skin structure; sexually transmitted diseases; prostatitis due to *Escherichia coli;* pelvic inflammatory disease (PID). **Ophthalmic:** Bacterial conjunctivitis, corneal ulcers. **Otic:** Otitis externa, acute/chronic otitis media.

PRECAUTIONS

CONTRAINDICATIONS: Hypersensitivity to any quinolones. Children <18 yrs. **CAUTIONS:** Renal impairment, CNS disorders, seizures, those taking theophylline or caffeine. May mask/delay symptoms of syphilis; serologic test for syphilis should be done at diagnosis and 3 mos after treatment.

LIFESPAN CONSIDERATIONS: Pregnancy/lactation: Distributed in breast milk; potentially serious adverse reactions in nursing infants. Risk of arthropathy to fetus. **Pregnancy Category C. Children:** Safety and efficacy not established (otic not established in those <1 yr). **Elderly:** No age-related precautions for otic. Age-related renal impairment may require dosage adjustment for oral/parenteral administration.

INTERACTIONS

DRUG: Antacids, sucralfate may decrease absorption, effect of ofloxacin. May increase **theophylline** concentrations, toxicity. **HERBAL:** None known. **FOOD:** None known. **LAB VALUES:** None known.

AVAILABILITY (Rx)

TABLETS: 200 mg, 300 mg, 400 mg. **PREMIX INJECTION:** 400 mg/100 D_5W. **OPHTHALMIC SOLUTION:** 0.3%. **OTIC SOLUTION:** 0.3%.

ADMINISTRATION/HANDLING

PO

• Do not give with food; preferred dosing time: 1 hr prior to or 2 hrs following meals. • Do not administer antacids (aluminum, magnesium) or iron/zinc-containing products within 2 hrs of ofloxacin. • Encourage cranberry juice, citrus fruits (to acidify urine). • Give with 8 oz of water, encourage fluid intake.

OPHTHALMIC

• Tilt pt's head back; place solution in conjunctival sac. • Have pt close eyes; press gently on lacrimal sac for 1 min. • Do not use ophthalmic solutions for injection. • Unless infection very superficial, systemic administration generally accompanies ophthalmic.

OTIC

• Instruct pt to lie down with head turned so affected ear is upright. • Instill toward canal wall, not directly on eardrum. • Pull the auricle down and posterior in children; up and posterior in adults.

IV

Storage • Store at room temperature. • After dilution, IV is stable for 72 hrs at room temperature; 14 days if refrigerated. • Discard unused portions. • Also available in premix ready-to-hang solutions.

Reconstitution • Must dilute each 200 mg with 50 ml D_5W or 0.9% NaCl (400 mg with 100 ml) to provide concentration of 4 mg/ml.

Rate of administration • Give only by IV infusion over at least 60 min; avoid rapid or bolus IV administration. • Do not add or infuse other medication through same IV line at same time.

IV INCOMPATIBILITIES

Amphotericin B complex (Abelcet, AmBisome, Amphotec), cefepime (Maxipime), doxorubicin liposome (Doxil).

IV COMPATIBILITY

Propofol (Diprivan).

INDICATIONS/ROUTES/DOSAGE

UTI

PO/IV infusion: ADULTS: 200 mg q12h.

LOWER RESPIRATORY TRACT, SKIN/SKIN STRUCTURE INFECTIONS
PO/IV infusion: ADULTS: 400 mg q12h for 10 days.

PROSTATITIS, SEXUALLY TRANSMITTED DISEASES (cervicitis, urethritis)
PO: ADULTS: 300 mg q12h.

PELVIC INFLAMMATORY DISEASE
PO: ADULTS: 400 mg q12h for 10–14 days.

PROSTATITIS
IV infusion: ADULTS: 300 mg q12h.

SEXUALLY TRANSMITTED DISEASES
IV infusion: ADULTS: 400 mg as single dose.

ACUTE, UNCOMPLICATED GONORRHEA
PO: ADULTS: 400 mg 1 time.

USUAL ELDERLY DOSAGE
PO: 200–400 mg q12–24h for 7 days up to 6 wks.

DOSAGE IN RENAL IMPAIRMENT
After a normal initial dose, dosage/interval based on creatinine clearance.

Creatinine Clearance	Adjusted Dosage	Dose Interval
>50 ml/min	None	12 hrs
10–50 ml/min	None	24 hrs
<10 ml/min	½	24 hrs

BACTERIAL CONJUNCTIVITIS
Ophthalmic: ADULTS, ELDERLY: 1–2 drops q2–4h for 2 days, then 4 times/day for 5 days.

CORNEAL ULCERS
Ophthalmic: ADULTS: 1–2 drops q30min while awake for 2 days, then q60min while awake for 5–7 days, then 4 times/day.

USUAL OTIC DOSAGE
ADULTS, ELDERLY, CHILDREN: Twice daily. Eardrops should be at body temperature (wrap hand around bottle).

SIDE EFFECTS

FREQUENT (7%–10%): Nausea, headache, insomnia. **OCCASIONAL (3%–5%):** Abdominal pain, diarrhea, vomiting, dry mouth, flatulence, dizziness, fatigue, drowsiness, rash, pruritus, fever. **RARE (<1%):** Constipation, numbness of hands/feet.

ADVERSE REACTIONS/ TOXIC EFFECTS

Superinfection, severe hypersensitivity reaction occur rarely. Arthropathy (joint disease with swelling, pain, clubbing of fingers/toes, degeneration of stress-bearing portion of a joint) may occur if given to children.

NURSING IMPLICATIONS

BASELINE ASSESSMENT

Question for history of hypersensitivity to ofloxacin, any quinolones.

INTERVENTION/EVALUATION

Monitor signs/symptoms of infection, WBC, mental status. Assess skin, discontinue medication at first sign of rash/other allergic reaction. Determine pattern of bowel activity, stool consistency. Assess during the night for insomnia. Check for dizziness, headache, visual difficulties, tremors; provide ambulation assistance as needed. Be alert for superinfection (genital pruritus, vaginitis, fever, sores, discomfort in mouth).

PATIENT/FAMILY TEACHING

Do not take antacids within 6 hrs before or 2 hrs after taking oflaxocan. Best taken 1 hr before or 2 hrs after meals. May cause insomnia, headache, drowsiness, dizziness. Avoid tasks requiring alertness, motor skills until response to drug is established.

olanzapine

oh-**lan**-sah-peen
(Zyprexa, Zyprexa Zydis)
Do not confuse with olsalazine, Zyrtec.

CLASSIFICATION

PHARMACOTHERAPEUTIC: Dibenzapin derivative. **CLINICAL:** Antipsychotic (see p. 56C).

ACTION

Antagonizes dopamine, serotonin, muscarinic, histamine, $alpha_1$-adrenergic receptors. Produces anticholinergic, histaminic, CNS depressant effects. **Therapeutic Effect:** Diminishes psychotic disorders.

PHARMACOKINETICS

Well absorbed following PO administration. Protein binding: 93%. Extensively distributed throughout body. Extensively metabolized by first-pass liver metabolism. Excreted in urine, with lesser amount eliminated in feces. Not removed by dialysis. **Half-life:** 21–54 hrs.

USES

Management of manifestations of psychotic disorders. Treatment of acute mania associated with bipolar disorder. **Unlabeled:** Anorexia, maintenance of treatment response in schizophrenic pts.

PRECAUTIONS

CONTRAINDICATIONS: None known. **CAUTIONS:** Hypersensitivity to clozapine, pts who should avoid anticholinergics (e.g., pts with benign prostatic hypertrophy), hepatic function impairment, elderly, concurrent potentially hepatotoxic drugs, dose escalation, known cardiovascular disease (history of MI, ischemia, heart failure, conduction abnormalities), cerebrovascular disease, conditions predisposing pts to hypotension (dehydration, hypovolemia, hypertensive medications), history of seizures, conditions lowering seizure threshold (e.g., Alzheimer's dementia), those at risk of aspiration pneumonia.

LIFESPAN CONSIDERATIONS: Pregnancy/lactation: Unknown if drug crosses placenta or is distributed in breast milk. **Pregnancy Category C. Children:** Safety and efficacy not established. **Elderly:** No age-related precautions noted.

INTERACTIONS

DRUG: Alcohol, CNS depressants may increase CNS depressant effects. **Antihypertensive agents** increase risk of hypotensive effect. May inhibit metabolism of **theophylline, imipramine. Fluvoxamine; ciprofloxacin (quinolone)** may increase olanzapine blood levels. Antagonizes effects of **levodopa, dopamine agonists. Carbamazepine** increases olanzapine clearance. **HERBAL:** None known. **FOOD:** None known. **LAB VALUES:** May significantly increase SGOT (AST), SGPT (ALT), GGT levels, prolactin levels.

AVAILABILITY (Rx)

TABLETS: 2.5 mg, 5 mg, 7.5 mg, 10 mg, 15 mg, 20 mg. **ORAL DISINTEGRATING TABLETS:** 5 mg, 10 mg, 15 mg, 20 mg.

ADMINISTRATION/HANDLING

PO

- Give without regard to meals.

INDICATIONS/ROUTES/DOSAGE

SCHIZOPHRENIA

PO: ADULTS: Initially, 5–10 mg once daily. May increase by 10 mg/day at 5- to 7-day intervals, then by 5–10 mg/day at 7-day intervals. RANGE: 10–30 mg/day. ELDERLY: Initially, 2.5 mg/day. May in-

O

crease as indicated. RANGE: 2.5–10 mg/day.

BIPOLAR MANIA

PO: ADULTS: Initially, 10–15 mg/day. May increase by 5 mg/day in intervals not less than 24 hrs. **Maximum:** 20 mg/day.

DEBILITATED, PREDISPOSITION TO HYPOTENSIVE REACTIONS, ELDERLY >65 YRS

PO: ADULTS, ELDERLY: Initially, 5 mg/day.

SIDE EFFECTS

FREQUENT: Somnolence (26%), agitation (23%), insomnia (20%), headache (17%), nervousness (16%), hostility (15%), dizziness (11%), rhinitis (10%). **OCCASIONAL:** Anxiety, constipation (9%); nonaggressive objectionable behavior (8%); dry mouth (7%); weight gain (6%); postural hypotension, fever, joint pain, restlessness, cough, pharyngitis, dimness of vision (5%). **RARE:** Tachycardia, back/chest/abdominal pain, tremor, extremity pain.

O

ADVERSE REACTIONS/ TOXIC EFFECTS

Seizures occur rarely. Neuroleptic malignant syndrome (NMS), a potentially fatal syndrome, occurs rarely and may present as hyperpyrexia, muscle rigidity, irregular pulse or B/P, tachycardia, diaphoresis, cardiac arrhythmias. Extrapyramidal symptoms may occur. Dysphagia (esophageal dysmotility, aspiration) may be noted. Overdosage (300 mg) produces drowsiness, slurred speech.

NURSING IMPLICATIONS

BASELINE ASSESSMENT

Obtain baseline hepatic function lab values prior to initiating treatment. Assess behavior, appearance, emotional status, response to environment, speech pattern, thought content.

INTERVENTION/EVALUATION

Monitor B/P. Assess for tremors; changes in gait; abnormal movements in trunk, neck, extremities; target behaviors. Supervise suicidal-risk pt closely during early therapy (as depression lessens, energy level improves, increasing suicide potential). Assess for therapeutic response (interest in surroundings, improvement in self-care, increased ability to concentrate, relaxed facial expression). Assist with ambulation if dizziness occurs. Assess sleep pattern. Notify physician if extrapyramidal symptoms occur.

PATIENT/FAMILY TEACHING

Avoid dehydration, particularly during exercise, exposure to extreme heat, concurrent use of medication causing dry mouth, other drying effects. Notify physician if pregnancy occurs or if there is intention to become pregnant during olanzapine therapy. Take medication as ordered; do not stop taking or increase dosage. Sugarless gum, sips of tepid water may relieve dry mouth. Drowsiness generally subsides during continued therapy. Avoid driving, performing tasks that require alertness, motor skills until response to drug is established. Watch diet/exercise to prevent weight gain.

olmesartan medoxomil

ol-**mess**-er-tan
(Benicar)

CLASSIFICATION

PHARMACOTHERAPEUTIC: Angiotensin II receptor antagonist. **CLINICAL:** Antihypertensive (see p. 7C).

ACTION

Potent vasodilator. An angiotensin II receptor (type AT_1) antagonist; blocks vasoconstrictor and aldosterone-secreting effects of angiotensin II, inhibiting the binding of angiotensin II to the AT_1 receptors. **Therapeutic Effect:** Produces vasodilation; decreases peripheral resistance, B/P.

PHARMACOKINETICS

Rapidly and completely absorbed after PO administration. Metabolized in the liver. Recovered primarily in feces and, to a lesser extent, in urine. Not removed by hemodialysis. **Half-life:** 13 hrs.

USES

Treatment of hypertension alone or in combination with other antihypertensives (diuretics, calcium channel blockers).

PRECAUTIONS

CONTRAINDICATIONS: Bilateral renal arterial stenosis. **CAUTIONS:** Renal/hepatic function impairment, renal arterial stenosis.

LIFESPAN CONSIDERATIONS: Pregnancy/lactation: Unknown if distributed in breast milk. May cause fetal/neonatal morbidity/mortality. **Pregnancy Category C** (**D** if used in second or third trimester). **Children:** Safety and efficacy not established. **Elderly:** No age-related precautions noted.

INTERACTIONS

DRUG: Diuretics produce further reduction in B/P. **HERBAL:** None known. **FOOD:** None known. **LAB VALUES:** May increase Hgb, Hct.

ADMINISTRATION/HANDLING

PO

- Give without regard to meals.

AVAILABILITY (Rx)

TABLETS: 5 mg, 20 mg, 40 mg.

INDICATIONS/ROUTES/DOSAGE

HYPERTENSION

PO: ADULTS, ELDERLY, MILDLY IMPAIRED RENAL/HEPATIC FUNCTION: 20 mg once daily in pts who are not volume depleted. After 2 wks of therapy, if further reduction in B/P is needed, may increase dosage to 40 mg/day.

SIDE EFFECTS

OCCASIONAL (3%): Dizziness. **RARE (<2%):** Headache, diarrhea, upper respiratory tract infection.

ADVERSE REACTIONS/ TOXIC EFFECTS

Overdosage may manifest as hypotension, tachycardia; bradycardia occurs less often. Institute supportive measures.

NURSING IMPLICATIONS

BASELINE ASSESSMENT

Obtain B/P, apical pulse immediately prior to each dose, in addition to regular monitoring (be alert to fluctuations). If excessive reduction in B/P occurs, place pt in supine position, feet slightly elevated. Question for possibility of pregnancy (see Pregnancy Category). Assess medication history (esp. diuretics).

INTERVENTION/EVALUATION

Maintain hydration (offer fluids frequently). Assess for evidence of upper respiratory infection. Assist with ambulation if dizziness occurs. Monitor all blood serum levels. Assess B/P for hypertension/hypotension.

PATIENT/FAMILY TEACHING

Inform female pts regarding consequences of second- and third-trimester exposure to olmesartan. Avoid tasks that require alertness, motor skills (possible dizziness effect). Report any signs of infection (sore throat, fever).

Need for lifelong control. Caution against exercise during hot weather (risk of dehydration, hypotension).

olsalazine sodium

ol-**sal**-ah-zeen
(Dipentum)

◆ CLASSIFICATION

PHARMACOTHERAPEUTIC: Salicylic acid derivative. **CLINICAL:** Anti-inflammatory.

ACTION

Converted in colon by bacterial action to mesalamine. Blocks prostaglandin production in bowel mucosa. **Therapeutic Effect:** Reduces colonic inflammation.

USES

Maintenance of remission of ulcerative colitis in pts intolerant of sulfasalazine medication. **Unlabeled:** Treatment of inflammatory bowel disease.

PRECAUTIONS

CONTRAINDICATIONS: History of hypersensitivity to salicylates. **CAUTIONS:** Preexisting renal disease. **Pregnancy Category C.**

INTERACTIONS

DRUG: None known. **HERBAL:** None known. **FOOD:** None known. **LAB VALUES:** May increase SGOT (AST), SGPT (ALT).

AVAILABILITY (Rx)

CAPSULES: 250 mg.

ADMINISTRATION/HANDLING

PO

- Give with food in evenly divided doses.

INDICATIONS/ROUTES/DOSAGE

MAINTENANCE OF CONTROLLED ULCERATIVE COLITIS

PO: ADULTS, ELDERLY: 1 g/day in 2 divided doses (preferably q12h).

SIDE EFFECTS

FREQUENT (5%–10%): Headache, diarrhea, abdominal pain/cramps, nausea. **OCCASIONAL (1%–5%):** Depression, fatigue, dyspepsia, upper respiratory infection, decreased appetite, rash, itching, arthralgia. **RARE (<1%):** Dizziness, vomiting, stomatitis.

ADVERSE REACTIONS/ TOXIC EFFECTS

Sulfite sensitivity in susceptible pts noted as cramping, headache, diarrhea, fever, rash, hives, itching, wheezing. Discontinue drug immediately. Excessive diarrhea associated with extreme fatigue noted rarely.

NURSING IMPLICATIONS

INTERVENTION/EVALUATION

Encourage adequate fluid intake. Assess bowel sounds for peristalsis. Monitor daily bowel activity/stool consistency (watery, loose, soft, semisolid, solid), record time of evacuation. Assess for abdominal disturbances. Assess skin for rash, hives. Medication should be discontinued if rash, fever, cramping, diarrhea occurs.

PATIENT/FAMILY TEACHING

Notify physician if diarrhea, cramping continues/increases, rash, fever, or pruritus occurs.

omalizumab

oh-mah-**liz**-uw-mab
(Xolair)

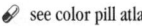

◆ CLASSIFICATION

PHARMACOTHERAPEUTIC: Monoclonal antibody. **CLINICAL:** Antiasthma.

ACTION

Selectively binds to human immunoglobulin E (IgE). Inhibits binding of IgE on the surface of mast cells, basophils. **Therapeutic Effect:** Reduction of surface-bound IgE limits the degree of release of mediators of the allergic response, reducing/preventing asthmatic attacks.

PHARMACOKINETICS

Following subcutaneous administration, absorbed slowly, with peak concentration in 7–8 days. Excreted in the liver, reticuloendothelial system and endothelial cells. **Half-life:** 26 days.

USES

Treatment of moderate to severe persistent asthma in pts reactive to a perennial allergen and inadequately controlled asthma symptoms with inhaled corticosteroids. **Unlabeled:** Treatment of seasonal allergic rhinitis.

PRECAUTIONS

CONTRAINDICATIONS: None known. **CAUTIONS:** Not for use in reversing acute bronchospasm, status asthmaticus.

LIFESPAN CONSIDERATIONS: Pregnancy/lactation: Because IgE is present in breast milk, is it expected omalizumab is present in breast milk. Use only if clearly needed. **Pregnancy Category B. Children:** Safety and efficacy not established in children <12 yrs. **Elderly:** No age-related precautions noted.

INTERACTIONS

DRUG: None known. **HERBAL:** None known. **FOOD:** None known. **LAB VALUES:** Total IgE levels did not return to pretreatment levels for up to 1 yr following omalizumab discontinuation.

AVAILABILITY (Rx)

POWDER FOR INJECTION: 202.5 mg (150 mg/1.2 ml following reconstitution).

ADMINISTRATION/HANDLING

Storage • Use only clear or slightly opalescent solution; solution is slightly viscous. • Refrigerate. • Reconstituted solution is stable for 8 hrs if refrigerated or within 4 hrs of reconstitution when stored at room temperature.

Reconstitution • Use only Sterile Water for Injection to prepare for subcutaneous administration. • Medication takes 15–20 min to dissolve. • Draw 1.4 ml Sterile Water for Injection into a 3-ml syringe with a 1-inch, 18-gauge needle; inject contents into powdered vial. • Swirl vial for approx. 1 min (do not shake) and again swirl vial for 5–10 sec every 5 min until no gel-like particles appear in the solution. • Do not use if contents do not dissolve completely by 40 min. • Invert the vial for 15 sec (allows solution to drain toward the stopper). Using a new 3-ml syringe with a 1-inch 18-gauge needle, obtain the required 1.2-ml dose, replace 18-gauge needle with a 25-gauge needle for subcutaneous administration.

Rate of administration • Subcutaneous administration may take 5–10 sec to administer due to its viscosity.

INDICATIONS/DOSAGE/ROUTES

Alert: Retesting of IgE levels during treatment cannot be used as a guide for dose determination (IgE levels remain elevated for up to 1 yr after discontinuation of treatment). Base dosage on IgE levels obtained at initiation of treatment.

ASTHMA

Subcutaneous: ADULTS, ELDERLY, CHILDREN >12 YRS: 150–375 mg every 2–4 wks, dosing/frequency depend on IgE level, body weight.

Subcutaneous dosage given every 4 wks:

Pretreatment IgE Serum Levels (units/ml)	Body Weight (kg) 30–60	61–70
>30–100	150	150
>100–200	300	300
>200–300	300	See every 2 wks table

Pretreatment IgE Serum Levels (units/ml)	Body Weight (kg) 71–90	91–150
>30–100	150	300
>100–200	300	See every 2 wks table
>200–300	See next table	See every 2 wks table

Subcutaneous dosage given every 2 wks:

Pretreatment IgE Serum Levels (units/ml)	Body Weight (kg) 30–60	61–70
>100–200	See every 4 wks table	See every 4 wks table
>200–300	See every 4 wks table	225
>300–400	225	225
>400–500	300	300
>500–600	300	375
>600–700	375	Do not dose

Pretreatment IgE Serum Levels (units/ml)	Body Weight (kg) 71–90	91–150
>100–200	See every 4 wks table	225
>200–300	225	300
>300–400	300	Do not dose
>400–500	375	Do not dose
>500–600	Do not dose	Do not dose
>600–700	Do not dose	Do not dose

SIDE EFFECTS

FREQUENT (11%–45%): Injection site reaction (bruising, redness, warmth, stinging, hive formation, stinging), viral infections, sinusitis, headache, pharyngitis. **OCCASIONAL (3%–8%):** Arthralgia, leg pain, fatigue, dizziness. **RARE (2%):** Arm pain, earache, dermatitis, pruritus.

ADVERSE REACTIONS/ TOXIC EFFECTS

Anaphylaxis, occurring within 2 hrs of the first or subsequent administration, occurs in 0.1% of pts. Malignant neoplasms occur in 0.5% of pts.

NURSING CONSIDERATIONS

BASELINE ASSESSMENT

Obtain baseline serum total IgE levels prior to initiation of treatment (dosage is based on pretreatment levels). Drug is not for treatment of acute exacerbations of asthma, acute bronchospasm, status asthmaticus.

INTERVENTION/EVALUATION

Monitor rate, depth, rhythm, type of respirations, quality/rate of pulse. Assess lung sounds for rhonchi, wheezing, rales. Observe lips, fingernails for blue/dusky color in light-skinned pts, gray in dark-skinned pts.

PATIENT/FAMILY TEACHING

Increase fluid intake (decreases lung secretion viscosity). Do not alter/stop other asthma medications.

omeprazole

oh-**mep**-rah-zole
(Losec, Prilosec, Prilosec DR)
Do not confuse with prilocaine, Prinivil, Prozac.

◆ **CLASSIFICATION**

PHARMACOTHERAPEUTIC: Benzimidazole. **CLINICAL:** Gastric acid pump inhibitor (see p. 128C).

ACTION

Converted to active metabolites that irreversibly bind to and inhibit H^+-K^+-ATPase (an enzyme on surface of gastric parietal cells). Inhibits hydrogen ion transport into gastric lumen. **Therapeutic Effect:** Increases gastric pH, reduces gastric acid production.

PHARMACOKINETICS

Onset	Peak	Duration
PO		
1 hr	2 hrs	72 hrs

Rapidly absorbed from GI tract. Protein binding: 99%. Primarily distributed into gastric parietal cells. Metabolized extensively in liver. Primarily excreted in urine. Unknown if removed by hemodialysis. **Half-life:** 0.5–1 hr (increased in decreased liver function).

USES

Short-term treatment (4–8 wks) of erosive esophagitis (diagnosed by endoscopy); symptomatic gastroesophageal reflux disease (GERD) poorly responsive to other treatment. Long-term treatment of pathologic hypersecretory conditions; treatment of active duodenal ulcer. Maintenance healing of erosive esophagitis. **Unlabeled:** Treatment of *H. pylori*–associated duodenal ulcer (with amoxicillin, clarithromycin), active benign gastric ulcers. Prevention/treatment of NSAID-induced ulcers.

PRECAUTIONS

CONTRAINDICATIONS: None known. **CAUTIONS:** None known.

LIFESPAN CONSIDERATIONS: Pregnancy/lactation: Unknown if drug crosses placenta or is distributed in breast milk. **Pregnancy Category C. Children:** Safety and efficacy not established. **Elderly:** No age-related precautions noted.

INTERACTIONS

DRUG: May increase concentration of **oral anticoagulants, diazepam, phenytoin.** **HERBAL:** None known. **FOOD:** None known. **LAB VALUES:** May increase SGOT (AST), SGPT (ALT), alkaline phosphatase.

AVAILABILITY (Rx)

CAPSULES (delayed-release): 10 mg, 20 mg, 40 mg.

ADMINISTRATION/HANDLING

PO

• Give before meals. • Do not crush/chew capsule; swallow whole.

INDICATIONS/ROUTES/DOSAGE

EROSIVE ESOPHAGITIS, POORLY RESPONSIVE GERD, ACTIVE DUODENAL ULCER, PREVENTION/TREATMENT OF NSAID-INDUCED ULCERS

PO: ADULTS, ELDERLY: 20 mg/day.

MAINTENANCE HEALING OF EROSIVE ESOPHAGITIS

PO: ADULTS, ELDERLY: 20 mg/day.

PATHOLOGIC HYPERSECRETORY CONDITIONS

PO: ADULTS, ELDERLY: Initially, 60 mg/day up to 120 mg, 3 times/day.

***H. PYLORI* DUODENAL ULCER**

PO: ADULTS, ELDERLY: 20 mg 2 times/day for 10 days.

ACTIVE BENIGN GASTRIC ULCER

PO: ADULTS, ELDERLY: 40 mg/day for 4–8 wks.

USUAL DOSAGE FOR CHILDREN >2 YRS

PO: (GERD, erosive gastritis): <20 KG: 10 mg/day. >20 KG: 20 mg/day.

O

SIDE EFFECTS

FREQUENT (7%): Headache. **OCCASIONAL (2%–3%):** Diarrhea, abdominal pain, nausea. **RARE (<2%):** Dizziness, asthenia (loss of strength), vomiting, constipation, upper respiratory infection, back pain, rash, cough.

ADVERSE REACTIONS/ TOXIC EFFECTS

None known.

NURSING IMPLICATIONS

INTERVENTION/EVALUATION

Evaluate for therapeutic response: relief of GI symptoms. Question if GI discomfort, nausea, diarrhea occurs.

PATIENT/FAMILY TEACHING

Report headache. Swallow capsules whole; do not chew/crush. Take prior to eating.

O

ondansetron hydrochloride

on-**dan**-sah-tron

(Zofran)

Do not confuse with Zantac, Zosyn.

CLASSIFICATION

PHARMACOTHERAPEUTIC: Selective receptor antagonist. **CLINICAL:** Antinausea, antiemetic.

ACTION

Blocks serotonin, both peripherally on vagal nerve terminals and centrally in chemoreceptor trigger zone. **Therapeutic Effect:** Prevents nausea, vomiting.

PHARMACOKINETICS

Readily absorbed from GI tract. Protein binding: 70%–76%. Metabolized in liver. Primarily excreted in urine. Unknown if removed by hemodialysis. **Half-life:** 4 hrs.

USES

Prevention, treatment of nausea/vomiting due to cancer chemotherapy, including high-dose cisplatin. Prevention of postop nausea/vomiting. Prevention of radiation-induced nausea/vomiting. **Unlabeled:** Treatment of postop nausea/vomiting.

PRECAUTIONS

CONTRAINDICATIONS: None known. **CAUTIONS:** None known.

LIFESPAN CONSIDERATIONS: Pregnancy/lactation: Unknown if drug crosses placenta or is distributed in breast milk. **Pregnancy Category B. Children:** Safety and efficacy not established. **Elderly:** No age-related precautions noted.

INTERACTIONS

DRUG: None known. **HERBAL:** None known. **FOOD:** None known. **LAB VALUES:** May transiently increase SGOT (AST), SGPT (ALT), bilirubin.

AVAILABILITY (Rx)

TABLETS: 4 mg, 8 mg, 24 mg. **ORAL DISINTEGRATING TABLETS:** 4 mg, 8 mg. **ORAL SOLUTION:** 4 mg/5 ml. **INJECTION:** 2 mg/ml. **INJECTION (Premix):** 32 mg/50 ml.

ADMINISTRATION/HANDLING

PO

- Give without regard to food.

IM

- Inject into large muscle mass.

IV

Storage • Store at room temperature. • Stable for 48 hrs following dilution.

Reconstitution • May give undiluted. • For IV infusion, dilute with 50 ml D_5W or 0.9% NaCl prior to administration.

Rate of administration • Give IV push over 2–5 min. • Give IV infusion over 15 min.

⌀ **IV INCOMPATIBILITIES**

Acyclovir (Zovirax), allopurinol (Aloprim), aminophylline, amphotericin B (Fungizone), amphotericin B complex (Abelcet, AmBisome, Amphotec), ampicillin (Polycillin), ampicillin/sulbactam (Unasyn), cefepime (Maxipime), cefoperazone (Cefobid), fluorouracil, lorazepam (Ativan), meropenem (Merrem IV), methylprednisolone (Solu-Medrol).

IV COMPATIBILITIES

Carboplatin (Paraplatin), cisplatin (Platinol), cyclophosphamide (Cytoxan), cytarabine (Cytosar), dacarbazine (DTIC-Dome), daunorubicin (Cerubidine), dexamethasone (Decadron), diphenhydramine (Benadryl), docetaxel (Taxoterc), dopamine (Intropin), etoposide (VePesid), gemcitabine (Gemzar), heparin, hydromorphone (Dilaudid), ifosfamide (Ifex), magnesium, mannitol, mesna (Mesnex), methotrexate, metoclopramide (Reglan), mitomycin (Mutamycin), mitoxantrone (Novantrone), morphine, paclitaxel (Taxol), potassium chloride, teniposide (Vumon), topotecan (Hycamptin), vinblastine (Velban), vincristine (Oncovin), vinorelbine (Navelbine).

INDICATIONS/ROUTES/DOSAGE

PREVENTION OF CHEMOTHERAPY INDUCED NAUSEA/VOMITING

IV: ADULTS, ELDERLY, CHILDREN 4–18 YRS: Single 32-mg dose or 0.15 mg/kg/dose given 30 min prior to chemotherapy, then 4 and 8 hrs following chemotherapy.

PO: ADULTS, ELDERLY, CHILDREN >11 YRS: 24 mg as a single dose 30 min prior to starting chemotherapy or 8 mg q8h (first dose 30 min prior to chemotherapy) then q12h for 1–2 days. CHILDREN 4–11 YRS: 4 mg 30 min prior to chemotherapy and 4 and 8 hrs following chemotherapy, then 4 mg q8h for 1–2 days.

POSTOP NAUSEA, VOMITING

IM/IV: ADULTS, ELDERLY: 4 mg undiluted over 2–5 min. CHILDREN <40 KG: 0.1 mg/kg. ≥40 KG: 4 mg.

NAUSEA/VOMITING DUE TO RADIATION THERAPY

PO: ADULTS, ELDERLY: 8 mg 3 times/day.

SIDE EFFECTS

FREQUENT (5%–13%): Anxiety, dizziness, drowsiness, headache, fatigue, constipation, diarrhea, hypoxia, urinary retention. **OCCASIONAL (2%–4%):** Abdominal pain, xerostomia (diminished saliva secretion), fever, feeling of cold, redness/pain at injection site, paresthesia, weakness. **RARE (<1%):** Hypersensitivity reaction (rash, itching), blurred vision.

ADVERSE REACTIONS/ TOXIC EFFECTS

Overdose may produce combination of CNS stimulation, depressant effects.

NURSING IMPLICATIONS

BASELINE ASSESSMENT

Assess for dehydration if excessive vomiting occurs (poor skin turgor, dry mucous membranes, longitudinal furrows in tongue). Provide emotional support.

INTERVENTION/EVALUATION

Monitor pt in environment. Assess bowel sounds for peristalsis. Provide supportive measures. Assess mental status. Monitor daily bowel activity, stool consistency (watery, loose, soft, semisolid, solid); record time of evacuation.

PATIENT/FAMILY TEACHING

Relief from nausea/vomiting generally occurs shortly after drug administra-

O

tion. Avoid alcohol, barbiturates. Report persistent vomiting. May cause drowsiness, dizziness.

oprelvekin (interleukin-2, IL-2)

oh-**prel**-vee-kinn
(Neumega)
Do not confuse with Neupogen.

CLASSIFICATION

PHARMACOTHERAPEUTIC: Hematopoietic. **CLINICAL:** Platelet growth factor.

ACTION

Stimulates production of blood platelets (essential in the blood-clotting process). **Therapeutic Effect:** Results in increased platelet production.

USES

Prevents severe thrombocytopenia, reduces need for platelet transfusions following myelosuppressive chemotherapy in pts with nonmyeloid malignancies.

PRECAUTIONS

CONTRAINDICATIONS: None known. **CAUTIONS:** CHF, those susceptible to developing CHF, history of heart failure, history of atrial arrhythmia. **Pregnancy Category C.**

INTERACTIONS

DRUG: None known. **HERBAL:** None known. **FOOD:** None known. **LAB VALUES:** May decrease Hgb, Hct (usually begins 3–5 days of initiation of therapy, reverses about 1 wk after discontinuance of therapy).

AVAILABILITY (Rx)

INJECTION: 5 mg.

ADMINISTRATION/HANDLING

SUBCUTANEOUS

Storage • Store in refrigerator. Once reconstituted, use within 3 hrs. • Give single injection in abdomen, thigh, hip, upper arm.

Reconstitution • Add 1 ml Sterile Water for Injection on side of vial; swirl contents gently (avoid excessive agitation) to provide concentration of 5 mg/ml oprelvekin). • Discard unused portion.

INDICATIONS/ROUTES/DOSAGE

Alert: Dosing should begin 6–24 hrs following completion of chemotherapy dosing.

PREVENTION OF THROMBOCYTOPENIA

Subcutaneous: ADULTS: 50 mcg/kg once daily. CHILDREN: 75–100 mcg/kg once daily. Continue for 14–28 days or until platelet count reaches 50,000 cell/mcl after its nadir.

SIDE EFFECTS

FREQUENT: Nausea/vomiting (77%); fluid retention (59%); neutropenic fever (48%); diarrhea (43%); rhinitis (42%); headache (41%); dizziness (38%); fever (36%); insomnia (33%); cough (29%); rash, pharyngitis (25%); tachycardia (20%); vasodilation (19%).

ADVERSE REACTIONS/ TOXIC EFFECTS

Transient atrial fibrillation/flutter occurs in 10% of pts (may be due to increased plasma volume; drug is not directly arrhythmogenic). Arrhythmias usually are brief in duration and convert to normal sinus rhythm spontaneously. Papilledema in children.

NURSING IMPLICATIONS

BASELINE ASSESSMENT

Obtain CBC prior to chemotherapy and at regular intervals thereafter.

INTERVENTION/EVALUATION

Monitor platelet counts. Closely monitor fluid/electrolyte status, particularly in pts receiving diuretic therapy. Assess for fluid retention evidenced by peripheral edema, dyspnea on exertion (generally occurs during first week of therapy and continues for duration of treatment). Monitor platelet count periodically to assess therapeutic duration of therapy. Dosing should continue until postnadir platelet count is >50,000 cell/mcl. Treatment should be stopped >2 days prior to starting next round of chemotherapy.

orlistat

ore-leh-stat
(Xenical)

CLASSIFICATION

PHARMACOTHERAPEUTIC: Gastric/pancreatic lipase inhibitor. **CLINICAL:** Obesity management agent (see p. 119C).

ACTION

Inhibits absorption of dietary fats by inactivating gastric and pancreatic enzymes. **Therapeutic Effect:** Results in a caloric deficit that may have a positive effect on weight control.

PHARMACOKINETICS

Minimal absorption after administration. Protein binding: >99%. Primarily eliminated unchanged in feces. Unknown if removed by hemodialysis. **Half-life:** 1–2 hrs.

USES

Management of obesity, including weight loss/maintenance, when used in conjunction with a reduced-calorie diet.

PRECAUTIONS

CONTRAINDICATIONS: Chronic malabsorption syndrome, cholestasis. **CAUTIONS:** None known.

LIFESPAN CONSIDERATIONS: Pregnancy/lactation: Unknown if excreted in breast milk. Not recommended during pregnancy or in breast-feeding women. **Pregnancy Category B. Children:** Safety and efficacy not established. **Elderly:** No age-related precautions noted.

INTERACTIONS

DRUG: May increase concentration, risk of rhabdomyolysis with **pravastatin. HERBAL:** None known. **FOOD:** None known. **LAB VALUES:** Decreases total cholesterol, LDL, glucose. Decreases absorption/levels of vitamins A and E.

AVAILABILITY (Rx)

CAPSULES: 120 mg.

ADMINISTRATION/HANDLING

PO

- Give without regard to food.

INDICATIONS/ROUTES/DOSAGE

WEIGHT REDUCTION

PO: ADULTS, ELDERLY: 120 mg 3 times/day.

SIDE EFFECTS

Alert: Side effects tend to be mild and transient in nature, gradually diminishing during treatment.

FREQUENT (20%–30%): Headache, abdominal discomfort, flatulence, fecal urgency, fatty/oily stool. **OCCASIONAL (5%–14%):** Back pain, menstrual irregularity, nausea, fatigue, diarrhea, dizziness. **RARE (<4%):** Anxiety, rash, myalgia, dry skin, vomiting.

ADVERSE REACTIONS/TOXIC EFFECTS

None known.

NURSING IMPLICATIONS

INTERVENTION/EVALUATION

Monitor cholesterol, LDL, glucose, changes in coagulation parameters.

PATIENT/FAMILY TEACHING

Maintain nutritionally balanced, reduced-calorie diet. Daily intake of fat, carbohydrates, protein to be distributed over the 3 main meals.

orphenadrine citrate

(Norflex)

See Classification section under: Skeletal muscle relaxants

oseltamivir

oh-sell-**tam**-ih-veer
(Tamiflu)

CLASSIFICATION

PHARMACOTHERAPEUTIC: Neuraminidase inhibitor. **CLINICAL:** Antiviral (see p. 59C).

ACTION

Selective inhibitor of influenza virus neuraminidase, an enzyme essential for viral replication. Acts against both influenza A and B viruses. **Therapeutic Effect:** Suppresses spread of infection within respiratory system, reduces duration of clinical symptoms.

PHARMACOKINETICS

Readily absorbed. Protein binding: 3%. Extensively converted to active drug in the liver. Primarily excreted in urine. **Half-life:** 6–10 hrs.

USES

Symptomatic treatment of uncomplicated acute illness caused by influenza A or B virus in adults and children >1 yr who are symptomatic no longer than 2 days. Prevention of influenza in adults, children >13 yrs.

PRECAUTIONS

CONTRAINDICATIONS: None known. **CAUTIONS:** Renal function impairment.

LIFESPAN CONSIDERATIONS: Pregnancy/lactation: Unknown if excreted in breast milk. **Pregnancy Category C. Children:** Safety and efficacy not established in those <1 yr. **Elderly:** No age-related precautions noted.

INTERACTIONS

DRUG: None known. **HERBAL:** None known. **FOOD:** None known. **LAB VALUES:** None known.

AVAILABILITY (Rx)

CAPSULES: 75 mg. **ORAL SUSPENSION:** 12 mg/ml.

ADMINISTRATION/HANDLING

PO

- Give without regard to food.

INDICATIONS/ROUTES/DOSAGE

INFLUENZA

PO: ADULTS, ELDERLY: 75 mg 2 times/day for 5 days. CHILDREN <15 KG: 30 mg twice daily. CHILDREN 15–23 KG: 45 mg twice daily. CHILDREN >23–40 KG: 60 mg twice daily. CHILDREN >40 KG: 75 mg twice daily.

DOSAGE IN RENAL IMPAIRMENT

PO: ADULTS, ELDERLY: 75 mg once daily for at least 7 days up to 6 wks.

PROPHYLAXIS AGAINST INFLUENZA

PO: ADULTS, ELDERLY: 75 mg once daily.

SIDE EFFECTS

FREQUENT (>5%): Nausea, vomiting, diarrhea. **OCCASIONAL (1%–5%):** Abdominal pain, bronchitis, dizziness, headache, cough, insomnia, fatigue, vertigo.

ADVERSE REACTIONS/ TOXIC EFFECTS

Colitis, pneumonia, pyrexia occur rarely.

NURSING IMPLICATIONS

INTERVENTION/EVALUATION

Monitor renal function, serum glucose in pts with diabetes.

PATIENT/FAMILY TEACHING

Begin as soon as possible from first appearance of flu symptoms. Avoid contact with those who are at high risk for influenza. Not a substitute for flu shot.

oxacillin

(Prostaphlin)

See Classification section under: Antibiotic: penicillins (p. 26C)

oxaliplatin

ox-**ale**-ee-plah-tin

(Eloxatin)

CLASSIFICATION

PHARMACOTHERAPEUTIC: Platinum-containing complex. **CLINICAL:** Antineoplastic (see p. 75C).

ACTION

Inhibits DNA replication by cross-linking with DNA strands. Cell cycle–phase nonspecific. **Therapeutic Effect:** Prevents cellular division.

PHARMACOKINETICS

Rapidly distributed. Undergoes rapid, extensive nonenzymatic biotransformation. Protein binding: >90%. Excreted in urine. **Half-life:** 70 hrs.

USES

Combination treatment of metastatic carcinoma of the colon or rectum with 5-fluorouracil (5-FU)/leucovorin in pts whose disease has recurred/progressed during or within 6 mos of completion of first-line therapy with bolus 5-FU/leucovorin and irinotrecan. **Unlabeled:** Treatment of ovarian cancer.

PRECAUTIONS

CONTRAINDICATIONS: History of allergy to platinum compounds. **CAUTIONS:** Previous therapy with other antineoplastic agents, radiation, impaired renal function, infection, pregnancy, immunosuppression, presence/history of peripheral neuropathy.

LIFESPAN CONSIDERATIONS: Pregnancy/lactation: If possible, avoid use during pregnancy, esp. first trimester. May cause fetal harm. Breast-feeding not recommended. **Pregnancy Category D. Children:** Safety and efficacy not established. **Elderly:** Increased incidence of diarrhea, dehydration, hypokalemia, fatigue.

INTERACTIONS

DRUG: Nephrotic agents may decrease clearance of oxaliplatin. **Live virus vaccines** may potentiate virus replication, increase vaccine side effects, decrease pt's antibody response to vaccine. **HERBAL:** None known. **FOOD:** None known. **LAB VALUES:** May alter SGOT (AST), SGPT (ALT), bilirubin. May decrease Hgb, Hct, platelet count.

ADMINISTRATION/HANDLING

Alert: Wear protective gloves during handling of oxaliplatin. If solution comes in contact with skin, wash skin immediately with soap, water. Do not use aluminum needles or administration sets that

O

may come in contact with drug; may cause degradation of platinum compounds.

IV

Storage • Following reconstitution, solution is stable for up to 24 hours if refrigerated and 6 hrs at room temperature.

Reconstitution

Alert: Pt to avoid ice or drinking, touching cold objects during infusion (can exacerbate acute neuropathy). Never reconstitute with sodium chloride solution or chloride-containing solutions.

• Reconstitute 50-mg vial with 10 ml Sterile Water for Injection or D_5W (20 ml for 100-mg vial). Further dilute with 150–500 ml D_5W.

Rate of administration • Administer differing infusion rates as a 2-hr or 22-hr rate, according to protocol orders.

⊘ **IV INCOMPATIBILITY**

Do not infuse with alkaline medications.

AVAILABILITY (Rx)

POWDER FOR INJECTION: 50-mg, 100-mg vials.

INDICATIONS/ROUTES/DOSAGE

Alert: Pretreat with antiemetics ($5\text{-}HT_3$ antagonists). Repeat courses should not be given more frequently than q2wks.

METASTATIC COLON/RECTAL CANCER

DAY 1

IV: ADULTS: Oxaliplatin 85 mg/m^2 in 250–500 ml D_5W and leucovorin 200 mg/m^2, both given >120 min at the same time in separate bags using a Y-line, followed by 5-FU 400 mg/m^2 IV bolus given over 2–4 min, followed by 5-FU 600 mg/m^2 IV infusion in 500 ml D_5W as a 22-hr continuous infusion.

DAY 2

IV: ADULTS: Leucovorin 200 mg/m^2 IV infusion given >120 min, followed by 5-FU 400 mg/m^2 IV bolus given over 2–4 min, followed by 5-FU 600 mg/m^2 IV infusion in 500 ml D_5W as a 22-hr continuous infusion.

OVARIAN CANCER

IV: ADULTS: Cisplatin 100 mg/m^2 and oxaliplatin 130 mg/m^2 q3wks.

SIDE EFFECTS

FREQUENT (20%–76%): Peripheral/sensory neuropathy usually occurs in hands, feet, perioral area, throat but may present as jaw spasm, abnormal tongue sensation, eye pain, chest pressure, difficulty walking, swallowing, writing; nausea (occurs in 64%), fatigue, diarrhea, vomiting, constipation, abdominal pain, fever, anorexia. **OCCASIONAL (10%–14%):** Stomatitis, earache, insomnia, cough, difficulty breathing, backache, edema. **RARE (3%–7%):** Dyspepsia (indigestion, heartburn), dizziness, rhinitis, flushing, alopecia.

ADVERSE REACTIONS/ TOXIC EFFECTS

Peripheral/sensory neuropathy can occur without any prior event, but ice or drinking, holding a glass of cold liquid during IV infusion phase can precipitate/exacerbate this neurotoxicity. Pulmonary fibrosis characterized as nonproductive cough, dyspnea, crackles, radiologic pulmonary infiltrates may warrant discontinuation of drug therapy. Hypersensitivity reaction (rash, hives, itching) occurs rarely.

NURSING IMPLICATIONS

BASELINE ASSESSMENT

Pt to avoid ice or drinking, holding a glass of cold liquid during IV infusion; can precipitate/exacerbate neurotoxicity (occurs within hours or 1–2 days of dosing, lasts up to 14 days). Assess baseline BUN, creatinine, WBC, platelet count.

INTERVENTION/EVALUATION

Monitor for decrease in WBC or platelets (myelosuppression is minimal). Monitor for diarrhea, GI bleeding (bright red/tarry stool). Maintain strict I&O. Assess oral mucosa for mucosal erythema, ulceration of inner margin of lips/mouth, sore throat (stomatitis).

PATIENT/FAMILY TEACHING

Avoid ice or drinking, holding a glass of cold liquid during IV infusion phase (can produce neuropathy). Promptly report fever, sore throat, signs of local infection, unusual bruising/bleeding from any site. Do not have immunizations without physician's approval (lowers body's resistance). Avoid contact with those who have recently taken oral polio vaccine. Avoid cold drinks, ice. Do not hold cold objects.

oxaprozin

ox-ah-**pro**-zin
(Daypro)
Do not confuse with oxazepam.

CLASSIFICATION

PHARMACOTHERAPEUTIC: Nonsteroidal anti-inflammatory. **CLINICAL:** Analgesic, anti-inflammatory (see p. 111C).

ACTIN

Produces analgesic, anti-inflammatory effect by inhibiting prostaglandin synthesis. **Therapeutic Effect:** Reduces inflammatory response, intensity of pain stimulus reaching sensory nerve endings.

PHARMACOKINETICS

Well absorbed from GI tract. Protein binding: >99%. Widely distributed. Metabolized in liver. Primarily excreted in urine; partially eliminated in feces. Not removed by hemodialysis. **Half-life:** 42–50 hrs.

USES

Acute, chronic treatment of osteoarthritis, rheumatoid arthritis.

PRECAUTIONS

CONTRAINDICATIONS: Active peptic ulcer, GI ulceration, chronic inflammation of GI tract, GI bleeding disorders, history of hypersensitivity to aspirin/NSAIDs. **CAUTIONS:** Impaired renal/hepatic function, history of GI tract disease, predisposition to fluid retention.

LIFESPAN CONSIDERATIONS: Pregnancy/lactation: Unknown if drug is excreted in breast milk. Avoid use during third trimester (may adversely affect fetal cardiovascular system: premature closure of ductus arteriosus). **Pregnancy Category C** (**D** if used third trimester or near delivery). **Children:** Safety and efficacy not established. **Elderly:** Age-related renal impairment may increase risk of liver/renal toxicity; decreased dosage recommended. GI bleeding or ulceration more likely to cause serious adverse effects.

INTERACTIONS

DRUG: May increase effects of **oral anticoagulants, heparin, thrombolytics.** May decrease effect of **antihypertensives, diuretics. Salicylates, aspirin** may increase risk of GI side effects, bleeding. **Bone marrow depressants** may increase risk of hematologic reactions. May increase concentration, toxicity of **lithium.** May increase **methotrexate** toxicity. **Probenecid** may increase concentration. **HERBAL: Ginkgo biloba** may increase risk of bleeding. May decrease **feverfew** effect. **FOOD:** None known. **LAB VALUES:** May increase SGOT (AST), SGPT (ALT), serum creatinine, BUN.

AVAILABILITY (Rx)

TABLETS: 600 mg.

ADMINISTRATION/HANDLING

PO

- May give with food, milk, antacids if GI distress occurs.

INDICATIONS/ROUTES/DOSAGE

OSTEOARTHRITIS

PO: ADULTS, ELDERLY: 1,200 mg once daily; 600 mg in pts with low body weight, mild disease. **Maximum:** 1,800 mg/day.

RHEUMATOID ARTHRITIS

PO: ADULTS, ELDERLY: 1,200 mg once daily. RANGE: 600–1,800 mg/day.

JUVENILE RHEUMATOID ARTHRITIS

Weight	Dose/day
22–31 kg	600 mg
32–54 kg	900 mg
>54 kg	1,200 mg

DOSAGE FOR RENAL IMPAIRMENT

PO: ADULTS, ELDERLY: 600 mg/day. May increase up to 1,200 mg/day.

SIDE EFFECTS

OCCASIONAL (3%–9%): Nausea, diarrhea, constipation, dyspepsia (heartburn, indigestion, epigastric pain). **RARE (<3%):** Vomiting, abdominal cramping/pain, flatulence, anorexia, confusion, ringing in ears, insomnia, drowsiness.

ADVERSE REACTIONS/ TOXIC EFFECTS

GI bleeding, coma may occur. Hypertension, acute renal failure, respiratory depression occur rarely.

NURSING IMPLICATIONS

BASELINE ASSESSMENT

Assess onset, type, location, duration of pain/inflammation.

INTERVENTION/EVALUATION

Observe for weight gain, edema, bleeding, bruising, mental confusion. Monitor renal/liver function tests. Evaluate for therapeutic response: relief of pain, stiffness, swelling; increase in joint mobility; reduced joint tenderness; improved grip strength.

PATIENT/FAMILY TEACHING

Avoid aspirin, alcohol during therapy (increases risk of GI bleeding). If gastric upset occurs, take with food, milk, antacids. If GI effects persist, inform physician. May cause drowsiness, confusion. Be cautious in performing tasks requiring mental alertness.

oxazepam

ox-**az**-eh-pam

(Apo-Oxazepam, Serax)

Do not confuse with Eurax, oxaprozin, Xerac.

CLASSIFICATION

PHARMACOTHERAPEUTIC: Benzodiazepine **(Schedule IV).** **CLINICAL:** Antianxiety (see p. 11C).

ACTION

Potentiates effects of GABA, other inhibitory neurotransmitters by binding to specific receptors in CNS. **Therapeutic Effect:** Produces anxiolytic effect, skeletal muscle relaxation.

PHARMACOKINETICS

Well absorbed from GI tract. Protein binding: >97%. Metabolized in liver. Primarily excreted in urine. Not removed by hemodialysis. **Half-life:** 5–20 hrs.

USES

Management of acute alcohol withdrawal symptoms (tremulousness, anxiety on withdrawal). Treatment of anxiety associated with depressive symptoms.

PRECAUTIONS

CONTRAINDICATIONS: Preexisting CNS depression, severe uncontrolled pain, narrow-angle glaucoma. **CAUTIONS:** History of drug dependence. **Pregnancy Category D.**

INTERACTIONS

DRUG: Potentiated effects when used with **other CNS depressants, including alcohol.** **HERBAL:** **Kava kava, valerian** may increase CNS depression. **FOOD:** None known. **LAB VALUES:** May produce abnormal renal function tests, elevate SGOT (AST), SGPT (ALT), LDH, alkaline phosphatase, serum bilirubin. Therapeutic blood serum level: 0.2–1.4 mcg/ml; toxic blood serum level: Not established.

AVAILABILITY (Rx)

CAPSULES: 10 mg, 15 mg, 30 mg.

INDICATIONS/ROUTES/DOSAGE

Alert: Use smallest effective dosage in elderly, debilitated, those with liver disease or low serum albumin.

MILD TO MODERATE ANXIETY

PO: ADULTS: 10–15 mg 3–4 times/day.

SEVERE ANXIETY

PO: ADULTS: 15–30 mg 3–4 times/day.

ALCOHOL WITHDRAWAL

PO: ADULTS: 15–30 mg 3–4 times/day.

USUAL ELDERLY DOSAGE

PO: Initially, 10–20 mg 3 times/day. May gradually increase up to 30–45 mg/day.

SIDE EFFECTS

FREQUENT: Mild, transient drowsiness at beginning of therapy. **OCCASIONAL:** Dizziness, headache. **RARE:** Paradoxical CNS hyperactivity/nervousness in children, excitement/restlessness in elderly/debilitated (generally noted during first 2 wks of therapy).

ADVERSE REACTIONS/ TOXIC EFFECTS

Abrupt or too rapid withdrawal may result in pronounced restlessness, irritability, insomnia, hand tremors, abdominal/muscle cramps, diaphoresis, vomiting, seizures. Overdose results in somnolence, confusion, diminished reflexes, coma.

NURSING IMPLICATIONS

BASELINE ASSESSMENT

Offer emotional support to anxious pt. Assess motor responses (agitation, trembling, tension), autonomic responses (cold/clammy hands, sweating).

INTERVENTION/EVALUATION

For those on long-term therapy, liver/renal function tests, blood counts should be performed periodically. Assess for paradoxical reaction, particularly during early therapy. Assist with ambulation if drowsiness, lightheadedness occurs. Evaluate for therapeutic response: a calm facial expression, decreased restlessness, insomnia. Therapeutic blood serum level: 0.2–1.4 mcg/ml; toxic blood serum level: Not established.

PATIENT/FAMILY TEACHING

Avoid alcohol, other CNS depressants. May cause drowsiness. Avoid tasks requiring mental alertness. Avoid abrupt discontinuation.

O

oxcarbazepine

ox-car-**bah**-zeh-peen
(Trileptal)

CLASSIFICATION

CLINICAL: Anticonvulsant (see p. 33C).

ACTION

Produces blockade of sodium channels, resulting in stabilization of hyperexcited neural membranes, inhibiting repetitive neuronal firing, diminishing synaptic impulses. **Therapeutic Effect:** Prevents seizures.

PHARMACOKINETICS

Completely absorbed and extensively metabolized to active metabolite in the liver. Protein binding: 40%. Primarily excreted in urine. **Half-life:** 2 hrs (metabolite: 6–10 hrs).

USES

O

Monotherapy and adjunctive therapy in adults, children 4–16 yrs for treatment of partial seizures. **Unlabeled:** Atypical panic disorder.

PRECAUTIONS

CONTRAINDICATIONS: None known. **CAUTIONS:** Renal function impairment, sensitivity to carbamazepine.

LIFESPAN CONSIDERATIONS: Pregnancy/lactation: Crosses placenta. Distributed in breast milk. **Pregnancy Category C. Children:** No age-related precautions in those >4 yrs. **Elderly:** Age-related renal impairment may require dosage adjustment.

INTERACTIONS

DRUG: Carbamazepine, phenobarbital, phenytoin, valproic acid, verapamil may decrease concentration, effect. May decrease concentration, effect of **felodipine, oral contraceptives.** May increase concentration, toxicity of **phenobarbital, phenytoin. HERBAL:** None known. **FOOD:** None known. **LAB VALUES:** May increase gamma G-T; increase or decrease blood glucose; increase liver function tests; decrease calcium, potassium, sodium.

AVAILABILITY (Rx)

TABLETS: 150 mg, 300 mg, 600 mg. **ORAL SUSPENSION:** 300 mg/5 ml.

ADMINISTRATION/HANDLING

PO

- Give without regard to food.

INDICATIONS/ROUTES/DOSAGE

Alert: Give all doses in a twice daily regimen.

ADJUNCTIVE THERAPY

PO: ADULTS, ELDERLY: Initially, 600 mg/day in 2 divided doses. May increase by a maximum of 600 mg/day at weekly intervals. **Maximum:** 2,400 mg/day. CHILDREN 4–16 YRS: 8–10 mg/kg. **Maximum:** 600 mg/day. Achieve maintenance dose over 2 wks based on pt's weight. 20–29 KG: 900 mg/day. 29.1–39 KG: 1,200 mg/day. >39 KG: 1,800 mg/day.

CONVERSION TO MONOTHERAPY

PO: ADULTS, ELDERLY: 600 mg/day in 2 divided doses (while decreasing concomitant antiepilepsy drug over 3–6 wks) increasing up to 2,400 mg/day over 2–4 wks. May increase by a maximum of 600 mg/day at weekly intervals.

INITIATION OF MONOTHERAPY

PO: ADULTS, ELDERLY: 600 mg/day in 2 divided doses. May increase by 300 mg/day q3days up to 1,200 mg/day.

DOSAGE FOR RENAL IMPAIRMENT

Creatine clearance <30 ml/min: Give 50% of normal starting dose, then titrate slowly to desired dose.

SIDE EFFECTS

FREQUENT (13%–22%): Dizziness, nausea, headache. **OCCASIONAL (5%–7%):** Vomiting, diarrhea, ataxia (muscular incoordination), nervousness, dyspepsia (heartburn, indigestion, epigastric pain), constipation. **RARE (4%):** Tremor, rash, back pain, nosebleed, sinusitis, diplopia (double vision).

ADVERSE REACTIONS/ TOXIC EFFECTS

May produce clinically significant hyponatremia.

NURSING IMPLICATIONS

BASELINE ASSESSMENT

Review history of seizure disorder (type, onset, intensity, frequency, duration, LOC), drug history (esp. other anticonvulsants). Provide safety precautions; quiet, dark environment. Initiate seizure precautions.

INTERVENTION/EVALUATION

Assist with ambulation if dizziness, ataxia occurs. Assess for visual abnormalities, headache. Monitor serum sodium levels. Assess for signs of hyponatremia (nausea, malaise, headache, lethargy, confusion). Assess for clinical improvement (decrease in intensity/ frequency of seizures).

PATIENT/FAMILY TEACHING

Do not abruptly stop (may increase seizure activity). Inform physician if rash, nausea, headache, dizziness occurs. May need periodic blood tests.

oxiconazole

(Oxistat)

See Classification section under: Antifungals: topical (p. 43C)

Oxistat

see oxycodone

oxybutynin

ox-ee-**byoo**-tih-nin

(Ditropan, Ditropan XL, Oxytrol)

Do not confuse with diazepam, Oxycontin.

◆CLASSIFICATION

PHARMACOTHERAPEUTIC: Anticholinergic. **CLINICAL:** Antispasmodic.

ACTION

Exerts antispasmodic (papaverine-like), antimuscarinic (atropine-like) action on detrusor smooth muscle of bladder. **Therapeutic Effect:** Increases bladder capacity, diminishes frequency of uninhibited detrusor muscle contraction, delays desire to void.

PHARMACOKINETICS

	Onset	Peak	Duration
PO	0.5–1 hr	3–6 hrs	6–10 hrs

Rapid absorption from GI tract. Metabolized in liver. Primarily excreted in urine. Unknown if removed by hemodialysis. **Half-life:** 1–2.3 hrs.

USES

Relief of symptoms (urgency, incontinence, frequency, nocturia, urge incontinence) associated with uninhibited neurogenic bladder, reflex neurogenic bladder.

PRECAUTIONS

CONTRAINDICATIONS: Glaucoma, myasthenia gravis, partial/complete GI obstruction, GU obstruction, ulcerative colitis, toxic megacolon. **CAUTIONS:** Renal/

liver impairment, cardiovascular disease, hyperthyroidism, reflux esophagitis, hypertension, prostatic hypertrophy, neuropathy.

LIFESPAN CONSIDERATIONS: Pregnancy/lactation: Unknown if drug crosses placenta or is distributed in breast milk. **Pregnancy Category B. Children:** No age-related precautions noted in those >5 yrs. **Elderly:** May be more sensitive to anticholinergic effects (e.g., dry mouth, urinary retention).

INTERACTIONS

DRUG: Medication with **anticholinergic effects (e.g., antihistamines)** may increase effects. **HERBAL:** None known. **FOOD:** None known. **LAB VALUES:** None known.

AVAILABILITY (Rx)

TABLETS: 5 mg. **SYRUP:** 5 mg/5 ml. **TABLETS (extended-release):** 5 mg, 10 mg, 15 mg. **TRANSDERMAL:** 3.9 mg.

ADMINISTRATION/HANDLING

PO

- Give without regard to meals.

O

INDICATIONS/ROUTES/DOSAGE

NEUROGENIC BLADDER

PO: ADULTS: 5 mg 2–3 times/day up to 5 mg 4 times/day. ELDERLY: 2.5–5 mg 2 times/day. May increase by 2.5 mg/day q1–2days. CHILDREN >5 YRS: 5 mg 2 times/day up to 5 mg 4 times/day. CHILDREN 1–5 YRS: 0.2 mg/kg/dose 2–4 times/day.

EXTENDED RELEASE

PO: ADULTS: 5–10 mg/day up to 30 mg/day.

Transdermal: ADULTS: 3.9 mg/day 2 times/wk (apply q3–4 days).

SIDE EFFECTS

FREQUENT: Constipation, dry mouth, drowsiness, decreased diaphoresis. **OCCASIONAL:** Decreased lacrimation, salivary/sweat gland secretion, sexual function. Urinary hesitancy/retention, suppressed lactation, blurred vision, mydriasis, nausea/vomiting, insomnia.

ADVERSE REACTIONS/ TOXIC EFFECTS

Overdosage produces CNS excitation (nervousness, restlessness, hallucinations, irritability), hypotension/hypertension, confusion, fast heartbeat/tachycardia, flushed/red face, respiratory depression (shortness of breath, troubled breathing).

NURSING IMPLICATIONS

BASELINE ASSESSMENT

Assess dysuria, urgency, frequency, incontinence.

INTERVENTION/EVALUATION

Monitor for symptomatic relief. Monitor I&O; palpate bladder for retention. Monitor bowel activity, stool consistency.

PATIENT/FAMILY TEACHING

Avoid alcohol. May cause drowsiness, dry mouth. Avoid driving, other tasks requiring alertness, coordination, manual dexterity until response to drug is established.

oxycodone

ox-ih-**koe**-doan

(Intensol, OxyContin, OxyFast, Oxy-IR, Percolone, Roxicodone, Supeudol♣)

Do not confuse with oxybutynin.

FIXED-COMBINATION(S)

Percocet, Roxicet, Tylox: oxycodone/acetaminophen (a non-narcotic analgesic): 5 mg/500 mg. **Percocet:** oxycodone/acetaminophen:

2.5 mg/325 mg; 5 mg/325 mg; 5 mg/500 mg; 7.5 mg/325 mg; 7.5 mg/500 mg; 10 mg/325 mg; 10 mg/650 mg. **Percodan:** oxycodone/aspirin (a non-narcotic analgesic): 2.25 mg/325 mg; 4.5 mg/325 mg.

◆ CLASSIFICATION

PHARMACOTHERAPEUTIC: Opioid analgesic **(Schedule II). CLINICAL:** Narcotic analgesic (see p. 121C).

ACTION

Binds with opioid receptors within CNS. **Therapeutic Effect:** Alters processes affecting pain perception, emotional response to pain.

PHARMACOKINETICS

Onset	Peak	Duration
Immediate-release		
—	—	4–5 hrs
Controlled-release		
—	—	12 hrs

Moderately absorbed from GI tract. Protein binding: 38%–45%. Widely distributed. Metabolized in liver. Excreted in urine. Unknown if removed by hemodialysis. **Half-life:** 2–3 hrs (controlled-release: 3.2 hrs).

USES

Relief of mild to moderately severe pain.

PRECAUTIONS

CONTRAINDICATIONS: None known. **EXTREME CAUTION:** CNS depression, anoxia, hypercapnia, respiratory depression, seizures, acute alcoholism, shock, untreated myxedema, respiratory dysfunction. **CAUTIONS:** Increased intracranial pressure, impaired hepatic function, acute abdominal conditions, hypothyroidism, prostatic hypertrophy, Addison's disease, urethral stricture, COPD.

LIFESPAN CONSIDERATIONS: Pregnancy/lactation: Readily crosses placenta. Distributed in breast milk. Respiratory depression may occur in neonate if mother received opiates during labor. Regular use of opiates during pregnancy may produce withdrawal symptoms in neonate (irritability, excessive crying, tremors, hyperactive reflexes, fever, vomiting, diarrhea, yawning, sneezing, seizures). **Pregnancy Category B (D** if used for prolonged periods or at high dosages at term). **Children:** Paradoxical excitement may occur. Those <2 yrs more susceptible to respiratory depressant effects. **Elderly:** Age-related renal impairment may increase risk of urinary retention. May be more susceptible to respiratory depressant effects.

INTERACTIONS

DRUG: Alcohol, CNS depressants may increase CNS or respiratory depression, hypotension. **MAOIs** may produce severe, fatal reaction (reduce dose to ¼ usual dose). **HERBAL:** None known. **FOOD:** None known. **LAB VALUES:** May increase amylase, lipase.

AVAILABILITY (Rx)

CAPSULES (immediate-release) (OxyIR): 5 mg. **ORAL CONCENTRATE** (OxyFast, Roxicodone, Intensol): 20 mg/ml. **ORAL SOLUTION** (Roxicodone): 5 mg/ml. **TABLETS (immediate-release)** (Percolone, Roxicodone): 5 mg, 15 mg, 30 mg. **TABLETS (controlled-release)** (Oxycontin): 10 mg, 20 mg, 40 mg, 80 mg, 160 mg.

ADMINISTRATION/HANDLING

PO

• Give without regard to meals. • Tablets may be crushed. • **Controlled-release:** Swallow whole; do not crush, break, chew.

INDICATIONS/ROUTES/DOSAGE

ANALGESIA

PO: ADULTS, ELDERLY (immediate-release): Initially, 5 mg q6h as needed. May increase up to 30 mg q4h. USUAL: 10–30

O

mg q4h as needed. CHILDREN: 0.05–0.15 mg/kg/dose q4–6h.

PO: ADULTS, ELDERLY (controlled-release): Initially, 10 mg q12h. May increase q1–2days by 25%–50%. USUAL: 40 mg/day (Cancer pain: 100 mg/day).

SIDE EFFECTS

Alert: Effects are dependent on dosage amount. Ambulatory pts, those not in severe pain may experience dizziness, nausea, vomiting, hypotension more frequently than those in supine position or having severe pain.

FREQUENT: Drowsiness, dizziness, hypotension, anorexia. **OCCASIONAL:** Confusion, diaphoresis, facial flushing, urinary retention, constipation, dry mouth, nausea, vomiting, headache. **RARE:** Allergic reaction, depression, paradoxical CNS hyperactivity/nervousness in children, excitement/restlessness in elderly/debilitated pts.

ADVERSE REACTIONS/ TOXIC EFFECTS

Overdose results in respiratory depression, skeletal muscle flaccidity, cold/clammy skin, cyanosis, extreme somnolence progressing to convulsions, stupor, coma. Hepatotoxicity may occur with overdosage of acetaminophen component. Tolerance to analgesic effect, physical dependence may occur with repeated use.

NURSING IMPLICATIONS

BASELINE ASSESSMENT

Assess onset, type, location, duration of pain. Effect of medication is reduced if full pain recurs before next dose. Obtain vital signs prior to giving medication. If respirations are ≤12/min (≤20/min in children), withhold medication, contact physician.

INTERVENTION/EVALUATION

Palpate bladder for urinary retention. Monitor pattern of daily bowel activity, stool consistency. Initiate deep breathing, coughing exercises, particularly in pts with impaired pulmonary function. Monitor pain relief, respiratory rate, mental status, B/P.

PATIENT/FAMILY TEACHING

May cause dry mouth, drowsiness. May affect ability to perform tasks requiring mental alertness, physical coordination. Avoid alcohol. May be habit forming. Do not crush, chew, break controlled-release tablets.

OxyContin

see oxycodone

OxyFast

see oxycodone

OxyIR

see oxycodone

oxytocin

ox-ih-**toe**-sin
(Pitocin)
Do not confuse with Pitressin.

◆ CLASSIFICATION

PHARMACOTHERAPEUTIC: Uterine smooth muscle stimulant. **CLINICAL:** Oxytocic.

ACTION

Acts on uterine myofibril activity. Stimulates mammary smooth muscle. **Therapeutic Effect:** Contracts uterine smooth muscle. Enhances milk ejection from breasts.

PHARMACOKINETICS

Onset	Peak	Duration
IM		
3–5 min	—	2–3 hrs
IV		
Immediate	—	1 hr
Intranasal		
Few minutes	—	20 min

Rapidly absorbed through nasal mucous membranes. Protein binding: 30%. Distributed in extracellular fluid. Metabolized in liver, kidney. Primarily excreted in urine. **Half-life:** 1–6 min.

USES

Parenteral (Antepartum): Initiates/improves uterine contraction to achieve early vaginal delivery; stimulate/reinforce labor; management of incomplete/inevitable abortion. **(Postpartum):** Produces uterine contractions during third stage of labor; controls uterine bleeding. **Nasal:** To promote breast milk ejection.

PRECAUTIONS

CONTRAINDICATIONS: Cephalopelvic disproportion, unfavorable fetal position/presentation, unengaged fetal head, fetal distress without imminent delivery, prematurity, when vaginal delivery is contraindicated (e.g., active genital herpes infection, placenta previa, cord presentation), obstetric emergencies that favor surgical intervention, grand multiparity, hypertonic/hyperactive uterus, adequate uterine activity that fails to progress. Nasal spray during pregnancy. **CAUTIONS:** Induction should be for medical, not elective, reasons.

LIFESPAN CONSIDERATIONS: Pregnancy/lactation: Used as indicated, not expected to present risk of fetal abnormalities. Small amounts in breast milk; breast-feeding not recommended. **Pregnancy Category X. Children/elderly:** Not used in these pt populations.

INTERACTIONS

DRUG: Caudal block anesthetics, vasopressors may increase pressor effects. **Other oxytocics** may cause uterine hypertonus, uterine rupture, cervical lacerations. **HERBAL:** None known. **FOOD:** None known. **LAB VALUES:** None known.

AVAILABILITY (Rx)

INJECTION: 10 units/ml.

ADMINISTRATION/HANDLING

IV

Storage • Store at room temperature.

Reconstitution • Dilute 10–40 units (1–4 ml) in 1,000 ml of 0.9% NaCl, lactated Ringer's, or D_5W to provide a concentration of 10–40 milliunits/ml solution.

Rate of administration • Give by IV infusion (use infusion device to carefully control rate of flow as ordered by physician).

IV INCOMPATIBILITY

No known incompatibilities via Y-site administration.

IV COMPATIBILITIES

Heparin, insulin, multivitamins, potassium chloride.

INDICATIONS/ROUTES/DOSAGE

INDUCTION/STIMULATION OF LABOR

IV infusion: ADULTS: Initially, 0.001–0.002 units/mins. May increase by

O

0.001–0.002 units q15-30min until contraction pattern has been established.

INCOMPLETE/INEVITABLE ABORTION
IV infusion: ADULTS: 10 units in 500 ml (20 milliunits/ml) D_5W or 0.9% NaCl infused at 20–40 mU/min.

CONTROL OF POSTPARTUM BLEEDING
IV infusion: ADULTS: 10–40 units (**Maximum:** 40 units/1,000 ml) infused at a rate sufficient to control uterine atony.

IM: ADULTS: 10 units after delivery of placenta.

POSTABORTION HEMORRHAGE
IV infusion: ADULTS: 10 units infused at rate of 20–100 milliunits/min.

SIDE EFFECTS

OCCASIONAL: Tachycardia, PVCs, hypotension, nausea, vomiting.

ADVERSE REACTIONS/ TOXIC EFFECTS

Hypertonicity with tearing of uterus, increased bleeding, abruptio placenta, cervical/vaginal lacerations. **FETAL:** Bradycardia, CNS/brain damage, trauma due to rapid propulsion, low Apgar at 5 min, retinal hemorrhage occur rarely. Prolonged IV infusion of oxytocin with excessive fluid volume has caused severe water intoxication with seizures, coma, death.

NURSING IMPLICATIONS

BASELINE ASSESSMENT

Assess baselines for vital signs, B/P, fetal heart rate. Determine frequency, duration, strength of contractions.

INTERVENTION/EVALUATION

Monitor B/P, pulse, respirations, fetal heart rate, intrauterine pressure, contractions (duration, strength, frequency) q15min. Notify physician of contractions that last >1 min, occur more frequently than every 2 min, or stop. Maintain careful I&O; be alert to potential water intoxication. Check for blood loss.

PATIENT/FAMILY TEACHING

Keep pt, family informed of labor progress.

Pacerone

see amiodarone

paclitaxel

pass-leh-**tax**-ell
(Onxol, Taxol)
Do not confuse with Paxil, Taxotere.

◆CLASSIFICATION

PHARMACOTHERAPEUTIC: Taxoid, antimitotic agent. **CLINICAL:** Antineoplastic (see p. 75C).

ACTION

Promotes assembly of microtubules, stabilizes microtubules by preventing depolymerization. **Therapeutic Effect:** Inhibits mitotic cellular functions, cell replication. Blocks cells in late G_2 phase/M phase of cell cycle.

PHARMACOKINETICS

Does not readily cross blood-brain barrier. Protein binding: 89%–98%. Metabolized in liver (active metabolites); eliminated via bile. Not removed by hemodialysis. **Half-life:** 1.3–8.6 hrs.

USES

First-line treatment of advanced ovarian cancer, treatment for metastatic ovarian cancer following failure of first-line or subsequent chemotherapy. Treatment of breast cancer, AIDS-related Kaposi's sarcoma, non–small cell lung cancer. **Unlabeled:** Treatment of head/neck cancer, small cell lung cancer, adenocarcinoma of upper GI tract, hormone-refractory prostate cancer, non-Hodgkin's lymphoma, transitional cell cancer of urothelium.

PRECAUTIONS

CONTRAINDICATIONS: Baseline neutropenia <1,500 cells/mm^3, hypersensitivity to drugs developed with Cremophor EL (polyoxyethylated castor oil). **CAUTIONS:** Liver impairment, severe neutropenia, peripheral neuropathy.

LIFESPAN CONSIDERATIONS: Pregnancy/lactation: May produce fetal harm. Unknown if distributed in breast milk. Avoid use in pregnancy. **Pregnancy Category D. Children:** Safety and efficacy not established. **Elderly:** No age-related precautions noted.

INTERACTIONS

DRUG: Bone marrow depressants may increase bone marrow depression. **Live virus vaccines** may potentiate virus replication, increase vaccine side effects, decrease pt's antibody response to vaccine. **HERBAL:** None known. **FOOD:** None known. **LAB VALUES:** May elevate alkaline phosphatase, SGOT (AST), SGPT (ALT), bilirubin. Decreases WBCs, RBCs, Hgb, Hct, platelets.

AVAILABILITY (Rx)

INJECTION: 30 mg/5 ml; 100 mg/17 ml; 150 mg/25 ml; 300 mg/50 ml.

ADMINISTRATION/HANDLING

IV

Alert: Wear gloves during handling; if contact with skin occurs, wash hands thoroughly with soap, water. If contact with mucous membranes occurs, flush with water.

Storage • Refrigerate unopened vials. • Prepared solution is stable at room temperature for 24 hrs. • Store diluted solutions in bottles or plastic bags and administer through polyethylene-lined administration sets (avoid plasticized PVC equipment or devices).

Reconstitution • Dilute with 0.9% NaCl, D_5W to final concentration of 0.3–1.2 mg/ml.

Rate of administration • Administer at rate as ordered by physician through in-line filter not greater than 0.22 microns. • Monitor vital signs during infusion, esp. during first hour. • Discontinue administration if severe hypersensitivity reaction occurs.

IV INCOMPATIBILITIES

Amphotericin B complex (Abelcet, AmBisome, Amphotec), chlorpromazine (Thorazine), doxorubicin liposome (Doxil), hydroxyzine (Vistaril), methylprednisolone (Solu-Medrol), mitoxantrone (Novantrone).

IV COMPATIBILITIES

Carboplatin (Paraplatin), cisplatin (Platinol AQ), cyclophosphamide (Cytoxan), cytarabine (Cytosar), dacarbazine (DTIC-Dome), dexamethasone (Decadron), diphenydramine (Benadryl), doxorubicin (Adriamycin), etoposide (VePesid), gemcitabine (Gemzar), granisetron (Kytril), hydromorphone (Dilaudid), magnesium sulfate, mannitol, methotrexate, morphine, ondansetron (Zofran), potassium chloride, vinblastine (Velban), vincristine (Oncovin).

P

INDICATIONS/ROUTES/DOSAGE

Alert: Pretreat with corticosteroids, diphenhydramine, H_2 antagonists.

OVARIAN CANCER
IV infusion: ADULTS: 135–175 mg/m²/dose over 1–24 hrs q3wks.

BREAST CARCINOMA
IV infusion: ADULTS, ELDERLY: 175 mg/m² over 3 hrs q3wks.

NON–SMALL CELL LUNG CARCINOMA
IV infusion: ADULTS, ELDERLY: 135 mg/m² over 24 hrs, then cisplatin 75 mg/m² q3wks.

KAPOSI'S SARCOMA
IV infusion: 135 mg/m²/dose over 3 hrs q3wks or 100 mg/m²/dose over 3 hrs q2wks.

DOSAGE IN LIVER IMPAIRMENT

Total Bilirubin	Total Dose
≤1.5 mg/dl	<135 mg/m²
1.6–3 mg/dl	<75 mg/m²
>3 mg/dl	<50 mg/m²

P

SIDE EFFECTS

COMMON (70%–90%): Diarrhea, alopecia, nausea, vomiting. **FREQUENT (46%–48%):** Myalgia/arthralgia, peripheral neuropathy. **OCCASIONAL (13%–20%):** Mucositis, hypotension (during infusion), pain/redness at injection site. **RARE (3%):** Bradycardia.

ADVERSE REACTIONS/ TOXIC EFFECTS

Neutropenic nadir occurs at median of 11 days. Anemia, leukopenia occur commonly; thrombocytopenia occurs occasionally. Severe hypersensitivity reaction (dyspnea, severe hypotension, angioedema, generalized urticaria) occurs rarely.

NURSING IMPLICATIONS

BASELINE ASSESSMENT

Give emotional support to pt, family. Use strict asepsis, protect pt from infection. Check blood counts, particularly neutrophil, platelet count prior to each course of therapy or as clinically indicated.

INTERVENTION/EVALUATION

Monitor CBC, platelets, vital signs, liver enzymes. Monitor for hematologic toxicity (fever, sore throat, signs of local infections, unusual bleeding/bruising), symptoms of anemia (excessive tiredness, weakness). Assess response to medication; monitor, report diarrhea. Avoid IM injections, rectal temperatures, other traumas that may induce bleeding. Put pressure to injection sites for full 5 min.

PATIENT/FAMILY TEACHING

Explain that alopecia is reversible, but new hair may have different color, texture. Do not have immunizations without physician's approval (drug lowers body's resistance). Avoid crowds, persons with known infections. Report signs of infection at once (fever, flulike symptoms). Contact physician if nausea/vomiting continues at home. Teach signs of peripheral neuropathy. Avoid pregnancy during therapy.

palivizumab

pal-iv-ih-zoo-mab
(Synagis)
Do not confuse with Synalgos-DC.

CLASSIFICATION

PHARMACOTHERAPEUTIC: Monoclonal antibody. **CLINICAL:** Pediatric lower respiratory tract infection agent.

ACTION

Exhibits neutralizing activity against respiratory syncytial virus (RSV) in infants. **Therapeutic Effect:** Inhibits RSV replication in the lower respiratory tract.

USES

Prevention of serious lower respiratory tract disease caused by RSV in pediatric pts at high risk for RSV disease (e.g., hemodynamically significant congenital heart disease).

PRECAUTIONS

CONTRAINDICATIONS: Children with cyanotic congenital heart disease. **CAUTIONS:** Thrombocytopenia, any coagulation disorder. Not to be used for treatment of established RSV disease. **Pregnancy Category C.**

INTERACTIONS

DRUG: None known. **HERBAL:** None known. **FOOD:** None known. **LAB VALUES:** None known.

AVAILABILITY (Rx)

LYOPHILIZED INJECTION: 50 mg, 100 mg.

INDICATIONS/ROUTES/DOSAGE

RESPIRATORY SYNCYTIAL VIRUS (RSV) PREVENTION

IM: CHILDREN: 15 mg/kg once a month during RSV season.

SIDE EFFECTS

FREQUENT (22%–49%): Upper respiratory tract infection, otitis media, rhinitis, rash. **OCCASIONAL (2%–10%):** Pain, pharyngitis. **RARE (<2%):** Cough, diarrhea, vomiting, injection site reaction.

ADVERSE REACTIONS/ TOXIC EFFECTS

Anaphylaxis, severe acute hypersensitivity reaction occur very rarely.

NURSING IMPLICATIONS

BASELINE ASSESSMENT

Assess for sensitivity to palivizumab.

INTERVENTION/EVALUATION

Monitor potential side effects, esp. otitis media, rhinitis, skin rash, upper respiratory tract infection.

PATIENT/FAMILY TEACHING

Discuss with family the purpose and potential side effects of medication.

palonosetron hydrochloride

pal-oh-**noe**-seh-tron
(Aloxi)

◆ CLASSIFICATION

PHARMACOTHERAPEUTIC: $5HT_3$ receptor antagonist. **CLINICAL:** Antinauseant, antiemetic.

P

ACTION

A $5HT_3$ receptor antagonist located centrally (CTZ) and peripherally (vagus nerve terminal). **Therapeutic Effect:** Prevents nausea/vomiting associated with cancer chemotherapy.

PHARMACOKINETICS

Protein binding: 52%. Eliminated in the urine. **Half-life:** 40 hrs.

USES

Prevention of acute, delayed nausea/vomiting associated with initial, repeated courses of moderately/highly ematogenic cancer chemotherapy.

PRECAUTIONS

CONTRAINDICATIONS: None known. **CAUTIONS:** History of cardiovascular disease.

LIFESPAN CONSIDERATIONS: Pregnancy/lactation: Unknown if excreted in breast milk. **Pregnancy Category B. Children:** Safety and efficacy not established. **Elderly:** No age-related precautions noted.

INTERACTIONS

DRUG: None known. **HERBAL:** None known. **FOOD:** None known. **LAB VALUES:** May transiently increase SGOT (AST), SGPT (ALT), bilirubin.

AVAILABILITY (Rx)

INJECTION: 0.25 mg/5 ml.

ADMINISTRATION/HANDLING

IV

Storage • Store at room temperature. Solution should appear colorless, clear. Discard if precipitate is present or solution appears cloudy.

Reconstitution • Give undiluted as an IV push.

Rate of administration • Give IV push over 30 sec. Flush infusion line with 0.9% NaCl prior to and following administration.

IV INCOMPATIBILITIES

Do not mix with any other drugs.

INDICATIONS/DOSAGE/ROUTES

NAUSEA, VOMITING: CHEMOTHERAPY

IV: ADULTS, ELDERLY: 0.25 mg given as a single dose 30 min prior to starting chemotherapy.

SIDE EFFECTS

OCCASIONAL (5%–9%): Headache, constipation. **RARE (<1%):** Diarrhea, dizziness, fatigue, abdominal pain, insomnia.

ADVERSE REACTIONS/ TOXIC EFFECTS

Overdose may produce combination of CNS stimulation, depressant effects.

NURSING IMPLICATIONS

BASELINE ASSESSMENT

Assess for dehydration if excessive vomiting occurs (poor skin turgor, dry mucous membranes, longitudinal furrows in tongue). Provide emotional support.

INTERVENTION/EVALUATION

Monitor pt in environment. Provide supportive measures. Assess mental status. Monitor daily bowel activity/stool consistency (watery, loose, soft, semisolid, solid); record time of evacuation.

PATIENT/FAMILY TEACHING

Relief from nausea/vomiting generally occurs shortly after drug administration. Avoid alcohol, barbiturates. Report persistent vomiting.

pamidronate disodium

pam-ih-**drow**-nate
(Aredia)

CLASSIFICATION

PHARMACOTHERAPEUTIC: Bisphosphonate. **CLINICAL:** Hypocalcemic.

ACTION

Binds to bone, inhibits osteoclast-mediated calcium resorption. **Therapeutic Effect:** Lowers serum calcium concentrations.

PHARMACOKINETICS

	Onset	Peak	Duration
IV	24–48 hrs	5–7 days	—

After IV administration, rapidly absorbed by bone. Slowly excreted unchanged in urine. Unknown if removed by hemodial-

P

ysis. **Bone half-life:** 300 days. **Unmetabolized half-life:** 2.5 hrs.

USES

Treatment of moderate to severe hypercalcemia associated with malignancy (with or without bone metastases). Treatment of moderate to severe Paget's disease, osteolytic bone lesions of multiple myeloma, breast cancer.

PRECAUTIONS

CONTRAINDICATIONS: Hypersensitivity to other bisphosphonates (etidronate, tiludronate, risedronate, alendronate). **CAUTIONS:** Cardiac failure, renal function impairment.

LIFESPAN CONSIDERATIONS: Pregnancy/lactation: There are no adequate and well-controlled studies in pregnant women; unknown if fetal harm can occur. Unknown if excreted in breast milk. **Pregnancy Category D. Children:** Safety and efficacy not established. **Elderly:** May become overhydrated. Careful monitoring of fluid/electrolytes; recommend diluted in smaller volume.

INTERACTIONS

DRUG: Calcium-containing medications, vitamin D may antagonize effects in treatment of hypercalcemia. **HERBAL:** None known. **FOOD:** None known. **LAB VALUES:** May decrease phosphate, potassium, magnesium, calcium levels.

AVAILABILITY (Rx)

POWDER FOR INJECTION: 30 mg, 90 mg.

ADMINISTRATION/HANDLING

IV

Storage • Store parenteral form at room temperature. • Reconstituted vial is stable for 24 hrs refrigerated; IV solution is stable for 24 hrs after dilution.

Reconstitution • Reconstitute each 30-mg vial with 10 ml Sterile Water for Injection to provide concentration of 3 mg/ml. • Allow drug to dissolve before withdrawing. • Further dilute with 1,000 ml sterile 0.45% or 0.9% NaCl or D_5W.

Rate of administration • Adequate hydration is essential in conjunction with pamidronate therapy (avoid overhydration in pts with potential for cardiac failure). • Administer as IV infusion over 2–24 hrs for treatment of hypercalcemia; over 2–4 hrs for other indications.

∅ IV INCOMPATIBILITY

Calcium-containing IV fluids.

INDICATIONS/ROUTES/DOSAGE

HYPERCALCEMIA

IV infusion: ADULTS, ELDERLY: Moderate (corrected serum calcium 12–13.5 mg/dl): 60–90 mg. Severe (corrected serum calcium >13.5 mg/dl): 90 mg.

PAGET'S DISEASE

IV infusion: ADULTS, ELDERLY: 30 mg/day for 3 days.

OSTEOLYTIC BONE LESION

IV infusion: ADULTS, ELDERLY: 90 mg over 2–4 hrs.

SIDE EFFECTS

FREQUENT (>10%): 27% of pts have temperature elevation (at least 1°C) 24–48 hrs after administration. Drug-related redness, swelling, induration, pain at catheter site (18% of pts receiving 90 mg). Anorexia, nausea, fatigue. **OCCASIONAL (1%–10%):** Constipation, rhinitis.

ADVERSE REACTIONS/ TOXIC EFFECTS

Hypophosphatemia, hypokalemia, hypomagnesemia, hypocalcemia occur more frequently with higher dosage. Anemia, hypertension, tachycardia, atrial fibrilla-

P

tion, somnolence occur more often with 90-mg dosages. GI hemorrhage occurs rarely.

NURSING IMPLICATIONS

INTERVENTION/EVALUATION

Monitor serum calcium, potassium, magnesium, creatinine, Hgb, Hct, CBC. Provide adequate hydration; avoid overhydration. Monitor I&O carefully; check lungs for rales, dependent body parts for edema. Monitor B/P, temperature, pulse. Assess catheter site for redness, swelling, pain. Monitor food intake, stool frequency. Be alert for potential GI hemorrhage with 90-mg dosage.

pancreatin

pan-kree-**ah**-tin
(Ku-Zyme, Pancreatin)

pancrelipase

pan-kree-**lie**-pace
(Cotazym, Creon, Pancrease, Pancrease MT, Ultrase, Viokase)

CLASSIFICATION

PHARMACOTHERAPEUTIC: Digestive enzyme. **CLINICAL:** Pancreatic enzyme replenisher.

ACTION

Replaces endogenous pancreatic enzymes. **Therapeutic Effect:** Assists in digestion of protein, starch, fats.

USES

Pancreatic enzyme replacement/supplement when enzymes are absent/deficient (chronic pancreatitis, cystic fibrosis, ductal obstruction from pancreatic cancer, common bile duct). Treatment of steatorrhea associated with postgastrectomy syndrome, bowel resection; reduces malabsorption.

PRECAUTIONS

CONTRAINDICATIONS: Hypersensitivity to pork protein, acute pancreatitis, exacerbation of chronic pancreatitis. **CAUTIONS:** Inhalation of powder may cause asthmatic attack.

LIFESPAN CONSIDERATIONS: Pregnancy/lactation: Unknown if drug crosses placenta or is distributed in breast milk. **Pregnancy Category C. Children:** Information not available. **Elderly:** No age-related precautions noted.

INTERACTIONS

DRUG: Antacids may decrease effect. May decrease absorption of **iron supplements. HERBAL:** None known. **FOOD:** None known. **LAB VALUES:** May increase uric acid.

AVAILABILITY (Rx)

TABLETS. CAPSULES.

ADMINISTRATION/HANDLING

PO

• Give before or with meals, snacks. • Tablets may be crushed. Do not crush enteric-coated form. • Instruct pt not to chew (minimizes irritation to mouth, lips, tongue). May open capsule and spread over applesauce, mashed fruit, rice cereal.

INDICATIONS/ROUTES/DOSAGE

USUAL ORAL DOSAGE

PO: ADULTS, ELDERLY: 1–3 capsules or tablets before or with meals, snacks. May increase up to 8 tablets/dose. CHILDREN: 1–2 tablets with meals, snacks.

SIDE EFFECTS

RARE: Allergic reaction, mouth irritation, shortness of breath, wheezing.

ADVERSE REACTIONS/ TOXIC EFFECTS

Excessive dosage may produce nausea, cramping, diarrhea. Hyperuricosuria, hyperuricemia reported with extremely high dosages.

NURSING IMPLICATIONS

BASELINE ASSESSMENT

Spilling powder on hands (Viokase) may irritate skin. Inhaling powder may irritate mucous membranes, produce bronchospasm.

INTERVENTION/EVALUATION

Question for therapeutic relief from GI symptoms. Do not change brands without consulting physician.

pancuronium bromide

(Pavulon)

See Classification section under: Neuromuscular blockers **(p. 107C)**

pantoprazole

pan-tow-**pray**-zoll

(Pantoloc✱, Protonix)

Do not confuse with Lotronex.

CLASSIFICATION

PHARMACOTHERAPEUTIC: Benzimidazole. **CLINICAL:** Proton pump inhibitor (see p. 128C).

ACTION

Converted to active metabolites that irreversibly bind to and inhibit H^+/K^+ ATPase (an enzyme on surface of gastric parietal cells). Inhibits hydrogen ion transport into gastric lumen. **Therapeutic Effect:** Increases gastric pH, reduces gastric acid production.

PHARMACOKINETICS

	Onset	Peak	Duration
PO	—	—	24 hrs

Rapidly absorbed from GI tract. Protein binding: >98%. Primarily distributed into gastric parietal cells. Metabolized extensively in liver. Primarily excreted in urine. Not removed by hemodialysis. **Half-life:** 1 hr.

USES

Treatment of erosive esophagitis associated with gastroesophageal reflux disease (GERD). Maintenance treatment of erosive esophagitis. **IV:** Short-term treatment of GERD, hypersecretion due to Zollinger-Ellison syndrome.

PRECAUTIONS

CONTRAINDICATIONS: None known. **CAUTIONS:** History of chronic/current hepatic disease.

LIFESPAN CONSIDERATIONS: Pregnancy/lactation: Unknown if drug crosses placenta or is distributed in breast milk. **Pregnancy Category B. Children:** Safety and efficacy not established. **Elderly:** No age-related precautions noted.

INTERACTIONS

DRUG: None known. **HERBAL:** None known. **FOOD:** None known. **LAB VALUES:** May increase creatinine, cholesterol, uric acid.

AVAILABILITY (Rx)

POWDER FOR INJECTION: 40 mg. **TABLETS (delayed-release):** 20 mg, 40 mg.

ADMINISTRATION/HANDLING

PO

• Give without regard to meals. • Tablet should not be crushed, chewed, split; swallow whole.

IV

Storage • Refrigerate vials, protect from light. • Do not freeze reconstituted vials. • Once diluted, stable for 12 hrs at room temperature.

Reconstitution • Mix 40-mg vial with 10 ml 0.9% NaCl injection. • Further dilute with 100 ml D_5W, 0.9% NaCl, or lactated Ringer's to concentration of 0.4 mg/ml.

Rate of administration • Infuse over 15 min using in-line filter provided. • Must position filter below the Y-site that is closest to the pt.

IV INCOMPATIBILITIES

Do not mix with other medications. Flush IV with D_5W, 0.9% NaCl, or lactated Ringer's before and after administration.

INDICATIONS/ROUTES/DOSAGE

EROSIVE ESOPHAGITIS

PO: ADULTS, ELDERLY: 40 mg/day for up to 8 wks. If not healed after 8 wks, may continue an additional 8 wks.

IV infusion: ADULTS, ELDERLY: 40 mg/day for 7–10 days.

HYPERSECRETORY CONDITIONS

IV: ADULTS, ELDERLY: 80 mg 2 times/day. May increase up to 80 mg q8h.

PO: ADULTS, ELDERLY: Initially, 40 mg 2 times/day. May increase up to 240 mg/day.

SIDE EFFECTS

RARE (<2%): Diarrhea, headache, dizziness, pruritus, skin rash.

ADVERSE REACTIONS/ TOXIC EFFECTS

None known.

NURSING IMPLICATIONS

BASELINE ASSESSMENT

Obtain baseline lab values, including serum creatinine, cholesterol.

INTERVENTION/EVALUATION

Evaluate for therapeutic response (i.e., relief of GI symptoms). Question if GI discomfort, nausea occur.

PATIENT/FAMILY TEACHING

Report headache. Swallow capsules whole; do not chew, crush. Take before eating.

paroxetine hydrochloride

pear-**ox**-eh-teen

(Asimia, Paxil, Paxil CR, Pexeva)

Do not confuse with Doxil, pyridoxine, Taxol.

CLASSIFICATION

PHARMACOTHERAPEUTIC: Serotonin uptake inhibitor. **CLINICAL:** Antidepressant, antiobsessive-compulsive, antianxiety (see pp. 11C, 36C).

ACTION

Selectively blocks uptake of neurotransmitter serotonin at CNS neuronal presynaptic membranes, thereby increasing availability at postsynaptic neuronal receptor sites. Results in enhancement of synaptic activity. **Therapeutic Effect:** Produces antidepressant effect, reduces obsessive-compulsive behavior, decreases anxiety.

PHARMACOKINETICS

Well absorbed from GI tract. Protein binding: 95%. Widely distributed. Metabolized in liver; excreted in urine. Not removed by hemodialysis. **Half-life:** 24 hrs.

USES

Treatment of major depression exhibited as persistent, prominent dysphoria (occurring nearly every day for at least 2 wks) manifested by 4 of 8 symptoms: change in appetite, change in sleep pattern, increased fatigue, impaired concentration, feelings of guilt/worthlessness, loss of interest in usual activities, psychomotor agitation/retardation, suicidal tendencies. Treatment of panic disorder, obsessive-compulsive disorder (OCD) manifested as repetitive tasks producing marked distress, time-consuming, or significant interference with social/occupational behavior. Treatment of social anxiety disorder (SAD), generalized anxiety disorder (GAD), premenstrual dysphoric disorder, post-traumatic stress disorder (PTSD).

PRECAUTIONS

CONTRAINDICATIONS: Within 14 days of MAOI therapy. **CAUTIONS:** History of seizures, mania, renal/liver impairment, cardiac disease, pts with suicidal tendencies, impaired platelet aggregation. Those who are volume depleted or using diuretics.

LIFESPAN CONSIDERATIONS: Pregnancy/lactation: May impair reproductive function. Not distributed in breast milk. **Pregnancy Category C. Children:** Safety and efficacy not established. **Elderly:** Age-related renal impairment may require dosage adjustment.

INTERACTIONS

DRUG: MAOIs may cause serotonergic syndrome (excitement, diaphoresis, rigidity, hyperthermia, autonomic hyperactivity, coma). **Cimetidine** may increase concentrations; **phenytoin** may decrease concentrations. Paroxetine can increase **risperidone** concentrations enough to cause extrapyramidal symptoms. **HERBAL: St. John's wort** may increase adverse effects. **FOOD:** None known. **LAB VALUES:** May increase liver enzymes. May decrease Hgb, Hct, WBC.

AVAILABILITY (Rx)

TABLETS: 10 mg, 20 mg, 30 mg, 40 mg. **TABLETS (controlled-release):** 12.5 mg, 25 mg, 37.5 mg. **ORAL SUSPENSION:** 10 mg/5 ml.

ADMINISTRATION/HANDLING

PO

- Give with food, milk if GI distress occurs.
- Scored tablet may be crushed.
- Best if given as single morning dose.

INDICATIONS/ROUTES/DOSAGE

Alert: Reduce dosage in elderly, pts with severe renal/hepatic impairment. Dose changes should occur at 1-wk intervals.

DEPRESSION

PO: ADULTS: Initially, 20 mg/day. May increase by 10 mg/day at ≥1-wk intervals. **Maximum:** 50 mg/day. **Controlled-release:** Initially, 25 mg/day. May increase by 12.5 mg/day at ≥1-wk intervals. **Maximum:** 62.5 mg/day.

GAD

PO: ADULTS: Initially, 20 mg/day. May increase by 10 mg/day at ≥1-wk intervals. RANGE: 20–50 mg/day.

OCD

PO: ADULTS: Initially, 20 mg/day. May increase by 10 mg/day at ≥1-wk intervals. RANGE: 20–60 mg/day.

PANIC DISORDER

PO: ADULTS: Initially, 10–20 mg/day. May increase by 10 mg/day at ≥1-wk intervals. RANGE: 10–60 mg/day.

SAD

PO: ADULTS: Initially, 20 mg/day. RANGE: 20–60 mg/day.

P

PTSD

PO: ADULTS: Initially, 20 mg/day. May increase by 10 mg/day at ≥1-wk intervals. RANGE: 20–50 mg/day.

USUAL ELDERLY DOSAGE

PO: Initially, 10 mg/day. May increase by 10 mg/day at ≥1-wk intervals. **Maximum:** 40 mg/day. **Controlled-release:** Initially, 12.5 mg/day. May increase by 12.5 mg/day at ≥1-wk intervals. **Maximum:** 50 mg/day.

SIDE EFFECTS

FREQUENT: Nausea (26%), somnolence (23%), headache, dry mouth (18%), weakness (15%), constipation (15%), dizziness, insomnia (13%), diarrhea (12%), excessive sweating (11%), tremor (8%). **OCCASIONAL:** Decreased appetite, respiratory disturbance (6%), anxiety, nervousness (5%), flatulence, paresthesia, yawning (4%), decreased libido/sexual dysfunction, abdominal discomfort (3%). **RARE:** Palpitations, vomiting, blurred vision, taste change, confusion.

P

ADVERSE REACTIONS/ TOXIC EFFECTS

None known.

NURSING IMPLICATIONS

BASELINE ASSESSMENT

Assess appearance, behavior, speech pattern, level of interest, mood.

INTERVENTION/EVALUATION

For those on long-term therapy, liver/renal function tests, blood counts should be performed periodically. Supervise suicidal-risk pt closely during early therapy (as depression lessens, energy level improves, increasing suicide potential). Assess appearance, behavior, speech pattern, level of interest, mood.

PATIENT/FAMILY TEACHING

May cause dry mouth. Avoid alcohol, St. John's wort. Therapeutic effect may be noted within 1–4 wks. Do not abruptly discontinue medication. Avoid tasks that require alertness, motor skills until response to drug is established. Inform physician of intention for pregnancy or if pregnancy occurs.

Paxil

see paroxetine

pegasparase

(Oncaspar)

See Classification section under: Cancer chemotherapeutic agents (p. 75C)

pegfilgrastim

peg-fill-**grass**-tim

(Neulasta)

CLASSIFICATION

PHARMACOTHERAPEUTIC: Colony-stimulating factor. **CLINICAL:** Hematopoietic, antineutropenic.

ACTION

Regulates production of neutrophils within bone marrow. A glycoprotein, primarily affects neutrophil progenitor proliferation, differentiation, selected end-cell functional activation. **Therapeutic Effect:** Increases phagocytic ability, antibody-dependent destruction.

PHARMACOKINETICS

Readily absorbed after subcutaneous administration. **Half-life:** 15–80 hrs.

USES

Decreases infection incidence in pts with nonmyeloid malignancies receiving myelosuppressive therapy associated with significant neutropenia, fever.

PRECAUTIONS

CONTRAINDICATIONS: Hypersensitivity to *Escherichia coli*–derived proteins, within 14 days before and 24 hrs after administration of cytotoxic chemotherapy. **CAUTIONS:** Concurrent use with medications having mycoloid properties, sickle cell disease.

LIFESPAN CONSIDERATIONS: Pregnancy/lactation: Unknown if drug crosses placenta or is distributed in breast milk. **Pregnancy Category C. Children:** Safety and efficacy not established. **Elderly:** No age-related precautions noted.

INTERACTIONS

DRUG: Lithium may potentiate release of neutrophils. **HERBAL:** None known. **FOOD:** None known. **LAB VALUES:** May increase alkaline phosphatase, LDH, uric acid, leukocyte (LAP) scores.

AVAILABILITY (Rx)

SOLUTION FOR INJECTION: 10 mg/ml.

ADMINISTRATION/HANDLING

SUBCUTANEOUS

Storage • Store in refrigerator, but may warm to room temperature up to a maximum of 48 hrs before use. Discard if left at room temperature for >48 hrs. • Protect from light. • Avoid freezing; but if accidentally frozen, may allow to thaw in refrigerator before administration. Discard if freezing takes place a second time. • Discard if discoloration, precipitate is present.

INDICATIONS

Alert: Do not administer in the period between 14 days before and 24 hrs after administration of cytotoxic chemotherapy. Do not use in infants, children, and adolescents <45 kg.

MYELOSUPPRESSION

Subcutaneous: ADULTS, ELDERLY: Give as a single 6-mg injection once per chemotherapy cycle.

SIDE EFFECTS

FREQUENT (15%–72%): Bone pain, nausea, fatigue, alopecia, diarrhea, vomiting, constipation, anorexia, abdominal pain, arthralgia, generalized weakness, peripheral edema, dizziness, stomatitis, mucositis, neutropenic fever.

ADVERSE REACTIONS/ TOXIC EFFECTS

Allergic reactions (anaphylaxis, rash, urticaria) occur rarely. Cytopenia resulting from an antibody response to growth factors occurs rarely. Splenomegaly occurs rarely (assess for left upper abdominal shoulder tip pain). Adult respiratory distress syndrome (ARDS) may occur in septic pts.

NURSING IMPLICATIONS

BASELINE ASSESSMENT

CBC, platelet count should be obtained prior to initiating therapy and routinely thereafter.

INTERVENTION/EVALUATION

Monitor for allergic-type reactions. Assess for peripheral edema, particularly behind medial malleolus (usually first area showing peripheral edema). Assess mucous membranes for evidence of stomatitis, mucositis (red mucous membranes, white patches, extreme mouth soreness). Assess muscle

P

strength. Monitor daily bowel activity, stool consistency (watery, loose, soft, semisolid, solid). ARDS may occur in septic pts.

PATIENT/FAMILY TEACHING

Inform pt of possible side effects, signs/symptoms of allergic reactions. Counsel pt on importance of compliance with pegfilgrastim treatment, including regular monitoring of blood counts.

peginterferon alfa-2a

peg-inn-ter-**fear**-on
(Pegasys)

CLASSIFICATION

PHARMACOTHERAPEUTIC: Immunomodulator. **CLINICAL:** Immunologic agent.

ACTION

Inhibits viral replication in virus-infected cells by binding to specific membrane receptors on cell surface. **Therapeutic Effect:** Suppresses cell proliferation, produces reversible decreases in leukocyte/platelet counts.

PHARMACOKINETICS

Readily absorbed after subcutaneous administration. Excreted in urine. **Half-life:** 80 hrs.

USES

Treatment of chronic hepatitis C in pts not previously treated with interferon-alfa who have compensated liver disease.

PRECAUTIONS

CONTRAINDICATIONS: Autoimmune hepatitis, decompensated liver disease, neonates, infants. **EXTREME CAUTION:** History of neuropsychiatric disorders. **CAUTIONS:** Renal impairment (creatinine clearance <50 ml/min), elderly, pulmonary disorders, compromised CNS function, cardiac diseases, autoimmune disorders, endocrine abnormalities, colitis, ophthalmologic disorders, myelosuppression.

LIFESPAN CONSIDERATIONS: Pregnancy/lactation: May have abortifacient potential. Unknown if distributed in breast milk. **Pregnancy Category C. Children:** Safety and efficacy not established in those <18 yrs. **Elderly:** CNS, cardiac, systemic effects may be more severe in the elderly, particularly in those with impaired renal function.

INTERACTIONS

DRUG: Bone marrow depressants may have additive effect. May increase **theophylline** serum level. **HERBAL:** None known. **FOOD:** None known. **LAB VALUES:** May increase SGPT (ALT). May decrease WBC, platelet counts, ANC; slight decrease in Hgb, Hct.

AVAILABILITY (Rx)

INJECTION: 180 mcg/ml.

ADMINISTRATION/HANDLING

SUBCUTANEOUS

• Refrigerate. • Vials are for single use only; discard unused portion. • Give subcutaneous in the abdomen, thigh.

INDICATIONS/ROUTES/DOSAGE

HEPATITIS C

Subcutaneous: ADULTS ≥18 YRS, ELDERLY: 180 mcg (1 ml) once weekly for 48 wks; given in the abdomen, thigh.

Alert: If moderate to severe adverse reactions occur, modify dose to 135 mcg (0.75 ml); dose reduction to 90 mcg (0.5 ml) may be necessary. Reduce dose to 135 mcg (0.75 ml) if neutrophil count is <750 cells/mm^3. In those with ANC <500 cells/mm^3, discontinue treatment until ANC returns to 1,000 cells/mm^3. Reduce dose to 90 mcg if platelet count is <50,000 cells/mm^3.

Renal function impairment requiring hemodialysis: Give 135 mcg.

Liver function impairment (progressive SGPT [ALT] increases above baseline): Give 90 mcg.

SIDE EFFECTS

FREQUENT (54%): Headache. **OCCASIONAL (13%–23%):** Alopecia, nausea, insomnia, anorexia, dizziness, diarrhea, abdominal pain, flulike symptoms (fever, body ache, fatigue), psychiatric reactions (depression, irritability, anxiety), injection site reaction. **RARE (5%–8%):** Impaired concentration, diaphoresis, dry mouth, nausea, vomiting.

ADVERSE REACTIONS/ TOXIC EFFECTS

Serious, acute hypersensitivity reactions (urticaria, angioedema, bronchoconstriction, anaphylaxis), pancreatitis, colitis, hyperthyroidism/hypothyroidism, ophthalmologic disorders, pulmonary abnormalities occur rarely.

NURSING IMPLICATIONS

BASELINE ASSESSMENT

CBC, platelet count, blood chemistry, urinalysis, renal/liver function tests, EKG should be performed prior to initial therapy and routinely thereafter. Pts with diabetes/hypertension should have an ophthalmologic exam before treatment begins.

INTERVENTION/EVALUATION

Monitor for evidence of depression. Offer emotional support. Monitor for abdominal pain, bloody diarrhea as evidence of colitis. Monitor chest x-ray for pulmonary infiltrates. Assess for pulmonary function impairment, hyperglycemia. Encourage ample fluid intake, particularly during early therapy. Assess serum hepatitis C virus RNA levels after 24 wks of treatment.

PATIENT/FAMILY TEACHING

Clinical response occurs in 1–3 mos. Flulike symptoms tend to diminish with continued therapy. Immediately report symptoms of depression, suicidal ideation. Avoid tasks requiring mental alertness, motor skills until response to drug is established.

peginterferon alfa-2b

peg-inn-ter-**fear**-on
(PEG-Intron)

◆CLASSIFICATION

PHARMACOTHERAPEUTIC: Immunomodulator. **CLINICAL:** Immunologic agent.

ACTION

Inhibits viral replication in virus-infected cells, suppresses cell proliferation by binding to specific membrane receptors on cell surface. **Therapeutic Effect:** Increases phagocytic action of macrophages, augmenting specific cytotoxicity of lymphocytes.

USES

As monotherapy or in combination with ribavirin for treatment of chronic hepatitis C in pts not previously treated with interferon alfa who have compensated liver disease and are ≥18 yrs.

PRECAUTIONS

CONTRAINDICATIONS: Autoimmune hepatitis, decompensated liver disease, history of psychiatric disorders. **CAUTIONS:** Renal impairment (creatinine clearance <50 ml/min), elderly, pulmonary disorders, compromised CNS

P

function, cardiac diseases, autoimmune disorders, endocrine abnormalities, ophthalmologic disorders, myelosuppression. **Pregnancy Category C.**

INTERACTIONS

DRUG: Bone marrow depressants may have additive effect. **HERBAL:** None known. **FOOD:** None known. **LAB VALUES:** May increase SGPT (ALT), blood glucose levels. May decrease neutrophil, platelet counts.

AVAILABILITY (Rx)

INJECTION: 50 mcg/0.5 ml; 80 mcg/0.5 ml; 120 mcg/0.5 ml; 150 mcg/0.5 ml.

ADMINISTRATION/HANDLING

SUBCUTANEOUS

Storage • Store at room temperature.

Reconstitution • Reconstitute with supplied diluent (5-ml vial). Use immediately or after reconstituted; may be refrigerated for ≤24 hrs before use.

INDICATIONS/ROUTES/DOSAGE

CHRONIC HEPATITIS C

Subcutaneous: ADULTS ≥18 YRS, ELDERLY: Administer once weekly for 1 yr on the same day each wk.

Alert: If severe adverse reactions occur, modify dose or temporarily discontinue. Dosage based on weight:

Vial Strength (mcg/ml)	Weight (kg)	mcg of Peginterferon to Administer	ml of Peginterferon to Administer
100	37–45	40	0.4
	46–56	50	0.5
160	57–72	64	0.4
	73–88	80	0.5
240	89–106	96	0.4
	107–136	120	0.5
300	137–160	150	0.5

SIDE EFFECTS

Alert: Dose-related effects.

FREQUENT (47%–50%): Flulike symptoms (fever, headache, rigors, body ache, fatigue, nausea); may decrease in severity as treatment continues. Injection site disorders (inflammation, bruising, itchiness, irritation). **OCCASIONAL (18%–29%):** Depression, anxiety, emotional lability, irritability, insomnia, alopecia, diarrhea. **RARE:** Rash, diaphoresis, dry skin, dizziness, flushing, vomiting, dyspepsia (heartburn, epigastric pain).

ADVERSE REACTIONS/ TOXIC EFFECTS

Serious, acute hypersensitivity reactions (urticaria, angioedema, bronchoconstriction, anaphylaxis), pancreatitis occur rarely. Ulcerative colitis may occur within 12 wks of initiation of treatment. Pulmonary disorders, hypothyroidism/ hyperthyroidism may occur.

NURSING IMPLICATIONS

BASELINE ASSESSMENT

CBC, platelet count, blood chemistry, urinalysis, renal/hepatic function tests, EKG should be performed prior to initial therapy and routinely thereafter. Pts with diabetes/hypertension should have an ophthalmologic exam before treatment begins.

INTERVENTION/EVALUATION

Monitor for evidence of depression; offer emotional support. Monitor for abdominal pain, bloody diarrhea as evidence of colitis. Monitor chest x-ray for pulmonary infiltrates. Assess for pulmonary function impairment, hyperglycemia. Encourage ample fluid intake, particularly during early therapy. Assess serum hepatitis C virus RNA levels after 24 wks of treatment.

PATIENT/FAMILY TEACHING

Maintain adequate hydration, avoid alcohol. May experience flulike syndrome: nausea, body ache, headache. Inform physician of persistent abdominal pain, bloody diarrhea, fever, signs of depression/infection, unusual bruising/bleeding.

pegvisomant

peg-**vis**-oh-mant
(Somavert)

◆ CLASSIFICATION

PHARMACOTHERAPEUTIC: Protein. **CLINICAL:** Acromegaly agent.

ACTION

Selectively binds to growth hormone receptors on cell surfaces, blocking the binding of endogenous growth hormones, interfering with growth hormone signal transduction. **Therapeutic Effect:** Decreases serum concentrations of IGF-1 serum protein, normalizing serum insulin-like growth factor-1 GF-1 levels.

PHARMACOKINETICS

Following subcutaneous administration, does not distribute extensively into tissues, and <1% is excreted in the urine. **Half-life:** 6 days.

USES

Treatment of acromegaly in pts with inadequate response to surgery/radiation/other medical therapies, or for whom these therapies are inappropriate.

PRECAUTIONS

CONTRAINDICATIONS: Latex allergy (stopper on the vial contains latex). **CAUTIONS:** Elderly, diabetes mellitus.

LIFESPAN CONSIDERATIONS: Pregnancy/lactation: Unknown if excreted in breast milk. **Pregnancy Category B. Children:** Safety and efficacy not established. **Elderly:** Initiation of treatment should begin at the low end of the dosage range.

INTERACTIONS

DRUG: Insulin, oral hypoglycemic agents dosing should be reduced at initiation of therapy. Pts on **opioid** therapy may require higher dosage of pegvisomant. **HERBAL:** None known. **FOOD:** None known. **LAB VALUES:** Interferes with measurement of serum growth hormone concentration. May increase SGOT (AST), SGPT (ALT), transaminase. Decreases effect of insulin on carbohydrate metabolism.

AVAILABILITY (Rx)

POWDER FOR INJECTION: 10-mg, 15-mg, 20-mg vials.

ADMINISTRATION/HANDLING

SUBCUTANEOUS

Storage • Refrigerate unreconstituted vials. • Administer within 6 hrs following reconstitution. • Solution should appear clear after reconstitution. Discard if particulate is present or solution appears cloudy.

Reconstitution • Withdraw 1 ml Sterile Water for Injection, inject into the vial of pegvisomant, aiming the stream against the glass wall. Hold the vial between the palms of both hands, roll to dissolve the powder (do not shake).

Rate of administration • Administer subcutaneously only 1 dose from each vial.

INDICATIONS/ROUTES/DOSAGE

ACROMEGALY

Subcutaneous: ADULTS, ELDERLY: Initially, 40 mg, given as a loading dose, and then 10 mg daily. After 4-6 wks, adjust dosage in 5-mg increments if serum IGF-1 concentration is still elevated (or 5-mg decrements if IGF-1 levels has decreased below the normal range). Do not exceed maximum daily dose of 30 mg.

SIDE EFFECTS

FREQUENT (23%): Infection characterized as cold symptoms, upper respiratory infection, blister, ear infection. **OCCASIONAL (5%–8%):** Back pain, dizziness, injection site reaction, peripheral edema, sinusitis, nausea. **RARE (<4%):** Diarrhea, paresthesia.

ADVERSE REACTIONS/ TOXIC EFFECTS

May produce marked elevation of liver enzymes, including serum transaminase level. Substantial weight gain occurs rarely.

NURSING IMPLICATIONS

BASELINE ASSESSMENT

Obtain baseline SGOT (AST), SGPT (ALT), alkaline phosphatase, total bilirubin serum levels.

INTERVENTION/EVALUATION

Monitor all pts with tumors that secrete growth hormone with periodic imaging scans of sella turcica for progressive tumor growth. Monitor diabetic pts for hypoglycemia. Obtain IGF-1 serum concentrations 4–6 wks after therapy begins and periodically thereafter; dosage adjustment based on results; dosage adjustment should not be based on growth hormone assays.

PATIENT/FAMILY TEACHING

Inform pt that routine monitoring of liver function tests is essential during treatment. Contact physician if jaundice (yellowing of eyes, skin) occurs.

pemoline

pem-oh-leen
(Cylert)

◆CLASSIFICATION

CLINICAL: CNS stimulant **(Schedule IV).**

ACTION

Blocks reuptake of dopaminergic neurons at cerebral cortex, subcortical structures. **Therapeutic Effect:** Reduces motor restlessness, increases mental alertness, provides mood elevation, reduces sense of fatigue.

USES

Treatment of attention deficit disorder in children with moderate to severe distraction, short attention span, hyperactivity, emotional impulsiveness.

PRECAUTIONS

CONTRAINDICATIONS: Impaired hepatic function, pts with motor tics, family history of Tourette's disorder. **CAUTIONS:** Renal impairment, hypertension, history of drug abuse, seizures, psychosis. **Pregnancy Category B.**

INTERACTIONS

DRUG: CNS-stimulating medications may increase CNS stimulation. **HERBAL:** None known. **FOOD:** None known. **LAB VALUES:** May increase SGOT (AST), SGPT (ALT), LDH.

AVAILABILITY (Rx)

TABLETS: 18.75 mg, 37.5 mg, 75 mg. **TABLETS (chewable):** 37.5 mg.

INDICATIONS/ROUTES/DOSAGE

ATTENTION DEFICIT DISORDER

PO: CHILDREN ≥6 YRS: Initially, 37.5 mg/day given as single dose in morning. May increase by 18.75 mg at weekly intervals until therapeutic response is achieved.

RANGE: 56.25–75 mg/day. **Maximum:** 112.5 mg/day.

SIDE EFFECTS

FREQUENT: Anorexia, insomnia. **OCCASIONAL:** Nausea, abdominal discomfort, diarrhea, headache, dizziness, drowsiness.

ADVERSE REACTIONS/ TOXIC EFFECTS

Dyskinetic movements of tongue/lips/ face/extremities, visual disturbances, rash have occurred. Large doses may produce extreme nervousness, tachycardia. Hepatic effects (hepatitis, jaundice) appear to be reversible when drug is discontinued. Prolonged administration to children with attention deficit disorder may produce a temporary suppression of weight and/or height patterns.

NURSING IMPLICATIONS

BASELINE ASSESSMENT

Liver function tests should be performed prior to beginning therapy and periodically during therapy.

PATIENT/FAMILY TEACHING

Avoid alcohol, caffeine. May cause dizziness, impair ability to perform tasks requiring mental alertness. May be habit forming; do not stop medication abruptly. Inform physician if dark urine, yellow skin, loss of appetite, GI complaints occur.

penbutolol

(Levatol)

See Classification section under: Beta-adrenergic blockers (p. 62C)

penciclovir

pen-**sigh**-klo-vear

(Denavir)

CLASSIFICATION

PHARMACOTHERAPEUTIC: Anti-infective. **CLINICAL:** Topical antiviral.

ACTION

Inhibits antiviral activity against herpes simplex virus (HSV). **Therapeutic Effect:** Prevents DNA synthesis, HSV replication.

USES

Treatment of recurrent herpes labialis (cold sores).

PRECAUTIONS

CONTRAINDICATIONS: None known. **CAUTIONS:** None known. **Pregnancy Category B.**

INTERACTIONS

DRUG: None known. **HERBAL:** None known. **FOOD:** None known. **LAB VALUES:** None known.

AVAILABILITY (Rx)

CREAM: 1%.

ADMINISTRATION/HANDLING

TOPICAL

• Store at room temperature. Do not freeze.

INDICATIONS/ROUTES/DOSAGE

Alert: Begin treatment as soon as possible (as soon as symptom indicating immediate onset of virus is evident or when lesions appear).

HERPES LABIALIS (cold sores)

Topical: ADULTS, ELDERLY: Apply q2h during waking hours for 4 days.

P

SIDE EFFECTS

FREQUENT (>5%): Headache, mild erythema. **OCCASIONAL** (1%–5%): Application site reaction. **RARE** (<1%): Altered taste, rash.

ADVERSE REACTIONS/ TOXIC EFFECTS

None known.

NURSING IMPLICATIONS

BASELINE ASSESSMENT

Use only on lips/face. Do not apply to oral mucous membranes. Avoid application in, near eyes (produces irritation).

PATIENT/FAMILY TEACHING

Observe precautions to avoid exposure of cold sores to direct sunlight.

penicillamine

pen-ih-**sill**-ah-mine
(Cuprimine, Depen)
Do not confuse with penicillin.

CLASSIFICATION

PHARMACOTHERAPEUTIC: Heavy metal antagonist. **CLINICAL:** Chelating agent, anti-inflammatory.

ACTION

Chelates with lead, copper, mercury, iron to form soluble complexes; depresses circulating IgM rheumatoid factor levels; depresses T-cell activity; combines with cystine to form more soluble compound. **Therapeutic Effect:** Promotes excretion of heavy metals, acts as anti-inflammatory drug, prevents renal calculi, may dissolve existing stones.

USES

Promotes excretion of copper in treatment of Wilson's disease, decreases excretion of cystine, prevents renal calculi in cystinuria associated with nephrolithiasis. Treatment of active rheumatoid arthritis not controlled with conventional therapy. **Unlabeled:** Treatment of rheumatoid vasculitis, heavy metal toxicity.

PRECAUTIONS

CONTRAINDICATIONS: History of penicillamine-related aplastic anemia or agranulocytosis, rheumatoid arthritis pts with history or evidence of renal insufficiency, pregnancy, breast-feeding. **CAUTIONS:** Elderly, debilitated, impaired renal/hepatic function, penicillin allergy. **Pregnancy Category D.**

INTERACTIONS

DRUG: **Iron supplements, antacids** may decrease absorption. **Bone marrow depressants, gold compounds, immunosuppressants** may increase risk of hematologic, renal adverse effects. **HERBAL:** None known. **FOOD:** Food may decrease absorption. **LAB VALUES:** None known.

AVAILABILITY (Rx)

CAPSULES (Cuprimine): 125 mg, 250 mg. **TABLETS (Depen):** 250 mg.

INDICATIONS/ROUTES/DOSAGE

RHEUMATOID ARTHRITIS

PO: ADULTS, ELDERLY: 125–250 mg/day. May increase at 1- to 3-mo intervals up to 1–1.5 g/day.

Alert: Dose >500 mg/day in divided doses.

CHILDREN: Initially, 3 mg/kg/day (**Maximum:** 250 mg) for 3 mos, then 6 mg/kg/day (**Maximum:** 500 mg) in 2 divided doses for 3 mos. **Maximum:** 10 mg/kg/day (1–1.5 g/day) in 3–4 divided doses.

WILSON'S DISEASE

PO: ADULTS, ELDERLY: 1 g/day in 4 divided doses. **Maximum:** 2 g/day. CHILDREN: 20 mg/kg/day in 2–4 doses. **Maximum:** 1 g/day.

Alert: Titrate to maintain urinary copper excretion >1 mg/day.

CYSTINURIA

Alert: Doses titrated to maintain urinary cystine excretion at 100–200 mg/day.

PO: ADULTS, ELDERLY: Initially, 2 g/day in divided doses q6h. RANGE: 1–4 g/day. CHILDREN: 30 mg/kg/day in 4 divided doses. **Maximum:** 4 g/day.

SIDE EFFECTS

FREQUENT: Rash (pruritic, erythematous, maculopapular, morbilliform), reduced/altered sense of taste (hypogeusia), GI disturbances (anorexia, epigastric pain, nausea, vomiting, diarrhea), oral ulcers, glossitis. **OCCASIONAL:** Proteinuria, hematuria, hot flashes, drug fever. **RARE:** Alopecia, tinnitus, pemphigoid rash (water blisters).

ADVERSE REACTIONS/ TOXIC EFFECTS

Aplastic anemia, agranulocytosis, thrombocytopenia, leukopenia, myasthenia gravis, bronchiolitis, erythematous-like syndrome, evening hypoglycemia, skin friability at sites of pressure/trauma producing extravasation or white papules at venipuncture, surgical sites reported. Iron deficiency (particularly children, menstruating women) may develop.

NURSING IMPLICATIONS

BASELINE ASSESSMENT

Baseline WBC, differential, Hgb, platelet count should be performed prior to beginning therapy, q2wks thereafter for first 6 mos, then monthly during therapy. Liver function tests (GGT, SGOT [AST], SGPT [ALT], LDH) and x-ray for renal stones should also be ordered. A 2-hr interval is necessary between iron and penicillamine therapy. In event of upcoming surgery, dosage should be reduced to 250 mg/day until wound healing is complete.

INTERVENTION/EVALUATION

Encourage copious amounts of water in pts with cystinuria. Monitor WBC, differential, platelet count. If WBC <3,500, neutrophils <2,000/mm^3, monocytes >500/mm^3, or platelet counts <100,000, or if a progressive fall in either platelet count or WBC in 3 successive determinations noted, inform physician (drug withdrawal necessary). Assess for evidence of hematuria. Monitor urinalysis for hematuria, proteinuria (if proteinuria exceeds 1 g/24 hrs, inform physician).

PATIENT/FAMILY TEACHING

Promptly report any missed menstrual periods/other indications of pregnancy, fever, sore throat, chills, bruising, bleeding, difficulty breathing on exertion, unexplained cough or wheezing. Take medication 1 hr before or 2 hrs after meals or at least 1 hr from any other drug, food, or milk.

penicillin G benzathine

pen-ih-**sil**-lin G **benz**-ah-thene
(Bicillin LA, Permapen)

FIXED COMBINATION(S)

Bicillin CR: penicillin G benzathine/penicillin procaine: 600,000 units benzathine/600,000 units procaine.

P

CLASSIFICATION

PHARMACOTHERAPEUTIC: Penicillin.
CLINICAL: Antibiotic (see p. 26C).

ACTION

Binds to one or more of the penicillin-binding proteins of bacteria. **Therapeutic Effect:** Inhibits bacterial cell wall synthesis. Bactericidal.

USES

Treatment of mild to moderate severe infections caused by organisms susceptible to low concentrations of penicillin. Prophylaxis of infections caused by susceptible organisms (e.g., rheumatic fever prophylaxis).

PRECAUTIONS

CONTRAINDICATIONS: Hypersensitivity to any penicillin. **CAUTIONS:** Impaired renal/cardiac function, seizure disorder, hypersensitivity to cephalosporins. **Pregnancy Category B.**

P

INTERACTIONS

DRUG: Probenecid increases serum concentration of penicillin. **Erythromycin** may antagonize effects of penicillin. **HERBAL:** None known. **FOOD:** None known. **LAB VALUES:** May cause positive Coombs' test.

AVAILABILITY (Rx)

INJECTION (prefilled syringe): 600,000 units/ml.

ADMINISTRATION/HANDLING

IM

- Store in refrigerator. Do not freeze.
- Administer undiluted by deep IM injection (upper outer quadrant of buttock for adolescents/adults; midlateral muscle of thigh for infants and children).

Alert: Do not give IV, intra-arterially, or subcutaneously (may cause thrombosis, severe neurovascular damage, cardiac arrest, death).

INDICATIONS/ROUTES/DOSAGE

GROUP A STREPTOCOCCAL INFECTION

IM: ADULTS, ELDERLY: 1.2 million units as a single dose. CHILDREN: 25–50,000 units/kg as a single dose.

PROPHYLAXIS FOR RHEUMATIC FEVER

IM: ADULTS, ELDERLY: 1.2 million units q3–4 wks or 600,000 units 2 times/mo. CHILDREN: 25–50,000 units/kg q3–4 wks.

EARLY SYPHILIS

IM: ADULTS, ELDERLY: 2.4 million units as a single dose in 2 injection sites.

CONGENITAL SYPHILIS

IM: CHILDREN: 50,000 units/kg qwk for 3 wks.

SYPHILIS >1 YRS' DURATION

IM: ADULTS, ELDERLY: 2.4 million units as a single dose in 2 injection sites qwk for 3 doses. CHILDREN: 50,000 units/kg qwk for 3 doses.

SIDE EFFECTS

OCCASIONAL: Lethargy, fever, dizziness, rash, pain at injection site. **RARE:** Seizures, interstitial nephritis.

ADVERSE REACTIONS/ TOXIC EFFECTS

Hypersensitivity reactions ranging from rash, fever/chills to anaphylaxis occur.

NURSING IMPLICATIONS

BASELINE ASSESSMENT

Question for history of allergies, particularly penicillins, cephalosporins, aspirin.

INTERVENTION/EVALUATION

Monitor CBC, urinalysis, renal function tests.

penicillin G potassium

pen-ih-**sil**-lin G
(Megacillin ✤, Novopen-G ✤, Pfizerpen)

◆CLASSIFICATION

PHARMACOTHERAPEUTIC: Penicillin.
CLINICAL: Antibiotic (see p. 26C).

ACTION

Binds to one or more of the penicillin-binding proteins of bacteria. **Therapeutic Effect:** Inhibits bacterial cell wall synthesis. Bactericidal.

USES

Treatment of sepsis, meningitis, pericarditis, endocarditis, pneumonia due to susceptible gram-positive organisms (not *Staphylococcus aureus*), some gram-negative organisms.

PRECAUTIONS

CONTRAINDICATIONS: Hypersensitivity to any penicillin. **CAUTIONS:** Impaired renal/liver function, seizure disorder, hypersensitivity to cephalosporins. **Pregnancy Category B.**

INTERACTIONS

DRUG: **Probenecid** increases serum concentration of penicillin. **Erythromycin** may antagonize effects of penicillin. **HERBAL:** None known. **FOOD:** **Food** or **milk** decreases absorption. **LAB VALUES:** May cause positive Coombs' test.

AVAILABILITY (Rx)

INJECTION: 5 million units. **PREMIXED DEXTROSE SOLUTION:** 1 million units, 2 million units, 3 million units.

ADMININSTRTION/HANDLING

IV

Storage • Reconstituted solution is stable for 7 days if refrigerated.

Reconstitution • Follow dilution guide per manufacturer. • After reconstitution, further dilute with 50–100 ml D_5W or 0.9% NaCl for a final concentration of 100–500,000 units/ml (50,000 units/ml for infants and neonates).

Rate of administration • Infuse over 15–60 min.

∅ IV INCOMPATIBILITIES

Amikacin (Amikin), aminophylline, amphotericin, dopamine (Intropin).

IV COMPATIBILITIES

Amiodarone (Cordarone), calcium gluconate, diltiazem (Cardizem), diphenhydramine (Benadryl), furosemide (Lasix), heparin, hydromorphone (Dilaudid), lidocaine, magnesium sulfate, methylprednisolone (Solu-Medrol), morphine, potassium chloride.

INDICATIONS/ROUTES/DOSAGE

USUAL DOSAGE

IM/IV: ADULTS, ELDERLY: 2–24 million units/day in divided doses q4–6h. CHILDREN: 100,000–400,000 units/kg/day in divided doses q4–6h.

DOSAGE IN RENAL IMPAIRMENT

Creatinine Clearance	Dosage Interval
10–30 ml/min	q8–12h
<10 ml/min	q12–18h

SIDE EFFECTS

OCCASIONAL: Lethargy, fever, dizziness, rash, electrolyte imbalance, diarrhea, thrombophlebitis. **RARE:** Seizures, interstitial nephritis.

ADVERSE REACTIONS/ TOXIC EFFECTS

Hypersensitivity reactions ranging from rash, fever/chills to anaphylaxis occur occasionally.

P

NURSING IMPLICATIONS

BASELINE ASSESSMENT

Question for history of allergies, particularly penicillins, cephalosporins, aspirin.

INTERVENTION/EVALUATION

Monitor CBC, urinalysis electrolytes, renal function tests.

penicillin G procaine

pen-ih-**sil**-lin G **pro**-cane
(Wycillin)

FIXED COMBINATION(S)

Bicillin CR: penicillin G procaine/penicillin G benzathine: 600,000 units benzathine/600,000 units procaine.

CLASSIFICATION

PHARMACOTHERAPEUTIC: Penicillin. **CLINICAL:** Antibiotic (see p. 26C).

P

ACTION

Binds to one or more of the penicillin-binding proteins of bacteria. **Therapeutic Effect:** Inhibits bacterial cell wall synthesis. Bactericidal.

USES

Treatment of mild to moderate infections caused by organisms susceptible to low concentrations of penicillin.

PRECAUTIONS

CONTRAINDICATIONS: Hypersensitivity to any penicillin. **CAUTIONS:** Impaired renal function, seizure disorder, hypersensitivity to cephalosporins. **Pregnancy Category B.**

INTERACTIONS

DRUG: Probenecid increases serum concentration of penicillin. **Erythromycin** may antagonize effects of penicillin. **HERBAL:** None known. **FOOD:** None known. **LAB VALUES:** May cause positive Coombs' test.

AVAILABILITY (Rx)

INJECTION (prefilled syringe): 600,000 units/ml.

ADMINISTRATION/HANDLING

IM

- Store in refrigerator. Do not freeze.
- Administer undiluted by deep IM injection (upper outer quadrant of buttock for adolescents/adults; midlateral muscle of thigh for infants and children.

Alert: Do not give IV, intra-arterially, or subcutaneously (may cause thrombosis, severe neurovascular damage, cardiac arrest, death).

INDICATIONS/ROUTES/DOSAGE

USUAL DOSAGE

IM: ADULTS, ELDERLY: 0.6–4.8 million units/day in divided doses q12–24h. CHILDREN: 25–50,000 units/kg/day in divided doses q12–24h.

SIDE EFFECTS

OCCASIONAL: Lethargy, fever, dizziness, rash, vasodilation, conduction disturbances, pain at injection site. **RARE:** Seizures, interstitial nephritis.

ADVERSE REACTIONS/ TOXIC EFFECTS

Hypersensitivity reactions ranging from rash, fever/chills to anaphylaxis occur occasionally.

NURSING IMPLICATIONS

BASELINE ASSESSMENT

Question for history of allergies, particularly penicillins, cephalosporins, aspirin.

INTERVENTION/EVALUATION

Monitor CBC, urinalysis, renal function tests. Observe for allergic reaction.

penicillin V potassium

(Apo-Pen-VK♣, Novo-Pen-VK♣, Pen-Vee K, V-Cillin-K)

CLASSIFICATION

PHARMACOTHERAPEUTIC: Penicillin. **CLINICAL:** Antibiotic (see p. 26C).

ACTION

Binds to bacterial membranes. **Therapeutic Effect:** Inhibits cell wall synthesis. Bactericidal.

PHARMACOKINETICS

Moderately absorbed from GI tract. Protein binding: 80%. Widely distributed. Metabolized in liver. Primarily excreted in urine. **Half-life:** 1 hr (half-life increased with impaired renal function).

USES

Treatment of mild to moderate infections of respiratory tract and skin/skin structure, otitis media, necrotizing ulcerative gingivitis; prophylaxis for rheumatic fever, dental procedures.

PRECAUTIONS

CONTRAINDICATIONS: Hypersensitivity to any penicillin. **CAUTIONS:** Renal impairment, history of allergies (particularly cephalosporins, aspirin), history of seizures.

LIFESPAN CONSIDERATIONS: Pregnancy/lactation: Readily crosses placenta; appears in cord blood, amniotic fluid. Distributed in breast milk in low concentrations. May lead to allergic sensitization, diarrhea, candidiasis, skin rash in infant. **Pregnancy Category B. Children:** Use caution in neonates/young infants (may delay renal elimination). **Elderly:** Age-related renal impairment may require dosage adjustment.

INTERACTIONS

DRUG: Probenecid may increase concentration, toxicity risk. **HERBAL:** None known. **FOOD:** None known. **LAB VALUES:** May cause positive Coombs' test.

AVAILABILITY (Rx)

TABLETS: 250 mg, 500 mg. **POWDER FOR ORAL SOLUTION:** 125 mg/5 ml, 250 mg/5 ml.

ADMINISTRATION/HANDLING

PO

• Store tablets at room temperature. Oral solution, after reconstitution, is stable for 14 days if refrigerated. • Space doses evenly around the clock. • Give without regard to meals.

INDICATIONS/ROUTES/DOSAGE

SYSTEMIC INFECTIONS

PO: ADULTS, ELDERLY, CHILDREN ≥12 YRS: 125–500 mg q6–8h. CHILDREN <12 YRS: 25–50 mg/kg/day in divided doses q6–8h. **Maximum:** 3 g/day.

PRIMARY PREVENTION OF RHEUMATIC FEVER

PO: ADULTS, ELDERLY: 500 mg 2–3 times/day for 10 days. CHILDREN: 250 mg 2–3 times/day for 10 days.

PROPHYLAXIS FOR RECURRENT RHEUMATIC FEVER

PO: ADULTS, ELDERLY, CHILDREN: 250 mg 2 times/day.

SIDE EFFECTS

FREQUENT: Mild hypersensitivity reaction (rash, fever/chills), nausea, vomiting, diarrhea. **RARE:** Bleeding, allergic reaction.

P

ADVERSE REACTIONS/ TOXIC EFFECTS

Severe hypersensitivity reaction, including anaphylaxis, may occur. Nephrotoxicity, antibiotic-associated colitis (severe abdominal pain/tenderness, fever, watery/severe diarrhea), other superinfections may result from high dosages, prolonged therapy.

NURSING IMPLICATIONS

BASELINE ASSESSMENT

Question for history of allergies, particularly penicillins, cephalosporins.

INTERVENTION/EVALUATION

Hold medication, promptly report rash (hypersensitivity) or diarrhea (with fever, abdominal pain, mucus/blood in stool may indicate antibiotic-associated colitis). Monitor I&O, urinalysis, renal function tests for nephrotoxicity. Be alert for superinfection: increased fever, sore throat, nausea, vomiting, diarrhea, ulceration/changes of oral mucosa, vaginal discharge, anal/genital pruritus. Review Hgb levels; check for bleeding: overt bleeding, bruising, swelling of tissue.

PATIENT/FAMILY TEACHING

Continue antibiotic for full length of treatment. Space doses evenly. Notify physician immediately in event of rash, diarrhea, bleeding, bruising, other new symptom.

pentaerythritol tetranitrate (P.E.T.N.)

(Duotrate, Peritrate)

See Classification section under: Nitrates

pentamidine isethionate

pen-**tam**-ih-deen

(NebuPent, Pentacarinat ♣, Pentam-300)

◆CLASSIFICATION

PHARMACOTHERAPEUTIC: Anti-infective. **CLINICAL:** Antiprotozoal.

ACTION

Interferes with nuclear metabolism, incorporation of nucleotides. **Therapeutic Effect:** Inhibits DNA, RNA, phospholipid, protein synthesis.

PHARMACOKINETICS

Minimal absorption after inhalation, well absorbed after IM administration. Widely distributed. Primarily excreted in urine. Minimally removed by hemodialysis. **Half-life:** 6.5 hrs (half-life increased with impaired renal function).

USES

Treatment of pneumonia caused by *Pneumocystis carinii* (PCP). Prevention of PCP in high-risk HIV-infected pts. **Unlabeled:** Treatment of visceral/cutaneous leishmaniasis, African trypanosomiasis.

PRECAUTIONS

CONTRAINDICATIONS: Do not use concurrently with didanosine. **CAUTIONS:** Diabetes mellitus, renal/liver impairment, hypertension/hypotension.

LIFESPAN CONSIDERATIONS: Pregnancy/lactation: Unknown if drug crosses placenta or is distributed in breast milk. **Pregnancy Category C. Children:** No age-related precautions noted. **Elderly:** Information not available.

INTERACTIONS

DRUG: Blood dyscrasia–producing medication, bone marrow depressants may increase abnormal hematologic effects. **Didanosine** may increase risk of pancreatitis. **Foscarnet** may increase hypocalcemia, hypomagnesemia, nephrotoxicity. **Nephrotoxic medications** may increase risk of nephrotoxicity. **HERBAL:** None known. **FOOD:** None known. **LAB VALUES:** May increase SGOT (AST), SGPT (ALT), alkaline phosphatase, bilirubin, BUN, creatinine. May decrease calcium, magnesium. May alter glucose levels.

AVAILABILITY (Rx)

INJECTION (Pentam-300): 300 mg. **POWDER FOR NEBULIZATION (NebuPent):** 300 mg.

ADMINISTRATION/HANDLING

Alert: Pt must be in supine position during administration, with frequent B/P checks until stable (potential for life-threatening hypotensive reaction). Have resuscitative equipment immediately available.

IM

- Reconstitute 300-mg vial with 3 ml Sterile Water for Injection to provide concentration of 100 mg/ml.

IV

Storage • Store vials at room temperature. • After reconstitution, IV solution is stable for 48 hrs at room temperature. • Discard unused portion.

Reconstitution • For intermittent IV infusion (piggyback), reconstitute each vial with 3–5 ml D_5W or Sterile Water for Injection. • Withdraw desired dose and further dilute with 50–250 ml D_5W.

Rate of administration • Infuse over 60 min. • Do not give by IV injection or rapid IV infusion (increases potential for severe hypotension).

AEROSOL (nebulizer)

- Aerosol stable for 48 hrs at room temperature. • Reconstitute 300-mg vial with 6 ml Sterile Water for Injection. Avoid NaCl (may cause precipitate).
- Do not mix with other medication in nebulizer reservoir.

∅ IV INCOMPATIBILITIES

Interleukin (Proleukin), cefazolin (Ancef), cefotaxime (Claforan), ceftazidime (Fortaz), ceftriaxone (Rocephin), fluconazole (Diflucan), foscarnet (Foscavir).

IV COMPATIBILITIES

Diltiazem (Cardizem), zidovudine (AZT, Retrovir).

INDICATIONS/ROUTES/DOSAGE

PCP TREATMENT

IV/IM: ADULTS, ELDERLY: 4 mg/kg/day once daily for 14–21 days. CHILDREN: 4 mg/kg/day once daily for 10–14 days.

PCP PREVENTION

Inhalation: ADULTS, ELDERLY: 300 mg q4wks. CHILDREN ≥5 YRS: 300 mg q3–4 wks. CHILDREN <5 YRS: 8 mg/kg/dose q3–4wks.

SIDE EFFECTS

FREQUENT: Injection (>10%): Abscess, pain at injection site. **Inhalation (>5%):** Fatigue, metallic taste, shortness of breath, decreased appetite, dizziness, rash, cough, nausea, vomiting, chills. **OCCASIONAL: Injection (1%–10%):** Nausea, decreased appetite, hypotension, fever, rash, bad taste, confusion. **Inhalation (1%–5%):** Diarrhea, headache, anemia, muscle pain. **RARE: Injection (<1%):** Neuralgia, thrombocytopenia, phlebitis, dizziness.

ADVERSE REACTIONS/ TOXIC EFFECTS

Life-threatening/fatal hypotension, arrhythmias, hypoglycemia, leukopenia,

P

nephrotoxicity/renal failure, anaphylactic shock, Stevens-Johnson syndrome, toxic epidural necrolysis occur rarely. Hyperglycemia, insulin-dependent diabetes mellitus (often permanent) may occur even months after therapy.

NURSING IMPLICATIONS

BASELINE ASSESSMENT

Avoid concurrent use of nephrotoxic drugs. Establish baseline for B/P, blood glucose. Obtain specimens for diagnostic tests prior to giving first dose.

INTERVENTION/EVALUATION

Monitor B/P during administration until stable for both IM and IV administration (pt should remain supine). Check glucose levels and clinical signs for hypoglycemia (diaphoresis, nervousness, tremor, tachycardia, palpitation, lightheadedness, headache, numbness of lips, double vision, incoordination), hyperglycemia (polyuria, polyphagia, polydipsia, malaise, visual changes, abdominal pain, headache, nausea/vomiting). Evaluate IM sites for pain, redness, induration; IV sites for phlebitis (heat, pain, red streaking over vein). Monitor renal, hepatic, hematology test results. Assess skin for rash. Evaluate equilibrium during ambulation. Be alert for respiratory difficulty when administering by inhalation route.

PATIENT/FAMILY TEACHING

Remain flat in bed during administration of medication; get up slowly with assistance only when B/P stable. Notify nurse immediately of diaphoresis, shakiness, lightheadedness, palpitations. Even several months after therapy stops, drowsiness, increased urination, thirst, anorexia may develop. Maintain adequate fluid intake. Inform physician if fever, cough, shortness of breath occurs. Avoid alcohol.

Pentasa

see mesalamine

pentazocine

(Talwin)

See Classification section under: Opioid analgesics

pentobarbital

(Nembutal)

See Classification section under: Sedative-hypnotics

pentostatin

(Nipent)

See Classification section under: Cancer chemotherapeutic agents (p. 75C)

pentoxifylline

pen-tox-ih-**fill**-in

(Pentoxyl, Trental)

Do not confuse with Tegretol.

CLASSIFICATION

PHARMACOTHERAPEUTIC: Blood viscosity-reducing agent. **CLINICAL:** Hemorheologic.

ACTION

Alters flexibility of RBCs; inhibits production of tumor necrosis factor, neutrophil activation, platelet aggregation. **Therapeutic Effect:** Reduces blood viscosity, improves blood flow.

PHARMACOKINETICS

Well absorbed after PO administration. Undergoes first-pass metabolism in liver. Primarily excreted in urine. Unknown if removed by hemodialysis. **Half-life:** 24–48 min; metabolite: 60–90 min.

USES

Symptomatic treatment of intermittent claudication associated with occlusive peripheral vascular disease, diabetic angiopathies.

PRECAUTIONS

CONTRAINDICATIONS: History of intolerance to xanthine derivatives (caffeine, theophylline, theobromine), recent cerebral/retinal hemorrhage. **CAUTIONS:** Renal/liver impairment, insulin-treated diabetes, chronic occlusive arterial disease, recent surgery, peptic ulcer disease.

LIFESPAN CONSIDERATIONS: Pregnancy/lactation: Unknown if drug crosses placenta. Distributed in breast milk. **Pregnancy Category C. Children:** Safety and efficacy not established. **Elderly:** Age-related renal impairment may require cautious use.

INTERACTIONS

DRUG: May increase effect of **antihypertensives. HERBAL:** None known. **FOOD:** None known. **LAB VALUES:** None known.

AVAILABILITY (Rx)

TABLETS (controlled-release): 400 mg.

ADMINISTRATION/HANDLING

PO

- Do not crush/break film-coated tablets.
- Give with meals to avoid GI upset.

INDICATIONS/ROUTES/DOSAGE

INTERMITTENT CLAUDICATION

PO: ADULTS, ELDERLY: 400 mg 3 times/day. Decrease to 400 mg 2 times/day if GI or CNS side effects occur. Continue for at least 8 wks.

SIDE EFFECTS

OCCASIONAL (2%–5%): Dizziness, nausea, bad taste, dyspepsia (heartburn, epigastric pain, indigestion). **RARE (<2%):** Rash, pruritus, anorexia, constipation, dry mouth, blurred vision, edema, nasal congestion, anxiety.

ADVERSE REACTIONS/ TOXIC EFFECTS

Angina, chest pain occur rarely. May be accompanied by palpitations, tachycardia, arrhythmias. Symptoms of overdosage (flushing, hypotension, nervousness, agitation, hand tremor, fever, somnolence) noted 4–5 hrs after ingestion, lasts 12 hrs.

NURSING IMPLICATIONS

INTERVENTION/EVALUATION

Assist with ambulation if dizziness occurs. Assess for hand tremor. Monitor for relief of symptoms of intermittent claudication (pain, aching, cramping in calf muscles, buttocks, thigh, feet). Symptoms generally occur while walking/exercising and not at rest or with weight bearing in absence of walking/exercising.

PATIENT/FAMILY TEACHING

Therapeutic effect generally noted in 2–4 wks. Avoid driving, tasks requiring mental alertness until response to drug is established. Do not smoke (causes constriction, occlusion of peripheral blood vessels). Limit caffeine.

P

Pepcid

see famotidine

pergolide mesylate

purr-go-lied
(Permax)

Do not confuse with Pentrax, Pernox.

CLASSIFICATION

PHARMACOTHERAPEUTIC: Dopamine agonist. **CLINICAL:** Antidyskinetic.

ACTION

Centrally active dopamine agonist. **Therapeutic Effect:** Assists in reduction in tremor, improvement in akinesia (absence of movement), posture/equilibrium disorders, rigidity of parkinsonism.

PHARMACOKINETICS

P

Well absorbed from GI tract. Protein binding: 90%. Metabolized in liver (undergoes extensive first-pass effect). Primarily excreted in urine. Unknown if removed by hemodialysis.

USES

Adjunctive treatment with levodopa/carbidopa in pts with Parkinson's disease.

PRECAUTIONS

CONTRAINDICATIONS: Hypersensitivity to pergolide or other ergot derivatives. **CAUTIONS:** Cardiac arrhythmias, history of confusion, hallucinations.

LIFESPAN CONSIDERATIONS: Pregnancy/lactation: Unknown if drug crosses placenta or is distributed in breast milk. May interfere with lactation. **Pregnancy Category B. Children:** Safety and efficacy not established. **Elderly:** No age-related precautions noted.

INTERACTIONS

DRUG: Haloperidol, loxapine, methyldopa, metoclopramide, phenothiazines may decrease effect. **Hypotension-producing medications** may increase hypotensive effect. **HERBAL:** None known. **FOOD:** None known. **LAB VALUES:** May increase plasma growth hormone.

AVAILABILITY (Rx)

TABLETS: 0.05 mg, 0.25 mg, 1 mg.

ADMINISTRATION/HANDLING

PO

- Scored tablets may be crushed.
- Give without regard to meals.

INDICATIONS/ROUTES/DOSAGE

Alert: Daily doses usually given in 3 divided doses.

PARKINSONISM

PO: ADULTS, ELDERLY: Initially, 0.05 mg/day for 2 days. Increase by 0.1–0.15 mg/day q3days over the following 12 days; then may increase by 0.25 mg/day q3days. **Maximum:** 5 mg/day. RANGE: 2–3 mg/day in 3 divided doses.

SIDE EFFECTS

FREQUENT (10%–24%): Nausea, dizziness, hallucinations, constipation, rhinitis, dystonia (impaired muscle tone), confusion, somnolence. **OCCASIONAL (3%–9%):** Postural hypotension, insomnia, dry mouth, peripheral edema, anxiety, diarrhea, dyspepsia, abdominal pain, headache, abnormal vision, anorexia, tremor, depression, rash. **RARE (<2%):** Urinary frequency, vivid dreams, neck pain, hypotension, vomiting.

ADVERSE REACTIONS/ TOXIC EFFECTS

Overdosage may require supportive measures to maintain arterial B/P (monitor cardiac function, vital signs, blood gases, serum electrolytes). Activated charcoal may be more effective than emesis or lavage.

NURSING IMPLICATIONS

INTERVENTION/EVALUATION

Be alert to neurologic effects: headache, lethargy, mental confusion, agitation. Monitor for evidence of dyskinesia (difficulty with movement). Monitor B/P. Assess for clinical reversal of Parkinson symptoms (improvement of tremor of head/hands at rest, masklike facial expression, shuffling gait, muscular rigidity).

PATIENT/FAMILY TEACHING

Tolerance to feeling of lightheadedness develops during therapy. To reduce hypotensive effect, rise slowly from lying to sitting position, permit legs to dangle momentarily before standing. Avoid tasks that require alertness, motor skills until response to drug is established. Dry mouth, drowsiness, dizziness may be expected responses of drug. Avoid alcoholic beverages during therapy.

perindopril erbumine

(Aceon)

See Classification section under: Angiotensin-converting enzyme (ACE) inhibitors (p. 6C)

perphenazine

(Trilafon)

See Classification section under: Antipsychotics

phenazopyridine hydrochloride

feen-ah-zoe-**peer**-ih-deen
(Azo-Gesic, Azo-Standard, Phenazo✤, Prodium, Pyridium, Pyronium✤, Uristat)

Do not confuse with pyridoxine.

CLASSIFICATION

PHARMACOTHERAPEUTIC: Interstitial cystitis agent. **CLINICAL:** Urinary tract analgesic.

ACTION

Exerts topical analgesic effect on urinary tract mucosa. **Therapeutic Effect:** Provides relief of urinary pain, burning, urgency, frequency.

PHARMACOKINETICS

Well absorbed from GI tract. Partially metabolized in liver. Primarily excreted in urine.

USES

Symptomatic relief of pain, burning, urgency, frequency resulting from lower urinary tract mucosa irritation (may be caused by infection, trauma, surgery).

PRECAUTIONS

CONTRAINDICATIONS: Renal/liver insufficiency. **CAUTIONS:** None known.

LIFESPAN CONSIDERATIONS: Pregnancy/lactation: Unknown if drug crosses placenta or is distributed in breast milk. **Pregnancy Category B. Children:** No age-related precautions noted in those >6 yrs. **Elderly:** Age-related renal impairment may increase toxicity.

INTERACTIONS

DRUG: None known. **HERBAL:** None known. **FOOD:** None known. **LAB VAL-**

P

UES: May interfere with urinalysis color reactions (e.g., urinary glucose, ketone tests, urinary protein, determination of urinary steroids).

AVAILABILITY (Rx)

TABLETS: 95 mg, 100 mg, 200 mg.

ADMINISTRATION/HANDLING

PO

- Give with meals.

INDICATIONS/ROUTES/DOSAGE

ANALGESIC

PO: ADULTS: 100–200 mg 3–4 times/day. CHILDREN >6 YRS: 12 mg/kg/day in 3 divided doses for 2 days.

DOSE INTERVAL IN RENAL IMPAIRMENT

Creatinine Clearance	Interval
50–80 ml/min	q8–16h
<50 ml/min	Avoid use

SIDE EFFECTS

OCCASIONAL: Headache, GI disturbance, rash, pruritus.

P

ADVERSE REACTIONS/ TOXIC EFFECTS

Overdosage levels in pts with impaired renal function or severe hypersensitivity may develop renal toxicity, hemolytic anemia, hepatic toxicity. Methemoglobinemia generally occurs as result of massive, acute overdosage.

NURSING IMPLICATIONS

INTERVENTION/EVALUATION

Assess for therapeutic response: relief of pain, burning, urgency, frequency of urination.

PATIENT/FAMILY TEACHING

A reddish orange discoloration of urine should be expected. May stain fabric. Take with meals (reduces possibility of GI upset).

phenelzine sulfate

fen-ell-zeen
(Nardil)

CLASSIFICATION

PHARMACOTHERAPEUTIC: MAOI. **CLINICAL:** Antidepressant (see p. 35C).

ACTION

Inhibits MAO enzyme system at CNS storage sites. The reduced MAO activity causes an increased concentration in epinephrine, norepinephrine, serotonin, dopamine at neuron receptor sites. **Therapeutic Effect:** Produces antidepressant effect.

USES

Treatment of depression refractory to other antidepressants, electroconvulsive therapy. **Unlabeled:** Treatment of panic disorder, vascular/tension headaches.

PRECAUTIONS

CONTRAINDICATIONS: Pheochromocytoma, renal/liver impairment, cerebrovascular/cardiovascular disease. **CAUTIONS:** Ingestion of tyramine-containing foods. **Pregnancy Category C.**

INTERACTIONS

DRUG: **Alcohol, CNS depressants** may increase CNS depressant effects. **Tricyclic antidepressants, fluoxetine, trazodone** may cause serotonin syndrome. May increase effect of **oral hypoglycemics, insulin.** B/P may increase with **buspirone. Caffeine-containing medications** may increase cardiac arrhythmias, hypertension. May precipitate hypertensive crises with **carbamazepine, cyclobenzaprine, maprotiline, other MAOIs. Meperidine, other opioid analgesics** may produce immediate excitation, diaphoresis, rigidity, severe hypertension/hypotension, severe respiratory distress, coma, convulsions, vascular collapse, death. May increase CNS stimulant effects of **methylphenidate. Sympathomimetics** may increase cardiac stimulant, vasopressor effects. **Tyramine, foods with pressor amines (e.g., aged cheese)** may cause sudden, severe hypertension. **HERBAL:** None known. **FOOD: Tyramine-containing foods, trytophan, dopamine, chocolate, caffeine** may increase B/P. **LAB VALUES:** None known.

AVAILABILITY (Rx)

TABLETS: 15 mg.

INDICATIONS/ROUTES/DOSAGE

DEPRESSION

PO: ADULTS: 15 mg 3 times/day. May increase to 60–90 mg/day. ELDERLY: Initially, 7.5 mg/day. May increase by 7.5–15 mg/day q3–4wks up to 60 mg/day in divided doses.

SIDE EFFECTS

FREQUENT: Postural hypotension, restlessness, GI upset, insomnia, dizziness, headache, lethargy, weakness, dry mouth, peripheral edema. **OCCASIONAL:** Flushing, diaphoresis, rash, urinary frequency, increased appetite, transient impotence. **RARE:** Visual disturbances.

ADVERSE REACTIONS/ TOXIC EFFECTS

Hypertensive crisis may be noted by severe hypertension, occipital headache radiating frontally, neck stiffness/soreness, nausea, vomiting, diaphoresis, fever/chilliness, clammy skin, dilated pupils, palpitations. Tachycardia, bradycardia, constricting chest pain may also be present. Antidote for hypertensive crisis: 5–10 mg phentolamine IV injection.

NURSING IMPLICATIONS

BASELINE ASSESSMENT

Periodic liver function tests should be performed in pts requiring high dosage who are undergoing prolonged therapy.

INTERVENTION/EVALUATION

Assess appearance, behavior, speech pattern, level of interest, mood. Monitor for occipital headache radiating frontally and/or neck stiffness/soreness (may be first signal of impending hypertensive crisis). Monitor B/P, heart rate, diet, weight, change in mood.

PATIENT/FAMILY TEACHING

Antidepressant relief may be noted during first week of therapy; maximum benefit noted in 2–6 wks. Report headache, neck stiffness/soreness immediately. Avoid foods that require bacteria/molds for their preparation/preservation or those that contain tyramine (e.g., cheese, sour cream, beer, wine, figs, raisins, bananas, avocados, soy sauce, yeast extracts, yogurt, papaya, broad beans, meat tenderizers, excessive amounts of caffeine [coffee, tea, chocolate]) or OTC preparations for hay fever, colds, weight reduction.

P

phenobarbital

feen-oh-**bar**-bih-tall

(Luminal)

FIXED-COMBINATION(S)

Dilantin with PB: phenobarbital/phenytoin (an anticonvulsant): 15 mg/100 mg; 30 mg/100 mg. **Bellergal-S:** phenobarbital/ergotamine/belladonna (an anticholinergic): 40 mg/0.6 mg/0.2 mg.

◆ **CLASSIFICATION**

PHARMACOTHERAPEUTIC: Barbiturate **(Schedule IV). CLINICAL:** Anticonvulsant, hypnotic (see p. 31C).

ACTION

Binds at GABA receptor complex, enhancing GABA activity. **Therapeutic Effect:** Depresses CNS activity, reticular activating system.

PHARMACOKINETICS

Onset	Peak	Duration
PO		
20–60 min	—	6–10 hrs
IV		
5 min	30 min	4–10 hrs

Well absorbed after PO, parenteral administration. Protein binding: 35%–50%. Rapidly, widely distributed. Metabolized in liver. Primarily excreted in urine. Removed by hemodialysis. **Half-life:** 53–118 hrs.

USES

Management of generalized tonic-clonic (grand mal) seizures, partial seizures, control of acute convulsive episodes (status epilepticus, eclampsia, febrile seizures). **Unlabeled:** Prophylaxis/treatment of hyperbilirubinemia.

PRECAUTIONS

CONTRAINDICATIONS: Preexisting CNS depression, severe pain, porphyria, severe respiratory disease. **CAUTIONS:** Renal/liver impairment.

LIFESPAN CONSIDERATIONS: Pregnancy/lactation: Readily crosses placenta. Distributed in breast milk. Produces respiratory depression in neonates during labor. May cause postpartum hemorrhage, hemorrhagic disease in newborn. Withdrawal symptoms may appear in neonates born to women receiving barbiturates during last trimester of pregnancy. Lowers serum bilirubin concentration in neonates. **Pregnancy Category D. Children:** May cause paradoxical excitement. **Elderly:** May exhibit excitement, confusion, mental depression.

INTERACTIONS

DRUG: May decrease effects of **glucocorticoids, digoxin, metronidazole, oral anticoagulants, quinidine, tricyclic antidepressants. Alcohol, CNS depressants** may increase effect. May increase metabolism of **carbamazepine. Valproic acid** decreases metabolism, increases concentration, toxicity. **HERBAL:** None known. **FOOD:** None known. **LAB VALUES:** May decrease bilirubin. Therapeutic blood serum level: 10–40 mcg/ml; toxic blood serum level: >40 mcg/ml.

AVAILABILITY (Rx)

TABLETS: 30 mg, 100 mg. **ELIXIR:** 20 mg/5 ml. **INJECTION:** 60 mg/ml, 130 mg/ml.

ADMINISTRATION/HANDLING

PO

• Give without regard to meals. Tablets may be crushed. • Elixir may be mixed with water, milk, fruit juice.

IM

• Do not inject more than 5 ml in any one IM injection site (produces tissue irritation). • Inject IM deep into gluteus maximus or lateral aspect of thigh.

IV

Storage • Store vials at room temperature.

Reconstitution • May give undiluted or may dilute with NaCl, D_5W, lactated Ringer's.

Rate of administration • Adequately hydrate pt before and immediately after (decreases risk of adverse renal effects). • Do not inject IV faster than 1 mg/kg/min and a maximum of 30 mg/min for

children and 60 mg/min for adults. (Too rapid IV may produce severe hypotension, marked respiratory depression.)
• Inadvertent intra-arterial injection may result in arterial spasm with severe pain, tissue necrosis. Extravasation in subcutaneous tissue may produce redness, tenderness, tissue necrosis. If either occurs, treat with 0.5% procaine solution into affected area, apply moist heat.

⊘ IV INCOMPATIBILITIES

Amphotericin B complex (Abelcet, AmBisome, Amphotec), hydrocortisone (Solu-Cortef), hydromorphone (Dilaudid), insulin.

IV COMPATIBILITIES

Calcium gluconate, enalapril (Vasotec), fentanyl (Sublimaze), fosphenytoin (Cerebyx), morphine, propofol (Diprivan).

INDICATIONS/ROUTES/DOSAGE

STATUS EPILEPTICUS

IV: ADULTS, ELDERLY, CHILDREN, NEONATES: (Loading dose): 15–20 mg/kg as single dose or in divided doses.

ANTICONVULSANT

Alert: Maintenance dose to begin 12 hrs after loading dose.

IV/PO: ADULTS, ELDERLY, CHILDREN >12 YRS: 1–3 mg/kg/day. CHILDREN 6–12 YRS: 4–6 mg/kg/day. CHILDREN 1–5 YRS: 6–8 mg/kg/day. CHILDREN <1 YR: 5–6 mg/kg/day. NEONATES: 3–4 mg/kg/day.

SEDATION

PO/IM: ADULTS, ELDERLY: 30–120 mg/day in 2–3 divided doses. CHILDREN: 2 mg/kg 3 times/day.

HYPNOTIC

PO/IM/IV/subcutaneous: ADULTS, ELDERLY: 100–320 mg at bedtime. CHILDREN: 3–5 mg/kg.

SIDE EFFECTS

OCCASIONAL (1%–3%): Somnolence. **RARE (<1%):** Confusion, paradoxical CNS hyperactivity/nervousness in children, excitement/restlessness in elderly (generally noted during first 2 wks of therapy, particularly noted in presence of uncontrolled pain).

ADVERSE REACTIONS/ TOXIC EFFECTS

Abrupt withdrawal after prolonged therapy may produce effects ranging from markedly increased dreaming, nightmares, insomnia, tremor, diaphoresis, vomiting, to hallucinations, delirium, seizures, status epilepticus. Skin eruptions appear as hypersensitivity reaction. Blood dyscrasias, liver disease, hypocalcemia occur rarely. Overdosage produces cold/clammy skin, hypothermia, severe CNS depression, cyanosis, rapid pulse, Cheyne-Stokes respirations. Toxicity may result in severe renal impairment.

NURSING IMPLICATIONS

BASELINE ASSESSMENT

Assess B/P, pulse, respirations immediately prior to administration. **Hypnotic:** Raise bed rails, provide environment conducive to sleep (back rub, quiet environment, low lighting). **Seizures:** Review history of seizure disorder (length, presence of auras, LOC). Observe frequently for recurrence of seizure activity. Initiate seizure precautions.

INTERVENTION/EVALUATION

Monitor CNS status, seizure activity, liver/renal function, respiratory rate, heart rate, B/P. Monitor for therapeutic serum level (10–30 mcg/ml). Therapeutic blood serum level: 10–40 mcg/ml; toxic blood serum level: >40 mcg/ml.

PATIENT/FAMILY TEACHING

Avoid alcohol, limit caffeine. May be habit forming. Do not discontinue

P

abruptly. May cause dizziness/drowsiness (avoid activities that require mental alertness, physical coordination).

phentolamine

fen-**toll**-ah-mean
(Rogitine)

Do not confuse with phentermine.

CLASSIFICATION

PHARMACOTHERAPEUTIC: Alpha-adrenergic blocking agent. **CLINICAL:** Pheochromocytoma agent.

ACTION

Blocks presynaptic ($alpha_2$) and postsynaptic ($alpha_1$) adrenergic receptors, acting on both arterial tree and venous bed. **Therapeutic Effect:** Decreases total peripheral resistance, diminishes venous return to heart.

PHARMACOKINETICS

Onset	Peak	Duration
IM		
15–20 min	20 min	30–45 min
IV		
Immediate	2 min	15–30 min

Metabolized in the liver. Excreted in urine. **Half-life:** 19 min.

USES

Diagnosis of pheochromocytoma. Control/prevention of hypertensive episodes immediately before, during surgical excision. Prevention/treatment of dermal necrosis, sloughing after IV administration of norepinephrine/dopamine. **Unlabeled:** Treatment of CHF.

PRECAUTIONS

CONTRAINDICATIONS: Epinephrine, MI, coronary insufficiency, angina, coronary artery disease. **CAUTIONS:** Gastritis, peptic ulcer, history of arrhythmias.

LIFESPAN CONSIDERATIONS: Pregnancy/lactation: Unknown if drug crosses placenta or is distributed in breast milk. **Pregnancy Category C. Children:** Safety and efficacy not established. **Elderly:** No age-related precautions noted.

INTERACTIONS

DRUG: May decrease effects of **sympathomimetics (e.g., dopamine, phenylephrine). HERBAL:** None known. **FOOD:** None known. **LAB VALUES:** None known.

AVAILABILITY (Rx)

INJECTION: 5-mg vials.

ADMINISTRATION/HANDLING

Alert: Maintain pt in supine position (preferably in quiet, darkened room) during pheochromocytoma testing. Decrease in B/P generally noted in <2 min.

IV

Storage • Store vials at room temperature. • After reconstitution, is stable for 48 hrs at room temperature or 1 wk if refrigerated.

Reconstitution • Reconstitute 5-mg vial with 1 ml Sterile Water for Injection to provide concentration of 5 mg/ml.

Rate of administration • Inject rapidly. Monitor B/P immediately after injection, q30sec for 3 min, then q60sec for 7 min.

IV INCOMPATIBILITY

Do not mix with any other medications.

IV COMPATIBILITIES

Amiodarone (Cordarone), dobutamine (Dobutrex).

INDICATIONS/ROUTES/DOSAGE

DIAGNOSIS OF PHEOCHROMOCYTOMA

IM/IV: ADULTS, ELDERLY: 2.5–5 mg.

CHILDREN: 0.05–0.1 mg/kg/dose. **Maximum:** 5 mg.

CONTROL/PREVENTION OF HYPERTENSION IN PHEOCHROMOCYTOMA

IV: ADULTS, ELDERLY: 5 mg 1–2 hrs before surgery. May repeat. CHILDREN: 0.05–0.1 mg/kg/dose 1–2 hrs before surgery. May repeat.

PREVENTION/TREATMENT OF NECROSIS/SLOUGHING

Infiltrate area with 1 ml of solution (reconstituted by diluting 5–10 mg in 0.9% NaCl) within 12 hrs of extravasation. **Maximum:** 0.1–0.2 mg/kg or 5 mg total.

SIDE EFFECTS

OCCASIONAL: Weakness, dizziness, flushing, nausea, vomiting, diarrhea, orthostatic hypotension.

ADVERSE REACTIONS/TOXIC EFFECTS

Tachycardia, arrhythmias, acute/prolonged hypotension may occur. Do not use epinephrine (will produce further drop in B/P).

NURSING IMPLICATIONS

BASELINE ASSESSMENT

Positive pheochromocytoma test indicated by decrease in B/P >35 mm Hg systolic, >25 mm Hg diastolic pressure. Negative test indicated by no B/P change, elevated B/P, or B/P elevated 35 mm Hg systolic and 25 mm Hg diastolic. Preinjection B/P generally occurs within 15–30 min following administration.

INTERVENTION/EVALUATION

Monitor B/P, heart rate. Assess for orthostatic hypotension. Monitor for extravasation (skin color streaking).

phenylephrine hydrochloride

fen-ill-**eh**-frin

(AK-Dilate, Neo-Synephrine, Prefrin)

◆ CLASSIFICATION

PHARMACOTHERAPEUTIC: Sympathomimetic, alpha receptor stimulant. **CLINICAL:** Nasal decongestant, mydriatic, vasopressor (see p. 134C).

ACTION

Acts on alpha-adrenergic receptors of vascular smooth muscle. **Therapeutic Effect:** Causes vasoconstriction of arterioles of nasal mucosa/conjunctiva, activates dilator muscle of the pupil to cause contraction, produces systemic arterial vasoconstriction.

PHARMACOKINETICS

	Onset	Peak	Duration
Subcutaneous	10–15 min	—	1 hr
IM	10–15 min	—	0.5–2 hrs
IV	Immediate	—	15–20 min

Minimal absorption after intranasal, ophthalmic administration. Metabolized in liver, GI tract. Primarily excreted in urine. **Half-life:** 2.5 hrs.

USES

Nasal: Topical application to nasal mucosa reduces nasal secretion, promoting drainage of sinus secretions. **Ophthalmic:** Topical application to conjunctiva relieves congestion, itching, minor irritation; whitens sclera of eye. **Parenteral:** Vascular failure in shock, drug-induced hypotension.

PRECAUTIONS

CONTRAINDICATIONS: Pheochromocytoma, severe hypertension, ventricular tachycardia, acute pancreatitis, hepatitis, thrombosis, heart disease, narrow-angle glaucoma. **CAUTIONS:** Hyperthyroidism, bradycardia, heart block, severe arteriosclerosis.

LIFESPAN CONSIDERATIONS: Pregnancy/lactation: Crosses placenta. Distributed in breast milk. **Pregnancy Category C. Children:** May exhibit increased absorption, toxicity with nasal preparation. No age-related precautions noted with systemic use. **Elderly:** More likely to experience adverse effects.

INTERACTIONS

DRUG: **Tricyclic antidepressants, maprotiline** may increase cardiovascular effects. May decrease effect of **methyldopa.** May have mutually inhibitory effects with **beta-blockers.** May increase risk of arrhythmias with **digoxin. Ergonovine, oxytocin** may increase vasoconstriction. **MAOIs** may increase vasopressor effects. **HERBAL: Ma huang (ephedra)** may increase CNS stimulation. **FOOD:** None known. **LAB VALUES:** None known.

AVAILABILITY (OTC)

INJECTION (Rx): 1% (10 mg/ml). **NASAL SOLUTION:** 0.25%, 0.5%. **NASAL SPRAY:** 0.25%, 0.5%, 1%. **OPHTHALMIC SOLUTION:** 0.12%, 2.5%, 10%.

P

ADMINISTRATION/HANDLING

NASAL

• Blow nose prior to administering medication. With head tilted back, apply drops in 1 nostril. Remain in same position and wait 5 min prior to applying drops in other nostril. • Sprays should be administered into each nostril with head erect. Sniff briskly while squeezing container. Wait 3–5 min before blowing nose gently. Rinse tip of spray bottle.

OPHTHALMIC

• Instruct pt to tilt head backward, look up. • Gently pull lower lid down to form pouch and instill medication. • Do not touch tip of applicator to lids or any surface. • When lower lid is released, have pt keep eye open without blinking for at least 30 sec. • Apply gentle finger pressure to lacrimal sac (bridge of the nose, inside corner of the eye) for 1–2 min. • Remove excess solution around eye with tissue. Wash hands immediately to remove medication on hands.

IV

Storage • Store vials at room temperature.

Reconstitution • For IV push, dilute 1 ml of 10 mg/ml solution with 9 ml Sterile Water for Injection to provide a concentration of 1 mg/ml. • For IV infusion, dilute 10-mg vial with 500 ml D_5W or 0.9% NaCl to provide a concentration of 2 mcg/ml. Maximum concentration: 500 mg/250 ml.

Rate of administration • For IV push, give over 20–30 sec. • For IV infusion, give as per physician order.

IV INCOMPATIBILITY

Thiopentothal (Pentothal).

IV COMPATIBILITIES

Amiodarone (Cordarone), dobutamine (Dobutrex), lidocaine, potassium chloride, propofol (Diprivan).

INDICATIONS/ROUTES/DOSAGE

NASAL DECONGESTANT

PO: ADULTS, ELDERLY, CHILDREN >12 YRS: 2–3 drops, 1–2 sprays of 0.25%–0.5% solution into each nostril. CHILDREN 6–12 YRS: 2–3 drops or 1–2 sprays of 0.25% solution in each nostril. CHILDREN <6 YRS: 2–3 drops of 0.125% solution in each nostril. Repeat q4h as needed. Do not use for >3 days.

OPHTHALMIC

Ophthalmic: ADULTS, ELDERLY, CHILDREN >12 YRS: 1–2 drops of 0.125% solution q3–4h.

HYPOTENSION/SHOCK

IM/subcutaneous: ADULTS, ELDERLY: 2–5 mg/dose q1–2h. CHILDREN: 0.1 mg/kg/dose q1–2h.

IV bolus: ADULTS, ELDERLY: 0.1–0.5 mg/dose q10–15min as needed. CHILDREN: 5–20 mcg/kg/dose q10–15min.

IV infusion: ADULTS, ELDERLY: 100–180 mcg/min. CHILDREN: 0.1–0.5 mcg/kg/min. Titrate to desired effect.

SIDE EFFECTS

FREQUENT: Nasal: Rebound nasal congestion due to overuse (>3 days). **OCCASIONAL:** Mild CNS stimulation (restlessness, nervousness, tremors, headache, insomnia), particularly in those hypersensitive to sympathomimetics (generally, elderly pts). **Nasal:** Stinging, burning, drying of nasal mucosa. **Ophthalmic:** Transient burning/stinging, brow ache, blurred vision.

ADVERSE REACTIONS/ TOXIC EFFECTS

Large doses may produce tachycardia, palpitations (particularly in those with cardiac disease), lightheadedness, nausea, vomiting. Overdosage in those >60 yrs may result in hallucinations, CNS depression, seizures. Prolonged nasal use may produce chronic swelling of nasal mucosa, rhinitis.

NURSING IMPLICATIONS

BASELINE ASSESSMENT

If phenylephrine 10% ophthalmic is instilled into denuded/damaged corneal epithelium, corneal clouding may result.

INTERVENTION/EVALUATION

Monitor B/P, heart rate.

PATIENT/FAMILY TEACHING

Discontinue drug if adverse reactions occur. Do not use for nasal decongestion for >3–5 days (rebound congestion). Discontinue drug if insomnia, dizziness, weakness, tremor, feeling of irregular heartbeat occurs. **Nasal:** Stinging/burning of inside nose may occur. **Ophthalmic:** Blurring of vision with eye instillation generally subsides with continued therapy. Discontinue medication if redness/swelling of eyelids, itching appears.

phenytoin

phen-ih-toyn
(Dilantin, Epamin✤)

Do not confuse with Dilaudid, mephenytoin.

phenytoin sodium

(Dilantin)

FIXED-COMBINATION(S)

Dilantin with PB: phenytoin/phenobarbital (a barbiturate): 100 mg/15 mg; 100 mg/30 mg.

◆ CLASSIFICATION

PHARMACOTHERAPEUTIC: Hydantoin. **CLINICAL:** Anticonvulsant, antiarrhythmic (see p. 32C).

P

ACTION

Anticonvulsant: Stabilizes neuronal membranes in motor cortex. **Therapeutic Effect:** Limits spread of seizure activity. Stabilizes threshold against hyperexcitability. Decreases post-tetanic potentiation, repetitive discharge. **Antiarrhythmic:** Decreases abnormal ventricular automaticity. **Therapeutic Effect:** Shortens refractory period, QT interval, action potential duration.

PHARMACOKINETICS

Slowly, variably absorbed after PO administration; slow but completely absorbed after IM administration. Protein binding: 90%–95%. Widely distributed. Metabolized in liver. Primarily excreted in urine. Not removed by hemodialysis. **Half-life:** 22 hrs.

USES

Management of generalized tonic-clonic seizures (grand mal), complex partial seizures (psychomotor), cortical focal seizures, status epilepticus. Ineffective in absence seizures, myoclonic seizures, atonic epilepsy when used alone. Treatment of cardiac arrhythmias due to digoxin intoxication. **Unlabeled:** Treatment of digoxin-induced arrhythmias, trigeminal neuralgia; muscle relaxant in treatment of muscle hyperirritability; adjunct in treatment of tricyclic antidepressant toxicity.

PRECAUTIONS

CONTRAINDICATIONS: Seizures due to hypoglycemia, hydantoin hypersensitivity. **IV Route Only:** Sinus bradycardia, sinoatrial block, second- and third-degree heart block, Adam-Stokes syndrome. **EXTREME CAUTION: IV Route Only:** Respiratory depression, MI, CHF, damaged myocardium. **CAUTIONS:** Impaired hepatic/renal function, severe myocardial insufficiency, hypotension, hyperglycemia.

P

LIFESPAN CONSIDERATIONS: Pregnancy/lactation: Crosses placenta. Is distributed in small amount in breast milk. Fetal hydantoin syndrome (craniofacial abnormalities, nail/digital hypoplasia, prenatal growth deficiency) has been reported. There is increased frequency of seizures in pregnant women due to altered absorption of metabolism of phenytoin. May increase risk of hemorrhage in neonate, maternal bleeding during delivery. **Pregnancy Category D. Children:** More susceptible to gingival hyperplasia, coarsening of facial features, excess body hair. **Elderly:** No age-related precautions noted but lower dosages recommended.

INTERACTIONS

DRUG: May decrease effect of **glucocorticoids. Alcohol, CNS depressants** may increase CNS depression. **Antacids** may decrease absorption. **Amiodarone, anticoagulants, cimetidine, disulfiram, fluoxetine, isoniazid, sulfonamides** may increase phenytoin concentration, effects, toxicity. **Fluconazole, ketoconazole, miconazole** may increase concentration. **Lidocaine, propranolol** may increase cardiac depressant effects. **Valproic acid** may increase concentration, decrease metabolism. May increase **xanthine** metabolism. **HERBAL:** None known. **FOOD:** None known. **LAB VALUES:** May increase alkaline phosphatase, GGT, glucose. Therapeutic blood serum level: 10–20 mcg/ml; toxic blood serum level: >20 mcg/ml.

AVAILABILITY (Rx)

CAPSULES: 30 mg, 100 mg. **TABLETS (chewable):** 50 mg. **ORAL SUSPENSION:** 125 mg/5 ml. **INJECTION:** 50 mg/ml.

ADMINISTRATION/HANDLING

PO

• Give with food if GI distress occurs. • Do not chew/break capsules. Tablets may be chewed. • Shake oral suspension well before using.

IV

Alert: Give by IV push.

Storage • Precipitate may form if parenteral form is refrigerated (will dissolve at room temperature). • Slight yellow discoloration of parenteral form does not affect potency, but do not use if solution is not clear or if precipitate is present.

Reconstitution • May give undiluted or may dilute with 0.9% NaCl.

Rate of administration • Administer 50 mg >2–3 min for elderly. In neonates, administer at rate not exceeding 1–3 mg/kg/min. • Severe hypotension, cardiovascular collapse occurs if rate of IV injection exceeds 50 mg/min for adults. IV push very painful (chemical irritation of vein due to alkalinity of solution). To minimize effect, flush vein with sterile saline solution through same IV needle/catheter after each IV push. • IV toxicity characterized by CNS depression, cardiovascular collapse.

IV INCOMPATIBILITIES

Diltiazem (Cardizem), dobutamine (Dobutrex), enalapril (Vasotec), heparin, hydromorphone (Dilaudid), insulin, lidocaine, morphine, nitrolgycerin, norepinephrine (Levophed), potassium chloride, propofol (Diprivan).

INDICATIONS/ROUTES/DOSAGE

Alert: Maintenance dose usually 12 hrs after loading dose.

STATUS EPILEPTICUS

IV: ADULTS, ELDERLY, CHILDREN: LOADING DOSE: 15–18 mg/kg. NEONATES: 15–20 mg/kg. ADULTS, ELDERLY: MAINTENANCE DOSE: 300 mg/day in 2–3 divided doses. CHILDREN 10–16 YRS: 6–7 mg/kg/day. CHILDREN 7–9 YRS: 7–8 mg/kg/day. CHILDREN 4–6 YRS: 7.5–9 mg/kg/day. CHILDREN 0.5–3 YRS: 8–10 mg/kg/day. NEONATES: 5–8 mg/kg/day.

ANTICONVULSANT

PO: ADULTS, ELDERLY, CHILDREN: LOADING DOSE: 15–20 mg/kg in 3 divided doses 2–4 hrs apart. MAINTENANCE DOSE: Same as above.

ARRHYTHMIAS

IV: ADULTS, ELDERLY, CHILDREN: LOADING DOSE: 1.25 mg/kg q5min. May repeat up to total dose of 15 mg/kg.

PO: ADULTS, ELDERLY: MAINTENANCE DOSE: 250 mg 4 times/day for 1 day, then 250 mg 2 times/day for 2 days, then 300–400 mg/day in divided doses 1–4 times/day.

PO/IV: CHILDREN: MAINTENANCE DOSE: 5–10 mg/kg/day in 2–3 divided doses.

SIDE EFFECTS

FREQUENT: Drowsiness, lethargy, confusion, slurred speech, irritability, gingival hyperplasia, hypersensitivity reaction (fever, rash, lymphadenopathy), constipation, dizziness, nausea. **OCCASIONAL:** Headache, hair growth, insomnia, muscle twitching.

ADVERSE REACTIONS/ TOXIC EFFECTS

Abrupt withdrawal may precipitate status epilepticus. Blood dyscrasias, lymphadenopathy, osteomalacia (due to interference of vitamin D metabolism) may occur. Phenytoin blood concentration of 25 mcg/ml (toxic) may produce ataxia (muscular incoordination), nystagmus (rhythmic oscillation of eyes), double vision. As level increases, extreme lethargy to comatose states occur.

P

NURSING IMPLICATIONS

BASELINE ASSESSMENT

Anticonvulsant: Review history of seizure disorder (intensity, frequency, duration, LOC). Initiate seizure precautions. Liver function tests, CBC, platelet count should be performed prior to beginning therapy and periodically during therapy. Repeat CBC, platelet count 2 wks following initiation of therapy and 2 wks following administration of maintenance dose.

INTERVENTION/EVALUATION

Observe frequently for recurrence of seizure activity. Assess for clinical improvement (decrease in intensity/frequency of seizures). Monitor CBC with differential, liver/renal function tests, B/P (with IV use). Assist with ambulation if drowsiness, lethargy occurs. Monitor for therapeutic serum level (10–20 mcg/ml). Therapeutic blood serum level: 10–20 mcg/ml; toxic blood serum level: >20 mcg/ml.

PATIENT/FAMILY TEACHING

Pain may occur with IV injection. To prevent gingival hyperplasia (bleeding, tenderness, swelling of gums), encourage good oral hygiene care, gum massage, regular dental visits. CBC should be performed every month for 1 yr after maintenance dose is established and q3mos thereafter. Urine may appear pink, red, red-brown. Report sore throat, fever, glandular swelling, skin reaction (hematologic toxicity). Drowsiness usually diminishes with continued therapy. Do not abruptly withdraw medication after long-term use (may precipitate seizures). Strict maintenance of drug therapy is essential for seizure control, arrhythmias. Avoid tasks that require alertness, motor skills until response to drug is established. Avoid alcohol.

P

PhosLo

see calcium acetate

phosphates

(Fleet enema, Fleet Phosphosoda, K-Phosphate, Neutra-Phos K, Uro KP)

CLASSIFICATION

PHARMACOTHERAPEUTIC: Electrolyte. **CLINICAL:** Mineral.

ACTION

Participates in bone deposition, calcium metabolism, utilization of B complex vitamins, buffer in acid-base equilibrium. **Laxative:** Exerts osmotic effect in small intestine. **Therapeutic Effect:** Produces distention; promotes peristalsis, evacuation of bowel.

PHARMACOKINETICS

Poorly absorbed after PO administration. PO form excreted in feces, IV forms excreted in urine.

USES

Prophylactic treatment of hypophosphatemia. Short-term treatment of constipation, for evacuation of colon for exams; urinary acidifier for reduction of formation of calcium stones. **Unlabeled:** Prevention of calcium renal calculi.

PRECAUTIONS

CONTRAINDICATIONS: Hyperphosphatemia, hyperkalemia, hypocalcemia, hypomagnesemia, hypernatremia, severe renal function impairment, CHF, abdominal pain (rectal dosage form), fecal impaction (rectal dosage form), phosphate kidney stones. **CAUTIONS:** Renal impairment, concomitant use of potassium-sparing drugs, adrenal insufficiency, cirrhosis.

LIFESPAN CONSIDERATIONS: Pregnancy/lactation: Unknown if drug crosses placenta or is distributed in breast milk. **Pregnancy Category C. Children/elderly:** No age-related precautions noted.

INTERACTIONS

DRUG: Glucocorticoids with sodium phosphate may cause edema. **Antacids** may decrease absorption. **Calcium-containing medications** may increase risk of calcium deposition in soft tissues, decrease phosphate absorption. **NSAIDs, ACE inhibitors, potassium-sparing diuretics, potassium-containing medications, salt substitutes with potassium phosphate** may increase potassium concentration. **Digoxin, potassium phosphate** may increase risk of heart block (due to hyperkalemia). **Phosphate-containing medications** may increase risk of hyperphosphatemia. **Sodium-containing medication with sodium phosphate** may increase risk of edema. **HERBAL:** None known. **FOOD:** None known. **LAB VALUES:** None known.

AVAILABILITY (Rx)

INJECTION: 3 mM/ml. **TABLETS. ORAL SOLUTION. ENEMA. POWDER.**

ADMINISTRATION/HANDLING

PO

• Dissolve tablets in water. • Take after meals or with food (decreases GI upset). • Maintain high fluid intake (prevents kidney stones).

IV

Storage • Store at room temperature.

Reconstitution • Must be diluted. Soluble in all commonly used IV solutions.

Rate of administration Maximum rate of infusion: 0.06 mmol phosphate/kg/hr.

IV INCOMPATIBILITY

Dobutamine (Dobutrex).

IV COMPATIBILITIES

Diltiazem (Cardizem), enalapril (Vasotec), famotidine (Pepcid), magnesium sulfate, metoclopramide (Reglan).

INDICATIONS/ROUTES/DOSAGE

HYPOPHOSPHATEMIA

IV: ADULTS, ELDERLY: 50–70 mmol/day. CHILDREN: 0.5–1.5 mmol/kg/day.

PO: ADULTS, ELDERLY: 50–150 mmol/day. CHILDREN: 2–3 mmol/kg/day.

LAXATIVE

PO: ADULTS, ELDERLY, CHILDREN ≥4 YRS: 1–2 capsules/packets 4 times/day. CHILDREN <4 YRS: 1 capsule/packet 4 times/day.

Rectal: ADULTS, ELDERLY, CHILDREN ≥12 YRS: 4.5-oz enema as single dose. May repeat. CHILDREN <12 YRS: 2.25-oz enema as single dose. May repeat.

URINARY ACIDIFICATION

PO: ADULTS, ELDERLY: 2 tablets 4 times/day.

SIDE EFFECTS

FREQUENT: Mild laxative effect first few days of therapy. **OCCASIONAL:** GI upset (diarrhea, nausea, abdominal pain, vomiting). **RARE:** Headache; dizziness; mental confusion; heaviness of legs; fatigue; muscle cramps; numbness/tingling of hands, feet, around lips; peripheral edema; irregular heartbeat; weight gain; thirst.

ADVERSE REACTIONS/TOXIC EFFECTS

High phosphate levels may produce extra-skeletal calcification.

NURSING IMPLICATIONS

INTERVENTION/EVALUATION

Monitor serum calcium, phosphorus, potassium, sodium, SGOT (AST), SGPT (ALT), alkaline phosphatase, bilirubin levels routinely.

PATIENT/FAMILY TEACHING

Report diarrhea, nausea, vomiting.

P

physostigmine

(Antilirium)

Do not confuse with Prostigmin, pyridostigmine.

◆CLASSIFICATION

PHARMACOTHERAPEUTIC: Parasympathomimetic (cholinergic). **CLINICAL:** Anticholinesterase agent (see p. 44C).

ACTION

Inhibits destruction of acetylcholine by enzyme acetylcholinesterase. **Therapeutic Effect:** Improves skeletal muscle tone, stimulates salivary/sweat gland secretion.

USES

Antidote for reversal of toxic CNS effects due to anticholinergic drugs, tricyclic antidepressants. **Unlabeled: Systemic:** Treatment of hereditary ataxia.

PRECAUTIONS

CONTRAINDICATIONS: Asthma, gangrene, diabetes, cardiovascular disease, mechanical obstruction of intestinal/urogenital tract, vagotonic state, pts receiving ganglionic-blocking agents. Hypersensitivity to cholinesterase inhibitors or any component of the preparation; active uveal inflammation; angle-closure (narrow-angle) glaucoma before iridectomy; glaucoma associated with iridocyclitis. **CAUTIONS:** Bronchial asthma, GI disturbances, peptic ulcer, bradycardia, hypotension, recent MI, epilepsy, parkinsonism, other disorders that may respond adversely to vagotonic effects. Use ophthalmic physostigmine only when shorter-acting miotics are not adequate, except in aphakics. **Pregnancy Category C.**

INTERACTIONS

DRUG: May increase effects of **cholinesterases (e.g., bethanechol, carbachol).** May prolong action of **succinylcholine. HERBAL:** None known. **FOOD:** None known. **LAB VALUES:** None known.

INDICATIONS/ROUTES/DOSAGE

ANTIDOTE

IM/IV: ADULTS, ELDERLY: Initially, 0.5–2 mg. If no response, repeat q20min until response occurs or adverse cholinergic effects occur. If initial response occurs, may give additional doses of 1–4 mg at 30- to 60-min intervals as life-threatening signs recur (arrhythmias, seizures, deep coma). CHILDREN: 0.01–0.03 mg/kg. May give additional doses at 5- to 10-min intervals until response occurs, adverse cholinergic effects occur, or total dose of 2 mg given.

SIDE EFFECTS

COMMON: Miosis, increased GI and skeletal muscle tone, reduced pulse rate. **OCCASIONAL:** Hypertensive pts may react with marked fall in B/P.

ADVERSE REACTIONS/ TOXIC EFFECTS

Parenteral overdosage produces a cholinergic reaction manifested as abdominal discomfort/cramping, nausea, vomiting, diarrhea, flushing, feeling of warmth/heat about face, excessive salivation/diaphoresis, urinary urgency, blurred vision. Requires a withdrawal of all anticholinergic drugs and immediate use of 0.6–1.2 mg atropine sulfate IM/IV for adults, 0.01 mg/kg in infants and children <12 yrs.

NURSING IMPLICATIONS

BASELINE ASSESSMENT

Have tissues readily available at pt's bedside.

INTERVENTION/EVALUATION

Parenteral: Assess vital signs immediately prior to and q15–30min following administration. Monitor diligently for cholinergic reaction (diaphoresis, irregular heartbeat, muscle weakness, abdominal pain, dyspnea, hypotension).

PATIENT/FAMILY TEACHING

Adverse effects often subside after the first few days of therapy. Avoid night driving, activities requiring visual acuity in dim light.

pilocarpine hydrochloride

pie-low-car-pine

(Adsorbocarpine, Akarpine, Carpine, Isopto, Ocu-Carpine, Pilocar, Pilopine, Piloptic, Pilostat, Salagen)

CLASSIFICATION

PHARMACOTHERAPEUTIC: Cholinergic parasympathomimetic. **CLINICAL:** Dry mouth agent.

See Classification section under: Antiglaucoma agents.

ACTION

Increases secretion by the exocrine glands by stimulating cholinergic receptors. **Therapeutic Effect:** Produces salivary gland production.

PHARMACOKINETICS

	Onset	Peak	Duration
PO	20 min	1 hr	3–5 hrs

Inactivation of pilocarpine thought to occur at neuronal synapses and probably in plasma. Excreted in the urine. Absorption is decreased if taken with a high-fat meal. **Half-life:** 4–12 hrs.

USES

Treatment of symptoms of dry mouth from salivary gland hypofunction caused by radiotherapy for cancer of the head/neck, treatment of symptoms of dry mouth in pts with Sjogren's syndrome.

PRECAUTIONS

CONTRAINDICATIONS: Uncontrolled asthma; when miosis is undesirable (acute iritis, narrow-angle [angle-closure] glaucoma). **CAUTIONS:** Significant cardiovascular/pulmonary disease, hepatic function impairment.

LIFESPAN CONSIDERATIONS: Pregnancy/lactation: May impair reproductive function. **Pregnancy Category C. Children:** Safety and efficacy not established. **Elderly:** Increased incidence of urinary frequency, diarrhea, dizziness.

INTERACTIONS

DRUG: May antagonize effects of **anticholinergics. Beta-blockers** may produce conduction disturbances. **HERBAL:** None known. **FOOD: High-fat meal** may decrease rate of pilocarpine absorption. **LAB VALUES:** None known.

AVAILABILITY (Rx)

TABLETS: 5 mg.

ADMINISTRATION/HANDLING

May give without regard to food.

INDICATIONS/DOSAGE/ROUTES

HEAD AND NECK CANCER

PO: ADULTS, ELDERLY: 5 mg 3 times daily. RANGE: 15–30 mg/day (do not exceed 2 tablets/dose).

SJOGREN'S SYNDROME

PO: ADULTS, ELDERLY: 5 mg 4 times daily. RANGE: 20–40 mg/day.

HEPATIC FUNCTION IMPAIRMENT

PO: ADULTS, ELDERLY: 5 mg twice daily.

SIDE EFFECTS

FREQUENT (29%): Diaphoresis. **OCCASIONAL (5%–11%):** Headache, dizziness, urinary frequency, flushing, dyspepsia

P

(heartburn, epigastric distress), nausea, asthenia (feeling of fatigue, weakness), lacrimation, visual disturbances. **RARE (<4%):** Diarrhea, abdominal pain, peripheral edema, chills.

ADVERSE REACTIONS/ TOXIC EFFECTS

Dehydration may develop if pt sweats excessively and does not drink enough fluids. There is a notable increase (2–3 times higher) in urinary frequency, diarrhea, dizziness in pts ≥ 65 yrs than compared to pts <65 yrs.

NURSING IMPLICATIONS

BASELINE ASSESSMENT

Assess oral mucosa for evidence of dryness. Encourage adequate daily fluid intake.

INTERVENTION/EVALUATION

Monitor daily bowel activity/stool consistency (watery, loose, soft, semisolid, solid). Assess for evidence of dizziness. Monitor for dehydration by checking skin for turgor, tenting. Monitor urinary frequency.

PATIENT/FAMILY TEACHING

Drink several glasses of water between meals. Caution pt that visual changes may occur, esp. at night. Avoid tasks that require alertness, motor skills until response to drug is established.

pimecrolimus

pim-eh-**crow**-leh-mus
(Elidel)

CLASSIFICATION

PHARMACOTHERAPEUTIC: Immunomodulator. **CLINICAL:** Anti-inflammatory.

ACTION

Inhibits release of cytokine, an enzyme that produces an inflammatory reaction. **Therapeutic Effect:** Produces anti-inflammatory activity.

USES

Treatment of mild to moderate atopic dermatitis (eczema).

PRECAUTIONS

CONTRAINDICATIONS: None known. **CAUTIONS:** None known.

INTERACTIONS

DRUG: None known. **HERBAL:** None known. **FOOD:** None known. **LAB VALUES:** None known.

AVAILABILITY (Rx)

TOPICAL: 1% cream.

INDICATIONS/ROUTES/DOSAGE

ATOPIC DERMATITIS (eczema)

Topical: ADULTS, ELDERLY, ADOLESCENTS, CHILDREN 2–17 YRS: Apply to affected area twice daily for up to 3 wks (up to 6 wks in adolescents, children 2–17 yrs). Rub in gently, completely.

SIDE EFFECTS

RARE: Transient application-site sensation of burning/feeling of heat.

ADVERSE REACTIONS/ TOXIC EFFECTS

Lymphadenopathy, phototoxicity occur rarely.

NURSING IMPLICATIONS

PATIENT/FAMILY TEACHING

Wash hands after application. May cause a mild to moderate feeling of warmth, sensation of burning at the site of application. Inform physician if application site reaction is severe or lasts for >1 wk. Avoid artificial sunlight, tanning beds. Contact physician if no improvement in the atopic dermatitis is seen following 6 wks of treatment or if condition worsens.

pindolol

(Novo-Pindol ✽, Visken)

Do not confuse with Panadol, Parlodel, Plendil.

See Classification section under: Beta-adrenergic blockers (p. 62C)

pioglitazone

pie-oh-**glit**-ah-zone
(Actos)

CLASSIFICATION

CLINICAL: Antidiabetic (see p. 40C).

ACTION

Improves target-cell response to insulin without increasing pancreatic insulin secretion. Decreases hepatic glucose output, increases insulin-dependent glucose utilization in skeletal muscle. **Therapeutic Effect:** Lowers blood glucose concentration.

PHARMACOKINETICS

Rapidly absorbed. Highly protein bound (>99%), primarily to albumin. Metabolized in liver. Excreted in urine. Unknown if removed by hemodialysis. **Half-life:** 16–24 hrs.

USES

Adjunct to diet, exercise to lower blood glucose in those with type 2 non–insulin-dependent diabetes mellitus (NIDDM). Used as monotherapy or in combination with a sulfonylurea or insulin to improve glycemic control.

PRECAUTIONS

CONTRAINDICATIONS: Diabetic ketoacidosis, type 1 diabetes mellitus, active liver disease, increased serum transaminase levels (SGPT [ALT] >2.5 times normal serum level). **CAUTIONS:** Hepatic function impairment, CHF, edematous pts.

LIFESPAN CONSIDERATIONS: Pregnancy/lactation: Unknown if drug crosses placenta or is distributed in breast milk. Not recommended in pregnant or breast-feeding women. **Pregnancy Category C. Children:** Safety and efficacy not established. **Elderly:** No age-related precautions noted.

INTERACTIONS

DRUG: May alter effects of **oral contraceptives. Ketoconazole** may significantly inhibit metabolism of pioglitazone. **HERBAL:** None known. **FOOD:** None known. **LAB VALUES:** May decrease Hgb levels by 2%–4%, bilirubin, SGOT (ALT), alkaline phosphatase. <1% experience SGPT (ALT) values = 3 times normal level. May increase CPK levels.

AVAILABILITY (Rx)

TABLETS: 15 mg, 30 mg, 45 mg.

ADMINISTRATION/HANDLING

PO

- Give without regard to meals.

INDICATIONS/ROUTES/DOSAGE

DIABETES MELLITUS, COMBINATION THERAPY

PO: ADULTS, ELDERLY: **Insulin:** Initially, 15–30 mg once/day. Initially, continue current insulin dose, then decrease insulin dose by 10%–25% if hypoglycemia or plasma glucose levels decrease to <100 mg/dl. **Maximum:** 45 mg/day.

Sulfonylureas: Initially, 15–30 mg/day. Decrease sulfonylurea if hypoglycemia occurs.

Metformin: Initially, 15–30 mg/day.

Monotherapy: Monotherapy is not to be used if pt is well controlled with diet and exercise alone. Initially, 15–30 mg/day. May increase dosage in increments up to 45 mg/day.

SIDE EFFECTS

FREQUENT (9%–13%): Headache, upper respiratory tract infection. **OCCASIONAL (5%–6%):** Sinusitis, myalgia (muscle aches), pharyngitis, aggravated diabetes mellitus.

ADVERSE REACTIONS/ TOXIC EFFECTS

None known.

NURSING IMPLICATIONS

BASELINE ASSESSMENT

Obtain liver enzyme levels prior to initiating therapy and periodically thereafter. Ensure follow-up instruction if pt/family do not thoroughly understand diabetes management or glucose-testing technique.

INTERVENTION/EVALUATION

Monitor blood glucose, Hgb, liver function tests, esp. SGOT (AST), SGPT (ALT). Assess for hypoglycemia (cool/wet skin, tremors, dizziness, anxiety, headache, tachycardia, numbness in mouth, hunger, diplopia), hyperglycemia (polyuria, polyphagia, polydipsia, nausea, vomiting, dim vision, fatigue, deep rapid breathing). Be alert to conditions that alter glucose requirements: fever, increased activity/stress, surgical procedures.

PATIENT/FAMILY TEACHING

Understand signs/symptoms of hypoglycemia and its management. Avoid alcohol. Inform physician of chest pain, palpitations, abdominal pain, fever, rash, hypoglycemic reactions, yellowing of skin/eyes, dark urine, light stool, nausea, vomiting.

pipecuronium

(Arduan)

See Classification section under: Neuromuscular blockers

piperacillin sodium

(Pipracil)

See Classification section under: Antibiotic: penicillins

piperacillin sodium/ tazobactam sodium

pip-ur-ah-**sill**-in/tay-zoe-**back**-tam

(Tazocin ✦, Zosyn)

Do not confuse with Zofran, Zyvox.

◆CLASSIFICATION

PHARMACOTHERAPEUTIC: Penicillin. **CLINICAL:** Antibiotic (see p. 27C).

ACTION

Piperacillin: Binds to bacterial membranes. **Therapeutic Effect:** Inhibits cell wall synthesis. Bactericidal. **Tazobactam:** Inactivates bacterial beta-lactamase enzymes. **Therapeutic Effect:** Protects piperacillin from inactivation by beta-lactamase–producing organisms, extends spectrum of activity, prevents bacterial overgrowth.

PHARMACOKINETICS

Protein binding: 16%–30%. Widely distributed. Primarily excreted unchanged in urine. Removed by hemodialysis. **Half-life:** 0.7–1.2 hrs (half-life increased with impaired renal function, hepatic cirrhosis).

USES

Treatment of appendicitis (complicated by rupture, abscess); peritonitis; uncomplicated and complicated skin/skin structure infections, including cellulitis, cutaneous abscesses, ischemic/diabetic foot infections; postpartum endometritis; pelvic inflammatory disease; community-acquired pneumonia (moderate severity only); moderate to severe nosocomial pneumonia.

PRECAUTIONS

CONTRAINDICATIONS: Hypersensitivity to any penicillin. **CAUTIONS:** History of allergies, esp. cephalosporins, other drugs, renal impairment, preexisting seizure disorder.

LIFESPAN CONSIDERATIONS: Pregnancy/lactation: Readily crosses placenta; appears in cord blood, amniotic fluid. Distributed in breast milk in low concentrations. May lead to allergic sensitization, diarrhea, candidiasis, skin rash in infant. **Pregnancy Category B. Children:** Dosage not established for those <12 yrs. **Elderly:** Age-related renal impairment may require dosage adjustment.

INTERACTIONS

DRUG: Probenecid may increase concentration, risk of toxicity. **Hepatotoxic** medications may increase hepatotoxicity. **HERBAL:** None known. **FOOD:** None known. **LAB VALUES:** May increase SGOT (AST), SGPT (ALT), alkaline phosphatase, bilirubin, LDH, sodium. May cause positive Coombs' test. May decrease potassium.

AVAILABILITY (Rx)

POWDER FOR INJECTION: 2.25 g, 3.375 g, 4.5 g. **PREMIX READY TO USE:** 2.25 g, 3.375 g, 4.5 g.

ADMINISTRATION/HANDLING

IV

Storage • Reconstituted vial is stable for 24 hrs at room temperature or 48 hrs if refrigerated. • After further dilution, is stable for 24 hrs at room temperature or 7 days if refrigerated.

Reconstitution • Reconstitute each 1 g with 5 ml D_5W or 0.9% NaCl. Shake vigorously to dissolve. • Further dilute with at least 50 ml D_5W, 0.9% NaCl, D_5W 0.9% NaCl, or lactated Ringer's.

Rate of administration • Infuse over 30 min.

IV INCOMPATIBILITIES

Amphotericin (Fungizone), amphotericin B complex (Abelcet, AmBisome, Amphotec), chlorpromazine (Thorazine), dacarbazine (DTIC), daunorubicin (Cerubidine), dobutamine (Dobutrex), doxorubicin (Adriamycin), doxorubicin liposome (Doxil), droperidol (Inapsine), famotidine (Pepcid), haloperidol (Haldol), hydroxyzine (Vistaril), idarubicin (Idamycin), minocycline (Minocin), nalbuphine (Nubain), prochlorpremazine (Compazine), promethazine (Phenergan), vancomycin (Vancocin).

IV COMPATIBILITIES

Aminophylline, bumetanide (Bumex), calcium gluconate, diphenhydramine (Benadryl), dopamine (Intropin), enalapril (Vasotec), furosemide (Lasix), granisetron (Kytril), heparin, hydrocortisone (Solu-Cortef), hydromorphone (Dilaudid), lorazepam (Ativan), magnesium sulfate, methylprednisolone (Solu-

P

Medrol), metoclopramide (Reglan), morphine, ondansetron (Zofran), potassium chloride.

INDICATIONS/ROUTES/DOSAGE

SEVERE INFECTIONS

IV: ADULTS, ELDERLY, CHILDREN >12 YRS: 4 g/0.5 g q8h or 3 g/0.375 g q6h. **Maximum:** 18 g/2.25 g daily.

MODERATE INFECTIONS

IV: ADULTS, ELDERLY, CHILDREN >12 YRS: 2 g/0.225 g q6–8h.

DOSAGE IN RENAL IMPAIRMENT

Dose and/or frequency based on creatinine clearance.

Creatinine Clearance	Dosage
20–40 ml/min	8 g/1 g/day (2.25 g q6h)
<20 ml/min	6 g/0.75 g/day (2.25 g q8h)

HEMODIALYSIS

IV: ADULTS, ELDERLY: 2.25 g q8h with additional dose of 0.75 g after each dialysis.

P

SIDE EFFECTS

FREQUENT: Diarrhea, headache, constipation, nausea, insomnia, rash. **OCCASIONAL:** Vomiting, dyspepsia, pruritus, fever, agitation, pain, moniliasis, dizziness, abdominal pain, edema, anxiety, dyspnea, rhinitis.

ADVERSE REACTIONS/ TOXIC EFFECTS

Antibiotic-associated colitis (severe abdominal pain/tenderness, fever, watery/ severe diarrhea) may result from altered bacterial balance. Overdosage, more often with renal impairment, may produce seizures, neurologic reactions. Severe hypersensitivity reactions, including anaphylaxis, occur rarely.

NURSING IMPLICATIONS

BASELINE ASSESSMENT

Question for history of allergies, esp. to penicillins, cephalosporins.

INTERVENTION/EVALUATION

Monitor bowel activity, stool consistency carefully; mild GI effects may be tolerable, but increasing severity may indicate onset of antibiotic-associated colitis. Be alert for superinfection: severe genital/anal pruritus, abdominal pain, severe mouth soreness, moderate to severe diarrhea. Monitor I&O, urinalysis, renal function tests. Monitor electrolytes, esp. potassium.

piroxicam

purr-**ox**-i-kam

(Apo-Piroxicam ✱, Feldene, Fexicam ✱, Novopirocam ✱)

CLASSIFICATION

PHARMACOTHERAPEUTIC: Nonsteroidal anti-inflammatory. **CLINICAL:** Anti-inflammatory, analgesic (see p. 111C).

ACTION

Produces analgesic, anti-inflammatory effect by inhibiting prostaglandin synthesis. **Therapeutic Effect:** Reduces inflammatory response, intensity of pain stimulus reaching sensory nerve endings.

USES

Symptomatic treatment of acute/chronic rheumatoid arthritis, osteoarthritis. **Unlabeled:** Treatment of ankylosing spondylitis, acute gouty arthritis, dysmenorrhea.

PRECAUTIONS

CONTRAINDICATIONS: Active peptic ulcer, GI ulceration, chronic inflammation of GI tract, GI bleeding disorders, history of hypersensitivity to aspirin/NSAIDs. **CAUTIONS:** Impaired renal/cardiac function, hypertension, GI disease, concomitant use of anticoagulants. **Pregnancy Category C** (**D** if used in third trimester).

INTERACTIONS

DRUG: May increase effects of **oral anticoagulants, heparin, thrombolytics.** May decrease effect of **antihypertensives, diuretics. Salicylates, aspirin** may increase risk of GI side effects, bleeding. **Bone marrow depressants** may increase risk of hematologic reactions. May increase concentration, toxicity of **lithium.** May increase toxicity of **methotrexate. Probenecid** may increase concentration. **HERBAL: St. John's wort** may increase risk of phototoxicity. May decrease effect of **feverfew. Ginkgo biloba** may increase risk of bleeding. **FOOD:** None known. **LAB VALUES:** May increase serum transaminase activity. May decrease uric acid.

AVAILABILITY (Rx)

CAPSULES: 10 mg, 20 mg.

ADMINISTRATION/HANDLING

PO

- Do not crush/break capsule form.
- May give with food, milk, antacids if GI distress occurs.

INDICATIONS/ROUTES/DOSAGE

ACUTE/CHRONIC RHEUMATOID ARTHRITIS, OSTEOARTHRITIS

PO: ADULTS, ELDERLY: Initially, 10–20 mg/day as single/divided doses. Some pts may require up to 30–40 mg/day. CHILDREN: 0.2–0.3 mg/kg/day. **Maximum:** 15 mg/day.

SIDE EFFECTS

FREQUENT (3%–9%): Dyspepsia, nausea, dizziness. **OCCASIONAL (1%–3%):** Diarrhea, constipation, abdominal cramping/pain, flatulence, stomatitis. **RARE (<1%):** Increased B/P, hives, painful/difficult urination, ecchymosis, blurred vision, insomnia.

ADVERSE REACTIONS/ TOXIC EFFECTS

Peptic ulcer, GI bleeding, gastritis, severe hepatic reaction (cholestasis, jaundice) occur rarely. Nephrotoxicity (dysuria, hematuria, proteinuria, nephrotic syndrome), severe hypersensitivity reaction (fever, chills, bronchospasm), hematologic toxicity (anemia, leukopenia, eosinophilia, thrombocytopenia) may occur rarely with long-term treatment.

NURSING IMPLICATIONS

BASELINE ASSESSMENT

Assess onset, type, location, duration of pain/inflammation. Inspect appearance of affected joints for immobility, deformities, skin condition.

INTERVENTION/EVALUATION

Monitor pattern of daily bowel activity, stool consistency. Monitor for evidence of nausea, GI distress. Evaluate for therapeutic response (relief of pain, stiffness, swelling; increased joint mobility; reduced joint tenderness; improved grip strength). Monitor CBC, renal/liver function tests.

PATIENT/FAMILY TEACHING

Avoid aspirin, alcohol during therapy (increases risk of GI bleeding). If GI upset occurs, take with food, milk, antacids. Avoid tasks that require alertness until response to drug is established.

Pitocin

see oxytocin

P

Plavix

see clopidogrel

Plendil

see felodipine

plicamycin

ply-kah-**my**-sin
(Mithracin)
Do not confuse with Minocin.

CLASSIFICATION

PHARMACOTHERAPEUTIC: Antibiotic. **CLINICAL:** Antihypercalcemic, antineoplastic (see p. 75C).

ACTION

Forms complexes with DNA, inhibiting DNA-directed RNA synthesis. May inhibit parathyroid hormone effect on osteoclasts, inhibit bone resorption. **Therapeutic Effect:** Lowers serum calcium concentration. Blocks hypercalcemic action of vitamin D, blocks action of parathyroid hormone. Decreases serum phosphate levels.

PHARMACOKINETICS

Onset	Peak	Duration
Reduces calcium		
1–2 days	2–3 days	3–15 days

Protein binding: None. Localized in liver, kidney, formed bone surfaces. Crosses blood-brain barrier, enters CSF. Primarily excreted in urine.

USES

Treatment of malignant testicular tumors, hypercalcemia, hypercalcuria associated with advanced neoplasms. **Unlabeled:** Treatment of Paget's disease refractory to other therapy.

PRECAUTIONS

CONTRAINDICATIONS: Existing thrombocytopenia, thrombocytopathy, coagulation disorders, tendency to hemorrhage, impaired bone marrow function. **EXTREME CAUTION:** Renal/hepatic impairment. **CAUTIONS:** Electrolyte imbalance.

LIFESPAN CONSIDERATIONS: Pregnancy/lactation: Contraindicated during pregnancy. Breast-feeding not recommended. **Pregnancy Category X. Children/elderly:** No information available.

INTERACTIONS

DRUG: May increase effect of **oral anticoagulants, heparin, thrombolytics.** May increase risk of hemorrhage with **NSAIDs, aspirin, dipyridamole, sulfinpyrazone, valproic acid. Bone marrow depressants, hepatotoxic and nephrotoxic medications** may increase toxicity. **Calcium-containing medications, vitamin D** may decrease effect. **Live virus vaccines** may potentiate virus replication, increase vaccine side effects, decrease pt's antibody response to vaccine. **HERBAL:** None known. **FOOD:** None known. **LAB VALUES:** None known.

AVAILABILITY (Rx)

POWDER FOR INJECTION: 2,500 mcg.

ADMINISTRATION/HANDLING

IV

Alert: May be carcinogenic, mutagenic, or teratogenic. Handle with extreme care during preparation/administration.

Storage • Refrigerate vials. • Solution must be freshly prepared before use; discard unused portions.

Reconstitution • Reconstitute 2,500-mcg (2.5-mg) vial with 4.9 ml Sterile Water for Injection to provide concentration of 500 mcg/ml (0.5 mg/ml). • Dilute with 500–1,000 ml D_5W or 0.9% NaCl.

Rate of administration • Infuse over 4–6 hrs. • Extravasation produces painful inflammation, induration. Sloughing may occur. Aspirate as much drug as possible. Apply warm compresses.

∅ IV INCOMPATIBILITY
Cefepime (Maxipime).

IV COMPATIBILITIES
Allopurinol (Aloprim), etoposide (VePesid), filgrastim (Neupogen), gemcitabine (Gemzar), granisetron (Kytril), teniposide (Vumon), vinorelbine (Navelbine).

INDICATIONS/ROUTES/DOSAGE

Alert: Dosage individualized based on clinical response, tolerance to adverse effects. Dose based on actual body weight. Use ideal body weight for obese/edematous pts. Do not exceed 30 mcg/kg/day or more than 10 daily doses (increases potential for hemorrhage).

TESTICULAR TUMORS
IV: ADULTS, ELDERLY: 25–30 mcg/kg/day for 8–10 days. Repeat at monthly intervals.

HYPERCALCEMIA/HYPERURICEMIA
IV: ADULTS, ELDERLY: 25 mcg/kg as a single dose. May repeat in 48 hrs if no response occurs or 25 mcg/kg/day for 3–4 days or 25–50 mcg/kg/dose every other day for 3–8 doses.

PAGET'S DISEASE
IV: ADULTS, ELDERLY: 15 mcg/kg/day for 10 days.

SIDE EFFECTS

FREQUENT: Nausea, vomiting, anorexia, diarrhea, stomatitis. **OCCASIONAL:** Fever, drowsiness, weakness, lethargy, malaise, headache, mental depression, nervousness, dizziness, rash, acne.

ADVERSE REACTIONS/ TOXIC EFFECTS

Hematologic toxicity noted by marked facial flushing, persistent nosebleeds, hemoptysis, purpura, ecchymoses, leukopenia, thrombocytopenia. Risk of bleeding tendencies increases with higher dosages and/or when >10 doses are given. May produce electrolyte imbalance.

NURSING IMPLICATIONS

BASELINE ASSESSMENT

Question for possibility of pregnancy prior to initiating therapy (Pregnancy Category X). Antiemetics may be effective in preventing, treating nausea. Discontinue therapy if platelet count falls below 150,000/mm^3, if WBC falls below 4,000/mm^3, or if prothrombin time is 4 sec higher than control test. Renal/hepatic studies should be performed daily in pts with impairment.

INTERVENTION/EVALUATION

Monitor hematologic, renal, hepatic function studies; platelet count; prothrombin, bleeding times; serum calcium, phosphorus, potassium levels. Assess pattern of daily bowel activity, stool consistency. Monitor for stomatitis (burning/erythema of oral mucosa at inner margin of lips, sore throat, difficulty swallowing, oral ulceration). Monitor for thrombocytopenia (bleeding from gums, tarry stool, petechiae, small subcutaneous hemorrhages). Avoid IM injections, rectal temperatures, any trauma that may induce bleeding.

P

PATIENT/FAMILY TEACHING

Maintain fastidious oral hygiene. Do not have immunizations without physician's approval (drug lowers body's resistance). Avoid crowds, those with infection. Contact physician if nausea/vomiting continues at home. Use nonhormonal contraception. Inform physician if fever, sore throat, signs of local infection, bleeding, bruising, shortness of breath, pain upon urination occur.

polycarbophil

polly-**car**-bow-fill
(Fibercon, Replens ✤)

CLASSIFICATION

CLINICAL: Bulk-forming laxative, antidiarrheal (see p. 104C).

ACTION

Laxative: Retains water in intestine, opposes dehydrating forces of the bowel. **Therapeutic Effect:** Promotes well-formed stools. **Antidiarrheal:** Absorbs fecal-free water, restores normal moisture level, provides bulk. **Therapeutic Effect:** Forms gel, produces formed stool.

PHARMACOKINETICS

	Onset	Peak	Duration
PO	12–72 hrs	—	—

Acts in small/large intestine.

USES

Treatment of diarrhea associated with irritable bowel syndrome, diverticulosis, acute nonspecific diarrhea. Relieves constipation associated with irritable/spastic bowel.

PRECAUTIONS

CONTRAINDICATIONS: Abdominal pain, nausea, vomiting, symptoms of appendicitis, partial bowel obstruction, dysphagia. **CAUTIONS:** None known.

LIFESPAN CONSIDERATIONS: Pregnancy/lactation: Safe for use in pregnancy. **Pregnancy Category C. Children:** Not recommended in those <6 yrs. **Elderly:** No age-related precautions noted.

INTERACTIONS

DRUG: May interfere with effects of **potassium-sparing diuretics, potassium supplements.** May decrease effect of **oral anticoagulants, digoxin, salicylates, tetracyclines** by decreasing absorption. **HERBAL:** None known. **FOOD:** None known. **LAB VALUES:** May increase glucose. May decrease potassium.

AVAILABILITY (OTC)

TABLETS: 500 mg, 625 mg. **TABLETS (chewable):** 500 mg.

INDICATIONS/ROUTES/DOSAGE

Alert: For severe diarrhea, give every half hour up to maximum daily dosage; for laxative, give with 8 oz liquid.

LAXATIVE, ANTIDIARRHEAL

PO: ADULTS, ELDERLY, CHILDREN >12 YRS: 1 g 1–4 times/day, or as needed. **Maximum:** 4 g/24 hrs. CHILDREN 6–12 YRS: 500 mg 1–4 times/day, or as needed. **Maximum:** 2 g/24 hrs. CHILDREN <6 YRS: Consult product labeling.

SIDE EFFECTS

RARE: Some degree of abdominal discomfort, nausea, mild cramps, griping, faintness.

ADVERSE REACTIONS/ TOXIC EFFECTS

Esophageal/bowel obstruction may occur if administered with insufficient liquid (<250 ml or 1 full glass).

NURSING IMPLICATIONS

INTERVENTION/EVALUATION

Encourage adequate fluid intake. Assess bowel sounds for peristalsis. Monitor daily bowel activity, stool consistency (watery, loose, soft, semisolid, solid), record time of evacuation. Monitor serum electrolytes in those exposed to prolonged, frequent, excessive use of medication.

PATIENT/FAMILY TEACHING

Institute measures to promote defecation (increase fluid intake, exercise, high-fiber diet). Drink 6–8 glasses of water/day when used as laxative (aids stool softening).

polyethylene glycol-electrolyte solution (PEG-ES)

poly-**eth**-ah-leen
(CoLyte, GoLYTELY, Klean-Prep ✦, MiraLax, NuLytely, Peglyte ✦, ProLax ✦)

CLASSIFICATION

PHARMACOTHERAPEUTIC: Laxative. **CLINICAL:** Bowel evacuant (see p. 105C).

ACTION

Osmotic effect. **Therapeutic Effect:** Induces diarrhea, cleanses bowel (electrolytes in solution prevent water/electrolyte imbalance).

PHARMACOKINETICS

Onset	Peak	Duration
Bowel cleansing		
1–2 hrs	—	—
Constipation		
2–4 days	—	—

USES

Bowel cleansing prior to GI examination, colon surgery. **MiraLax:** Treatment of occasional constipation.

PRECAUTIONS

CONTRAINDICATIONS: GI obstruction, gastric retention, bowel perforation, toxic colitis, toxic megacolon, ileus. **CAUTIONS:** Ulcerative colitis.

LIFESPAN CONSIDERATIONS: Pregnancy/lactation: Unknown if drug crosses placenta or is distributed in breast milk. **Pregnancy Category C. Children/elderly:** No age-related precautions noted.

INTERACTIONS

DRUG: May decrease absorption of **oral medications** if given within 1 hr (may be flushed from GI tract). **HERBAL:** None known. **FOOD:** None known. **LAB VALUES:** None known.

AVAILABILITY (Rx)

POWDER FOR ORAL SOLUTION. ORAL SOLUTION.

ADMINISTRATION/HANDLING

PO

• Refrigerate reconstituted solutions; use within 48 hrs. • May use tap water to prepare solution. Shake vigorously several minutes to ensure complete dissolution of powder. • Fasting should occur ≥3 hrs before ingestion of solution (solid food should always be avoided <2 hrs prior to administration). • Only clear liquids permitted after administration. • May give via NG tube. • Rapid drinking preferred. Chilled solution is more palatable.

INDICATIONS/ROUTES/DOSAGE

BOWEL EVACUANT

PO: ADULTS, ELDERLY: 4 liters prior to GI examination: 240 ml (8 oz) q10min until 4 liters consumed or rectal effluent clear. NG tube: 20–30 ml/min until 4 liters given. CHILDREN: 25–40 ml/kg/hr until rectal effluent clear.

CONSTIPATION

PO: ADULTS (MiraLax): 17 g (or 1 heaping tbs) daily.

SIDE EFFECTS

FREQUENT (50%): Some degree of abdominal fullness, nausea, bloating. **OCCASIONAL (1%–10%):** Abdominal cramping, vomiting, anal irritation. **RARE (<1%):** Urticaria, rhinorrhea, dermatitis.

ADVERSE REACTIONS/ TOXIC EFFECTS

None known.

NURSING IMPLICATIONS

BASELINE ASSESSMENT

Do not give oral medication within 1 hr of start of therapy (may not adequately be absorbed before GI cleansing).

INTERVENTION/EVALUATION

Assess bowel sounds for peristalsis. Monitor bowel activity, stool consistency (watery, loose, soft, semisolid, solid), record time of evacuation. Assess for abdominal disturbances. Monitor electrolytes, BUN, glucose, urine osmolality.

P

polymyxin B sulfate

polly-**mix**-in

FIXED-COMBINATION(S)

Neosporin: polymyxin/neomycin (an anti-infective)/bacitracin (an anti-infective): 5,000 units/3.5 mg/4,000 units/g. **Neosporin GU Irrigant:** polymyxin/neomycin: 200,000 units/40 mg/ml. **Dexacidin, Maxitrol:** polymyxin/neomycin/dexamethasone (a corticosteroid): 10,000 units/0.35%/0.1%/g.

◆CLASSIFICATION

PHARMACOTHERAPEUTIC: Polypeptide. **CLINICAL:** Antibiotic.

ACTION

Binds to phospholipids, altering permeability and damaging the bacterial membrane allowing leakage of intracellular contents. **Therapeutic Effect:** Produces bactericidal activity.

USES

Topically for wound irrigation, bladder irrigation.

PRECAUTIONS

CONTRAINDICATIONS: None known. **CAUTIONS:** Renal impairment, neuromuscular disorders. **Pregnancy Category B.**

INTERACTIONS

DRUG: May produce muscle paralysis, prolonged/increased skeletal muscle relaxation with **neuromuscular blocking agents** or **anesthetics. Aminoglycosides, other nephrotoxic drugs** may increase nephrotoxicity. **HERBAL:** None known. **FOOD:** None known. **LAB VALUES:** None known.

AVAILABILITY (Rx)

POWDER FOR INJECTION: 500,000 units.

INDICATIONS/ROUTES/DOSAGE

USUAL IRRIGATION DOSAGE

Continuous bladder irrigation: ADULTS, ELDERLY: 1 ml urogenital concentrate (contains 200,000 units polymyxin B, 57 mg neomycin) added to 1,000 ml 0.9% NaCl. Give each 1,000 ml

>24 hrs for up to 10 days (may increase to 2,000 ml/day when urine output >2 L/day).

SIDE EFFECTS

OCCASIONAL: Fever, urticaria.

ADVERSE REACTIONS/ TOXIC EFFECTS

Nephrotoxicity, esp. with concurrent/sequential use of other nephrotoxic drugs; renal impairment; concurrent/sequential use of muscle relaxants. Superinfection, esp. with fungi, may occur.

NURSING IMPLICATIONS

BASELINE ASSESSMENT

Assess for hypersensitivity to polymyxin.

poractant alfa

pour-**act**-tant
(Curosurf, Curosurg✱)

CLASSIFICATION

CLINICAL: Pulmonary surfactant.

ACTION

Reduces surface tension of alveoli during ventilation; stabilizes alveoli against collapse that may occur at resting transpulmonary pressures. **Therapeutic Effect:** Prevents alveoli from collapsing during expiration by lowering surface tension between air and alveolar surfaces.

USES

Treatment (rescue) of respiratory distress syndrome (RDS—hyaline membrane disease) in premature infants. **Unlabeled:** Prophylaxis for RDS; adult RDS due to viral pneumonia, HIV-infected infants with *Pneumocystis carinii* pneumonia, treatment in adult RDS following near-drowning.

PRECAUTIONS

CONTRAINDICATIONS: None known. **CAUTIONS:** Pts at risk for circulatory overload. Correct acidosis, hypotension, anemia, hypoglycemia, hypothermia prior to administration.

LIFESPAN CONSIDERATIONS: Neonate: No age-related precautions noted for neonate.

INTERACTIONS

DRUG: None known. **HERBAL:** None known. **FOOD:** None known. **LAB VALUES:** None known.

AVAILABILITY (Rx)

INTRATRACHEAL SUSPENSION: 1.5 ml (120 mg), 3 ml (240 mg).

ADMINISTRATION/HANDLING

INTRATRACHEAL

Storage • Refrigerate vials. • Warm by standing vial at room temperature for 20 min or warm in hand 8 min. • To obtain uniform suspension, turn upside down gently, swirl vial (do not shake). • After warming, may return to refrigerator one time only. • Withdraw entire contents of vial into a 3- or 5-ml plastic syringe through large-gauge needle (≥20 gauge).

Administration

• Attach syringe to catheter and instill through catheter inserted into infant's endotracheal tube. Monitor for bradycardia, decreased O_2 saturation during administration. Stop dosing procedure if these effects occur; begin appropriate measures before reinstituting therapy.

INDICATIONS/ROUTES/DOSAGE

RDS

Endotracheal: INFANTS: Initially, 2.5 ml/kg birth weight (BW). Up to 2 sub-

P

see also www.elsevierhealth.com/EVOLVE/SaundersNDH

sequent doses of 1.25 ml/kg BW at 12-hr intervals. **Maximum Total Dose:** 5 ml/kg.

SIDE EFFECTS

FREQUENT: Transient bradycardia, O_2 desaturation; increased CO_2 tension. **OCCASIONAL:** Endotracheal tube reflux. **RARE:** Apnea, endotracheal tube blockage, hypotension/hypertension, pallor, vasoconstriction.

ADVERSE REACTIONS/ TOXIC EFFECTS

Pneumonia (17%), septicemia (14%), bronchopulmonary dysplasia (18%), intracranial hemorrhage (51%), patent ductus arteriosus (60%), pneumothorax (21%), pulmonary interstitial emphysema (21%) may occur.

NURSING IMPLICATIONS

BASELINE ASSESSMENT

Immediately prior to administration, change ventilator setting to 40–60 breaths/min, inspiratory time 0.5 sec, supplemental O_2 sufficient to maintain Sao_2 >92%. Drug must be administered in highly supervised setting. Clinicians in care of neonate must be experienced with intubation, ventilator management. Offer emotional support to parents.

INTERVENTION/EVALUATION

Monitor infant with arterial or transcutaneous measurement of systemic O_2 and CO_2. Assess lung sounds for rales, moist breath sounds. Monitor heart rate.

porfimer

(Photofrin)

See Classification section under: Cancer chemotherapeutic agents

potassium acetate

(Potassium acetate)

potassium bicarbonate/citrate

(K-Lyte)

potassium chloride

(Apo-K, Kaochlor, K-Dur, K-Lor, Klor-Con M15, Klotrix, K-Lyte-Cl, Micro-K, Slow-K)

potassium gluconate

(Kaon)

Do not confuse with Cardura, Slow-FE.

CLASSIFICATION

PHARMACOTHERAPEUTIC: Electrolyte. **CLINICAL:** Potassium replenisher.

ACTION

Necessary for multiple cellular metabolic processes. Primary action intracellular. **Therapeutic Effect:** Is necessary for nerve impulse conduction, contraction of cardiac, skeletal, smooth muscle; maintains normal renal function, acid-base balance.

PHARMACOKINETICS

Well absorbed from GI tract. Enters cells via active transport from extracellular fluid. Primarily excreted in urine.

USES

Treatment of potassium deficiency found in severe vomiting, diarrhea, loss of GI fluid, malnutrition, prolonged diuresis, debilitated, poor GI absorption, metabolic alkalosis, prolonged parenteral alimentation. Prevention of hypokalemia in at-risk pts.

PRECAUTIONS

CONTRAINDICATIONS: Severe renal impairment, untreated Addison's disease, postop oliguria, shock with hemolytic reaction and/or dehydration, hyperkalemia, pts receiving potassium-sparing diuretics, digitalis toxicity, heat cramps, severe burns. **CAUTIONS:** Cardiac disease, tartrazine sensitivity (mostly noted in those with aspirin hypersensitivity).

LIFESPAN CONSIDERATIONS: Pregnancy/lactation: Unknown if drug crosses placenta or is distributed in breast milk. **Pregnancy Category C (A for potassium chloride). Children:** No age-related precautions noted. **Elderly:** May be at increased risk for hyperkalemia. Age-related ability to excrete potassium is reduced.

INTERACTIONS

DRUG: ACE inhibitors, NSAIDs, beta-adrenergic blockers, potassium-sparing diuretics, heparin, potassium-containing medications, salt substitutes may increase potassium concentration. **Anticholinergics** may increase risk of GI lesions. **HERBAL:** None known. **FOOD:** None known. **LAB VALUES:** None known.

AVAILABILITY (Rx)

ACETATE: **INJECTION:** 2 mEq/ml.

BICARBONATE/CITRATE: **EFFERVESCENT TABLETS:** 25 mEq, 50 mEq.

CHLORIDE: **TABLETS:** 6.7 mEq, 8 mEq, 10 mEq, 20 mEq. **LIQUID:** 20 mEq/15 ml, 30 mEq/15 ml, 40 mEq/15 ml. **ORAL POWDER:** 20 mEq, 25 mEq. **INJECTION:** 2 mEq/ml.

GLUCONATE: **LIQUID:** 20 mEq/15 ml.

ADMINISTRATION/HANDLING

PO

• Take with or after meals and with full glass of water (decreases GI upset). • Liquids, powder, effervescent tablets: Mix, dissolve with juice, water before administering. • Do not chew, crush tablets; swallow whole.

IV

Storage • Store at room temperature.

Reconstitution • For IV infusion only, must dilute before administration, mix well, infuse slowly. • Avoid adding potassium to hanging IV.

Rate of administration • Give at rate no more than 40 mEq/L; no faster than 20 mEq/hr. (Higher concentrations/faster rates may sometimes be necessary.) • Check IV site closely during infusion for evidence of phlebitis (heat, pain, red streaking of skin over vein, hardness to vein), extravasation (swelling, pain, cool skin, little/no blood return).

IV INCOMPATIBILITIES

Amphotericin B complex (Abelcet, AmBisome, Amphotec), methylprednisolone (solu-Medrol), phenytoin (Dilantin).

IV COMPATIBILITIES

Aminophylline, amiodarone (Cordarone), atropine, aztreonam (Azactam), calcium gluconate, cefepime (Maxipime), ciprofloxacin (Cipro), clindamycin (Cleocin), dexamethasone (Decadron), digoxin (Lanoxin), diltiazem (Cardizem), diphenhydramine (Benadryl), dobutamine (Dobutrex), dopamine (Intropin), enalapril (Vasotec), famotidine (Pepcid), fluconazole (Diflucan), furosemide (Lasix), granisetron (Kytril), heparin, hydrocortisone (Solu-Cortef), insulin, lidocaine, lorazepam (Ativan), magnesium sulfate, methylprednisolone (Solu-Medrol), midazolam (Versed), milrinone (Primacor), metoclopramide (Reglan), morphine, norepinephrine (Levophed), ondansetron (Zofran), oxytocin (Pitocin), piperacillin/tazobactam

P

(Zosyn), procainamide (Pronestyl), propofol (Diprivan), propranolol (Inderal).

INDICATIONS/ROUTES/DOSAGE

PREVENTION OF HYPOKALEMIA (ON DIURETIC THERAPY)

PO: ADULTS, ELDERLY: 20–40 mEq/day in 1–2 divided doses. CHILDREN: 1–2 mEq/kg in 1–2 divided doses.

TREATMENT OF HYPOKALEMIA

IV: ADULTS, ELDERLY: 5–10 mEq/hr. **Maximum:** 400 mEq/day. CHILDREN: 1 mEq/kg over 1–2 hrs.

PO: ADULTS, ELDERLY: 40–80 mEq/day. Further doses based on laboratory values. CHILDREN: 1–2 mEq/day. Further doses based on laboratory values.

SIDE EFFECTS

OCCASIONAL: Nausea, vomiting, diarrhea, flatulence, abdominal discomfort with distention, phlebitis with IV administration (particularly when potassium concentration of >40 mEq/L is infused). **RARE:** Rash.

ADVERSE REACTIONS/ TOXIC EFFECTS

Hyperkalemia (observed particularly in elderly or in pts with impaired renal function) manifested as paresthesia of extremities, heaviness of legs, cold skin, grayish pallor, hypotension, mental confusion, irritability, flaccid paralysis, cardiac arrhythmias.

NURSING IMPLICATIONS

BASELINE ASSESSMENT

PO should be given with food or after meals with full glass of water, fruit juice (minimizes GI irritation).

INTERVENTION/EVALUATION

Monitor serum potassium level (particularly in renal function impairment). If GI disturbance is noted, dilute preparation further or give with meals. Be alert to decrease in urinary output (may be indication of renal insufficiency). Monitor daily bowel activity, stool consistency. Assess I&O diligently during diuresis, IV site for extravasation, phlebitis. Be alert to evidence of hyperkalemia (skin pallor/coldness, complaints of paresthesia of extremities, feeling of heaviness of legs).

PATIENT/FAMILY TEACHING

Foods rich in potassium include beef, veal, ham, chicken, turkey, fish, milk, bananas, dates, prunes, raisins, avocados, watermelon, cantaloupe, apricots, molasses, beans, yams, broccoli, brussel sprouts, lentils, potatoes, spinach. Report paresthesia of extremities, feeling of heaviness of legs.

pramipexole

pram-ih-**pecks**-all
(Mirapex)

Do not confuse with Mifeprex, MiraLax.

CLASSIFICATION

PHARMACOTHERAPEUTIC: Dopamine receptor agonist. **CLINICAL:** Antiparkinson agent.

ACTION

Stimulates dopamine receptors in the striatum. **Therapeutic Effect:** Relieves signs/symptoms of Parkinson's disease.

PHARMACOKINETICS

Rapid, extensive absorption following PO administration. Protein binding: 15%. Widely distributed. Steady-state concentrations achieved within 2 days. Primarily eliminated in urine. Not removed by hemodialysis. **Half-life:** 8 hrs (12 hrs in those >65 yrs).

USES

Treatment of signs/symptoms of idiopathic Parkinson's disease.

PRECAUTIONS

CONTRAINDICATIONS: History of hypersensitivity to medication. **CAUTIONS:** History of orthostatic hypotension, syncope, hallucinations, renal function impairment, concomitant use of CNS depressants.

LIFESPAN CONSIDERATIONS: Pregnancy/lactation: Unknown if distributed in breast milk. **Pregnancy Category C. Children:** Safety and efficacy not established. **Elderly:** Increased risk of hallucinations.

INTERACTIONS

DRUG: Cimetidine increases pramipexole's plasma concentration and increases its half-life. Combined use of **cimetidine, ranitidine, diltiazem, triamterene, verapamil, quinidine, quinine** may decrease pramipexole clearance. May increase plasma levels of **carbidopa** or **levodopa** combinations. **HERBAL:** None known. **FOOD:** Time to maximum plasma levels is increased by 1 hr when taken with **food** (extent of absorption not affected). **LAB VALUES:** None known.

AVAILABILITY (Rx)

TABLETS: 0.125 mg, 0.25 mg, 0.5 mg, 1 mg, 1.5 mg.

ADMINISTRATION/HANDLING

PO

- Give without regard to food.

INDICATIONS/ROUTES/DOSAGE

PARKINSON'S DISEASE

PO: ADULTS, ELDERLY: Initially, 0.375 mg/day in 3 divided doses. Do not increase dose more frequently than q5–7days. MAINTENANCE: 1.5–4.5 mg/day in equally divided doses 3 times/day.

RENAL FUNCTION IMPAIRMENT

PO: ADULTS, ELDERLY, CREATININE CLEARANCE >60 ML/MIN: Initially, 0.125 mg 3 times/day. **Maximum:** 1.5 mg 3 times/day. CREATININE CLEARANCE 35–59 ML/MIN: Initially, 0.125 mg 2 times/day. **Maximum:** 1.5 mg twice daily. CREATININE CLEARANCE 15–34 ML/MIN: Initially, 0.125 mg 1 time/day. **Maximum:** 1.5 mg once daily.

SIDE EFFECTS

FREQUENT: Early Parkinson's disease (10%–28%): Nausea, asthenia (weakness), dizziness, somnolence, insomnia, constipation. **Advanced Parkinson's disease (17%–53%):** Postural hypotension, extrapyramidal signs, insomnia, dizziness, hallucinations. **OCCASIONAL: Early Parkinson's disease (2%–5%):** Edema, malaise, confusion, amnesia, akathisia (restlessness), anorexia, dysphagia, peripheral edema, altered vision, impotence. **Advanced Parkinson's disease (7%–10%):** Asthenia, somnolence, confusion, constipation, gait abnormality, dry mouth. **RARE: Advanced Parkinson's disease (2%–6%):** General edema, malaise, chest pain, amnesia, tremors, urinary frequency/incontinence, dyspnea, rhinitis, vision changes.

ADVERSE REACTIONS/ TOXIC EFFECTS

None known.

NURSING IMPLICATIONS

INTERVENTION/EVALUATION

Instruct pt to rise from lying to sitting or sitting to standing position slowly to prevent risk of postural hypotension. Assess for clinical improvement. Assist

P

with ambulation if dizziness occurs. Assess for constipation; encourage fiber, fluids, exercise.

PATIENT/FAMILY TEACHING

Inform pt that hallucinations may occur, esp. in the elderly. Postural hypotension may occur more frequently during initial therapy. Avoid tasks that require alertness, motor skills until response to drug is established. If nausea occurs, take medication with food. Avoid abrupt withdrawal.

Prandin

see repaglinide

Pravachol

see pravastatin

pravastatin

pra-vah-sta-tin
(Pravachol)

Do not confuse with Prevacid, propranolol.

FIXED-COMBINATION(S)

Pravigard: pravastatin/aspirin (anticoagulant): 20 mg/81 mg; 40 mg/81 mg; 80 mg/81 mg; 20 mg/325 mg; 40 mg/325 mg; 80 mg/325 mg.

CLASSIFICATION

PHARMACOTHERAPEUTIC: HMG-CoA reductase inhibitor. **CLINICAL:** Antihyperlipidemic (see p. 50C).

ACTION

Interferes with cholesterol biosynthesis by preventing the conversion of HMG-CoA reductase to mevalonate, a precursor to cholesterol. **Therapeutic Effect:** Lowers LDL cholesterol, VLDL, plasma triglycerides; increases HDL concentration.

PHARMACOKINETICS

Poorly absorbed from GI tract. Protein binding: 50%. Metabolized in liver (minimal active metabolites). Primarily excreted in feces via biliary system. Not removed by hemodialysis. **Half-life:** 2.7 hrs.

USES

Treatment of hypercholesterolemia by reducing total and LDL cholesterol, apo B, triglycerides, increasing HDL cholesterol. Preventive therapy to reduce risks of the following in pts with previous MI and normal cholesterol levels: recurrent MI, undergoing myocardial revascularization procedures; stroke/transient ischemic attack. Prevention of CV events in pts with elevated cholesterol levels.

PRECAUTIONS

CONTRAINDICATIONS: Active liver disease; unexplained, persistent elevations of liver function tests. **CAUTIONS:** History of liver disease, substantial alcohol consumption. Withholding/discontinuing pravastatin may be necessary when pt at risk for renal failure secondary to rhabdomyolysis. Severe metabolic, endocrine, electrolyte disorders.

LIFESPAN CONSIDERATIONS: Pregnancy/lactation: Contraindicated in pregnancy (suppression of cholesterol biosynthesis may cause fetal toxicity) and lactation. Unknown if drug is distributed in breast milk, but there is risk of serious adverse reactions in nursing infants. **Pregnancy Category X. Children:** Safety and efficacy not established. **Elderly:** No age-related precautions noted.

INTERACTIONS

DRUG: Increased risk of rhabdomyolysis, acute renal failure with **cyclosporine, erythromycin, gemfibrozil, niacin, other immunosuppressants.** **HERBAL:** None known. **FOOD:** None known. **LAB VALUES:** May increase creatinine kinase, serum transaminase concentrations.

AVAILABILITY (Rx)

TABLETS: 10 mg, 20 mg, 40 mg, 80 mg.

ADMINISTRATION/HANDLING

PO

• Give without regard to meals. • Administer in evening.

INDICATIONS/ROUTES/DOSAGE

Alert: Prior to initiating therapy, pt should be on standard cholesterol-lowering diet for minimum of 3–6 mos. Continue diet throughout pravastatin therapy.

USUAL DOSAGE

PO: ADULTS, ELDERLY: Initially, 40 mg/day. Titrate to desired response. RANGE: 10–80 mg/day. CHILDREN 14–18 YRS: 40 mg/day. CHILDREN 8–13 YRS: 20 mg/day.

DOSAGE IN RENAL/LIVER IMPAIRMENT

Initially, 10 mg/day. Titrate to desired response.

SIDE EFFECTS

Generally well tolerated. Side effects usually mild, transient. **OCCASIONAL (4%–7%):** Nausea, vomiting, diarrhea, constipation, abdominal pain, headache, rhinitis, rash, pruritus. **RARE (2%–3%):** Heartburn, myalgia, dizziness, cough, fatigue, flulike symptoms.

ADVERSE REACTIONS/ TOXIC EFFECTS

Potential for malignancy, cataracts. Hypersensitivity occurs rarely.

NURSING IMPLICATIONS

BASELINE ASSESSMENT

Question for possibility of pregnancy prior to initiating therapy (Pregnancy Category X). Assess baseline lab results: cholesterol, triglycerides, liver function tests.

INTERVENTION/EVALUATION

Monitor cholesterol, triglyceride lab results for therapeutic response. Monitor liver function tests. Determine pattern of bowel activity. Check for headache, dizziness (provide assistance as needed). Assess for rash, pruritus. Be alert for malaise, muscle cramping/weakness; if accompanied by fever, may require discontinuation of medication.

PATIENT/FAMILY TEACHING

Follow special diet (important part of treatment). Periodic lab tests are essential part of therapy. Report promptly any muscle pain/weakness, esp. if accompanied by fever, malaise. Do not drive, perform activities that require alert response if dizziness occurs. Use nonhormonal contraception.

P

prazosin hydrochloride ⓔ

pray-zoe-sin
(Minipress)

FIXED-COMBINATION(S)

Minizide: prazosin/polythiazide (a diuretic): 1 mg/0.5 mg; 2 mg/0.5 mg; 5 mg/0.5 mg.

◆ CLASSIFICATION

PHARMACOTHERAPEUTIC: Alpha-adrenergic blocker. **CLINICAL:** Antihypertensive, antidote, vasodilator (see p. 53C).

ACTION

Selectively blocks alpha$_1$-adrenergic receptors, decreasing peripheral vascular resistance. **Therapeutic Effect:** Produces vasodilation of veins, arterioles; decreases total peripheral resistance; relaxes smooth muscle in bladder neck, prostate.

USES

Treatment of mild to moderate hypertension. Used alone or in combination with other antihypertensives. **Unlabeled:** Treatment of CHF, ergot alkaloid toxicity, pheochromocytoma, Raynaud's phenomena, benign prostate hypertrophy.

PRECAUTIONS

CONTRAINDICATIONS: None known. **CAUTIONS:** Chronic renal failure, impaired hepatic function. **Pregnancy Category C.**

INTERACTIONS

DRUG: **Estrogen, NSAIDs, sympathomimetics** may decrease effect. **Hypotension-producing medications** may increase antihypertensive effect. **HERBAL:** **Licorice** causes sodium and water retention, potassium loss. **FOOD:** None known. **LAB VALUES:** None known.

AVAILABILITY (Rx)

CAPSULES: 1 mg, 2 mg, 5 mg.

ADMINISTRATION/HANDLING

PO

• Give without regard to food. • Administer first dose at bedtime (minimizes risk of fainting due to "first-dose syncope").

INDICATIONS/ROUTES/DOSAGE

HYPERTENSION

PO: ADULTS, ELDERLY: Initially, 1 mg 2–3 times/day. MAINTENANCE: 3–15 mg/day in divided doses. **Maximum:** 20 mg/day. CHILDREN: 5 mcg/kg/dose q6h. Gradually increase up to 25 mcg/kg/dose. **Maximum:** 15 mg or 400 mcg/kg/day.

SIDE EFFECTS

FREQUENT (7%–10%): Dizziness, drowsiness, headache, asthenia (loss of strength, energy). **OCCASIONAL (4%–5%):** Palpitations, nausea, dry mouth, nervousness. **RARE (<1%):** Angina, urinary urgency.

ADVERSE REACTIONS/ TOXIC EFFECTS

"First-dose syncope" (hypotension with sudden loss of consciousness) generally occurs 30–90 min following initial dose of ≥2 mg, a too rapid increase in dosage, or addition of another hypotensive agent to therapy. May be preceded by tachycardia (120–160 beats/min).

NURSING IMPLICATIONS

BASELINE ASSESSMENT

Give first dose at bedtime. If initial dose is given during daytime, pt must remain recumbent for 3–4 hrs. Assess B/P, pulse immediately prior to each dose and q15–30min until stabilized (be alert to B/P fluctuations).

INTERVENTION/EVALUATION

Monitor B/P, pulse diligently (first-dose syncope may be preceded by tachycardia). Monitor pattern of daily bowel activity, stool consistency. Assist with ambulation if dizziness occurs.

PATIENT/FAMILY TEACHING

Avoid driving for 12–24 hrs after first dose or increase in dosage. Use caution driving or operating machinery and when rising from sitting or lying position. Report dizziness or palpitations if bothersome.

prednicarbate

(Dermatop)
See Classification section under: Corticosteroids: topical (p. 85C)

prednisolone

pred-**niss**-oh-lone
(AK-Pred, AK-Tate ✤, Econopred, Inflamase, Minims-Prednisolone ✤, Novo-Prednisolone ✤, Pediapred, Pred Mild, Prelone)

FIXED-COMBINATION(S)

Blephamide: prednisolone/sulfacetamide (an anti-infective): 0.2%/10%. **Vasocidin:** prednisolone/sulfacetamide: 0.25%/10%.

CLASSIFICATION

PHARMACOTHERAPEUTIC: Adrenal corticosteroid. **CLINICAL:** Glucocorticoid (see p. 82C).

ACTION

Inhibits accumulation of inflammatory cells at inflammation sites, phagocytosis, lysosomal enzyme release/synthesis, release of mediators of inflammation. **Therapeutic Effect:** Prevents/suppresses cell-mediated immune reactions. Decreases/prevents tissue response to inflammatory process.

USES

Substitution Therapy in Deficiency States: Acute/chronic adrenal insufficiency, congenital adrenal hyperplasia, adrenal insufficiency secondary to pituitary insufficiency. **Nonendocrine Disorders:** Arthritis; rheumatic carditis; allergic, collagen, intestinal tract, liver, ocular, renal, skin diseases; bronchial asthma; cerebral edema; malignancies.

PRECAUTIONS

CONTRAINDICATIONS: Acute superficial herpes simplex keratitis, systemic fungal infections, varicella. **CAUTIONS:** Hyperthyroidism, cirrhosis, ocular herpes simplex, peptic ulcer disease, osteoporosis, myasthenia gravis, hypertension, CHF, ulcerative colitis, thromboembolic disorders. **Pregnancy Category C** (**D** if used in first trimester).

INTERACTIONS

DRUG: **Amphotericin** may increase hypokalemia. May decrease effect of **oral hypoglycemics, insulin, diuretics, potassium supplements.** May increase **digoxin** toxicity (due to hypokalemia). **Hepatic enzyme inducers** may decrease effect. **Live virus vaccines** may potentiate virus replication, increase vaccine side effects, decrease pt's antibody response to vaccine. **HERBAL:** None known. **FOOD:** None known. **LAB VALUES:** May decrease calcium, potassium, thyroxine. May increase cholesterol, lipids, glucose, sodium, amylase.

AVAILABILITY (Rx)

OPHTHALMIC SUSPENSION: 0.12%, 1%. **OPHTHALMIC SOLUTION:** 0.125%, 1%. **ORAL SOLUTION:** 5 mg/5 ml, 15 mg/5 ml. **TABLETS:** 5 mg, 20 mg.

INDICATIONS/ROUTES/DOSAGE

USUAL ADULT DOSAGE

PO: 5–60 mg/day.

ACUTE ASTHMA

PO: CHILDREN: 1–2 mg/kg/day in divided doses.

P

ANTI-INFLAMMATION/ IMMUNOSUPPRESSION

PO: CHILDREN: 0.1–2 mg/kg/day in divided doses.

USUAL OPHTHALMIC DOSAGE

Ophthalmic: ADULTS, ELDERLY: *Solution:* 1–2 drops qh during day; q2h during night; after response, decrease dosage to 1 drop q4h, then 1 drop 3–4 times/day.

SIDE EFFECTS

FREQUENT: Insomnia, heartburn, nervousness, abdominal distention, diaphoresis, acne, mood swings, increased appetite, facial flushing, delayed wound healing, increased susceptibility to infection, diarrhea/constipation. **OCCASIONAL:** Headache, edema, change in skin color, frequent urination. **RARE:** Tachycardia, allergic reaction (rash, hives), psychic changes, hallucinations, depression. **Ophthalmic:** Stinging/burning, posterior subcapsular cataracts.

ADVERSE REACTIONS/ TOXIC EFFECTS

LONG-TERM THERAPY: Hypocalcemia, hypokalemia, muscle wasting (esp. arms, legs), osteoporosis, spontaneous fractures, amenorrhea, cataracts, glaucoma, peptic ulcer, CHF. **ABRUPT WITHDRAWAL FOLLOWING LONG-TERM THERAPY:** Anorexia, nausea, fever, headache, sudden/severe joint pain, rebound inflammation, fatigue, weakness, lethargy, dizziness, orthostatic hypotension. Sudden discontinuance may be fatal.

NURSING IMPLICATIONS

BASELINE ASSESSMENT

Obtain baselines for height, weight, B/P, glucose, electrolytes. Check results of initial tests (e.g., TB skin test, x-rays, EKG). Never give live virus vaccine (e.g., smallpox).

INTERVENTION/EVALUATION

Monitor B/P, weight, electrolytes, glucose, height, weight in children. Be alert to infection (sore throat, fever, vague symptoms); assess mouth daily for signs of candida infection (white patches, painful tongue/mucous membranes).

PATIENT/FAMILY TEACHING

Notify physician of fever, sore throat, muscle aches, sudden weight gain/ swelling. Avoid alcohol, minimize use of caffeine. Do not abruptly discontinue without physician's approval. Avoid exposure to chickenpox, measles.

prednisone

pred-nih-sewn

(Apo-Prednisone♣, Deltasone, Meticorten, Winpred♣)

Do not confuse with prednisolone, Primidone.

◆ CLASSIFICATION

PHARMACOTHERAPEUTIC: Adrenal corticosteroid. **CLINICAL:** Glucocorticoid (see p. 82C).

ACTION

Inhibits accumulation of inflammatory cells at inflammation sites, phagocytosis, lysosomal enzyme release/synthesis, release of mediators of inflammation. **Therapeutic Effect:** Prevents/suppresses cell-mediated immune reactions. Decreases/prevents tissue response to inflammatory process.

PHARMACOKINETICS

Well absorbed from GI tract. Protein binding: 70%–90%. Widely distributed. Metabolized in liver (converted to prednisolone). Primarily excreted in urine. Not removed by hemodialysis. **Half-life:** 3.4–3.8 hrs.

USES

Substitution Therapy in Deficiency States: Acute/chronic adrenal insufficiency, congenital adrenal hyperplasia, adrenal insufficiency secondary to pituitary insufficiency. **Nonendocrine Disorders:** Arthritis; rheumatic carditis; allergic, collagen, intestinal tract, liver, ocular, renal, skin diseases; bronchial asthma; cerebral edema; malignancies.

PRECAUTIONS

CONTRAINDICATIONS: Acute superficial herpes simplex keratitis, systemic fungal infections, varicella. **CAUTIONS:** Hyperthyroidism, cirrhosis, ocular herpes simplex, peptic ulcer disease, osteoporosis, myasthenia gravis, hypertension, CHF, ulcerative colitis, thromboembolic disorders.

LIFESPAN CONSIDERATIONS: Pregnancy/lactation: Crosses placenta. Distributed in breast milk. Cleft palate generally occurs with chronic use, first trimester. **Pregnancy Category C (D** if used in first trimester). **Children:** Prolonged treatment or high dosages may decrease short-term growth rate, cortisol secretion. **Elderly:** May be more susceptible to developing hypertension or osteoporosis.

INTERACTIONS

DRUG: Amphotericin may increase hypokalemia. May decrease effect of **oral hypoglycemics, insulin, diuretics, potassium supplements.** May increase **digoxin** toxicity (due to hypokalemia). **Hepatic enzyme inducers** may decrease effect. **Live virus vaccines** may potentiate virus replication, increase vaccine side effects, decrease pt's antibody response to vaccine. **HERBAL:** None known. **FOOD:** None known. **LAB VALUES:** May decrease calcium, potassium, thyroxine. May increase cholesterol, lipids, glucose, sodium, amylase.

AVAILABILITY (Rx)

TABLETS: 1 mg, 2.5 mg, 5 mg, 10 mg, 20 mg, 50 mg. **ORAL SOLUTION:** 5 mg/5 ml, 5 mg/ml.

ADMINISTRATION/HANDLING

PO

• Give without regard to meals (give with food if GI upset occurs). • Give single doses before 9 AM, multiple doses at evenly spaced intervals.

INDICATIONS/ROUTES/DOSAGE

USUAL ADULT DOSAGE

PO: 5–60 mg/day.

ACUTE ASTHMA

PO: CHILDREN: 1–2 mg/kg/day in divided doses.

ANTI-INFLAMMATION/ IMMUNOSUPPRESSION

PO: CHILDREN: 0.05–2 mg/kg/day in divided doses.

SIDE EFFECTS

FREQUENT: Insomnia, heartburn, nervousness, abdominal distention, diaphoresis, acne, mood swings, increased appetite, facial flushing, delayed wound healing, increased susceptibility to infection, diarrhea/constipation. **OCCASIONAL:** Headache, edema, change in skin color, frequent urination. **RARE:** Tachycardia, allergic reaction (rash, hives), psychic changes, hallucinations, depression.

ADVERSE REACTIONS/ TOXIC EFFECTS

LONG-TERM THERAPY: Muscle wasting (esp. arms, legs), osteoporosis, spontaneous fractures, amenorrhea, cataracts, glaucoma, peptic ulcer, CHF. **ABRUPT WITHDRAWAL FOLLOWING LONG-TERM THERAPY:** Anorexia, nausea, fever, head-

P

ache, sudden/severe joint pain, rebound inflammation, fatigue, weakness, lethargy, dizziness, orthostatic hypotension. Sudden discontinuance may be fatal.

NURSING IMPLICATIONS

BASELINE ASSESSMENT

Obtain baselines for height, weight, B/P, glucose, electrolytes. Check results of initial tests (e.g., TB skin test, x-rays, EKG). Never give live virus vaccine (e.g., smallpox).

INTERVENTION/EVALUATION

Monitor B/P, weight, electrolytes, glucose, height, weight in children. Be alert to infection (sore throat, fever, vague symptoms); assess mouth daily for signs of candida infection (white patches, painful tongue/mucous membranes).

PATIENT/FAMILY TEACHING

Notify physician of fever, sore throat, muscle aches, sudden weight gain/swelling. Avoid alcohol, minimize use of caffeine. Do not abruptly discontinue without physician's approval. Avoid exposure to chickenpox, measles.

P

Premarin

see conjugated estrogens

Prevacid

see lansoprazole

Prilosec

see omeprazole

Primacor

see milrinone

Primaxin

see imipenem-cilastatin

primidone

prih-mih-doan
(Apo-Primidone ♣, Mysoline)
Do not confuse with prednisone.

CLASSIFICATION

PHARMACOTHERAPEUTIC: Barbiturate. **CLINICAL:** Anticonvulsant (see p. 31C).

ACTION

Decreases motor activity to electrical/chemical stimulation, stabilizes threshold against hyperexcitability. **Therapeutic Effect:** Produces anticonvulsant effect.

USES

Management of partial seizures with complex symptomatology (psychomotor seizures), generalized tonic-clonic (grand mal) seizures. **Unlabeled:** Treatment of essential tremor.

PRECAUTIONS

CONTRAINDICATIONS: History of porphyria, bronchopneumonia. **CAUTIONS:** Renal/liver impairment. **Pregnancy Category D.**

INTERACTIONS

DRUG: May decrease effects of **glucocorticoids, digoxin, metronidazole,**

oral anticoagulants, quinidine, tricyclic antidepressants. Alcohol, CNS depressants may increase effect. May increase metabolism of **carbamazepine. Valproic acid** decreases metabolism, increases concentration, toxicity. **HERBAL:** None known. **FOOD:** None known. **LAB VALUES:** May decrease bilirubin. Therapeutic blood serum level: 4–12 mcg/ml; toxic blood serum level: >12 mcg/ml.

AVAILABILITY (Rx)

TABLETS: 50 mg, 250 mg.

INDICATIONS/ROUTES/DOSAGE

ANTICONVULSANT

PO: ADULTS, ELDERLY, CHILDREN ≥8 YRS: 125–150 mg/day at bedtime. May increase by 125–250 mg/day q3–7days. **Maximum:** 2 g/day. CHILDREN <8 YRS: Initially, 50–125 mg/day at bedtime. May increase by 50–125 mg/day q3–7days. USUAL DOSE: 10–25 mg/kg/day in divided doses. NEONATES: 12–20 mg/kg/day in divided doses.

SIDE EFFECTS

FREQUENT: Ataxia, dizziness. **OCCASIONAL:** Loss of appetite, drowsiness, mental changes, nausea, vomiting, paradoxical excitement. **RARE:** Skin rash.

ADVERSE REACTIONS/ TOXIC EFFECTS

Abrupt withdrawal after prolonged therapy may produce effects ranging from markedly increased dreaming, nightmares, insomnia, tremor, diaphoresis, vomiting to hallucinations, delirium, seizures, status epilepticus. Skin eruptions may appear as hypersensitivity reaction. Blood dyscrasias, liver disease, hypocalcemia occur rarely. Overdosage produces cold/clammy skin, hypothermia, severe CNS depression followed by high fever, coma.

NURSING IMPLICATIONS

BASELINE ASSESSMENT

Review history of seizure disorder (intensity, frequency, duration, LOC). Observe frequently for recurrence of seizure activity. Initiate seizure precautions.

INTERVENTION/EVALUATION

Monitor serum concentrations; CBC; neurologic status; frequency, duration, severity of seizures. Monitor for therapeutic serum level: 4–12 mcg/ml; toxic serum level: >12 mcg/ml.

PATIENT/FAMILY TEACHING

Do not abruptly withdraw medication after long-term use (may precipitate seizures). Strict maintenance of drug therapy is essential for seizure control. Drowsiness usually disappears during continued therapy. If dizziness occurs, change positions slowly from recumbent to sitting position before standing. Avoid tasks that require alertness, motor skills until response to drug is established. Avoid alcohol.

P

Prinivil

see lisinopril

probenecid

pro-**ben**-ah-sid

(Benuryl✤)

Do not confuse with procainamide.

◆CLASSIFICATION

PHARMACOTHERAPEUTIC: Uricosuric. **CLINICAL:** Antigout.

ACTION

Competitively inhibits reabsorption of uric acid at proximal convoluted tobule. Inhibits renal tubular secretion of weak organic acids (e.g., penicillins). **Therapeutic Effect:** Promotes uric acid excretion, reduces serum uric acid levels, increases plasma levels of penicillins, cephalosporins.

USES

Treatment of hyperuricemia associated with gout, gouty arthritis. Adjunctive therapy with penicillins or cephalosporins to elevate/prolong antibiotic plasma levels.

PRECAUTIONS

CONTRAINDICATIONS: Concurrent high-dose aspirin therapy, severe renal impairment, blood dyscrasias, uric acid kidney stones, children <2 yrs. **CAUTIONS:** Peptic ulcer, hematuria, renal colic. **Pregnancy Category C.**

INTERACTIONS

DRUG: May increase concentrations of **cephalosporins, methotrexate, NSAIDs, nitrofurantoin, penicillins, zidovudine. Antineoplastics** may increase risk of uric acid nephropathy. **Salicylates** may decrease uricosuric effect. May increase/prolong effects of **heparin. HERBAL:** None known. **FOOD:** None known. **LAB VALUES:** May inhibit renal excretion of PSP (phenolsulfonphthalein), 17-ketosteroids, BSP (sulfobromophthalein) tests.

AVAILABILITY (Rx)

TABLETS: 500 mg.

ADMINISTRATION/HANDLING

PO

• Give with or immediately after meals or milk. • Instruct pt to drink at least 6–8 glasses (8 oz) of water/day (prevents kidney stone development).

INDICATIONS/ROUTES/DOSAGE

GOUT

Alert: Do not start until acute gout attack subsides; continue if acute attack occurs during therapy.

PO: ADULTS, ELDERLY: Initially, 250 mg 2 times/day for 1 wk; then 500 mg 2 times/day. May increase by 500 mg q4wks. **Maximum:** 2–3 g/day. MAINTENANCE: Dosage that maintains normal uric acid levels.

PENICILLIN/CEPHALOSPORIN THERAPY

Alert: Do not use in presence of renal impairment.

PO: ADULTS, ELDERLY: 2 g/day in divided doses. CHILDREN 2–14 YRS: Initially, 25 mg/kg. MAINTENANCE: 40 mg/kg/day in 4 divided doses. CHILDREN >50 KG: Receive adult dosage.

GONORRHEA

PO: ADULTS, ELDERLY: 1 g 30 min prior to penicillin, ampicillin, amoxicillin.

SIDE EFFECTS

FREQUENT (5%–10%): Headache, anorexia, nausea, vomiting. **OCCASIONAL (1%–5%):** Lower back/side pain, rash, hives, itching, dizziness, flushed face, frequent urge to urinate, gingivitis.

ADVERSE REACTIONS/ TOXIC EFFECTS

Severe hypersensitivity reactions (including anaphylaxis) occur rarely (usually within a few hours after readministration following previous use). Discontinue immediately, contact physician. Pruritic maculopapular rash should be considered a toxic reaction. May be accompanied by malaise, fever, chills, joint pain, nausea, vomiting, leukopenia, aplastic anemia.

NURSING IMPLICATIONS

BASELINE ASSESSMENT

Do not initiate therapy until acute gouty attack has subsided. Question for hypersensitivity to probenecid or if taking penicillin or cephalosporin antibiotics.

INTERVENTION/EVALUATION

If exacerbation of gout recurs after therapy, use other agents for gout. Discontinue medication immediately if rash or other evidence of allergic reaction appears. Encourage high fluid intake (3,000 ml/day). Monitor I&O (output should be at least 2,000 ml/day). Assess CBC, serum uric acid levels. Assess urine for cloudiness, unusual color, odor. Assess for therapeutic response (reduced joint tenderness, swelling, redness, limitation of motion).

PATIENT/FAMILY TEACHING

Drink plenty of fluids to decrease risk of uric acid kidney stones. Avoid alcohol, large doses of aspirin/other salicylates. Encourage low-purine food intake (reduce/omit meat, fowl, fish; use eggs, cheese, vegetables). Foods high in purine: kidneys, liver, sweetbreads, sardines, anchovies, meat extracts. May take ≥1 wk for full therapeutic effect. Drink 6–8 glasses (8 oz) of fluid daily while on medication.

procainamide hydrochloride

pro-**cane**-ah-myd
(Apo-Procainamide✤, Procanbid, Procan-SR, Pronestyl)

Do not confuse with Ponstel, probenecid.

◆ CLASSIFICATION

CLINICAL: Antiarrhythmic (see p. 13C).

ACTION

Increases electrical stimulation threshold of ventricle, His-Purkinje system. Possesses direct cardiac effects. **Therapeutic Effect:** Decreases myocardial excitability, conduction velocity, depresses myocardial contractility. Produces antiarrhythmic effect.

PHARMACOKINETICS

Rapidly, completely absorbed from GI tract. Protein binding: 15%–20%. Widely distributed. Metabolized in liver to active metabolite. Primarily excreted in urine. Removed by hemodialysis. **Half-life:** 2.5–4.5 hrs; metabolite: 6 hrs.

USES

Prophylactic therapy to maintain normal sinus rhythm after conversion of atrial fibrillation/flutter. Treatment of premature ventricular contractions, paroxysmal atrial tachycardia, atrial fibrillation, ventricular tachycardia. **Unlabeled:** Conversion/management of atrial fibrillation.

PRECAUTIONS

CONTRAINDICATIONS: Complete heart block, second- or third-degree heart block, torsades de pointes, preexisting QT prolongation, myasthenia gravis, systemic lupus erythematosus. **CAUTIONS:** Marked AV conduction disturbances, bundle-branch block, severe digoxin toxicity, CHF, supraventricular tachyarrhythmias, renal/liver impairment.

LIFESPAN CONSIDERATIONS: Pregnancy/lactation: Crosses placenta. Unknown if distributed in breast milk. **Pregnancy Category C. Children:** No age-related precautions noted. **Elderly:** More susceptible to hypotensive

P

effect. Age-related renal impairment may require dosage adjustment.

INTERACTIONS

DRUG: **Pimozide, other antiarrhythmics** may increase cardiac effects. May increase effects of **antihypertensives (IV procainamide), neuromuscular blockers.** May decrease antimyasthenic effect on skeletal muscle. **HERBAL**: None known. **FOOD**: None known. **LAB VALUES**: May cause positive ANA, Coombs' test, EKG changes. May increase SGOT (AST), SGPT (ALT), alkaline phosphatase, bilirubin, LDH. Therapeutic blood serum level: 4–8 mcg/ml; toxic blood serum level: >10 mcg/ml.

AVAILABILITY (Rx)

CAPSULES: 250 mg, 375 mg, 500 mg. **TABLETS**: 250 mg, 375 mg, 500 mg. **TABLETS (extended-release)**: 500 mg, 750 mg, 1,000 mg. **INJECTION**: 100 mg/ml, 500 mg/ml.

ADMINISTRATION/HANDLING

PO

• Do not crush/break sustained-release tablets.

IM/IV

Alert: May give by IM injection, IV push, or IV infusion.

Storage • Solution appears clear, colorless to light yellow. • Discard if solution darkens/appears discolored or if precipitate forms. • When diluted with D_5W, solution is stable for 24 hrs at room temperature or for 7 days if refrigerated.

Reconstitution • For IV push, dilute with 5–10 ml D_5W. • For initial loading IV infusion, add 1 g to 50 ml D_5W to provide a concentration of 20 mg/ml. • For IV infusion, add 1 g to 250–500 ml D_5W to provide concentration of 2–4 mg/ml. Maximum concentration: 4 g/250 ml.

Rate of administration • For IV push, with pt in supine position, administer at rate not exceeding 25–50 mg/min. • For initial loading infusion, infuse 1 ml/min for up to 25–30 min. • For IV infusion, infuse at 1–3 ml/min. • Check B/P q5–10min during infusion. If fall in B/P exceeds 15 mm Hg, discontinue drug, contact physician. • Monitor EKG for cardiac changes, particularly widening of QRS, prolongation of PR and QT intervals. Notify physician of any significant interval changes. • B/P, EKG should be monitored continuously during IV administration and rate of infusion adjusted to eliminate arrhythmias.

⊘ IV INCOMPATIBILITY

Milrinone (Primacor).

IV COMPATIBILITIES

Amiodarone (Cordarone), dobutamine (Dobutrex), heparin, lidocaine, potassium chloride.

INDICATIONS/ROUTES/DOSAGE

Alert: Dose, interval of administration individualized based on underlying myocardial disease, pt's age, renal function, clinical response. Extended-release capsules used for maintenance therapy.

ARRHYTHMIAS

IV: ADULTS, ELDERLY: LOADING DOSE: 50–100 mg/dose. May repeat q5–10min or 15–18 mg/kg. (**Maximum:** 1–1.5 g) then maintenance infusion of 3–4 mg/min. RANGE: 1–6 mg/min. CHILDREN: LOADING DOSE: 3–6 mg/kg/dose over 5 min (**Maximum:** 100 mg). May repeat q5–10min to maximum total dose of 15 mg/kg then maintenance dose of 20–80 mcg/kg/min. **Maximum:** 2 g/day.

PO: ADULTS, ELDERLY: **(Immediate-release)**: 250–500 mg q3–6h. **(Sustained-release)**: 0.5–1 g q6h. **(Procanbid)**: 1–2 g q12h. CHILDREN: **(Immediate-release)**: 15–50 mg/kg/

P

day in divided doses q3–6h. **Maximum:** 4 g/day.

DOSAGE IN RENAL IMPAIRMENT

Creatinine Clearance	Dosage Interval
10–50 ml/min	q6–12h
<10 ml/min	q8–24h

SIDE EFFECTS

FREQUENT: PO: Abdominal pain/cramping, nausea, diarrhea, vomiting. **OCCASIONAL:** Dizziness, giddiness, weakness, hypersensitivity reaction (rash, urticaria, pruritus, flushing). **INFREQUENT: IV:** Transient, but at times, marked hypotension. **RARE:** Confusion, mental depression, psychosis.

ADVERSE REACTIONS/ TOXIC EFFECTS

Paradoxical, extremely rapid ventricular rate may occur during treatment of atrial fibrillation/flutter. Systemic lupus erythematosus–like syndrome (fever, joint pain, pleuritic chest pain) with prolonged therapy. Cardiotoxic effects occur most commonly with IV administration, observed as conduction changes (50% widening of QRS complex, frequent ventricular premature contractions, ventricular tachycardia, complete AV block). Prolonged PR and QT intervals, flattened T waves occur less frequently (discontinue drug immediately).

NURSING IMPLICATIONS

BASELINE ASSESSMENT

Check B/P, pulse for 1 full min (unless pt is on continuous monitor) prior to giving medication.

INTERVENTION/EVALUATION

Monitor EKG for cardiac changes, particularly widening of QRS, prolongation of PR and QT intervals. Assess pulse for strength/weakness, irregular rate. Monitor I&O, electrolyte serum level (potassium, chloride, sodium). Assess for complaints of GI upset, headache, dizziness, joint pain. Monitor pattern of daily bowel activity, stool consistency. Assess for dizziness. Monitor B/P for hypotension. Assess skin for evidence of hypersensitivity reaction (esp. in pts on high-dose therapy). Monitor for therapeutic serum level (3–10 mcg/ml). Therapeutic blood serum level: 4–8 mcg/ml; toxic blood serum level: >10 mcg/ml.

PATIENT/FAMILY TEACHING

Take medication at evenly spaced doses around the clock. Contact physician if fever, joint pain/stiffness, signs of upper respiratory infection occur. Do not abruptly discontinue medication. Compliance with therapy regimen is essential to control arrhythmias. Do not use nasal decongestants, OTC cold preparations (stimulants) without physician approval. Restrict salt, alcohol intake.

procaine hydrochloride

(Novocain)

See Classification section under: Anesthetics: local (p. 4C)

procarbazine hydrochloride

pro-**car**-bah-zeen

(Matulane, Natulan ✤)

Do not confuse with dacarbazine.

CLASSIFICATION

PHARMACOTHERAPEUTIC: Methylhydrazine derivative. **CLINICAL:** Antineoplastic (see p. 75C).

ACTION

Inhibits DNA, RNA, protein synthesis. May also directly damage DNA. Cell cycle–specific for S phase of cell division.

USES

Treatment of advanced Hodgkin's disease. **Unlabeled:** Treatment of non-Hodgkin's lymphoma, primary brain tumors, lung carcinoma, malignant melanoma, multiple myeloma, polycythemia vera.

PRECAUTIONS

CONTRAINDICATIONS: Inadequate bone marrow reserve. **CAUTIONS:** Impaired renal/hepatic function. **Pregnancy Category D.**

INTERACTIONS

DRUG: Alcohol may cause disulfiram reaction. **Anticholinergics, antihistamines** may increase anticholinergic effects. **Tricyclic antidepressants** may increase anticholinergic effects, cause hyperpyretic crisis, convulsions. May increase effects of **oral hypoglycemics, insulin. Bone marrow depressants** may increase bone marrow depression. May increase B/P with **buspirone, caffeine-containing medications.** May cause hyperpyretic crisis, seizures, death with **carbamazepine, cyclobenzaprine, maprotiline, MAOIs. CNS depressants** may increase CNS depression. **Meperidine** may produce immediate excitation, diaphoresis, rigidity, severe hypertension/hypotension, severe respiratory distress, coma, convulsions, vascular collapse. **Sympathomimetics** may increase cardiac stimulant, vasopressor effects. **HERBAL:** None known. **FOOD:** None known. **LAB VALUES:** None known.

AVAILABILITY (Rx)

CAPSULES: 50 mg.

INDICATIONS/ROUTES/DOSAGE

HODGKIN'S DISEASE

PO: ADULTS, ELDERLY: Initially, 2–4 mg/kg daily as single or divided dose for 1 wk, then 4–6 mg/kg day. MAINTENANCE: 1–2 mg/kg/day. CHILDREN: 50–100 mg/m^2/day once daily for 10–14 days of a 28-day cycle. Continue until maximum response, leukocyte count falls below 4,000/mm^3, or platelets fall below 100,000/mm^3. MAINTENANCE: 50 mg/m^2 daily.

SIDE EFFECTS

FREQUENT: Severe nausea, vomiting, respiratory disorders (cough, effusion), myalgia, arthralgia, drowsiness, nervousness, insomnia, nightmares, diaphoresis, hallucinations, seizures. **OCCASIONAL:** Hoarseness, tachycardia, nystagmus, retinal hemorrhage, photophobia, photosensitivity, urinary frequency, nocturia, hypotension, diarrhea, stomatitis, paresthesia, unsteadiness, confusion, decreased reflexes, foot drop. **RARE:** Hypersensitivity reaction (dermatitis, pruritus, rash, urticaria), hyperpigmentation, alopecia.

ADVERSE REACTIONS/ TOXIC EFFECTS

Major toxic effects are bone marrow depression manifested as hematologic toxicity (principally leukopenia, thrombocytopenia, anemia), hepatotoxicity manifested by jaundice, ascites. UTI secondary to leukopenia may occur. Therapy should be discontinued if stomatitis, diarrhea, paresthesia, neuropathies, confusion, hypersensitivity reaction occurs.

NURSING IMPLICATIONS

BASELINE ASSESSMENT

Obtain bone marrow tests, Hgb, Hct, leukocyte, differential, reticulocyte, platelet, urinalysis, serum transaminase, serum alkaline phosphatase, BUN results prior to therapy and periodically thereafter. Therapy should be interrupted if WBC falls below 4,000/ mm^3 or platelet count falls below 100,000/mm^3.

INTERVENTION/EVALUATION

Monitor hematologic status, renal, hepatic function studies. Assess for stomatitis (burning/erythema of oral mucosa at inner margin of lips, sore throat, difficulty swallowing, oral ulceration). Monitor for hematologic toxicity (fever, sore throat, signs of local infection, unusual bruising/bleeding from any site), symptoms of anemia (excessive tiredness, weakness).

PATIENT/FAMILY TEACHING

Inform physician of fever, sore throat, bleeding, bruising. Avoid alcohol (may cause disulfiram reaction: nausea, vomiting, headache, sedation, visual disturbances).

prochlorperazine

pro-klor-**pear**-ah-zeen
(Compazine, Stemetil ✤)

Do not confuse with chlorpromazine, Copaxone.

CLASSIFICATION

PHARMACOTHERAPEUTIC: Phenothiazine. **CLINICAL:** Antiemetic.

ACTION

Acts centrally to inhibit/block dopamine receptors in chemoreceptor trigger zone and peripherally to block vagus nerve in GI tract. **Therapeutic Effect:** Relieves nausea and vomiting.

PHARMACOKINETICS

(Antiemetic)	Onset	Peak	Duration
Tablets, syrup	30–40 min	—	3–4 hrs
Extended-release	30–40 min	—	10–12 hrs
Rectal	60 min	—	3–4 hrs

Variably absorbed following PO administration. Widely distributed. Metabolized in liver, GI mucosa. Primarily excreted in urine. Unknown if removed by hemodialysis. **Half-life:** 23 hrs.

USES

Control of severe nausea/vomiting.

PRECAUTIONS

CONTRAINDICATIONS: Narrow-angle glaucoma, bone marrow suppression, severe liver/cardiac impairment, severe hypotension/hypertension, CNS depression, coma. **CAUTIONS:** Seizures, Parkinson's disease, children <2 yrs.

LIFESPAN CONSIDERATIONS: Pregnancy/lactation: Crosses placenta. Distributed in breast milk. **Pregnancy Category C. Children:** Safety and efficacy not established in those <9 kg or <2 yrs. **Elderly:** More susceptible to orthostatic hypotension, anticholinergic effects (e.g., dry mouth), sedation, extrapyramidal symptoms (EPS); lower dosage recommended.

INTERACTIONS

DRUG: Alcohol, CNS depressants may increase CNS, respiratory depression; hypotensive effects. **Tricyclic antidepressants, MAOIs** may increase sedative, anticholinergic effects. **Antithyroid agents** may increase risk of agranulocytosis. EPS may increase with **EPS-producing medications. Antihypertensives** may increase hypotension. May decrease **levodopa** effects. **Lithium** may decrease absorption, produce adverse neurologic effects. **HERBAL:** None

P

known. **FOOD:** None known. **LAB VALUES:** None known.

AVAILABILITY (Rx)

TABLETS: 5 mg, 10 mg. **CAPSULES (sustained-release):** 10 mg, 15 mg. **SUPPOSITORY:** 2.5 mg, 5 mg, 25 mg.

ADMINISTRATION/HANDLING

PO

- Give without regard to meals.

RECTAL

- Moisten suppository with cold water before inserting well into rectum.

INDICATIONS/ROUTES/DOSAGE

ANTIEMETIC

PO: ADULTS, ELDERLY: 5–10 mg 3–4 times/day. CHILDREN: 0.4 mg/kg/day in 3–4 divided doses.

PO (extended-release): ADULTS, ELDERLY: 10 mg 2 times/day or 15 mg once/day.

Rectal: ADULTS, ELDERLY: 25 mg 2 times/day. CHILDREN: 0.4 mg/kg/day in 3–4 divided doses.

P

PSYCHOSIS

PO: ADULTS, ELDERLY: 5–10 mg 3–4 times/day. **Maximum:** 150 mg/day. CHILDREN: 2.5 mg 2–3 times/day. **Maximum:** 2–5 yrs: 20 mg. 6–12 yrs: 25 mg.

SIDE EFFECTS

FREQUENT: Drowsiness, hypotension, dizziness, fainting occur frequently after first dose, occasionally after subsequent dosing, rarely with oral dosage. **OCCASIONAL:** Dry mouth, blurred vision, lethargy, constipation/diarrhea, muscular aches, nasal congestion, peripheral edema, urinary retention.

ADVERSE REACTIONS/ TOXIC EFFECTS

EPS appear dose related (particularly with high dosage) and are divided into three categories: akathisia (inability to sit still, tapping of feet, urge to move around); parkinsonian symptoms (mask-like face, tremors, shuffling gait, hypersalivation); acute dystonias: torticollis (neck muscle spasm), opisthotonos (rigidity of back muscles), oculogyric crisis (rolling back of eyes). Dystonic reaction may also produce diaphoresis, pallor. Tardive dyskinesia (protrusion of tongue, puffing of cheeks, chewing/puckering of the mouth) occurs rarely (may be irreversible). Abrupt withdrawal after long-term therapy may precipitate nausea, vomiting, gastritis, dizziness, tremors. Blood dyscrasias, particularly agranulocytosis, mild leukopenia (sore mouth/gums/throat) may occur. May lower seizure threshold.

NURSING IMPLICATIONS

BASELINE ASSESSMENT

Avoid skin contact with solution (contact dermatitis). **Antiemetic:** Assess for dehydration (poor skin turgor, dry mucous membranes, longitudinal furrows in tongue). **Antipsychotic:** Assess behavior, appearance, emotional status, response to environment, speech pattern, thought content.

INTERVENTION/EVALUATION

Monitor B/P for hypotension. Assess for EPS. Monitor WBC, differential count for blood dyscrasias. Monitor for fine tongue movement (may be early sign of tardive dyskinesia). Supervise suicidal-risk pt closely during early therapy (as depression lessens, energy level improves, increasing suicide potential). Assess for therapeutic response (interest in surroundings, improvement in self-care, increased ability to concentrate, relaxed facial expression).

PATIENT/FAMILY TEACHING

Limit caffeine. Avoid alcohol. May impair ability to perform tasks requiring mental alertness, physical coordination (e.g., driving).

Procrit

see epoetin alfa

progesterone

proe-**jess**-ter-one
(Crinone, Gesterol, Gesterol LA, Prochieve, Prometrium)

◆CLASSIFICATION

PHARMACOTHERAPEUTIC: Progestin. **CLINICAL:** Hormone.

ACTION

Natural steroid hormone. **Therapeutic Effect:** Transforms endometrium from proliferative to secretory (in estrogen-primed endometrium), promotes mammary gland development, relaxes uterine smooth muscle.

USES

Treatment of primary or secondary amenorrhea, abnormal uterine bleeding due to hormonal imbalance, endometriosis. Prevention of endometrial hyperplasia in estrogen recipients. **Vaginal Gel (8%):** Treatment of infertility. **Unlabeled:** Treatment of corpus luteum dysfunction.

PRECAUTIONS

CONTRAINDICATIONS: Thrombophlebitis, thromboembolic disorders, cerebral apoplexy or history of these conditions; severe liver dysfunction; breast cancer; undiagnosed vaginal bleeding; missed abortion; use as a diagnostic test for pregnancy. **CAUTIONS:** Diabetes, conditions aggravated by fluid retention (e.g., asthma, epilepsy, migraine, cardiac/renal dysfunction), history of mental depression. **Pregnancy Category D.**

INTERACTIONS

DRUG: May interfere with effects of **bromocriptine. HERBAL:** None known. **FOOD:** None known. **LAB VALUES:** May increase alkaline phosphatase, LDL. May decrease HDL. May cause abnormal thyroid, metapyrone, liver, endocrine function tests; decrease glucose tolerance.

AVAILABILITY (Rx)

INJECTION: 50 mg/ml. **(Gesterol LA):** 250 mg/ml. **CAPSULES:** 100 mg, 200 mg. **VAGINAL GEL:** 4%, 8%.

INDICATIONS/ROUTES/DOSAGE

AMENORRHEA

IM: ADULTS: 5–10 mg for 6–8 days. Withdrawal bleeding expected in 48–72 hrs if ovarian activity produced proliferative endometrium.

Vaginal: ADULTS: Apply every other day for ≤6 doses.

PO: ADULTS: 400 mg daily in evening for 10 days.

ABNORMAL UTERINE BLEEDING

IM: ADULTS: 5–10 mg for 6 days. (When estrogen given concomitantly, begin progesterone after 2 wks of estrogen therapy; discontinue when menstrual flow begins.)

PREVENTION OF ENDOMETRIAL HYPERPLASIA

PO: ADULTS: 200 mg in evening for 12 days per 28-day cycle in combination with daily conjugated estrogen.

SIDE EFFECTS

FREQUENT: Breakthrough bleeding/spotting at beginning of therapy. Amenorrhea, change in menstrual flow, breast tenderness. **OCCASIONAL:** Edema, weight gain/loss, rash, pruritus, photosensitivity, skin pigmentation. **RARE:**

P

Pain/swelling at injection site, acne, mental depression, alopecia, hirsutism.

ADVERSE REACTIONS/ TOXIC EFFECTS

Thrombophlebitis, cerebrovascular disorders, retinal thrombosis, pulmonary embolism occur rarely.

NURSING IMPLICATIONS

BASELINE ASSESSMENT

Question for possibility of pregnancy or hypersensitivity to progestins prior to initiating therapy. Obtain baseline weight, blood glucose level, B/P.

INTERVENTION/EVALUATION

Check weight daily; report weekly gain of ≥5 lbs. Assess skin for rash, hives. Immediately report the development of chest pain, sudden shortness of breath, sudden decrease in vision, migraine headache, pain (esp. with swelling, warmth, redness) in calves, numbness of an arm/leg (thrombotic disorders). Check B/P periodically. Note progesterone therapy on pathology specimens.

PATIENT/FAMILY TEACHING

Use sunscreens, protective clothing to protect from sunlight/ultraviolet light until tolerance determined. Notify physician of abnormal vaginal bleeding, other symptoms. Stop taking medication and contact physician at once if pregnancy suspected.

promethazine hydrochloride

pro-**meth**-ah-zeen

(Histantil ✤, Phenergan)

Do not confuse with promazine.

FIXED-COMBINATION(S)

Phenergan with codeine: promethazine/codeine (a cough suppressant): 6.25 mg/10 mg/5 ml. **Phenergan VC:** promethazine/phenylephrine (a vasoconstrictor): 6.25 mg/5 mg/5 ml. **Phenergan VC with codeine:** promethazine/phenylephrine/codeine: 6.25 mg/5 mg/10 mg/5 ml.

◆CLASSIFICATION

PHARMACOTHERAPEUTIC: Phenothiazine. **CLINICAL:** Antihistamine, antiemetic, sedative-hypnotic (see p. 49C).

ACTION

Antihistamine: Inhibits histamine at histamine receptor sites. **Therapeutic Effect:** Prevents, antagonizes most allergic effects (e.g., urticaria, pruritus). **Antiemetic:** Diminishes vestibular stimulation, depresses labyrinthine function, acts on chemoreceptor trigger zone. **Therapeutic Effect:** Produces antiemetic effect. **Sedative-Hypnotic:** Decreases stimulation to brainstem reticular formation. **Therapeutic Effect:** Produces CNS depression.

PHARMACOKINETICS

	Onset	Peak	Duration
PO	20 min	—	2–8 hrs
IM	20 min	—	2–8 hrs
Rectal	20 min	—	2–8 hrs
IV	3–5 min	—	2–8 hrs

Well absorbed from GI tract following IM administration. Widely distributed. Metabolized in liver. Primarily excreted in urine. Not removed by hemodialysis. **Half-life:** 16–19 hrs.

USES

Symptomatic relief of allergic symptoms; sedative/antiemetic in surgery/labor; decreases postop nausea/vomiting; adjunct to analgesics in control of pain; management of motion sickness.

PRECAUTIONS

CONTRAINDICATIONS: Narrow-angle glaucoma, severe CNS depression/coma, GI/GU obstruction. **CAUTIONS:** Impaired cardiovascular disease, liver function impairment, asthma, peptic ulcer, history of seizures, sleep apnea, pts suspected of Reye's syndrome.

LIFESPAN CONSIDERATIONS: Pregnancy/lactation: Readily crosses placenta. Unknown if drug is excreted in breast milk. May inhibit platelet aggregation in neonates if taken within 2 wks of birth. May produce jaundice, extrapyramidal symptoms in neonates if taken during pregnancy. **Pregnancy Category C. Children:** May experience increased excitement. Not recommended for those <2 yrs. **Elderly:** More sensitive to dizziness, sedation, confusion, hypotension, hyperexcitability, anticholinergic effects (e.g., dry mouth).

INTERACTIONS

DRUG: Alcohol, CNS depressants may increase CNS depressant effects. **Anticholinergics** may increase anticholinergic effects. **MAOIs** may prolong, intensify anticholinergic, CNS depressant effects. **HERBAL:** None known. **FOOD:** None known. **LAB VALUES:** May suppress wheal/flare reactions to antigen skin testing, unless discontinued 4 days before testing.

AVAILABILITY (Rx)

TABLETS: 12.5 mg, 25 mg, 50 mg. **SYRUP:** 6.25 mg/5 ml. **SUPPOSITORY:** 12.5 mg, 25 mg, 50 mg. **INJECTION:** 25 mg/ml, 50 mg/ml.

ADMINISTRATION/HANDLING

PO

- Give without regard to meals.
- Scored tablets may be crushed.

IM

Alert: Significant tissue necrosis may occur if given subcutaneously. Inadvertent intra-arterial injection may produce severe arteriospasm, resulting in severe circulation impairment.

- Inject deep IM.

IV

Storage • Store at room temperature.

Reconstitution • May be given undiluted or dilute with 0.9% NaCl. Final dilution should not exceed 25 mg/ml.

Rate of administration • Administer at 25 mg/min rate through IV infusion tube. • A too rapid rate of infusion may result in transient fall in B/P, producing orthostatic hypotension, reflex tachycardia. • If pt complains of pain at IV site, stop injection immediately (possibility of intra-arterial needle placement/perivascular extravasation).

RECTAL

• Refrigerate suppository. • Moisten suppository with cold water before inserting well into rectum.

IV INCOMPATIBILITIES

Allopurinol (Aloprim), amphotericin B complex (Abelcet, AmBisome, Amphotec), heparin, ketorolac (Toradol), nalbuphine (Nubain), piperacillin tazobactam (Zosyn).

IV COMPATIBILITIES

Atropine, diphenhydramine (Benadryl), glycopyrrolate (Robinul), hydromorphone (Dilaudid), hydroxyzine (Vistaril), midazolam (Versed), morphine.

INDICATIONS/ROUTES/DOSAGE

ALLERGIC SYMPTOMS

IV/IM: ADULTS, ELDERLY: 25 mg. May repeat in 2 hrs.

PO: ADULTS, ELDERLY: 6.25–12.5 mg 3 times/day plus 25 mg at bedtime. CHILDREN: 0.1 mg/kg/dose (**Maximum:**

P

12.5 mg) 3 times/day plus 0.5 mg/kg/ dose (**Maximum:** 25 mg) at bedtime.

MOTION SICKNESS
PO: ADULTS, ELDERLY: 25 mg 30–60 min before departure; may repeat in 8–12 hrs, then every morning on rising and before evening meal. CHILDREN: 0.5 mg/kg (same regimen).

PREVENTION OF NAUSEA, VOMITING
PO/IM/IV/rectal: ADULTS, ELDERLY: 12.5–25 mg q4–6h as needed. CHILDREN: 0.25–1 mg/kg q4–6h as needed.

PREOP AND POSTOP SEDATION; ADJUNCT TO ANALGESICS
IM/IV: ADULTS, ELDERLY: 25–50 mg. CHILDREN: 12.5–25 mg.

SIDE EFFECTS

HIGH INCIDENCE: Drowsiness, disorientation. Hypotension, confusion, syncope more likely noted in elderly. **FREQUENT:** Dry mouth, urinary retention, thickening of bronchial secretions. **OCCASIONAL:** Epigastric distress, flushing, visual disturbances, hearing disturbances, wheezing, paresthesia, sweating, chills. **RARE:** Dizziness, urticaria, photosensitivity, nightmares. Fixed-combination form with pseudoephedrine may produce mild CNS stimulation.

ADVERSE REACTIONS/ TOXIC EFFECTS

Paradoxical reaction (particularly in children) manifested as excitation, nervousness, tremor, hyperactive reflexes, convulsions. CNS depression has occurred in infants, young children (respiratory depression, sleep apnea, SIDS). Long-term therapy may produce extrapyramidal symptoms noted as dystonia (abnormal movements), pronounced motor restlessness (most frequently occurs in children), parkinsonian symptoms (esp. noted in elderly). Blood dyscrasias, particularly agranulocytosis, have occurred.

NURSING IMPLICATIONS

BASELINE ASSESSMENT

Assess B/P, pulse for bradycardia/ tachycardia if pt is given parenteral form. If used as an antiemetic, assess for dehydration (poor skin turgor, dry mucous membranes, longitudinal furrows in tongue).

INTERVENTION/EVALUATION

Monitor serum electrolytes in pts with severe vomiting. Assist with ambulation if drowsiness, lightheadedness occurs.

PATIENT/FAMILY TEACHING

Drowsiness, dry mouth may be an expected response to drug. Sugarless gum, sips of tepid water may relieve dry mouth. Coffee/tea may help reduce drowsiness. Report visual disturbances. Avoid tasks that require alertness, motor skills until response to drug is established. Avoid alcohol, other CNS depressants.

propafenone hydrochloride

pro-**pah**-phen-own
(Rythmol)

CLASSIFICATION

CLINICAL: Antiarrhythmic (see p. 14C).

ACTION

Decreases the fast sodium current in Purkinje/myocardial cells. **Therapeutic Effect:** Decreases excitability, automaticity; prolongs conduction velocity, refractory period.

USES

Treatment of documented, life-threatening ventricular arrhythmias (e.g., sustained ventricular tachycardias). **Unlabeled:** Treatment of supraventricular arrhythmias.

PRECAUTIONS

CONTRAINDICATIONS: Uncontrolled CHF; cardiogenic shock; sinoatrial, AV, intraventricular disorders of impulse/conduction (sick sinus syndrome [bradycardia-tachycardia], AV block) without presence of pacemaker; bradycardia; marked hypotension, bronchospastic disorders; manifest electrolyte imbalance. **CAUTIONS:** Impaired renal/hepatic function, recent MI, CHF, conduction disturbances. **Pregnancy Category C.**

INTERACTIONS

DRUG: May increase concentrations of **digoxin, propranolol.** May increase effects of **warfarin.** **HERBAL:** None known. **FOOD:** None known. **LAB VALUES:** May cause EKG changes (e.g., QRS widening, PR prolongation), positive ANA titers.

AVAILABILITY (Rx)

TABLETS: 150 mg.

INDICATIONS/ROUTES/DOSAGE

USUAL DOSAGE

PO: ADULTS, ELDERLY: Initially, 150 mg q8h, may increase at 3- to 4-day intervals to 225 mg q8h, then to 300 mg q8h. **Maximum:** 900 mg/day.

SIDE EFFECTS

FREQUENT (7%–13%): Dizziness, nausea, vomiting, unusual taste, constipation. **OCCASIONAL (3%–6%):** Headache, dyspnea, blurred vision, dyspepsia (heartburn, indigestion, epigastric pain). **RARE (<2%):** Rash, weakness, dry mouth, diarrhea, rash, edema, hot flashes.

ADVERSE REACTIONS/ TOXIC EFFECTS

May produce/worsen existing arrhythmias. Overdosage may produce hypotension, somnolence, bradycardia, intra-atrial/intraventricular conduction disturbances.

NURSING IMPLICATIONS

BASELINE ASSESSMENT

Correct electrolyte imbalance prior to administering medication.

INTERVENTION/EVALUATION

Assess pulse for strength/weakness, irregular rate. Monitor EKG for cardiac performance/changes, particularly widening of QRS, prolongation of PR interval. Question for visual disturbances, headache, GI upset. Monitor fluid, electrolyte serum levels. Monitor pattern of daily bowel activity, stool consistency. Assess for dizziness, unsteadiness. Monitor liver enzymes results. Monitor for therapeutic serum level (0.06–1 mcg/ml).

PATIENT/FAMILY TEACHING

Compliance with therapy regimen is essential to control arrhythmias. Unusual taste sensation may occur. Report headache, blurred vision, fever. Use caution performing tasks requiring mental alertness, physical coordination (e.g., driving).

propofol

pro-**poe**-foal
(Diprivan)

CLASSIFICATION

PHARMACOTHERAPEUTIC: Rapid-acting general anesthetic. **CLINICAL:** Sedative-hypnotic (see p. 3C).

P

ACTION

Inhibits sympathetic vasoconstrictor nerve activity, decreases vascular resistance. **Therapeutic Effect:** Produces hypnosis rapidly.

PHARMACOKINETICS

	Onset	Peak	Duration
IV	40 sec	—	3–10 min

Protein binding: 97%–99%. Rapidly, extensively distributed. Metabolized in liver. Primarily excreted in urine. Unknown if removed by hemodialysis. **Half-life:** 3–12 hrs.

USES

Induction/maintenance of anesthesia. Continuous sedation in intubated/respiratory controlled adult pts in ICU.

PRECAUTIONS

CONTRAINDICATIONS: Increased intracranial pressure, impaired cerebral circulation. **CAUTIONS:** Debilitated; impaired respiratory, circulatory, renal, hepatic, lipid metabolism disorders; seizures; history of epilepsy.

P

LIFESPAN CONSIDERATIONS: Pregnancy/lactation: Unknown if drug crosses placenta. Distributed in breast milk. Not recommended for obstetrics, nursing mothers. **Pregnancy Category B. Children:** Safety and efficacy not established. FDA approved for use in those >3 yrs. **Elderly:** No age-related precautions noted; lower dosages recommended.

INTERACTIONS

DRUG: Alcohol, CNS depressants may increase CNS, respiratory, depression, hypotensive effect. **HERBAL:** None known. **FOOD:** None known. **LAB VALUES:** None known.

AVAILABILITY (Rx)

INJECTION: 10 mg/ml.

ADMINISTRATION/HANDLING

IV

Alert: Do not give through same IV line with blood or plasma.

Storage • Store at room temperature. • Discard unused portions. • Do not use if emulsion separates. • Shake well before using.

Reconstitution • May give undiluted, or dilute only with D_5W. • Do not dilute to concentration <2 mg/ml (4 ml D_5W to 1 ml propofol yields 2 mg/ml).

Rate of administration • A too rapid IV may produce marked severe hypotension, respiratory depression, irregular muscular movements. • Observe for signs of intra-arterial injection (pain, discolored skin patches, white/blue color to hand, delayed onset of drug action). • Inadvertent intra-arterial injection may result in arterial spasm with severe pain, thrombosis, gangrene.

IV INCOMPATIBILITIES

Amikacin (Amikin), amphotericin B complex (Abelcet, AmBisome, Amphotec), bretylium (Bretylol), calcium chloride, ciprofloxacin (Cipro), diazepam (Valium), digoxin (Lanoxin), doxorubicin (Adriamycin), gentamicin (Garamycin), methylprednisolone (Solu-Medrol), minocycline (Minocin), phenytoin (Dilantin), tobramycin (Nebcin), verapamil (Isoptin).

IV COMPATIBILITIES

Acyclovir (Zovirax), bumetanide (Bumex), calcium gluconate, ceftazidime (Fortaz), dobutamine (Dobutrex), dopamine (Intropin), enalapril (Vasotec), fentanyl, heparin, insulin, labetalol (Normodyne, Trandate), lidocaine, lorazepam

(Ativan), magnesium, milrinone (Primacor), nitroglycerin, norepinephrine (Levophed), potassium chloride, vancomycin (Vancocin).

INDICATIONS/ROUTES/DOSAGE

ICU SEDATION

IV infusion: ADULTS: Initially, 0.3 mg/kg/hr. May increase by 0.3–0.6 mg/kg/hr q5–10min until desired effect obtained. MAINTENANCE: 0.3–3 mg/kg/hr.

ANESTHESIA

IV: ADULTS ASA I & II: 2–2.5 mg/kg (about 40 mg q10sec until onset of anesthesia). ELDERLY, DEBILITATED, HYPOVOLEMIC, ASA III OR IV: 1–1.5 mg/kg q10sec until onset of anesthesia. CHILDREN >3 YRS ASA I OR II: 2.5–3.5 mg/kg (lower dosage in ASA III or IV).

MAINTENANCE

IV: ADULTS ASA I & II: 0.1–0.2 mg/kg/min. ELDERLY, DEBILITATED, HYPOVOLEMIC, ASA III OR IV: 0.05–0.1 mg/kg/min. CHILDREN >2 MOS–16 YRS: 0.125–0.15 mg/kg/min.

SIDE EFFECTS

FREQUENT: Involuntary muscular movement, apnea (common during induction; lasts >60 sec), hypotension, nausea, vomiting, burning/stinging at IV site. **OCCASIONAL:** Twitching, bucking, jerking, thrashing, headache, dizziness, bradycardia, hypertension, fever, abdominal cramping, tingling, numbness, coldness, cough, hiccups, facial flushing. **RARE:** Rash, dry mouth, agitation, confusion, myalgia, thrombophlebitis.

ADVERSE REACTIONS/ TOXIC EFFECTS

Continuous/repeated intermittent infusion may result in extreme somnolence, respiratory/circulatory depression. A too rapid IV may produce marked severe hypotension, respiratory depression, irregular muscular movements. Acute allergic reaction (erythema, pruritus, urticaria, rhinitis, dyspnea, hypotension, restlessness, anxiety, abdominal pain) may occur.

NURSING IMPLICATIONS

BASELINE ASSESSMENT

Resuscitative equipment, endotracheal tube, suction, O_2 must be available. Obtain vital signs prior to administration.

INTERVENTION/EVALUATION

Monitor respiratory rate, B/P, heart rate, O_2 saturation, ABGs, depth of sedation, lipid/triglycerides if used >24 hrs. May change urine color to green.

propoxyphene hydrochloride

pro-**pox**-ih-feen
(Darvon)

propoxyphene napsylate

(Darvon-N ✤)

FIXED-COMBINATION(S)

Darvocet-N: propoxyphene/acetaminophen: 50 mg/325 mg; 100 mg/650 mg. **Darvocet A500:** propoxyphene/acetaminophen: 100 mg/500 mg.

◆CLASSIFICATION

PHARMACOTHERAPEUTIC: Opioid agonist **(Schedule IV). CLINICAL:** Analgesic (see p. 121C).

ACTION

Binds with opioid receptors within CNS. **Therapeutic Effect:** Alters processes affecting pain perception, emotional response to pain.

P

PHARMACOKINETICS

	Onset	Peak	Duration
PO	15–60 min	—	4–6 hrs

Well absorbed from GI tract. Protein binding: High. Widely distributed. Metabolized in liver. Primarily excreted in urine. Not removed by hemodialysis. **Half-life:** 6–12 hrs; metabolite: 30–36 hrs.

USES

Relief of mild to moderate pain.

PRECAUTIONS

CONTRAINDICATIONS: None known. **CAUTIONS:** Renal/liver impairment, substitution for opiates in narcotic-dependent pts.

LIFESPAN CONSIDERATIONS: Pregnancy/lactation: Crosses placenta. Minimal amount distributed in breast milk. Respiratory depression may occur in neonate if mother received opiates during labor. Regular use of opiates during pregnancy may produce withdrawal symptoms in neonate (irritability, excessive crying, tremors, hyperactive reflexes, fever, vomiting, diarrhea, yawning, sneezing, seizures). **Pregnancy Category C** (**D** if used for prolonged periods). **Children:** Dosage not established. **Elderly:** May be more susceptible to CNS effects, constipation. Avoid use if possible.

INTERACTIONS

DRUG: **Alcohol, CNS depressants** may increase CNS/respiratory depression, risk of hypotension. May increase concentration, toxicity of **carbamazepine.** Effects may be decreased with **buprenorphine. MAOIs** may produce severe, fatal reaction (reduce dose to ¼ usual dose). **HERBAL:** None known. **FOOD:** None known. **LAB VALUES:** May increase amylase, lipase, SGOT (AST), SGPT (ALT), LDH, alkaline phosphatase, bilirubin. Therapeutic blood serum level: 100–400 ng/ml; toxic blood serum level: >500 ng/ml.

AVAILABILITY (Rx)

CAPSULES (Hydrochloride): 65 mg. **TABLETS (Napsylate):** 100 mg.

ADMINISTRATION/HANDLING

PO

• Give without regard to meals. • Capsules may be emptied and mixed with food. • Shake oral suspension well. • Do not crush/break film-coated tablets.

INDICATIONS/ROUTES/DOSAGE

Alert: Reduce initial dosage in pts with hypothyroidism, concurrent CNS depressants, Addison's disease, renal insufficiency, elderly/debilitated.

PROPOXYPHENE HYDROCHLORIDE

PO: ADULTS, ELDERLY: 65 mg q4h, as needed. **Maximum:** 390 mg/day.

PROPOXYPHENE NAPSYLATE

PO: ADULTS, ELDERLY: 100 mg q4h, as needed. **Maximum:** 600 mg/day.

SIDE EFFECTS

Alert: Effects dependent on dosage amount. Ambulatory pts and those not in moderate pain may experience dizziness, nausea, vomiting, hypotension more frequently than those in supine position or having moderate pain.

FREQUENT: Dizziness, drowsiness, dry mouth, euphoria, hypotension, nausea, vomiting, unusual tiredness. **OCCASIONAL:** Histamine reaction (decreased B/P, diaphoresis, flushing, wheezing),

P

trembling, decreased urination, altered vision, constipation, headache. **RARE:** Confusion, increased B/P, depression, stomach cramps, anorexia.

ADVERSE REACTIONS/ TOXIC EFFECTS

Overdosage results in respiratory depression, skeletal muscle flaccidity, cold/clammy skin, cyanosis, extreme somnolence progressing to convulsions, stupor, coma. Hepatotoxicity may occur with overdosage of acetaminophen component. Tolerance to analgesic effect, physical dependence may occur with repeated use.

NURSING IMPLICATIONS

BASELINE ASSESSMENT

Obtain vital signs prior to giving medication. If respirations are ≤12/min (≤20/min in children), withhold medication, contact physician. Assess onset, type, location, duration of pain. Effect of medication is reduced if full pain recurs prior to next dose.

INTERVENTION/EVALUATION

Palpate bladder for urinary retention. Monitor pattern of daily bowel activity, stool consistency. Initiate deep breathing/coughing exercises, particularly in pts with impaired pulmonary function. Assess for clinical improvement, record onset of relief of pain. Contact physician if pain is not adequately relieved. Therapeutic blood serum level: 100–400 ng/ml; toxic blood serum level: >500 ng/ml.

PATIENT/FAMILY TEACHING

Avoid alcohol. May be habit forming. May impair ability to perform tasks requiring mental alertness, physical coordination (e.g., driving). Do not discontinue abruptly.

propranolol hydrochloride

pro-**pran**-oh-lol

(Apo-Propranolol ✤, Inderal, Inno-Pran XL)

Do not confuse with Adderall, Isordil, Pravachol.

FIXED-COMBINATION(S)

Inderide: propranolol/hydrochlorothiazide (a diuretic): 40 mg/25 mg; 80 mg/25 mg. **Inderide LA:** propranolol/hydrochlorothiazide (a diuretic): 80 mg/50 mg; 120 mg/50 mg; 160 mg/50 mg.

◆CLASSIFICATION

PHARMACOTHERAPEUTIC: Beta-adrenergic blocker. **CLINICAL:** Antihypertensive, antianginal, antiarrhythmic, antimigraine (see pp. 14C, 62C).

ACTION

Blocks $beta_1$- and $beta_2$-adrenergic receptors. Decreases O_2 requirements. Slows AV conduction, increases refractory period in AV node. **Therapeutic Effect:** Slows sinus heart rate, decreases cardiac output, decreases B/P. Increases airway resistance. Decreases myocardial ischemia severity. Exhibits antiarrhythmic activity.

PHARMACOKINETICS

	Onset	Peak	Duration
PO	1–2 hrs	—	6 hrs

Well absorbed from GI tract. Protein binding: 93%. Widely distributed. Metabolized in liver. Primarily excreted in urine. Not removed by hemodialysis. **Half-life:** 3–5 hrs.

USES

Treatment of hypertension, angina, various cardiac arrhythmias, hypertrophic subaortic stenosis, migraine headache, essential tremor, and as an adjunct to alpha-blocking agents in the treatment of pheochromocytoma. Used to reduce risk of cardiovascular mortality and reinfarction in pts who have previously suffered an MI. **Unlabeled:** Treatment of adjunct anxiety, thyrotoxicosis, mitral valve prolapse syndrome.

PRECAUTIONS

CONTRAINDICATIONS: Uncompensated CHF, cardiogenic shock, bradycardia, heart block, asthma, COPD, Raynaud's syndrome. **CAUTIONS:** Diabetes, renal/liver impairment, concurrent use of calcium blockers when using IV administration.

LIFESPAN CONSIDERATIONS: Pregnancy/lactation: Crosses placenta. Distributed in breast milk. Avoid use during first trimester. May produce bradycardia, apnea, hypoglycemia, hypothermia during delivery, low birth-weight infants. **Pregnancy Category C** (**D** if used in second or third trimester). **Children:** No age-related precautions noted. **Elderly:** Age-related peripheral vascular disease may increase susceptibility to decreased peripheral circulation.

INTERACTIONS

DRUG: Diuretics, other hypotensives may increase hypotensive effect. **Sympathomimetics, xanthines** may mutually inhibit effects. May mask symptoms of hypoglycemia, prolong hypoglycemic effect of **insulin, oral hypoglycemics. NSAIDs** may decrease antihypertensive effect. May increase cardiac depressant effect with **IV phenytoin. HERBAL:** None known. **FOOD:** None known. **LAB VALUES:** May increase ANA titer, SGOT (AST), SGPT (ALT), alkaline phosphatase, LDH, bilirubin, BUN, creatinine, potassium, uric acid, lipoproteins, triglycerides.

AVAILABILITY (Rx)

TABLETS: 10 mg, 20 mg, 40 mg, 60 mg, 80 mg. **CAPSULES (sustained-release):** 60 mg, 80 mg, 120 mg, 160 mg. **ORAL SOLUTION:** 4 mg/ml, 8 mg/ml. **SOLUTION (concentrate):** 80 mg/ml. **INJECTION:** 1 mg/ml.

ADMINISTRATION/HANDLING

PO

• May crush scored tablets. • Give at same time each day.

IV

Storage • Store at room temperature.

Reconstitution • Give undiluted for IV push. • For IV infusion, may dilute each 1 mg in 10 ml D_5W.

Rate of administration • Do not exceed 1 mg/min injection rate. • For IV infusion, give 1 mg over 10–15 min.

IV INCOMPATIBILITIES

Amphotericin B complex (Abelcet, AmBisome, Amphotec).

IV COMPATIBILITIES

Alteplase (Activase), heparin, milrinone (Primacor), potassium chloride, propofol (Diprivan).

INDICATIONS/ROUTES/DOSAGE

HYPERTENSION

PO: ADULTS, ELDERLY: Initially, 40 mg 2 times/day. May increase dose q3–7days. RANGE: Up to 320 mg/day in divided doses. **Maximum:** 640 mg/day. CHILDREN: Initially, 0.5–1 mg/kg/day in divided doses q6–12h. May increase at 3- to 5-day interval. Usual dose: 1–5 mg/kg/day. **Maximum:** 8 mg/kg/day.

ANGINA

PO: ADULTS, ELDERLY: 80–320 mg/day in divided doses.

P

PO (long-acting): Initially, 80 mg/day. **Maximum:** 320 mg/day.

ARRHYTHMIAS

IV: ADULTS, ELDERLY: 1 mg/dose. May repeat q5min. **Maximum:** 5 mg total dose. CHILDREN: 0.01–0.1 mg/kg. **Maximum:** 3 mg. INFANTS: **Maximum:** 1 mg.

PO: ADULTS, ELDERLY: Initially, 10–20 mg q6–8h. May gradually increase dose. RANGE: 40–320 mg/day. CHILDREN: Initially, 0.5–1 mg/kg/day in divided doses q6–8h. May increase q3–5days. Usual dosage: 2–4 mg/kg/day. **Maximum:** 16 mg/kg/day or 60 mg/day.

HYPERTROPHIC SUBAORTIC STENOSIS

PO: ADULTS, ELDERLY: 20–40 mg in 3–4 divided doses or 80–160 mg/day as extended-release capsule.

PHEOCHROMOCYTOMA

PO: ADULTS, ELDERLY: 60 mg/day in divided doses with alpha-blocker for 3 days before surgery. MAINTENANCE (inoperable tumor): 30 mg/day with alpha-blocker.

MIGRAINE HEADACHE

PO: ADULTS, ELDERLY: 80 mg/day in divided doses or 80 mg once daily as extended-release capsule. Increase up to 160–240 mg/day in divided doses. CHILDREN: 0.6–1.5 mg/kg/day in divided doses q8h. **Maximum:** 4 mg/kg/day.

MI

PO: ADULTS, ELDERLY: 180–240 mg/day in divided doses.

ESSENTIAL TREMOR

PO: ADULTS, ELDERLY: Initially, 40 mg 2 times/day increased up to 120–320 mg/day in 3 divided doses.

SIDE EFFECTS

FREQUENT: Decreased sexual function, drowsiness, difficulty sleeping, unusual tiredness/weakness. **OCCASIONAL:** Bradycardia, depression, cold hands/feet, diarrhea, constipation, anxiety, nasal congestion, nausea, vomiting. **RARE:** Altered taste; dry eyes; itching; numbness of fingers, toes, scalp.

ADVERSE REACTIONS/ TOXIC EFFECTS

May produce profound bradycardia, hypotension. Abrupt withdrawal may result in diaphoresis, palpitations, headache, tremulousness. May precipitate CHF, MI in those with cardiac disease; thyroid storm in those with thyrotoxicosis; peripheral ischemia in those with existing peripheral vascular disease. Hypoglycemia may occur in pts with previously controlled diabetes.

NURSING IMPLICATIONS

BASELINE ASSESSMENT

Assess baseline renal/liver function tests. Assess B/P, apical pulse immediately prior to administering the drug (if pulse is ≤60/min or systolic B/P is <90 mm Hg, withhold medication, contact physician). **Anginal:** Record onset, type (sharp, dull, squeezing), radiation, location, intensity, duration of anginal pain, precipitating factors (exertion, emotional stress).

INTERVENTION/EVALUATION

Assess pulse for strength/weakness, irregular rate, bradycardia. Monitor EKG for cardiac arrhythmias. Assess fingers for color, numbness (Raynaud's). Assess for evidence of CHF (dyspnea [particularly on exertion or lying down], night cough, peripheral edema, distended neck veins). Monitor I&O (increase in weight, decrease in urine output may indicate CHF). Assess for rash, fatigue, behavioral changes. Therapeutic response ranges from a few days to several weeks. Measure B/P near end of dosing interval (determines if B/P is controlled throughout day).

P

PATIENT/FAMILY TEACHING

Do not abruptly discontinue medication. Compliance with therapy regimen is essential to control hypertension, arrhythmia, anginal pain. To avoid hypotensive effect, rise slowly from lying to sitting position, wait momentarily before standing. Avoid tasks that require alertness, motor skills until response to drug is established. Report excessively slow pulse rate (<60 beats/min), peripheral numbness, dizziness. Do not use nasal decongestants, OTC cold preparations (stimulants) without physician approval. Restrict salt, alcohol intake.

propylthiouracil

pro-pill-thye-oh-**your**-ah-sill
(Propylthiouracil, Propyl-Thyracil ✱)

◆CLASSIFICATION

PHARMACOTHERAPEUTIC: Thiourea derivative. **CLINICAL:** Antithyroid.

ACTION

Blocks oxidation of iodine in the thyroid gland, blocks synthesis of thyroxine, triiodothyronine. **Therapeutic Effect:** Inhibits synthesis of thyroid hormone.

USES

Palliative treatment of hyperthyroidism; adjunct to ameliorate hyperthyroidism in preparation for surgical treatment, radioactive iodine therapy.

PRECAUTIONS

CONTRAINDICATIONS: None known. **CAUTIONS:** Pts >40 yrs or in combination with other agranulocytosis-inducing drugs. **Pregnancy Category D.**

INTERACTIONS

DRUG: **Amiodarone, iodinated glycerol, iodine, potassium iodide** may decrease response. May decrease effect of **oral anticoagulants.** May increase concentration of **digoxin** (as pt becomes euthyroid). May decrease thyroid uptake of **^{131}I.** **HERBAL:** None known. **FOOD:** None known. **LAB VALUES:** May increase SGOT (AST), SGPT (ALT), alkaline phosphatase, LDH, bilirubin, prothrombin time.

AVAILABILITY (Rx)

TABLETS: 50 mg.

INDICATIONS/ROUTES/DOSAGE

HYPERTHYROIDISM

PO: ADULTS, ELDERLY: Initially: 300–450 mg/day in divided doses q8h. MAINTENANCE: 100–150 mg/day in divided doses q8–12h. CHILDREN: Initially, 5–7 mg/kg/day in divided doses q8h. MAINTENANCE: ⅓–⅔ of initial dose in divided doses q8–12h. NEONATES: 5–10 mg/kg/day in divided doses q8h.

SIDE EFFECTS

FREQUENT: Urticaria, rash, pruritus, nausea, skin pigmentation, hair loss, headache, paresthesia. **OCCASIONAL:** Drowsiness, lymphadenopathy, vertigo. **RARE:** Drug fever, lupus-like syndrome.

ADVERSE REACTIONS/ TOXIC EFFECTS

Agranulocytosis (may occur as long as 4 mos after therapy), pancytopenia, fatal hepatitis have occurred.

NURSING IMPLICATIONS

BASELINE ASSESSMENT

Obtain baseline weight, pulse.

INTERVENTION/EVALUATION

Monitor pulse, weight daily. Check for skin eruptions, itching, swollen lymph glands. Be alert to hepatitis (nausea, vomiting, drowsiness, jaundice). Monitor hematology results for bone marrow suppression; check for signs of infection/bleeding.

PATIENT/FAMILY TEACHING

Space evenly around the clock. Take resting pulse daily (teach pt/family), report as directed. Seafood, iodine products may be restricted. Report illness, unusual bleeding/bruising immediately. Inform physician of sudden/continuous weight gain, cold intolerance, depression.

Proscar

see finasteride

protamine sulfate

pro-tah-meen

(Protamine✤, Protamine sulfate)

Do not confuse with ProAmatine, Protopam, Protropin.

◆CLASSIFICATION

PHARMACOTHERAPEUTIC: Protein. **CLINICAL:** Heparin antagonist.

ACTION

Complexes with heparin to form a stable salt. **Therapeutic Effect:** Results in reduction of anticoagulant activity of heparin.

USES

Treatment of severe heparin overdose (causing hemorrhage). Neutralizes effects of heparin administered during extracorporeal circulation. **Unlabeled:** Treatment of enoxaparin toxicity.

PRECAUTIONS

CONTRAINDICATIONS: None known. **CAUTIONS:** History of allergy to fish; vasectomized/infertile men; those on isophane (NPH), insulin, or previous protamine therapy (propensity to hypersensitivity reaction). **Pregnancy Category C.**

INTERACTIONS

DRUG: None known. **HERBAL:** None known. **FOOD:** None known. **LAB VALUES:** None known.

ADMINISTRATION/HANDLING

IV

Storage • Store vials at room temperature.

Rate of administration • May give undiluted over 10 min. Do not exceed 5 mg/min (50 mg in any 10-min period).

AVAILABILITY (Rx)

INJECTION: 10 mg/ml.

INDICATIONS/ROUTES/DOSAGE

ANTIDOTE

IV: ADULTS, ELDERLY: 1 mg protamine sulfate neutralizes 90–115 units of heparin. Heparin disappears rapidly from circulation, reducing the dosage demand for protamine as time elapses.

SIDE EFFECTS

FREQUENT: Decreased B/P, dyspnea. **OCCASIONAL:** Hypersensitivity reaction: urticaria, angioedema; nausea, vomiting (generally occurs in those sensitive to fish, men who have undergone a vasectomy, infertile men, those on isophane [NPH], insulin, or previous protamine therapy). **RARE:** Back pain.

ADVERSE REACTIONS/TOXIC EFFECTS

A too rapid IV administration may produce acute hypotension, bradycardia, pulmonary hypertension, dyspnea, transient flushing, feeling of warmth. Heparin

P

rebound may occur several hours after heparin has been neutralized by protamine (usually evident 8–9 hrs after protamine administration). Occurs most often after arterial/cardiac surgery.

NURSING IMPLICATIONS

BASELINE ASSESSMENT

Check prothrombin time, activated partial thromboplastin time (aPTT), Hct; assess for bleeding.

INTERVENTION/EVALUATION

Monitor coagulation tests, aPTT or ACT, B/P, cardiac function.

Protonix

see pantoprazole

protriptyline hydrochloride

(Vivactil)

See Classification section under: Antidepressants (p. 35C)

Prozac

see fluoxetine

pseudoephedrine hydrochloride

su-do-eh-**fed**-rin
(Eltor♣, Sudafed)

pseudoephedrine sulfate

(Afrinol Repetabs)

FIXED-COMBINATION(S)

Claritin-D: pseudoephedrine/loratadine (an antihistamine): 120 mg/5 mg; 240 mg/10 mg. **Zyrtec-D:** pseudoephedrine/cetirizine (an antihistamine): 120 mg/5 mg. **Allegra-D:** pseudoephedrine/fexofenadine (an antihistamine): 120 mg/60 mg.

◆CLASSIFICATION

PHARMACOTHERAPEUTIC: Sympathomimetic. **CLINICAL:** Nasal decongestant.

ACTION

Directly stimulates alpha-adrenergic and beta-adrenergic receptors. **Therapeutic Effect:** Produces vasoconstriction of respiratory tract mucosa; shrinks nasal mucous membranes; reduces edema, nasal congestion.

PHARMACOKINETICS

Onset	Peak	Duration
Tablets, syrup		
15–30 min	—	4–6 hrs
Extended-release		
—	—	8–12 hrs

Well absorbed from GI tract. Partially metabolized in liver. Primarily excreted in urine. Not removed by hemodialysis. **Half-life:** 9–16 hrs (3.1 hrs in children).

USES

Temporary relief of nasal congestion due to the common cold, upper respiratory allergies, sinusitis. Enhances nasal, sinus drainage.

PRECAUTIONS

CONTRAINDICATIONS: Severe hypertension, coronary artery disease, lactating women, MAOI therapy. **CAUTIONS:** Elderly, hyperthyroidism, diabetes, ischemic heart disease, prostatic hypertrophy.

LIFESPAN CONSIDERATIONS: Pregnancy/lactation: Crosses placenta. Distributed in breast milk. **Pregnancy Category C. Children:** Safety and efficacy not established in those <2 yrs. **Elderly:** Age-related prostatic hypertrophy may require dosage adjustment.

INTERACTIONS

DRUG: May decrease effects of **antihypertensive, diuretics, beta-adrenergic blockers. MAOIs** may increase cardiac stimulant, vasopressor effects. **HERBAL: Ma huang (ephedra)** may increase CNS stimulation. **FOOD:** None known. **LAB VALUES:** None known.

AVAILABILITY (OTC)

GELCAPS: 30 mg. **LIQUID:** 15 mg/5 ml. **ORAL DROPS:** 7.5 mg/0.8 ml. **SYRUP:** 30 mg/5 ml. **TABLETS:** 30 mg, 60 mg. **TABLETS (chewable):** 15 mg. **TABLETS (extended-release):** 120 mg, 240 mg.

ADMINISTRATION/HANDLING

PO

- Do not crush, chew extended-release tablets; swallow whole.

INDICATIONS/ROUTES/DOSAGE

DECONGESTANT

PO: ADULTS, CHILDREN >12 YRS: 60 mg q4–6h. **Maximum:** 240 mg/day. CHILDREN 6–12 YRS: 30 mg q6h. **Maximum:** 120 mg/day. CHILDREN 2–5 YRS: 15 mg q6h. **Maximum:** 60 mg/day. CHILDREN <2 YRS: 4 mg/kg/day in divided doses q6h.

USUAL ELDERLY DOSE

PO: 30–60 mg q6h as needed.

EXTENDED-RELEASE

PO: ADULTS, CHILDREN >12 YRS: 120 mg q12h.

SIDE EFFECTS

OCCASIONAL (5%–10%): Nervousness, restlessness, insomnia, trembling, headache. **RARE (1%–4%):** Diaphoresis, weakness.

ADVERSE REACTIONS/ TOXIC EFFECTS

Large doses may produce tachycardia, palpitations (particularly in pts with cardiac disease), lightheadedness, nausea, vomiting. Overdosage in those >60 yrs may result in hallucinations, CNS depression, seizures.

NURSING IMPLICATIONS

PATIENT/FAMILY TEACHING

Discontinue drug if adverse reactions occur. Report insomnia, dizziness, tremors, rapid/irregular heartbeat.

P

psyllium

sill-ee-um

(Fiberall, Hydrocil, Konsyl, Metamucil, Perdiem, Prodiem Plain ✤)

CLASSIFICATION

PHARMACOTHERAPEUTIC: Bulk-forming laxative (see p. 104C).

ACTION

Powder, wafer dissolves and swells in water (provides increased bulk, moisture content in stool). **Therapeutic Effect:** Increased bulk promotes peristalsis, bowel motility.

PHARMACOKINETICS

	Onset	Peak	Duration
PO	12–24 hrs	2–3 days	—

Acts in small/large intestine.

USES

Treatment of chronic constipation, constipation associated with rectal disorders, management of irritable bowel syndrome, adjunct with low-cholesterol or saturated-fat diet to reduce risk of coronary artery disease.

PRECAUTIONS

CONTRAINDICATIONS: Fecal impaction, GI obstruction. **CAUTIONS:** Esophageal strictures, ulcers, stenosis, intestinal adhesions.

LIFESPAN CONSIDERATIONS: Pregnancy/lactation: Safe for use in pregnancy. **Pregnancy Category B. Children:** Safety and efficacy not established for those <6 yrs. **Elderly:** No age-related precautions noted.

INTERACTIONS

DRUG: May interfere with effects of **potassium-sparing diuretics, potassium supplements.** May decrease effect of **oral anticoagulants, digoxin, salicylates** by decreasing absorption. **HERBAL:** None known. **FOOD:** None known. **LAB VALUES:** May increase glucose. May decrease potassium.

AVAILABILITY (OTC)

POWDER. WAFER.

ADMINISTRATION/HANDLING

PO

• Drink 6–8 glasses of water/day (aids stool softening). • Do not swallow in dry form; mix with at least 1 full glass (8 oz) of liquid.

INDICATIONS/ROUTES/DOSAGE

LAXATIVE

PO: ADULTS, ELDERLY: 1–2 rounded tsp, packet, or wafer in water 1–4 times/day. CHILDREN 6–11 YRS: ½–1 tsp in water 1–3 times/day.

SIDE EFFECTS

RARE: Some degree of abdominal discomfort, nausea, mild cramps, griping, faintness.

ADVERSE REACTIONS/ TOXIC EFFECTS

Esophageal/bowel obstruction may occur if administered with insufficient liquid (<250 ml or 1 full glass).

NURSING IMPLICATIONS

INTERVENTION/EVALUATION

Encourage adequate fluid intake. Assess bowel sounds for peristalsis. Monitor daily bowel activity, stool consistency (watery, loose, soft, semisolid, solid). Monitor serum electrolytes in pts exposed to prolonged, frequent, excessive use of medication.

PATIENT/FAMILY TEACHING

Take each dose with a full glass of water. Inadequate fluid intake may cause swelling in throat, choking. Institute measures to promote defecation (increase fluid intake, exercise, high-fiber diet).

pyrazinamide

peer-a-**zin**-a-mide
(Pyrazinamide, Tebrazid)

FIXED-COMBINATION(S)

Rifater: pyrazinamide/isoniazid/rifampin (an antitubercular): 300 mg/50 mg/120 mg.

◆ CLASSIFICATION

CLINICAL: Antitubercular.

ACTION

Exact mechanism unknown. **Therapeutic Effect:** Is either bacteriostatic or bactericidal, depending on its concentration at infection site and susceptibility of infecting bacteria.

USES

In conjunction with at least one other antitubercular agent in treatment of clinical tuberculosis after failure of primary agents (isoniazid, rifampin).

PRECAUTIONS

CONTRAINDICATIONS: Severe hepatic dysfunction. **CAUTIONS:** Diabetes mellitus, renal impairment, history of gout, children (safety not established). Possible cross-sensitivity with isoniazid, ethionamide, niacin. **Pregnancy Category C.**

INTERACTIONS

DRUG: May decrease effects of **allopurinol, colchicine, probenecid, sulfinpyrazone. HERBAL:** None known. **FOOD:** None known. **LAB VALUES:** May increase SGOT (AST), SGPT (ALT), uric acid concentrations.

AVAILABILITY (Rx)

TABLETS: 500 mg.

INDICATIONS/ROUTES/DOSAGE

TUBERCULOSIS

PO: ADULTS: 15–30 mg/kg/day in 1–4 doses. **Maximum:** 3 g/day. CHILDREN: 20–40 mg/kg/day in 1 or 2 doses. **Maximum:** 2 g/day.

SIDE EFFECTS

FREQUENT: Arthralgia, myalgia (usually mild and self-limiting). **RARE:** Hypersensitivity (rash, urticaria, pruritus), photosensitivity.

ADVERSE REACTIONS/ TOXIC EFFECTS

Hepatotoxicity, thrombocytopenia, anemia occurs rarely.

NURSING IMPLICATIONS

BASELINE ASSESSMENT

Question for hypersensitivity to pyrazinamide, isoniazid, ethionamide, niacin. Ensure collection of specimens for culture, sensitivity. Evaluate results of initial CBC, hepatic function tests, uric acid levels.

INTERVENTION/EVALUATION

Monitor hepatic function results; be alert for hepatic reactions: jaundice, malaise, fever, liver tenderness, anorexia/nausea/vomiting (stop drug, notify physician promptly). Check serum uric acid levels; assess for hot, painful, swollen joints, esp. big toe, ankle, knee (gout). Evaluate blood sugar levels, diabetic status carefully (pyrazinamide makes management difficult). Assess for rash, skin eruptions. Monitor CBC for thrombocytopenia, anemia.

PATIENT/FAMILY TEACHING

Do not skip doses; complete full length of therapy (may be months or years). Office visits, lab tests are essential part of treatment. Take with food to reduce GI upset. Avoid excessive exposure to sun, ultraviolet light until photosensitivity is determined. Notify physician of any new symptom, immediately for yellow eyes/skin; unusual tiredness; fever; loss of appetite; hot, painful, swollen joints.

P

pyridostigmine bromide

pier-id-oh-**stig**-meen
(Mestinon, Regonol)

Do not confuse with Mesantoin, Metatensin, physostigmine, Renagel, Reglan, Regroton.

◆CLASSIFICATION

PHARMACOTHERAPEUTIC: Anticholinesterase. **CLINICAL:** Cholinergic muscle stimulant (see p. 80C).

ACTION

Prevents destruction of acetylcholine by enzyme, anticholinesterase. **Therapeutic Effect:** Produces miosis; increases tone of intestinal, skeletal muscles; stimulates salivary, sweat gland secretions.

USES

Improvement of muscle strength in control of myasthenia gravis, reversal of effects of nondepolarizing neuromuscular blocking agents after surgery.

PRECAUTIONS

CONTRAINDICATIONS: Mechanical GI, urinary obstruction. **CAUTIONS:** Bronchial asthma, bradycardia, epilepsy, recent coronary occlusion, vagotonia, hyperthyroidism, cardiac arrhythmias, peptic ulcer. **Pregnancy Category C.**

INTERACTIONS

DRUG: Anticholinergics reverse/prevent effects. **Cholinesterase inhibitors** may increase toxicity. Antagonizes **neuromuscular blocking agents. Quinidine, procainamide** may antagonize action. **HERBAL:** None known. **FOOD:** None known. **LAB VALUES:** None known.

AVAILABILITY (Rx)

TABLETS: 60 mg. **TABLETS (sustained-release):** 180 mg. **SYRUP:** 60 mg/5 ml. **INJECTION:** 5 mg/ml.

ADMINISTRATION/HANDLING

PO

• Give with food, milk. • Tablets may be crushed; do not chew, crush extended-release tablets (may be broken). • Give larger dose at times of increased fatigue (e.g., for those with difficulty in chewing, 30–45 min before meals).

IM/IV

• Give large parenteral doses concurrently with 0.6–1.2 mg atropine sulfate IV to minimize side effects.

IV INCOMPATIBILITY

Do not mix with any other medications.

INDICATIONS/ROUTES/DOSAGE

Alert: Dosage, frequency of administration dependent on daily clinical pt response (remissions, exacerbations, physical/emotional stress).

MYASTHENIA GRAVIS

PO: ADULTS, ELDERLY: Initially, 60 mg 3 times/day. Increase dose at intervals of ≥48 hrs until therapeutic response is achieved. When increased dosage does not produce further increase in muscle strength, reduce dose to previous dosage level. MAINTENANCE: 60–1,500 mg/day. CHILDREN: Initially, 7 mg/kg/day in 5–6 divided doses. NEONATE: 5 mg q4–6h.

Extended-release: ADULTS, ELDERLY: 180–540 mg 1–2 times/day (must maintain at least 6 hrs between doses).

IM/IV: ADULTS, ELDERLY: 2 mg q2–3h.

IM: NEONATE: 0.05–0.15 mg/kg q4–6h.

REVERSAL OF NONDEPOLARIZING MUSCLE RELAXANTS

IV: ADULTS, ELDERLY: 10–20 mg with, or shortly after, 0.6–1.2 mg atropine sulfate or 0.3–0.6 mg glycopyrrolate. CHILDREN:

P

0.1–0.25 mg/kg/dose preceded by atropine or glycopyrrolate.

SIDE EFFECTS

FREQUENT: Miosis, increased GI/skeletal muscle tone, reduced pulse rate, constriction of bronchi/ureters, increased salivary/sweat gland secretion. **OCCASIONAL:** Headache, rash, slight temporary decrease in diastolic B/P with mild reflex tachycardia, short periods of atrial fibrillation in hyperthyroid pts. Hypertensive pts may react with marked fall in B/P.

ADVERSE REACTIONS/ TOXIC EFFECTS

Overdosage may produce a cholinergic crisis, manifested by increasingly severe muscle weakness (appears first in muscles involving chewing, swallowing, followed by muscular weakness of shoulder girdle, upper extremities), respiratory muscle paralysis followed by pelvis girdle/leg muscle paralysis. Requires withdrawal of all cholinergic drugs and immediate use of 1–4 mg atropine sulfate IV for adults, 0.01 mg/kg in infants and children <12 yrs.

NURSING IMPLICATIONS

BASELINE ASSESSMENT

Larger doses should be given at time of greatest fatigue. Assess muscle strength prior to testing for diagnosis of myasthenia gravis and following drug administration. Avoid large doses in pts with megacolon or reduced GI motility.

INTERVENTION/EVALUATION

Have tissues readily available at pt's bedside. Monitor respirations closely during myasthenia gravis testing or if dosage is increased. Assess diligently for cholinergic reaction, as well as bradycardia in the myasthenic pt in crisis. Coordinate dosage time vs. periods of fatigue and increased/decreased muscle strength. Monitor for therapeutic response to medication (increased muscle strength, decreased fatigue, improved chewing/swallowing functions).

PATIENT/FAMILY TEACHING

Report nausea, vomiting, diarrhea, diaphoresis, increased salivary secretions, irregular heartbeat, muscle weakness, severe abdominal pain, difficulty breathing.

pyridoxine hydrochloride (vitamin B_6)

pie-rih-**docks**-in

(Hexa-Betalin ✤, Pyridoxine)

Do not confuse with paroxetine, pralidoxime, Pyridium.

◆CLASSIFICATION

PHARMACOTHERAPEUTIC: Coenzyme. **CLINICAL:** Vitamin (B_6) (see p. 137C).

ACTION

Coenzyme for various metabolic functions. **Therapeutic Effect:** Maintains metabolism of proteins, carbohydrates, fats. Aids in release of liver/muscle glycogen and in the synthesis of GABA in the CNS.

PHARMACOKINETICS

Readily absorbed primarily in jejunum. Stored in liver, muscle, brain. Metabolized in liver. Primarily excreted in urine. Removed by hemodialysis. **Half-life:** 15–20 days.

USES

Prevention, treatment of pyridoxine deficiency caused by inadequate diet, drug-induced (e.g., isoniazid [INH], penicillamine, cyclosporine), congenital error of metabolism. Treatment of INH poisoning. Treatment of seizures in neonate unresponsive to conventional therapy. Treatment of sideroblastic anemia associated with increased serum iron concentrations.

PRECAUTIONS

CONTRAINDICATIONS: None known. **CAUTIONS:** None known.

LIFESPAN CONSIDERATIONS: Pregnancy/lactation: Crosses placenta. Distributed in breast milk. High dosages in utero may produce seizures in neonates. **Pregnancy Category A. Children/elderly:** No age-related precautions noted.

INTERACTIONS

DRUG: Immunosuppressants, isoniazid, penicillamine may antagonize pyridoxine (may cause anemia/peripheral neuritis). Reverses effects of **levodopa. HERBAL:** None known. **FOOD:** None known. **LAB VALUES:** None known.

P

AVAILABILITY (OTC)

CAPSULES: 100 mg, 150 mg, 200 mg, 250 mg, 500 mg. **INJECTION:** 100 mg/ml. **TABLETS:** 10 mg, 25 mg, 50 mg, 100 mg, 250 mg, 500 mg. **TABLETS (time-release):** 500 mg.

ADMINISTRATION/HANDLING

Alert: Give PO unless nausea, vomiting, malabsorption occurs. Avoid IV use in cardiac pts.

IV

- Give undiluted or add to IV solutions and give as infusion.

IV INCOMPATIBILITY

Do not mix with any other medications.

INDICATIONS/ROUTES/DOSAGE

PYRIDOXINE DEFICIENCY

PO: ADULTS, ELDERLY: **(Diet):** 2.5–10 mg/day; after signs of deficiency decrease, 2.5–5 mg/day for several wks. **(Drug-induced):** 10–50 mg/day (INH, penicillamine); 100–300 mg/day (cyclosporine). **(Error of metabolism):** 100–500 mg/day. CHILDREN: 5–25 mg/day for 3 wks, then 1.5–2.5 mg/day.

SEIZURES IN NEONATES

IM/IV: NEONATES: 10–100 mg/day, then PO 50–100 mg/day for life.

DRUG-INDUCED NEURITIS

PO: ADULTS: 100–300 mg/day in divided doses for 3 wks, then 25–100 mg/day. CHILDREN: 50–100 mg/day as treatment, then 1–2 mg/kg/day as prophylaxis.

SIDEROBLASTIC ANEMIA

PO: ADULTS, ELDERLY: 200–600 mg/day. After adequate response, 30–50 mg/day for life.

SIDE EFFECTS

OCCASIONAL: Stinging at IM injection site. **RARE:** Headache, nausea, somnolence; high dosages cause sensory neuropathy (paresthesia, unstable gait, clumsiness of hands).

ADVERSE REACTIONS/ TOXIC EFFECTS

Long-term megadoses (2–6 g >2 mos) may produce sensory neuropathy (reduced deep tendon reflex, profound impairment of sense of position in distal limbs, gradual sensory ataxia). Toxic symptoms reverse with drug discontinuance. Seizures have occurred following IV megadoses.

NURSING IMPLICATIONS

INTERVENTION/EVALUATION

Observe for improvement of deficiency symptoms, including nervous system abnormalities (anxiety, depression, insomnia, motor difficulty, peripheral numbness, tremors), skin lesions (glossitis, seborrhea-like lesions around mouth, nose, eyes). Evaluate for nutritional adequacy.

PATIENT/FAMILY TEACHING

Discomfort may occur with IM injection. Encourage foods rich in pyridoxine (legumes, soybeans, eggs, sunflower seeds, hazelnuts, organ meats, tuna, shrimp, carrots, avocado, banana, wheat germ, bran).

quazepam

(Doral)

See Classification section under: Sedative-hypnotics (p. 129C)

quetiapine

kwe-**tie**-ah-peen

(Seroquel)

CLASSIFICATION

PHARMACOTHERAPEUTIC: Dibenzapin derivative. **CLINICAL:** Antipsychotic (see p. 57C).

ACTION

Interacts with neurotransmitter receptors, including dopamine, serotonin, histamine, alpha$_1$-adrenergic receptors. **Therapeutic Effect:** Diminishes psychotic disorders. Produces moderate sedation, few extrapyramidal effects, no anticholinergic effects.

PHARMACOKINETICS

Well absorbed following PO administration. Protein binding: 83%. Widely distributed in tissues; CNS concentration exceeds plasma concentration. Extensively metabolized by first-pass liver metabolism. Primarily excreted in the urine. **Half-life:** 6 hrs.

USES

Management of manifestations of psychotic disorders.

PRECAUTIONS

CONTRAINDICATIONS: None known. **CAUTIONS:** Alzheimer's dementia, history of breast cancer, cardiovascular disease (e.g., CHF, history of MI), cerebrovascular disease, impaired liver function, dehydration, hypovolemia, history of drug abuse/dependence, seizures, hypothyroidism.

LIFESPAN CONSIDERATIONS: Pregnancy/lactation: Unknown if distributed in breast milk. Not recommended for nursing mothers. **Pregnancy Category C. Children:** Safety and efficacy not established. **Elderly:** No age-related precautions noted, but lower initial and target dosages may be necessary.

INTERACTIONS

DRUG: Alcohol, CNS depressants may increase CNS depression. May increase effects of **antihypertensives. Hepatic enzyme inducers (e.g., phenytoin),** may increase drug clearance. **HERBAL:** None known. **FOOD:** None known. **LAB VALUES:** May produce false-positive pregnancy test. May decrease total and free thyroxine (T_4) levels. May increase cholesterol, triglycerides, transaminase levels (e.g., SGOT [AST], SGPT [ALT]).

AVAILABILITY (Rx)

TABLETS: 25 mg, 100 mg, 200 mg, 300 mg.

Q

ADMINISTRATION/HANDLING

PO

• Dosage adjustments should occur at 2-day intervals. • Initial dose and dosage titration should occur at a lower dosage in elderly, pts with hepatic impairment, debilitated, or those predisposed to hypotensive reactions. • When restarting pts who have been off quetiapine for <1 wk, titration is not required and maintenance dose can be reinstituted. • When restarting pts who have been off quetiapine for >1 wk, follow initial titration schedule. • Give without regard to food.

INDICATIONS/ROUTES/DOSAGE

PSYCHOTIC DISORDER

PO: ADULTS, ELDERLY: Initially, 25 mg 2 times/day, then 25–50 mg 2–3 times daily on second and third days, up to 300–400 mg/day by the fourth day, given 2–3 times daily. Further adjustments of 25–50 mg 2 times/day made at ≥2-day intervals. MAINTENANCE: (ADULTS): 300–800 mg/day. (ELDERLY): 50–200 mg/day.

SIDE EFFECTS

FREQUENT (10%–19%): Headache, somnolence/drowsiness, dizziness. **OCCASIONAL (3%–9%):** Constipation, postural hypotension, tachycardia, dry mouth, dyspepsia, rash, weakness, abdominal pain, rhinitis. **RARE (2%):** Back pain, fever, weight gain.

ADVERSE REACTIONS/ TOXIC EFFECTS

Overdosage produces heart block (slow, irregular pulse), decreased B/P, hypokalemia (weakness), tachycardia.

NURSING IMPLICATIONS

BASELINE ASSESSMENT

Assess behavior, appearance, emotional status, response to environment, speech pattern, thought content. Obtain baseline CBC, hepatic function serum levels prior to initiating treatment and periodically thereafter.

INTERVENTION/EVALUATION

Assist with ambulation if dizziness occurs. Supervise suicidal-risk pt closely during early therapy (as psychosis, depression lessens, energy level improves, increasing suicide potential). Monitor B/P for hypotension. Assess pulse for tachycardia (esp. with rapid increase in dosage). Monitor CBC for evidence of blood dyscrasias. Question about bowel activity for evidence of constipation. Assess for therapeutic response (improved thought content, increased ability to concentrate, improvement in self-care).

PATIENT/FAMILY TEACHING

Avoid exposure to extreme heat. Drink fluids often, esp. during physical activity. Take medication as ordered; do not stop taking or increase dosage. Drowsiness generally subsides during continued therapy. Avoid driving or performing tasks that require alertness, motor skills until response to drug is established. Avoid alcohol. Change positions slowly to reduce hypotensive effect.

quinapril hydrochloride

quin-ah-prill
(Accupril)

Do not confuse with Accolate, Accutane.

FIXED-COMBINATION(S)

Accuretic: quinapril/hydrochlorothiazide (a diuretic): 10 mg/12.5 mg; 20 mg/12.5 mg; 20 mg/25 mg.

◆ **CLASSIFICATION**

PHARMACOTHERAPEUTIC: Angiotensin-converting enzyme (ACE) inhibitor. **CLINICAL:** Antihypertensive (see p. 6C).

ACTION

Suppresses renin-angiotensin-aldosterone system (prevents conversion of angiotensin I to angiotensin II, a potent vasoconstrictor; may also inhibit angiotensin II at local vascular and renal sites). **Therapeutic Effect:** Reduces peripheral arterial resistance, B/P, pulmonary capillary wedge pressure; improves cardiac output.

PHARMACOKINETICS

	Onset	Peak	Duration
PO	1 hr	—	24 hrs

Readily absorbed from GI tract. Protein binding: 97%. Metabolized in liver, GI tract, extravascular tissue to active metabolite. Primarily excreted in urine. Minimal removal by hemodialysis. **Half-life:** 1–2 hrs; metabolite: 3 hrs (half-life increased with impaired renal function).

USES

Treatment of hypertension. Used alone or in combination with other antihypertensives. Adjunctive therapy in management of heart failure. **Unlabeled:** Treatment of hypertension/renal crisis in scleroderma.

PRECAUTIONS

CONTRAINDICATIONS: Bilateral renal stenosis. **CAUTIONS:** Renal impairment, CHF, collagen vascular disease, hypovolemia, renal stenosis, hyperkalemia.

LIFESPAN CONSIDERATIONS: Pregnancy/lactation: Crosses placenta. Unknown if distributed in breast milk. May cause fetal/neonatal mortality/morbidity. **Pregnancy Category C** (**D** if used in second or third trimester). **Children:** Safety and efficacy not established. **Elderly:** May be more sensitive to hypotensive effects.

INTERACTIONS

DRUG: **Alcohol, diuretics, hypotensive agents** may increase effects. **NSAIDs** may decrease effect. **Potassium-sparing diuretics, potassium supplements** may cause hyperkalemia. May increase **lithium** concentration, toxicity. **HERBAL:** **Ephedra, yohimbe, ginseng** may worsen hypertension. **Garlic** may increase antihypertensive effect. **FOOD:** None known. **LAB VALUES:** May increase potassium, SGOT (AST), SGPT (ALT), alkaline phosphatase, bilirubin, BUN, creatinine. May decrease sodium. May cause positive ANA titer.

AVAILABILITY (Rx)

TABLETS: 5 mg, 10 mg, 20 mg, 40 mg.

ADMINISTRATION/HANDLING

PO

• Give without regard to food. • Tablets may be crushed.

INDICATIONS/ROUTES/DOSAGE

HYPERTENSION (used alone)

PO: ADULTS: Initially, 10–20 mg/day. May adjust dosage after at least 2-wk intervals. MAINTENANCE: 20–80 mg/day as single or 2 divided doses. **Maximum:** 80 mg/day.

HYPERTENSION (combination therapy)

Alert: Discontinue diuretic 2–3 days before initiating quinapril therapy.

PO: ADULTS: Initially, 5 mg/day titrated to pt's needs.

USUAL ELDERLY DOSE

PO: Initially, 2.5–5 mg/day. May increase by 2.5–5 mg q1–2wks.

HEART FAILURE

PO: ADULTS, ELDERLY: Initially, 5 mg 2 times/day. RANGE: 20–40 mg/day.

Q

DOSAGE IN RENAL IMPAIRMENT

Titrate to pt need after initial doses:

Creatinine Clearance	Initial Dose
>60 ml/min	10 mg
30–60 ml/min	5 mg
10–29 ml/min	2.5 mg

SIDE EFFECTS

FREQUENT (5%–7%): Headache, dizziness. **OCCASIONAL (2%–4%):** Fatigue, vomiting, nausea, hypotension, chest pain, cough, syncope. **RARE (<2%):** Diarrhea, cough, dyspnea, rash, palpitations, impotence, insomnia, drowsiness, malaise.

ADVERSE REACTIONS/ TOXIC EFFECTS

Excessive hypotension ("first-dose syncope") may occur in those with CHF, severely salt/volume depleted. Angioedema (swelling of face/lips), hyperkalemia occur rarely. Agranulocytosis, neutropenia may be noted in those with impaired renal function, collagen vascular disease (systemic lupus erythematosus, scleroderma). Nephrotic syndrome may be noted in pts with history of renal disease.

NURSING IMPLICATIONS

BASELINE ASSESSMENT

Obtain B/P immediately prior to each dose in addition to regular monitoring (be alert to fluctuations). If excessive reduction in B/P occurs, place pt in supine position with legs slightly elevated. Renal function tests should be performed prior to beginning therapy. In pts with prior renal disease, urine test for protein by dipstick method should be made with first urine of day prior to beginning therapy and periodically thereafter. In those with renal impairment, autoimmune disease or in those taking drugs that affect leukocytes/immune response, CBC, differential count should be performed prior to beginning therapy and q2wks for 3 mos, then periodically thereafter.

INTERVENTION/EVALUATION

Monitor renal function, potassium, WBC. Assist with ambulation if dizziness occurs. Question for evidence of headache. Noncola carbonated beverage, unsalted crackers, dry toast may relieve nausea.

PATIENT/FAMILY TEACHING

To reduce hypotensive effect, rise slowly from lying to sitting position, permit legs to dangle from bed momentarily before standing. Full therapeutic effect may take 1–2 wks. Report any sign of infection (sore throat, fever). Skipping doses or voluntarily discontinuing drug may produce severe rebound hypertension. Avoid driving, other tasks that require alertness, motor skills until response to drug is known.

quinidine

kwin-ih-deen

(Apo-Quinidine ♣, Quinate ♣, Quinidex)

Do not confuse with clonidine, quinine.

◆CLASSIFICATION

CLINICAL: Antiarrhythmic (see p. 13C).

ACTION

Decreases sodium influx during depolarization, potassium efflux during repolarization, reduces calcium transport across cell membrane. **Therapeutic Effect:** Decreases myocardial excitability, conduction velocity, contractility.

USES

Prophylactic therapy to maintain normal sinus rhythm following conversion of atrial fibrillation/flutter. Prevention of premature atrial, AV, ventricular contractions, paroxysmal atrial tachycardia, paroxysmal AV junctional rhythm, atrial fibrillation, atrial flutter, paroxysmal ventricular tachycardia not associated with complete heart block. **Unlabeled:** Treatment of malaria (IV only).

PRECAUTIONS

CONTRAINDICATIONS: Complete AV block, intraventricular conduction defects (widening of QRS complex). **CAUTIONS:** Myocardial depression, sick sinus syndrome, incomplete AV block, digoxin toxicity, renal/liver impairment, myasthenia gravis. **Pregnancy Category C.**

INTERACTIONS

DRUG: May increase concentration of **digoxin. Pimozide, other antiarrhythmics** may increase cardiac effects. **Urinary alkalizers (e.g., antacids)** may decrease excretion. May increase effects of **oral anticoagulants, neuromuscular blockers.** May decrease effects of **antimyasthenics** on skeletal muscle. **HERBAL:** None known. **FOOD:** None known. **LAB VALUES:** None known. Therapeutic blood serum level: 2–5 mcg/ml; toxic blood serum level: >5 mcg/ml.

AVAILABILITY (Rx)

GLUCONATE: **TABLETS (sustained-release):** 324 mg. **INJECTION:** 80 mg/ml (50 mg/ml quinidine).

SULFATE: **TABLETS:** 200 mg, 300 mg. **TABLETS (sustained-release):** 300 mg.

ADMINISTRATION/HANDLING

PO

• Do not crush/chew sustained-release tablets. • GI upset can be reduced if given with food.

IV

Alert: B/P, EKG should be monitored continuously during IV administration and rate of infusion adjusted to minimize arrhythmias and hypotension.

Storage • Use only clear, colorless solution. • Solution is stable for 24 hrs at room temperature when diluted with D_5W.

Reconstitution • For IV infusion, dilute 800 mg with 40 ml D_5W to provide concentration of 16 mg/ml.

Rate of administration • Administer with pt in supine position. • For IV infusion, give at rate of 1 ml (16 mg)/min (a too rapid rate may markedly decrease arterial pressure). • Monitor EKG for cardiac changes, particularly prolongation of PR, QT intervals, widening of QRS complex. Notify physician of any significant interval changes.

IV INCOMPATIBILITIES

Furosemide (Lasix), heparin.

IV COMPATIBILITY

Milrinone (Primacor).

INDICATIONS/ROUTES/DOSAGE

USUAL DOSAGE

IV: ADULTS, ELDERLY: 200–400 mg/dose. CHILDREN: 2–10 mg/kg/dose.

PO: ADULTS, ELDERLY: 100–600 mg/dose q4–6h. **(Long-acting):** 324–972 mg q8–12h. CHILDREN: 30 mg/kg/day in divided doses q4–6h.

SIDE EFFECTS

FREQUENT: Abdominal pain/cramps, nausea, diarrhea, vomiting (can be immediate, intense). **OCCASIONAL:** Mild cinchonism (ringing in ears, blurred vision, hearing loss), severe cinchonism (headache, vertigo, diaphoresis, lightheadedness, photophobia, confusion, delirium). **RARE:** Hypotension (particularly with IV administration), hypersensitivity reaction (fever, anaphylaxis, photosensitivity reaction).

ADVERSE REACTIONS/ TOXIC EFFECTS

Cardiotoxic effects occur most commonly with IV administration, particularly at high concentration, observed as conduction changes (50% widening of QRS complex, prolonged QT interval, flattened T waves, disappearance of P wave), ventricular tachycardia/flutter, frequent PVCs, complete AV block. Quinidine-induced syncope may occur with usual dosage (discontinue drug). Severe hypotension may result from high dosages. Atrial flutter/fibrillation pts may experience a paradoxical, extremely rapid ventricular rate (may be prevented by prior digitalization). Hepatotoxicity with jaundice due to drug hypersensitivity.

NURSING IMPLICATIONS

BASELINE ASSESSMENT

Check B/P, pulse (for 1 full min unless pt is on continuous monitor) prior to giving medication. For those on long-term therapy, CBC, liver/renal function tests should be performed periodically.

INTERVENTION/EVALUATION

Monitor EKG for cardiac changes, particularly prolongation of PR, QT intervals, widening of QRS complex. Monitor I&O, CBC, serum potassium, hepatic/renal function tests. Monitor pattern of daily bowel activity, stool consistency. Monitor B/P for hypotension (esp. in pts on high-dose therapy). If cardiotoxic effect occurs (see Adverse Reactions/Toxic Effects), notify physician immediately. Therapeutic blood serum level: 2–5 mcg/ml; toxic blood serum level: >5 mcg/ml.

PATIENT/FAMILY TEACHING

Inform physician of fever, rash, unusual bleeding/bruising, ringing in the ears, visual disturbances. May cause photosensitivity reaction; avoid direct sunlight, artificial light.

quinine sulfate

kwye-nine

(Quinine)

Do not confuse with quinidine.

FIXED-COMBINATION(S)

With vitamin E for nocturnal leg cramps **(M-KYA, Q-vel).**

◆CLASSIFICATION

PHARMACOTHERAPEUTIC: Cinchona alkaloid. **CLINICAL:** Antimalarial, antimyotonic.

ACTION

Myotonia: Increases the refractory period, decreases excitability of motor end plates, affects distribution of calcium with muscle fiber. **Therapeutic Effect:** Relaxes skeletal muscle. **Antimalaria:** Depresses O_2 uptake, carbohydrate metabolism, elevates pH in intracellular organelles of parasites. **Therapeutic Effect:** Produces parasitic death.

USES

Prevention, treatment of nocturnal recumbency leg cramps. Used alone, with pyrimethamine and sulfonamide (or with oral tetracycline) for treatment of chloroquine-resistant falciparum malaria.

PRECAUTIONS

CONTRAINDICATIONS: Ringing in ears, optic neuritis, G6PD deficiency, pregnancy. **CAUTIONS:** Arrhythmias, myasthenia gravis, liver function impairment. **Pregnancy Category D.**

INTERACTIONS

DRUG: May increase concentration of **digoxin. Mefloquine** may increase seizures, EKG abnormalities. **HERBAL:** None known. **FOOD:** None known. **LAB VALUES:** May interfere with 17-OH steroid determinations.

AVAILABILITY (Rx)

CAPSULES: 200 mg, 325 mg. **TABLETS:** 260 mg.

INDICATIONS/ROUTES/DOSAGE

NOCTURNAL LEG CRAMPS

PO: ADULTS, ELDERLY: 200–300 mg at bedtime as needed.

TREATMENT OF MALARIA

PO: ADULTS, ELDERLY: 260–650 mg 3 times a day for 6–12 days. CHILDREN: 10 mg/kg q8h for 5–7 days.

SIDE EFFECTS

FREQUENT: Nausea, headache, tinnitus, slight visual disturbances (mild cinchonism). **OCCASIONAL:** Extreme flushing of skin with intense generalized pruritus is most typical hypersensitivity reaction; also rash, wheezing, dyspnea, angioedema. Prolonged therapy: cardiac conduction disturbances, decreased hearing.

ADVERSE REACTIONS/ TOXIC EFFECTS

Overdosage (severe cinchonism): cardiovascular effects, severe headache, intestinal cramps with vomiting/diarrhea, apprehension, confusion, seizures, blindness, respiratory depression. Hypoprothrombinemia, thrombocytopenic purpura, hemoglobinuria, asthma, agranulocytosis, hypoglycemia, deafness, optic atrophy occur rarely.

NURSING IMPLICATIONS

BASELINE ASSESSMENT

Question for possibility of pregnancy prior to initiating therapy (Pregnancy Category D). Question for hypersensitivity to quinine, quinidine. Evaluate initial EKG, CBC results.

INTERVENTION/EVALUATION

Check for hypersensitivity: flushing, rash/urticaria, itching, dyspnea, wheezing. Assess level of hearing, visual acuity, presence of headache/tinnitus, nausea. Report adverse effects promptly (possible cinchonism). Monitor CBC results for blood dyscrasias. Be alert to infection (fever, sore throat), bleeding/ bruising, unusual tiredness/weakness. Assess pulse, EKG for arrhythmias. Check fasting blood sugar levels; watch for hypoglycemia (cold sweating, tremors, tachycardia, hunger, anxiety).

PATIENT/FAMILY TEACHING

Report ringing in ears, hearing loss, rash, any visual disturbances. Periodic lab tests are part of therapy.

quinupristin-dalfopristin

quin-you-pris-tin/**dal**-foh-pris-tin (Synercid)

CLASSIFICATION

PHARMACOTHERAPEUTIC: Streptogramin. **CLINICAL:** Antimicrobial.

ACTION

Bactericidal (in combination). Two chemically distinct compounds that, when given together, bind to different sites on bacterial ribosomes forming a drug-ribosome complex. Protein synthesis is interrupted. **Therapeutic Effect:** Results in bacterial cell death.

PHARMACOKINETICS

Following IV administration, both are extensively metabolized in the liver with

Q

dalfopristin to active metabolite. Protein binding: (quinupristin) 23%–32%, (dalfopristin) 50%–56%. Primarily eliminated in feces. **Half-life:** quinupristin: 0.85 hr; dalfopristin: 0.7 hr.

USES

Treatment of intra-abdominal, skin/skin structure, urinary tract, central line catheter, bone, joint, respiratory infections; endocarditis; bacteremia.

PRECAUTIONS

CONTRAINDICATIONS: None known. **CAUTIONS:** Liver/renal dysfunction.

LIFESPAN CONSIDERATIONS: Pregnancy/lactation: Unknown if drug crosses placenta or is distributed in breast milk. **Pregnancy Category B. Children:** Safety and efficacy not established. **Elderly:** No age-related precautions noted.

INTERACTIONS

DRUG: None known. **HERBAL:** None known. **FOOD:** None known. **LAB VALUES:** May increase SGOT (AST), SGPT (ALT), LDH, serum creatinine, bilirubin.

Q

AVAILABILITY (Rx)

INJECTION: 500-mg vial (350 mg dalfopristin/150 mg quinupristin).

ADMINISTRATION/HANDLING

IV

Storage • Refrigerate unopened vials. • Reconstituted vials are stable for 1 hr at room temperature. Diluted infusion bag is stable for 6 hrs at room temperature or 54 hrs if refrigerated.

Reconstitution • Reconstitute vial by slowly adding 5 ml D_5W or Sterile Water for Injection to make a 100 mg/ml solution. • Gently swirl vial contents to minimize foaming. • Further dilute with D_5W to final concentration of 2 mg/ml (5 mg/ml using central line).

Rate of administration • Infuse over 60 min. • After infusion, flush line with D_5W to minimize vein irritation. Do **not** flush with 0.9% NaCl (incompatible).

IV INCOMPATIBILITIES
Heparin, sodium chloride.

IV COMPATIBILITIES
Aztreonam (Azactam), ciprofloxacin (Cipro), fluconazole (Diflucan), haloperidol (Haldol), metoclopramide (Reglan), morphine, potassium chloride.

INDICATIONS/ROUTES/DOSAGE

VANOMYCIN-RESISTANT ENTEROCOCCUS

IV infusion: ADULTS, ELDERLY: 7.5 mg/kg/dose q8h.

SKIN/SKIN STRUCTURE INFECTIONS

IV infusion: ADULTS, ELDERLY: 7.5 mg/kg/dose q12h.

SIDE EFFECTS

Generally well tolerated. **FREQUENT:** Mild erythema, itching, pain, burning at infusion site for doses ≥7 mg/kg. **OCCASIONAL:** Headache, diarrhea. **RARE:** Vomiting, arthralgia, myalgia.

ADVERSE REACTIONS/ TOXIC EFFECTS

Superinfection, including antibiotic-associated colitis, may result from bacterial imbalance. Liver function abnormalities, peripheral venous intolerability may occur.

NURSING IMPLICATIONS

BASELINE ASSESSMENT

Assess temperature, B/P, respiratory rate, pulse. Obtain baseline liver function tests, BUN, CBC, urinalysis.

INTERVENTION/EVALUATION

Monitor CBC, liver function tests. Observe infusion site for redness, vein irritation. Hold medication and promptly inform physician of diarrhea (with fever, abdominal pain, mucus/blood in stool may indicate antibiotic-associated colitis). Evaluate IV site for erythema, itching, pain, burning. Be alert for superinfection: increased fever, onset of sore throat, nausea, vomiting, diarrhea, ulceration/changes of oral mucosa, anal/genital pruritus.

rabeprazole sodium

rah-**bep**-rah-zole
(Aciphex)
Do not confuse with Accupril, Aricept.

CLASSIFICATION

PHARMACOTHERAPEUTIC: Proton pump inhibitor. **CLINICAL:** Gastric acid inhibitor (see p. 128C).

ACTION

Converts to active metabolites that irreversibly binds to and inhibits H^+/K^+ ATPase (an enzyme on surface of gastric parietal cells). Actively secretes hydrogen ions for potassium ions, resulting in an accumulation of H^+ in gastric lumen. **Therapeutic Effect:** Increases gastric pH, reducing gastric acid production.

PHARMACOKINETICS

Rapidly absorbed from GI tract after passing through stomach relatively intact. Protein binding: 96%. Metabolized extensively in liver. Primarily excreted in urine. Unknown if removed by hemodialysis. **Half-life:** 1–2 hrs (half-life increased with impaired liver function).

USES

Short-term treatment (4–8 wks) in healing/maintenance of erosive/ulcerative gastroesophageal reflux disease (GERD). Treatment of daytime/nighttime heartburn, other symptoms of GERD. Short-term treatment (≤4 wks) in healing, symptomatic relief of duodenal ulcers. Long-term treatment of pathologic hypersecretory conditions, including Zollinger-Ellison syndrome. Treatment of NSAID-induced ulcers. Treatment of *H. pylori* (in combination with other medication).

PRECAUTIONS

CONTRAINDICATIONS: None known. **CAUTIONS:** Impaired hepatic function.

LIFESPAN CONSIDERATIONS: Pregnancy/lactation: Unknown if drug crosses placenta or is distributed in breast milk. **Pregnancy Category B. Children:** Safety and efficacy not established. **Elderly:** No age-related precautions noted.

INTERACTIONS

DRUG: May decrease concentration of **ketoconazole.** May increase plasma concentration of **digoxin. HERBAL:** None known. **FOOD:** None known. **LAB VALUES:** May increase SGOT (AST), SGPT (ALT), alkaline phosphatase.

AVAILABILITY (Rx)

TABLETS (delayed-release): 20 mg.

ADMINISTRATION/HANDLING

PO

• Give before meals. • Do not crush, chew, split tablet; swallow whole.

INDICATIONS/ROUTES/DOSAGE

GERD

PO: ADULTS, ELDERLY: 20 mg/day for 4–8 wks. MAINTENANCE: 20 mg/day.

DUODENAL ULCER

PO: ADULTS, ELDERLY: 20 mg/day after morning meal for 4 wks.

PATHOLOGIC HYPERSECRETORY CONDITIONS

PO: ADULTS, ELDERLY: Initially, 60 mg once daily. May increase up to 60 mg 2 times/day.

R

H. PYLORI

PO: ADULTS, ELDERLY: 20 mg 2 times a day for 7 days (given in combination with amoxicillin 1,000 mg and clarithromycin 500 mg).

SIDE EFFECTS

RARE (≤2%): Headache, nausea, dizziness, rash, diarrhea, malaise.

ADVERSE REACTIONS/ TOXIC EFFECTS

Hyperglycemia, hypokalemia, hyponatremia, hyperlipidemia occur rarely.

NURSING IMPLICATIONS

BASELINE ASSESSMENT

Obtain baseline lab values, esp. blood chemistries.

INTERVENTION/EVALUATION

Monitor ongoing laboratory results. Evaluate for therapeutic response (i.e., relief of GI symptoms). Question if GI discomfort, nausea, diarrhea, headache occurs. Assess skin for evidence of rash. Observe for evidence of dizziness; utilize appropriate safety precautions.

PATIENT/FAMILY TEACHING

Swallow tablets whole; do not chew, split, crush tablets. Report headache.

R

raloxifene

rah-**lock**-sih-feen

(Evista)

CLASSIFICATION

PHARMACOTHERAPEUTIC: Selective estrogen receptor modulator. **CLINICAL:** Osteoporosis preventive.

ACTION

Selective estrogen receptor modulator that affects some receptors as estrogen. **Therapeutic Effect:** Like estrogen, prevents bone loss, improves lipid profiles.

PHARMACOKINETICS

Rapidly absorbed following PO administration. Highly bound to plasma proteins (>95%), albumin. Undergoes extensive first-pass metabolism in liver. Excreted mainly in feces with a lesser amount in urine. Unknown if removed by hemodialysis. **Half-life:** 27.7 hrs.

USES

Prevention/treatment of osteoporosis in postmenopausal women. **Unlabeled:** Prevents fractures, breast cancer in postmenopausal women.

PRECAUTIONS

CONTRAINDICATIONS: Pregnancy, those who may become pregnant, active or history of venous thromboembolic events (deep vein thrombosis, pulmonary embolism, retinal vein thrombosis). **CAUTIONS:** Cardiovascular disease, history of cervical/uterine cancer, renal/liver impairment.

LIFESPAN CONSIDERATIONS: Pregnancy/lactation: Unknown if distributed in breast milk. Not recommended for nursing mothers. **Pregnancy Category X. Children:** Not used in this population. **Elderly:** No age-related precautions noted.

INTERACTIONS

DRUG: Cholestyramine, ampicillin reduces raloxifene peak levels, extent of absorption. May decrease effect of **warfarin** (decreases prothrombin time). Do not use concurrently with systemic **estrogen or hormone replacement therapy. HERBAL:** None known. **FOOD:** None known. **LAB VALUES:** Lowers serum total and LDL cholesterol (does not affect HDL cholesterol or triglycerides). Slight decrease in serum total calcium, inorganic phosphate, total protein, albumin, platelet count.

AVAILABILITY (Rx)

TABLETS: 60 mg.

ADMINISTRATION/HANDLING

PO

- Give at any time of day without regard to meals.

INDICATIONS/ROUTES/DOSAGE

PREVENTION/TREATMENT OF OSTEOPOROSIS

PO: ADULTS, ELDERLY: 60 mg daily.

SIDE EFFECTS

FREQUENT (10%–25%): Hot flashes, flu syndrome, arthralgia, sinusitis. **OCCASIONAL (5%–9%):** Weight gain, nausea, myalgia, pharyngitis, cough, dyspepsia, leg cramps, rash, depression. **RARE (3%–4%):** Vaginitis, urinary tract infection, peripheral edema, flatulence, vomiting, fever, migraine, diaphoresis.

ADVERSE REACTIONS/ TOXIC EFFECTS

Pneumonia, gastroenteritis, chest pain, vaginal bleeding, breast pain occur rarely.

NURSING IMPLICATIONS

BASELINE ASSESSMENT

Question for possibility of pregnancy (Pregnancy Category X). Drug should be discontinued 72 hrs prior to and during prolonged immobilization (postop recovery, prolonged bed rest). Therapy may be resumed only after pt is fully ambulatory. Determine total and LDL cholesterol serum blood levels prior to therapy and routinely thereafter.

INTERVENTION/EVALUATION

Monitor total and LDL cholesterol, total calcium, inorganic phosphate, total protein, albumin, bone mineral density, platelet count.

PATIENT/FAMILY TEACHING

Avoid prolonged restriction of movement during travel (increased risk of venous thromboembolic events). Take supplemental calcium, vitamin D if daily dietary intake is inadequate. Encourage regular exercise. Recommend modification/discontinuation of cigarette smoking, alcohol consumption.

ramipril

ram-ih-prill

(Altace)

Do not confuse with Alteplase, Artane.

CLASSIFICATION

PHARMACOTHERAPEUTIC: Renin-angiotensin system antagonist. **CLINICAL:** Antihypertensive (see p. 6C).

ACTION

Suppresses renin-angiotensin-aldosterone system. Decreases plasma angiotensin II, increases plasma renin activity, decreases aldosterone secretion. **Therapeutic Effect:** Reduces peripheral arterial resistance, decreasing B/P.

PHARMACOKINETICS

	Onset	Peak	Duration
PO	1–2 hrs	3–6 hrs	24 hrs

Well absorbed from GI tract. Protein binding: 73%. Metabolized in liver to active metabolite. Primarily excreted in urine. Not removed by hemodialysis. **Half-life:** 5.1 hrs.

USES

Treatment of hypertension. Used alone or in combination with other antihypertensives. Treatment of CHF. **Unlabeled:** Treatment of hypertension/renal crisis in scleroderma. Prevention of heart attacks, stroke.

PRECAUTIONS

CONTRAINDICATIONS: Bilateral renal stenosis. **CAUTIONS:** Renal impairment, CHF, collagen vascular disease, hypovolemia, renal stenosis, hyperkalemia.

LIFESPAN CONSIDERATIONS: Pregnancy/lactation: Crosses placenta. Distributed in breast milk. May cause fetal/neonatal mortality/morbidity. **Pregnancy Category C** (**D** if used in second or third trimester). **Children:** Safety and efficacy not established. **Elderly:** May be more sensitive to hypotensive effects.

INTERACTIONS

DRUG: Alcohol, diuretics, hypotensive agents may increase effects. **NSAIDs** may decrease effect. **Potassium-sparing diuretics, potassium supplements** may cause hyperkalemia. May increase **lithium** concentration, toxicity. **HERBAL: Ephedra, yohimbe, ginseng** may worsen hypertension. **Garlic** may increase antihypertensive effect. **FOOD:** None known. **LAB VALUES:** May increase potassium, SGOT (AST), SGPT (ALT), alkaline phosphatase, bilirubin, BUN, creatinine. May decrease sodium. May cause positive ANA titer.

AVAILABILITY (Rx)

CAPSULES: 1.25 mg, 2.5 mg, 5 mg, 10 mg.

ADMINISTRATION/HANDLING

PO

• Give without regard to food. • Do not chew/break capsules. • May mix with water, apple juice/sauce.

INDICATIONS/ROUTES/DOSAGE

HYPERTENSION (used alone)

PO: ADULTS, ELDERLY: Initially, 2.5 mg/day. MAINTENANCE: 2.5–20 mg/day as single or in 2 divided doses.

HYPERTENSION (combination therapy)

Alert: Discontinue diuretic 2–3 days prior to initiating ramipril therapy.

PO: ADULTS, ELDERLY: Initially, 1.25 mg/day titrated to pt's needs.

CHF

PO: ADULTS, ELDERLY: Initially, 1.25–2.5 mg 2 times/day. **Maximum:** 5 mg 2 times/day.

RISK REDUCTION FOR MI/STROKE

PO: ADULTS, ELDERLY: Initially, 2.5 mg/day for 7 days, then 5 mg/day for 21 days, then 10 mg/day as a single dose or in divided doses.

DOSAGE IN RENAL IMPAIRMENT

Creatinine clearance <40 ml/min: 25% of normal dose.

Hypertension: Initially, 1.25 mg/day, titrate upward.

CHF: 1.25 mg/day, titrate up to 2.5 mg twice daily.

SIDE EFFECTS

FREQUENT (5%–12%): Cough, headache. **OCCASIONAL (2%–4%):** Dizziness, fatigue, nausea, asthenia (loss of strength). **RARE (<2%):** Palpitations, insomnia, nervousness, malaise, abdominal pain, myalgia.

ADVERSE REACTIONS/ TOXIC EFFECTS

Excessive hypotension ("first-dose syncope") may occur in those with CHF, se-

R

verely salt/volume depleted. Angioedema (swelling of face/lips), hyperkalemia occur rarely. Agranulocytosis, neutropenia may be noted in pts with impaired renal function, collagen vascular disease (systemic lupus erythematosus, scleroderma). Nephrotic syndrome may be noted in pts with history of renal disease.

NURSING IMPLICATIONS

BASELINE ASSESSMENT

Obtain B/P immediately prior to each dose, in addition to regular monitoring (be alert to fluctuations). If excessive reduction in B/P occurs, place pt in supine position with legs elevated. Renal function tests should be performed prior to beginning therapy. In pts with prior renal disease, urine test for protein (by dipstick method) should be made with first urine of day prior to beginning therapy and periodically thereafter. In pts with renal impairment, autoimmune disease, or taking drugs that affect leukocytes/immune response, CBC, differential count should be performed prior to beginning therapy and q2wks for 3 mos, then periodically thereafter.

INTERVENTION/EVALUATION

Monitor renal function, potassium, WBC. Assess for cough (frequent effect). Assist with ambulation if dizziness occurs. Assess lung sounds for rales, wheezing in pts with CHF. Monitor urinalysis for proteinuria. Monitor serum potassium levels in those on concurrent diuretic therapy.

PATIENT/FAMILY TEACHING

Do not discontinue medication without physician approval. Report palpitations, cough, chest pain. Dizziness, lightheadedness may occur in the first few days (avoid tasks that require alertness, motor skills until response to drug is established.

ranitidine

rah-**nih**-tih-deen

(Apo-Ranitidine ♣, Novo-Ranidine ♣, Zantac, Zantac-75, Zantac EFFERdose)

Do not confuse with Xanax, Ziac, Zyrtec.

ranitidine bismuth citrate

(Tritec)

CLASSIFICATION

PHARMACOTHERAPEUTIC: Histamine H_2 receptor antagonist. **CLINICAL:** Antiulcer (see p. 92C).

ACTION

Inhibits histamine action at H_2 receptors of gastric parietal cells. **Therapeutic Effect:** Inhibits gastric acid secretion (fasting, nocturnal, or when stimulated by food, caffeine, insulin). Reduces volume, hydrogen ion concentration of gastric juice.

PHARMACOKINETICS

Rapidly absorbed from GI tract. Protein binding: 15%. Widely distributed. Metabolized in liver. Primarily excreted in urine. Not removed by hemodialysis. **Half-life:** PO: 2.5 hrs; IV: 2–2.5 hrs (half-life increased with impaired renal function).

USES

Short-term treatment of active duodenal ulcer. Prevention of duodenal ulcer recurrence. Treatment of active benign gastric ulcer, pathologic GI hypersecretory conditions, acute gastroesophageal reflux disease (GERD), including erosive esophagitis. Maintenance of healed erosive esophagitis. **Bismuth Citrate:** Treatment of duodenal ulcers associated with *H. pylori*. **Unlabeled:** Prophylaxis of aspiration pneumonia.

PRECAUTIONS

CONTRAINDICATIONS: History of acute porphyria. **CAUTIONS:** Impaired renal/hepatic function, elderly.

LIFESPAN CONSIDERATIONS: Pregnancy/lactation: Unknown if drug crosses placenta or is distributed in breast milk. **Pregnancy Category B. Children:** No age-related precautions noted. **Elderly:** Confusion more likely in pts with liver/renal impairment.

INTERACTIONS

DRUG: **Antacids** may decrease absorption (do not give within 1 hr). May decrease absorption of **ketoconazole** (give at least 2 hrs after). **HERBAL:** None known. **FOOD:** None known. **LAB VALUES:** Interferes with skin tests using allergen extracts. May increase liver enzymes, creatinine, gamma-glutamyl transpeptidase.

AVAILABILITY (Rx)

TABLETS: 75 mg (OTC), 150 mg, 300 mg. **TABLETS (effervescent):** 150 mg. **CAPSULES:** 150 mg, 300 mg. **SYRUP:** 15 mg/ml. **GRANULES (effervescent):** 150 mg. **INJECTION (vial):** 25 mg/ml. **INJECTION (infusion premix):** 0.5 mg/ml, 50 ml infusion.

BISMUTH CITRATE: **TABLETS:** 400 mg.

ADMINISTRATION/HANDLING

PO

• Give without regard to meals. Best given after meals or at bedtime. • Do not administer within 1 hr of magnesium- or aluminum-containing antacids (decreases absorption by 33%).

IM

• May be given undiluted. • Give deep IM into large muscle mass.

IV

Storage • IV solutions appear clear, colorless to yellow (slight darkening does not affect potency). • IV infusion (piggyback) is stable for 48 hrs at room temperature (discard if discolored or precipitate forms).

Reconstitution • For IV push, dilute each 50 mg with 20 ml 0.9% NaCl, D_5W. • For intermittent IV infusion (piggyback), dilute each 50 mg with 50 ml 0.9% NaCl, D_5W. • For IV infusion, dilute with 250–1,000 ml 0.9% NaCl, D_5W.

Rate of administration • Administer IV push over minimum of 5 min (prevents arrhythmias, hypotension). • Infuse IV piggyback over 15–20 min. • Infuse IV infusion over 24 hrs.

IV INCOMPATIBILITIES

Amphotericin B complex (Abelcet, AmBisome, Amphotec).

IV COMPATIBILITIES

Diltiazem (Cardizem), dobutamine (Dobutrex), dopamine (Intropin), heparin, hydromorphone (Dilaudid), insulin, lidocaine, lorazepam (Ativan), morphine, norepinephrine (Levophed), potassium chloride, propofol (Diprivan).

INDICATIONS/ROUTES/DOSAGE

DUODENAL, GASTRIC ULCERS, GERD

PO: ADULTS, ELDERLY: 150 mg 2 times/day or 300 mg at hs. MAINTENANCE: 150 mg at bedtime. CHILDREN: 2–4 mg/kg/day in divided doses 2 times/day. **Maximum:** 300 mg/day.

EROSIVE ESOPHAGITIS

PO: ADULTS, ELDERLY: 150 mg 4 times/day. MAINTENANCE: 150 mg 2 times/day or 300 mg at bedtime. CHILDREN: 4–10 mg/kg/day in 2 divided doses. **Maximum:** 600 mg/day.

HYPERSECRETORY CONDITIONS

PO: ADULTS, ELDERLY: 150 mg 2 times/day. May increase up to 6 g/day.

R

USUAL PARENTERAL DOSAGE

IV/IM: ADULTS, ELDERLY: 50 mg/dose q6–8h. **Maximum:** 400 mg/day. CHILDREN: 2–4 mg/kg/day in divided doses q6–8h. **Maximum:** 200 mg/day.

USUAL NEONATAL DOSAGE

IV: Initially, 1.5 mg/kg/dose, then 1.5–2 mg/kg/day in divided doses q12h.

PO: 2 mg/kg/day in divided doses q12h.

DOSAGE IN RENAL IMPAIRMENT (creatinine clearance <50 ml/min)

PO: 150 mg q24h.

IM/IV: 50 mg q18–24h.

SIDE EFFECTS

OCCASIONAL (2%): Diarrhea. **RARE (1%):** Constipation, headache (may be severe).

ADVERSE REACTIONS/ TOXIC EFFECTS

Reversible hepatitis, blood dyscrasias occur rarely.

NURSING IMPLICATIONS

BASELINE ASSESSMENT

Obtain baseline hepatic/renal function tests.

INTERVENTION/EVALUATION

Monitor serum SGOT (AST), SGPT (ALT) levels. Assess mental status in elderly.

PATIENT/FAMILY TEACHING

Smoking decreases effectiveness of medication. Do not take medicine within 1 hr of magnesium- or aluminum-containing antacids. Transient burning/itching may occur with IV administration. Report headache. Avoid alcohol, aspirin.

rasburicase

raz-**beur**-ih-case
(Elitek)

◆ CLASSIFICATION

PHARMACOTHERAPEUTIC: Urate oxidase inhibitor. **CLINICAL:** Antihyperuricemic.

ACTION

Recombinant form of urate oxidase that rapidly catalyzes oxidation of uric acid into an inactive and soluble metabolite. **Therapeutic Effect:** Controls hyperuricemia after chemotherapy treatment in children.

USES

Initial management of increased plasma uric acid levels in pediatric pts with leukemia, lymphoma, solid tumor malignancies receiving anticancer therapy expected to result in tumor lysis, elevation of plasma uric acid.

PRECAUTIONS

CONTRAINDICATIONS: Existing hemolysis, methemoglobinemia, G6PD deficiency. **CAUTIONS:** History of asthma, allergies, hypersensitivity reaction to other medications, children <2 yrs. **Pregnancy Category C.**

R

INTERACTIONS

DRUG: None known. **HERBAL:** None known. **FOOD:** None known. **LAB VALUES:** May decrease uric acid assay readings.

AVAILABILITY (Rx)

POWDER FOR INJECTION: 1.5 mg/vial.

ADMINISTRATION/HANDLING

Storage • Refrigerate powder and diluent provided by manufacturer; do not freeze. • Protect from light. • Reconstituted or diluted solution is stable up to 24 hrs if refrigerated. Discard unused portion.

Reconstitution • Reconstitute powder with diluent (1 ml). • Dissolve the powder by gently swirling (do not shake). Further reconstitute with 50 ml 0.9% NaCl.

Rate of administration • Infuse diluted solution over 30 min. • Do not use filter during infusion.

⌀ **IV INCOMPATIBILITIES**

Do not administer via the same line as other medications.

INDICATIONS/ROUTES/DOSAGE

HYPERURICEMIA

IV infusion: CHILDREN: 0.15–0.2 mg/kg once daily as a 30-min infusion for 5 days. Chemotherapy should begin 4–24 hrs after first dose of rasburicase is administered.

SIDE EFFECTS

FREQUENT: Headache, diarrhea, mucositis, rash, fever. **OCCASIONAL:** Nausea, vomiting, myalgia. **RARE:** Edema, arrhythmias.

ADVERSE REACTIONS/ TOXIC EFFECTS

Severe hypersensitivity reaction is characterized by rash, urticaria, pruritus, chest pain, dyspnea, hypotension, bronchospasm. Blood dyscrasias present as hemolytic anemia, methemoglobinemia, neutropenia. Heart failure, MI occur rarely.

NURSING IMPLICATIONS

BASELINE ASSESSMENT

Obtain baseline uric acid serum level.

INTERVENTION/EVALUATION

Monitor uric acid, serum creatinine, phosphorus, calcium, potassium. Assess vital signs during and for several hours after completion of infusion. Monitor stool consistency, frequency. Assess oral mucous membranes for evidence of mucositis (redness, pain, bleeding).

PATIENT/FAMILY TEACHING

Report possible hypersensitivity reaction (rash, itching, hives, difficulty breathing). Contact physician if oral ulcers, nausea, diarrhea develops.

Reglan

see metoclopramide

Remeron

see mirtazapine

Remicade

see infliximab

remifentanil hydrochloride

(Ultiva)

See Classification section under: Opioid analgesics

repaglinide

reh-**pah**-glih-nide

(Prandin)

R

◆ **CLASSIFICATION**

PHARMACOTHERAPEUTIC: Antihyperglycemic. **CLINICAL:** Antidiabetic (see p. 40C).

ACTION

Stimulates release of insulin from beta cells of the pancreas by depolarizing beta cells, leading to an opening of calcium channels. Resulting calcium influx induces insulin secretion. **Therapeutic Effect:** Lowers glucose concentration.

PHARMACOKINETICS

Rapidly, completely absorbed from GI tract. Protein binding: 98%. Metabolized in liver to inactive metabolites. Excreted primarily in feces with a lesser amount in urine. Unknown if removed by hemodialysis. **Half-life:** 1 hr.

USES

Adjunct to diet/exercise to lower blood glucose in pts with type 2 diabetes mellitus. Used as monotherapy or in combination with metformin, pioglitazone, or rosiglitazone.

PRECAUTIONS

CONTRAINDICATIONS: Diabetic ketoacidosis, type 1 diabetes mellitus. **CAUTIONS:** Hepatic/renal function impairment.

LIFESPAN CONSIDERATIONS: Pregnancy/lactation: Unknown if distributed in breast milk. **Pregnancy Category C. Children:** Safety and efficacy not established. **Elderly:** No age-related precautions noted, but hypoglycemia more difficult to recognize.

INTERACTIONS

DRUG: NSAIDs, salicylates, sulfonamides, chloramphenicol, gemfibrozil, warfarin, probenecid, MAOIs, beta-blockers may increase effect. **HERBAL:** None known. **FOOD:** Food decreases repaglinide plasma concentration. **LAB VALUES:** None known.

AVAILABILITY (Rx)

TABLETS: 0.5 mg, 1 mg, 2 mg.

ADMINISTRATION/HANDLING

PO

- Ideally, give within 15 min of a meal but may be given immediately before a meal to as long as 30 min before a meal.

INDICATIONS/ROUTES/DOSAGE

DIABETES MELLITUS

PO: ADULTS, ELDERLY: 0.5–4 mg 2–4 times/day. **Maximum:** 16 mg/day.

SIDE EFFECTS

FREQUENT (6%–10%): Upper respiratory infection, headache, rhinitis, bronchitis, back pain. **OCCASIONAL (3%–5%):** Diarrhea, dyspepsia, sinusitis, nausea, arthralgia, urinary tract infection. **RARE (2%):** Constipation, vomiting, paresthesia, allergic reaction.

ADVERSE REACTIONS/ TOXIC EFFECTS

Hypoglycemia occurs in 16% of pts. Chest pain occurs rarely.

NURSING IMPLICATIONS

BASELINE ASSESSMENT

Check fasting blood glucose and glycosylated Hgb (HbA_1C) levels periodically to determine minimum effective dose. Ensure follow-up instruction if pt/family do not thoroughly understand diabetes management or glucose-testing technique. At least 1 wk should elapse to assess response to drug before new dosage adjustment is made.

INTERVENTION/EVALUATION

Monitor fasting blood glucose, glycosylated Hgb (HbA_1C) levels, food intake. Assess for hypoglycemia (cool/wet skin, tremors, dizziness, anxiety, headache, tachycardia, numbness in mouth,

R

hunger, diplopia), hyperglycemia (polyuria, polyphagia, polydipsia, nausea, vomiting, dim vision, fatigue, deep/rapid breathing). Be alert to conditions that alter glucose requirements: fever, increased activity/stress, surgical procedures.

PATIENT/FAMILY TEACHING

Diabetes mellitus requires lifelong control. Prescribed diet/exercise is principal part of treatment; do not skip, delay meals. Continue to adhere to dietary instructions, a regular exercise program, regular testing of urine or blood glucose. When taking combination drug therapy with a sulfonylurea or insulin, have a source of glucose available to treat symptoms of low blood sugar.

Requip

see ropinicole

respiratory syncytial immune globulin

(Respigam)

CLASSIFICATION

PHARMACOTHERAPEUTIC: Immune serum. **CLINICAL:** Respiratory agent.

ACTION

High concentration of neutralizing, protective antibodies specific for respiratory syncytial virus (RSV).

USES

Prevents serious lower respiratory tract infections caused by RSV in children <24 mos with bronchopulmonary dysplasia, history of premature birth.

PRECAUTIONS

CONTRAINDICATIONS: IgA deficiency. **CAUTIONS:** Pulmonary disease. **Pregnancy Category C.**

AVAILABILITY (Rx)

INJECTION: 50 mg/ml, 50-ml vial.

ADMINISTRATION/HANDLING

IV

Storage • Refrigerate vials. Do not freeze. • Do not shake. • Start infusion within 6 hrs and completed within 12 hrs of vial entry.

Rate of administration • Initial infusion rate of 1.5 ml/kg/hr for first 15 min, then increase to 3 ml/kg/hr next 15 min. Infusion rate of 6 ml/kg/hr 30 min to end of infusion. • Maximum infusion rate: 6 ml/kg/hr.

INDICATIONS/ROUTES/DOSAGE

RSV

IV infusion: CHILDREN (<24 MO): 750 mg/kg (15 ml/kg). Initially, 1.5 ml/kg/hr for first 15 min, increase to 3 ml/kg/hr for next 15 min, then 6 ml/kg/hr for remainder of infusion. Administer monthly during RSV season (starting in November through April).

SIDE EFFECTS

OCCASIONAL (2%–6%): Fever, vomiting, wheezing. **RARE (<1%):** Diarrhea, rash, tachycardia, hypertension, hypoxia, injection site inflammation.

NURSING IMPLICATIONS

INTERVENTION/EVALUATION

Monitor heart rate, B/P, temperature, respiratory rate. Observe for rales, wheezing, retractions.

Restoril

see temazepam

Ritalin

see methylphenidate

reteplase, recombinant

rhet-eh-place
(Retavase)
Do not confuse with Restasis.

CLASSIFICATION

PHARMACOTHERAPEUTIC: Tissue plasminogen activator. **CLINICAL:** Thrombolytic (see p. 30C).

ACTION

Activates fibrinolytic system by directly cleaving plasminogen to generate plasmin, an enzyme that degrades the fibrin of the thrombus. **Therapeutic Effect:** Exerts thrombolytic action.

PHARMACOKINETICS

Rapidly cleared from plasma. Eliminated primarily by the liver and kidney. **Half-life:** 13–16 min.

USES

Management of acute myocardial infarction (AMI) for improvement of ventricular function following AMI, reduction of incidence of CHF, reduction of mortality associated with AMI.

PRECAUTIONS

CONTRAINDICATIONS: Active internal bleeding, history of CVA, recent intracranial/intraspinal surgery/trauma, intracranial neoplasm, arteriovenous malformation/aneurysm, bleeding diathesis, severe uncontrolled hypertension (increases risk of bleeding). **CAUTIONS:** Recent major surgery (coronary artery bypass graft, OB delivery, organ biopsy), cerebrovascular disease, recent GI/GU bleeding, hypertension, mitral stenosis with atrial fibrillation, acute pericarditis, bacterial endocarditis, hepatic/renal impairment, diabetic retinopathy, ophthalmic hemorrhage, septic thrombophlebitis, occluded AV cannula at an infected site, advanced age, pts receiving oral anticoagulants.

LIFESPAN CONSIDERATIONS: Pregnancy/lactation: Unknown if distributed in breast milk. **Pregnancy Category C. Children:** Safety and efficacy not established. **Elderly:** More susceptible to bleeding; caution advised.

INTERACTIONS

DRUG: Heparin, warfarin platelet aggregation antagonists (e.g., aspirin, dipyridamole, abciximab) increases risk of bleeding. **HERBAL: Ginkgo biloba** may increase risk of bleeding. **FOOD:** None known. **LAB VALUES:** Plasminogen, fibrinogen levels may decrease.

AVAILABILITY (Rx)

POWDER FOR INJECTION: 10.8 units (18.8 mg).

ADMINISTRATION/HANDLING

IV

Storage • Use within 4 hrs of reconstitution. • Discard any unused portion.

Reconstitution • Reconstitute only with Sterile Water for Injection immediately prior to use. • Reconstituted solution contains 1 unit/ml. • Slight foaming may occur; let stand for a few minutes to allow bubbles to dissipate.

Rate of administration • Give through a dedicated IV line. • Give as a 10 unit plus 10 unit double bolus, with each IV bolus administered over 2-min period. • Give the second bolus 30 min after the first bolus injection. • Do not add other medications to the bolus injection solution. • Do not give second bolus if serious bleeding occurs after first IV bolus is given.

IV INCOMPATIBILITY

Do not mix with any other medications.

INDICATIONS/ROUTES/DOSAGE

ACUTE MI

IV bolus: ADULTS, ELDERLY: 10 units over 2 min, then repeat 10 units 30 min after administration of first bolus injection. **Alert:** Withhold second dose if bleeding, anaphylaxis occurs.

SIDE EFFECTS

FREQUENT: Bleeding at superficial sites (venous injection sites, catheter insertion sites, venous cutdowns, arterial punctures, sites of recent surgical procedures).

ADVERSE REACTIONS/ TOXIC EFFECTS

Bleeding at internal sites (intracranial, retroperitoneal, GI, GU, respiratory) occurs occasionally. Lysis of coronary thrombi may produce atrial/ventricular arrhythmias, stroke.

NURSING IMPLICATIONS

BASELINE ASSESSMENT

Obtain baseline B/P, apical pulse. Evaluate 12-lead EKG, CPK, CPK-MB, electrolytes. Assess Hct, platelet count, thrombin (TT), activated partial thromboplastin time (aPTT), prothrombin time (PT), plasminogen, fibrinogen level before therapy is instituted. Type, hold blood.

INTERVENTION/EVALUATION

Carefully monitor all needle puncture sites, catheter insertion sites for bleeding. Continuous cardiac monitoring for arrhythmias, B/P, pulse, respiration is essential until pt is stable. Check peripheral pulses, lung sounds. Monitor for chest pain relief; notify physician of continuation/recurrence of chest pain (note location, type, intensity). Avoid any trauma that may increase risk of bleeding (injections, shaving).

Rh_o(D) immune globulin

(BayRho-D full dose, Bay-Rho Mini-dose, MICRhogam, RhoGAM, Win-Rho SDF)

CLASSIFICATION

CLINICAL: Immune globulin.

ACTION

The Rh_o(D) antigen is responsible for most cases of Rh sensitization (occurs when Rh-positive fetal RBCs enter the maternal circulation of an Rh-negative woman). Injection of anti-D globulin results in opsonization of the fetal RBCs, which are then phagocytized in the spleen, preventing immunization of the mother. Injection of anti-D into an Rh-positive pt with idiopathic thrombocytopenic purpura (ITP) coats the pt's own D-positive RBCs with antibody and, as they are cleared by the spleen, they saturate the capacity of the spleen to clear antibody-coated cells, sparing antibody-coated platelets.

USES

Treatment of Rh_o(D)-positive children and adults (without splenectomy) with chronic ITP, children with acute ITP, children and adults with ITP secondary to HIV infection; prevention of isoimmunization in Rh-negative individuals exposed to Rh-positive blood during delivery of an Rh-positive infant, within 72 hrs of an abortion, following amniocentesis or abdominal trauma, following a transfusion accident; prevention of hemolytic disease of the newborn if there is a subsequent pregnancy with an Rh-positive infant.

PRECAUTIONS

CONTRAINDICATIONS: Hypersensitivity to any component, IgA deficiency, Rh_o(D)-positive mother or pregnant woman, transfusion of Rh_o(D)-positive blood in previous 3 mos, prior sensitization to Rh_o(D), mothers whose Rh group or immune status is uncertain. **CAUTIONS:** Thrombocytopenia, bleeding disorders. Hgb <8 g/dl. **Pregnancy Category C.**

INTERACTIONS

DRUG: May interfere with immune response to **live virus vaccines. HERBAL:** None known. **FOOD:** None known. **LAB VALUES:** None known.

AVAILABILITY (Rx)

INJECTION, POWDER FOR RECONSTITUTION (WinRho SDF): 120 mcg, 300 mcg, 1,000 mcg. **INJECTION SOLUTION:** 50 mcg, 300 mcg.

ADMINISTRATION/HANDLING

IV

Storage • Refrigerate vials (do not freeze). • Once reconstituted, stable for 12 hrs at room temperature.

Reconstitution • Reconstitute 120 mcg and 300 mcg with 2.5 ml NaCl (8.5 ml for 1,000-mcg vial). • Gently swirl; do not shake.

Rate of administration • Infuse over 3–5 min.

IM

• Reconstitute 120 mcg and 300 mcg with 2.5 ml NaCl (8.5 ml for 1,000-mcg vial). • Administer into deltoid muscle of upper arm or anterolateral aspect of upper thigh.

INDICATIONS/ROUTES/DOSAGE

ITP

IV: ADULTS, ELDERLY, CHILDREN: *(WinRho SDF):* Initially, 50 mcg/kg as a single dose (reduce to 25–40 mcg/kg if Hgb <10 g/dl). MAINTENANCE: 25–60 mcg/kg based on platelet, Hgb levels.

PREGNANCY

IM: *(BayRho-D Full Dose, RhoGAM):* 300 mcg preferably within 72 hrs of delivery.

IV/IM: *(WinRho SDF):* 300 mcg at 28 wks. Following delivery: 120 mcg preferably within 72 hrs.

THREATENED ABORTION

IM: *(BayRho-D Full Dose, RhoGAM):* 300 mcg as soon as possible.

IV/IM: *(WinRho SDF):* 300 mcg as soon as possible.

ABORTION, MISCARRIAGE, TERMINATION OF ECTOPIC PREGNANCY

IM: *(Bay-Rho-D, RhoGAM):* 300 mcg if >13 wks, 50 mcg if <13 wks.

IM/IV: *(WinRho SDF):* 120 mcg after 34 wks gestation.

TRANSFUSION INCOMPATIBILITY

Alert: Within 72 hrs after exposure of incompatible blood transfusion or massive fetal hemorrhage.

IV: ADULTS: 3,000 international units (600 mcg) q8h until total dose given.

IM: ADULTS: 6,000 international units (1,200 mcg) q12h until total dose given.

SIDE EFFECTS

Hypotension, pallor, vasodilation (IV formulation), fever, headache, chills, dizziness, somnolence, lethargy, rash, pruritus, abdominal pain, diarrhea, discomfort/swelling at injection site, back pain, myalgia, arthralgia, weakness.

ADVERSE REACTIONS/ TOXIC EFFECTS

None known.

ribavirin

rye-bah-**vi**-rin
(Copegus, Rebetol, Virazole)
Do not confuse with riboflavin.

FIXED-COMBINATION(S)

With interferon, alfa 2b **(Rebetron).** Individually packaged.

◆CLASSIFICATION

PHARMACOTHERAPEUTIC: Synthetic nucleoside. **CLINICAL:** Antiviral (see p. 59C).

R

ACTION

Inhibits replication of RNA, DNA viruses. Inhibits influenza virus RNA polymerase activity and interferes with expression of messenger RNA. **Therapeutic Effect:** Inhibits viral protein synthesis.

USES

Inhalation: Treatment of respiratory syncytial virus (RSV) infections (esp. in pts with underlying compromising conditions such as chronic lung disorders, congenital heart disease, recent transplant recipients). **Capsule/Tablet:** Treatment of chronic hepatitis C in pts with compensated hepatic disease. **Unlabeled:** Treatment of West Nile virus, treatment of influenza A or B.

PRECAUTIONS

CONTRAINDICATIONS: Pregnancy, women of childbearing age who will not use contraception reliably. **CAUTIONS: Inhalation:** Pts requiring assisted ventilation, COPD, asthma. **Oral:** Cardiac, pulmonary disease, elderly, history of psychiatric disorders. **Pregnancy Category X.**

INTERACTIONS

DRUG: Nucleoside analogues **(adefovir, didanosine, lamivudine, stavudine, zalcitabine, zidovudine)** may increase risk of lactic acidosis. **Didanosine** may increase risk of pancreatitis or peripheral neuropathy. May decrease effect of **didanosine. HERBAL:** None known. **FOOD:** None known. **LAB VALUES:** None known.

AVAILABILITY (Rx)

POWDER FOR RECONSTITUTION (AEROSOL): 6 g/100 ml. **CAPSULES:** 200 mg. **TABLETS:** 200 mg.

ADMINISTRATION/HANDLING

INHALATION

Alert: May be given via nasal or oral inhalation.

• Solution appears clear and colorless, is stable for 24 hrs at room temperature. Discard solution for nebulization after 24 hrs. • Discard if discolored or cloudy. • Add 50–100 ml Sterile Water for Injection or inhalation to 6-g vial. • Transfer to a flask, serving as reservoir for aerosol generator. • Further dilute to final volume of 300 ml, giving a solution concentration of 20 mg/ml. • Use only aerosol generator available from manufacturer of drug. • Do not give concomitantly with other drug solutions for nebulization. • Discard reservoir solution when fluid levels are low and at least q24h. • Controversy over safety in ventilator-dependent pts; only experienced personnel should administer.

PO

• Capsules may be taken without regard to food. • Tablets should be given with food.

INDICATIONS/ROUTES/DOSAGE

SEVERE LOWER RESPIRATORY TRACT INFECTION CAUSED BY RSV

Inhalation: CHILDREN, INFANTS: Use with Viratek small-particle aerosol generator at a concentration of 20 mg/ml (6 g reconstituted with 300 ml sterile water) 12–18 hrs/day for 3 days or up to 7 days.

CHRONIC HEPATITIS C

CAPSULE (IN COMBINATION WITH INTERFERON ALFA-2b)

PO: ADULTS, ELDERLY: 1,000–1,200 mg/day in 2 divided doses.

CAPSULE (IN COMBINATION WITH PEG-INTERFERON ALFA-2b)

PO: ADULTS, ELDERLY: 800 mg/day in 2 divided doses.

TABLETS (IN COMBINATION WITH PEG-INTERFERON ALFA-2b)

PO: ADULTS, ELDERLY: 800–1,200 mg/day in 2 divided doses.

SIDE EFFECTS

FREQUENT (>10%): Dizziness, headache, fatigue, fever, insomnia, irritability, depression, emotional lability, impaired concentration, alopecia, rash, pruritus, nausea, anorexia, dyspepsia, vomiting, decreased hemoglobin, hemolysis, arthralgia, musculoskeletal pain, dyspnea, sinusitis, flu-like symptoms. **OCCASIONAL (1%–10%):** Nervousness, altered taste, weakness.

ADVERSE REACTIONS/ TOXIC EFFECTS

Cardiac arrest, apnea, ventilator dependence, bacterial pneumonia, pneumonia, pneumothorax occur rarely. If therapy exceeds 7 days, anemia may occur.

NURSING IMPLICATIONS

BASELINE ASSESSMENT

Obtain respiratory tract secretions prior to giving first dose or at least during first 24 hrs of therapy. Assess respiratory status for baseline. **Oral:** CBC with differential, pretreatment and monthly pregnancy test for women of childbearing age.

INTERVENTION/EVALUATION

Monitor I&O, fluid balance carefully. Check hematology reports for anemia due to reticulocytosis when therapy exceeds 7 days. For ventilator-assisted pts, watch for "rainout" in tubing and empty frequently; be alert to impaired ventilation/gas exchange due to drug precipitate. Assess skin for rash. Monitor B/P, respirations; assess lung sounds.

PATIENT/FAMILY TEACHING

Report immediately any difficulty breathing, itching/swelling/redness of eyes. Educate females about prevention of pregnancy and need for pregnancy testing. Educate males about protection of female partners from pregnancy.

rifabutin

rye-fah-**byew**-tin
(Mycobutin)
Do not confuse with rifampin.

CLASSIFICATION

PHARMACOTHERAPEUTIC: Antitubercular. **CLINICAL:** Antibacterial (antimycobacterial).

ACTION

Inhibits DNA-dependent RNA polymerase, an enzyme in susceptible strains of *E. coli* and *Bacillus subtilis*. **Thera-**

R

peutic Effect: Prevents *M. avium* complex (MAC) disease.

PHARMACOKINETICS

Readily absorbed from GI tract (high-fat meals slow absorption). Protein binding: 85%. Widely distributed. Crosses blood-brain barrier. Extensive intracellular tissue uptake. Metabolized in liver to active metabolite. Excreted in urine; eliminated in feces. Unknown if removed by hemodialysis. **Half-life:** 16–69 hrs.

USES

Prevention of disseminated *M. avium* complex (MAC) disease in those with advanced HIV infection.

PRECAUTIONS

CONTRAINDICATIONS: Hypersensitivity to other rifamycins (e.g., rifampin). Active tuberculosis. **CAUTIONS:** Safety in children not established. Renal/liver impairment.

LIFESPAN CONSIDERATIONS: Pregnancy/lactation: Unknown if drug crosses placenta or is excreted in breast milk. **Pregnancy Category B. Children/elderly:** No age-related precautions noted.

INTERACTIONS

DRUG: May decrease effects of **oral contraceptives.** May decrease concentration of **zidovudine** (does not affect inhibition of HIV by zidovudine). **HERBAL:** None known. **FOOD:** None known. **LAB VALUES:** May increase SGOT (AST), SGPT (ALT), alkaline phosphatase. May cause anemia, neutropenia, leukopenia, thrombocytopenia.

AVAILABILITY (Rx)

CAPSULES: 150 mg.

ADMINISTRATION/HANDLING

PO

• Give without regard to food. Give with food if GI irritation occurs. • May mix with applesauce if pt is unable to swallow capsules whole.

INDICATIONS/ROUTES/DOSAGE

PROPHYLAXIS (FIRST EPISODE MAC)

PO: ADULTS, ELDERLY: 300 mg as a single or in 2 divided doses.

PROPHYLAXIS (RECURRENT MAC)

PO: ADULTS, ELDERLY: 300 mg/day (in combination).

DOSAGE IN RENAL IMPAIRMENT

Creatinine clearance <30 ml/min: Reduce dose by 50%.

SIDE EFFECTS

FREQUENT (30%): Red-orange/red-brown discoloration of urine, feces, saliva, skin, sputum, sweat, tears. **OCCASIONAL (3%–11%):** Rash, nausea, abdominal pain, diarrhea, dyspepsia (heartburn, indigestion, epigastric pain), belching, headache, altered taste, uveitis, corneal deposits. **RARE (≤2%):** Anorexia, flatulence, fever, myalgia, vomiting, insomnia.

ADVERSE REACTIONS/ TOXIC EFFECTS

Hepatitis, thrombocytopenia occur rarely.

NURSING IMPLICATIONS

BASELINE ASSESSMENT

Obtain chest x-ray, sputum/blood cultures. Biopsy of suspicious node(s) must be done to rule out active tuberculosis. Obtain baseline CBC, hepatic function tests.

INTERVENTION/EVALUATION

Monitor hepatic function tests, CBC, platelet count, Hgb, Hct. Avoid IM injections, rectal temperatures, other trauma that may induce bleeding. Check temperature; notify physician of flulike syndrome, rash, GI intolerance.

PATIENT/FAMILY TEACHING

Urine, feces, saliva, sputum, perspiration, tears, skin may be discolored brown-orange. Soft contact lenses may be permanently discolored. Rifabutin may decrease efficacy of oral contraceptives; nonhormonal methods should be considered. Avoid crowds, those with infection. Report flulike symptoms, nausea, vomiting, dark urine, unusual bleeding/bruising, any visual disturbances.

rifampin

rif-**am**-pin
(Rifadin, Rimactane, Rofact✱)

Do not confuse with rifabutin, Rifamate, rifapentine, Ritalin.

FIXED-COMBINATION(S)

Rifamate: rifampin/isoniazid (an antitubercular): 300 mg/150 mg. **Rifater:** rifampin/isoniazid/pyrazinamide (an antitubercular): 120 mg/50 mg/300 mg.

◆ CLASSIFICATION

PHARMACOTHERAPEUTIC: Antitubercular.

ACTION

Interferes with bacterial RNA synthesis by binding to DNA-dependent RNA polymerase, preventing attachment of the enzyme to DNA, thereby blocking RNA transcription. **Therapeutic Effect:** Bactericidal activity occurs in susceptible microorganisms.

PHARMACOKINETICS

Well absorbed from GI tract (food delays absorption). Protein binding: 80%. Widely distributed. Metabolized in liver to active metabolite. Primarily eliminated via biliary system. Not removed by hemodialysis. **Half-life:** 3–5 hrs (half-life increased in liver impairment).

USES

In conjunction with at least one other antitubercular agent for initial treatment and retreatment of clinical tuberculosis. Eliminates *Neisseria* meningococci from the nasopharynx of asymptomatic carriers in situations with high risk of meningococcal meningitis (prophylaxis, not cure). Recommended by WHO as adjunctive therapy with dapsone for leprosy. **Unlabeled:** Prophylaxis of *H. influenzae* type b infection; treatment of atypical mycobacterial infection, serious infections caused by *Staphylococcus* species.

PRECAUTIONS

CONTRAINDICATIONS: Hypersensitivity to rifampin or any rifamycins, concomitant therapy with amprenavir. **CAUTIONS:** Hepatic dysfunction, active/treated alcoholism.

LIFESPAN CONSIDERATIONS: Pregnancy/lactation: Crosses placenta. Distributed in breast milk. **Pregnancy Category C. Children/elderly:** No age-related precautions noted.

INTERACTIONS

DRUG: Alcohol, hepatotoxic medications may increase risk of hepatotoxicity. May increase clearance of **aminophylline, theophylline.** May decrease effects of **oral anticoagulants, oral hypoglycemics, chloramphenicol, digoxin, disopyramide, mexiletine, quinidine, tocainide, fluconazole, methadone, phenytoin, verapamil. HERBAL:** None known. **FOOD:** None known. **LAB VALUES:** May increase SGOT (AST), SGPT (ALT), alkaline phosphatase, bilirubin, BUN, uric acid.

R

AVAILABILITY (Rx)

CAPSULES: 150 mg, 300 mg. **POWDER FOR INJECTION:** 600 mg.

ADMINISTRATION/HANDLING

PO

• Preferably give 1 hr prior to or 2 hrs following meals with 8 oz of water (may give with food to decrease GI upset; will delay absorption). • For those unable to swallow capsules, contents may be mixed with applesauce, jelly. • Administer at least 1 hr prior to antacids, esp. those containing aluminum.

IV

Storage • Reconstituted vial is stable for 24 hrs. • Once reconstituted vial is further diluted, it is stable for 4 hrs in D_5W or 24 hrs in 0.9% NaCl.

Reconstitution • Reconstitute 600-mg vial with 10 ml Sterile Water for Injection to provide concentration of 60 mg/ml. • Withdraw desired dose and further dilute with 500 ml D_5W.

Rate of administration • For IV infusion only. Avoid IM, subcutaneous administration. • Avoid extravasation (local irritation, inflammation). • Infuse over 3 hrs (may dilute with 100 ml D_5W and infuse over 30 min).

R

IV INCOMPATIBILITY

Diltiazem (Cardizem).

INDICATIONS/ROUTES/DOSAGE

TUBERCULOSIS

IV/PO: ADULTS, ELDERLY: 10 mg/kg/day. **Maximum:** 600 mg/day. CHILDREN: 10–20 mg/kg/day in divided doses q12–24h.

MENINGOCOCCAL PROPHYLAXIS

IV/PO: ADULTS, ELDERLY: 600 mg q12h for 2 days. CHILDREN: 20 mg/kg/day in divided doses q12–24h. **Maximum:** 600 mg/dose. INFANTS <1 MO: 10 mg/kg/day in divided doses q12h for 2 days.

STAPHYLOCOCCAL INFECTIONS

IV/PO: ADULTS, ELDERLY: 600 mg once daily. CHILDREN: 15 mg/kg/day in divided doses q12h.

SYNERGY FOR *S. AUREUS* INFECTIONS

PO: ADULTS, ELDERLY: 300–600 mg 2 times/day (in combination). NEONATES: 5–20 mg/kg/day in divided doses q12h (in combination).

***H. INFLUENZAE* PROPHYLAXIS**

PO: ADULTS, ELDERLY: 600 mg/day for 4 days. CHILDREN ≥1 MO: 20 mg/kg/day in divided doses q12h for 5–10 days. CHILDREN <1 MO: 10 mg/kg/day in divided doses q12h for 2 days.

SIDE EFFECTS

EXPECTED: Red-orange/red-brown discoloration of urine, feces, saliva, skin, sputum, sweat, tears. **OCCASIONAL (2%–5%):** Hypersensitivity reaction (pruritus, flushing, rash). **RARE (1%–2%):** Diarrhea, dyspepsia, nausea, fungal overgrowth (sore mouth/tongue).

ADVERSE REACTIONS/ TOXIC EFFECTS

Hepatotoxicity (risk increased with isoniazid combination), hepatitis, blood dyscrasias, Stevens-Johnson syndrome, antibiotic-associated colitis occur rarely.

NURSING IMPLICATIONS

BASELINE ASSESSMENT

Question for hypersensitivity to rifampin, rifamycins. Ensure collection of diagnostic specimens. Evaluate initial hepatic/renal function, CBC results.

INTERVENTION/EVALUATION

Assess IV site at least hourly during infusion; restart at another site at the first sign of irritation/inflammation. Monitor hepatic function tests and assess for hepatitis: jaundice, anorexia, nausea, vomiting, fatigue, weakness (hold rifampin and inform physician at once). Report hypersensitivity reactions promptly: any type of skin eruption, pruritus, flulike syndrome with high dosage. Monitor frequency, consistency of stools (potential for antibiotic-associated colitis). Monitor CBC results for blood dyscrasias, be alert for infection (fever, sore throat), bleeding/bruising, unusual tiredness/weakness.

PATIENT/FAMILY TEACHING

Preferably take on empty stomach with 8 oz of water 1 hr before or 2 hrs after meal (with food if GI upset). Avoid alcohol during treatment. Do not take **any** other medications without consulting physician, including antacids; must take rifampin at least 1 hr before antacid. Urine, feces, sputum, sweat, tears may become red-orange; soft contact lenses may be permanently stained. Notify physician of **any** new symptom, immediately for yellow eyes/skin, fatigue, weakness, nausea/vomiting, sore throat, fever, flu, unusual bruising/bleeding. If taking oral contraceptives, check with physician (reliability may be affected).

rifapentine

rif-ah-**pen**-teen
(Priftin)

◆ CLASSIFICATION

PHARMACOTHERAPEUTIC: Antitubercular.

ACTION

Inhibits DNA-dependent RNA polymerase in *M. tuberculosis.* Interferes with bacterial RNA synthesis, preventing attachment of enzyme to DNA, thereby blocking RNA transcription. **Therapeutic Effect:** Bactericidal activity.

USES

Treatment of pulmonary tuberculosis in combination with at least one other antituberculosis medication.

PRECAUTIONS

CONTRAINDICATIONS: None known. **CAUTIONS:** Alcoholism, liver function impairment. **Pregnancy Category C.**

INTERACTIONS

DRUG: None known. **HERBAL:** None known. **FOOD:** None known. **LAB VALUES:** None known.

AVAILABILITY (Rx)

TABLETS: 150 mg.

INDICATIONS/ROUTES/DOSAGE

Alert: Use only in combination with another antituberculosis agent.

TUBERCULOSIS

PO: ADULTS, ELDERLY: Intensive phase: 600 mg 2 times/wk for 2 mos (interval no less than 3 days). Continuation phase: 600 mg weekly for 4 mos.

SIDE EFFECTS

RARE (<4%): Red-orange/red-brown discoloration of urine, feces, saliva, skin, sputum, sweat, tears, arthralgia, pain, nausea, vomiting, headache, dyspepsia (heartburn, indigestion, epigastric pain), hypertension, dizziness, diarrhea.

ADVERSE REACTIONS/ TOXIC EFFECTS

Hyperuricemia, neutropenia, proteinuria, hematuria occur rarely.

R

NURSING IMPLICATIONS

BASELINE ASSESSMENT

Evaluate initial hepatic function, CBC results.

INTERVENTION/EVALUATION

Monitor liver function tests; frequency, consistency of stools. Assess for nausea, vomiting, GI upset, diarrhea.

PATIENT/FAMILY TEACHING

Urine, feces, sputum, sweat, tears may become red-orange; soft contact lenses may be permanently stained. If taking oral contraceptives, check with physician (reliability may be affected). Report fever, decreased appetite, nausea, vomiting, dark urine, yellow skin/eyes, pain/swelling of joints.

rimantadine hydrochloride

rye-**man**-tah-deen
(Flumadine)

Do not confuse with flunisolide, flutamide, ranitidine.

◆CLASSIFICATION

CLINICAL: Antiviral.

R

ACTION

Appears to exert inhibitory effect early in viral replication cycle. May inhibit uncoating of virus. **Therapeutic Effect:** Prevents replication of influenza A virus.

USES

Adults: Prophylaxis/treatment of illness due to influenza A virus. **Children:** Prophylaxis against influenza A virus.

PRECAUTIONS

CONTRAINDICATIONS: Hypersensitivity to amantadine, rimantadine. **CAUTIONS:** Liver disease, seizures, history of recurrent eczematoid dermatitis, uncontrolled psychosis, renal impairment, concomitant use of CNS stimulant medications. **Pregnancy Category C.**

INTERACTIONS

DRUG: Acetaminophen, aspirin may decrease concentrations. **Cimetidine** may increase concentrations. **Anticholinergics, CNS stimulants** may increase side effects. **HERBAL:** None known. **FOOD:** None known. **LAB VALUES:** None known.

AVAILABILITY (Rx)

TABLETS: 100 mg. **SYRUP:** 50 mg/5 ml.

ADMINISTRATION/HANDLING

PO

- Give without regard to food.

INDICATIONS/ROUTES/DOSAGE

PROPHYLAXIS AGAINST INFLUENZA A VIRUS

PO: ADULTS, ELDERLY, CHILDREN ≥10 YRS: 100 mg 2 times/day for at least 10 days after known exposure (usually 6–8 wks). SEVERE HEPATIC/RENAL IMPAIRMENT, ELDERLY NURSING HOME PTS: 100 mg/day. CHILDREN <10 YRS: 5 mg/kg once daily. **Maximum:** 150 mg.

TREATMENT OF INFLUENZA A VIRUS

PO: ADULTS, ELDERLY: 100 mg 2 times/day for 7 days. SEVERE HEPATIC/RENAL IMPAIRMENT, ELDERLY NURSING HOME PTS: 100 mg/day for 7 days.

SIDE EFFECTS

OCCASIONAL (2%–3%): Insomnia, nausea, nervousness, impaired concentration, dizziness. **RARE (<2%):** Vomiting, anorexia, dry mouth, abdominal pain, asthenia (loss of strength, energy), fatigue.

ADVERSE REACTIONS/ TOXIC EFFECTS

None known.

NURSING IMPLICATIONS

INTERVENTION/EVALUATION

Assess for nervousness, evaluate sleep pattern for insomnia. Provide assistance if dizziness occurs.

PATIENT/FAMILY TEACHING

Avoid contact with those who are at high risk for influenza A (rimantadine-resistant virus may be shed during therapy). Do not drive, perform tasks that require alert response if dizziness or decreased concentration occurs. Do not take aspirin, acetaminophen, compounds containing these drugs. May cause dry mouth.

risedronate sodium

rize-droe-nate

(Actonel)

◆ CLASSIFICATION

PHARMACOTHERAPEUTIC: Bisphosphonate. **CLINICAL:** Calcium regulator.

ACTION

Binds to bone hydroxyapatite, inhibits osteoclasts. **Therapeutic Effect:** Reduces bone turnover (number of sites at which bone is remodeled), bone resorption.

USES

Treatment of Paget's disease of bone (osteitis deformans). Treatment/prophylaxis for postmenopausal, glucocorticoid-induced osteoporosis.

PRECAUTIONS

CONTRAINDICATIONS: Hypersensitivity to other bisphosphonates (etidronate, tiludronate, risedronate, alendronate), renal impairment when serum creatinine clearance >5 mg/dl hypocalcemia. Inability to stand or sit upright for at least 30 min. **CAUTIONS:** GI diseases (duodenitis, dysphagia, esophagitis, gastritis, ulcers [drug may exacerbate these conditions]), severe renal impairment. **Pregnancy Category C.**

INTERACTIONS

DRUG: **Antacids** with **calcium, magnesium, aluminum**, **vitamin D** may decrease absorption. **HERBAL:** None known. **FOOD:** None known. **LAB VALUES:** None known.

AVAILABILITY (Rx)

TABLETS: 5 mg, 30 mg, 35 mg.

ADMINISTRATION/HANDLING

PO

• Administer 30–60 min before taking any food, drink, other medications orally to avoid interference with absorption. • Take on empty stomach with full glass of water (not mineral water). • Avoid lying down for 30 min after swallowing tablet (helps delivery to stomach).

INDICATIONS/ROUTES/DOSAGE

PAGET'S DISEASE

PO: ADULTS, ELDERLY: 30 mg/day for 2 mos. Retreatment may occur after 2-mo post-treatment observation period.

OSTEOPOROSIS (Postmenopausal, prevention/treatment)

PO: ADULTS, ELDERLY: 5 mg/day or 35 mg once weekly.

OSTEOPOROSIS (glucocorticoid induced)

PO: ADULTS, ELDERLY: 5 mg/day.

SIDE EFFECTS

FREQUENT (30%): Arthralgia. **OCCASIONAL (8%–12%):** Rash, flulike symptoms, peripheral edema. **RARE (3%–5%):**

R

Bone pain, sinusitis, asthenia, (loss of strength, energy), dry eye, tinnitus.

ADVERSE REACTIONS/ TOXIC EFFECTS

Hypocalcemia, hypophosphatemia, significant GI disturbances result from overdosage.

NURSING IMPLICATIONS

BASELINE ASSESSMENT

Hypocalcemia, vitamin D deficiency must be corrected before therapy. Obtain lab baselines, esp. electrolytes, renal function.

INTERVENTION/EVALUATION

Check electrolytes (esp. calcium, alkaline phosphatase serum levels). Monitor I&O, BUN, creatinine in pts with impaired renal function.

PATIENT/FAMILY TEACHING

Instruct pt that expected benefits occur only when medication is taken with full glass (6–8 oz) of plain water, first thing in the morning and at least 30 min before first food, beverage, medication of the day. Any other beverage (mineral water, orange juice, coffee) significantly reduces absorption of medication. Do not lie down for at least 30 min after taking medication (potentiates delivery to stomach, reduces risk of esophageal irritation). Consider weight-bearing exercises, modify behavioral factors (e.g., cigarette smoking, alcohol consumption).

risperidone

ris-**pear**-ih-doan
(Risperdal, Risperdal M-TABS, Risperdal Consta)
Do not confuse with reserpine.

CLASSIFICATION

PHARMACOTHERAPEUTIC: Benzisoxazole derivative. **CLINICAL:** Antipsychotic (see p. 57C).

ACTION

Action may be due to dopamine, serotonin receptor antagonism. **Therapeutic Effect:** Suppresses behavioral response in psychosis.

PHARMACOKINETICS

Well absorbed from GI tract (unaffected by food). Protein binding: 90%. Extensively metabolized in liver to active metabolite. Primarily excreted in urine. **Half-life:** 3–20 hrs; metabolite: 21–30 hrs (half-life increased in elderly).

USES

Management of manifestations of psychotic disorders. Delays relapse in long-term treatment of schizophrenia.

PRECAUTIONS

CONTRAINDICATIONS: None known. **CAUTIONS:** Renal/liver impairment, seizure disorders, cardiac disease, recent MI, breast cancer, suicidal patients, those at risk for aspiration pneumonia. May increase risk of stroke in pts with dementia.

LIFESPAN CONSIDERATIONS: Pregnancy/lactation: Unknown if drug crosses placenta or is excreted in breast milk. Recommend against breast-feeding. **Pregnancy Category C. Children:** Safety and efficacy not established. **Elderly:** More susceptible to postural hypotension. Age-related renal or hepatic impairment may require dosage adjustment.

INTERACTIONS

DRUG: May decrease effects of **levodopa, dopamine agonists. Carbamazepine** may decrease concentration. **Clozapine** may increase concentration.

Alcohol, CNS depressants may increase CNS depression. **Paroxetine** can increase concentration, risk of extrapyramidal symptoms. **HERBAL:** None known. **FOOD:** None known. **LAB VALUES:** May increase creatine phosphatase, uric acid, triglycerides, SGOT (AST), SGPT (ALT), prolactin. May decrease potassium, sodium, protein, glucose. May cause EKG changes.

AVAILABILITY (Rx)

INJECTION: 25 mg, 37.5 mg, 50 mg. **TABLETS:** 0.25 mg, 0.5 mg, 1 mg, 2 mg, 3 mg, 4 mg. **(M-TABS):** 0.5 mg, 1 mg, 2 mg. **ORAL SOLUTION:** 1 mg/ml.

ADMINISTRATION/HANDLING

PO

• Give without regard to food. • May mix oral solution with water, coffee, orange juice, low-fat milk. Do not mix with cola, tea.

INDICATIONS/ROUTES/DOSAGE

PSYCHOTIC DISORDER

PO: ADULTS: Initially, 0.5–1 mg 2 times/day. May increase slowly. ELDERLY: Initially, 0.25–2 mg/day in 1–2 divided doses. May increase slowly. RANGE: 2–6 mg/day.

DOSAGE IN RENAL IMPAIRMENT

PO: ADULTS, ELDERLY: Initially, 0.25–0.5 mg 2 times/day. Titrate slowly to desired effect.

USUAL IM DOSAGE

IM: ADULTS, ELDERLY: 25 mg q 2 wks. **Maximum:** 50 mg q 2 wks.

SIDE EFFECTS

FREQUENT (13%–26%): Agitation, anxiety, insomnia, headache, constipation. **OCCASIONAL (4%–10%):** Dyspepsia, rhinitis, drowsiness, dizziness, nausea, vomiting, rash, abdominal pain, dry skin, tachycardia. **RARE (2%–3%):** Visual disturbances, fever, back pain, pharyngitis, cough, arthralgia, angina, aggressive reaction.

ADVERSE REACTIONS/ TOXIC EFFECTS

Neuroleptic malignant syndrome (NMS): hyperpyrexia, muscle rigidity, change in mental status, irregular pulse or B/P, tachycardia, diaphoresis, cardiac arrhythmias, rhabdomyolysis, acute renal failure. Tardive dyskinesia (protrusion of tongue, puffing of cheeks, chewing/puckering of the mouth).

NURSING IMPLICATIONS

BASELINE ASSESSMENT

Renal/liver function tests should be done before therapy. Assess behavior, appearance, emotional status, response to environment, speech pattern, thought content.

INTERVENTION/EVALUATION

Monitor B/P, heart rate, weight, liver function tests, EKG. Monitor for fine tongue movement (may be first sign of tardive dyskinesia, which may be irreversible). Supervise suicidal-risk pt closely during early therapy (as depression lessens, energy level improves, increasing suicide potential). Assess for therapeutic response (greater interest in surroundings, improved self-care, increased ability to concentrate, relaxed facial expression). Monitor for potential neuroleptic malignant syndrome: fever, muscle rigidity, irregular B/P or pulse, altered mental status.

PATIENT/FAMILY TEACHING

May cause dizziness/drowsiness. Avoid tasks that may require mental alertness or physical coordination (e.g., driving). Avoid alcohol. Use caution when changing position from lying or sitting to standing. Inform physician of trembling in fingers, altered gait, unusual muscle/skeletal movements, palpita-

R

tions, severe dizziness/fainting, swelling/pain in breasts, visual changes, rash, difficulty in breathing.

ritonavir

rih-**tone**-ah-vir
(Norvir)
Do not confuse with Retrovir.

CLASSIFICATION

PHARMACOTHERAPEUTIC: Protease inhibitor. **CLINICAL:** Antiviral (see pp. 59C, 100C).

ACTION

Inhibits HIV-1, HIV-2 proteases, rendering the enzymes incapable of processing the polypeptide precursor that leads to production of immature HIV particles. **Therapeutic Effect:** Slows HIV replication, reducing progression of HIV infection.

PHARMACOKINETICS

Well absorbed following PO administration (extent of absorption increased with food). Protein binding: 98%–99%. Extensively metabolized by liver to active metabolite. Primarily eliminated in feces. Unknown if removed by hemodialysis. **Half-life:** 2.7–5 hrs.

USES

Used in combination with nucleoside analogues or as monotherapy for treatment of HIV infection.

PRECAUTIONS

CONTRAINDICATIONS: Due to potential serious and/or life-threatening drug interactions, the following medications should not be given concomitantly with ritonavir: amiodarone, astemizole, bepridil, bupropion, cisapride, clozapine, encainide, flecainide, meperidine, piroxicam, propafenone, propoxyphene, quinidine, rifabutin, terfenadine (increase risk of arrhythmias, hematologic abnormalities, seizures). Alprazolam, clorazepate, diazepam, estazolam, flurazepam, midazolam, triazolam, zolpidem may produce extreme sedation, respiratory depression. **CAUTIONS:** Impaired hepatic function.

LIFESPAN CONSIDERATIONS: Pregnancy/lactation: Breast-feeding not recommended (possibility of HIV transmission). **Pregnancy Category B. Children:** No age-related precautions noted in those >2 yrs. **Elderly:** None known.

INTERACTIONS

DRUG: May produce disulfiram-like reaction if taken with **disulfiram** or drugs causing disulfiram-like reaction **(e.g., metronidazole). Enzyme inducers (e.g., nevirapine, phenobarbital, carbamazepine, dexamethasone, phenytoin, rifampin, rifabutin)** may increase metabolism, decrease efficacy. May decrease effectiveness of **theophylline, oral contraceptives.** May increase concentration of **desipramine, fluoxetine, other antidepressants. HERBAL: St. John's wort** may decrease concentration, effect. **FOOD:** None known. **LAB VALUES:** May alter SGOT (AST), SGPT (ALT), creatinine clearance, GGT, CPK, uric acid, triglycerides.

AVAILABILITY (Rx)

SOFT GELATIN CAPSULES: 100 mg. **ORAL SOLUTION:** 80 mg/ml.

ADMINISTRATION/HANDLING

PO

• Store capsules, solution in refrigerator. • Protect from light. • Refrigeration of oral solution is recommended but not necessary if used within 30 days and stored below 77°F. • Give without regard to meals (preferably give with food). • May improve taste of oral solu-

R

tion by mixing with chocolate milk, Ensure, Advera within 1 hr of dosing.

INDICATIONS/ROUTES/DOSAGE

HIV INFECTION

PO: ADULTS, CHILDREN ≥12 YRS: 600 mg 2 times/day. If nausea becomes apparent upon initiation of 600 mg twice daily, give 300 mg twice daily for 1 day, 400 mg twice daily for 2 days, 500 mg twice daily for 1 day, then 600 mg twice daily thereafter. CHILDREN <12 YRS: Initially, 250 mg/m^2/dose 2 times/day. Increase by 50 mg/m^2/dose up to 400 mg/m^2/dose. **Maximum:** 600 mg/dose 2 times/day.

SIDE EFFECTS

FREQUENT: GI disturbances (nausea, diarrhea, vomiting, anorexia, abdominal pain), neurologic disturbances (taste perversion; circumoral and peripheral paresthesias, esp. around lips, hands, feet), headache, dizziness, fatigue, weakness. **OCCASIONAL:** Allergic reaction, flu syndrome, hypotension.

ADVERSE REACTIONS/ TOXIC EFFECTS

None known.

NURSING IMPLICATIONS

BASELINE ASSESSMENT

Pts beginning combination therapy with ritonavir and nucleosides may promote GI tolerance by beginning ritonavir alone and subsequently adding nucleosides prior to completing 2 wks of ritonavir monotherapy. Obtain baseline laboratory testing, esp. liver function tests, triglycerides prior to beginning ritonavir therapy and at periodic intervals during therapy. Offer emotional support.

INTERVENTION/EVALUATION

Closely monitor for evidence of GI disturbances, neurologic abnormalities (particularly paresthesias). Monitor liver function tests, blood glucose, CD4 cell count, plasma levels of HIV RNA.

PATIENT/FAMILY TEACHING

Continue therapy for full length of treatment. Doses should be evenly spaced. Ritonavir is not a cure for HIV infection, nor does it reduce risk of transmission to others. Pts may continue to acquire illnesses associated with advanced HIV infection. If possible, take ritonavir with food. Taste of solution may be improved when mixed with chocolate milk, Ensure, Advera. Inform physician of increased thirst, frequent urination, nausea, vomiting, abdominal pain.

rituximab

rye-**tucks**-ih-mab
(Rituxan)

CLASSIFICATION

PHARMACOTHERAPEUTIC: Monoclonal antibody. **CLINICAL:** Antineoplastic (see p. 75C).

ACTION

Binds to CD20, the antigen found on surface of B lymphocytes and B-cell non-Hodgkin's lymphomas. **Therapeutic Effect:** Produces cytotoxicity, reducing tumor size.

PHARMACOKINETICS

Rapidly depletes B cells. **Half-life:** 59.8 hrs after first infusion, 174 hrs after fourth infusion.

USES

Treatment of relapsed or refractory low-grade or follicular B-cell non-Hodgkin's lymphoma.

PRECAUTIONS

CONTRAINDICATIONS: Hypersensitivity to murine proteins. **CAUTIONS:** Those with history of cardiac disease.

LIFESPAN CONSIDERATIONS: Pregnancy/lactation: Has potential to cause fetal B-cell depletion. Unknown if distributed in breast milk. Those with childbearing potential should use contraceptive methods during treatment and up to 12 mos following therapy. **Pregnancy Category C. Children:** Safety and efficacy not established. **Elderly:** No age-related precautions noted.

INTERACTIONS

DRUG: None known. **HERBAL:** None known. **FOOD:** None known. **LAB VALUES:** None known.

AVAILABILITY (Rx)

INJECTION: 10 mg/ml.

ADMINISTRATION/HANDLING

IV

Storage

Alert: Do not give by IV push or bolus.

• Refrigerate vials. • Diluted solution is stable for 24 hrs if refrigerated and at room temperature for an additional 12 hrs.

Reconstitution • Dilute with 0.9% NaCl or D_5W to provide a final concentration of 1–4 mg/ml into infusion bag.

Rate of administration • Infuse at rate of 50 mg/hr. May increase infusion rate in 50 mg/hr increments q30min to maximum 400 mg/hr. • Subsequent infusion can be given at 100 mg/hr and increased by 100 mg/hr increments q30min to maximum 400 mg/hr.

IV INCOMPATIBILITY

Do not mix with any other medications.

INDICATIONS/ROUTES/DOSAGE

Alert: Pretreatment with acetaminophen and diphenhydramine before each infusion may prevent infusion-related effects.

NON-HODGKIN'S LYMPHOMA

IV infusion: ADULTS: 375 mg/m^2 given once weekly for 4–8 wks. May be retreated with second 4-wk course.

SIDE EFFECTS

FREQUENT: Fever (49%), chills (32%), asthenia (16%), headache (14%), angioedema (13%), hypotension (10%), nausea (18%), rash/pruritus (10%). **OCCASIONAL (<10%):** Myalgia, dizziness, abdominal pain, throat irritation, vomiting, neutropenia, rhinitis, bronchospasm, urticaria.

ADVERSE REACTIONS/ TOXIC EFFECTS

Hypersensitivity reaction produces hypotension, bronchospasm, angioedema. Cardiac arrhythmias may occur, particularly in pts with history of preexisting cardiac conditions.

NURSING IMPLICATIONS

BASELINE ASSESSMENT

Pretreatment with acetaminophen and diphenhydramine prior to each infusion may prevent infusion-related effects. CBC, platelet count should be obtained at regular interval during therapy.

INTERVENTION/EVALUATION

Monitor for an infusion-related symptoms complex consisting mainly of fever, chills, rigors that generally occurs 30 min–2 hrs of beginning first infusion. Slowing infusion resolves symptoms.

rivastigmine tartrate

rye-vah-**stig**-meen
(Exelon)

CLASSIFICATION

PHARMACOTHERAPEUTIC: Cholinesterase inhibitor. **CLINICAL:** Anti-Alzheimer's dementia agent.

ACTION

Increases the concentration of acetylcholine through reversible inhibition of its hydrolysis by cholinesterase. **Therapeutic Effect:** Enhances cholinergic function.

PHARMACOKINETICS

Rapidly and completely absorbed. Protein binding: 60%. Widely distributed throughout the body. Rapidly and extensively metabolized. Primarily excreted in urine. **Half-life:** 1.5 hrs.

USES

Treatment of mild to moderate dementia of the Alzheimer's type.

PRECAUTIONS

CONTRAINDICATIONS: None known. **CAUTIONS:** Peptic ulcer disease, concurrent use of NSAIDs, sick sinus syndrome, bradycardia, urinary obstruction, seizure disorders, asthma, COPD.

LIFESPAN CONSIDERATIONS: Pregnancy/lactation: Unknown if distributed in breast milk. **Pregnancy Category B. Children:** Not indicated for use in children. **Elderly:** No age-related precautions.

INTERACTIONS

DRUG: May interfere with **anticholinergic medications.** May have additive effect with **bethanecol. HERBAL:** None known. **FOOD:** None known. **LAB VALUES:** None known.

AVAILABILITY (Rx)

CAPSULES: 1.5 mg, 3 mg, 4.5 mg, 6 mg. **ORAL SOLUTION:** 2 mg/ml.

ADMINISTRATION/HANDLING

PO

- Give with food in divided doses morning and evening.

ORAL SOLUTION

- Using oral syringe (provided by manufacturer), withdraw prescribed amount rivastigmine from container. • May be swallowed directly from syringe or mixed in small glass of water, cold fruit juice, soda (use within 4 hrs of mixing).

INDICATIONS/ROUTES/DOSAGE

ALZHEIMER'S DISEASE

PO: ADULTS, ELDERLY: Initially, 1.5 mg twice daily. May increase after minimum of 2 wks to 3 mg twice daily. Subsequent increases to 4.5 mg and 6 mg twice daily may be made after a minimum of 2 wks at the previous dose. **Maximum:** 6 mg twice daily.

SIDE EFFECTS

FREQUENT (17%–47%): Nausea, vomiting, dizziness, diarrhea, headache, anorexia. **OCCASIONAL (6%–13%):** Abdominal pain, insomnia, dyspepsia (heartburn, indigestion, epigastric pain), confusion, urinary tract infection, depression. **RARE (3%–5%):** Anxiety, somnolence, constipation, malaise, hallucinations, tremor, flatulence, rhinitis, hypertension, flulike symptoms, weight decrease, syncope.

ADVERSE REACTIONS/ TOXIC EFFECTS

Overdosage can produce cholinergic crisis characterized by severe nausea, vom-

R

iting, salivation, diaphoresis, bradycardia, hypotension, respiratory depression, seizures.

NURSING IMPLICATIONS

BASELINE ASSESSMENT

Obtain baseline vital signs. Assess history for peptic ulcer, urinary obstruction, asthma, COPD. Assess cognitive, behavioral, functional deficits.

INTERVENTION/EVALUATION

Monitor for cholinergic reaction: GI discomfort/cramping, feeling of facial warmth, excessive salivation and diaphoresis, lacrimation, pallor, urinary urgency, dizziness. Assess eyes for pupillary contraction. Monitor for nausea, diarrhea, headache, insomnia.

PATIENT/FAMILY TEACHING

Take with meals (at breakfast, dinner). Swallow capsule whole. Do not chew, break, crush capsules. Report nausea, vomiting, diarrhea, sweating, increased salivary secretions, severe abdominal pain, dizziness.

R

rizatriptan benzoate

rise-ah-**trip**-tan
(Maxalt, Maxalt-MLT)

CLASSIFICATION

PHARMACOTHERAPEUTIC: Serotonin receptor agonist. **CLINICAL:** Antimigraine (see p. 54C).

ACTION

Binds selectively to vascular receptors, producing a vasoconstrictive effect on cranial blood vessels. **Therapeutic Effect:** Produces relief of migraine headache.

PHARMACOKINETICS

Well absorbed following PO administration. Protein binding: 14%. Crosses blood-brain barrier. Metabolized by the liver to inactive metabolite. Eliminated primarily in urine with lesser amount excreted in feces. **Half-life:** 2–3 hrs.

USES

Treatment of acute migraine attack with or without aura.

PRECAUTIONS

CONTRAINDICATIONS: Coronary artery disease, uncontrolled hypertension, ischemic heart disease (angina pectoris, history of MI, silent ischemia), Prinzmetal's angina, concurrent use (or within 24 hrs) of ergotamine-containing preparations, concurrent (or within 2 wks) of MAO therapy, hemiplegic or basilar migraine, within 24 hrs of another serotonin receptor agonist. **CAUTIONS:** Mild to moderate renal/hepatic impairment, pt profile suggesting cardiovascular risks.

LIFESPAN CONSIDERATIONS: Pregnancy/lactation: Unknown if distributed in breast milk. **Pregnancy Category C. Children:** Safety and efficacy not established. **Elderly:** No age-related precautions noted.

INTERACTIONS

DRUG: Ergotamine-containing drugs may produce vasospastic reaction. **MAOIs, propranolol** may dramatically increase plasma concentration of rizatriptan. Combined use of **fluoxetine, fluvoxamine, paroxetine, sertraline** may produce weakness, hyper-reflexia, incoordination. **HERBAL:** None known. **FOOD:** Food delays peak drug concentrations by 1 hr. **LAB VALUES:** None known.

AVAILABILITY (Rx)

TABLETS: 5 mg, 10 mg. **ORAL DISINTEGRATING TABLETS:** 5 mg, 10 mg.

ADMINISTRATION/HANDLING

PO

- The oral disintegrating tablet is packaged in an individual aluminum pouch.
- Open packet with dry hands. Place tablet onto tongue to be dissolved and swallowed with saliva. Administration with water is not necessary.

INDICATIONS/ROUTES/DOSAGE

MIGRAINE

PO: ADULTS >18 YRS, ELDERLY: 5–10 mg. Separate doses by at least 2 hrs. **Maximum:** 30 mg/24 hrs.

SIDE EFFECTS

FREQUENT (7%–9%): Dizziness, somnolence, tingling in extremities, fatigue. **OCCASIONAL (3%–6%):** Nausea, paresthesia, sensation of chest pressure, dry mouth. **RARE (2%):** Headache, neck/throat/jaw pressure, photosensitivity.

ADVERSE REACTIONS/ TOXIC EFFECTS

Cardiac events (ischemia, coronary artery vasospasm, MI), noncardiac vasospasm-related reactions (hemorrhage, stroke) occur rarely but particularly in those with hypertension, obesity, smokers, diabetes, strong family history of coronary artery disease, males >40 yrs, postmenopausal women.

NURSING IMPLICATIONS

BASELINE ASSESSMENT

Question for history of peripheral vascular disease, renal/hepatic impairment. Question pt regarding onset, location, duration of migraine and possible precipitating symptoms.

INTERVENTION/EVALUATION

Monitor for evidence of dizziness. Assess for relief of migraine headache and potential for photophobia, phonophobia (sound sensitivity, nausea, vomiting).

PATIENT/FAMILY TEACHING

Take a single dose as soon as symptoms of an actual migraine attack appear. Medication is intended to relieve migraine, not to prevent or reduce number of attacks. Avoid tasks that require alertness, motor skills until response to drug is established. If palpitations, pain/tightness in chest/throat, pain/weakness of extremities occurs, contact physician immediately. Do not remove the blister from the orally disintegrating tablet until just before dosing. Use protective measures (e.g., sunscreen, protective clothing) against exposure to UV/sunlight.

Rocephin

see ceftriaxone

rocuronium bromide

(Zemuron)

See Classification section under: Neuromuscular blockers (p. 107C)

R

rofecoxib

row-feh-**cox**-ib

(Vioxx)

Do not confuse with Zyvox.

◆CLASSIFICATION

PHARMACOTHERAPEUTIC: Nonsteroidal anti-inflammatory. **CLINICAL:** Antiarthritic, analgesic, antidysmenorrheal (see p. 111C).

ACTION

Produces analgesic, anti-inflammatory effect by inhibiting prostaglandin synthesis. **Therapeutic Effect:** Reduces inflammatory response, intensity of pain stimulus reaching sensory nerve endings.

PHARMACOKINETICS

Rapid, complete absorption from GI tract. Protein binding: 87%. Primarily metabolized in liver. Primarily eliminated in urine with a lesser amount excreted in feces. Not removed by hemodialysis. **Half-life:** 17 hrs.

USES

Relief of signs/symptoms of osteoarthritis. Treatment of rheumatoid arthritis. Management of acute pain in adults. Treatment of primary dysmenorrhea.

PRECAUTIONS

CONTRAINDICATIONS: History of hypersensitivity to aspirin, NSAIDs. **CAUTIONS:** Impaired renal/hepatic function, history of GI tract disease, predisposition to fluid retention.

LIFESPAN CONSIDERATIONS: Pregnancy/lactation: Unknown if drug is distributed in breast milk. Avoid use during third trimester (may adversely affect fetal cardiovascular system: premature closure of ductus arteriosus). **Pregnancy Category C (D** if used in third trimester or near delivery). **Children:** Safety and efficacy not established. **Elderly:** GI bleeding/ulceration more likely to cause serious adverse effects. Age-related renal impairment may increase risk of hepatic/renal toxicity; decreased dosage recommended.

R

INTERACTIONS

DRUG: May increase effects of **anticoagulants. Aspirin** may increase risk of GI side effects, bleeding. **HERBAL:** May decrease effects of **feverfew. Ginkgo biloba** may increase risk of bleeding. **FOOD:** None known. **LAB VALUES:** May prolong bleeding time. May increase alkaline phosphatase, LDH, liver function tests. May decrease sodium, Hgb, Hct.

AVAILABILITY (Rx)

TABLETS: 12.5 mg, 25 mg, 50 mg. **SUSPENSION:** 12.5 mg/5 ml, 25 mg/5 ml.

ADMINISTRATION/HANDLING

PO

- Give without regard to meals.

INDICATIONS/ROUTES/DOSAGE

OSTEOARTHRITIS

PO: ADULTS: Initially, 12.5 mg/day. May increase dosage to 25 mg/day. **Maximum:** 25 mg/day.

RHEUMATOID ARTHRITIS

PO: ADULTS, ELDERLY: 25 mg/day.

ACUTE PAIN, DYSMENORRHEA

PO: ADULTS: Initially, 50 mg/day.

SIDE EFFECTS

FREQUENT (5%–6%): Nausea (with or without vomiting), diarrhea, abdominal distress. **OCCASIONAL (3%):** Dyspepsia (heartburn, indigestion, epigastric pain). **RARE (<2%):** Constipation, flatulence.

ADVERSE REACTIONS/ TOXIC EFFECTS

None known.

NURSING IMPLICATIONS

BASELINE ASSESSMENT

Assess onset, type, location, duration of pain, inflammation. Inspect appearance of affected joints for immobility, deformities, skin condition.

INTERVENTION/EVALUATION

Monitor for evidence of nausea, dyspepsia. Monitor pattern of daily bowel activity, stool consistency. Evaluate for therapeutic response: relief of pain, stiffness, swelling; increase in joint mobility; reduced joint tenderness; improved grip strength. Monitor B/P.

PATIENT/FAMILY TEACHING

Avoid aspirin, alcohol during therapy (increase risk of GI bleeding). If GI upset occurs, take with food, milk, antacid. If GI upset persists, contact physician.

ropinirole hydrochloride

roh-**pin**-ih-role
(Requip)

CLASSIFICATION

PHARMACOTHERAPEUTIC: Dopamine agonist. **CLINICAL:** Antiparkinson agent.

ACTION

Stimulates dopamine receptors in the striatum. **Therapeutic Effect:** Relieves signs/symptoms of Parkinson's disease.

PHARMACOKINETICS

Rapidly absorbed following PO administration. Protein binding: 40%. Extensively distributed throughout the body. Extensively metabolized. Steady-state concentrations achieved within 2 days. Eliminated in urine. Unknown if removed by hemodialysis. **Half-life:** 6 hrs.

USES

Treatment of signs/symptoms of idiopathic Parkinson's disease.

PRECAUTIONS

CONTRAINDICATIONS: None known. **CAUTIONS:** History of orthostatic hypotension, syncope, hallucinations, esp. in elderly. Concurrent use of CNS depressants.

LIFESPAN CONSIDERATIONS: Pregnancy/lactation: Distributed in breast milk. Drug activity possible in nursing infant. **Pregnancy Category C. Children:** Safety and efficacy not established. **Elderly:** No age-related precautions noted, but hallucinations appear to occur more frequently.

INTERACTIONS

DRUG: Additive side effects with **CNS depressants.** Increases **levodopa** concentration. **Estrogens** reduce ropinirole clearance. **Ciprofloxacin** increases ropinirole concentration. **Cimetidine, diltiazem, enoxacin, erythromycin, fluvoxamine, mexiletine, norfloxacin, tacrine** alter ropinirole's concentration. **Phenothiazines, butyrophenones, thioxanthenes, metoclopramide** diminish effectiveness of ropinirole. **HERBAL:** None known. **FOOD:** Time to maximum plasma levels is increased by 2.5 hrs when taken with food (extent of absorption not affected). Food may decrease the occurrence of nausea. **LAB VALUES:** May increase alkaline phosphatase.

AVAILABILITY (Rx)

TABLETS: 0.25 mg, 0.5 mg, 1 mg, 2 mg, 4 mg, 5 mg.

ADMINISTRATION/HANDLING

PO

• Ascending-dose schedule should increase very gradually at weekly intervals: **Week 1:** 0.25 mg 3 times/day to total daily dose 0.75 mg. **Week 2:** 0.5 mg 3 times/day to total daily dose 1.5 mg. **Week 3:** 0.75 mg 3 times/day to total daily dose 2.25 mg. **Week 4:** 1 mg 3 times/day to total daily dose 3 mg. • Discontinue medication gradually at 7-day intervals. Decrease frequency from 3 times/day to 2 times/day for 4 days.

For the remaining 3 days, decrease frequency to once daily prior to complete withdrawal.

INDICATIONS/ROUTES/DOSAGE

PARKINSON'S DISEASE

PO: ADULTS, ELDERLY: Initially, 0.25 mg 3 times/day. Do not increase dosage more frequently than q7days. After week 4, daily dosage may be increased, if needed, by 1.5–3 mg/day per week to total daily dose of 24 mg/day.

SIDE EFFECTS

FREQUENT (40%–60%): Nausea, dizziness, excessive drowsiness. **OCCASIONAL (5%–12%):** Syncope, vomiting, fatigue, viral infection, dyspepsia, diaphoresis, weakness, orthostatic hypotension, abdominal discomfort, pharyngitis, abnormal vision, dry mouth, hypertension, hallucinations, confusion. **RARE (≤4%):** Anorexia, peripheral edema, memory loss, rhinitis, sinusitis, palpitations, impotence.

ADVERSE REACTIONS/ TOXIC EFFECTS

None known.

NURSING IMPLICATIONS

INTERVENTION/EVALUATION

Assess for clinical improvement, clinical reversal of symptoms (improvement of tremor of head/hands at rest, masklike facial expression, shuffling gait, muscular rigidity). Assist with ambulation if dizziness occurs.

PATIENT/FAMILY TEACHING

Drowsiness, dizziness may be an initial response to drug. Postural hypotension may occur more frequently during initial therapy. Instruct pt to rise from lying to sitting or sitting to standing position slowly to prevent risk of postural hypotension. Avoid tasks that require alertness, motor skills until response to drug is established. If nausea occurs, take medication with food. Inform pt that hallucinations may occur, more so in the elderly than in younger pts with Parkinson's disease.

rosiglitazone maleate

rose-ih-**glit**-ah-zone

(Avandia)

FIXED-COMBINATION(S)

Avandamet: rosiglitazone/metformin: 1 mg/500 mg; 2 mg/500 mg; 4 mg/500 mg; 2 mg/1 g; 4 mg/1 g.

◆CLASSIFICATION

CLINICAL: Antidiabetic (see p. 40C).

ACTION

Improves target-cell response to insulin without increasing pancreatic insulin secretion. Decreases hepatic glucose output, increases insulin-dependent glucose utilization in skeletal muscle. **Therapeutic Effect:** Lowers blood glucose concentration.

PHARMACOKINETICS

Rapidly absorbed. Protein binding: >99%. Metabolized in liver. Excreted primarily in urine with a lesser amount in feces. Not removed by hemodialysis. **Half-life:** 3–4 hrs.

USES

Adjunct to diet/exercise to lower blood glucose in those with type 2 non–insulin-dependent diabetes mellitus (NIDDM). Used as monotherapy or in combination with metformin or insulin to improve glycemic control.

PRECAUTIONS

CONTRAINDICATIONS: Diabetic ketoacidosis, type 1 diabetes mellitus, active liver disease, increased serum transami-

R

nase levels (SGPT [ALT] >2.5 times the normal serum level). **CAUTIONS:** Hepatic function impairment, CHF, edematous pts.

LIFESPAN CONSIDERATIONS: Pregnancy/lactation: Unknown if drug crosses placenta or is distributed in breast milk. Not recommended in pregnant or breast-feeding women. **Pregnancy Category C. Children:** Safety and efficacy not established. **Elderly:** No age-related precautions noted in the elderly.

INTERACTIONS

DRUG: None known. **HERBAL:** None known. **FOOD:** None known. **LAB VALUES:** May decrease Hgb, Hct, bilirubin, SGOT (AST), alkaline phosphatase. <1% of pts experience SGPT (ALT) values ≤3 times normal level.

AVAILABILITY (Rx)

TABLETS: 2 mg, 4 mg, 8 mg.

ADMINISTRATION/HANDLING

PO

- Give without regard to meals.

INDICATIONS/ROUTES/DOSAGE

DIABETES MELLITUS, COMBINATION THERAPY

PO: ADULTS, ELDERLY: Initially, 4 mg as a single daily dose or in divided doses twice daily. May increase to 8 mg/day after 12 wks of therapy if fasting glucose is not adequately controlled.

Monotherapy: Initially, 4 mg as single daily dose or in divided doses twice daily. May increase to 8 mg/day after 12 wks of therapy.

SIDE EFFECTS

FREQUENT (9%): Upper respiratory tract infection. **OCCASIONAL (2%–4%):** Headache, edema, back pain, fatigue, sinusitis, diarrhea.

ADVERSE REACTIONS/ TOXIC EFFECTS

None known.

NURSING IMPLICATIONS

BASELINE ASSESSMENT

Obtain liver enzyme levels prior to initiation of therapy and periodically thereafter. Ensure follow-up instruction if pt/family do not thoroughly understand diabetes management or glucose-testing technique.

INTERVENTION/EVALUATION

Monitor blood glucose, Hgb, liver function tests, esp. SGOT (AST), SGPT (ALT). Assess for hypoglycemia (cool/wet skin, tremors, dizziness, anxiety, headache, tachycardia, numbness in mouth, hunger, diplopia), hyperglycemia (polyuria, polyphagia, polydipsia, nausea, vomiting, dim vision, fatigue, deep/rapid breathing). Be alert to conditions that alter glucose requirements: fever, increased activity/stress, surgical procedures.

PATIENT/FAMILY TEACHING

Diabetes mellitus requires lifelong control. Prescribed diet, exercise are principal part of treatment; do not skip/delay meals. Wear medical alert identification. Continue to adhere to dietary instructions, a regular exercise program, regular testing of urine or blood glucose. When taking combination drug therapy with a sulfonylurea or insulin, have a source of glucose available to treat symptoms of low blood sugar.

R

rosuvastatin calcium

ross-uh-vah-**stah**-tin
(Crestor)

◆ **CLASSIFICATION**

PHARMACOTHERAPEUTIC: HMG-CoA reductase inhibitor. **CLINICAL:** Antihyperlipidemic.

ACTION

Interferes with cholesterol biosynthesis by inhibiting the conversion of the enzyme HMG-CoA to mevalonate, a precursor to cholesterol. **Therapeutic Effect:** Decreases LDL cholesterol, VLDL, plasma triglycerides; increases HDL concentration.

PHARMACOKINETICS

Protein binding: 88%. Minimal hepatic metabolism. Primarily eliminated in the feces. **Half-life:** 19 hrs (half-life increased with severe renal function).

USES

Adjunct to diet therapy to decrease elevated total and LDL cholesterol concentrations in pts with primary hypercholesterolemia (types IIa and IIb), lowers serum triglyceride levels, increases HDL.

PRECAUTIONS

CONTRAINDICATIONS: Pregnancy, breast-feeding, active liver disease, unexplained, persistent elevations of serum transaminase. **CAUTIONS:** Anticoagulant therapy, history of liver disease; substantial alcohol consumption; major surgery; severe acute infection; trauma; hypotension; severe metabolic, endocrine, electrolyte disorders; uncontrolled seizures.

LIFESPAN CONSIDERATIONS: Pregnancy/lactation: Contraindicated in pregnancy (suppression of cholesterol biosynthesis may cause fetal toxicity), lactation. Risk of serious adverse reactions in nursing infants. **Pregnancy Category X. Children:** Safety and efficacy not established. **Elderly:** No age-related precautions noted.

R

INTERACTIONS

DRUG: Increased risk of myopathy with **cyclosporine, gemfibrozil, niacin.** Concurrent use of **warfarin** enhances anticoagulant effect. Increases **norgestrel, ethinylestradiol** plasma concentrations. Reduces **erythromycin** plasma concentration. **HERBAL:** None known. **FOOD:** None known. **LAB VALUES:** May increase creatinine kinase, serum transaminase concentrations. M... produce urine protein, hematuria.

AVAILABILITY (Rx)

TABLETS: 5 mg, 10 mg, 20 mg, 40 mg.

ADMINISTRATION/HANDLING

PO

- Give without regard to meals. Usually administered in the evening.

INDICATIONS/ROUTES/DOSAGE

Alert: Prior to initiating therapy, pt should be on standard cholesterol-lowering diet for minimum of 3–6 mos. Continue diet throughout rosuvastatin therapy.

HYPERLIPIDEMIA, DYSLIPIDEMIA

PO: ADULTS, ELDERLY: 5–40 mg/day. Usual starting dosage is 10 mg/day, with adjustments based on lipid levels, monitored q2–4wks until desired level is achieved.

RENAL IMPAIRMENT

PO: ADULTS, ELDERLY: 5 mg/day; do not exceed 10 mg/day.

CONCURRENT CYCLOSPORINE USE

PO: ADULTS, ELDERLY: 5 mg/day.

CONCURRENT LIPID-LOWERING THERAPY

PO: ADULTS, ELDERLY: 10 mg/day.

SIDE EFFECTS

Generally well tolerated. Side effects usually mild and transient. **OCCASIONAL**

(3%–9%): Pharyngitis, headache, diarrhea, dyspepsia (heartburn, epigastric distress), nausea. **RARE (<3%):** Myalgia, asthenia (unusual fatigue, weakness), back pain.

ADVERSE REACTIONS/ TOXIC EFFECTS

Potential for lens opacities. Hypersensitivity reaction, hepatitis occurs rarely.

NURSING IMPLICATIONS

BASELINE ASSESSMENT

Question for possibility of pregnancy prior to initiating therapy (Pregnancy Category X). Assess baseline lab results: cholesterol, triglycerides, liver function tests.

INTERVENTION/EVALUATION

Monitor cholesterol, triglyceride lab results for therapeutic response. Monitor liver function tests. Determine pattern of bowel activity. Assess for headache, sore throat. Be alert for muscle aches/weakness.

PATIENT/FAMILY TEACHING

Use appropriate contraceptive measures (Pregnancy Category X). Periodic lab tests are essential part of therapy. Continue to follow diet (important part of treatment).

Roxanol

see morphine

salmeterol

sal-**met**-er-all
(Serevent Diskus)
Do not confuse with Serentil.

FIXED-COMBINATION(S)

Advair: salmeterol/fluticasone (a corticosteroid): 50 mcg/100 mcg; 50 mcg/250 mcg; 50 mcg/500 mcg.

CLASSIFICATION

PHARMACOTHERAPEUTIC: Sympathomimetic (adrenergic agonist). **CLINICAL:** Bronchodilator (see p. 65C).

ACTION

Stimulates $beta_2$-adrenergic receptors in the lungs resulting in relaxation of bronchial smooth muscle. **Therapeutic Effect:** Relieves bronchospasm, reducing airway resistance.

PHARMACOKINETICS

Onset	Peak	Duration
Inhalation		
10–20 min	3 hrs	12 hrs

Primarily acts in lung; low systemic absorption. Protein binding: 95%. Metabolized by hydroxylation. Primarily eliminated in feces. **Half-life:** 3–4 hrs.

USES

Maintenance of asthma; prevention of exercise-induced bronchospasm, bronchospasm in pts with reversible obstructive airway disease. Long-term maintenance treatment of bronchospasm associated with COPD, including emphysema, chronic bronchitis.

PRECAUTIONS

CONTRAINDICATIONS: History of hypersensitivity to sympathomimetics. **CAUTIONS:** Not for acute symptoms. May cause paradoxical bronchospasm. Pts with cardiovascular disorders (e.g., coronary insufficiency, arrhythmias, hypertension), seizure disorder, thyrotoxicosis.

LIFESPAN CONSIDERATIONS: Pregnancy/lactation: Unknown if excreted

S

in breast milk. **Pregnancy Category C. Children:** No age-related precautions in those >4 yrs. **Elderly:** Lower dosages may be needed due to increased sympathetic sensitivity (may be more susceptible to tachycardia or tremors).

INTERACTIONS

DRUG: May decrease effects of **beta-adrenergic blockers. HERBAL: Ma huang (ephedra)** may increase CNS stimulation. **FOOD:** None known. **LAB VALUES:** May decrease serum potassium levels.

AVAILABILITY (Rx)

AEROSOL POWDER: 50 mcg.

ADMINISTRATION/HANDLING

INHALATION

• Shake container well, exhale completely through mouth; place mouthpiece into mouth and close lips, holding inhaler upright. • Inhale deeply through mouth while fully depressing the top of canister. Hold breath as long as possible before exhaling slowly. • Wait 2 min before inhaling second dose (allows for deeper bronchial penetration). • Rinse mouth with water immediately after inhalation (prevents mouth/throat dryness).

INDICATIONS/ROUTES/DOSAGE

MAINTENANCE/PREVENTION ASTHMA

Inhalation: ADULTS, ELDERLY, CHILDREN >4 YRS: *Diskus:* 1 activation (50 mcg) q12h.

PREVENT EXERCISE-INDUCED BRONCHOSPASM

Inhalation: ADULTS, ELDERLY, CHILDREN >4 YRS: 1 inhalation at least 30 min prior to exercise.

COPD

Inhalation: ADULTS, ELDERLY: 1 inhalation q12h.

SIDE EFFECTS

FREQUENT (28%): Headache. **OCCASIONAL (≤3%–7%):** Cough, tremor, dizziness, vertigo, throat dryness/irritation, pharyngitis. **RARE (<3%):** Palpitations, tachycardia, shakiness, nausea, heartburn, GI distress, diarrhea.

ADVERSE REACTIONS/ TOXIC EFFECTS

May prolong QT interval (may lead to ventricular arrhythmias). May cause hypokalemia, hyperglycemia.

NURSING IMPLICATIONS

INTERVENTION/EVALUATION

Monitor rate, depth, rhythm, type of respiration; quality/rate of pulse, B/P. Assess lungs for wheezing, rales, rhonchi. Periodically evaluate potassium levels.

PATIENT/FAMILY TEACHING

Not for relief of acute episodes. Keep canister at room temperature (cold decreases effects). Do not stop medication or exceed recommended dosage. Notify physician promptly of chest pain, dizziness. Wait at least 1 full min prior to second inhalation. Administer dose 30–60 min prior to exercise when used to prevent exercise-induced bronchospasm. Avoid excessive use of caffeine derivatives: coffee, tea, colas, chocolate.

salsalate

sal-sah-late
(Disalcid, Mono-Gesic)

CLASSIFICATION

PHARMACOTHERAPEUTIC: Nonsteroidal anti-inflammatory. **CLINICAL:** Analgesic, anti-inflammatory.

ACTION

Inhibits prostaglandin synthesis. Reduces inflammatory response, intensity of pain stimulus reaching sensory nerve endings. **Therapeutic Effect:** Produces analgesic, anti-inflammatory response.

USES

Treatment of mild to moderate pain, inflammation, fever, acute and/or chronic rheumatoid arthritis, osteoarthritis.

PRECAUTIONS

CONTRAINDICATIONS: Bleeding disorders, hypersensitivity to salicylates, NSAIDs. **CAUTIONS:** Platelet or bleeding disorders, liver/renal impairment, history of gastric irritation, peptic ulcer, gastritis, asthma. **Pregnancy Category C.**

INTERACTIONS

DRUG: **Alcohol, NSAIDs** may increase risk of GI effects (e.g., ulceration). **Urinary alkalinizers, antacids** increase excretion. **Anticoagulants, heparin, thrombolytics** increase risk of bleeding. Large dose may increase effect of **insulin, oral hypoglycemics. Valproic acid, platelet aggregation inhibitors** may increase risk of bleeding. May increase toxicity of **methotrexate, zidovudine. Ototoxic medications, vancomycin** may increase ototoxicity. May decrease effect of **probenecid, sulfinpyrazone.** **HERBAL:** **Ginkgo biloba** may increase risk of bleeding. **FOOD:** None known. **LAB VALUES:** May alter SGOT (AST), SGPT (ALT), alkaline phosphatase, uric acid; prolong prothrombin time, bleeding time. May decrease cholesterol, potassium, T_3, T_4.

AVAILABILITY (Rx)

CAPSULES: 500 mg. **TABLETS:** 500 mg, 750 mg.

INDICATIONS/ROUTES/DOSAGE

RHEUMATOID ARTHRITIS, OSTEOARTHRITIS

PO: ADULTS, ELDERLY: Initially, 3 g/day in 2–3 divided doses. MAINTENANCE: 2–4 g/day.

SIDE EFFECTS

OCCASIONAL: Nausea, dyspepsia (heartburn, indigestion, epigastric pain).

ADVERSE REACTIONS/ TOXIC EFFECTS

Tinnitus may be the first sign that serum salicylic acid concentration is reaching/exceeding upper therapeutic range. May also produce vertigo, headache, confusion, drowsiness, diaphoresis, hyperventilation, vomiting, diarrhea. Severe overdosage may result in electrolyte imbalance, hyperthermia, dehydration, blood pH imbalance. Low incidence of GI bleeding, peptic ulcer.

NURSING IMPLICATIONS

BASELINE ASSESSMENT

Do not give to children/teenagers who have flu/chickenpox (increases risk of Reye's syndrome). Assess type, location, duration of pain, inflammation. Inspect appearance of affected joints for immobility, deformities, skin condition.

INTERVENTION/EVALUATION

Assess for evidence of nausea, dyspepsia. Evaluate for therapeutic response: relief of pain/stiffness/swelling, increase in joint mobility, reduced joint tenderness, improved grip strength.

PATIENT/FAMILY TEACHING

Avoid alcohol. Avoid use of aspirin-containing products. Use antacids or take with food to relieve stomach upset. Report ringing in ears, persistent GI pain.

saquinavir

sah-**quin**-ah-vir
(Fortovase, Invirase)
Do not confuse with Sinequan.

CLASSIFICATION

PHARMACOTHERAPEUTIC: Protease inhibitor. **CLINICAL:** Antiretroviral (see pp. 60C, 100C).

ACTION

Inhibits HIV protease, rendering the enzyme incapable of processing the polyprotein precursor to generate functional proteins in HIV-infected cells. **Therapeutic Effect:** Slows HIV replication, reducing progression of HIV infection.

PHARMACOKINETICS

Poorly absorbed following PO administration (high-calorie/high-fat meal increases absorption). Protein binding: 99%. Metabolized in liver to inactive metabolite. Primarily eliminated in feces. Unknown if removed by hemodialysis. **Half-life:** 13 hrs.

USES

Treatment of HIV infection in combination with other antiretroviral agents.

S

PRECAUTIONS

CONTRAINDICATIONS: Clinically significant hypersensitivity to drug. Concurrent use with midazolam, triazolam, ergot medications, simvastatin, lovastatin. **CAUTIONS:** Diabetes mellitus, liver impairment.

LIFESPAN CONSIDERATIONS: Pregnancy/lactation: Breast-feeding not recommended (possibility of HIV transmission). **Pregnancy Category B. Children:** Safety and efficacy not established. **Elderly:** Information not available.

INTERACTIONS

DRUG: Ketoconazole increases saquinavir concentration. **Rifampin, phenobarbital, phenytoin, dexamethasone, carbamazepine** may reduce saquinavir plasma concentration. May increase **calcium channel blocker, clindamycin, dapsone, quinidine, triazolam** plasma concentrations. **HERBAL: St. John's wort, garlic** may decrease concentration, effect. **FOOD: Grapefruit juice** may increase saquinavir concentrations. **LAB VALUES:** May elevate serum transaminase, lower glucose level, alter CPK.

AVAILABILITY (Rx)

CAPSULES (Invirase): 200 mg. **CAPSULES (gelatin) (Fortovase):** 200 mg.

ADMINISTRATION/HANDLING

PO

- Give within 2 hrs after a full meal (if taken without food in stomach, may result in no antiviral activity).

INDICATIONS/ROUTES/DOSAGE

HIV INFECTION (combination therapy)

PO: ADULTS, ELDERLY: *Fortovase:* 1,200 mg 3 times/day. *Saquinavir:* Three 200-mg capsules given 3 times daily within 2 hrs after a full meal. Do not give <600 mg/day (does not produce antiviral activity). *Recommended daily doses of ddC or AZT:* ddC 0.75 mg 3 times daily; AZT 200 mg 3 times daily.

SIDE EFFECTS

OCCASIONAL: Diarrhea, abdominal discomfort/pain, nausea, photosensitivity, buccal mucosa ulceration. **RARE:** Confusion, ataxia, weakness, headache, rash.

ADVERSE REACTIONS/ TOXIC EFFECTS

None known.

NURSING IMPLICATIONS

BASELINE ASSESSMENT

Obtain baseline laboratory testing, esp. liver function tests, prior to beginning saquinavir therapy and at periodic intervals during therapy. Offer emotional support. Obtain medication history.

INTERVENTION/EVALUATION

Monitor liver function tests, triglycerides, glucose, CD4 cell count, HIV RNA levels. Closely monitor for evidence of GI discomfort. Monitor stool frequency, consistency (watery, loose, soft). Inspect mouth for signs of mucosal ulceration. Monitor clinical chemistry tests for marked laboratory abnormalities. If serious or severe toxicities occur, interrupt therapy, contact physician.

PATIENT/FAMILY TEACHING

Report numbness, tingling, persistent abdominal pain, nausea, vomiting. Avoid exposure to sunlight, artificial light sources. Continue therapy for full length of treatment. Doses should be evenly spaced. Saquinavir is not a cure for HIV infection, nor does it reduce risk of transmission to others. Pts may continue to acquire illnesses associated with advanced HIV infection. Take within 2 hrs after a full meal. Avoid coadministration with grapefruit products.

sargramostim (granulocyte macrophage colony-stimulating factor; GM-CSF)

sar-gra-**moh**-stim
(Leukine)
Do not confuse with Leukeran.

CLASSIFICATION

PHARMACOTHERAPEUTIC: Colony-stimulating factor. **CLINICAL:** Hematopoietic, antineutropenic.

ACTION

Stimulates proliferation/differentiation of hematopoietic cells to activate mature granulocytes and macrophages. **Therapeutic Effect:** Assists bone marrow in making new WBCs; increases chemotactic, antifungal, antiparasitic activity. Increases cytoneoplastic cells, activates neutrophils to inhibit tumor cell growth.

PHARMACOKINETICS

Onset	Peak	Duration
Increase WBCs		
7–14 days	—	1 wk

Detected in serum within 5 min following subcutaneous administration. **Half-life:** IV: 1 hr; subcutaneous: 3 hrs.

USES

Accelerates myeloid recovery in pts with non-Hodgkin's lymphoma, acute lymphoblastic leukemia, Hodgkin's disease undergoing autologous bone marrow transplantation. Used in pts with allogenic or autologous bone marrow transplantation where engraftment is delayed or has failed. Shortens time of neutrophil recovery after induction chemotherapy in pts with AML. Mobilizes autologous peripheral blood progenitor cells (PBPCs) after induction of chemotherapy in pts >55 yrs with acute myelogenous leukemia; used in myeloid reconstitution after allogenic bone marrow transplantation. **Unlabeled:** Treatment of AIDS-related neutropenia; chronic, severe neutropenia; drug-induced neutropenia; myelodysplastic syndrome.

PRECAUTIONS

CONTRAINDICATIONS: Excessive leukemic myeloid blasts in bone marrow or

S

peripheral blood (>10%), known hypersensitivity to GM-CSF, yeast-derived products, any component of drug, 24 hrs before/after chemotherapy, 12 hrs before/after radiation therapy. **CAUTIONS:** Preexisting cardiac disease, hypoxia, preexisting fluid retention, pulmonary infiltrates, CHF, impaired renal/hepatic function.

LIFESPAN CONSIDERATIONS: Pregnancy/lactation: Unknown if drug crosses placenta or is distributed in breast milk. **Pregnancy Category C. Children:** Safety and efficacy not established. **Elderly:** No age-related precautions noted.

INTERACTIONS

DRUG: Lithium, steroids may increase effect. **HERBAL:** None known. **FOOD:** None known. **LAB VALUES:** May decrease albumin. May increase bilirubin, creatinine, liver enzymes.

AVAILABILITY (Rx)

POWDER FOR INJECTION: 250 mcg, 500 mcg. **LIQUID FOR INJECTION:** 500 mcg/ml.

ADMINISTRATION/HANDLING

IV

Storage • Refrigerate powder, reconstituted solution, diluted solution for injection. Do not shake. Do not use past expiration date. • Reconstituted solutions are clear, colorless. • Use within 6 hrs; discard unused portions. Use 1 dose/vial; do not reenter vial.

Reconstitution • To 250 mcg/500 mcg vial, add 1 ml Sterile Water for Injection (preservative free). • Direct Sterile Water for Injection to side of vial, gently swirl contents to avoid foaming; do not shake/vigorously agitate. • After reconstitution, further dilute with 0.9% NaCl. If final concentration <10 mcg/ml, add 1 mg albumin/ml 0.9% NaCl to provide a final albumin concentration of 0.1%.

Alert: Albumin is added before addition of sargramostim (prevents drug adsorption to components of drug delivery system).

Rate of administration • Give each single dose over 2, 4, or 24 hrs as directed by physician.

IV INCOMPATIBILITIES

Amphotericin B complex (Abelcet, AmBisome, Amphotec), hydromorphone (Dilaudid), lorazepam (Ativan), morphine.

IV COMPATIBILITIES

Calcium gluconate, dopamine (Intropin), heparin, magnesium, potassium chloride.

INDICATIONS/ROUTES/DOSAGE

USUAL PARENTERAL DOSAGE

IV infusion: ADULTS, ELDERLY: 250 mcg/m^2/day for 21 days (as a 2-hr infusion). Begin 2–4 hrs after autologous bone marrow infusion and not less than 24 hrs after last dose of chemotherapy or not less than 12 hrs after last radiation treatment. Discontinue if blast cells appear or underlying disease progresses.

BONE MARROW TRANSPLANTATION FAILURE/ENGRAFTMENT DELAY

IV infusion: ADULTS, ELDERLY: 250 mcg/m^2/day for 14 days. Infuse over 2 hrs. May repeat after 7 days of therapy if engraftment has not occurred with 500 mcg/m^2/day for 14 days.

MOBILIZATION OR POST PBPC TRANSPLANT

IV/subcutaneous: ADULTS: 250 mcg/m^2/day.

ALLOGENIC TRANSPLANTATION

IV infusion: ADULTS: 250 mcg/m^2/day for 21 days starting 2–4 hrs after bone marrow infusion and not less than 24 hrs after last chemotherapy dose or 12 hrs after last radiation dose.

APLASTIC ANEMIA
IV/subcutaneous: ADULTS, ELDERLY: 15–480 mcg/m²/day.

CANCER CHEMOTHERAPY RECOVERY
IV/subcutaneous: 3–15 mcg/kg/day for 10 days.

SIDE EFFECTS

FREQUENT: GI disturbances (nausea, diarrhea, vomiting, stomatitis, anorexia, abdominal pain), arthralgia/myalgia, headache, malaise, rash, pruritus. **OCCASIONAL:** Peripheral edema, weight gain, dyspnea, asthenia (loss of strength), fever, leukocytosis, capillary leak syndrome (e.g., fluid retention, irritation at local injection site, peripheral edema). **RARE:** Rapid/irregular heartbeat, thrombophlebitis.

ADVERSE REACTIONS/ TOXIC EFFECTS

Pleural/pericardial effusion occurs rarely after infusion.

NURSING IMPLICATIONS

BASELINE ASSESSMENT

Monitor for supraventricular arrhythmias during administration (particularly in pts with history of cardiac arrhythmias). Assess closely for dyspnea during and immediately following infusion (particularly in pts with history of lung disease). If dyspnea occurs during infusion, cut infusion rate by half. If dyspnea continues, stop infusion immediately. If neutrophil count exceeds 20,000 cells/mm³ or platelet count exceeds 500,000/mm³, stop infusion or reduce dose by half, based on clinical condition of pt. Blood counts return to normal or baseline 3–7 days after discontinuation of therapy.

INTERVENTION/EVALUATION

Monitor CBC with differential, platelets, renal/liver function, pulmonary function, vital signs, weight.

saw palmetto

Also known as American dwarf palm tree, cabbage palm, sabal, zu-zhong

CLASSIFICATION

HERBAL.

ACTION

Appears to inhibit 5-alpha-reductase and prevent conversion of testosterone to dihydrotestosterone (DHT). **Effect:** Reduces prostate growth. Contains antiandrogenic, antiproliferative, anti-inflammatory properties.

USES

Symptoms of benign prostate hyperplasia (BPH). Also used as a mild diuretic, sedative, anti-inflammatory agent, antiseptic.

PRECAUTIONS

CONTRAINDICATIONS: Pregnancy, lactation due to antiandrogenic and estrogenic activity. **CAUTIONS:** None known.

LIFESPAN CONSIDERATIONS: Pregnancy/lactation: Contraindicated. **Children:** Safety and efficacy not established. **Elderly:** No age-related precautions noted.

INTERACTIONS

DRUG: May interfere with **oral contraceptives, hormone therapy.** **HERBAL:** None known. **FOOD:** None known. **LAB VALUES:** None known.

AVAILABILITY (OTC)

CAPSULES: 80 mg, 160 mg, 500 mg. **BERRIES. FLUID EXTRACT. TEA.**

INDICATIONS/ROUTES/DOSAGE

BPH
PO: ADULTS, ELDERLY: 160 mg 2 times/day or 320 mg once/day.

S

SIDE EFFECTS

Mild anorexia, dizziness, nausea, vomiting, constipation, diarrhea, headache, impotence, hypersensitivity reactions, back pain.

ADVERSE REACTIONS/ TOXIC EFFECTS

None known.

NURSING IMPLICATIONS

BASELINE ASSESSMENT

Determine use of oral contraceptives, hormone replacement therapy (may interfere). Assess pt's urinary patterns.

INTERVENTION/EVALUATION

Assess for hypersensitivity reactions. Monitor symptoms of BHP (e.g., frequent/painful urination, hesitancy, urgency). Observe for decreased nocturia, improved urinary flow, decreased residual urine volume.

PATIENT/FAMILY TEACHING

Should be taken with food. Obtain a prostate-specific antigen (PSA) level before using.

scopolamine

sko-**poll**-ah-meen
(Trans-Derm Scop, Transderm-V)

CLASSIFICATION

PHARMACOTHERAPEUTIC: Anticholinergic. **CLINICAL:** Antinausea, antiemetic.

ACTION

Reduces excitability of labyrinthine receptors, depressing conduction in vestibular cerebellar pathway. **Therapeutic Effect:** Prevents nausea/vomiting induced by motion.

USES

Prevention of motion sickness.

PRECAUTIONS

CONTRAINDICATIONS: Narrow-angle glaucoma, GI/GU obstruction, thyrotoxicosis, tachycardia, paralytic ileus, myasthenia gravis. **CAUTIONS:** Liver/renal impairment, cardiac disease, seizures, psychoses. **Pregnancy Category C.**

INTERACTIONS

DRUG: **CNS depressants** may increase CNS depression. **Antihistamines, tricyclic antidepressants** may increase anticholinergic effects. **HERBAL:** None known. **FOOD:** None known. **LAB VALUES:** May interfere with gastric secretion test.

AVAILABILITY (Rx)

TRANSDERMAL SYSTEM: 1.5 mg.

ADMINISTRATION/HANDLING

TRANSDERMAL

• Apply patch to hairless area behind one ear. • If dislodged or on >72 hrs, replace with fresh patch.

INDICATIONS/ROUTES/DOSAGE

PREVENTION OF MOTION SICKNESS

Transdermal: ADULTS: 1 system q72h.

SIDE EFFECTS

FREQUENT (>15%): Dry mouth, drowsiness, blurred vision. **RARE (1%–5%):** Dizziness, restlessness, hallucinations, confusion, difficulty urinating, rash.

ADVERSE REACTION/TOXIC EFFECTS

None known.

NURSING IMPLICATIONS

BASELINE ASSESSMENT

Assess for use of other CNS depressants, drugs with anticholinergic action, history of narrow-angle glaucoma.

INTERVENTION/EVALUATION

Monitor liver/renal function.

PATIENT/FAMILY TEACHING

Avoid tasks requiring alertness, motor skills until response to drug is established (may cause drowsiness, disorientation, confusion). Teach proper application of patch. Use only 1 patch at a time; do not cut. Wash hands after administration.

secobarbital sodium

(Seconal)

See Classification section under: Sedative-hypnotics

selegiline hydrochloride

sell-**eh**-geh-leen

(Eldepryl, Novo-Selegiline ✤)

Do not confuse with enalapril, Stelazine.

CLASSIFICATION

CLINICAL: Antiparkinson agent.

ACTION

Irreversibly inhibits MAO type B activity. Increases dopaminergic action. **Therapeutic Effect:** Assists in reduction of tremor, akinesia (absence of sense of movement), posture/equilibrium disorders, rigidity of parkinsonism.

PHARMACOKINETICS

Rapidly absorbed from GI tract. Crosses blood-brain barrier. Metabolized in liver to active metabolites. Primarily excreted in urine. **Half-life:** amphetamine: 17 hrs; methamphetamine: 20 hrs.

USES

Adjunct to levodopa/carbidopa in treatment of Parkinson's disease.

PRECAUTIONS

CONTRAINDICATIONS: None known. **CAUTIONS:** History of peptic ulcer disease, dementia, psychosis, tardive dyskinesia, profound tremor, cardiac dysrhythmias.

LIFESPAN CONSIDERATIONS: Pregnancy/lactation: Unknown if drug crosses placenta or is distributed in breast milk. **Pregnancy Category C. Children:** Safety and efficacy not established. **Elderly:** No age-related precautions noted.

INTERACTIONS

DRUG: Fluoxetine may cause mania, serotonin syndrome (mental changes, restlessness, diaphoresis, diarrhea, fever). **Meperidine** may cause a potentially fatal reaction (e.g., excitation, diaphoresis, rigidity, hypertension/hypotension, coma, death). **HERBAL:** None known. **FOOD: Tyramine-rich foods** may produce hypertensive reactions. **LAB VALUES:** None known.

AVAILABILITY (Rx)

CAPSULES: 5 mg. **TABLETS:** 5 mg.

ADMINISTRATION/HANDLING

PO

- Give without meals.

INDICATIONS/ROUTES/DOSAGE

Alert: Therapy should begin with lowest dosage, then increase in gradual increments over 3–4 wks.

PARKINSONISM

PO: ADULTS: 10 mg/day in divided doses (5 mg at breakfast and lunch). EL-

DERLY: Initially, 5 mg in morning. May increase up to 10 mg/day.

SIDE EFFECTS

FREQUENT (4%–10%): Nausea, dizziness, lightheadedness, faintness, abdominal discomfort. **OCCASIONAL (2%–3%):** Confusion, hallucinations, dry mouth, vivid dreams, dyskinesia (impairment of voluntary movement). **RARE (1%):** Headache, generalized aches, anxiety, diarrhea, insomnia.

ADVERSE REACTIONS/ TOXIC EFFECTS

Overdosage may vary from CNS depression (sedation, apnea, cardiovascular collapse, death) to severe paradoxical reaction (hallucinations, tremor, seizures). Impaired motor coordination (loss of balance, blepharospasm [blinking], facial grimace, feeling of heavy leg/stiff neck, involuntary movements), hallucinations, confusion, depression, nightmares, delusions, overstimulation, sleep disturbance, anger occurs in some pts.

NURSING IMPLICATIONS

INTERVENTION/EVALUATION

Be alert to neurologic effects (headache, lethargy, mental confusion, agitation). Monitor for evidence of dyskinesia (difficulty with movement). Assess for clinical reversal of symptoms (improvement of tremor of head/hands at rest, masklike facial expression, shuffling gait, muscular rigidity).

PATIENT/FAMILY TEACHING

Tolerance to feeling of lightheadedness develops during therapy. To reduce hypotensive effect, rise slowly from lying to sitting position, permit legs to dangle momentarily before standing. Avoid tasks that require alertness, motor skills until response to drug is established. Dry mouth, drowsiness, dizziness may be an expected response of drug. Avoid alcohol during therapy. Coffee/tea may help reduce drowsiness.

senna

sen-ah
(Senokot, Senolax)

FIXED-COMBINATION(S)

Gentlax-S, Senokot-S: senna/docusate (a laxative) 8.6 mg/50 mg.

CLASSIFICATION

PHARMACOTHERAPEUTIC: GI stimulant. **CLINICAL:** Laxative (see p. 105C).

ACTION

Direct effect on intestinal smooth musculature (stimulates intramural nerve plexi). **Therapeutic Effect:** Increases peristalsis, promotes laxative effect.

PHARMACOKINETICS

	Onset	Peak	Duration
PO	6–12 hrs	—	—
Rectal	0.5–2 hrs	—	—

Minimal absorption following PO administration. Hydrolyzed to active form by enzymes of colonic flora. Absorbed drug metabolized in liver; eliminated in feces via biliary system.

USES

Short-term use in constipation, to evacuate the colon prior to bowel/rectal examinations.

PRECAUTIONS

CONTRAINDICATIONS: Abdominal pain, nausea, vomiting, appendicitis, intestinal obstruction. **CAUTIONS:** Prolonged use (>1 wk).

S

LIFESPAN CONSIDERATIONS: Pregnancy/lactation: Unknown if distributed in breast milk. **Pregnancy Category C. Children:** Safety and efficacy not established in those <6 yrs. **Elderly:** No age-related precautions noted; monitor for signs of dehydration/electrolyte loss.

INTERACTIONS

DRUG: May decrease transit time of concurrently administered **oral medication,** decreasing absorption. **HERBAL:** None known. **FOOD:** None known. **LAB VALUES:** May increase glucose, may decrease potassium.

AVAILABILITY (OTC)

GRANULES: 15 mg/3 g. **LIQUID:** 25 mg/15 ml, 33.3 mg/ml. **SYRUP:** 8.8 mg/5 ml. **TABLETS:** 8.6 mg. **TABLETS (chewable):** 10 mg, 15 mg.

ADMINISTRATION/HANDLING

PO

• Give on an empty stomach (faster results). • Offer at least 6–8 glasses of water/day (aids stool softening). • Avoid giving within 1 hr of other oral medication (decreases drug absorption).

INDICATIONS/ROUTES/DOSAGE

CONSTIPATION:

Tablets: ADULTS, ELDERLY, CHILDREN >12 YRS: 2 at bedtime up to 4 tablets 2 times/day. CHILDREN 6–12 YRS: 1 at bedtime up to 2 tablets 2 times/day. CHILDREN 2–<6 YRS: ½ tablet at bedtime up to 1 tablet 2 times/day.

Syrup: ADULTS, ELDERLY, CHILDREN >12 YRS: 10–15 ml at bedtime up to 15 ml 2 times/day. CHILDREN 6–12 YRS: 5–7.5 ml at bedtime up to 7.5 ml 2 times/day. CHILDREN 2–<6 YRS: 2.5–3.75 ml at bedtime up to 3.75 ml 2 times/day.

Granules: ADULTS, ELDERLY, CHILDREN >12 YRS: 1 tsp at bedtime up to 2 tsp 2 times/day. CHILDREN 6–12 YRS: ½ tsp at bedtime up to 1 tsp 2 times/day. CHILDREN 2–<6 YRS: ¼ tsp at bedtime up to ½ tsp 2 times/day.

SIDE EFFECTS

FREQUENT: Pink-red, red-violet, red-brown, yellow-brown discoloration of urine. **OCCASIONAL:** Some degree of abdominal discomfort, nausea, mild cramps, griping, faintness.

ADVERSE REACTIONS/ TOXIC EFFECTS

Long-term use may result in laxative dependence, chronic constipation, loss of normal bowel function. Chronic use/overdosage may result in electrolyte disturbances (hypokalemia, hypocalcemia, metabolic acidosis/alkalosis), persistent diarrhea, malabsorption, weight loss. Electrolyte disturbance may produce vomiting, muscle weakness.

NURSING IMPLICATIONS

INTERVENTION/EVALUATION

Encourage adequate fluid intake. Assess bowel sounds for peristalsis. Monitor stool frequency, consistency (watery, loose, soft, semisolid, solid). Assess for GI disturbances. Monitor serum electrolytes in pts exposed to prolonged, frequent, excessive use of medication.

PATIENT/FAMILY TEACHING

Urine may turn pink-red, red-violet, red-brown, yellow-brown (only temporary and not harmful). Institute measures to promote defecation (increase fluid intake, exercise, high-fiber diet). Laxative effect generally occurs in 6–12 hrs but may take 24 hrs. Suppository produces evacuation in 30 min–2 hrs. Do not take other oral medication within 1 hr of taking this medicine (decreased effectiveness).

S

Septra

see co-trimoxazole

sertraline hydrochloride

sir-trah-leen
(Zoloft)
Do not confuse with Serentil.

CLASSIFICATION

PHARMACOTHERAPEUTIC: Serotonin reuptake inhibitor. **CLINICAL:** Antidepressant, antipanic, obsessive-compulsive adjunct (see p. 36C).

ACTION

Blocks reuptake of the neurotransmitter serotonin at CNS neuronal presynaptic membranes, increasing availability at postsynaptic receptor sites. **Therapeutic Effect:** Produces antidepressant effect, reduces obsessive-compulsive behavior, decreases anxiety.

PHARMACOKINETICS

Incompletely, slowly absorbed from GI tract (food increases absorption). Protein binding: 98%. Widely distributed. Undergoes extensive first-pass metabolism in liver to active compound. Excreted in urine, eliminated in feces. Not removed by hemodialysis. **Half-life:** 26 hrs.

USES

Treatment of major depressive disorders, panic disorder, obsessive-compulsive disorder (OCD), post-traumatic stress disorder, premenstrual dysphoric disorder (PMDD), social anxiety disorder.

PRECAUTIONS

CONTRAINDICATIONS: During or within 14 days of MAOI antidepressant therapy. **CAUTIONS:** Seizure disorders, cardiac disease, recent MI, liver impairment, suicidal pts.

LIFESPAN CONSIDERATIONS: Pregnancy/lactation: Unknown if drug crosses placenta or is distributed in breast milk. **Pregnancy Category B. Children:** No age-related precautions in those >6 yrs. **Elderly:** No age-related precautions noted, but lower initial dosages recommended.

INTERACTIONS

DRUG: May increase concentration, toxicity of **highly protein-bound medications (e.g., digoxin, warfarin). MAOIs** may cause serotonin syndrome (mental changes, restlessness, diaphoresis, shivering, diarrhea, fever), confusion, agitation, hyperpyretic convulsions. **HERBAL: St. John's wort** may increase risk of adverse effects. **FOOD:** None known. **LAB VALUES:** May increase SGOT (AST), SGPT (ALT), total cholesterol, triglycerides. May decrease uric acid.

AVAILABILITY (Rx)

TABLETS: 25 mg, 50 mg, 100 mg. **ORAL CONCENTRATE:** 20 mg/ml.

ADMINISTRATION/HANDLING

PO

• Give with food, milk if GI distress occurs.

INDICATIONS/ROUTES/DOSAGE

ANTIDEPRESSANT, OCD

PO: ADULTS, CHILDREN 13–17 YRS: Initially, 50 mg/day with morning or evening meal. May increase by 50 mg/day at 7-day intervals. ELDERLY, CHILDREN 6–12

YRS: Initially, 25 mg/day. May increase by 25–50 mg/day at 7-day intervals. **Maximum:** 200 mg/day.

PANIC DISORDER, POST-TRAUMATIC STRESS DISORDER, SOCIAL ANXIETY DISORDER

PO: ADULTS, ELDERLY: Initially, 25 mg/day. May increase by 50 mg/day at 7-day intervals. RANGE: 50–200 mg/day. **Maximum:** 200 mg/day.

PMDD

PO: ADULTS: Initially, 50 mg/day. May increase up to 150 mg/day in 50-mg increments.

SIDE EFFECTS

FREQUENT (12%–26%): Headache, nausea, diarrhea, insomnia, drowsiness, dizziness, fatigue, rash, dry mouth. **OCCASIONAL (4%–6%):** Anxiety, nervousness, agitation, tremor, dyspepsia, diaphoresis, vomiting, constipation, abnormal ejaculation, change in vision, change in taste. **RARE (<3%):** Flatulence, urinary frequency, paresthesia, hot flashes, chills.

ADVERSE REACTIONS/ TOXIC EFFECTS

None known.

NURSING IMPLICATIONS

BASELINE ASSESSMENT

For those on long-term therapy, liver/renal function tests, blood counts should be performed periodically.

INTERVENTION/EVALUATION

Supervise suicidal-risk pt closely during early therapy (as depression lessens, energy level improves, increasing suicide potential). Assess appearance, behavior, speech pattern, level of interest, mood. Monitor pattern of daily bowel activity, stool consistency. Assist with ambulation if dizziness occurs.

PATIENT/FAMILY TEACHING

Dry mouth may be relieved by sugarless gum, sips of tepid water. Report headache, fatigue, tremor, sexual dysfunction. Avoid tasks that require alertness, motor skills until response to drug is established. Take with food if nausea occurs. Inform physician if pregnancy occurs. Avoid alcohol. Do not take OTC medications without consulting physician.

sevelamer hydrochloride

seh-**vell**-ah-mur

(Renagel)

Do not confuse with Reglan, Regonol.

◆CLASSIFICATION

PHARMACOTHERAPEUTIC: Polymeric phosphate binder. **CLINICAL:** Antihyperphosphatemia.

ACTION

Binds/removes dietary phosphorus in GI tract and eliminates phosphorus through normal digestive process. **Therapeutic Effect:** Decreases incidence of hypercalcemic episodes in pts receiving calcium acetate treatment.

PHARMACOKINETICS

Not absorbed systemically. Unknown if removed by hemodialysis.

USES

Reduction of serum phosphorus in pts with end-stage renal disease (ESRD).

PRECAUTIONS

CONTRAINDICATIONS: Bowel obstruction, hypophosphatemia. **CAUTIONS:** Dysphagia, severe GI tract motility disorders, major GI tract surgery, swallowing disorders.

LIFESPAN CONSIDERATIONS: Pregnancy/lactation: Not distributed in breast milk. **Pregnancy Category C. Children:** Safety and efficacy not established. **Elderly:** No age-related precautions noted.

INTERACTIONS

DRUG: None known. **HERBAL:** None known. **FOOD:** None known. **LAB VALUES:** None known.

AVAILABILITY (Rx)

CAPSULES: 403 mg. **TABLETS:** 400 mg, 800 mg.

ADMINISTRATION/HANDLING

PO

• Give with meals. • Do not break capsule apart before administration (contents expand in water). • Space other medication by ≥1 hr before or 3 hrs after sevelamer.

INDICATIONS/ROUTES/DOSAGE

HYPERPHOSPHATEMIA

PO: ADULTS, ELDERLY: 800–1,600 mg with each meal depending on severity of hyperphosphatemia.

SIDE EFFECTS

FREQUENT (11%–20%): Infection, pain, hypotension, diarrhea, dyspepsia, nausea, vomiting. **OCCASIONAL (1%–10%):** Headache, constipation, hypertension, thrombosis, increased coughing.

ADVERSE REACTIONS/ TOXIC EFFECTS

None known.

NURSING IMPLICATIONS

BASELINE ASSESSMENT

Obtain baseline serum phosphorus level; assess for any bowel obstruction.

INTERVENTION/EVALUATION

Monitor serum phosphorus, bicarbonate, chloride, calcium levels.

PATIENT/FAMILY TEACHING

Take with meals, swallow whole. Report persistent headache, nausea, vomiting, diarrhea, hypotension.

sibutramine

sigh-**bew**-trah-meen

(Meridia)

See Classification section under: Obesity management (p. 119C)

sildenafil citrate

sill-**den**-ah-fill

(Viagra)

Do not confuse with Vaniqa.

CLASSIFICATION

CLINICAL: Erectile dysfunction adjunct.

ACTION

Inhibits type V cyclic GMP, a specific phosphodiesterase, the predominant isoenzyme in human corpus cavernosum in the penis. **Therapeutic Effect:** Relaxes smooth muscle, increases blood flow, facilitating an erection.

USES

Treatment of male erectile dysfunction. **Unlabeled:** Treatment of sexual dysfunction from SSRI (antidepressants), diabetic gastroparesis.

PRECAUTIONS

CONTRAINDICATIONS: Pts concurrently using sodium nitroprusside or organic nitrates in any form. **CAUTIONS:** Renal, cardiac, hepatic function impairment; anatomic deformation of the penis; pts who may be predisposed to priapism (sickle cell anemia, multiple myeloma, leukemia). **Pregnancy Category B.**

INTERACTIONS

DRUG: **Cimetidine, erythromycin, itraconazole, ketoconazole** may increase sildenafil plasma concentration. Potentiates hypotensive effects of **nitrates.** **HERBAL:** None known. **FOOD:** Rate of absorption is reduced and time to maximum effectiveness is delayed by 1 hr when taken with a high-fat meal. **LAB VALUES:** None known.

AVAILABILITY (Rx)

TABLETS: 25 mg, 50 mg, 100 mg.

ADMINISTRATION/HANDLING

PO

- May take approx. 1 hr before sexual activity but may be taken anywhere from 4 hrs–30 min before sexual activity.

INDICATIONS/ROUTES/DOSAGE

ERECTILE DYSFUNCTION

PO: ADULTS: 50 mg (½–4 hrs before sexual activity). RANGE: 25–100 mg.

SIDE EFFECTS

OCCASIONAL: Headache, flushing (10%–16%); dyspepsia (heartburn, indigestion, epigastric pain), nasal congestion, urinary tract infection, abnormal vision, diarrhea (3%–7%). **RARE (2%):** Dizziness, rash.

ADVERSE REACTIONS/ TOXIC EFFECTS

None known.

NURSING IMPLICATIONS

BASELINE ASSESSMENT

Assess cardiovascular status before initiating treatment for erectile dysfunction.

PATIENT/FAMILY TEACHING

Sildenafil has no effect in the absence of sexual stimulation.

silver sulfadiazine

sul-fah-**dye**-ah-zeen
(Demazin ✤, Flamazine ✤, Silvadene, SSD, Thermazene)

◆CLASSIFICATION

PHARMACOTHERAPEUTIC: Anti-infective. **CLINICAL:** Burn preparation.

ACTION

Acts on cell wall/cell membrane in concentrations selectively toxic to bacteria. **Therapeutic Effect:** Produces bactericidal effect.

USES

Prevention, treatment of infection in second- and third-degree burns; protection against conversion from partial- to full-thickness wounds (infection causes extended tissue destruction). **Unlabeled:** Treatment of minor bacterial skin infection, dermal ulcer.

PRECAUTIONS

CONTRAINDICATIONS: None known. **CAUTIONS:** Impaired renal/hepatic function, G6PD deficiency, premature neonates, infants <2 mos. **Pregnancy Category B.**

INTERACTIONS

DRUG: **Collagenase, papain, sutilains** may be inactivated. **HERBAL:**

S

None known. **FOOD:** None known. **LAB VALUES:** None known.

AVAILABILITY (Rx)

CREAM: 10 mg/g.

ADMINISTRATION/HANDLING

TOPICAL

• Apply to cleansed, debrided burns using sterile glove. • Keep burn areas covered with silver sulfadiazine cream at all times; reapply to areas where removed by pt activity. • Dressings may be ordered on individual basis.

INDICATIONS/ROUTES/DOSAGE

USUAL TOPICAL DOSAGE

Topical: ADULTS, ELDERLY, CHILDREN: Apply 1–2 times/day.

SIDE EFFECTS

Side effects characteristic of all sulfonamides may occur when systemically absorbed, (e.g., extensive burn areas [>20% of body surface]): anorexia, nausea, vomiting, headache, diarrhea, dizziness, photosensitivity, joint pain. **FREQUENT:** Burning feeling at treatment site. **OCCASIONAL:** Brown-gray skin discoloration, rash, itching. **RARE:** Increased sensitivity of skin to sunlight.

ADVERSE REACTIONS/ TOXIC EFFECTS

Hemolytic anemia, hypoglycemia, diuresis, peripheral neuropathy, Stevens-Johnson syndrome, agranulocytosis, disseminated lupus erythematosus, anaphylaxis, hepatitis, toxic nephrosis possible with significant systemic absorption. Fungal superinfections may occur. Interstitial nephritis occurs rarely.

NURSING IMPLICATIONS

BASELINE ASSESSMENT

Determine initial CBC, renal/hepatic function test results.

INTERVENTION/EVALUATION

Monitor electrolytes, urinalysis, renal function, CBC if burns are extensive, therapy prolonged.

PATIENT/FAMILY TEACHING

For external use only; may discolor skin.

simethicone

sye-**meth**-ih-cone

(Alka-Seltzer Gas Relief, Gas-X, Genasym, Maalox AntiGas, Mylanta Gas, Ovol, Phazyme)

FIXED-COMBINATION(S)

Mylanta, Extra Strength Maalox, Aludrox: simethicone/magnesium and aluminum hydroxide (antacids): 20 mg/200 mg/200 mg; 40 mg/400 mg/400 mg.

CLASSIFICATION

CLINICAL: Antiflatulent.

ACTION

Changes surface tension of gas bubbles, allowing easier elimination of gas. **Therapeutic Effect:** Disperses, prevents formation of gas pockets in GI tract.

PHARMACOKINETICS

Does not appear to be absorbed from GI tract. Excreted unchanged in feces.

USES

Treatment of flatulence, gastric bloating, postop gas pain, when gas retention may be problem (i.e., peptic ulcer, spastic colon, air swallowing). **Unlabeled:** Adjunct to gastroscopy, bowel radiography.

S

PRECAUTIONS

CONTRAINDICATIONS: None known. **CAUTIONS:** None known.

LIFESPAN CONSIDERATIONS: Pregnancy/lactation: Unknown if drug crosses placenta or is distributed in breast milk. **Pregnancy Category C. Children/elderly:** None known.

INTERACTIONS

DRUG: None known. **HERBAL:** None known. **FOOD:** None known. **LAB VALUES:** None known.

AVAILABILITY (OTC)

SOFTGEL: 125 mg, 180 mg. **ORAL SUSPENSION DROPS:** 40 mg/0.6 ml. **TABLETS (chewable):** 80 mg, 125 mg.

ADMINISTRATION/HANDLING

PO

- Give after meals and at bedtime as needed. Chewable tablets are to be chewed thoroughly before swallowing.
- Shake suspension well before using.

INDICATIONS/ROUTES/DOSAGE

ANTIFLATULENT

PO: ADULTS, ELDERLY, CHILDREN >12 YRS: 40–250 mg after meals and at bedtime. **Maximum:** 500 mg/day. CHILDREN 2–12 YRS: 40 mg 4 times/day. CHILDREN <2 YRS: 20 mg 4 times/day.

SIDE EFFECTS

None known.

ADVERSE REACTIONS/ TOXIC EFFECTS

None known.

NURSING IMPLICATIONS

INTERVENTION/EVALUATION

Evaluate for therapeutic response: relief of flatulence, abdominal bloating.

PATIENT/FAMILY TEACHING

Avoid carbonated beverages.

simvastatin

sim-vah-**stay**-tin

(Zocor)

Do not confuse with Cozaar.

CLASSIFICATION

PHARMACOTHERAPEUTIC: HMG-CoA reductase inhibitor. **CLINICAL:** Antihyperlipidemic (see p. 51C).

ACTION

Interferes with cholesterol biosynthesis by inhibiting the conversion of the enzyme HMG-CoA to mevalonate. **Therapeutic Effect:** Decreases LDL, cholesterol, VLDL, plasma triglycerides; slight increase in HDL concentration.

PHARMACOKINETICS

Onset	Peak	Duration
PO to reduce cholesterol		
>3 days	14 days	—

Well absorbed from GI tract. Protein binding: 95%. Undergoes extensive first-pass metabolism. Hydrolyzed to active metabolite. Primarily eliminated in feces. Unknown if removed by hemodialysis.

USES

Adjunct to diet therapy to decrease elevated total and LDL cholesterol concentrations in those with primary hypercholesterolemia (types IIa and IIb), lowers triglyceride levels, increases HDL. Reduces deaths, prevents heart attacks in pts with heart disease, high cholesterol. Decreases risk of mortality by decreasing coronary death, risk of nonfatal MI, need for myocardial revascularization procedures. Decreases risk for stroke/TIA.

PRECAUTIONS

CONTRAINDICATIONS: Pregnancy; active liver disease; and unexplained, persistent elevations of liver function tests, <18 yrs. **CAUTIONS:** History of liver disease, substantial alcohol consumption. Withholding/discontinuing simvastatin may be necessary when pt is at risk for renal failure secondary to rhabdomyolysis. Severe metabolic, endocrine, electrolyte disorders.

LIFESPAN CONSIDERATIONS: Pregnancy/lactation: Contraindicated in pregnancy (suppression of cholesterol biosynthesis may cause fetal toxicity), lactation. Risk of serious adverse reactions in nursing infants. **Pregnancy Category X. Children:** Safety and efficacy not established. **Elderly:** No age-related precautions noted.

INTERACTIONS

DRUG: Increased risk of rhabdomyolysis, acute renal failure with **cyclosporine, erythromycin, gemfibrozil, niacin, other immunosuppressants. Erythromycin, itraconazole, ketoconazole** may increase concentration; cause muscle pain, inflammation, or weakness. **HERBAL:** None known. **FOOD:** None known. **LAB VALUES:** May increase creatinine kinase, serum transaminase concentrations.

S

AVAILABILITY (Rx)

TABLETS: 5 mg, 10 mg, 20 mg, 40 mg, 80 mg.

ADMINISTRATION/HANDLING

PO

• Give without regard to meals. • Administer in evening.

INDICATIONS/ROUTES/DOSAGE

Alert: Prior to initiating therapy, pt should be on standard cholesterol-lowering diet for minimum of 3–6 mos. Continue diet throughout simvastatin therapy.

HYPERLIPIDEMIA/DECREASED MORTALITY

PO: ADULTS: Initially, 10–40 mg/day in evening. Dosage adjustment at 4-wk intervals. ELDERLY: Initially, 10 mg/day. May increase by 5–10 mg/day q4wks. RANGE: 5–80 mg/day. **Maximum:** 80 mg/day.

SIDE EFFECTS

Generally well tolerated. Side effects usually mild and transient. **OCCASIONAL (2%–3%):** Headache, abdominal pain/cramps, constipation, upper respiratory infection. **RARE (<2%):** Diarrhea, flatulence, asthenia (loss of strength, energy), nausea/vomiting.

ADVERSE REACTIONS/ TOXIC EFFECTS

Potential for lens opacities. Hypersensitivity reaction, hepatitis occurs rarely.

NURSING IMPLICATIONS

BASELINE ASSESSMENT

Question for possibility of pregnancy before initiating therapy (Pregnancy Category X). Question for history of hypersensitivity to simvastatin. Assess baseline lab results: cholesterol, triglycerides, liver function tests.

INTERVENTION/EVALUATION

Monitor cholesterol, triglyceride lab results for therapeutic response. Monitor liver function tests. Determine pattern of bowel activity. Assess for headache.

PATIENT/FAMILY TEACHING

Use appropriate contraceptive measures (Pregnancy Category X). Periodic lab tests are essential part of therapy.

Sinemet

see carbidopa-levodopa

Singulair

see montelukast

sirolimus

sigh-row-**lie**-mus
(Rapamune)

✦ CLASSIFICATION

CLINICAL: Immunosuppressant (see p. 102C).

ACTION

Inhibits T-lymphocyte proliferation induced by stimulation of cell surface receptors, mitogens, alloantigens, lymphokines. Prevents activation of enzyme TOR, a key regulatory kinase in cell cycle progression. **Therapeutic Effect:** Inhibits T- and B-cell proliferation (essential components of immune response).

USES

Prophylaxis of organ rejection in pts after renal transplant in combination with cyclosporine and corticosteroids.

PRECAUTIONS

CONTRAINDICATIONS: Hypersensitivity to sirolimus, current malignancy. **CAUTIONS:** Chickenpox, herpes zoster, impaired liver function, infection. **Pregnancy Category C.**

INTERACTIONS

DRUG: **Cyclosporine, diltiazem, ketoconazole** may increase concentration, toxicity. **Rifampin** may decrease concentration effect. **HERBAL:** None known. **FOOD:** **Grapefruit juice** may decrease metabolism. **LAB VALUES:** May decrease Hct, Hgb, platelets. May increase serum creatinine, cholesterol, triglycerides.

AVAILABILITY (Rx)

ORAL SOLUTION: 1 mg/ml. **TABLETS:** 1 mg, 2 mg.

INDICATIONS/ROUTES/DOSAGE

PROPHYLAXIS OF ORGAN REJECTION

PO: ADULTS: LOADING DOSE: 6 mg. MAINTENANCE: 2 mg/day. CHILDREN ≥13 YRS <40 KG: 3 mg/m^2 loading dose, then 1 mg/m^2/day.

SIDE EFFECTS

OCCASIONAL: Hypercholesterolemia, hyperlipidemia, hypertension, rash. **High dose (5 mg/day):** Anemia, arthralgia, diarrhea, hypokalemia, thrombocytopenia.

ADVERSE REACTIONS/ TOXIC EFFECTS

None known.

NURSING IMPLICATIONS

BASELINE ASSESSMENT

Obtain baseline hepatic profile. Assess for pregnancy, lactation. Question for medication usage (esp. cyclosporine, diltiazem, ketoconazole, rifampin). Determine if pt has chickenpox, herpes zoster, malignancy, infection.

INTERVENTION/EVALUATION

Monitor hepatic function periodically.

PATIENT/FAMILY TEACHING

Avoid those with colds, other infections. Avoid grapefruit juice/grapefruit. Close monitoring by physician is important.

S

sodium bicarbonate

CLASSIFICATION

PHARMACOTHERAPEUTIC: Alkalinizing agent. **CLINICAL:** Antacid.

ACTION

Dissociates to provide bicarbonate ion. **Therapeutic Effect:** Neutralizes hydrogen ion concentration, raises blood/urinary pH.

PHARMACOKINETICS

	Onset	Peak	Duration
PO	15 min	—	1–3 hrs
IV	Immediate	—	8–10 min

Following administration, sodium bicarbonate dissociates to sodium and bicarbonate ions. Forms/excretes CO_2 (with increased hydrogen ions combines to form carbonic acid, then dissociates to CO_2, which is excreted by lungs). Plasma concentration regulated by kidney (ability to form/excrete bicarbonate).

USES

Management of metabolic acidosis, antacid, alkalinization of urine, stabilizes acid-base balance, cardiac arrest, life-threatening hyperkalemia.

PRECAUTIONS

CONTRAINDICATIONS: Metabolic/respiratory alkalosis, hypocalcemia, excessive chloride loss due to vomiting/diarrhea/GI suction. **CAUTIONS:** CHF, edematous states, renal insufficiency, pts on corticosteroid therapy.

LIFESPAN CONSIDERATIONS: Pregnancy/lactation: May produce hypernatremia, increase tendon reflexes in neonate/fetus whose mother is a chronic, high-dose user. May be distributed in breast milk. **Pregnancy Category C. Children:** No age-related precautions noted. Do not use as antacid in those <6 yrs. **Elderly:** Age-related renal impairment may require caution.

INTERACTIONS

DRUG: May decrease excretion of **quinidine, ketoconazole, tetracyclines. Calcium-containing products** may result in milk-alkali syndrome. May increase excretion of **salicylates, lithium.** May decrease effect of **methenamine. HERBAL:** None known. **FOOD: Milk, milk products** may result in milk-alkali syndrome. **LAB VALUES:** May increase serum, urinary pH.

AVAILABILITY (OTC)

TABLETS: 325 mg, 650 mg. **INJECTION (Rx):** 0.5 mEq/ml (4.2%), 0.6 mEq/ml (5%), 0.9 mEq/ml (7.5%), 1 mEq/ml (8.4%).

ADMINISTRATION/HANDLING

PO

- Give 1–3 hrs after meals.

IV

Storage • Store at room temperature.

Reconstitution • May give undiluted.

Rate of administration

Alert: For direct IV administration in neonates/infants, use 0.5 mEq/ml concentration.

• For IV push, give up to 1 mEq/kg over 1–3 min for cardiac arrest. • For IV infusion, do not exceed rate of infusion of 50 mEq/hr. For children <2 yrs, premature infants, neonates, administer by slow infusion, up to 8 mEq/min.

IV INCOMPATIBILITIES

Ascorbic acid, diltiazem (Cardizem), dobutamine (Dobutrex), dopamine (Intropin), hydromorphone (Dilaudid), magnesium sulfate, midazolam (Versed), morphine, norepinephrine (Levophed).

IV COMPATIBILITIES

Aminophylline, calcium chloride, furosemide (Lasix), heparin, insulin, lidocaine, mannitol, milrinone (Primacor), morphine, phenylephrine (Neo-Synephrine), phenytoin (Dilantin), potassium chloride, propofol (Diprivan), vancomycin (Vancocin).

INDICATIONS/ROUTES/DOSAGE

Alert: May give by IV push, IV infusion, or orally. Dose individualized based on severity of acidosis; laboratory values; pt age, weight, clinical conditions. Do not fully correct bicarbonate deficit during first 24 hrs (may cause metabolic alkalosis).

CARDIAC ARREST

IV: ADULTS, ELDERLY: Initially, 1 mEq/kg (as 7.5%–8.4% solution). May repeat with 0.5 mEq/kg q10min during continued cardiopulmonary arrest. Use in the postresuscitation phase based on arterial blood pH, $Paco_2$ base deficit. CHILDREN, INFANTS: Initially, 1 mEq/kg.

METABOLIC ACIDOSIS (less severe)

IV infusion: ADULTS, ELDERLY, OLDER CHILDREN: 2–5 mEq/kg over 4–8 hrs. May repeat based on laboratory values.

ACIDOSIS (associated with chronic renal failure)

Alert: Give when plasma bicarbonate <15 mEq/L.

PO: ADULTS, ELDERLY: Initially, 20–36 mEq/day in divided doses.

RENAL TUBULAR ACIDOSIS

PO (Distal): ADULTS, ELDERLY: 0.5–2 mEq/kg/day in 4–6 divided doses. CHILDREN: 2–3 mEq/kg/day in divided doses. **(Proximal):** ADULTS, ELDERLY, CHILDREN: 5–10 mEq/kg/day in divided doses.

ALKALINIZATION OF URINE

PO: ADULTS, ELDERLY: Initially, 4 g, then 1–2 g q4h. **Maximum:** 16 g/day. CHILDREN: 84–840 mg/kg/day in divided doses.

ANTACID

PO: ADULTS, ELDERLY: 300 mg–2 g 1–4 times/day.

SIDE EFFECTS

FREQUENT: Abdominal distention, flatulence, belching.

ADVERSE REACTIONS/ TOXIC EFFECTS

Excessive/chronic use may produce metabolic alkalosis (irritability, twitching, numbness/tingling of extremities, cyanosis, slow/shallow respiration, headache, thirst, nausea). Fluid overload results in headache, weakness, blurred vision, behavioral changes, incoordination, muscle twitching, rise in B/P, decrease in pulse rate, rapid respirations, wheezing, coughing, distended neck veins. Extravasation may occur at IV site, resulting in necrosis, ulceration.

NURSING IMPLICATIONS

BASELINE ASSESSMENT

Do not give other PO medication within 1–2 hrs of antacid administration.

INTERVENTION/EVALUATION

Monitor blood/urine pH, CO_2 level, serum electrolytes, plasma bicarbonate, $Paco_2$ levels. Watch for signs of metabolic alkalosis, fluid overload. Assess for clinical improvement of metabolic acidosis (relief from hyperventilation, weakness, disorientation). Assess pattern of daily bowel activity, stool consistency. Monitor serum phosphate, calcium, uric acid levels. Assess for relief of gastric distress.

S

sodium chloride

(Ocean Mist, Salinex, Sodium chloride❋)

CLASSIFICATION

CLINICAL: Electrolyte, ophthalmic adjunct, bronchodilator.

ACTION

Sodium is a major cation of extracellular fluid. **Therapeutic Effect:** Controls water distribution, fluid/electrolyte balance, osmotic pressure of body fluids; maintains acid-base balance.

PHARMACOKINETICS

Well absorbed from GI tract. Widely distributed. Primarily excreted in urine.

USES

Parenteral: Source of hydration; prevention/treatment of sodium and chloride deficiencies (hypertonic for severe deficiencies). Prevention of muscle cramps/heat prostration occurring with excessive perspiration. **Hypotonic:** Hydrating solution used to assess renal function status, manage hyperosmolar diabetes. Diluent for reconstitution. **Nasal:** Restores moisture, relieves dry/inflamed nasal membranes. **Ophthalmic:** Therapy in reduction of corneal edema, diagnostic aid in ophthalmoscopic exam.

S

PRECAUTIONS

CONTRAINDICATIONS: Hypernatremia, fluid retention. **CAUTIONS:** CHF, renal impairment, cirrhosis, hypertension. Do not use NaCl preserved with benzyl alcohol in neonates.

LIFESPAN CONSIDERATIONS: Pregnancy/lactation: Pregnancy Category C. Children/elderly: No age-related precautions noted.

INTERACTIONS

DRUG: Hypertonic saline and oxytocics may cause uterine hypertonus, possible uterine ruptures or lacerations. **HERBAL:** None known. **FOOD:** None known. **LAB VALUES:** None known.

AVAILABILITY (OTC)

TABLETS: 1 g. **NASAL SOLUTION:** 0.4%, 0.6%, 0.75%. **OPHTHALMIC SOLUTION:** 2%, 5%. **OPHTHALMIC OINTMENT:** 5%. **INJECTION (concentrate) (Rx):** 14.6%, 23.4%. **INJECTION (infusion) (Rx):** 0.45%, 0.9%, 3%, 5%. **IRRIGATION (Rx):** 0.45%, 0.9%.

ADMINISTRATION/HANDLING

PO

• Do not crush/break enteric-coated or extended-release tablets. • Administer with full glass of water.

NASAL

• Instruct pt to begin inhaling slowly just before releasing medication into nose. • Inhale slowly, then release air gently through mouth. • Continue technique for 20–30 sec.

OPHTHALMIC

• Place finger on lower eyelid, pull out until pocket is formed between eye and lower lid. Hold dropper above pocket, place prescribed number of drops (or apply thin strip of ointment) in pocket. Instruct pt to close eyes gently so that medication will not be squeezed out of sac. • When lower lid is released, have pt keep eye open without blinking for at least 30 sec for solution; for ointment have pt close eye, roll eyeball around to distribute medication. • When using drops, apply gentle finger pressure to lacrimal sac (bridge of the nose, inside corner of the eye) for 1–2 min after administration of solution (reduces systemic absorption).

IV

• Hypertonic solutions (3% or 5%) are administered via large vein; avoid infiltration; do not exceed 100 ml/hr. • Vials containing 2.5–4 mEq/ml (concentrated NaCl) must be diluted with D_5W or $D_{10}W$ before administration.

INDICATIONS/ROUTES/DOSAGE

USUAL PARENTERAL DOSAGE

Alert: Dosage based on age, weight, clinical condition; fluid, electrolyte, acid-base status.

IV infusion: ADULTS, ELDERLY: (0.9% or 0.45%): 1–2 L/day. (3% or 5%): 100 ml over 1 hr; assess serum electrolyte concentration before additional fluid is given.

USUAL ORAL DOSAGE

PO: ADULTS, ELDERLY: 1–2 g 3 times/day.

USUAL NASAL DOSAGE

Intranasal: ADULTS, ELDERLY: Take as needed.

USUAL OPHTHALMIC DOSAGE

Ophthalmic: ADULTS, ELDERLY: *Solution:* 1–2 drops q3–4h. *Ointment:* Once/day or as directed.

SIDE EFFECTS

FREQUENT: Facial flushing. **OCCASIONAL:** Fever, irritation/phlebitis/extravasation at injection site. **Ophthalmic:** Temporary burning/irritation.

ADVERSE REACTIONS/ TOXIC EFFECTS

Too rapid administration may produce peripheral edema, CHF, pulmonary edema. Excessive dosage produces hypokalemia, hypervolemia, hypernatremia.

NURSING IMPLICATIONS

BASELINE ASSESSMENT

Assess fluid balance (I&O, daily weight, lung sounds, edema).

INTERVENTION/EVALUATION

Monitor fluid balance (e.g., I&O, daily weight, edema, lung sounds), IV site for extravasation. Monitor serum electrolytes, acid-base balance, B/P. Hypernatremia associated with edema, weight gain, elevated B/P; hyponatremia associated with muscle cramps, nausea, vomiting, dry mucous membranes.

PATIENT/FAMILY TEACHING

Temporary burning, irritation may occur upon instillation of eye medication. Discontinue eye medication and contact physician if severe pain, headache, rapid change in vision (side and straight ahead), sudden appearance of floating spots, acute redness of eyes, pain on exposure to light, double vision occurs.

sodium ferric gluconate complex

(Ferrlecit)

CLASSIFICATION

PHARMACOTHERAPEUTIC: Trace element. **CLINICAL:** Hematinic.

ACTION

Repletes total body content of iron. **Therapeutic Effect:** Replaces iron found in Hgb, myoglobin, specific enzymes; allows oxygen transport via Hgb.

USES

Treatment of iron deficiency anemia in pts undergoing chronic hemodialysis who are receiving supplemental erythropoietin therapy.

PRECAUTIONS

CONTRAINDICATIONS: All anemias not associated with iron deficiency. **CAUTIONS:** Pts with iron overload, significant allergies, asthma, liver impairment, rheumatoid arthritis.

LIFESPAN CONSIDERATIONS: Pregnancy/lactation: Unknown if distributed in breast milk. **Pregnancy Category B. Children:** Safety and efficacy not established. **Elderly:** No age-related precautions noted; lower initial dosages recommended.

INTERACTIONS

DRUG: None known. **HERBAL:** None known. **FOOD:** None known. **LAB VALUES:** None known.

AVAILABILITY (Rx)

AMPOULES: 12.5 mg/ml elemental iron.

ADMINISTRATION/HANDLING

IV

Storage • Store at room temperature. • Use immediately after dilution.

Reconstitution • Must be diluted. • Test dose: dilute 25 mg (2 ml) with 50 ml 0.9% NaCl. • Recommended dose: dilute 125 mg (10 ml) with 100 ml 0.9% NaCl.

Rate of administration • Infuse test dose and recommended dose over 1 hr.

IV INCOMPATIBILITY
Do not mix with any other medications.

INDICATIONS/ROUTES/DOSAGE

Alert: Initially, a 25-mg test dose is diluted in 50 ml 0.9% NaCl and given over 60 min. May give IV undiluted without test dose.

IV infusion: ADULTS, ELDERLY: 125 mg in 100 ml 0.9% NaCl infused over 1 hr. Minimum cumulative dose 1 g elemental iron given over 8 sessions at sequential dialysis treatment. (May be given during dialysis session itself.)

SIDE EFFECTS

FREQUENT (>3%): Flushing, hypotension, hypersensitivity reaction. **OCCASIONAL (1%–3%):** Injection site reaction, headache, abdominal pain, chills, flulike syndrome, dizziness, leg cramps, dyspnea, nausea, vomiting, diarrhea, myalgia, pruritus, edema.

ADVERSE REACTIONS/ TOXIC EFFECTS

Rarely, potentially fatal hypersensitivity reaction characterized by cardiovascular collapse, cardiac arrest, dyspnea, bronchospasm, angioedema, urticaria. Hypotension associated with flushing, lightheadedness, fatigue, weakness, severe pain in chest, back, groin with rapid administration of iron.

NURSING IMPLICATIONS

BASELINE ASSESSMENT

Do not give concurrently with oral iron form (excessive iron may produce excessive iron storage [hemosiderosis]). Be alert to pts with rheumatoid arthritis or iron deficiency anemia (acute exacerbation of joint pain, swelling may occur).

INTERVENTION/EVALUATION

Monitor vital signs, lab tests, esp. CBC, serum iron concentrations (may not be meaningful for 3 wks after administration).

PATIENT/FAMILY TEACHING

Stools frequently become black with iron therapy; this is harmless unless accompanied by red streaking, sticky consistency of stool, abdominal pain/cramping, which should be reported to physician.

sodium oxybate (gamma hydroxybutyrate)

(GHB)

CLASSIFICATION

PHARMACOTHERAPEUTIC: Neurotransmitter. **CLINICAL:** Antinarcolepsy.

ACTION

Mechanism of action unknown.

USES

Treatment of adult with cataplexy associated with narcolepsy.

PRECAUTIONS

CONTRAINDICATIONS: Metabolic/respiratory alkalosis, current treatment with sedative-hypnotics, succinic semialdehyde dehydrogenase deficient. **CAUTIONS:** Hepatic insufficiency; history of depression; hypertension; pregnancy; concurrent ingestion of alcohol, other CNS depressants.

INTERACTIONS

DRUG: **Barbiturates, benzodiazepines, centrally acting muscle relaxants, opioid analgesics** may have additive CNS and respiratory depressant effects. **HERBAL:** None known. **FOOD:** **Alcohol** may have additive CNS and respiratory depressant effects. **LAB VALUES:** May increase sodium, glucose level.

ADMINISTRATION/HANDLING

PO

- Store at room temperature. • Give first of two daily dosages at bedtime while pt is in bed and the second dosage 2.5–4 hrs later.

AVAILABILITY (Rx)

ORAL SOLUTION.

INDICATIONS/ROUTES/DOSAGE

NARCOLEPSY

PO: ADULTS, ELDERLY: 4.5 g/day in 2 equal doses of 2.25 g, the first taken at bedtime while in bed and the second 2.5–4 hrs later. **Maximum:** 9 g/day in 2 weekly increments of 1.5 g/day.

SIDE EFFECTS

FREQUENT (58%): Mild bradycardia. **OCCASIONAL:** Headache, vertigo, dizziness, restless legs, abdominal pain, muscle weakness. **RARE:** Dreamlike state of confusion.

ADVERSE REACTIONS/TOXIC EFFECTS

Metabolic alkalosis (irritability, twitching, numbness/tingling of extremities, cyanosis, slow/shallow respiration, headache, thirst, nausea) has been noted, particularly in pts with head trauma before treatment. Concurrent use of alcohol may result in respiratory depression, apnea, comatose state. Severe dependence, craving produces a high potential for abuse.

NURSING IMPLICATIONS

INTERVENTION/EVALUATION

Watch for signs of metabolic alkalosis (irritability, twitching, numbness/tingling of extremities, cyanosis, slow/shallow respiration, headache, thirst, nausea). Monitor serum glucose, sodium levels.

S

PATIENT/FAMILY TEACHING

Avoid alcohol due to high potential for comatose state. Severe dependence may occur.

sodium polystyrene sulfonate

(Kayexalate, SPS)

CLASSIFICATION

PHARMACOTHERAPEUTIC: Cation exchange resin. **CLINICAL:** Antihyperkalemic.

ACTION

Ion exchange resin that releases sodium ions in exchange primarily for potassium ions. **Therapeutic Effect:** Removes potassium in the intestine before the resin is passed from the body.

USES

Treatment of hyperkalemia.

PRECAUTIONS

CONTRAINDICATIONS: Hypernatremia, intestinal obstruction/perforation. **CAUTIONS:** Severe CHF, hypertension, edema.

LIFESPAN CONSIDERATIONS: Pregnancy/lactation: Unknown if drug crosses placenta or is distributed in breast milk. **Pregnancy Category C. Children:** No age-related precautions noted. **Elderly:** May be at increased risk for fecal impaction.

INTERACTIONS

DRUG: Cation-donating antacids, laxatives (e.g., magnesium hydroxide) may decrease effect, cause systemic alkalosis (pts with renal impairment). **HERBAL:** None known. **FOOD:** None known. **LAB VALUES:** May decrease magnesium, calcium.

AVAILABILITY (Rx)

SUSPENSION: 15 g/60 ml. **POWDER.**

ADMINISTRATION/HANDLING

PO

• Give with 20–100 ml sorbitol (facilitates passage of resin through intestinal tract, prevents constipation, aids in potassium removal, increases palatability). • Do not mix with foods, liquids containing potassium.

RECTAL

• After initial cleansing enema, insert large rubber tube into rectum well into sigmoid colon, tape in place. • Introduce suspension (with 100 ml sorbitol) via gravity. • Flush with 50–100 ml fluid and clamp. • Retain for several hrs if possible. • Irrigate colon with non–sodium-containing solution to remove resin.

INDICATIONS/ROUTES/DOSAGE

HYPERKALEMIA

PO: ADULTS, ELDERLY: 60 ml (15 g) 1–4 times/day. CHILDREN: 1 g/kg/dose q6h. **Rectal:** ADULTS, ELDERLY: 30–50 g as needed q6h. CHILDREN: 1 g/kg/dose q2–6h.

SIDE EFFECTS

FREQUENT: High dosage: Anorexia, nausea, vomiting, constipation. **High dosage in elderly:** Fecal impaction (severe stomach pain with nausea/vomiting). **OCCASIONAL:** Diarrhea, sodium retention (decreased urination, peripheral edema, increased weight).

ADVERSE REACTIONS/ TOXIC EFFECTS

Serious potassium deficiency may occur. Early signs of hypokalemia: extreme weakness, irritability, confusion, delayed thought processes, EKG changes (often associated with lengthened QT interval;

S

widening, flattening, conversion of T wave, prominent U waves). Hypocalcemia (abdominal/muscle cramps) occurs occasionally. Arrhythmias, severe muscle weakness may be noted.

NURSING IMPLICATIONS

BASELINE ASSESSMENT

Does not rapidly correct severe hyperkalemia (may take hours to days). Consider other measures in medical emergency (IV calcium, IV sodium bicarbonate/glucose/insulin, dialysis).

INTERVENTION/EVALUATION

Monitor potassium levels frequently. Assess pt's clinical condition, EKG (valuable in determining when treatment should be discontinued). In addition to checking serum potassium, monitor magnesium, calcium levels. Monitor daily bowel activity, stool consistency (fecal impaction may occur in pts on high dosages, particularly in elderly).

Solu-Medrol

see methylprednisolone

somatrem

soe-ma-trem

(Protropin)

Do not confuse with Proloprim, Protamine, Protopam, somatropin.

✤ CLASSIFICATION

PHARMACOTHERAPEUTIC: Polypeptide hormone. **CLINICAL:** Growth stimulator.

ACTION

Increases number, size of muscle cells; increases RBC mass. Affects carbohydrate metabolism (antagonizes action of insulin), fats (increases mobilization of fats), proteins (increases cellular protein synthesis). **Therapeutic Effect:** Stimulates linear growth.

USES

Long-term treatment of children who have growth failure due to endogenous growth hormone deficiency, treatment of AIDS-wasting syndrome.

PRECAUTIONS

CONTRAINDICATIONS: None known. **CAUTIONS:** Diabetes mellitus, untreated hypothyroidism, malignancy. **Pregnancy Category C.**

INTERACTIONS

DRUG: **Corticosteroids** may inhibit growth response. **HERBAL:** None known. **FOOD:** None known. **LAB VALUES:** May increase alkaline phosphatase, serum inorganic phosphorus, parathyroid hormone.

AVAILABILITY (Rx)

POWDER FOR INJECTION: 5 mg, 10 mg.

INDICATIONS/ROUTES/DOSAGE

USUAL PARENTERAL DOSAGE

IM/subcutaneous: Up to 0.1 mg/kg (0.26 international units/kg) 3 times/wk.

SIDE EFFECTS

FREQUENT: 30% of pts develop persistent antibodies to growth hormone (generally does not cause failure to respond to somatrem). **OCCASIONAL:** Headache, muscle pain, weakness, mild hyperglycemia, allergic reaction (rash, itching),

S

pain/swelling at injection site, pain in hip/knee.

NURSING IMPLICATIONS

BASELINE ASSESSMENT

Obtain baseline thyroid function, blood glucose levels.

INTERVENTION/EVALUATION

Monitor bone age, calcium, parathyroid, phosphorus, renal function, glucose, growth rate, thyroid function: Observe for decreased wasting in AIDS.

PATIENT/FAMILY TEACHING

Teach correct procedure to reconstitute for IM/subcutaneous administration, safe handling/disposal of needles. Inform of need for regular follow-up with physician.

somatropin

soe-mah-**troe**-pin

(Humatrope, Norditropin, Nutropin, Nutropin AQ, Nutropin Depot)

Do not confuse with somatrem, sumatriptan.

CLASSIFICATION

PHARMACOTHERAPEUTIC: Polypeptide hormone. **CLINICAL:** Growth stimulator.

ACTION

Increases number, size of muscle cells; increases RBC mass. Affects carbohydrate metabolism (antagonizes action of insulin), fats (increases mobilization of fats), proteins (increases cellular protein synthesis). **Therapeutic Effect:** Stimulates linear growth.

USES

Long-term treatment of children who have growth failure due to endogenous growth hormone deficiency or associated with chronic renal insufficiency (Nutropin only). Long-term therapy in adults with growth hormone deficiency. Long-term treatment of short stature associated with Turner's syndrome, treatment of AIDS-wasting syndrome.

PRECAUTIONS

CONTRAINDICATIONS: None known. **CAUTIONS:** Diabetes mellitus, untreated hypothyroidism, malignancy. **Pregnancy Category C.**

INTERACTIONS

DRUG: Corticosteroids may inhibit growth response. **HERBAL:** None known. **FOOD:** None known. **LAB VALUES:** May increase alkaline phosphatase, serum inorganic phosphorus, parathyroid hormone.

AVAILABILITY (Rx)

INJECTION: 4 mg, 5 mg, 8 mg, 10 mg. **Depot:** 13.5 mg, 18 mg, 22.5 mg.

INDICATIONS/ROUTES/DOSAGE

GROWTH HORMONE DEFICIENCY

IM/subcutaneous: (Humatrope): Up to 0.06 mg/kg 3 times/wk.

Subcutaneous: (Nutropin): 0.3 mg/kg/wk.

Subcutaneous: (Nutropin Depot): 1.5 mg/kg/mo or 0.75 mg/kg 2 times/mo.

Subcutaneous: ADULTS: 0.04 mg/kg/wk in 6–7 injections/wk. **Maximum:** 0.08 mg/kg/wk.

CHRONIC RENAL INSUFFICIENCY

Subcutaneous: (Nutropin): 0.35 mg/kg/wk.

TURNER'S SYNDROME

Subcutaneous: 0.375 mg/kg/wk divided into 3–7 equal doses/wk.

AIDS-WASTING SYNDROME

Subcutaneous: 4–6 mg at bedtime.

SIDE EFFECTS

FREQUENT: Development of persistent antibodies to growth hormone (generally does not cause failure to respond to somatropin); hypercalciuria during first 2–3 mos of therapy. **OCCASIONAL:** Headache, muscle pain, weakness, mild hyperglycemia, allergic reaction (rash, itching), pain/swelling at injection site, pain in hip/knee.

NURSING IMPLICATIONS

BASELINE ASSESSMENT

Obtain baseline thyroid function, blood glucose levels.

INTERVENTION/EVALUATION

Monitor bone age, calcium, parathyroid, phosphorus, renal function, glucose, growth rate, thyroid function. Observe for decreased wasting in AIDS.

PATIENT/FAMILY TEACHING

Teach correct procedure to reconstitute for IM/subcutaneous administration, safe handling/disposal of needles. Inform of need for regular follow-up with physician.

sotalol hydrochloride

sew-tah-lol

(Betapace, Sotacor✤)

Do not confuse with Stadol.

CLASSIFICATION

PHARMACOTHERAPEUTIC: Beta-adrenergic blocking agent. **CLINICAL:** Antiarrhythmic (see pp. 15C, 63C).

ACTION

Prolongs action potential, effective refractory period, QT interval. Decreases heart rate, AV nodal conduction; increases AV nodal refractoriness. **Therapeutic Effect:** Produces antiarrhythmic activity.

PHARMACOKINETICS

Well absorbed from GI tract. Protein binding: None. Widely distributed. Primarily excreted unchanged in urine. Removed by hemodialysis. **Half-life:** 12 hrs (half-life increased in elderly, pts with impaired renal function).

USES

Treatment of documented, life-threatening ventricular arrhythmias. **Unlabeled:** Treatment of chronic angina pectoris, hypertension, hypertrophic cardiomyopathy, MI, pheochromocytoma, tremors, anxiety, thyrotoxicosis, mitral valve prolapse syndrome. Maintenance of normal heart rhythm in chronic/recurring atrial fibrillation/flutter.

PRECAUTIONS

CONTRAINDICATIONS: Bronchial asthma, uncontrolled cardiac failure, sinus bradycardia, second- and third-degree heart block, cardiogenic shock, prolonged QT syndrome (unless functioning pacemaker present). **CAUTIONS:** Pts with history of ventricular tachycardia, ventricular fibrillation, cardiomegaly, CHF, diabetes mellitus, excessive prolongation of QT interval, hypokalemia, hypomagnesemia. Severe, prolonged diarrhea. Pts with sick sinus syndrome, pts at risk of developing thyrotoxicosis. Avoid abrupt withdrawal.

LIFESPAN CONSIDERATIONS: Pregnancy/lactation: Crosses placenta. Excreted in breast milk. **Pregnancy Category B** (**D** if used in second or third trimester). **Children:** Safety and efficacy not established. **Elderly:** Age-related peripheral vascular disease may increase susceptibility to decreased peripheral circulation.

S

INTERACTIONS

DRUG: **Antiarrhythmics, phenothiazine, tricyclic antidepressants** may increase prolonged QT interval. May increase proarrhythmia with **digoxin. Calcium channel blockers** may increase effect on AV conduction, B/P. May mask signs of hypoglycemia, prolong effect of **insulin, oral hypoglycemics.** May inhibit effects of **sympathomimetics.** May potentiate rebound hypertension noted after discontinuing **clonidine.** **HERBAL:** None known. **FOOD:** None known. **LAB VALUES:** May increase glucose, alkaline phosphatase, LDH, SGOT (AST), SGPT (ALT), lipoproteins, triglycerides.

AVAILABILITY (Rx)

TABLETS: 80 mg, 120 mg, 160 mg, 240 mg.

ADMINISTRATION/HANDLING

PO

- Give without regard to food.

INDICATIONS/ROUTES/DOSAGE

ANTIARRHYTHMIC

PO: ADULTS, ELDERLY: Initially, 80 mg 2 times/day. May increase gradually at 2- to 3-day intervals. RANGE: 240–320 mg/day.

Alert: Some pts may require 480–640 mg/day. Dosing more than 2 times/day usually not necessary due to long half-life.

DOSAGE IN RENAL IMPAIRMENT

Creatinine Clearance	Dosage Interval
30–60 ml/min	24 hrs
10–29 ml/min	36–48 hrs
<10 ml/min	Individualized

SIDE EFFECTS

FREQUENT: Decreased sexual function, drowsiness, insomnia, unusual tiredness/weakness. **OCCASIONAL:** Depression, cold hands/feet, diarrhea, constipation, anxiety, nasal congestion, nausea, vomiting. **RARE:** Altered taste, dry eyes, itching, numbness of fingers, toes, scalp.

ADVERSE REACTIONS/ TOXIC EFFECTS

Bradycardia, CHF, hypotension, bronchospasm, hypoglycemia, prolonged QT interval, torsades de pointes, ventricular tachycardia, premature ventricular complexes.

NURSING IMPLICATIONS

BASELINE ASSESSMENT

Pt must be on continuous cardiac monitoring upon initiation of therapy. Do not administer without consulting physician if pulse is ≤60 beats/min.

INTERVENTION/EVALUATION

Diligently monitor for arrhythmias. Assess B/P for hypotension, pulse for bradycardia. Assess for CHF: dyspnea, peripheral edema, jugular vein distention, increased weight, rales in lungs, decreased urine output.

PATIENT/FAMILY TEACHING

Do not discontinue or change dose without physician approval. May cause drowsiness, impair ability to perform tasks requiring mental alertness or physical coordination (e.g., driving). Periodic lab tests, EKGs are a necessary part of therapy.

spironolactone

spear-own-oh-**lak**-tone
(Aldactone, Novospiroton)

FIXED-COMBINATION(S)

Aldactazide: spironolactone/hydrochlorothiazide (a thiazide diuretic): 25 mg/25 mg; 50 mg/50 mg.

CLASSIFICATION

PHARMACOTHERAPEUTIC: Aldosterone antagonist. **CLINICAL:** Potassium-sparing diuretic, antihypertensive, antihypokalemic (see p. 87C).

ACTION

Competitively inhibits action of aldosterone. Interferes with sodium reabsorption in distal tubule. **Therapeutic Effect:** Increases potassium retention while promoting sodium and water excretion.

PHARMACOKINETICS

Onset	Peak	Duration
PO		
24–48 hrs	48–72 hrs	48–72 hrs

Well absorbed from GI tract (increased with food). Protein binding: 91%–98%. Metabolized in liver to active metabolite. Primarily excreted in urine. Unknown if removed by hemodialysis. **Half-life:** 0–24 hrs; metabolite: 13–24 hrs.

USES

Treatment of excessive aldosterone production, essential hypertension, edema due to CHF, CHF, cirrhosis of liver/nephrotic syndrome. Adjunct to potassium-losing diuretics or to potentiate action of other diuretics. Diagnosis of hyperaldosteronism. **Unlabeled:** Treatment of polycystic ovary syndrome, female hirsutism.

PRECAUTIONS

CONTRAINDICATIONS: Acute renal insufficiency/impairment, anuria, BUN/creatinine over twice normal value levels, hyperkalemia. **CAUTIONS:** Dehydration, hyponatremia, impaired renal/liver function, concurrent use of supplemental potassium.

LIFESPAN CONSIDERATIONS: Pregnancy/lactation: Active metabolite excreted in breast milk; breast-feeding not advised. **Pregnancy Category C (D** if used in pregnancy-induced hypertension). **Children:** No age-related precautions noted. **Elderly:** May be more susceptible to develop hyperkalemia. Age-related renal impairment may require cautious use.

INTERACTIONS

DRUG: May decrease effect of **anticoagulants, heparin. NSAIDs** may decrease antihypertensive effect. **ACE inhibitors (e.g., captopril), potassium-containing medications, potassium supplements** may increase potassium. May decrease **lithium** clearance, increase toxicity. May increase **digoxin** half-life. **HERBAL:** None known. **FOOD:** None known. **LAB VALUES:** May increase BUN, calcium excretion, creatinine, glucose, magnesium, potassium, uric acid. May decrease sodium.

AVAILABILITY (Rx)

TABLETS: 25 mg, 50 mg, 100 mg.

ADMINISTRATION/HANDLING

PO

- Oral suspension containing crushed tablets in cherry syrup is stable for up to 30 days if refrigerated.
- Drug absorption enhanced if taken with food.
- Scored tablets may be crushed.

INDICATIONS/ROUTES/DOSAGE

DIURETIC, HYPERTENSION

PO: ADULTS, ELDERLY: 25–200 mg/day in 1–2 divided doses. CHILDREN: 1.5–3.3 mg/kg/day in divided doses q6–12h. NEONATES (Diuretic): 1–3 mg/kg/day q12–24h.

CHF

PO: ADULTS, ELDERLY: 25 mg/day.

DIAGNOSIS OF PRIMARY ALDOSTERONISM

PO: ADULTS, ELDERLY: 100–400 mg/day in 1–2 divided doses. CHILDREN: 100–400 mg/m^2/day in 1–2 divided doses.

DOSAGE IN RENAL IMPAIRMENT

Creatinine Clearance	Interval
10–50 ml/min	12–24 hrs
<10 ml/min	Avoid

SIDE EFFECTS

FREQUENT: Hyperkalemia for pts on supplemental potassium or those with renal insufficiency, dehydration, hyponatremia, lethargy. **OCCASIONAL:** Nausea, vomiting, anorexia, cramping, diarrhea, headache, ataxia, drowsiness, confusion, fever. **Male:** Gynecomastia, impotence, decreased libido. **Female:** Menstrual irregularities/amenorrhea, postmenopausal bleeding, breast tenderness. **RARE:** Rash, urticaria, hirsutism.

ADVERSE REACTIONS/ TOXIC EFFECTS

Severe hyperkalemia may produce arrhythmias, bradycardia, EKG changes (tented T-waves, widening QRS, ST depression). May proceed to cardiac standstill or ventricular fibrillation. Cirrhosis pts at risk for hepatic decompensation if dehydration/hyponatremia occurs. Pts with primary aldosteronism may experience rapid weight loss, severe fatigue during high-dose therapy.

NURSING IMPLICATIONS

BASELINE ASSESSMENT

Weigh pt; initiate strict I&O. Evaluate hydration status by assessing mucous membranes, skin turgor. Obtain baseline electrolytes, renal/hepatic functions, urinalysis. Assess for edema; note location, extent. Check baseline vital signs, note pulse rate/regularity.

INTERVENTION/EVALUATION

Monitor electrolyte values, esp. for increased potassium. Monitor B/P levels. Monitor for hyponatremia: mental confusion, thirst, cold/clammy skin, drowsiness, dry mouth. Monitor for hyperkalemia: colic, diarrhea, muscle twitching followed by weakness/paralysis, arrhythmias. Obtain daily weight. Note changes in edema, skin turgor.

PATIENT/FAMILY TEACHING

Expect increase in volume, frequency of urination. Therapeutic effect takes several days to begin and can last for several days when drug is discontinued. This may not apply if pt is on a potassium-losing drug concomitantly (diet and use of supplements should be established by physician). Notify physician for irregular/slow pulse, electrolyte imbalance (signs noted previously). Avoid foods high in potassium such as whole grains (cereals), legumes, meat, bananas, apricots, orange juice, potatoes (white, sweet), raisins. May cause drowsiness, impair ability to perform tasks requiring mental alertness or physical coordination.

stavudine (d4T)

stay-view-deen
(Zerit)

CLASSIFICATION

PHARMACOTHERAPEUTIC: Nucleoside reverse transcriptase inhibitor. **CLINICAL:** Antiviral (see pp. 60C, 98C).

ACTION

Inhibits HIV reverse transcriptase via viral DNA chain termination. Also inhibits RNA- and DNA-dependent DNA polymerase, an enzyme necessary for viral HIV replication. **Therapeutic Effect:** Slows HIV replication, reducing progression of HIV infection.

PHARMACOKINETICS

Rapidly, completely absorbed following PO administration. Undergoes minimal metabolism. Excreted in urine. **Half-life:** 1.5 hrs (half-life increased with impaired renal function).

USES

Treatment of HIV infection in combination with other antiretroviral agents.

PRECAUTIONS

CONTRAINDICATIONS: None known. **CAUTIONS:** History of peripheral neuropathy, renal/liver impairment.

LIFESPAN CONSIDERATIONS: Pregnancy/lactation: Breast-feeding not recommended (possibility of HIV transmission). **Pregnancy Category C. Children:** No age-related precautions noted. **Elderly:** Information not available.

INTERACTIONS

DRUG: None known. **HERBAL:** None known. **FOOD:** None known. **LAB VALUES:** Commonly increases SGOT (AST), SGPT (ALT). May decrease neutrophil count.

AVAILABILITY (Rx)

CAPSULES: 15 mg, 20 mg, 30 mg, 40 mg. **ORAL SOLUTION:** 1 mg/ml.

ADMINISTRATION/HANDLING

PO

- Give without regard to meals.

INDICATIONS/ROUTES/DOSAGE

HIV INFECTION

PO: ADULTS ≥60 KG: 40 mg twice daily. ADULTS <60 KG: 30 mg twice daily. If peripheral neuropathy or elevated hepatic transaminases present, stop therapy. If symptoms resolve completely, resume treatment using following schedule: ADULTS ≥60 KG: 20 mg twice daily. ADULTS <60 KG: 15 mg twice daily. CHILDREN ≥30 KG: Same as adults. CHILDREN <30 KG: 2 mg/kg/day.

DOSAGE IN RENAL IMPAIRMENT

Dose and/or frequency is modified based on creatinine clearance, pt weight.

Creatinine Clearance	≥60 kg	<60 kg
>50	40 mg q12h	30 mg q12h
26–50	20 mg q12h	15 mg q12h
10–25	20 mg q24h	15 mg q24h

SIDE EFFECTS

FREQUENT: Headache (55%), diarrhea (50%), chills/fever (38%), nausea/vomiting; myalgia (35%), rash (33%), asthenia (loss of strength, energy) (28%), insomnia, abdominal pain (26%), anxiety (22%), arthralgia (18%), back pain (20%), sweating (19%), malaise (17%), depression (14%). **OCCASIONAL:** Anorexia, weight loss, nervousness, dizziness, conjunctivitis, dyspepsia, dyspnea. **RARE:** Constipation, vasodilation, confusion, migraine, urticaria, abnormal vision.

ADVERSE REACTIONS/ TOXIC EFFECTS

Peripheral neuropathy, characterized by numbness, tingling, pain in hands/feet, occurs frequently (15%–21%). Ulcerative stomatitis (erythema/ulcers of oral mucosa, glossitis, gingivitis), pneumonia, benign skin neoplasms occur occasionally. Pancreatitis, lactic acidosis occur rarely.

S

NURSING IMPLICATIONS

BASELINE ASSESSMENT

Obtain baseline laboratory testing, esp. liver function tests, prior to beginning stavudine therapy and at periodic intervals during therapy. Offer emotional support. Question for previous history of peripheral neuropathy.

INTERVENTION/EVALUATION

Monitor for peripheral neuropathy (characterized by numbness, tingling, pain in hands/feet). Symptoms resolve promptly if therapy is discontinued (symptoms may worsen temporarily after drug is withdrawn). If symptoms resolve completely, reduced dosage may be resumed. Assess for headache, nausea, vomiting, myalgia. Monitor skin for evidence of rash, signs of chills/fever. Determine pattern of bowel activity, stool consistency. Assess for muscle/joint aches, dizziness, sleep pattern. Assess eating pattern; monitor for weight loss. Check eyes for signs of conjunctivitis. Monitor CBC, Hgb, renal/liver function, CD4 cell count, HIV RNA levels.

PATIENT/FAMILY TEACHING

Continue therapy for full length of treatment. Doses should be evenly spaced. Do not take any medications, including OTC drugs, without consulting physician. Stavudine is not a cure for HIV infection, nor does it reduce risk of transmission to others. Pt may continue to experience illnesses, including opportunistic infections. Report tingling, burning, pain, numbness, abdominal discomfort, nausea, vomiting, fatigue, dyspnea, weakness.

St. John's wort

Also known as amber, demon chaser, goatweed, hardhay, rosin rose, tipton weed

CLASSIFICATION

HERBAL.

S

ACTION

Inhibits COMT (catechol-*O*-methyl transferase), MAO (monoamine oxidase); modulates effects of serotonin by inhibiting serotonin reuptake and 5-HT_3 and 5-HT_4 antagonism. **Effect:** Produces antidepressant effect.

USES

Treatment of depression, including secondary effects of depression (fatigue, loss of appetite, anxiety, nervousness, insomnia).

PRECAUTIONS

CONTRAINDICATIONS: Pregnancy, breastfeeding (may cause increased muscle tone of uterus; infants may experience colic, drowsiness, lethargy). **CAUTIONS:** Bipolar disorder, schizophrenia. **Pregnancy Category C.**

LIFESPAN CONSIDERATIONS: Pregnancy/lactation: Contraindicated. **Children:** Safety and efficacy not established. Avoid use. **Elderly:** No age-related precautions noted.

INTERACTIONS

DRUG: Antidepressants may increase therapeutic effect. **Cyclosporine** may cause organ rejection. **Digoxin** may cause CHF exacerbation. **ACE inhibitors** may cause hypertension. May decrease concentration/effect of **indinavir. HERBAL: Ginseng, chamomile, goldenseal, kava kava, valerian** may increase therapeutic and adverse effects. **FOOD:** Large doses with **tyramine-containing food** may cause hypertensive crisis. **LAB VALUES:** May increase INR/PT in pts treated with warfarin.

AVAILABILITY

CAPSULES: 150 mg, 300 mg. **LIQUID EXTRACT. TINCTURE.**

INDICATIONS/ROUTES/DOSAGE

DEPRESSION

PO: ADULTS, ELDERLY: 300 mg 3 times/day is the most common.

SIDE EFFECTS

Abdominal cramps, insomnia, vivid dreams, restlessness, anxiety, agitation, irritability, fatigue, dry mouth, headache, dizziness, photosensitivity, confusion.

ADVERSE REACTIONS/ TOXIC EFFECTS

None known.

NURSING IMPLICATIONS

BASELINE ASSESSMENT

Assess if pt is pregnant or breast-feeding, has history of psychiatric disease. Determine medication usage (many potential interactions). Assess mental status: mood, memory, anxiety level.

INTERVENTION/EVALUATION

Monitor changes in depressive state, behavior, signs of side effects.

PATIENT/FAMILY TEACHING

Do not abruptly discontinue (may increase adverse effects). Check with physician before taking other medications (many interactions). Avoid foods high in tyramine (e.g., aged cheese, pickled products, beer, wine). Therapeutic effect may take 4–6 wks. Avoid the sun, use sunscreen/protective clothing (increased photosensitivity).

streptokinase

strep-toe-**kine**-ace
(Streptase)

CLASSIFICATION

PHARMACOTHERAPEUTIC: Enzyme. **CLINICAL:** Thrombolytic (see p. 30C).

ACTION

Activates fibrinolytic system by converting plasminogen to plasmin (enzyme that degrades fibrin clots). Acts indirectly by forming complex with plasminogen, which converts plasminogen to plasmin. Action occurs within thrombus, on its surface, and in circulating blood. **Therapeutic Effect:** Resultant effect destroys thrombi.

PHARMACOKINETICS

Rapidly cleared from plasma by antibodies, reticuloendothelial system. Route of elimination unknown. Duration of action continues for several hours after discontinuing medication. **Half-life:** 23 min.

USES

Management of acute MI (lyses thrombi obstructing coronary arteries, decreases infarct size, improves ventricular function after MI, decreases CHF, mortality associated with MI). Lysis of diagnosed pulmonary emboli, acute/extensive thrombi of deep veins, acute arterial thrombi/emboli. Clears totally/partially occluded arteriovenous (AV) cannulae.

PRECAUTIONS

CONTRAINDICATIONS: Recent streptococcal infection, internal bleeding, CVA, intracranial surgery, severe hypertension, carcinoma of brain. **CAUTIONS:** Major surgery within 10 days, GI bleeding, recent trauma.

LIFESPAN CONSIDERATIONS: Pregnancy/lactation: Use only when benefit outweighs potential risk to fetus. Unknown if drug crosses placenta or is distributed in breast milk. **Pregnancy Category C. Children:** Safety and efficacy not established. **Elderly:** May have increased risk of intracranial hemorrhage; caution recommended.

INTERACTIONS

DRUG: Anticoagulants, heparin may increase risk of hemorrhage. **Platelet aggregation inhibitors (e.g., aspirin)** may increase risk of bleeding. **HERBAL:** None known. **FOOD:** None known. **LAB VALUES:** Decreases plas-

S

minogen and fibrinogen level during infusion, decreasing clotting time (confirms presence of lysis).

AVAILABILITY (Rx)

POWDER FOR INJECTION: 250,000 international units, 600,000 international units, 750,000 international units, 1.5 million international units.

ADMINISTRATION/HANDLING

Alert: Must be administered within 12–14 hrs of clot formation (little effect on older, organized clots).

IV

Storage • Store unopened vials at room temperature. Refrigerate reconstituted solution. Use within 24 hrs.

Reconstitution

AV CANNULA OCCLUSION

• Dilute 250,000 international unit vial with 2 ml 0.9% NaCl. Add diluent slowly to side of vial, roll and tilt to avoid foaming. Do not shake vial.

USES OTHER THAN CANNULA OCCLUSION

• Reconstitute vial with 5 ml D_5W or 0.9% NaCl (preferred). Add diluent slowly to side of vial, roll and tilt to avoid foaming. Do not shake vial. • May further dilute with 50–500 ml in 45-ml increments of D_5W or 0.9% NaCl.

Rate of administration

AV CANNULA OCCLUSION

• Give IV push slowly into each occluded limb of cannula. • Clamp for 2 hrs, then aspirate contents, flush with 0.9% NaCl.

IV INJECTION FOR CORONARY ARTERY THROMBI

• Give 1.5 million international units over 60 min.

CORONARY ARTERY THROMBI

• Give bolus dose over 25–30 sec using coronary catheter. Follow with 2,000 international units/min for 60 min.

DEEP VEIN THROMBOSIS, PULMONARY ARTERIAL EMBOLISM ARTERIAL THROMBI

• Give single dose over 25–30 min. Follow with maintenance dose of 100,000 or more every hr for 24–72 hrs. • Monitor B/P during infusion (hypotension may be severe, occurs in 1%–10%). Decrease of infusion rate may be necessary. • If uncontrolled hemorrhage occurs, discontinue infusion immediately (slowing rate of infusion may produce worsening hemorrhage). Do not use dextran to control hemorrhage.

∅ IV INCOMPATIBILITY

Do not mix with any other medications.

IV COMPATIBILITIES

Dobutamine (Dobutrex), dopamine (Intropin), heparin, lidocaine, nitroglycerin.

INDICATIONS/ROUTES/DOSAGE

Alert: Do not use from 5 days to 6 mos of previous streptokinase treatment or streptococcal infection (pharyngitis, rheumatic fever, acute glomerulonephritis secondary to streptococcal infection).

ACUTE EVOLVING TRANSMURAL MI (give as soon as possible after symptoms occur)

IV infusion: ADULTS, ELDERLY: (1.5 million units diluted to 45 ml): 1.5 million international units infused over 60 min.

Intracoronary infusion: ADULTS, ELDERLY: (250,000 units diluted to 125 ml): Initially, 20,000 international units (10 ml) bolus; then, 2,000 international units/min for 60 min. TOTAL DOSE: 140,000 international units.

PULMONARY EMBOLISM, DEEP VEIN THROMBOSIS, ARTERIAL THROMBOSIS/EMBOLISM (give within 7 days after onset)

IV infusion: ADULTS, ELDERLY: (1.5 million units diluted to 90 ml): Initially, 250,000 international units infused over 30 min; then, 100,000 international units/hr for 24–72 hrs for arterial thrombosis/embolism, 24–72 hrs for pulmonary embolism, 72 hrs for deep vein thrombosis.

Intracoronary infusion: ADULTS, ELDERLY: (1.5 million units diluted to 45 ml): Initially, 250,000 international units infused over 30 min; then, 100,000 international units/hr for maintenance.

SIDE EFFECTS

FREQUENT: Fever, superficial bleeding at puncture sites, decreased B/P. **OCCASIONAL:** Allergic reaction (rash, wheezing), bruising.

ADVERSE REACTIONS/ TOXIC EFFECTS

Severe internal hemorrhage may occur. Lysis of coronary thrombi may produce atrial or ventricular arrhythmias.

NURSING IMPLICATIONS

BASELINE ASSESSMENT

Assess Hct, platelet count, thrombin (TT), activated partial thromboplastin time (aPTT), prothrombin time (PT), fibrinogen level before therapy is instituted. If heparin is component of treatment, discontinue before streptokinase is instituted (TT/aPTT should be less than twice normal value before institution of therapy).

INTERVENTION/EVALUATION

Assess clinical response, vital signs per protocol. Handle pt carefully and as infrequently as possible to prevent bruising/bleeding. Do not obtain B/P in lower extremities (possible deep vein thrombi). Monitor TT, PT, aPTT, fibrinogen level q4h after initiation of therapy. Check stool for occult blood. Assess for decrease in B/P, increase in pulse rate, complaint of abdominal/back pain, severe headache (may be evidence of hemorrhage). Question for increase in amount of discharge during menses. Assess area of thromboembolus for color, temperature. Assess peripheral pulses, skin for bruises, petechiae. Check for excessive bleeding from minor cuts, scratches. Assess urine output for hematuria. Monitor B/P, platelets, Hgb, Hct, signs of bleeding.

streptomycin sulfate

(Streptomycin)

See Classification section under: Antibiotic: aminoglycosides (p. 19C)

streptozocin

strep-toe-**zoe**-sin

(Zanosar)

◆CLASSIFICATION

PHARMACOTHERAPEUTIC: Nitrosourea. **CLINICAL:** Antineoplastic (see p. 75C).

ACTION

Inhibits DNA synthesis without significantly affecting RNA or protein synthesis by cross-linking strands of DNA. Cell cycle–phase nonspecific. **Therapeutic Effect:** Promotes cell death.

PHARMACOKINETICS

Rapidly distributed primarily in liver, kidneys, intestine, pancreas. Metabolized in liver. Primarily excreted in urine. **Half-life:** 35 min; metabolite: 40 min.

USES

Treatment of metastatic islet cell carcinoma of pancreas. **Unlabeled:** Treatment of carcinoid tumor.

S

PRECAUTIONS

CONTRAINDICATIONS: None known. **EXTREME CAUTION:** Impaired renal function. **CAUTIONS:** Impaired hepatic function.

LIFESPAN CONSIDERATIONS: Pregnancy/lactation: If possible, avoid use during pregnancy, esp. first trimester. Unknown if distributed in breast milk. Breast-feeding not recommended. **Pregnancy Category C. Children:** Safety and efficacy not established. **Elderly:** Age-related renal impairment may require caution.

INTERACTIONS

DRUG: Nephrotoxic medications may increase nephrotoxicity. May decrease effects of **phenytoin. Live virus vaccines** may potentiate virus replication, increase vaccine side effects, decrease pt's antibody response to vaccine. **HERBAL:** None known. **FOOD:** None known. **LAB VALUES:** May increase SGOT (AST), SGPT (ALT), alkaline phosphatase, bilirubin, LDH, BUN, creatinine, urinary protein. May decrease albumin, phosphate concentrations.

AVAILABILITY (Rx)

POWDER FOR INJECTION: 1 g.

ADMINISTRATION/HANDLING

Alert: May give by IV injection or infusion. Wear gloves when preparing solution (topical contact may be carcinogenic hazard). If powder or solution comes in contact with skin, wash immediately, thoroughly with soap, water. May be carcinogenic, mutagenic, or teratogenic. Handle with extreme care during preparation/administration.

IV

Storage • Refrigerate unopened vials. • Solution appears clear to pale gold. Discard if color changes to dark brown (indicates decomposition). • Discard solution within 12 hrs after reconstitution.

Reconstitution • Reconstitute 1-g vial with 9.5 ml D_5W or 0.9% NaCl to provide concentration of 100 mg/ml. • For IV infusion, further dilute with 10–200 ml D_5W or 0.9% NaCl solution.

Rate of administration • For IV push, administer over 10–15 min. • Infuse piggyback over 15 min–6 hrs. • Extravasation may produce severe tissue necrosis. Apply warm compresses to reduce severity of irritation at IV site.

IV INCOMPATIBILITIES

Allopurinol (Aloprim), aztreonam (Azactam), cefepime (Maxipime), piperacillin/tazobactam (Zosyn).

IV COMPATIBILITIES

Granisetron (Kytril), ondansetron (Zofran).

INDICATIONS/ROUTES/DOSAGE

Alert: Dosage individualized based on clinical response, tolerance to adverse effects. When used in combination therapy, consult specific protocols for optimum dosage, sequence of drug administration. Dosage based on body surface area (BSA).

DAILY

IV: ADULTS, ELDERLY: 500 mg/m^2 of BSA for 5 consecutive days q6wks.

WEEKLY

IV: ADULTS, ELDERLY: Initially, 1 g/m^2 BSA weekly for 2 wks. May increase up to 1.5 g/m^2 BSA.

SIDE EFFECTS

FREQUENT (>90%): Severe nausea, vomiting (usually begins 1–4 hrs after administration; may persist over 24 hrs). **OCCASIONAL:** A burning sensation originating at IV site and moving up arm (occurs particularly with rapid IV injection),

S

diarrhea, confusion, lethargy, depression, particularly in pts receiving continuous IV infusion over 5 days.

ADVERSE REACTIONS/ TOXIC EFFECTS

High incidence of nephrotoxicity manifested by azotemia, anuria, proteinuria, hyperchloremia, hypophosphatemia. Proximal renal tubular acidosis evidenced by glycosuria, acetonuria, aminoaciduria. Mild to moderate bone marrow depression manifested as hematologic toxicity (leukopenia, thrombocytopenia, anemia). Severe myelosuppression, hepatotoxicity occur rarely.

NURSING IMPLICATIONS

BASELINE ASSESSMENT

Phenothiazine antiemetics are only minimally effective in preventing/reducing nausea, vomiting; droperidol, metoclopramide appear to be more effective. Obtain renal function tests, electrolytes, CBC prior to and weekly during therapy. Obtain hepatic function tests before therapy.

INTERVENTION/EVALUATION

Monitor urinalysis, creatinine clearance, BUN, serum creatinine, electrolyte, CBC. (Earliest sign of renal toxicity is mild proteinuria, glycosuria.) Inform physician if urine is positive for proteinuria or if vomiting exceeds 600–800 ml/8 hrs. Monitor for hematologic toxicity (fever, sore throat, signs of local infection, unusual bruising/bleeding from any site), symptoms of anemia (excessive tiredness, weakness).

PATIENT/FAMILY TEACHING

Do not have immunizations without physician's approval (drug lowers body's resistance). Avoid contact with those who have recently received live virus vaccine. Promptly report fever, sore throat, signs of local infection, unusual bruising/bleeding from any site. Increase fluid intake (decreases risk of nephrotoxicity).

succinylcholine chloride

(Anectine, Quelicin)

See Classification section under: Neuromucular blockers **(p. 107C)**

sucralfate

sue-**kral**-fate

(Carafate, Novo-Sucralate✱, Sulcrate✱)

Do not confuse with Cafergot.

CLASSIFICATION

CLINICAL: Antiulcer.

ACTION

Forms an ulcer-adherent complex with proteinaceous exudate (e.g., albumin) at ulcer site. Also forms a viscous, adhesive barrier on surface of intact mucosa of stomach/duodenum. **Therapeutic Effect:** Protects damaged mucosa from further destruction by absorbing gastric acid, pepsin, bile salts.

PHARMACOKINETICS

Minimally absorbed from GI tract. Eliminated in feces with small amount excreted in urine. Not removed by hemodialysis.

S

USES

Short-term treatment (8 wks) of duodenal ulcer. Maintenance therapy of duodenal ulcer after healing of acute ulcers. **Unlabeled:** Treatment of gastric ulcer, rheumatoid arthritis (relieves GI symptoms associated with NSAIDs). Prevention/treatment of stress-related mucosal damage, esp. acutely ill pts; treatment of gastroesophageal reflux.

PRECAUTIONS

CONTRAINDICATIONS: None known. **CAUTIONS:** None known.

LIFESPAN CONSIDERATIONS: Pregnancy/lactation: Unknown if drug crosses placenta or is distributed in breast milk. **Pregnancy Category B. Children:** Safety and efficacy not established. **Elderly:** No age-related precautions noted.

INTERACTIONS

DRUG: Antacids may interfere with binding (do not give within 30 min). May decrease absorption of **digoxin, phenytoin, quinolones (e.g., ciprofloxacin), theophylline** (do not give within 2–3 hrs of sucralfate). **HERBAL:** None known. **FOOD:** None known. **LAB VALUES:** None known.

S

AVAILABILITY (Rx)

TABLETS: 1 g. **ORAL SUSPENSION:** 500 mg/5 ml.

ADMINISTRATION/HANDLING

PO

• Administer 1 hr before meals and at bedtime. • Tablets may be crushed/dissolved in water. • Avoid antacids ½ hr before or after giving sucralfate.

INDICATIONS/ROUTES/DOSAGE

Alert: 1 g = 10 ml suspension.

DUODENAL ULCERS, ACTIVE

PO: ADULTS, ELDERLY: 1 g 4 times/day (before meals and at bedtime) for up to 8 wks.

DUODENAL ULCERS, MAINTENANCE

PO: ADULTS, ELDERLY: 1 g 2 times/day.

SIDE EFFECTS

FREQUENT (2%): Constipation. **OCCASIONAL (<2%):** Dry mouth, backache, diarrhea, dizziness, drowsiness, nausea, indigestion, skin rash/hives/itching, stomach discomfort.

ADVERSE REACTIONS/ TOXIC EFFECTS

None known.

NURSING IMPLICATIONS

INTERVENTION/EVALUATION

Monitor stool consistency, frequency.

PATIENT/FAMILY TEACHING

Take medication on an empty stomach. Antacids may be given as an adjunct but should not be taken for 30 min before or after sucralfate (formation of sucralfate gel is activated by stomach acid). Dry mouth may be relieved by sour hard candy, sips of tepid water.

Sudafed

see pseudoephedrine

sufentanil citrate

(Sufenta)

See Classification section under: Opioid analgesics

sulconazole nitrate

(Exelderm)

See Classification section under: Antifungals: topical

sulfacetamide sodium

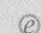

sul-fah-**see**-tah-mide

(AK-Sulf, Bleph-10, Cetamide✤, Diosulf✤, Isopto Cetamide, Sulfair)

◆CLASSIFICATION

PHARMACOTHERAPEUTIC: Sulfonamide. **CLINICAL:** Ophthalmic, topical agent.

ACTION

Interferes with synthesis of folic acid that bacteria require for growth. **Therapeutic Effect:** Prevents further bacterial growth. Bacteriostatic.

USES

Treatment of corneal ulcers, conjunctivitis and other superficial infections of the eye, prophylaxis after injuries to the eye/removal of foreign bodies, adjunctive therapy for trachoma and inclusion conjunctivitis. **Unlabeled:** Treatment of bacterial blepharitis, blepharoconjunctivitis, bacterial keratitis, keratoconjunctivitis.

PRECAUTIONS

CONTRAINDICATIONS: Infants <2 mos, herpes simplex keratitis, varicella, other viral diseases of cornea/conjunctiva, fungal disease. **CAUTIONS:** Severe dry eye, G6PD deficiency. **Pregnancy Category C.**

INTERACTIONS

DRUG: **Silver-containing preparations.** **HERBAL:** None known. **FOOD:** None known. **LAB VALUES:** None known.

AVAILABILITY (Rx)

OPHTHALMIC OINTMENT: 10%. **OPHTHALMIC SOLUTION:** 10%, 15%, 30%.

INDICATIONS/ROUTES/DOSAGE

USUAL OPHTHALMIC DOSAGE

Ophthalmic: ADULTS, ELDERLY, CHILDREN >2 MOS: **Ointment:** Apply small amount in lower conjunctival sac 1–4 times/day and at bedtime. **Solution:** 1–3 drops to lower conjunctival sac q2–3h.

SIDE EFFECTS

FREQUENT: Transient ophthalmic burning, stinging. **OCCASIONAL:** Headache. **RARE:** Hypersensitivity: erythema, rash, itching, swelling, photosensitivity.

ADVERSE REACTIONS/ TOXIC EFFECTS

Superinfection, drug-induced lupus erythematosus, Stevens-Johnson syndrome occur rarely.

NURSING IMPLICATIONS

BASELINE ASSESSMENT

Question for hypersensitivity to sulfonamides, any ingredients of preparation (e.g., sulfite).

INTERVENTION/EVALUATION

Withhold medication, notify physician at once of hypersensitivity reaction (redness, itching, urticaria, rash). Assess for fever, joint pain, ulcers in mouth—hold drug, inform physician.

PATIENT/FAMILY TEACHING

May have transient burning, stinging upon ophthalmic application; may cause sensitivity to light; wear sunglasses, avoid bright light. Notify physi-

S

cian of **any** new symptom, esp. swelling, itching, rash, joint pain, fever.

sulfasalazine

sul-fah-**sal**-ah-zeen
(Azulfidine, Azulfidine EN-tabs, Salazopyrin*, SAS-500*)

Do not confuse with azathioprine, sulfadiazine, sulfisoxazole.

CLASSIFICATION

PHARMACOTHERAPEUTIC: Sulfonamide. **CLINICAL:** Anti-inflammatory.

ACTION

Inhibits prostaglandin synthesis. Acts locally in colon. **Therapeutic Effect:** Decreases inflammatory response, interferes with secretion. Effect may be result of antibacterial action with change in intestinal flora.

PHARMACOKINETICS

Poorly absorbed from GI tract. Cleaved in colon by intestinal bacterial forming sulfapyridine and mesalamine (5-ASA). Absorbed in colon. Widely distributed. Metabolized in liver. Primarily excreted in urine. **Half-life:** sulfapyridine: 6–14 hrs; 5-ASA: 0.6–1.4 hrs.

S

USES

Treatment of ulcerative colitis, inflammatory bowel disease, rheumatoid arthritis. **Unlabeled:** Treatment of ankylosing spondylitis.

PRECAUTIONS

CONTRAINDICATIONS: Hypersensitivity to salicylates, sulfonamides, sulfonylureas, thiazide or loop diuretics, carbonic anhydrase inhibitors, sunscreens containing PABA, local anesthetics, pregnancy at term, severe hepatic/renal dysfunction, porphyria, intestinal/urinary tract obstruction, children <2 yrs. **CAUTIONS:** Severe allergies, bronchial asthma, impaired hepatic/renal function, G6PD deficiency.

LIFESPAN CONSIDERATIONS: Pregnancy/lactation: May produce infertility, oligospermia in men while on medication. Readily crosses placenta; if given near term, may produce jaundice, hemolytic anemia, kernicterus. Excreted in breast milk. Do not breast-feed premature infant or those with hyperbilirubinemia or G6PD deficiency. **Pregnancy Category B (D** if given near term). **Children/elderly:** No age-related precautions noted in those >2 yrs.

INTERACTIONS

DRUG: May increase effects of **oral anticoagulants, anticonvulsants, oral hypoglycemics, methotrexate. Hemolytics** may increase toxicity. **Hepatotoxic medications** may increase hepatotoxicity. **HERBAL:** None known. **FOOD:** None known. **LAB VALUES:** None known.

AVAILABILITY (Rx)

TABLETS (Azulfidine): 500 mg. **TABLETS (delayed-release) (Azulfidine EN-Tabs):** 500 mg.

ADMINISTRATION/HANDLING

PO

- Space doses evenly (intervals not to exceed 8 hrs).
- Administer after meals if possible (prolong intestinal passage).
- Swallow enteric-coated tablets whole; do not chew.
- Give with 8 oz of water; encourage several glasses of water between meals.

INDICATIONS/ROUTES/DOSAGE

ULCERATIVE COLITIS

PO: ADULTS, ELDERLY: 1 g 3–4 times/day in divided doses q4–6h. **Maximum:** 6 g/day. MAINTENANCE: 2 g/day in divided doses q6–12h. CHILDREN: 40–75 mg/kg/day in divided doses q4–6h.

Maximum: 6 g/day. MAINTENANCE: 30–50 mg/kg/day in divided doses q4–8h. **Maximum:** 2 g/day.

RHEUMATOID ARTHRITIS

PO: ADULTS, ELDERLY: Initially, 0.5–1 g/day for 1 wk. Increase by 0.5 g/wk, up to 3 g/day.

JUVENILE RHEUMATOID ARTHRITIS

PO: CHILDREN: Initially, 10 mg/kg/day. May increase by 10 mg/kg/day at weekly intervals. RANGE: 30–50 mg/kg/day. **Maximum:** 2 g/day.

SIDE EFFECTS

FREQUENT (33%): Anorexia, nausea, vomiting, headache, oligospermia (generally reversed by withdrawal of drug). **OCCASIONAL (3%):** Hypersensitivity reaction: rash, urticaria, pruritus, fever, anemia. **RARE (<1%):** Tinnitus, hypoglycemia, diuresis, photosensitivity.

ADVERSE REACTIONS/ TOXIC EFFECTS

Anaphylaxis, Stevens-Johnson syndrome, hematologic toxicity (leukopenia, agranulocytosis); hepatotoxicity, nephrotoxicity occur rarely.

NURSING IMPLICATIONS

BASELINE ASSESSMENT

Question for hypersensitivity to medications (see Contraindications). Check initial urinalysis, CBC, hepatic/renal function tests.

INTERVENTION/EVALUATION

Monitor I&O, urinalysis, renal function tests; ensure adequate hydration (minimum output 1,500 ml/24 hr) to prevent nephrotoxicity. Assess skin for rash (discontinue drug/notify physician at first sign). Check pattern of bowel activity, stool consistency (dosage may need to be increased if diarrhea continues/recurs). Monitor CBC closely; assess for/report immediately hematologic effects: bleeding, bruising, fever, sore throat, pallor, weakness, purpura, jaundice.

PATIENT/FAMILY TEACHING

May cause orange-yellow discoloration of urine, skin. Space doses evenly around the clock. Take after food with 8 oz of water; drink several glasses of water between meals. Continue for full length of treatment; may be necessary to take drug even after symptoms relieved. Follow-up, lab tests are essential. In event of dental/other surgery inform dentist/surgeon of sulfasalazine therapy. Avoid exposure to sun, ultraviolet light until photosensitivity determined (may last for months after last dose).

sulindac

suel-**in**-dak

(Apo-Sulin✤, Clinoril, Novo Sundac✤)

Do not confuse with Clozaril.

◆ CLASSIFICATION

PHARMACOTHERAPEUTIC: Nonsteroidal anti-inflammatory. **CLINICAL:** Anti-inflammatory, antigout (see p. 111C).

ACTION

Produces analgesic, anti-inflammatory effect by inhibiting prostaglandin synthesis. **Therapeutic Effect:** Reduces inflammatory response, intensity of pain stimulus reaching sensory nerve endings.

PHARMACOKINETICS

Onset	Peak	Duration
PO (antirheumatic)		
7 days	2–3 wks	—

Well absorbed from GI tract. Metabolized in liver to active metabolite. Primarily excreted in urine. Not removed by hemodialysis. **Half-life:** 7.8 hrs; metabolite: 16.4 hrs.

USES

Treatment of pain of rheumatoid arthritis, osteoarthritis, ankylosing spondylitis, acute painful shoulder, bursitis/tendinitis, acute gouty arthritis.

PRECAUTIONS

CONTRAINDICATIONS: Active peptic ulcer, GI ulceration, chronic inflammation of GI tract, GI bleeding disorders, history of hypersensitivity to aspirin/NSAIDs, concurrent anticoagulant use. **CAUTIONS:** Impaired renal/hepatic function, history of GI tract disease, predisposition to fluid retention.

LIFESPAN CONSIDERATIONS: Pregnancy/lactation: Unknown if drug is excreted in breast milk. Avoid use during third trimester (may adversely affect fetal cardiovascular system: premature closure of ductus arteriosus). **Pregnancy Category B** (**D** if used in third trimester or near delivery). **Children:** Safety and efficacy not established. **Elderly:** GI bleeding/ulceration more likely to cause serious adverse effects. Age-related renal impairment may increase risk of liver/renal toxicity; lower dosage recommended.

INTERACTIONS

DRUG: May increase effects of **oral anticoagulants, heparin, thrombolytics.** May decrease effect of **antihypertensives, diuretics. Salicylates, aspirin** may increase risk of GI side effects, bleeding. **Bone marrow depressants** may increase risk of hematologic reactions. May increase concentration, toxicity of **lithium.** May increase toxicity of **methotrexate. Probenecid** may increase concentration. **Antacids** may decrease concentration. **HERBAL: Ginkgo biloba** may increase risk of bleeding. May reduce effects of **feverfew. FOOD:** None known. **LAB VALUES:** May increase alkaline phosphatase, liver function tests.

AVAILABILITY (Rx)

TABLETS: 150 mg, 200 mg.

ADMINISTRATION/HANDLING

PO

- Give with food, milk, antacids if GI distress occurs.

INDICATIONS/ROUTES/DOSAGE

RHEUMATOID ARTHRITIS, OSTEOARTHRITIS, ANKYLOSING SPONDYLITIS

PO: ADULTS, ELDERLY: Initially, 150 mg 2 times/day, up to 400 mg/day.

ACUTE PAINFUL SHOULDER, GOUTY ARTHRITIS, BURSITIS, TENDINITIS

PO: ADULTS, ELDERLY: 200 mg 2 times/day.

SIDE EFFECTS

FREQUENT (3%–9%): Diarrhea/constipation, indigestion, nausea, maculopapular rash, dermatitis, dizziness, headache. **OCCASIONAL (1%–3%):** Anorexia, GI cramps, flatulence.

ADVERSE REACTIONS/ TOXIC EFFECTS

GI bleeding, peptic ulcer occur infrequently. Nephrotoxicity (glomerular nephritis, interstitial nephritis, nephrotic syndrome) may occur in pts with preexisting impaired renal function. Acute hypersensitivity reaction (fever, chills, joint pain) occurs rarely.

NURSING IMPLICATIONS

BASELINE ASSESSMENT

Assess onset, type, location, duration of pain, fever, inflammation. Inspect appearance of affected joints for immobility, deformities, skin condition.

INTERVENTION/EVALUATION

Assist with ambulation if dizziness occurs. Monitor pattern of daily bowel activity, stool consistency. Assess for evidence of rash. Evaluate for therapeutic response: relief of pain, stiffness, swelling; increase in joint mobility; reduced joint tenderness; improved grip strength. Monitor renal/liver function, CBC, platelets.

PATIENT/FAMILY TEACHING

Therapeutic antiarthritic effect noted 1–3 wks after therapy begins. Avoid aspirin, alcohol during therapy (increases risk of GI bleeding). If GI upset occurs, take with food, milk.

sumatriptan

sue-mah-**trip**-tan
(Imitrex)
Do not confuse with somatropin.

CLASSIFICATION

PHARMACOTHERAPEUTIC: Serotonin receptor agonist. **CLINICAL:** Antimigraine (see p. 54C).

ACTION

Binds selectively to serotonin (5-HT) receptor in cranial arteries. **Therapeutic Effect:** Causes vasoconstriction, reduces inflammation, relieves migraine.

PHARMACOKINETICS

	Onset	Peak	Duration
Subcutaneous	<10 min	<2 hrs	—
PO	1–1.5 hrs	2–4 hrs	—

Rapidly absorbed following subcutaneous administration. Widely distributed, protein binding: 10%–21% undergoes first-pass hepatic metabolism; excreted in urine. **Half-life:** 2 hrs.

USES

Acute treatment of migraine headache with or without aura; treatment of cluster headaches.

PRECAUTIONS

CONTRAINDICATIONS: Ischemic heart disease, Prinzmetal angina, stroke, TIA, severe liver impairment, uncontrolled hypertension, concomitant use of ergotamine medications, vasoconstrictive medications, MAOIs within 14 days. **CAUTIONS:** Liver/renal impairment, epilepsy, hypersensitivity to sulfonamides.

LIFESPAN CONSIDERATIONS: Pregnancy/lactation: Unknown if distributed in breast milk. **Pregnancy Category C. Children:** Safety and efficacy not established. **Elderly:** No age-related precautions noted.

INTERACTIONS

DRUG: Ergotamine-containing drugs may produce vasospastic reaction. **MAOIs** may increase concentration, half-life. **HERBAL:** None known. **FOOD:** None known. **LAB VALUES:** None known.

AVAILABILITY (Rx)

TABLETS: 25 mg, 50 mg, 100 mg. **INJECTION:** 6 mg/0.5 ml. **NASAL SPRAY:** 5 mg, 20 mg.

S

ADMINISTRATION/HANDLING

PO

• Swallow tablets whole. • Take with full glass of water.

NASAL

• Unit contains only one spray—do not test before use. • Gently blow nose to clear nasal passages. • With head upright, close one nostril with index finger. Breathe out gently through mouth. • Insert nozzle into open nostril about ½ inch. • Close mouth, and while taking a breath through nose, release spray dos-

age by firmly pressing the blue plunger.
• Remove nozzle from nose and gently breathe in through nose and out through mouth for 10–20 sec. Do not breathe in deeply.

SUBCUTANEOUS

• Follow pt instructions provided by manufacturer using autoinjection device.

INDICATIONS/ROUTES/DOSAGE

VASCULAR HEADACHE

Subcutaneous: ADULTS, ELDERLY: 6 mg. **Maximum:** No more than two 6-mg injections within a 24-hr period separated by at least 1 hr between injections.

PO: ADULTS, ELDERLY: 25–50 mg. **Maximum single dose:** 100 mg. May repeat no sooner than 2 hrs. **Maximum:** 200 mg/24 hrs.

Nasal: ADULTS, ELDERLY: 5–20 mg; may repeat in 2 hrs. **Maximum:** 40 mg/24 hrs.

SIDE EFFECTS

FREQUENT: Oral (5%–10%): Tingling, nasal discomfort. **Subcutaneous (>10%):** Injection site reactions, tingling, warm/hot sensation, dizziness, vertigo. **Nasal (>10%):** Bad/unusual taste, nausea, vomiting. **OCCASIONAL: Oral (1%–5%):** Flushing, weakness, visual disturbances. **Subcutaneous (2%–10%):** Burning sensation, numbness, chest discomfort, drowsiness, weakness. **Nasal (1%–5%):** Discomfort of nasal cavity/throat, dizziness. **RARE: Oral (<1%):** Agitation, eye irritation, dysuria. **Subcutaneous (<2%):** Anxiety, fatigue, sweating, muscle cramps, muscle pain. **Nasal (<1%):** Burning sensation.

ADVERSE REACTIONS/ TOXIC EFFECTS

Excessive dosage may produce tremor, redness of extremities, reduced respirations, cyanosis, convulsions, paralysis. Serious arrhythmias occur rarely, but particularly in those with hypertension, obesity, smokers, diabetics, and those with strong family history of coronary artery disease.

NURSING IMPLICATIONS

BASELINE ASSESSMENT

Question for history of peripheral vascular disease, renal/hepatic impairment, possibility of pregnancy. Question regarding onset, location, duration of migraine and possible precipitating symptoms.

INTERVENTION/EVALUATION

Evaluate for relief of migraine headache and resulting photophobia, phonophobia (sound sensitivity), nausea, vomiting.

PATIENT/FAMILY TEACHING

Teach pt proper loading of autoinjector, injection technique, and discarding of syringe. Do not use >2 injections during any 24-hr period and allow at least 1 hr between injections. If wheezing, heart throbbing, skin rash, swelling of eyelids/face/lips, pain/tightness in chest or throat occurs, contact physician immediately.

Synthroid

see levothyroxine

tacrine hydrochloride

tay-crin
(Cognex)

◆ CLASSIFICATION

PHARMACOTHERAPEUTIC: Cholinesterase inhibitor. **CLINICAL:** Antidementia.

S

ACTION

Elevates acetylcholine concentrations in cerebral cortex by slowing degeneration of acetylcholine released by still intact cholinergic neurons (Alzheimer's disease involves degeneration of cholinergic neuronal pathways). **Therapeutic Effect:** Resultant effect slows Alzheimer's disease process.

USES

Symptomatic treatment of pts with Alzheimer's disease.

PRECAUTIONS

CONTRAINDICATIONS: Known hypersensitivity to cholinergics; current treatment with other cholinesterase inhibitors; active liver disease, active or untreated gastric/duodenal ulcers, mechanical obstruction of intestine/urinary tract, pregnancy, breast-feeding, or childbearing potential. **CAUTIONS:** Known hepatic dysfunction, asthma, COPD, seizure disorders, bradycardia, hyperthyroidism, cardiac arrhythmias, history of gastric/intestinal ulcers, alcohol abuse. **Pregnancy Category C.**

INTERACTIONS

DRUG: May increase **theophylline** concentration. **Cimetidine** may increase tacrine concentration. May interfere with **anticholinergics.** May increase adverse effects of **NSAIDs. HERBAL:** None known. **FOOD:** None known. **LAB VALUES:** Increases SGOT (AST), SGPT (ALT). Alters Hgb, Hct, electrolytes.

AVAILABILITY (Rx)

CAPSULES: 10 mg, 20 mg, 30 mg, 40 mg.

ADMINISTRATION/HANDLING

PO

- Give without regard to food.

INDICATIONS/ROUTES/DOSAGE

ALZHEIMER'S DISEASE

PO: ADULTS, ELDERLY: Initially, 10 mg 4 times/day for 6 wks; then 20 mg 4 times/day for 6 wks; then 30 mg 4 times/day for 12 wks; then to maximum of 40 mg 4 times/day if needed.

DOSAGE IN HEPATIC IMPAIRMENT

ALT >3 to 5 times normal: Decrease dose by 40 mg/day. Resume when ALT returns to normal.

ALT >5 times normal: Stop treatment, restart when ALT returns to normal.

Alert: If medication is stopped for >14 days, must retitrate as noted above.

SIDE EFFECTS

FREQUENT (11%–28%): Headache, nausea, vomiting, diarrhea, dizziness. **OCCASIONAL (4%–9%):** Fatigue, chest pain, dyspepsia, anorexia, abdominal pain, flatulence, constipation, confusion, agitation, rash, depression, ataxia (muscular incoordination), insomnia, rhinitis, myalgia. **RARE (<3%):** Weight loss, anxiety, cough, facial flushing, urinary frequency, back pain, tremor.

ADVERSE REACTIONS/ TOXIC EFFECTS

Overdose can cause cholinergic crisis (increased salivation, lacrimation, urination, defecation, bradycardia, hypotension, increased muscle weakness). Treatment aimed at general supportive measures, use of anticholinergics (e.g., atropine).

NURSING IMPLICATIONS

BASELINE ASSESSMENT

Assess cognitive, behavioral, functional deficits of pt. Assess hepatic function.

INTERVENTION/EVALUATION

Monitor cognitive, behavioral, functional status of pt. Monitor SGOT (AST), SGPT (ALT). EKG evaluation,

S

periodic rhythm strips in pts with underlying arrhythmias. Monitor for symptoms of ulcer, GI bleeding.

PATIENT/FAMILY TEACHING

Take at regular intervals, between meals (may take with meals if GI upset occurs). Do not reduce or stop medication; do not increase dosage without physician direction. Do not smoke (reduces plasma concentration of tacrine). Inform family of local chapter of Alzheimer's Disease Association (provides a guide to services for these pts).

tacrolimus

tack-row-**lee**-mus
(Prograf, Protopic)

◆ CLASSIFICATION

PHARMACOTHERAPEUTIC: Immunologic agent. **CLINICAL:** Immunosuppressant (see p. 102C).

ACTION

Binds to intracellular protein, forming a complex, inhibiting phosphatase activity. Inhibits T-lymphocyte activation. **Therapeutic Effect:** Suppresses immunologically mediated inflammatory response. Assists in preventing organ transplant rejection.

S

PHARMACOKINETICS

Variably absorbed following PO administration (food reduces absorption). Protein binding: 75%–97%. Extensively metabolized in the liver. Excreted in urine. Not removed by hemodialysis. **Half-life:** 11.7 hrs.

USES

Prophylaxis of organ rejection in pts receiving allogeneic liver transplants, kidney transplants. Should be used concurrently with adrenal corticosteroids. **Topical:** Atopic dermatitis. **Unlabeled:** Prophylaxis of organ rejection in pts receiving allogeneic bone marrow, cardiac, pancreas, pancreatic island cell, and small bowel transplantation. Treatment of autoimmune disease, severe recalcitrant psoriasis.

PRECAUTIONS

CONTRAINDICATIONS: Hypersensitivity to tacrolimus, hypersensitivity to HCO-60 polyoxyl 60 hydrogenated castor oil (used in vehicle for injection), concurrent use with cyclosporine (increased risk of ototoxicity). **CAUTIONS:** Immunosuppressed pts, renal/hepatic function impairment.

LIFESPAN CONSIDERATIONS: Pregnancy/lactation: Crosses placenta. Neonatal hyperkalemia, renal dysfunction noted in neonates. Excreted in breast milk. Avoid breast-feeding. **Pregnancy Category C. Children:** May require higher dosages (decreased bioavailability, increased clearance). May make post-transplant lymphoproliferative disorder more common (esp. those <3 yrs). **Elderly:** Age-related renal impairment may require dosage adjustment.

INTERACTIONS

DRUG: Aminoglycosides, amphotericin B, cisplatin increase risk of renal dysfunction. **Cyclosporine** increases risk of nephrotoxicity. **Antifungals, bromocriptine, calcium channel blockers, cimetidine, clarithromycin, cyclosporine, danazol, diltiazem, erythromycin, methylprednisolone, metoclopramide** increase tacrolimus blood levels. **Carbamazepine, phenobarbital, phenytoin, rifamycins** decrease tacrolimus blood levels. **Other immunosuppressants** may increase risk of infection or development of lymphomas. **Live virus**

vaccines may potentiate virus replication, increase vaccine side effects, decrease pt's antibody response to vaccine. **HERBAL: Echinacea** may decrease effects. **FOOD:** None known. **LAB VALUES:** May increase creatinine, BUN, WBCs, glucose. May decrease thrombocytes, RBCs, magnesium. Alters potassium level.

AVAILABILITY (Rx)

CAPSULES: 0.5 mg, 1 mg, 5 mg. **INJECTION:** 5 mg/ml. **OINTMENT:** 0.03%, 0.1%.

ADMINISTRATION/HANDLING

PO

• Administer on empty stomach. • Use polyethylene oral syringe or glass container when giving (avoid plastic). • Do not give with grapefruit/grapefruit juice or within 2 hrs of antacids.

TOPICAL

• For external use only. • Do not cover with occlusive dressing. • Rub in gently and completely onto clean, dry skin.

IV

Storage • Store diluted infusion solution in glass or polyethylene containers and discard after 24 hrs. • Do not store in a PVC container (decreased stability, potential for extraction).

Reconstitution • Dilute with an appropriate amount (250–1,000 ml, depending on desired dose) 0.9% NaCl or D_5W to provide a concentration between 0.004 and 0.02 mg/ml.

Rate of administration • Give as continuous IV infusion. • Continuously monitor pt for anaphylaxis for at least 30 min after start of infusion. • Stop infusion immediately at first sign of hypersensitivity reaction.

∅ IV INCOMPATIBILITY

No known specific drug incompatibilities. Do not mix with other medications if possible (see IV Compatibilities).

IV COMPATIBILITIES

Calcium gluconate, dexamethasone (Decadron), diphenhydramine (Benadryl), dobutamine (Dobutrex), dopamine (Intropin), furosemide (Lasix), heparin, hydromorphone (Dilaudid), insulin, leucovorin, lorazepam (Ativan), morphine, nitroglycerin, potassium chloride.

INDICATIONS/ROUTES/DOSAGE

Alert: In pts unable to take capsules, initiate therapy with IV infusion. Give oral dose 8–12 hrs after discontinuing IV infusion. Titrate dosing based on clinical assessments of rejection and tolerability. In pts with hepatic/renal function impairment, give lowest IV and oral dosing range (delay dosing up to 48 hrs or longer in pts with postop oliguria).

TRANSPLANT REJECTION

IV infusion: ADULTS, ELDERLY: 0.03–0.1 mg/kg/day. CHILDREN: 0.03–0.15 mg/kg/day.

PO: ADULTS, ELDERLY: 0.15–0.3 mg/kg/day in 2 divided doses 12 hrs apart. CHILDREN: 0.15–0.4 mg/kg/day in 2 divided doses 12 hrs apart.

PEDIATRIC DOSAGE (without preexisting renal/hepatic dysfunction)

IV infusion: 0.05–1.5 mg/kg/day.

PO: 0.3 mg/kg/day.

ATOPIC DERMATITIS

Topical: ADULTS, ELDERLY, CHILDREN ≥2 YRS: 0.03% ointment to affected area 2 times/day. Continue for 1 wk after symptoms have cleared.

SIDE EFFECTS

FREQUENT (>30%): Headache, tremor, insomnia, paresthesia, diarrhea, nausea, constipation, vomiting, abdominal pain, hypertension. **OCCASIONAL (10%–29%):** Rash, pruritus, anorexia, asthenia, peripheral edema, photosensitivity.

T

ADVERSE REACTIONS/ TOXIC EFFECTS

Nephrotoxicity, pleural effusion occur frequently. Overt nephrotoxicity characterized by increasing serum creatinine, decrease in urine output. Thrombocytopenia, leukocytosis, anemia, atelectasis occur occasionally. Neurotoxicity, including tremor, headache, mental status changes, occur commonly. Sepsis, infection occur occasionally. Significant anemia, thrombocytopenia, leukocytosis may occur.

NURSING IMPLICATIONS

BASELINE ASSESSMENT

Assess medical history, esp. renal function, and drug history, esp. other immunosuppressants. Have aqueous solution of epinephrine 1:1,000 available at bedside as well as O_2 prior to beginning IV infusion. Assess pt continuously for first 30 min following start of infusion and at frequent intervals thereafter.

INTERVENTION/EVALUATION

Closely monitor pts with impaired renal function. Monitor lab values, esp. serum creatinine, serum potassium levels, CBC with differential, hepatic function tests. Monitor I&O closely. CBC should be performed weekly during first month of therapy, twice monthly during second and third months of treatment, then monthly throughout the first year. Report any major change in assessment of pt.

PATIENT/FAMILY TEACHING

Take dose at same time each day. Avoid crowds, those with infection. Inform physician if decreased urination, chest pain, headache, dizziness, respiratory infection, rash, unusual bleeding/bruising occurs. Avoid exposure to sun, artificial light (may cause photosensitivity reaction).

tadalafil

tah-**dal**-ah-fil
(Cialis)

◆ CLASSIFICATION

PHARMACOTHERAPEUTIC: Phosphodiesterase inhibitor. **CLINICAL:** Erectile dysfunction adjunct.

ACTION

Increases cyclic guanosine monophosphate in smooth muscle cells by inhibiting a specific enzyme, phosphodiesterase type 5, the predominant isoenzyme in human corpus cavernosum in the penis. **Therapeutic Effect:** Relaxes smooth muscle, increases blood flow, resulting in penile rigidity.

PHARMACOKINETCS

	Onset	Peak	Duration
PO	16 min	2 hrs	36 hrs

Rapidly absorbed following PO administration. No effect on penile blood flow without sexual stimulation. **Half-life:** 17.5 hours.

USES

Treatment of erectile dysfunction.

PRECAUTIONS

CONTRAINDICATIONS: Pts concurrently using sodium nitroprusside or nitrates in any form (potentiates hypotensive effects of these medications), any alpha-blocker other than 0.4 mg once daily tamsulosin, severe hepatic impairment. **CAUTIONS:** Renal/hepatic function impairment, anatomical deformation of the penis, pts who may be predisposed to priapism (sickle cell anemia, multiple myeloma, leukemia).

LIFESPAN CONSIDERATIONS: Elderly: No age-related precautions noted.

T

INTERACTIONS

DRUG: **Ritonavir, indinivir, erythromycin, itraconazole, ketoconazole** may increase tadalafil concentration. Potentiates hypotensive effects of **nitrates** (contraindicated). **Doxazosin** may produce additive hypotensive effect. **Alcohol** increases potential for postural hypotension. **HERBAL:** None known. **FOOD:** None known. **LAB VALUES:** None known.

AVAILABILITY (Rx)

TABLETS: 5 mg, 10 mg, 20 mg.

ADMINISTRATION/HANDLING

PO

- May give without regard to food. Do not crush/break film-coated tablets.

INDICATIONS/ROUTES/DOSAGE

ERECTILE DYSFUNCTION

PO: ADULTS, ELDERLY: 10 mg prior to sexual activity. Dose may be increased to 20 mg or decreased to 5 mg, based on tolerability. Maximum dosing frequency is once daily.

MODERATE RENAL FUNCTION IMPAIRMENT (Ccr 31–50 ml/min)

PO: ADULTS, ELDERLY: 5 mg prior to sexual activity. **Maximum dose:** 10 mg not more than once every 48 hrs.

MILD OR MODERATE HEPATIC FUNCTION IMPAIRMENT (Child-Pugh class A or B)

PO: ADULTS, ELDERLY: No more than 10 mg once daily.

SIDE EFFECTS

OCCASIONAL: Headache, dyspepsia (heartburn, indigestion, epigastric pain), back pain, myalgia, nasal congestion, flushing.

ADVERSE REACTIONS/ TOXIC EFFECTS

Prolonged erections (over 4 hrs), priapism (painful erections over 6 hrs in duration) occur rarely.

NURSING IMPLICATIONS

BASELINE ASSESSMENT

Assess cardiovascular status prior to initiating treatment for erectile dysfunction.

PATIENT/FAMILY TEACHING

Has no effect in the absence of sexual stimulation. Seek treatment immediately if an erection persists for over 4 hrs.

Tagamet

see cimetidine

tamoxifen citrate

tam-**ox**-ih-fen

(Apo-Tamox ✤, Istubol, Nolvadex, Nolvadex-D ✤, Novo-Tamoxifen ✤, Tamofen ✤, Tamone ✤)

◆ CLASSIFICATION

PHARMACOTHERAPEUTIC: Nonsteroidal antiestrogen. **CLINICAL:** Antineoplastic (see p. 76C).

ACTION

Competes with estradiol for binding to estrogen in tissues containing high concentration of receptors (e.g., breasts, uterus, vagina). **Therapeutic Effect:** Reduces DNA synthesis, inhibits estrogen response.

PHARMACOKINETICS

Well absorbed from GI tract. Metabolized in liver. Primarily eliminated in feces via biliary system. **Half-life:** 7 days.

USES

Treatment of metastatic breast carcinoma in women/men. Effective in delaying recurrence after total mastectomy and axil-

T

lary dissection or segmental mastectomy, axillary dissection and breast irradiation in women with axillary node-negative breast carcinoma. Prevention of breast cancer in high-risk women. **Unlabeled:** Induction of ovulation.

PRECAUTIONS

CONTRAINDICATIONS: None known. **CAUTIONS:** Leukopenia, thrombocytopenia.

LIFESPAN CONSIDERATIONS: Pregnancy/lactation: If possible, avoid use during pregnancy, esp. first trimester. May cause fetal harm. Unknown if distributed in breast milk. Breast-feeding not recommended. **Pregnancy Category D. Children:** Safe and effective in girls 2–10 yrs with McCune Albright syndrome and precocius puberty. **Elderly:** No age-related precautions noted.

INTERACTIONS

DRUG: Estrogens may decrease effect. **HERBAL:** None known. **FOOD:** None known. **LAB VALUES:** May increase calcium, cholesterol, triglycerides.

AVAILABILITY (Rx)

TABLETS: 10 mg, 20 mg.

ADMINISTRATION/HANDLING

PO

- Give without regard to food.

INDICATIONS/ROUTES/DOSAGE

BREAST CANCER

PO: ADULTS, ELDERLY: 20–40 mg/day. Give doses >20 mg/day in divided doses.

PREVENTION OF BREAST CANCER

PO: ADULTS, ELDERLY: 20 mg/day.

SIDE EFFECTS

FREQUENT: Women (>10%): Hot flashes, nausea, vomiting. **OCCASIONAL: Women (1%–9%):** Changes in menstrual period, genital itching, vaginal discharge, endometrial hyperplasia/polyps. **Males:** Impotence, decreased libido. **Men/women:** Headache, nausea, vomiting, rash, bone pain, confusion, weakness, sleepiness.

ADVERSE REACTIONS/ TOXIC EFFECTS

Retinopathy, corneal opacity, decreased visual acuity noted in pts receiving extremely high dosages (240–320 mg/day) for >17 mos.

NURSING IMPLICATIONS

BASELINE ASSESSMENT

An estrogen receptor assay should be done before therapy is begun. CBC, platelet count, serum calcium levels should be checked prior to and periodically during therapy.

INTERVENTION/EVALUATION

Be alert to increased bone pain and ensure adequate pain relief. Monitor I&O, weight. Observe for edema, esp. of dependent areas. Assess for hypercalcemia (increased urine volume, excessive thirst, nausea, vomiting, constipation, hypotonicity of muscles, deep bone/flank pain, renal stones).

PATIENT/FAMILY TEACHING

Report vaginal bleeding/discharge/itching, leg cramps, weight gain, shortness of breath, weakness. May initially experience increase in bone, tumor pain (appears to indicate good tumor response). Contact physician if nausea/vomiting continues at home. Nonhormonal contraceptives are recommended during treatment.

tamsulosin hydrochloride

tam-sul-**owe**-sin

(Flomax)

Do not confuse with Fosamax, Volmax.

CLASSIFICATION

PHARMACOTHERAPEUTIC: Alpha$_1$-adrenergic blocker. **CLINICAL:** Benign prostatic hyperplasia agent.

ACTION

An alpha$_1$ antagonist, targets receptors around bladder neck and prostate capsule. **Therapeutic Effect:** Results in relaxation of smooth muscle with improvement in urinary flow, symptoms of prostate hyperplasia.

PHARMACOKINETICS

Well absorbed following PO administration. Protein binding: 94%–99%. Widely distributed. Metabolized in liver. Primarily excreted in urine. Unknown if removed by hemodialysis. **Half-life:** 9–13 hrs.

USES

Treatment of symptoms of benign prostatic hyperplasia.

PRECAUTIONS

CONTRAINDICATIONS: History of sensitivity to tamsulosin. **CAUTIONS:** Renal function impairment.

LIFESPAN CONSIDERATIONS: Pregnancy/lactation: Not indicated for use in women. **Pregnancy Category B. Children:** Not indicated in this pt population. **Elderly:** No age-related precautions noted.

INTERACTIONS

DRUG: Other **alpha-adrenergic blocking agents (prazosin, cimetidine, terazosin, doxazosin)** may have additive effect. May alter effects of **warfarin. HERBAL:** None known. **FOOD:** None known. **LAB VALUES:** None known.

AVAILABILITY (Rx)

CAPSULES: 0.4 mg.

ADMINISTRATION/HANDLING

PO

• Give at the same time each day, 30 min after the same meal. • Do not crush/open capsule unless directed by physician.

INDICATIONS/ROUTES/DOSAGE

BENIGN PROSTATIC HYPERTROPHY

PO: ADULTS: 0.4 mg once daily, approx. 30 min after same meal each day. May increase dosage if inadequate response in 2–4 wks.

SIDE EFFECTS

FREQUENT: (7%–9%): Dizziness, drowsiness. **OCCASIONAL (3%–5%):** Headache, anxiety, insomnia, postural hypotension. **RARE (<2%):** Nasal congestion, pharyngitis, rhinitis, nausea, vertigo, impotence.

ADVERSE REACTIONS/TOXIC EFFECTS

First-dose syncope (hypotension with sudden LOC) may occur 30–90 min after giving initial dose. May be preceded by tachycardia (120–160 beats/min).

NURSING IMPLICATIONS

BASELINE ASSESSMENT

Question for sensitivity to tamsulosin, use of other alpha-adrenergic blocking agents, warfarin.

INTERVENTION/EVALUATION

Assist with ambulation if dizziness occurs. Monitor renal function, B/P.

PATIENT/FAMILY TEACHING

Take at the same time each day, 30 min after the same meal. Use caution when getting up from sitting or lying position. Avoid tasks that require alertness, motor skills until response to drug is established. Do not chew, crush, open capsule.

T

Taxol

see paclitaxel

Taxotere

see docetaxel

tazarotene

tay-zah-**row**-teen
(Avage, Tazorac)

CLASSIFICATION

PHARMACOTHERAPEUTIC: Retinoid. **CLINICAL:** Antipsoriasis, antiacne.

ACTION

Modulates differentiation/proliferation of epithelial tissue; binds selectively to retinoic acid receptors. **Therapeutic Effect:** Restores normal differentiation of the epidermis, reduces epidermal inflammation.

USES

Treatment of stable plaque psoriasis in pts with at least 20% body surface area involvement. Treatment of mild to moderate facial acne.

T

AVAILABILITY (Rx)

GEL: Acne: 0.1% gel. **Psoriasis:** 0.05% gel. **CREAM:** 0.05%, 0.1%.

INDICATIONS/ROUTES/DOSAGE

ACNE

Topical: ADULTS, ELDERLY, CHILDREN >12 YRS: *(Cream, gel 0.1%):* Cleanse face. After skin is dry, apply thin film once daily in the evening.

PSORIASIS

Topical: ADULTS, ELDERLY, CHILDREN >12 YRS: *(Gel 0.05%, 0.1%):* Apply once daily in evening (no more than 20% of body surface area). ADULTS, ELDERLY: *(Cream 0.05%, 0.1%):* Apply once daily in evening (no more than 20% of body surface area).

SIDE EFFECTS

FREQUENT (10%–30%): Acne: Desquamation, burning/stinging, dry skin, itching, erythema. **Psoriasis:** Itching, burning/stinging, erythema, worsening of psoriasis, irritation, skin pain. **OCCASIONAL (1%–9%): Acne:** Irritation, skin pain, fissuring, localized edema, skin discoloration. **Psoriasis:** Rash, desquamation, contact dermatitis, skin inflammation, fissuring, bleeding, dry skin.

NURSING IMPLICATIONS

BASELINE ASSESSMENT

Assess for sensitivity to tazarotene. Determine whether pt is taking medications that may increase risk of photosensitivity (e.g., sulfa, fluoroquinolones).

INTERVENTION/EVALUATION

Monitor for improvement of psoriasis, acne. Assess skin for irritation, burning, stinging.

PATIENT/FAMILY TEACHING

Discontinue if skin irritation, pruritus, skin redness is excessive; contact physician. For external use only. Avoid contact with eyes, eyelids, mouth. Photosensitization may occur; use sunscreen, protective clothing.

tegaserod

te-**gas**-err-odd
(Zelnorm)

◆CLASSIFICATION

PHARMACOTHERAPEUTIC: 5-HT_4 receptor partial agonist. **CLINICAL:** Anti-irritable bowel syndrome (IBS) agent.

ACTION

Binds to 5-HT_4 receptors in GI tract. **Therapeutic Effect:** Triggers a peristaltic reflex in the gut, increasing bowel motility.

PHARMACOKINETICS

Rapidly absorbed. Widely distributed. Protein binding: 98%. Metabolized by hydrolysis in the stomach and oxidation and conjugation of the primary metabolite. Primarily excreted in feces. **Half-life:** 11 hrs.

USES

Short-term treatment of women with irritable bowel syndrome (IBS) whose primary bowel symptom is constipation.

PRECAUTIONS

CONTRAINDICATIONS: Severe renal impairment, moderate to severe hepatic impairment, history of bowel obstruction, symptomatic gallbladder disease, suspected sphincter of Oddi dysfunction, abdominal adhesions, diarrhea. **CAUTIONS:** None known.

LIFESPAN CONSIDERATIONS: Pregnancy/lactation: Unknown if distributed in breast milk. **Pregnancy Category B. Children:** Safety and efficacy not established. **Elderly:** No age-related precautions noted.

INTERACTIONS

DRUG: None known. **HERBAL:** None known. **FOOD:** None known. **LAB VALUES:** None known.

AVAILABILITY (Rx)

TABLETS: 2 mg, 6 mg.

ADMINISTRATION/HANDLING

PO

• Give before meals. • Tablets may be crushed.

INDICATIONS/ROUTES/DOSAGE

IBS

PO: ADULTS, ELDERLY WOMEN: 6 mg 2 times/day for 4–6 wks.

SIDE EFFECTS

FREQUENCY (>5%): Headache, abdominal pain, diarrhea, nausea, flatulence. **OCCASIONAL (2%–5%):** Dizziness, migraine, back pain, leg pain.

ADVERSE REACTIONS/ TOXIC EFFECTS

None known.

NURSING IMPLICATIONS

BASELINE ASSESSMENT

Assess for diarrhea (avoid use in these pts).

INTERVENTION/EVALUATION

Assess for improvement in symptoms (relief from bloating, cramping, urgency, abdominal discomfort).

PATIENT/FAMILY TEACHING

Take before meals. Inform physician of new/worsening episodes of abdominal pain.

Tegretol

see carbamazepine

T

telmisartan

tell-mih-**sar**-tan
(Micardis)

FIXED-COMBINATION(S)

Micardis HCT: telmisartan/hydrochlorothiazide (a diuretic): 40 mg/12.5 mg; 80 mg/12.5 mg.

CLASSIFICATION

PHARMACOTHERAPEUTIC: Angiotensin II receptor antagonist. **CLINICAL:** Antihypertensive (see p. 7C).

ACTION

Potent vasodilator. An angiotensin II receptor (type AT_1) antagonist; blocks vasoconstrictor and aldosterone-secreting effects of angiotensin II, inhibiting the binding of angiotensin II to the AT_1 receptors. **Therapeutic Effect:** Causes vasodilation, decreased peripheral resistance, decrease in B/P.

PHARMACOKINETICS

Rapidly and completely absorbed after PO administration. Protein binding: >99%. Undergoes hepatic metabolism to inactive metabolite. Excreted in feces. Unknown if removed by hemodialysis. **Half-life:** 24 hrs.

USES

Treatment of hypertension alone or in combination with other antihypertensives. **Unlabeled:** Treatment of congestive heart failure.

PRECAUTIONS

CONTRAINDICATIONS: None known. **CAUTIONS:** Volume-depleted pts, hepatic/renal impairment, renal artery stenosis (unilateral or bilateral).

LIFESPAN CONSIDERATIONS: Pregnancy/lactation: May cause fetal harm. Unknown if excreted in breast milk. **Pregnancy Category C (D** if used in second or third trimester). **Children:** Safety and efficacy not established. **Elderly:** No age-related precautions noted.

INTERACTIONS

DRUG: Increases **digoxin** plasma concentration. Slightly decreases **warfarin** plasma concentration. **HERBAL:** None known. **FOOD:** None known. **LAB VALUES:** May increase serum creatinine. May decrease Hgb, Hct.

AVAILABILITY (Rx)

TABLETS: 20 mg, 40 mg, 80 mg.

ADMINISTRATION/HANDLING

PO

- Give without regard to meals.

INDICATIONS/ROUTES/DOSAGE

Alert: May be given concurrently with other antihypertensives. If B/P is not controlled by telmisartan alone, a diuretic may be added.

HYPERTENSION

PO: ADULTS, ELDERLY: 40 mg once daily. RANGE: 20–80 mg.

SIDE EFFECTS

OCCASIONAL (3%–7%): Upper respiratory tract infection, sinusitis, back/leg pain, diarrhea. **RARE (1%):** Dizziness, headache, fatigue, nausea, heartburn, myalgia, cough, peripheral edema.

ADVERSE REACTIONS/ TOXIC EFFECTS

Overdosage may manifest as hypotension and tachycardia; bradycardia occurs less often.

NURSING IMPLICATIONS

BASELINE ASSESSMENT

Obtain B/P, apical pulse immediately prior to each dose, in addition to regular monitoring (be alert to fluctuations). If excessive reduction in B/P occurs, place pt in supine position, feet slightly elevated. Assess medication history (esp. diuretic). Question for history of hepatic/renal impairment, renal artery stenosis. Obtain BUN, serum creatinine, Hgb, vital signs, particularly B/P, pulse rate.

INTERVENTION/EVALUATION

Monitor B/P, pulse, electrolytes, renal function.

PATIENT/FAMILY TEACHING

Monitor during initial doses for hypotension. Maintain proper fluid intake. Inform female pt regarding consequences of second- and third-trimester exposure to telmisartan. Report pregnancy to physician as soon as possible. Avoid tasks that require alertness, motor skills (possible dizziness effect) until response to drug is established. Report any sign of infection (sore throat, fever). Discuss need for lifelong B/P control. Caution against excessive exertion during hot weather (risk of dehydration, hypotension).

temazepam

tem-**az**-eh-pam

(Apo-Temazepam ♣, Novo-Temazepam ♣, PMS-Temazepam ♣, Restoril)

Do not confuse with Vistaril, Zestril.

CLASSIFICATION

PHARMACOTHERAPEUTIC: Benzodiazepine **(Schedule IV). CLINICAL:** Sedative-hypnotic (see p. 129C).

ACTION

Enhances action of inhibitory neurotransmitter gamma-aminobutyric acid (GABA). **Therapeutic Effect:** Produces hypnotic effect due to CNS depression.

PHARMACOKINETICS

Well absorbed from GI tract. Protein binding: 96%. Widely distributed. Crosses blood-brain barrier. Metabolized in liver. Primarily excreted in urine. Not removed by hemodialysis. **Half-life:** 4–18 hrs.

USES

Short-term treatment of insomnia (≤5 wks). Reduces sleep-induction time, number of nocturnal awakenings; increases length of sleep.

PRECAUTIONS

CONTRAINDICATIONS: Severe uncontrolled pain, CNS depression, narrow-angle glaucoma, sleep apnea. **CAUTIONS:** Mental impairment, pts with drug dependence potential.

LIFESPAN CONSIDERATIONS: Pregnancy/lactation: Crosses placenta. May be distributed in breast milk. Chronic ingestion during pregnancy may produce withdrawal symptoms, CNS depression in neonates. **Pregnancy Category X. Children:** Not recommended in those <18 yrs. **Elderly:** Use small initial doses with gradual dosage increases to avoid ataxia, excessive sedation.

INTERACTIONS

DRUG: Alcohol, CNS depressants may increase CNS depressant effect. **HERBAL: Kava kava, valerian** may increase CNS effects. **FOOD:** None known. **LAB VALUES:** None known.

AVAILABILITY (Rx)

CAPSULES: 7.5 mg, 15 mg, 30 mg.

T

ADMINISTRATION/HANDLING

PO

• Give without regard to meals. • Capsules may be emptied and mixed with food.

INDICATIONS/ROUTES/DOSAGE

INSOMNIA

PO: ADULTS >18 YRS: 15–30 mg at bedtime. ELDERLY/DEBILITATED: 7.5–15 mg at bedtime.

SIDE EFFECTS

FREQUENT: Drowsiness, sedation, rebound insomnia (may occur for 1–2 nights after drug is discontinued), dizziness, confusion, euphoria. **OCCASIONAL:** Weakness, anorexia, diarrhea. **RARE:** Paradoxical CNS excitement, restlessness (particularly noted in elderly/debilitated).

ADVERSE REACTIONS/ TOXIC EFFECTS

Abrupt or too rapid withdrawal may result in pronounced restlessness, irritability, insomnia, hand tremors, abdominal/muscle cramps, diaphoresis, vomiting, seizures. Overdosage results in somnolence, confusion, diminished reflexes, respiratory depression, coma.

NURSING IMPLICATIONS

BASELINE ASSESSMENT

Question for possibility of pregnancy before initiating therapy (Pregnancy Category X). Assess B/P, pulse, respirations immediately prior to administration. Raise bed rails. Provide environment conducive to sleep (back rub, quiet environment, low lighting).

INTERVENTION/EVALUATION

Assess sleep pattern of pt. Assess elderly/debilitated for paradoxical reaction, particularly during early therapy. Monitor respiratory, cardiovascular, mental status. Evaluate for therapeutic response: decrease in number of nocturnal awakenings, increase in length of sleep.

PATIENT/FAMILY TEACHING

Avoid alcohol, other CNS depressants. May cause daytime drowsiness. Avoid tasks that require alertness, motor skills until response to drug is established. Take about 30 min before bedtime. Inform physician if you are or are planning to become pregnant.

temozolomide

teh-moe-**zoll**-oh-mide
(Temodal ❋, Temodar)

◆CLASSIFICATION

PHARMACOTHERAPEUTIC: Imidazotetrazine derivative. **CLINICAL:** Antineoplastic (see p. 76C).

ACTION

Prodrug, converted to highly active cytotoxic metabolite. Cytotoxic effect associated with methylation of DNA. **Therapeutic Effect:** Inhibits DNA replication, causing cell death.

PHARMACOKINETICS

Rapidly, completely absorbed following PO administration. Protein binding: 15%. Peak plasma concentration occurs in 1 hr. Weakly bound to plasma proteins. Penetrates across blood-brain barrier. Primarily eliminated in urine and, to a much lesser extent, in feces. **Half-life:** 1.6–1.8 hrs.

USES

Treatment of active vs. primary or recurrent gliomas, metastatic melanoma. Treatment of refractory anaplastic astrocytoma in adults whose disease has relapsed after initial therapy with other agents.

PRECAUTIONS

CONTRAINDICATIONS: Hypersensitivity to dacarbazine, pregnancy. **CAUTIONS:** Severe renal/hepatic impairment.

LIFESPAN CONSIDERATIONS: Pregnancy/lactation: May cause fetal harm. May produce malformation of external organs, soft tissue, skeleton. If possible, avoid use during pregnancy. Unknown if drug is excreted in breast milk. **Pregnancy Category D. Children:** Safety and efficacy not established. **Elderly:** In those >70 yrs, may experience a higher risk of developing grade 4 neutropenia and grade 4 thrombocytopenia.

INTERACTIONS

DRUG: **Valproic acid** decreases temozolomide clearance. **Live virus vaccines** may potentiate virus replication, increase vaccine side effects, decrease pt's antibody response to vaccine. **HERBAL:** None known. **FOOD:** Food decreases rate of absorption. **LAB VALUES:** May decrease Hgb, WBCs, platelets, neutrophils.

AVAILABILITY (Rx)

CAPSULES: 5 mg, 20 mg, 100 mg, 250 mg.

ADMINISTRATION/HANDLING

• Food reduces rate, extent of absorption; increases risk of nausea, vomiting. • For best results, administer at bedtime. • Swallow capsule whole with glass of water. If unable to swallow, open capsule and mix with applesauce, apple juice. Avoid exposure to medication during handling (cytotoxic).

INDICATIONS/ROUTES/DOSAGE

ANAPLASTIC ASTROCYTOMA

PO: ADULTS: Initially, 150 mg/m^2 daily for 5 consecutive days of a 28-day treatment cycle. If myelosuppression is not severe on day 22, may increase dose to 200 mg/m^2 and repeat at 4-wk intervals.

SIDE EFFECTS

FREQUENT (33%–53%): Nausea, vomiting, headache, fatigue, constipation. **OCCASIONAL (10%–16%):** Diarrhea, asthenia (loss of strength, energy), fever, dizziness, peripheral edema, incoordination, insomnia. **RARE (5%–9%):** Paresthesia, drowsiness, anorexia, urinary incontinence, anxiety, pharyngitis, cough.

ADVERSE REACTIONS/ TOXIC EFFECTS

Myelosuppression is characterized by neutropenia and thrombocytopenia, with elderly and women showing the higher incidence of developing severe myelosuppression. Usually occurs within the first few cycles; is not cumulative. Nadir occurs approximately 26–28 days, with recovery 14 days of nadir.

NURSING IMPLICATIONS

BASELINE ASSESSMENT

Prior to dosing, absolute neutrophil count (ANC) must be ≥1,500 and platelet count ≥100,000. Potential for nausea, vomiting readily controlled with antiemetic therapy.

INTERVENTION/EVALUATION

Obtain CBC on day 22 (21 days after the first dose) or within 48 hrs of that day and weekly until ANC is ≥1,500 and platelet count is ≥100,000. Monitor for hematologic toxicity (fever, sore throat, signs of local infection, unusual bruising/bleeding from any site), symptoms of anemia (excessive tiredness, weakness).

PATIENT/FAMILY TEACHING

To reduce nausea/vomiting, take temozolomide on an empty stomach. Do not open capsules. Promptly report fever, sore throat, signs of local infection, unusual bruising/bleeding from any site.

T

Avoid crowds, those with infection. Do not have immunizations without physician's approval. Avoid pregnancy.

tenecteplase

ten-**eck**-teh-place
(TNKase)

CLASSIFICATION

PHARMACOTHERAPEUTIC: Tissue plasminogen activator. **CLINICAL:** Thrombolytic (see p. 30C).

ACTION

A tissue plasminogen activator (tPA) produced by recombinant DNA, binds to fibrin and converts plasminogen to plasmin. **Therapeutic Effect:** Initiates fibrinolysis (degrades fibrin clots, fibrinogen, other plasma proteins).

PHARMACOKINETICS

Extensively distributed to tissues. Completely eliminated by hepatic metabolism. **Half-life:** 11–20 min.

USES

Treatment and reduction of mortality associated with acute myocardial infarction (AMI).

PRECAUTIONS

CONTRAINDICATIONS: Active internal bleeding, history of CVA, intracranial/intraspinal surgery/trauma within 2 mos, intracranial neoplasm, AV malformation, aneurysm, known bleeding diathesis, severe uncontrolled hypertension. **CAUTIONS:** Pts who previously received tenecteplase, severe hepatic impairment.

LIFESPAN CONSIDERATIONS: Pregnancy/lactation: Unknown if distributed in breast milk. **Pregnancy Category C. Children:** Safety and efficacy not established. **Elderly:** May have increased risk of intracranial hemorrhage, stroke, major bleeding; caution advised.

INTERACTIONS

DRUG: Anticoagulants (e.g., heparin, warfarin), aspirin, dipyridamole, GP IIb/IIIa inhibitors increased risk of bleeding. **HERBAL: Ginkgo biloba** may increase risk of bleeding. **FOOD:** None known. **LAB VALUES:** Decreases plasminogen and fibrinogen levels during infusion, decreasing clotting time (confirms presence of lysis). Decreases Hgb, Hct.

AVAILABILITY (Rx)

POWDER FOR INJECTION: 50 mg.

ADMINISTRATION/HANDLING

IV

Storage • Store at room temperature. • If possible, use immediately but may refrigerate up to 8 hrs after reconstitution. • Appears as colorless to pale yellow solution. Do not use if discolored or contains particulates. • Discard after 8 hrs.

Reconstitution • Add 10 ml Sterile Water for Injection without preservative to vial to provide concentration of 5 mg/ml. Gently swirl until dissolved. Do not shake. • If foaming occurs, vial should be left undisturbed for several minutes.

Rate of administration • Administer as IV push over 5 sec.

IV INCOMPATIBILITY

Do not mix with any other medications.

INDICATIONS/ROUTES/DOSAGE

Alert: Give as a single IV bolus over 5 sec. Precipitate may occur when given in an IV line containing dextrose. Flush with saline before and after administration.

ACUTE MI

IV: ADULTS: Dosage is based on the weight of the pt. Treatment to be initiated

T

as soon as possible after onset of AMI symptoms.

Weight (kg)	(mg)	(ml)
<60	30	6
≥60 to <70	35	7
≥70 to <80	40	8
≥80 to <90	45	9
≥90	50	10

SIDE EFFECTS

FREQUENT: Bleeding (major: 4.7%; minor 21.8%).

ADVERSE REACTIONS/ TOXIC EFFECTS

Bleeding at internal sites (intracranial, retroperitoneal, GI, GU, respiratory) may occur. Lysis of coronary thrombi may produce atrial or ventricular dysrhythmias, stroke.

NURSING IMPLICATIONS

BASELINE ASSESSMENT

Obtain baseline B/P, apical pulse. Record weight. Evaluate 12-lead EKG, cardiac enzymes, electrolytes. Assess Hgb, Hct, platelet count, thrombin (TT), activated partial thromboplastin time (aPTT), prothrombin time (PT), fibrinogen level before therapy is instituted. Type and hold blood.

INTERVENTION/EVALUATION

Continuous cardiac monitoring for arrhythmias, B/P, pulse, respirations q15min until stable, then hourly. Check peripheral pulses, heart/lung sounds. Monitor chest pain relief; notify physician of continuation/recurrence (note location, type, intensity). Assess for bleeding: overt blood, blood in any body substance. Monitor PTT per protocol. Maintain B/P. Avoid any trauma that might increase risk of bleeding (e.g., injections, shaving). Assess neurologic status with vital signs.

teniposide

ten-**ih**-poe-side
(Vumon)
See Classification section under: Cancer chemotherapeutic agents (p. 76C)

tenofovir

ten-**oh**-fah-vir
(Viread)

◆ CLASSIFICATION

PHARMACOTHERAPEUTIC: Nucleotide analogue. **CLINICAL:** Antiviral (see pp. 60C, 99C).

ACTION

Inhibits HIV viral reverse transcriptase by being incorporated into viral DNA causing chain termination. **Therapeutic Effect:** Slows HIV replication, reduces viral load.

USES

Treatment of HIV-1 infection in combination with other antiretroviral agents.

PRECAUTIONS

CONTRAINDICATIONS: None known. **CAUTIONS:** Impaired hepatic/renal function. **Pregnancy Category B.**

INTERACTIONS

DRUG: May increase **didanosine** concentrations. May decrease concentration of **lamivudine, indinavir, lopinavir, ritonavir.** **HERBAL:** None known. **FOOD: High-fat food** increases bioavailability. **LAB VALUES:** May elevate serum transaminase. May alter SGOT (AST), SGPT (ALT), creatinine clearance, GGT, CPK, uric acid, triglycerides.

T

AVAILABILITY (Rx)

TABLETS: 300 mg.

ADMINISTRATION/HANDLING

PO

- Give with food.

INDICATIONS/ROUTES/DOSAGE

HIV INFECTION

PO: ADULTS, ELDERLY, CHILDREN ≥18 YRS: 300 mg once daily.

SIDE EFFECTS

OCCASIONAL: GI disturbances (nausea, diarrhea, vomiting, flatulence).

ADVERSE REACTIONS/ TOXIC EFFECTS

Lactic acidosis, hepatomegaly with steatosis (excess fat in liver) occur rarely; may be severe.

NURSING IMPLICATIONS

BASELINE ASSESSMENT

Obtain baseline laboratory testing, esp. liver function tests, triglycerides prior to beginning tenofovir therapy and at periodic intervals during therapy. Offer emotional support.

INTERVENTION/EVALUATION

Closely monitor for evidence of GI discomfort. Monitor stool frequency, consistency (watery, loose, soft). Monitor CBC, Hgb, reticulocyte count, liver function, CD4 cell count, HIV, RNA plasma levels.

PATIENT/FAMILY TEACHING

Continue therapy for full length of treatment. Tenofovir is not a cure for HIV infection, nor does it reduce risk of transmission to others. Take with a meal (increases absorption). Inform physician if persistent abdominal pain, nausea, vomiting occurs.

Tenormin

see atenolol

Tequin

see gatifloxacin

terazosin hydrochloride

tear-**aye**-zoe-sin

(Apo-Terazosin ✤, Hytrin)

◆CLASSIFICATION

PHARMACOTHERAPEUTIC: Alpha-adrenergic blocker. **CLINICAL:** Antihypertensive, benign prostatic hyperplasia agent (see p. 53C).

ACTION

Blocks alpha-adrenergic receptors. **Hypertension:** Produces vasodilation, decreases peripheral resistance. **Therapeutic Effect:** Results in decreased B/P. **Benign prostatic hypertrophy:** Targets receptors around bladder neck and prostate. **Therapeutic Effect:** Results in relaxation of smooth muscle, improvement in urinary flow.

PHARMACOKINETICS

	Onset	Peak	Duration
PO	15 min	1–2 hrs	12–24 hrs

Rapidly, completely absorption from GI tract. Protein binding: 90%–94%. Metabolized in liver to active metabolite. Primarily eliminated in feces via biliary system; excreted in urine. Not removed by hemodialysis. **Half-life:** 12 hrs.

USES

Treatment of mild to moderate hypertension. Used alone or in combination with other antihypertensives. Treatment of benign prostatic hypertrophy.

PRECAUTIONS

CONTRAINDICATIONS: None known. **CAUTIONS:** Confirmed or suspected coronary artery disease.

LIFESPAN CONSIDERATIONS: Pregnancy/lactation: Unknown if drug croses placenta or is distributed in breast milk. **Pregnancy Category C. Children:** Safety and efficacy not established. **Elderly:** No age-related precautions noted but may be more sensitive to hypotensive effects.

INTERACTIONS

DRUG: Estrogen, NSAIDs, sympathomimetics may decrease effect. **Hypotension-producing medications** may increase antihypertensive effect. **HERBAL: Dong quai, ephedra, yohimbe, ginseng, garlic** may decrease antihypertensive effect. **FOOD:** None known. **LAB VALUES:** May decrease albumin, total protein, Hgb, Hct, WBC.

AVAILABILITY (Rx)

CAPSULES: 1 mg, 2 mg, 5 mg, 10 mg. **TABLETS:** 2 mg, 5 mg, 10 mg.

ADMINISTRATION/HANDLING

PO

• Give without regard to food. • Tablets may be crushed. • Administer first dose at bedtime (minimizes risk of fainting due to "first-dose syncope").

INDICATIONS/ROUTES/DOSAGE

Alert: If medication is discontinued for several days, retitrate initially using 1-mg dose at bedtime.

HYPERTENSION

PO: ADULTS, ELDERLY: Initially, 1 mg at bedtime. Slowly increase dosage to desired levels. RANGE: 1–5 mg/day as single or 2 divided doses. **Maximum:** 20 mg.

BENIGN PROSTATIC HYPERTROPHY

PO: ADULTS, ELDERLY: Initially, 1 mg at bedtime. May increase up to 10 mg/day. **Maximum:** 20 mg/day.

SIDE EFFECTS

FREQUENT (5%–9%): Dizziness, headache, unusual tiredness. **RARE (<2%):** Peripheral edema, orthostatic hypotension, back/joint pain, blurred vision, nausea, vomiting, nasal congestion, drowsiness.

ADVERSE REACTIONS/ TOXIC EFFECTS

"First-dose syncope" (hypotension with sudden LOC) generally occurs 30–90 min after giving initial dose of ≥2 mg, a too rapid increase in dose, or addition of another hypotensive agent to therapy. May be preceded by tachycardia (120–160 beats/min).

NURSING IMPLICATIONS

BASELINE ASSESSMENT

Give first dose at bedtime. If initial dose is given during daytime, pt must remain recumbent for 3–4 hrs. Assess B/P, pulse immediately prior to each dose, and q15–30min until stabilized (be alert to B/P fluctuations).

INTERVENTION/EVALUATION

Monitor pulse diligently ("first-dose syncope" may be preceded by tachycardia). Assist with ambulation if dizziness occurs. Assess for peripheral edema (usually, first area of swelling is behind medial malleolus in ambulatory, sacral area in bedridden). Monitor B/P, GU function.

PATIENT/FAMILY TEACHING

Noncola carbonated beverage, unsalted crackers, dry toast may relieve nausea. Nasal congestion may occur. Full therapeutic effect may not occur for 3–4 wks. Avoid tasks requiring alertness, motor skills until response to drug is established. Use caution rising from sitting position. Report dizziness, palpitations.

terbinafine hydrochloride

tur-**bin**-ah-feen
(Lamisil, Lamisil Derma Gel)
Do not confuse with Lamictal, terbutaline.

◆CLASSIFICATION

CLINICAL: Antifungal (see p. 43C).

ACTION

Fungicidal. Inhibits the enzyme, squalene epoxidase, interfering with biosynthesis in fungi. **Therapeutic Effect:** Results in fungal cell death.

USES

Systemic: Treatment of onychomycosis (fungal disease of nails due to dermatophytes). **Topical:** Treatment of tinea cruris (jock itch), t. pedis (athlete's foot), t. corporis (ringworm). **Derma Gel:** Treatment of t. corporis, t. pedis, t. versicolor.

T

PRECAUTIONS

CONTRAINDICATIONS: **Oral:** Preexisting hepatic disease or renal impairment (creatinine clearance ≤50 ml/min). Safety in children <12 yrs not established. **CAUTIONS:** None known. **Pregnancy Category B.**

INTERACTIONS

DRUG: **Alcohol, other hepatotoxic medications** may increase risk of hepatotoxicity. **Liver enzyme inhibitors** may decrease clearance **(e.g., cimetidine). Liver enzyme inducers** may increase clearance **(e.g., rifampin).** **HERBAL:** None known. **FOOD:** None known. **LAB VALUES:** May increase SGOT (AST), SGPT (ALT).

AVAILABILITY (Rx)

TABLETS: 250 mg. **CREAM:** 1%. **TOPICAL SOLUTION:** 1%.

INDICATIONS/ROUTES/DOSAGE

Alert: Topical therapy used for minimum 1 wk, not to exceed 4 wks.

T. PEDIS

Topical: ADULTS, ELDERLY, CHILDREN ≥12 YRS: Apply 2 times/day until signs/symptoms significantly improved.

T. CRURIS, T. CORPORIS

Topical: ADULTS, ELDERLY, CHILDREN ≥12 YRS: Apply 1–2 times/day until signs/symptoms significantly improved.

ONYCHOMYCOSIS

PO: ADULTS, ELDERLY, CHILDREN ≥12 YRS: 250 mg/day for 6 wks (fingernails), 12 wks (toenails).

T. VERSICOLOR

Topical: ADULTS, ELDERLY: *(Solution):* Apply to affected area 2 times/day for 7 days.

SYSTEMIC MYCOSIS

PO: ADULTS, ELDERLY: 250–500 mg/day for up to 16 mos.

SIDE EFFECTS

FREQUENT (13%): Oral: Headache. **OCCASIONAL (3%–6%): Oral:** Diarrhea, rash, dyspepsia, pruritus, taste disturbance, nausea. **RARE: Oral:** Abdominal pain, flatulence, urticaria, visual disturbance. **Topical:** Irritation, burning, itching, dryness.

ADVERSE REACTIONS/ TOXIC EFFECTS

Hepatobiliary dysfunction (including cholestatic hepatitis), serious skin reactions, severe neutropenia occur rarely. Ocular lens and retinal changes have been noted.

NURSING IMPLICATIONS

BASELINE ASSESSMENT

Hepatic function tests should be obtained in pts receiving treatment for >6 wks.

INTERVENTION/EVALUATION

Check for therapeutic response. Discontinue medication, notify physician if local reaction occurs (irritation, redness, swelling, itching, oozing, blistering, burning). Monitor hepatic function in pts receiving treatment for >6 wks.

PATIENT/FAMILY TEACHING

Keep areas clean, dry; wear light clothing to promote ventilation. Separate personal items. Avoid topical cream contact with eyes, nose, mouth, other mucous membranes. Rub well into affected, surrounding area. Do not cover with occlusive dressing. Notify physician if skin irritation, diarrhea occurs.

terbutaline sulfate

tur-**byew**-ta-leen
(Brethine)
Do not confuse with Brethaire, terbinafine, tolbutamide.

CLASSIFICATION

PHARMACOTHERAPEUTIC: Sympathomimetic (adrenergic agonist). **CLINICAL:** Bronchodilator, premature labor inhibitor (see p. 65C).

ACTION

Stimulates $beta_2$-adrenergic receptors. **Therapeutic Effect: Bronchospasm:** Relaxes bronchial smooth muscle, relieves bronchospasm, reduces airway resistance. **Labor:** Relaxes uterine muscle, inhibiting uterine contractions.

USES

Symptomatic relief of reversible bronchospasm due to bronchial asthma, bronchitis, emphysema. Delays premature labor in pregnancies between 20 and 34 wks.

PRECAUTIONS

CONTRAINDICATIONS: History of hypersensitivity to sympathomimetics. **CAUTIONS:** Impaired cardiac function, diabetes mellitus, hypertension, hyperthyroidism, history of seizures. **Pregnancy Category B.**

INTERACTIONS

DRUG: Tricyclic antidepressants may increase cardiovascular effects. **MAOIs** may increase risk of hypertensive crises. May decrease effects of **beta-blockers. Digoxin, sympathomimetics** may increase risk of dysrhythmias. **HERBAL:** None known. **FOOD:** None known. **LAB VALUES:** May decrease serum potassium levels.

AVAILABILITY (Rx)

TABLETS: 2.5 mg, 5 mg. **INJECTION:** 1 mg/ml.

ADMINISTRATION/HANDLING

PO

• Give without regard to food (give with food if GI upset occurs). • Tablets may be crushed.

SUBCUTANEOUS

• Do not use if solution appears discolored. • Inject subcutaneously into lateral deltoid region.

INDICATIONS/ROUTES/DOSAGE

BRONCHOSPASM

PO: ADULTS, ELDERLY, CHILDREN >15 YRS: Initially, 2.5 mg 3–4 times/day. MAINTE-

T

NANCE: 2.5–5 mg 3 times/day q6h while awake. **Maximum:** 15 mg/day. CHILDREN 12–15 YRS: 2.5 mg 3 times/day. **Maximum:** 7.5 mg/day. CHILDREN <12 YRS: Initially, 0.05 mg/kg/dose q8h. May increase up to 0.15 mg/kg/dose. **Maximum:** 5 mg.

Subcutaneous: ADULTS: Initially, 0.25 mg. Repeat in 15–30 min if substantial improvement does not occur. **Maximum:** No more than 0.5 mg/4 hrs. CHILDREN <12 YRS: 0.005–0.01 mg/kg/dose to a maximum of 0.4 mg/dose q15–20min for 2 doses.

PRETERM LABOR

IV: ADULTS: 2.5–10 mcg/min. May increase gradually q15–20min up to 17.5–30 mcg/min.

PO: ADULTS: 2.5–10 mg q4–6h.

SIDE EFFECTS

FREQUENT (23%–38%): Tremor, shakiness, nervousness. **OCCASIONAL (10%–11%):** Drowsiness, headache, nausea, heartburn, dizziness. **RARE (1%–3%):** Flushing, weakness, drying/irritation of oropharynx noted with inhalation therapy.

ADVERSE REACTIONS/ TOXIC EFFECTS

Too frequent or excessive use may lead to loss of bronchodilating effectiveness and/or severe, paradoxical bronchoconstriction. Excessive sympathomimetic stimulation may cause palpitations, extrasystoles, tachycardia, chest pain, slight increase in B/P followed by a substantial decrease, chills, diaphoresis, blanching of skin.

NURSING IMPLICATIONS

BASELINE ASSESSMENT

Bronchospasm: Offer emotional support (high incidence of anxiety due to difficulty in breathing, sympathomimetic response to drug). **Preterm labor:** Assess baseline maternal pulse, B/P, frequency/duration of contractions, fetal heart rate.

INTERVENTION/EVALUATION

Bronchospasm: Monitor rate, depth, rhythm, type of respiration; quality/rate of pulse. Assess lung sounds for rhonchi, wheezing, rales. Monitor ABGs. Observe lips, fingernails for blue or dusky color in light-skinned pts; gray in dark-skinned pts. Observe for clavicular retractions, hand tremor. Evaluate for clinical improvement (quieter, slower respirations, relaxed facial expression, cessation of clavicular retractions). **Preterm labor:** Monitor for frequency, duration, strength of contractions. Diligently monitor fetal heart rate.

PATIENT/FAMILY TEACHING

Inform physician if palpitations, chest pain, muscle tremors, dizziness, headache, flushing, breathing difficulties continue. May cause nervousness, shakiness. Avoid excessive use of caffeine derivatives (chocolate, coffee, tea, cola, cocoa).

terconazole

ter-**con**-ah-zole
(Terazol)
Do not confuse with tioconazole.

CLASSIFICATION

CLINICAL: Antifungal.

ACTION

Disrupts fungal cell membrane permeability. **Therapeutic Effect:** Produces antifungal activity.

USES

Treatment of vulvovaginal candidiasis (moniliasis).

AVAILABILITY (Rx)

VAGINAL TABLETS: 80 mg. **VAGINAL CREAM:** 0.4%, 0.8%.

INDICATIONS/ROUTES/DOSAGE

VULVOVAGINAL CANDIDIASIS

Tablet (intravaginal): ADULTS, ELDERLY: 1 suppository vaginally at bedtime for 3 days.

Cream (0.4%): ADULTS, ELDERLY: 1 applicatorful at bedtime for 7 days; 0.8% for 3 days.

SIDE EFFECTS

FREQUENT (>10%): Headache, vulvovaginal burning. **OCCASIONAL (1%–10%):** Dysmenorrhea, pain in female genitalia, abdominal pain, fever, itching. **RARE (<1%):** Chills.

teriparatide acetate

tear-ee-**pear**-ah-tide
(Forteo)

CLASSIFICATION

PHARMACOTHERAPEUTIC: Synthetic hormone. **CLINICAL:** Osteoporosis agent.

ACTION

Acts on bone to mobilize calcium; also acts on kidney to reduce calcium clearance, increase phosphate excretion. **Therapeutic Effect:** Promotes an increased rate of release of calcium from bone into blood, stimulates new bone formation.

USES

Treatment of postmenopausal women with osteoporosis who are at increased risk for fractures, increase bone mass in men with primary or hypogonadal osteoporosis who are at high risk for fractures. High-risk pts include those with a history of osteoporotic fractures, those who have failed previous osteoporosis therapy or are intolerant to previous osteoporosis therapy.

PRECAUTIONS

CONTRAINDICATIONS: Serum calcium above normal level, those at increased risk for osteosarcoma (Paget's disease, unexplained elevations of alkaline phosphatase, open epiphyses, prior radiation therapy that include the skeleton), hypercalcemic disorders (e.g., hyperparathyroidism). **CAUTIONS:** Bone metastases, history of skeletal malignancies, metabolic bone diseases other than osteoporosis, concurrent therapy with digoxin. **Pregnancy Category C.**

INTERACTIONS

DRUG: May increase serum **digoxin** concentration. **HERBAL:** None known. **FOOD:** None known. **LAB VALUES:** May increase serum calcium.

AVAILABILITY (Rx)

INJECTION: 3-ml prefilled pen containing 750 mcg teriparatide.

ADMINISTRATION/HANDLING

SUBCUTANEOUS

• Refrigerate, minimizing the time out of the refrigerator. Do not freeze; discard if frozen. • Administer into the thigh or abdominal wall.

INDICATIONS/ROUTES/DOSAGE

OSTEOPOROSIS

Subcutaneous: ADULTS, ELDERLY: 20 mcg once daily into the thigh or abdominal wall.

SIDE EFFECTS

OCCASIONAL: Leg cramps, nausea, dizziness, headache, orthostatic hypotension, tachycardia.

T

ADVERSE REACTIONS/ TOXIC EFFECTS

None known.

NURSING IMPLICATIONS

BASELINE ASSESSMENT

Check urinary and serum calcium levels, blood parathyroid hormone levels.

INTERVENTION/EVALUATION

Monitor bone mineral density, urinary and serum calcium levels, parathyroid hormone levels, symptoms of hypercalcemia. Monitor B/P for hypotension, pulse for tachycardia.

PATIENT/FAMILY TEACHING

Immediately sit/lie down if symptoms of orthostatic hypotension occur. Inform physician if persistent symptoms of hypercalcemia occur (e.g., nausea, vomiting, constipation, lethargy, asthenia [loss of strength, energy]).

testosterone

tess-**toss**-ter-own
(Andronaq, Delatestryl✤, Histerone, Striant)

testosterone cypionate

(Depotest, Depo-Testosterone)

testosterone enanthate

(Delatest)

testosterone propionate

(Testex)

testosterone transdermal

(Androderm, Testim, Testoderm, Testoderm TTS)

Do not confuse with testolactone.

◆CLASSIFICATION

PHARMACOTHERAPEUTIC: Androgen. **CLINICAL:** Sex hormone.

ACTION

Primary endogenous androgen. **Therapeutic Effect:** Promotes growth/development of male sex organs, maintains secondary sex characteristics in androgen-deficient males.

PHARMACOKINETICS

Well absorbed following IM administration. Protein binding: 98%. Metabolized in liver (undergoes first-pass metabolism). Primarily excreted in urine. Unknown if removed by hemodialysis. **Half-life:** 10–20 min.

USES

Male hypogonadism, inoperable breast cancer, replacement therapy in treatment of delayed male puberty.

PRECAUTIONS

CONTRAINDICATIONS: Severe renal/hepatic disease, cardiac impairment, prostatic or breast cancer in males, hypercalcemia, pregnancy. **CAUTIONS:** Renal/hepatic dysfunction, diabetes.

LIFESPAN CONSIDERATIONS: Pregnancy/lactation: Contraindicated during lactation. **Pregnancy Category X. Children:** Safety and efficacy not established; use with caution. **Elderly:** May increase risk of hyperplasia or stimulate growth of occult prostate carcinoma.

INTERACTIONS

DRUG: May increase effect of **oral anticoagulants. Hepatotoxic medications** may increase hepatotoxicity. **HERBAL:** None known. **FOOD:** None known. **LAB VALUES:** May increase SGOT (AST), alkaline phosphatase, bilirubin, calcium, potassium, sodium, Hgb, Hct, LDL. May decrease HDL.

AVAILABILITY (Rx)

INJECTION: Aqueous suspension: 50 mg/ml, 100 mg/ml. **Cypionate:** 100 mg/ml, 200 mg/ml. **Enanthate:** 200 mg/ml. **Propionate:** 100 mg/ml. **Pellets for subcutaneous implantation:** 75 mg. **TRANSDERMAL GEL:** 25 mg (2.5 g gel/pack), 50 mg (5 g gel/pack). **TRANSDERMAL SYSTEM:** 2.5 mg/day, 4 mg/day, 5 mg/day, 6 mg/day. **BUCCAL SYSTEM:** 30 mg.

ADMINISTRATION/HANDLING

IM

• Give deep in gluteal muscle. • Do **not** give IV. • Warming/shaking redissolves crystals that may form in long-acting preparations. • Wet needle of syringe may cause solution to become cloudy; this does not affect potency.

TRANSDERMAL

Testoderm

• Apply to clean, dry scrotal skin that has been dry-shaved (optimal skin contact). Testoderm TTS may be applied to arm, back, upper buttock.

Androderm

• Apply to clean, dry area on skin on back, abdomen, upper arms, thighs. • Do not apply to bony prominences (e.g., shoulder) or oily, damaged, irritated skin. Do not apply to scrotum. • Rotate application site with 7-day interval to same site.

TRANSDERMAL GEL

(Androgel, Testim)

• Apply (morning preferred) to clean, dry, intact skin of shoulder, upper arms (Androgel may also be applied to abdomen). • Upon opening packet(s), squeeze entire contents into palm of hand and immediately apply to application site. • Allow to dry. • Do not apply to genitals.

BUCCAL

(Striant)

• Apply to gum area (above incisor tooth). • Not affected by food, tooth brushing, gum, chewing, alcoholic beverages. • Remove prior to placing new system.

INDICATIONS/ROUTES/DOSAGE

MALE HYPOGONADISM

IM: ADULTS, ELDERLY: *(Aqueous/propionate):* 10–25 mg 2–3 times/wk. *(Cypionate/enanthate):* 50–400 mg q2–4wks. CHILDREN: *(Cypionate/enanthate): Initial pubertal growth:* 40–50 mg/m^2/dose qmo. *Terminal growth phase:* 100 mg/m^2/dose qmo. MAINTENANCE VIRILIZING DOSE: 100 mg/m^2/dose 2 times/mo.

Transdermal Patches: *(Testoderm):* Start therapy with 6 mg/day patch. Apply to scrotal skin. *(Testoderm TTS):* Apply to arm, back, or upper buttocks. *(Androderm):* Start therapy with 5 mg/day patch applied at night. Apply to back, abdomen, upper arms, or thighs.

Transdermal Gel: *(Androgel):* Initial dose 5 g (delivers 50 mg testosterone) applied once daily to shoulders, upper arms, or abdomen. May increase to 7.5 g then to 10 g if necessary. *(Testim):* Initial dose 5 g (delivers 50 mg testosterone) applied once daily to shoulders, or upper arms. May increase to 10 g.

Subcutaneous: *(Pellets):* ADULTS, ELDERLY: 150–450 mg q3–6mos.

T

DELAYED PUBERTY
IM: 40–50 mg/m^2/dose qmo for 6 mos.

BREAST CARCINOMA
IM: ADULTS: *(Aqueous):* 50–100 mg 3 times/wk. *(Cypionate/enanthate):* 200–400 mg q2–4wks. *(Propionate):* 50–100 mg 3 times/wk.

SIDE EFFECTS

FREQUENT: Gynecomastia, acne, amenorrhea, other menstrual irregularities. **Females:** Hirsutism, deepening of voice, clitoral enlargement (may not be reversible when drug discontinued). **OCCASIONAL:** Edema, nausea, insomnia, oligospermia, priapism, male pattern of baldness, bladder irritability, hypercalcemia in immobilized pts or those with breast cancer, hypercholesterolemia, inflammation/pain at IM injection site. **Transdermal:** Itching, erythema, skin irritation. **RARE:** Polycythemia with high dosage, hypersensitivity.

ADVERSE REACTIONS/ TOXIC EFFECTS

Peliosis hepatitis (liver, spleen replaced with blood-filled cysts), hepatic neoplasms, hepatocellular carcinoma have been associated with prolonged high-dosage, anaphylactoid reactions.

NURSING IMPLICATIONS

BASELINE ASSESSMENT

Establish baseline weight, B/P, Hgb, Hct. Check hepatic function test results, electrolytes, cholesterol if ordered. Wrist x-rays may be ordered to determine bone maturation in children.

INTERVENTION/EVALUATION

Weigh daily and report weekly gain of >5 lbs; evaluate for edema. Monitor I&O. Check B/P at least 2 times/day. Assess electrolytes, cholesterol, Hgb, Hct (periodically for high dosage), hepatic function test results, radiologic exam of wrist/hand (when using in prepubertal children). With breast cancer or immobility, check for hypercalcemia (lethargy, muscle weakness, confusion, irritability). Ensure adequate intake of protein, calories. Assess for virilization. Monitor sleep patterns. Check injection site for redness, swelling, pain.

PATIENT/FAMILY TEACHING

Regular visits to physician and monitoring tests are necessary. Do not take any other medications without consulting physician. Teach diet high in protein, calories. Food may be better tolerated in small, frequent feedings. Weigh daily, report 5 lbs/gain/wk. Notify physician if nausea, vomiting, acne, pedal edema occurs. **Females:** Promptly report menstrual irregularities, hoarseness, deepening of voice. **Males:** Report frequent erections, difficulty urinating, gynecomastia.

tetracaine

(Pontocaine)
See Classification section under: Anesthetics: local (p. 4C)

tetracycline hydrochloride

tet-rah-**sigh**-klin
(Achromycin, Apo-Tetra✦, Novotetra✦, Sumycin)

◆ CLASSIFICATION

PHARMACOTHERAPEUTIC: Tetracycline. **CLINICAL:** Antibiotic.

ACTION

Inhibits bacterial protein synthesis by binding to ribosomes. **Therapeutic Effect:** Prevents bacterial cell growth. Bacteriostatic.

PHARMACOKINETICS

Readily absorbed from GI tract. Protein binding: 30%–60%. Widely distributed. Excreted in urine; eliminated in feces via biliary system. Not removed by hemodialysis. **Half-life:** 6–11 hrs (half-life increased with impaired renal function).

USES

Treatment of inflammatory acne vulgaris, Lyme disease, mycoplasma disease, *Legionella,* Rocky Mountain spotted fever, chlamydial infection in pts with gonorrhea.

PRECAUTIONS

CONTRAINDICATIONS: Hypersensitivity to tetracyclines, sulfite, children ≤8 yrs. **CAUTIONS:** Sun, ultraviolet light exposure (severe photosensitivity reaction).

LIFESPAN CONSIDERATIONS: Pregnancy/lactation: Readily crosses placenta. Distributed in breast milk. Avoid use in women during last half of pregnancy. May produce permanent tooth discoloration/enamel hypoplasia, inhibit fetal skeletal growth in children ≤8 yrs. **Pregnancy Category D** (**B** with topical). **Children:** Not recommended in those ≤8 yrs; may cause permanent staining of teeth, enamel hypoplasia, decreased linear skeletal growth rate. **Elderly:** No age-related precautions noted.

INTERACTIONS

DRUG: Cholestyramine, colestipol may decrease absorption. May decrease effect of **oral contraceptives. Carbamazepine, phenytoin** may decrease concentrations. **HERBAL: St. John's wort** may increase risk of photosensitivity. **FOOD: Dairy products** inhibit absorption. **LAB VALUES:** May increase BUN, SGOT (AST), SGPT (ALT), alkaline phosphatase, amylase, bilirubin concentrations.

AVAILABILITY (Rx)

CAPSULES: 250 mg, 500 mg. **TABLETS:** 250 mg, 500 mg. **SUSPENSION:** 125 mg/5 ml. **TOPICAL SOLUTION. TOPICAL OINTMENT:** 3%.

ADMINISTRATION/HANDLING

PO

• Give capsules, tablets with full glass of water 1 hr before or 2 hrs after meals.

TOPICAL

• Cleanse area gently before application. • Apply only to affected area.

INDICATIONS/ROUTES/DOSAGE

Alert: Space doses evenly around the clock.

USUAL DOSAGE

PO: ADULTS, ELDERLY: 250–500 mg q6–12h. CHILDREN >8 YRS: 25–50 mg/kg/day in 4 divided doses. **Maximum:** 3 g/day.

H. PYLORI

PO: ADULTS, ELDERLY: 500 mg 2–4 times/day (in combination).

DOSAGE IN RENAL IMPAIRMENT

Creatinine Clearance	Dosage Interval
50–80 ml/min	q8–12h
10–49 ml/min	q12–24h
<10 ml/min	q24h

USUAL TOPICAL DOSAGE

Topical: ADULTS, ELDERLY: Apply 2 times/day in morning, evening.

SIDE EFFECTS

FREQUENT: Dizziness, lightheadedness, diarrhea, nausea, vomiting, stomach cramps, increased sensitivity of skin to sunlight. **Topical:** Dry scaly skin, stinging, burning sensation. **OCCASIONAL:** Pigmentation of skin, mucous membranes, itching in rectal/genital area,

T

sore mouth/tongue. **Topical:** Pain, redness, swelling, other skin irritation.

ADVERSE REACTIONS/ TOXIC EFFECTS

Superinfection (esp. fungal), anaphylaxis, increased intracranial pressure, bulging fontanelles occur rarely in infants.

NURSING IMPLICATIONS

BASELINE ASSESSMENT

Question for history of allergies, esp. tetracyclines, sulfite.

INTERVENTION/EVALUATION

Assess skin for rash. Determine pattern of bowel activity, stool consistency. Monitor food intake, tolerance. Be alert for superinfection: diarrhea, ulceration/changes of oral mucosa, anal/genital pruritus. Monitor B/P, LOC (potential for increased intracranial pressure).

PATIENT/FAMILY TEACHING

Continue antibiotic for full length of treatment. Space doses evenly. Take oral doses on empty stomach (1 hr before or 2 hrs after food, beverages). Drink full glass of water with capsules; avoid bedtime doses. Notify physician if diarrhea, rash, other new symptom occurs. Protect skin from sun, ultraviolet light exposure. Consult physician before taking any other medication. **Topical:** Skin may turn yellow with topical application (washing removes solution); fabrics may be stained by heavy application. Do not apply to deep/open wounds.

Teveten

see eprosartan

thalidomide

thah-**lid**-owe-mide
(Thalomid)

CLASSIFICATION

PHARMACOTHERAPEUTIC: Immunomodulator. **CLINICAL:** Immunosuppressive agent.

ACTION

Exact mechanism unknown. Has sedative, anti-inflammatory, immunosuppressive activity. Action may be due to selective inhibition of the production of tumor necrosis factor alpha. **Therapeutic Effect:** Reduces local and systemic effects of leprosy.

USES

Treatment of leprosy. **Unlabeled:** Wasting syndrome of HIV or cancer, recurrent aphthous ulcers in HIV pts, multiple myeloma, Crohn's disease.

PRECAUTIONS

CONTRAINDICATIONS: Sensitivity to thalidomide, neutropenia, peripheral neuropathy, pregnancy. **CAUTIONS:** History of seizures. **Pregnancy Category X.**

INTERACTIONS

DRUG: **Alcohol, CNS depressants** may increase sedative effects. **Medication associated with peripheral neuropathy (e.g., INH, lithium, metronidazole, phenytoin)** may increase peripheral neuropathy. **Medications decreasing effectiveness of hormonal contraceptives (e.g., carbamazepine, protease inhibitors, rifampin)** may decrease effectiveness of the contraceptive (must use 2 other methods of contraception). **HERBAL:** None known. **FOOD:** None known. **LAB VALUES:** None known.

AVAILABILITY (Rx)

CAPSULES: 50 mg, 100 mg, 200 mg.

T

INDICATIONS/ROUTES/DOSAGE

AIDS-RELATED MUSCLE WASTING

PO: ADULTS: 100–300 mg daily.

SIDE EFFECTS

FREQUENT: Drowsiness, dizziness, mood changes, constipation, xerostomia, peripheral neuropathy. **OCCASIONAL:** Increased appetite, weight gain, headache, loss of libido, edema of face/limbs, nausea, hair loss, dry skin, skin rash, hypothyroidism.

ADVERSE REACTIONS/ TOXIC EFFECTS

Neutropenia, peripheral neuropathy, thromboembolism occur rarely.

NURSING IMPLICATIONS

BASELINE ASSESSMENT

Assess for hypersensitivity to thalidomide. Assess for pregnancy in females (contraindicated). Determine use of other medications (many interactions).

INTERVENTION/EVALUATION

Monitor WBC, nerve conduction studies, HIV viral load. Observe for signs/ symptoms of peripheral neuropathy.

PATIENT/FAMILY TEACHING

Avoid use of alcoholic beverages, other drugs causing drowsiness. Pregnancy test within 24 hrs before starting thalidomide, then q2–4wks in women of childbearing age. Discontinue and call physician if symptoms of peripheral neuropathy occur.

thiamine hydrochloride (vitamin B_1)

thigh-ah-min

(Betalin, Betaxin ✤)

◆CLASSIFICATION

PHARMACOTHERAPEUTIC: Water-soluble vitamin. **CLINICAL:** Vitamin B complex (see p. 136C).

ACTION

Combines with adenosine triphosphate (ATP) in liver, kidney, leukocytes to form thiamine diphosphate. **Therapeutic Effect:** Necessary for carbohydrate metabolism.

PHARMACOKINETICS

Readily absorbed from GI tract, primarily in duodenum, following IM administration. Widely distributed. Metabolized in liver. Primarily excreted in urine.

USES

Prevention/treatment of thiamine deficiency (e.g., beriberi, Wernicke's encephalopathy syndrome, peripheral neuritis associated with pellegra), alcoholic pts with altered sensorium.

PRECAUTIONS

CONTRAINDICATIONS: None known. **CAUTIONS:** None known.

LIFESPAN CONSIDERATIONS: Pregnancy/lactation: Crosses placenta. Unknown if excreted in breast milk. **Pregnancy Category A** (**C** if used in doses above RDA). **Children/elderly:** No age-related precautions noted.

INTERACTIONS

DRUG: None known. **HERBAL:** None known. **FOOD:** None known. **LAB VALUES:** None known.

AVAILABILITY (OTC)

TABLETS: 50 mg, 100 mg, 250 mg. **INJECTION (Rx):** 100 mg/ml.

ADMINISTRATION/HANDLING

Alert: IM/IV administration used only in acutely ill or those unresponsive to PO

T

route (GI malabsorption syndrome). IM route preferred to IV use. Give by IV push, or add to most IV solutions and give as infusion.

IV COMPATIBILITIES

Famotidine (Pepcid), multivitamins.

INDICATIONS/ROUTES/DOSAGE

DIETARY SUPPLEMENT

PO: ADULTS, ELDERLY: 1–2 mg/day. CHILDREN: 0.5–1 mg/day. INFANTS: 0.3–0.5 mg/day.

THIAMINE DEFICIENCY

PO: ADULTS, ELDERLY: 5–30 mg/day, in single or 3 divided doses, for 1 mo. CHILDREN: 10–50 mg/day in 3 divided doses.

CRITICALLY ILL/MALABSORPTION SYNDROME

IM/IV: ADULTS, ELDERLY: 5–100 mg, 3 times/day. CHILDREN: 10–25 mg/day.

METABOLIC DISORDERS

PO: ADULTS, ELDERLY, CHILDREN: 10–20 mg/day; up to 4 g in divided doses/day.

SIDE EFFECTS

FREQUENT: Pain, induration, tenderness at IM injection site.

ADVERSE REACTIONS/ TOXIC EFFECTS

Rare, severe hypersensitivity reaction with IV administration may result in feeling of warmth, pruritus, urticaria, weakness, diaphoresis, nausea, restlessness, tightness in throat, angioedema (swelling of face/lips), cyanosis, pulmonary edema, GI tract bleeding, cardiovascular collapse.

T

NURSING IMPLICATIONS

INTERVENTION/EVALUATION

Monitor lab values for erythrocyte activity, EKG readings. Assess for clinical improvement (improved sense of well-being, weight gain). Observe for reversal of deficiency symptoms (**neurologic:** peripheral neuropathy, hyporeflexia, nystagmus, ophthalmoplegia, ataxia, muscle weakness; **cardiac:** venous hypertension, bounding arterial pulse, tachycardia, edema; **mental:** confused state).

PATIENT/FAMILY TEACHING

Discomfort may occur with IM injection. Foods rich in thiamine include pork, organ meats, whole grain and enriched cereals, legumes, nuts, seeds, yeast, wheat germ, rice bran. Urine may appear bright yellow.

thioguanine

thigh-oh-**guan**-een

(Thioguanine)

See Classification section under: Cancer chemotherapeutic agents (p. 76C)

thiopental sodium

(Pentothal)

See Classification section under: Anesthetics: general (p. 3C)

thioridazine

thigh-oh-**rid**-ah-zeen

(Apo-Thioridazine✱, Mellaril)

Do not confuse with Mebaral, thiothixene, Thorazine.

CLASSIFICATION

PHARMACOTHERAPEUTIC: Phenothiazine. **CLINICAL:** Antipsychotic, sedative, antidyskinetic (see p. 57C).

ACTION

Blocks dopamine at postsynaptic receptor sites. Possesses strong anticholinergic, sedative effects. **Therapeutic Effect:** Suppresses behavioral response in psychosis, reducing locomotor activity, aggressiveness and suppressing conditioned responses.

USES

Treatment of refractory schizophrenic pts. **Unlabeled:** Depressive neurosis, dementia, behaviorial problems in children.

PRECAUTIONS

CONTRAINDICATIONS: Drugs that prolong QT interval, cardiac arrhythmias, severe CNS depression, narrow-angle glaucoma, blood dyscrasias, hepatic/cardiac impairment. **CAUTIONS:** Seizures. **Pregnancy Category C.**

INTERACTIONS

DRUG: **Alcohol, CNS depressants** may increase respiratory depression, hypotensive effects. **Tricyclic antidepressants, MAOIs** may increase sedative, anticholinergic effects. **Antithyroid agents** may increase risk of agranulocytosis. Extrapyramidal symptoms (EPS) may increase with **EPS-producing medications. Hypotensives** may increase hypotension. May decrease **levodopa** effects. **Lithium** may decrease absorption, produce adverse neurologic effects. **HERBAL:** None known. **FOOD:** None known. **LAB VALUES:** May cause EKG changes. Therapeutic blood serum level: 0.2–2.6 mcg/ml; toxic blood serum level: N/E.

AVAILABILITY (Rx)

TABLETS: 10 mg, 15 mg, 100 mg, 150 mg, 200 mg. **ORAL CONCENTRATE:** 30 mg/ml.

INDICATIONS/ROUTES/DOSAGE

PSYCHOSIS

PO: ADULTS, ELDERLY, CHILDREN >12 YRS: Initially, 25–100 mg 3 times/day. Gradually increase. **Maximum:** 800 mg/day. CHILDREN 2–12 YRS: Initially, 0.5 mg/kg/day in 2–3 divided doses. **Maximum:** 3 mg/kg/day.

SIDE EFFECTS

Generally well tolerated with only mild and transient effects. **OCCASIONAL:** Drowsiness during early therapy, dry mouth, blurred vision, lethargy, constipation, diarrhea, nasal congestion, peripheral edema, urinary retention. **RARE:** Ocular changes, skin pigmentation (those taking high dosages for prolonged periods), photosensitivity.

ADVERSE REACTIONS/ TOXIC EFFECTS

Prolongation of QT interval may produce torsades de pointes (a form of ventricular tachycardia), sudden death.

NURSING IMPLICATIONS

BASELINE ASSESSMENT

Avoid skin contact with solution (contact dermatitis). Assess behavior, appearance, emotional status, response to environment, speech pattern, thought content.

INTERVENTION/EVALUATION

Assess for extrapyramidal symptoms. Monitor EKG, potassium, CBC, B/P, hepatic function, eye exams. Monitor for fine tongue movement (may be early sign of tardive dyskinesia). Supervise suicidal-risk pt closely during early therapy (as depression lessens, energy level improves, and suicide potential increases). Assess for therapeutic response (interest in surroundings, improvement in self-care, increased ability to concentrate, relaxed facial

T

expression). Therapeutic blood serum level: 0.2–2.6 mcg/ml; toxic blood serum level: not established.

PATIENT/FAMILY TEACHING

Full therapeutic effect may take up to 6 wks. Urine may darken. Do not abruptly withdraw from long-term drug therapy. Report visual disturbances. Sugarless gum, sips of tepid water may relieve dry mouth. Drowsiness generally subsides during continued therapy. Avoid tasks that require alertness, motor skills until response to drug is established. Avoid alcohol. Avoid exposure to sunlight, artificial light.

thiotepa

thigh-oh-**teh**-pah
(Thiotepa)

CLASSIFICATION

PHARMACOTHERAPEUTIC: Alkylating agent. **CLINICAL:** Antineoplastic (see p. 76C).

ACTION

Binds with many intracellular structures. Cross-links strands of DNA, RNA. Cell cycle–phase nonspecific. **Therapeutic Effect:** Disrupts protein synthesis, producing cell death.

USES

Treatment of superficial papillary carcinoma of urinary bladder, adenocarcinoma of breast and ovary, Hodgkin's disease, lymphosarcoma. Intracavitary injection to control pleural, pericardial, peritoneal effusions due to metastatic tumors. **Unlabeled:** Treatment of lung carcinoma.

PRECAUTIONS

CONTRAINDICATIONS: Severe myelosuppression (leukocytes <3,000/mm^3 or platelets <150,000 mm^3), pregnancy. **CAUTIONS:** Hepatic/renal impairment, bone marrow dysfunction. **Pregnancy Category D.**

INTERACTIONS

DRUG: May decrease effect of **antigout medications. Bone marrow depressants** may increase bone marrow depression. **Live virus vaccines** may potentiate virus replication, increase vaccine side effects, decrease pt's antibody response to vaccine. **HERBAL:** None known. **FOOD:** None known. **LAB VALUES:** May increase uric acid levels.

AVAILABILITY (Rx)

POWDER FOR INJECTION: 15 mg, 30 mg.

ADMINISTRATION/HANDLING

Alert: May be carcinogenic, mutagenic, teratogenic. Handle with extreme care during preparation/administration.

IV

Alert: Give by IV, intrapleural, intraperitoneal, intrapericardial, or intratumor injection; intravesical instillation.

Storage • Refrigerate unopened vials. • Reconstituted solution appears clear to slightly opaque; is stable for 5 days if refrigerated. Discard if solution appears grossly opaque or precipitate forms.

Reconstitution • Reconstitute 15-mg vial with 1.5 ml Sterile Water for Injection to provide concentration of 10 mg/ml. Shake solution gently; let stand to clear.

Rate of administration Withdraw reconstituted drug through a 0.22-micron filter prior to administration. For IV push, give over 5 min at concentration of 10 mg/ml. Give IV infusion at concentration of 1 mg/ml.

∅ IV INCOMPATIBILITIES

Cisplatin (Platinol AQ), filgrastim (Neupogen).

IV COMPATIBILITIES

Allopurinol (Aloprim), bumetanide (Bumex), calcium gluconate, carboplatin (Paraplatin), cyclophosphamide (Cytoxan), dexamethasone (Decadron), diphenhydramine (Benadryl), doxorubicin (Adriamycin), etoposide (VePesid), fluorouracil, gemcitabine (Gemzar), granisetron (Kytril), heparin, hydromorphone (Dilaudid), leucovorin, lorazepam (Ativan), magnesium sulfate, morphine, ondansetron (Zofran), paclitaxel (Taxol), potassium chloride, vincristine (Oncovin), vinorelbine (Navelbine).

INDICATIONS/ROUTES/DOSAGE

Alert: Dosage individualized based on clinical response, tolerance to adverse effects. When used in combination therapy, consult specific protocols for optimum dosage, sequence of drug administration.

INITIAL TREATMENT

IV: ADULTS, ELDERLY: 0.3–0.4 mg/kg q1–4wks. Maintenance dose adjusted weekly on basis of blood counts. CHILDREN: 25–65 mg/m^2 as a single dose q3–4wks.

Intracavitary: ADULTS, ELDERLY: 0.6–0.8 mg/kg q1–4wks.

SIDE EFFECTS

OCCASIONAL: Pain at injection site, headache, dizziness, hives, rash, nausea, vomiting, anorexia, stomatitis. **RARE:** Alopecia, cystitis, hematuria following intravesical dosing.

ADVERSE REACTIONS/ TOXIC EFFECTS

Hematologic toxicity manifested as leukopenia, anemia, thrombocytopenia, pancytopenia due to bone marrow depression. Although WBC falls to lowest point at 10–14 days after initial therapy, bone marrow effects not evident for 30 days. Stomatitis, ulceration of intestinal mucosa may be noted.

NURSING IMPLICATIONS

BASELINE ASSESSMENT

Obtain hematologic status at least weekly during therapy and for 3 wks after therapy discontinued.

INTERVENTION/EVALUATION

Interrupt therapy if WBC falls below 3,000/mm^3, platelet count below 150,000/mm^3, WBC or platelet count declines rapidly. Monitor uric acid serum levels, hematology tests. Assess for stomatitis (burning/erythema of oral mucosa at inner margin of lips, sore throat, difficulty swallowing, oral ulceration). Monitor for hematologic toxicity: infection (fever, sore throat, signs of local infection), unusual bruising/bleeding from any site, symptoms of anemia (excessive tiredness, weakness). Assess skin for rash, hives.

PATIENT/FAMILY TEACHING

Maintain fastidious oral hygiene. Do not have immunizations without physician's approval (drug lowers body's resistance). Avoid crowds, those with infection. Promptly report fever, sore throat, signs of local infection, unusual bruising/bleeding from any site.

T

thiothixene

thigh-oh-**thicks**-een
(Navane)
Do not confuse with thioridazine.

◆ CLASSIFICATION

CLINICAL: Antipsychotic (see p. 57C).

ACTION

Blocks postsynaptic dopamine receptor sites in brain. Has alpha-adrenergic blocking effects; depresses release of hypothalamic, hypophyseal hormones. **Therapeutic Effect:** Suppresses behavioral response in psychosis.

PHARMACOKINETICS

Well absorbed from GI tract following IM administration. Widely distributed. Metabolized in liver. Primarily excreted in urine. Unknown if removed by hemodialysis. **Half-life:** 34 hrs.

USES

Symptomatic management of psychotic disorders.

PRECAUTIONS

CONTRAINDICATIONS: Comatose states, circulatory collapse, CNS depression, blood dyscrasias, history of seizures. **CAUTIONS:** Severe cardiovascular disorders, alcoholic withdrawal, pt exposure to extreme heat, glaucoma, prostatic hypertrophy.

LIFESPAN CONSIDERATIONS: Pregnancy/lactation: Crosses placenta. Distributed in breast milk. **Pregnancy Category C. Children:** May develop neuromuscular or extrapyramidal symptoms, esp. dystonias. **Elderly:** More prone to orthostatic hypotension, anticholinergic effects (e.g., dry mouth), sedation, extrapyramidal symptoms (EPS).

T

INTERACTIONS

DRUG: Alcohol, CNS depressants may increase CNS, respiratory depression, increase hypotension. **Extrapyramidal symptom (EPS)–producing medications** may increase risk of EPS. May inhibit effects of **levodopa.** May increase cardiac effects with **quinidine. HERBAL: Kava kava, valerian, St. John's wort** may increase CNS depression. **FOOD:** None known. **LAB VALUES:** May decrease uric acid.

AVAILABILITY (Rx)

CAPSULES: 1 mg, 2 mg, 5 mg, 10 mg, 20 mg. **ORAL CONCENTRATE:** 5 mg/ml.

ADMINISTRATION/HANDLING

PO

• Give without regard to meals. • Avoid skin contact with oral solution (contact dermatitis).

INDICATIONS/ROUTES/DOSAGE

PSYCHOSIS

PO: ADULTS, ELDERLY, CHILDREN >12 YRS: Initially, 2 mg 3 times/day. **Maximum:** 60 mg/day.

SIDE EFFECTS

Hypotension, dizziness, fainting occur frequently after first injection, occasionally after subsequent injections, rarely with oral dosage. **FREQUENT:** Transient drowsiness, dry mouth, constipation, blurred vision, nasal congestion. **OCCASIONAL:** Diarrhea, peripheral edema, urinary retention, nausea. **RARE:** Ocular changes, skin pigmentation (those taking high dosage for prolonged periods), photosensitivity.

ADVERSE REACTIONS/ TOXIC EFFECTS

Akathisia (motor restlessness, anxiety) is the most frequently noted extrapyramidal symptom. Akinesia (rigidity, tremor, salivation, masklike facial expression, reduced voluntary movements) occurs less frequently. Infrequently noted are dystonias: torticollis (neck muscle spasm), opisthotonos (rigidity of back muscles), and oculogyric crisis (rolling back of eyes). Tardive dyskinesia (protrusion of tongue, puffing of cheeks, chewing/puckering of mouth) occurs rarely but may be irreversible. Risk is greater in female geriatric pts. Grand mal seizures may occur in epileptic pts (risk higher with IM administration). Neuroleptic malignant syndrome occurs rarely.

NURSING IMPLICATIONS

BASELINE ASSESSMENT

Assess behavior, appearance, emotional status, response to environment, speech pattern, thought content.

INTERVENTION/EVALUATION

Supervise suicidal-risk pt closely during early therapy (as depression lessens, energy level improves, increasing suicide potential). Monitor B/P for hypotension. Assess for peripheral edema. Assess stools for frequency, consistency. Prevent constipation. Monitor for EPS, tardive dyskinesia (see Adverse Reactions/Toxic Effects) and potentially fatal, rare neuroleptic malignant syndrome: fever, irregular pulse or B/P, muscle rigidity, altered mental status. Assess for therapeutic response (interest in surroundings, improvement in self-care, increased ability to concentrate, relaxed facial expression).

PATIENT/FAMILY TEACHING

Full therapeutic effect may take up to 6 wks. Report visual disturbances. Sugarless gum, sips of tepid water may relieve dry mouth. Drowsiness generally subsides during continued therapy. Avoid tasks that require alertness, motor skills until response to drug is established. Avoid alcohol, other CNS depressants. Avoid exposure to direct sunlight, artificial light.

thyroid

(Armour Thyroid, S-P-T, Thyrar)

See Classification section under: Thyroid (p. 135C)

tiagabine

tie-**ag**-ah-bean
(Gabitril)

◆CLASSIFICATION

CLINICAL: Anticonvulsant (see p. 33C).

ACTION

Blocks reuptake of gamma-aminobutyric acid (GABA) in the presynaptic neurons, the major inhibitory neurotransmitter in the CNS, increasing GABA levels at postsynaptic neurons. **Therapeutic Effect:** Inhibits seizures.

USES

Adjunctive therapy for treatment of partial seizures.

PRECAUTIONS

CONTRAINDICATIONS: None known. **CAUTIONS:** Hepatic function impairment. Concurrent use of alcohol, other CNS depressants. **Pregnancy Category C.**

INTERACTIONS

DRUG: May alter **valproate** effect. **Carbamazepine, phenytoin, phenobarbital** may increase tiagabine clearance. **HERBAL:** None known. **FOOD:** None known. **LAB VALUES:** None known.

AVAILABILITY (Rx)

TABLETS: 2 mg, 4 mg, 12 mg, 16 mg.

INDICATIONS/ROUTES/DOSAGE

PARTIAL SEIZURES

PO: ADULTS, ELDERLY: Initially, 4 mg once daily. May increase by 4–8 mg/day at weekly intervals. **Maximum:** 56 mg/day. CHILDREN 12–18 YRS: Initially, 4 mg

T

once daily, may increase by 4 mg at week 2 and by 4–8 mg/wk thereafter. **Maximum:** 32 mg/day.

SIDE EFFECTS

FREQUENT (20%–34%): Dizziness, asthenia (loss of strength, energy), somnolence, nervousness, confusion, headache, infection, tremor. **OCCASIONAL:** Nausea, diarrhea, stomach pain, difficulty concentrating, weakness.

ADVERSE REACTIONS/ TOXIC EFFECTS

Overdosage characterized by agitation, confusion, hostility, weakness. Full recovery occurs within 24 hrs.

NURSING IMPLICATIONS

BASELINE ASSESSMENT

Review history of seizure disorder (intensity, frequency, duration, LOC). Observe frequently for recurrence of seizure activity. Initiate seizure precautions.

INTERVENTION/EVALUATION

For those on long-term therapy, hepatic/renal function tests, CBC should be performed periodically. Assist with ambulation if dizziness occurs. Assess for clinical improvement (decrease in intensity/frequency of seizures).

PATIENT/FAMILY TEACHING

If dizziness occurs, change positions slowly from recumbent to sitting position before standing. Avoid tasks that require alertness, motor skills until response to drug is established. Avoid alcohol.

Tiazac

see diltiazem

ticarcillin disodium

(Ticar)

See Classification section under: Antibiotic: penicillins

ticarcillin disodium/ clavulanate potassium

tie-car-**sill**-in/klah-view-**lan**-ate (Timentin)

CLASSIFICATION

PHARMACOTHERAPEUTIC: Penicillin. **CLINICAL:** Antibiotic (see p. 27C).

ACTION

Ticarcillin: Binds to bacterial cell wall, inhibiting bacterial cell wall synthesis. **Therapeutic Effect:** Causes cell lysis, death. Bactericidal. **Clavulanate:** Inhibits action of bacterial beta-lactamase. **Therapeutic Effect:** Protects ticarcillin from enzymatic degradation.

PHARMACOKINETICS

Widely distributed. Protein binding: **Ticarcillin:** 45%–60%. **Clavulanate:** 9%–30%. Minimal metabolism in liver. Primarily excreted unchanged in urine. Removed by hemodialysis. **Half-life:** 1–1.2 hrs (half-life increased with impaired renal function).

USES

Treatment of septicemia; skin/skin structure, bone, joint, lower respiratory tract, urinary tract infections; endometritis.

PRECAUTIONS

CONTRAINDICATIONS: Hypersensitivity to any penicillin. **CAUTIONS:** History of allergies, esp. cephalosporins, renal impairment.

LIFESPAN CONSIDERATIONS: Pregnancy/lactation: Readily crosses placenta; appears in cord blood, amniotic fluid. Distributed in breast milk in low concentrations. May lead to allergic sensitization, diarrhea, candidiasis, skin rash in infant. **Pregnancy Category B. Children:** Safety and efficacy not established in those <3 mos. **Elderly:** Age-related renal impairment may require dosage adjustment.

INTERACTIONS

DRUG: Anticoagulants, heparin, thrombolytics, NSAIDs may increase risk of hemorrhage with high dosages of ticarcillin. **Probenecid** may increase concentration, risk of toxicity. **HERBAL:** None known. **FOOD:** None known. **LAB VALUES:** May cause positive Coombs' test. May increase SGOT (AST), SGPT (ALT), alkaline phosphatase, bilirubin, creatinine, LDH, bleeding time. May decrease potassium, sodium, uric acid.

AVAILABILITY (Rx)

POWDER FOR INJECTION: 3.1 g. **SOLUTION FOR INFUSION:** 3.1 g/100 ml.

ADMINISTRATION/HANDLING

IV

Storage • Solution appears colorless to pale yellow (if solution darkens, indicates loss of potency). • Reconstituted IV infusion (piggyback) is stable for 24 hrs at room temperature, 3 days if refrigerated. • Discard if precipitate forms.

Reconstitution • Available in ready-to-use containers. • For IV infusion (piggyback), reconstitute each 3.1-g vial with 13 ml Sterile Water for Injection or 0.9% NaCl to provide concentration of 200 mg ticarcillin and 6.7 mg clavulanic acid per ml. • Shake vial to assist reconstitution. • Further dilute with 50–100 ml D_5W or 0.9% NaCl.

Rate of administration • Infuse over 30 min. • Because of potential for hypersensitivity/anaphylaxis, start initial dose at few drops/min, increase slowly to ordered rate. Monitor pt first 10–15 min, then check q10min.

IV INCOMPATIBILITIES

Amphotericin B complex (Abelcet, AmBisome, Amphotec), vancomycin (Vancocin).

IV COMPATIBILITIES

Diltiazem (Cardizem), heparin, insulin, morphine, propofol (Diprivan).

INDICATIONS/ROUTES/DOSAGE

SYSTEMIC INFECTIONS

IV: ADULTS, ELDERLY: 3.1 g (3 g ticarcillin) q4–6h. **Maximum:** 18–24 g/day. CHILDREN >3 MOS: 200–300 mg (as ticarcillin) q4–6h.

UTI

IV: ADULTS, ELDERLY: 3.1 g q6–8h.

DOSAGE IN RENAL IMPAIRMENT

Creatinine Clearance	Dosage Interval
10–30 ml/min	q8h
<10 ml/min	q12h

SIDE EFFECTS

FREQUENT: Phlebitis, thrombophlebitis with IV dose, rash, urticaria, pruritus, taste/smell disturbances. **OCCASIONAL:** Nausea, diarrhea, vomiting. **RARE:** Headache, fatigue, hallucinations, bruising/bleeding.

ADVERSE REACTIONS/ TOXIC EFFECTS

Overdosage may produce seizures, neurologic reactions. Superinfections, potentially fatal antibiotic-associated colitis

T

may result from bacterial imbalance. Severe hypersensitivity reactions, including anaphylaxis, occur rarely.

NURSING IMPLICATIONS

BASELINE ASSESSMENT

Question for history of allergies, esp. penicillins, cephalosporins.

INTERVENTION/EVALUATION

Hold medication and promptly report rash (hypersensitivity), diarrhea (fever, abdominal pain, mucus and blood in stool may indicate antibiotic-associated colitis). Assess food tolerance. Provide mouth care, sugarless gum, hard candy to offset taste, smell effects. Evaluate IV site for phlebitis (heat, pain, red streaking over vein). Monitor I&O, urinalysis, renal function tests. Assess for overt bleeding, bruising, swelling. Monitor hematology reports, electrolytes, particularly potassium. Be alert for superinfection: increased fever, sore throat, diarrhea, vomiting, ulceration or other oral changes, anal/genital pruritus.

ticlopidine hydrochloride

tie-**clow**-pih-deen

(Apo-Ticlopidine✤, Ticlid)

CLASSIFICATION

PHARMACOTHERAPEUTIC: Aggregation inhibitor. **CLINICAL:** Antiplatelet (see p. 29C).

ACTION

Inhibits ADP-induced platelet-fibrinogen binding, further platelet-platelet interactions. **Therapeutic Effect:** Inhibits platelet aggregation.

USES

To reduce risk of stroke in those who have experienced stroke-like symptoms (transient ischemic attacks) or those with history of thrombotic stroke. **Unlabeled:** Treatment of intermittent claudication, subarachnoid hemorrhage, sickle cell disease.

PRECAUTIONS

CONTRAINDICATIONS: Hematopoietic disorders (neutropenia, thrombocytopenia), presence of hemostatic disorder, active pathologic bleeding (e.g., bleeding peptic ulcer, intracranial bleeding), severe hepatic impairment. **CAUTIONS:** Those at increased risk of bleeding, severe hepatic/renal disease. **Pregnancy Category B.**

INTERACTIONS

DRUG: May increase risk of bleeding with **oral anticoagulants, heparin, thrombolytics, aspirin.** **HERBAL:** None known. **FOOD:** None known. **LAB VALUES:** May increase alkaline phosphatase, bilirubin, liver function tests, cholesterol, triglycerides. May prolong bleeding time. May decrease neutrophil, platelet count.

AVAILABILITY (Rx)

TABLETS: 250 mg.

ADMINISTRATION/HANDLING

PO

- Give with food or just after meals (bioavailability increased, GI discomfort decreased).

INDICATIONS/ROUTES/DOSAGE

PREVENTION OF STROKE

PO: ADULTS, ELDERLY: 250 mg 2 times/day.

SIDE EFFECTS

FREQUENT (5%–13%): Diarrhea, nausea, dyspepsia (heartburn, indigestion, GI discomfort, bloating). **RARE (1%–2%):** Vomiting, flatulence, pruritus, dizziness.

T

ADVERSE REACTIONS/ TOXIC EFFECTS

Neutropenia occurs in approx. 2% of pts. Thrombotic thrombocytopenia purpura (TTP), agranulocytosis, hepatitis, cholestatic jaundice, tinnitus occur rarely.

NURSING IMPLICATIONS

BASELINE ASSESSMENT

Drug should be discontinued 10–14 days prior to surgery if antiplatelet effect is not desired.

INTERVENTION/EVALUATION

Monitor bowel activity, stool consistency. Assist with ambulation if dizziness occurs. Monitor heart sounds by auscultation. Assess B/P for hypotension. Assess skin for flushing, rash. Observe for signs of bleeding. Monitor CBC, hepatic function tests.

PATIENT/FAMILY TEACHING

Take with food to decrease GI symptoms. Periodic blood tests are essential. Inform physician if fever, sore throat, chills, unusual bleeding occurs.

tiludronate

tie-**lew**-dro-nate
(Skelid)

◆ CLASSIFICATION

PHARMACOTHERAPEUTIC: Bone resorption inhibitor. **CLINICAL:** Calcium regulator.

ACTION

Inhibits functioning osteoclasts through disruption of cytoskeletal ring structure and inhibition of osteoclastic proton pump. **Therapeutic Effect:** Inhibits bone resorption.

USES

Treatment of Paget's disease of bone (osteitis deformans).

PRECAUTIONS

CONTRAINDICATIONS: GI disease (e.g., dysphagia, gastric ulcer), impaired renal function. **CAUTIONS:** Hyperparathyroidism, hypocalcemia, vitamin D deficiency. **Pregnancy Category C.**

INTERACTIONS

DRUG: Aluminium- or magnesium-containing antacids, calcium, salicylates may interfere with tiludronate absorption. **HERBAL:** None known. **FOOD:** None known. **LAB VALUES:** None known.

AVAILABILITY (Rx)

TABLETS: 200 mg.

INDICATIONS/ROUTES/DOSAGE

PAGET'S DISEASE

PO: ADULTS, ELDERLY: 400 mg once daily for 3 mos. Must take with 6–8 oz plain water. Do not take within 2 hrs of food intake. Avoid taking aspirin, calcium supplements, mineral supplements, antacids within 2 hrs of taking tiludronate.

SIDE EFFECTS

FREQUENT (6%–9%): Nausea, diarrhea, generalized body pain, back pain, headache. **OCCASIONAL:** Rash, dyspepsia, vomiting, rhinitis, sinusitis, dizziness.

NURSING IMPLICATIONS

BASELINE ASSESSMENT

Assess if pt is pregnant, using medications (esp. aluminum, magnesium, calcium, salicylates). Determine baseline renal function. Assess for GI disease.

INTERVENTION/EVALUATION

Monitor alkaline phosphatase, urinary hydroxyproline, adjusted calcium, serum osteocalcin to assess effectiveness of medication.

T

PATIENT/FAMILY TEACHING

Take with 6–8 oz water. Avoid other medication for 2 hrs before or after taking tiludronate. Check with physician if calcium and vitamin D supplements are necessary.

timolol maleate

tim-oh-lol

(Apo-Timol ♣, Apo-Timop ♣, Betimol, Blocadren, Gen-Timolol ♣, Novo-Timol, Timoptic, Timoptic XE)

Do not confuse with atenolol, Viroptic.

FIXED-COMBINATION(S)

Timolide: timolol/hydrochlorothiazide (a diuretic): 10 mg/25 mg. **Cosopt:** timolol/dorzolamide (a carbonic anhydrase inhibitor): 0.5%/2%.

◆CLASSIFICATION

PHARMACOTHERAPEUTIC: Beta-adrenergic blocker. **CLINICAL:** Antihypertensive, antimigraine, antiglaucoma (see pp. 46C, 63C).

ACTION

Blocks $beta_1$-, $beta_2$-adrenergic receptors. **Therapeutic Effect:** Reduces intraocular pressure (IOP) by reducing aqueous humor production, reduces B/P, produces negative chronotropic and inotropic activity.

PHARMACOKINETICS

Onset	Peak	Duration
Eyedrops		
30 min	1–2 hrs	12–24 hrs

Well absorbed from GI tract. Protein binding: <10%. Minimal absorption following ophthalmic administration. Metabolized in liver. Primarily excreted in urine. Not removed by hemodialysis. **Half-life:** 4 hrs. **Ophthalmic:** Systemic absorption may occur.

USES

Management of mild to moderate hypertension. Used alone or in combination with diuretics, esp. thiazide type. Reduces cardiovascular mortality in those with definite/suspected acute MI. Prophylaxis of migraine headache. **Ophthalmic:** Reduces IOP in management of open-angle glaucoma, aphakic glaucoma, ocular hypertension, secondary glaucoma. **Unlabeled: Systemic:** Treatment of chronic angina pectoris, cardiac arrhythmias, hypertrophic cardiomyopathy, pheochromocytoma, tremors, anxiety, thyrotoxicosis, migraines. **Ophthalmic:** With miotics, decreases IOP in acute/chronic angle-closure glaucoma, treatment of secondary glaucoma, malignant glaucoma, angle-closure glaucoma during/after iridectomy.

PRECAUTIONS

CONTRAINDICATIONS: Bronchial asthma, COPD, uncontrolled cardiac failure, sinus bradycardia, heart block greater than first degree, cardiogenic shock, CHF unless secondary to tachyarrhythmias, those on MAOIs. Precautions also apply to oral and ophthalmic administration (due to systemic absorption of ophthalmic). **CAUTIONS:** Inadequate cardiac function, impaired renal/hepatic function, hyperthyroidism.

LIFESPAN CONSIDERATIONS: Pregnancy/lactation: Distributed in breast milk; not for use in nursing women because of potential for serious adverse effect on breast-feeding infant. Avoid use during first trimester. May produce bradycardia, apnea, hypoglycemia, hypothermia during delivery, low birth-weight infants. **Pregnancy Category C** (**D** if used in second or third trimester). **Children:** Safety and efficacy not established. **Elderly:** Age-related peripheral vascular disease increases susceptibility to decreased peripheral circulation.

INTERACTIONS

DRUG: Diuretics, other hypotensives may increase hypotensive effect. **Sympathomimetics, xanthines** may mutually inhibit effects. May mask symptoms of hypoglycemia, prolong hypoglycemic effect of **insulin, oral hypoglycemics. NSAIDs** may decrease antihypertensive effect. **HERBAL:** None known. **FOOD:** None known. **LAB VALUES:** May increase ANA titer, SGOT (AST), SGPT (ALT), alkaline phosphatase, LDH, bilirubin, BUN, creatinine, potassium, uric acid, lipoproteins, triglycerides.

AVAILABILITY (Rx)

TABLETS: 5 mg, 10 mg, 20 mg. **OPHTHALMIC SOLUTION:** 0.25%, 0.5%. **OPHTHALMIC GEL:** 0.25%, 0.5%.

ADMINISTRATION/HANDLING

PO

• Give without regard to meals. • Tablets may be crushed.

OPHTHALMIC

Alert: When using gel, invert container, shake once prior to each use.

• Place finger on lower eyelid, pull out until pocket is formed between eye and lower lid. • Hold dropper above pocket, place prescribed number of drops or amount of prescribed gel into pocket. Instruct pt to close eyes gently so that medication will not be squeezed out of sac. • Apply gentle finger pressure to the lacrimal sac at inner canthus for 1 min following installation (lessens risk of systemic absorption).

INDICATIONS/ROUTES/DOSAGE

HYPERTENSION

PO: ADULTS, ELDERLY: Initially, 10 mg 2 times/day, alone or in combination with other therapy. Gradually increase at intervals of not less than 1 wk. MAINTENANCE: 20–60 mg/day in 2 divided doses.

MI

PO: ADULTS, ELDERLY: 10 mg 2 times/day, beginning within 1–4 wks after infarction.

MIGRAINE PROPHYLAXIS

PO: ADULTS, ELDERLY: Initially, 10 mg 2 times/day. RANGE: 10–30 mg/day.

GLAUCOMA

Ophthalmic: ADULTS, ELDERLY, CHILDREN: 1 drop of 0.25% solution in affected eye(s) 2 times/day. May be increased to 1 drop of 0.5% solution in affected eye(s) 2 times/day. When IOP is controlled, dosage may be reduced to 1 drop 1 time/day. If pt is transferred to timolol from another antiglaucoma agent, administer concurrently for 1 day. Discontinue other agent on following day. **Timoptic XE:** ADULTS, ELDERLY: 1 drop/day.

SIDE EFFECTS

FREQUENT: Decreased sexual function, drowsiness, difficulty sleeping, unusual tiredness/weakness. **Ophthalmic:** Eye irritation, visual disturbances. **OCCASIONAL:** Depression, cold hands/feet, diarrhea, constipation, anxiety, nasal congestion, nausea, vomiting. **RARE:** Altered taste, dry eyes, itching, numbness of fingers, toes, scalp.

ADVERSE REACTIONS/ TOXIC EFFECTS

Oral form may produce profound bradycardia, hypotension, bronchospasm. Abrupt withdrawal may result in diaphoresis, palpitations, headache, tremulousness. May precipitate CHF, MI in those with cardiac disease; thyroid storm in those with thyrotoxicosis; peripheral ischemia in those with existing peripheral vascular disease. Hypoglycemia may occur in pts with previously controlled diabetes. Ophthalmic overdosage may produce bradycardia, hypotension, bronchospasm, acute cardiac failure.

NURSING IMPLICATIONS

BASELINE ASSESSMENT

Assess B/P, apical pulse immediately prior to drug is administered (if pulse is ≤60/min or systolic B/P is <90 mm Hg, withhold medication, contact physician).

INTERVENTION/EVALUATION

Assess pulse for quality, irregular rate, bradycardia. Monitor EKG for cardiac arrhythmias, particularly PVCs. Monitor stool frequency, consistency. Monitor heart rate, B/P, hepatic and renal function, intraocular pressure (ophthalmic preparation).

PATIENT/FAMILY TEACHING

Do not abruptly discontinue medication. Compliance with therapy regimen is essential to control glaucoma, hypertension, angina, arrhythmias. Avoid tasks that require alertness, motor skills until response to drug is established. Report shortness of breath, excessive fatigue, prolonged dizziness/headache. Do not use nasal decongestants, OTC cold preparations (stimulants) without physician approval. Restrict salt, alcohol intake. **Ophthalmic:** Teach pt how to instill drops correctly, how to take pulse. Transient stinging, discomfort may occur upon instillation.

T

tinzaparin sodium

tin-zah-**pare**-inn
(Innohep)

CLASSIFICATION

PHARMACOTHERAPEUTIC: Low-molecular-weight heparin. **CLINICAL:** Anticoagulant (see p. 29C).

ACTION

Inhibits factor Xa. Tinzaparin causes less inactivation of thrombin, inhibition of platelets, and bleeding than standard heparin. Does not significantly influence bleeding time, prothrombin time (PT), activated partial thromboplastin time (aPTT). **Therapeutic Effect:** Produces anticoagulation.

PHARMACOKINETICS

Well absorbed following subcutaneous administration. Primarily eliminated in urine. **Half-life:** 3–4 hrs.

USES

Treatment of acute symptomatic deep vein thrombosis (DVT) with or without pulmonary embolism, when given in conjunction with warfarin.

PRECAUTIONS

CONTRAINDICATIONS: Active major bleeding, concurrent heparin therapy, thrombocytopenia associated with positive in vitro test for antiplatelet antibody, hypersensitivity to heparin or pork products. **CAUTIONS:** Conditions with increased risk of hemorrhage, history of heparin-induced thrombocytopenia, impaired renal function, elderly, uncontrolled arterial hypertension, history of recent GI ulceration/hemorrhage.

LIFESPAN CONSIDERATIONS: Pregnancy/lactation: Use with caution, particularly during last trimester, immediate postpartum period (increased risk of maternal hemorrhage). Unknown if distributed in breast milk. **Pregnancy Category B. Children:** Safety and efficacy not established. **Elderly:** May be more susceptible to bleeding.

INTERACTIONS

DRUG: Anticoagulants, platelet inhibitors may increase bleeding (use with caution). **HERBAL: Ginkgo biloba** may increase risk of bleeding. **FOOD:**

None known. **LAB VALUES:** Reversible increases in SGOT (AST), SGPT (ALT), alkaline phosphatase, LDH.

AVAILABILITY (Rx)

INJECTION: 20,000 anti-Xa international units/ml.

ADMINISTRATION/HANDLING

Alert: Do not mix with other injections or infusions. Do not give IM.

SUBCUTANEOUS

• Parenteral form appears clear and colorless to pale yellow. • Store at room temperature. • Instruct pt to lie down before administering by deep subcutaneous injection. • Introduce entire length of needle (½ inch) into skin fold held between thumb and forefinger, holding skin fold during injection. • Inject between left and right anterolateral and left and right posterolateral abdominal wall.

INDICATIONS/ROUTES/DOSAGE

DEEP VEIN THROMBOSIS (DVT)

Subcutaneous: ADULTS, ELDERLY: 175 anti-Xa international units/kg given once daily. Continue at least 6 days and until pt is sufficiently anticoagulated with warfarin (INR ≥2 for 2 consecutive days).

SIDE EFFECTS

FREQUENT (16%): Injection site reaction (inflammation, oozing, nodules, skin necrosis). **RARE (<2%):** Nausea, asthenia (unusual tiredness/weakness), constipation, epistaxis (nosebleed).

ADVERSE REACTIONS/ TOXIC EFFECTS

Accidental overdosage may lead to bleeding complications ranging from local ecchymoses to major hemorrhage. **ANTIDOTE:** Dose of protamine sulfate (1% solution) should be equal to the dose of tinzaparin injected. One mg protamine sulfate neutralizes 100 international units of tinzaparin. A second dose of 0.5 mg/mg protamine sulfate may be given if aPTT tested 2–4 hrs after the first infusion remains prolonged.

NURSING IMPLICATIONS

BASELINE ASSESSMENT

Assess CBC, including platelet count. Determine initial B/P.

INTERVENTION/EVALUATION

Periodically monitor CBC, platelet count. Assess for any sign of bleeding: bleeding at surgical site, hematuria, blood in stool, bleeding from gums, petechiae, bruising, bleeding from injection sites.

PATIENT/FAMILY TEACHING

Administer only subcutaneously. May have tendency to bleed easily, use precautions (e.g., use electric razor, soft toothbrush). Inform physician if chest pain, unusual bleeding/bruising, pain, numbness, tingling, swelling in joints, injection site reaction (oozing, nodules, inflammation) occurs.

tioconazole

tie-oh-**con**-ah-zole

(Gynecure ✤, Trosyd ✤, Vagistat)

Do not confuse with terconazole.

CLASSIFICATION

PHARMACOTHERAPEUTIC: Imidazole derivative. **CLINICAL:** Antifungal.

ACTION

Inhibits synthesis of ergosterol (vital component of fungal cell formation). **Therapeutic Effect:** Damages fungal cell membrane. Fungistatic.

USES

Treatment of vulvovaginal candidiasis (moniliasis).

T

INTERACTIONS

DRUG: None known. **HERBAL:** None known. **FOOD:** None known. **LAB VALUES:** None known.

AVAILABILITY (OTC)

VAGINAL OINTMENT: 6.5%.

INDICATIONS/ROUTES/DOSAGE

VULVOVAGINAL CANDIDIASIS

Intravaginal: ADULTS, ELDERLY: 1 applicatorful just before bedtime as a single dose.

SIDE EFFECTS

FREQUENT (25%): Headache. **OCCASIONAL (1%–6%):** Burning, itching. **RARE (<1%):** Irritation, vaginal pain, dysuria, dryness of vaginal secretions, vulvar edema/swelling.

tirofiban

tie-**row**-fih-ban

(Aggrastat)

Do not confuse with Aggrenox.

CLASSIFICATION

PHARMACOTHERAPEUTIC: Glycoprotein (GP) IIb/IIIa inhibitor. **CLINICAL:** Antiplatelet, antithrombotic (see p. 30C).

ACTION

Binds to platelet receptor glycoprotein IIb/IIIa, preventing binding of fibrinogen. **Therapeutic Effect:** Inhibits platelet aggregation.

PHARMACOKINETICS

Poorly bound to plasma proteins; unbound fraction in plasma: 35%. Limited metabolism. Primarily eliminated in the urine (65%) and, to a lesser amount, in the feces. **Half-life:** 2 hrs. Clearance is significantly decreased in severe renal impairment (creatinine clearance <30 ml/min). Removed by hemodialysis.

USES

In combination with heparin, treatment of acute coronary syndrome, including those to be managed medically and those undergoing percutaneous transluminal coronary angioplasty (PTCA) or atherectomy.

PRECAUTIONS

CONTRAINDICATIONS: Active internal bleeding or a history of bleeding diathesis within previous 30 days, history of thrombocytopenia after prior exposure to tirofiban, stroke, major surgical procedure within previous 30 days, severe hypertension, history of intracranial hemorrhage, intracranial neoplasm, arteriovenous malformation or aneurysm. **CAUTIONS:** Pts with platelets <150,000/mm^3, hemorrhagic retinopathy. Concomitant use of drugs affecting hemostasis (e.g., warfarin), renal function impairment.

LIFESPAN CONSIDERATIONS: Pregnancy/lactation: Unknown if distributed in breast milk. **Pregnancy Category B. Children:** Safety and efficacy not established. **Elderly:** Increased risk of bleeding; caution advised.

INTERACTIONS

DRUG: Drugs that affect hemostasis **(e.g., aspirin, NSAIDs, heparin, thrombolytics, warfarin). HERBAL:** None known. **FOOD:** None known. **LAB VALUES:** Decreases Hgb, Hct, platelets.

AVAILABILITY (Rx)

INJECTION PREMIX: 12.5 mg/250 ml, 25 mg/500 ml (50 mcg/ml). **VIAL:** 250 mcg/ml.

ADMINISTRATION/HANDLING

IV

Storage • Store at room temperature. • Protect from light. • Use only clear solution. • Discard unused solution 24 hrs after start of infusion.

Reconstitution

Alert: Heparin and tirofiban can be administered through the same IV line.

INJECTION FOR SOLUTION (250 mcg/ml) • Withdraw and discard 100 ml from a 500-ml bag 0.9% NaCl or D_5W and replace this volume with 100 ml of tirofiban (from two 50-ml vials) or withdraw and discard 50 ml from a 250-ml bag and replace with 50 ml of tirofiban (from one 50-ml vial) to achieve a final concentration of 50 mcg/ml. • Mix well before administration.

INJECTION (50 MCG/ML) PREMIX IN 500-ML INTRAVIA CONTAINER
• To open the IntraVia container, tear off the dust cover. • Check for leaks by squeezing the inner bag firmly; if any leak is found or if the solution is not clear, discard the solution. • Do not add other drugs or remove solution directly from the bag with a syringe. Do not use plastic containers in series connections (may result in air embolism by drawing air from the first container if it is empty of solution).

Rate of administration • For loading dose, give 0.4 mcg/kg/min for 30 min. • For maintenance infusion, give 0.1 mcg/kg/min.

⊘ IV INCOMPATIBILITY
Do not mix with any other medications.

INDICATIONS/ROUTES/DOSAGE

INHIBITION OF PLATELET AGGREGATION
IV: ADULTS, ELDERLY: Give at initial rate of 0.4 mcg/kg/min for 30 min and then continue at 0.1 mcg/kg/min through procedure and for 12–24 hrs following procedure.

SEVERE RENAL INSUFFICIENCY (creatinine clearance <30 ml/min)
Half the usual rate of infusion.

SIDE EFFECTS

OCCASIONAL (3%–6%): Pelvis pain, bradycardia, dizziness, leg pain. **RARE (1%–2%):** Edema/swelling, vasovagal reaction, diaphoresis, nausea, fever, headache.

ADVERSE REACTIONS/ TOXIC EFFECTS

Overdosage manifested as primarily minor mucocutaneous bleeding and bleeding at the femoral artery access site. Thrombocytopenia occurs rarely.

NURSING IMPLICATIONS

BASELINE ASSESSMENT

Assess platelet count, Hgb, Hct, aPTT, renal function prior to treatment, within 6 hrs following the loading dose, and at least daily thereafter during therapy. If platelet count is $<90,000/mm^3$, additional platelet counts should be obtained routinely to avoid thrombocytopenia. If thrombocytopenia occurs, drug therapy and heparin should be discontinued.

INTERVENTION/EVALUATION

Monitor aPTT 6 hrs following the beginning of the heparin infusion. Adjust heparin dosage to maintain aPTT at approx. 2 times control. Diligently monitor for potential bleeding, particularly at other arterial and venous puncture sites, IM injection site. If possible, urinary catheters, NG tubes should be avoided. Maintain complete bed rest with head of the bed elevated at 30°.

T

tizanidine

tih-**zan**-ih-deen
(Zanaflex)

CLASSIFICATION

PHARMACOTHERAPEUTIC: Skeletal muscle relaxant. **CLINICAL:** Antispastic.

ACTION

Increases presynaptic inhibition of spinal motor neurons mediated by $alpha_2$-adrenergic agonists, reducing facilitation to postsynaptic motor neurons. **Therapeutic Effect:** Reduces muscle spasticity.

USES

Acute and intermittent management of muscle spasticity (spasms, stiffness, rigidity). **Unlabeled:** Spasticity associated with multiple sclerosis, spinal cord injury.

PHARMACOKINETICS

	Onset	Peak	Duration
PO	—	1–2 hrs	3–6 hrs

Metabolized in liver: **Half-life:** 4–8 hrs.

PRECAUTIONS

CONTRAINDICATIONS: None known. **CAUTIONS:** Renal/hepatic disease, hypotension, cardiac disease.

LIFESPAN CONSIDERATIONS: Pregnancy/lactation: Pregnancy Category C. Children: Safety and efficacy not established. **Elderly:** Age-related renal impairment may warrant caution.

INTERACTIONS

DRUG: Oral contraceptives may reduce tizanidine clearance. May increase serum levels/toxicity of **phenytoin. Alcohol, CNS depressants** may increase CNS depressant effects. **Antihypertensives** may increase tizanidine's hypotensive potential. **HERBAL:** None known. **FOOD:** None known. **LAB VALUES:** May increase SGOT (AST), SGPT (ALT), alkaline phosphatase.

AVAILABILITY (Rx)

TABLETS: 2 mg, 4 mg.

INDICATIONS/ROUTES/DOSAGE

MUSCLE SPASTICITY

PO: ADULTS, ELDERLY: Initially 2–4 mg, gradually increased in 2- to 4-mg increments and repeated q6–8h. **Maximum:** 3 doses/day or 36 mg total in 24 hrs.

SIDE EFFECTS

FREQUENT (41%–49%): Dry mouth, somnolence, asthenia (loss of strength, weakness). **OCCASIONAL (4%–16%):** Dizziness, urinary tract infection, constipation. **RARE (3%):** Nervousness, amblyopia (dimness of vision), pharyngitis, rhinitis, vomiting, urinary frequency.

ADVERSE REACTIONS/ TOXIC EFFECTS

Hypotension with a reduction in either diastolic or systolic B/P and may be associated with bradycardia, orthostatic hypotension, and, rarely, syncope. As dosage increases, risk of hypotension increases and is noted within 1 hr after dosing.

NURSING IMPLICATIONS

BASELINE ASSESSMENT

Record onset, type, location, duration of muscular spasm. Check for immobility, stiffness, swelling. Obtain baseline hepatic function tests, alkaline phosphatase, total bilirubin.

INTERVENTION/EVALUATION

Assist with ambulation at all times. For those on long-term therapy, hepatic/renal function tests should be performed periodically. Evaluate for therapeutic response (decreased intensity of skeletal muscle pain/tenderness, improved mobility, decrease in spasticity). For those at increased risk of orthostatic hypotension, instruct pt to rise slowly from lying to sitting and from sitting to supine position.

PATIENT/FAMILY TEACHING

Avoid tasks that require alertness, motor skills until response to drug is established. Avoid sudden changes. May cause hypotension, sedation, impaired coordination.

tobramycin sulfate

tow-bra-**my**-sin
(Nebcin, Tobi, Tobrex)

FIXED-COMBINATION(S)

TobraDex: tobramycin/dexamethasone (a steroid): 0.3%/0.1% per ml or per g.

CLASSIFICATION

PHARMACOTHERAPEUTIC: Aminoglycoside. **CLINICAL:** Antibiotic (see p. 19C).

ACTION

Irreversibly binds to protein on bacterial ribosome. **Therapeutic Effect:** Interferes in protein synthesis of susceptible microorganisms.

PHARMACOKINETICS

Rapid, complete absorption following IM administration. Protein binding: <30%. Widely distributed (does not cross blood-brain barrier, low concentrations in CSF). Excreted unchanged in urine. Removed by hemodialysis. **Half-life:** 2–4 hrs (half-life increased with impaired renal function, neonates; decreased in cystic fibrosis, burn or febrile pts).

USES

Skin/skin structure, bone, joint, respiratory tract infections; postop, burn, intra-abdominal infections; complicated urinary tract infections; septicemia; meningitis. **Ophthalmic:** Superficial eye infections: blepharitis, conjunctivitis, keratitis, corneal ulcers. **Inhalation:** Bronchopulmonary infections in pts with cystic fibrosis.

PRECAUTIONS

CONTRAINDICATIONS: Hypersensitivity to aminoglycosides (cross-sensitivity). **CAUTIONS:** Impaired renal function, preexisting auditory/vestibular impairment, concomitant use of neuromuscular blocking agents.

LIFESPAN CONSIDERATIONS: Pregnancy/lactation: Readily crosses placenta. Distributed in breast milk. May cause fetal nephrotoxicity. **Pregnancy Category C.** Ophthalmic form should not be used in nursing mothers and only when specifically indicated in pregnancy. **Pregnancy Category B. Children:** Immature renal function in neonates and premature infants may increase risk of toxicity. **Elderly:** Age-related renal impairment may increase risk of toxicity; dosage adjustment recommended.

INTERACTIONS

DRUG: Other aminoglycosides, nephrotoxic, ototoxic-producing medications may increase toxicity. May increase effects of **neuromuscular blocking agents. HERBAL:** None known. **FOOD:** None known. **LAB VALUES:** May increase BUN, SGOT (AST), SGPT (ALT), bilirubin, creatinine, LDH concentrations; may decrease serum calcium, magnesium, potassium, sodium concentrations. Therapeutic blood serum level: Peak: 5–20 mcg/ml; trough: 0.5–2 mcg/ml. Toxic blood serum level: Peak: >20 mcg/ml; trough: >2 mcg/ml.

AVAILABILITY (Rx)

INJECTION: 10 mg/ml, 40 mg/ml. **POWDER FOR INJECTION:** 1.2 g. **OPHTHALMIC SOLUTION:** 0.3%. **OPHTHALMIC OINTMENT:** 3 mg/g. **INHALATION SOLUTION:** 300 mg/5 ml.

T

ADMINISTRATION/HANDLING

Alert: Coordinate peak and trough lab draws with administration times.

IM

• To minimize discomfort, give deep IM slowly. • Less painful if injected into gluteus maximus rather than lateral aspect of thigh.

IV

Storage • Store vials at room temperature. • Solutions may be discolored by light/air (does not affect potency).

Reconstitution • Dilute with 50–200 ml D_5W, 0.9% NaCl. Amount of diluent for infants, children depends on individual need.

Rate of administration • Infuse over 20–60 min.

OPHTHALMIC

• Place finger on lower eyelid, pull out until a pocket is formed between eye and lower lid. • Hold dropper above pocket, place correct number of drops (¼–½ inch ointment) into pocket. Have pt close eye gently. • **Solution:** Apply digital pressure to lacrimal sac for 1–2 min (minimizes drainage into nose and throat, reducing risk of systemic effects.) • **Ointment:** Close eye for 1–2 min, rolling eyeball (increases contact area of drug to eye). • Remove excess solution or ointment around eye with tissue.

T

IV INCOMPATIBILITIES

Amphotericin B complex (Abelcet, AmBisome, Amphotec), heparin, hetastarch (Hespan), indomethacin (Indocin), propofol (Diprivan), sargramostim (Leukine, Prokine).

IV COMPATIBILITIES

Amiodarone (Cordarone), calcium gluconate, diltiazem (Cardizem), furosemide (Lasix), hydromorphone (Dilaudid), insulin, magnesium sulfate, midazolam (Versed), morphine, theophylline.

INDICATIONS/ROUTES/DOSAGE

Alert: Space parenteral doses evenly around the clock. Dosage based on ideal body weight. Peak, trough levels determined periodically to maintain desired serum concentrations (minimizes risk of toxicity). Recommended peak level: 4–10 mcg/ml; trough level: 1–2 mcg/ml.

USUAL PARENTERAL DOSAGE

IM/IV: ADULTS, ELDERLY: 3–6 mg/kg/day in 3 divided doses (may use 4–6.6 mg/kg once daily).

USUAL DOSAGE FOR CHILDREN, INFANTS

IM/IV: 6–7.5 mg/kg/day in 3–4 divided doses.

DOSAGE IN RENAL IMPAIRMENT

Dose and/or frequency is modified based on degree of renal impairment, serum concentration of drug. Following loading dose of 1–2 mg/kg, maintenance dose/frequency based on serum creatinine/creatinine clearance.

USUAL OPHTHALMIC DOSAGE

Ophthalmic ointment: ADULTS, ELDERLY: Thin strip to conjunctiva q8–12h (q3–4h for severe infections).

Ophthalmic solution: ADULTS, ELDERLY: 1–2 drops q4h (2 drops every hour for severe infections).

USUAL INHALATION DOSAGE

ADULTS: 60–80 mg twice daily for 28 days, then off for 28 days. CHILDREN: 40–80 mg 2–3 times/day.

SIDE EFFECTS

OCCASIONAL: Pain, induration at IM injection site, phlebitis, thrombophlebitis with IV administration, hypersensitivity reaction (rash, fever, urticaria, pruritus). **Ophthalmic:** Tearing, itching, redness, swelling of eyelid. **RARE:** Hypotension, nausea, vomiting.

ADVERSE REACTIONS/ TOXIC EFFECTS

Nephrotoxicity (evidenced by increased BUN and serum creatinine, decreased creatinine clearance) may be reversible if drug stopped at first sign of symptoms; irreversible ototoxicity (tinnitus, dizziness, ringing/roaring in ears, reduced hearing), neurotoxicity (headache, dizziness, lethargy, tremors, visual disturbances) occur occasionally. Risk is greater with higher dosages, with prolonged therapy, or if solution is applied directly to mucosa. Superinfections, particularly with fungi, may result from bacterial imbalance via any route of administration; anaphylaxis.

NURSING IMPLICATIONS

BASELINE ASSESSMENT

Dehydration must be treated prior to beginning parenteral therapy. Question for history of allergies, esp. aminoglycosides and sulfite (and parabens for topical/ophthalmic routes). Establish baseline for hearing acuity.

INTERVENTION/EVALUATION

Monitor I&O (maintain hydration), urinalysis (casts, RBCs, WBCs, decrease in specific gravity). Monitor results of peak/trough blood tests. Therapeutic blood serum level: Peak: 5–20 mcg/ml; trough: 0.5–2 mcg/ml. Toxic blood serum level: Peak: >20 mcg/ml; trough: >2 mcg/ml. Be alert to ototoxic and neurotoxic symptoms (see Adverse Reactions/Toxic Effects). Evaluate IV site for phlebitis (heat, pain, red streaking over vein). Assess for rash. Be alert for superinfection, particularly genital/anal pruritus, changes of oral mucosa, diarrhea. When treating pts with neuromuscular disorders, assess respiratory response carefully. **Ophthalmic:** Assess for redness, swelling, itching, tearing.

PATIENT/FAMILY TEACHING

Notify physician in event of any hearing, visual, balance, urinary problems, even after therapy is completed. **Ophthalmic:** Blurred vision/tearing may occur briefly after application. Contact physician if tearing, redness, irritation continues.

tocainide hydrochloride

toe-**kay**-nied
(Tonocard)

CLASSIFICATION

PHARMACOTHERAPEUTIC: Amide-type local anesthetic. **CLINICAL:** Antiarrhythmic (see p. 13C).

ACTION

Shortens action potential duration, decreases effective refractory period, automaticity in His-Purkinje system of myocardium by blocking sodium transport across myocardial cell membranes. **Therapeutic Effect:** Suppresses ventricular arrhythmias.

USES

Suppression, prevention of ventricular arrhythmias, including frequent unifocal/multifocal coupled premature ventricular contractions, paroxysmal ventricular tachycardia.

PRECAUTIONS

CONTRAINDICATIONS: Hypersensitivity to local anesthetics, second- or third-degree AV block. **CAUTIONS:** Renal/hepatic impairment, preexisting arrhythmias, bone marrow failure, CHF. **Pregnancy Category C.**

INTERACTIONS

DRUG: Other **antiarrhythmics** may increase risk of adverse cardiac effects. **Beta-adrenergic blockers** may increase pulmonary wedge pressure, decrease cardiac index. **HERBAL:** None known. **FOOD:** None known. **LAB VALUES:** None known. Therapeutic blood serum level: 4–10 mcg/ml; toxic blood serum level: not established.

AVAILABILITY (Rx)

TABLETS: 400 mg, 600 mg.

INDICATIONS/ROUTES/DOSAGE

Alert: When giving tocainide in those receiving IV lidocaine, give single 600-mg dose 6 hrs prior to cessation of lidocaine and repeat in 6 hrs. Then give standard tocainide maintenance doses.

VENTRICULAR ARRHYTHMIAS

PO: ADULTS, ELDERLY: Initially, 400 mg q8h. MAINTENANCE: 1.2–1.8 g/day in divided doses q8h. **Maximum:** 2,400 mg/day.

SIDE EFFECTS

Generally well tolerated. **FREQUENT (3%–10%):** Minor, transient lightheadedness, dizziness, nausea, paresthesia, rash, tremor. **OCCASIONAL (1%–3%):** Clammy skin, night sweats, joint pain. **RARE (<1%):** Restlessness, nervousness, disorientation, mood changes, ataxia (muscular incoordination), visual disturbances.

ADVERSE REACTIONS/ TOXIC EFFECTS

High dosage may produce bradycardia/ tachycardia, hypotension, palpitations, increased ventricular arrhythmias, PVCs, chest pain, exacerbation of CHF, altered sensorium, paresthesias.

NURSING IMPLICATIONS

BASELINE ASSESSMENT

Assess baseline EKG, pulse for quality, irregular rate.

INTERVENTION/EVALUATION

Monitor EKG for cardiac changes, particularly shortening of QT interval. Notify physician of any significant interval changes. Monitor fluid status and serum electrolyte levels. Assess hand movement for sign of tremor (usually first clinical sign that maximum dose is being reached). Assess sleeping pt for night sweats. Question for tingling/ numbness in hands/feet. Assess skin for rash, clamminess. Observe for CNS disturbances (restlessness, disorientation, mood changes, incoordination). Assess for evidence of CHF: dyspnea (particularly on exertion or lying down), night cough, peripheral edema, distended neck veins. Monitor I&O (increase in weight, decrease in urine output may indicate CHF). Monitor for therapeutic serum level (3–10 mcg/ml). Therapeutic blood serum level: 4–10 mcg/ml; toxic blood serum level: not established.

PATIENT/FAMILY TEACHING

Avoid tasks that require alertness, motor skills until response to drug is established. Inform physician if any unusual bleeding, cough, tremor, palpitations, chills, fever, sore throat, breathing difficulties occur. May take with food.

tolazamide

(Tolamide, Tolinase)

See Classification section under: Antidiabetics (p. 39C)

tolbutamide

(Oramide, Orinase)

See Classification section under: Antidiabetics (p. 39C)

tolcapone

toll-cah-pone

(Tasmar)

CLASSIFICATION

PHARMACOTHERAPEUTIC: Antidyskinetic. **CLINICAL:** Antiparkinson agent.

ACTION

Inhibits the enzyme COMT, sustaining plasma levels and thereby increasing the duration of action of levodopa, resulting in greater effect. **Therapeutic Effect:** Relieves signs/symptoms of Parkinson's disease.

PHARMACOKINETICS

Rapidly absorbed following PO administration. Protein binding: 99%. Metabolized in liver. Eliminated primarily in urine (60%) and to a lesser amount (40%) in feces. Unknown if removed by hemodialysis. **Half-life:** 2–3 hrs.

USES

Adjunctive therapy to levodopa and carbidopa for treatment of signs/symptoms of idiopathic Parkinson's disease.

PRECAUTIONS

CONTRAINDICATIONS: None known. **CAUTIONS:** Severe renal/hepatic impairment, those with history of hallucinations, baseline hypotension, history of orthostatic hypotension.

LIFESPAN CONSIDERATIONS: Pregnancy/lactation: Unknown if distributed in breast milk. **Pregnancy Category C. Children:** Not used in children. **Elderly:** May have increased risk of hallucinations.

INTERACTIONS

DRUG: Increases **levodopa** duration of action. **HERBAL:** None known. **FOOD:** Food given 1 hr before or 2 hrs after tolcapone administration decreases bioavailability by 10%–20%. **LAB VALUES:** May increase SGOT (AST), SGPT (ALT).

AVAILABILITY (Rx)

TABLETS: 100 mg, 200 mg.

ADMINISTRATION/HANDLING

PO

- Give without regard to food.

INDICATIONS/ROUTES/DOSAGE

Alert: May combine tolcapone with both the immediate and sustained-release form of levodopa/carbidopa.

PARKINSON'S DISEASE

PO: ADULTS, ELDERLY: Initially, 100–200 mg 3 times/day. **Maximum:** 600 mg/day. For those with moderate to severe cirrhosis of liver, do not increase to >200 mg 3 times/day.

SIDE EFFECTS

Alert: Frequency of occurrence increases with dosage amount. Following is based on 200-mg dose.

T

FREQUENT: Nausea (35%), insomnia, somnolence, anorexia, diarrhea, muscle cramps, orthostatic hypotension, excessive dreaming (16%–25%). **OCCASIONAL (4%–11%):** Headache, vomiting, confusion, hallucinations, constipation, diaphoresis, urine discoloration (bright yellow), dry eyes, abdominal pain, dizziness, flatulence. **RARE (2%–3%):** Dyspepsia, neck pain, hypotension, fatigue, chest discomfort.

ADVERSE REACTIONS/ TOXIC EFFECTS

Upper respiratory infection, urinary tract infection occur occasionally (5%–7%). Too rapid withdrawal from therapy may produce withdrawal emergent hyperpyrexia characterized by elevated temperature, muscular rigidity, altered consciousness. An increase in dyskinesia (impaired voluntary movement) or dystonia (impaired muscular tone) occurs frequently.

NURSING IMPLICATIONS

BASELINE ASSESSMENT

Serum transaminase levels should be monitored q2wks for the first year, q4wks for the next 6 mos, and q8wks thereafter. Treatment should be discontinued if SGPT (ALT) exceeds the upper limit of normal or clinical signs of onset of hepatic failure occur. If hallucinations occur, may be eliminated if levodopa dosage is reduced. Hallucinations generally are accompanied by confusion and, to a lesser extent, insomnia.

INTERVENTION/EVALUATION

Instruct pt to rise from lying to sitting or sitting to standing position slowly to prevent risk of postural hypotension. Assist with ambulation if dizziness occurs. Assess for clinical reversal of symptoms (improvement of tremor of head/hands at rest, masklike facial expression, shuffling gait, muscular rigidity).

PATIENT/FAMILY TEACHING

If nausea occurs, take medication with food. Drowsiness, dizziness, nausea may be an initial response of drug but diminishes/disappears with continued treatment. Postural hypotension may occur more frequently during initial therapy. Avoid tasks that require alertness, motor skills until response to drug is established. Hallucinations may occur, more so in the elderly, typically within the first 2 wks of therapy. Inform physician if possibility of pregnancy occurs. Urine will change color to a bright yellow. Inform physician if persistent nausea, fatigue, anorexia, jaundice, itching, dark urine, falls, abnormal contractions of head, neck, trunk occur.

tolmetin sodium

toll-meh-tin
(Tolectin)

◆ CLASSIFICATION

PHARMACOTHERAPEUTIC: Nonsteroidal anti-inflammatory. **CLINICAL:** Antiarthritic (see p. 111C).

ACTION

Produces analgesic, anti-inflammatory effects by inhibiting prostaglandin synthesis. **Therapeutic Effect:** Reduces inflammatory response, intensity of pain stimulus reaching sensory nerve endings.

USES

Relief of pain, disability associated with rheumatoid arthritis, juvenile rheumatoid arthritis, osteoarthritis. **Unlabeled:** Treatment of ankylosing spondylitis, psoriatic arthritis.

PRECAUTIONS

CONTRAINDICATIONS: History of hypersensitivity to aspirin or other NSAIDs; those severely incapacitated, bedridden, wheelchair bound. **CAUTIONS:** Impaired renal/cardiac function, coagulation disorders, history of upper GI disease. **Pregnancy Category C (D** if used in third trimester).

INTERACTIONS

DRUG: May increase effects of **oral anticoagulants, heparin, thrombolytics.** May decrease effect of **antihypertensives, diuretics. Salicylates, aspirin** may increase risk of GI side effects, bleeding. **Bone marrow depressants** may increase risk of hematologic reactions. May increase concentration, toxicity of **lithium.** May increase toxicity of **methotrexate. Probenecid** may increase concentration. **Antacids** may decrease concentration. **HERBAL: Ginkgo biloba** may increase risk of bleeding. May decrease **feverfew** effect. **FOOD:** None known. **LAB VALUES:** May increase BUN, potassium, hepatic function tests. May decrease Hgb, Hct. May prolong bleeding time.

AVAILABILITY (Rx)

TABLETS: 200 mg, 600 mg. **CAPSULES:** 400 mg.

ADMINISTRATION/HANDLING

PO

- May give with food, milk, antacids if GI distress occurs.

INDICATIONS/ROUTES/DOSAGE

RHEUMATOID ARTHRITIS, OSTEOARTHRITIS

PO: ADULTS, ELDERLY: Initially, 400 mg 3 times/day (including 1 dose upon arising, 1 dose at bedtime). Adjust dosage at 1- to 2-wk intervals. MAINTENANCE: 600–1,800 mg/day in 3–4 divided doses. **Maximum:** 2 g/day.

JUVENILE RHEUMATOID ARTHRITIS

PO: CHILDREN >2 YRS: Initially, 20 mg/kg/day in 3–4 divided doses. MAINTENANCE: 15–30 mg/kg/day in 3–4 divided doses. **Maximum:** 1,800 mg/day.

SIDE EFFECTS

OCCASIONAL (3%–11%): Nausea, vomiting, diarrhea, abdominal cramping, dyspepsia (heartburn, indigestion, epigastric pain), flatulence, dizziness, headache, weight decrease or increase. **RARE (<3%):** Constipation, anorexia, rash, pruritus.

ADVERSE REACTIONS/ TOXIC EFFECTS

Peptic ulcer, GI bleeding, gastritis, severe hepatic reaction (cholestasis, jaundice) occur rarely. Nephrotoxicity (dysuria, hematuria, proteinuria, nephrotic syndrome), severe hypersensitivity reaction (fever, chills, bronchospasm) occur rarely.

NURSING IMPLICATIONS

BASELINE ASSESSMENT

Assess onset, type, location, duration of pain, inflammation. Inspect appearance of affected joints for immobility, deformities, skin condition.

INTERVENTION/EVALUATION

Monitor for weight gain, edema, bleeding/bruising, mental confusion, renal/hepatic function. Monitor pattern of daily bowel activity, stool consistency. Assist with ambulation if dizziness occurs. Monitor for evidence of GI distress. Evaluate for therapeutic response (relief of pain, stiffness, swelling; increase in joint mobility; reduced joint tenderness; improved grip strength).

PATIENT/FAMILY TEACHING

Therapeutic effect noted in 1–3 wks. Avoid tasks that require alertness, motor skills until response to drug is established. If GI upset occurs, take with food, milk. Avoid aspirin, alcohol during therapy (increases risk of GI bleeding). Report headache, GI distress.

tolnaftate

(Aftate, Tinactin)

See Classification section under: Antifungals: topical (p. 43C)

T

tolterodine tartrate

toll-**tear**-oh-deen
(Detrol, Detrol LA)

CLASSIFICATION

PHARMACOTHERAPEUTIC: Muscarinic receptor antagonist. **CLINICAL:** Antispasmodic.

ACTION

Exhibits potent antimuscarinic activity by interceding via cholinergic muscarinic receptors, thereby relaxing urinary bladder contraction. **Therapeutic Effect:** Decreases urinary frequency, urgency.

PHARMACOKINETICS

Rapidly, well absorbed following PO administration. Protein binding: 96%. Extensive first-pass hepatic metabolism to active metabolite. Primarily excreted in urine. Unknown if removed by hemodialysis. **Half-life:** 1.9–3.7 hrs.

USES

Treatment of overactive bladder in pts with symptoms of urinary frequency, urgency, incontinence.

PRECAUTIONS

CONTRAINDICATIONS: Urinary retention, uncontrolled narrow-angle glaucoma. **CAUTIONS:** Renal function impairment, clinically significant bladder outflow obstruction (risk of urinary retention), GI obstructive disorders (e.g., pyloric stenosis [risk of gastric retention]), treated narrow-angle glaucoma.

LIFESPAN CONSIDERATIONS: Pregnancy/lactation: Unknown if distributed in breast milk. Recommended to discontinue during breast-feeding. **Pregnancy Category C. Children:** Safety and efficacy not established. **Elderly:** No age-related precautions noted.

T

INTERACTIONS

DRUG: **Clarithromycin, erythromycin, itraconazole, ketoconazole, miconazole** may increase concentration of tolterodine. **Fluoxetine** may inhibit metabolism of tolterodine. **HERBAL:** None known. **FOOD:** None known. **LAB VALUES:** None known.

AVAILABILITY (Rx)

TABLETS: 1 mg, 2 mg. **CAPSULES (extended-release):** 2 mg, 4 mg.

ADMINISTRATION/HANDLING

PO

- May give without regard to food.

INDICATIONS/ROUTES/DOSAGE

OVERACTIVE BLADDER

PO: ADULTS, ELDERLY: 1–2 mg twice daily. SEVERE HEPATIC IMPAIRMENT: 1 mg twice daily. **Extended-release:** 2–4 mg once daily.

SIDE EFFECTS

FREQUENT: (40%): Dry mouth. **OCCASIONAL (4%–11%):** Headache, dizziness, fatigue, constipation, dyspepsia (heartburn, indigestion, epigastric discomfort), upper respiratory infection, urinary tract infection, abnormal vision (including accommodation, dry eyes), nausea, diarrhea. **RARE (3%):** Somnolence, chest/back pain, arthralgia, rash, weight gain, dry skin.

ADVERSE REACTIONS/ TOXIC EFFECTS

Overdosage can result in severe anticholinergic effects, including GI cramping, feeling of facial warmth, excessive salivation, diaphoresis, lacrimation, pallor, urinary urgency, blurred vision, QT interval prolongation.

NURSING IMPLICATIONS

INTERVENTION/EVALUATION

Assist with ambulation if dizziness occurs. Question for change in vision. Monitor incontinence, postvoid residuals.

PATIENT/FAMILY TEACHING

May cause blurred vision, dry eyes/mouth, constipation. Inform physician of any confusion, change in mental status.

Topamax

see topiramate

topiramate

toe-**pie**-rah-mate
(Topamax)

CLASSIFICATION

CLINICAL: Anticonvulsant (see p. 33C).

ACTION

Blocks repetitive, sustained firing of neurons by enhancing the ability of gamma-aminobutyric acid (GABA) to induce a flux of chloride ions into the neurons; may block sodium channels. **Therapeutic Effect:** Decreases spread of seizure activity.

PHARMACOKINETICS

Rapidly absorbed following PO administration. Protein binding: 13%–17%. Not extensively metabolized. Primarily excreted unchanged in the urine. Removed by hemodialysis. **Half-life:** 21 hrs.

USES

Adjunctive therapy for the treatment of partial-onset seizures, tonic-clonic seizures, seizures associated with Lennox-Gastaut syndrome. **Unlabeled:** Prevention of migraine.

PRECAUTIONS

CONTRAINDICATIONS: None known. **CAUTIONS:** Sensitivity to topiramate, impaired hepatic/renal function, predisposition to renal calculi.

LIFESPAN CONSIDERATIONS: Pregnancy/lactation: Unknown if distributed in breast milk. **Pregnancy Category C. Children:** No age-related precautions noted in those >2 yrs. **Elderly:** Age-related renal impairment may require dosage adjustment.

INTERACTIONS

DRUG: Phenytoin, valproic acid, carbamazepine may decrease topiramate concentration. **Carbonic anhydrase inhibitors** may increase risk of renal calculi. May decrease effectiveness of **oral contraceptives. Alcohol, CNS depressants** may increase CNS depression. **HERBAL:** None known. **FOOD:** None known. **LAB VALUES:** None known.

AVAILABILITY (Rx)

TABLETS: 25 mg, 100 mg, 200 mg. **SPRINKLE CAPSULES:** 15 mg, 25 mg.

ADMINISTRATION/HANDLING

PO

- Do not break tablets (bitter taste).
- Give without regard to meals.
- Capsules may be swallowed whole or contents sprinkled on a teaspoonful of soft food and swallowed immediately; do not chew.

INDICATIONS/ROUTES/DOSAGE

PARTIAL SEIZURES

PO: ADULTS, ELDERLY, CHILDREN >17 YRS: Initially, 25–50 mg for 1 wk. May increase by 25–50 mg/day at weekly inter-

T

vals. **Maximum:** 1,600 mg/day. CHILDREN 2–16 YRS: Initially, 1–3 mg/kg/day (**Maximum:** 25 mg). May increase by 1–3 mg/kg/day at weekly intervals. MAINTENANCE: 5–9 mg/kg/day in 2 divided doses.

TONIC-CLONIC SEIZURES

PO: ADULTS, ELDERLY, CHILDREN: Individual and titrated.

Alert: Reduce dosage by 50% if creatinine clearance <70 ml/min.

SIDE EFFECTS

FREQUENT (10%–30%): Somnolence, dizziness, ataxia, nervousness, nystagmus (involuntary eye movement), diplopia (double vision), paresthesia, nausea, tremor. **OCCASIONAL (3%–9%):** Confusion, breast pain, dysmenorrhea, dyspepsia, depression, asthenia (loss of strength), pharyngitis, weight loss, anorexia, rash, back/abdominal/leg pain, difficulty with coordination, sinusitis, agitation, flulike symptoms. **RARE (2%–3%):** Mood disturbances (irritability, depression), dry mouth, aggressive reaction.

ADVERSE REACTIONS/ TOXIC EFFECTS

Psychomotor slowing, difficulty with concentration, language problems (esp. word-finding difficulties), memory disturbances occur occasionally. These events are generally mild to moderate but may be severe enough to require withdrawal from drug therapy.

T

NURSING IMPLICATIONS

BASELINE ASSESSMENT

Review history of seizure disorder (intensity, frequency, duration, LOC). Initiate seizure precautions. Provide quiet, dark environment. Question for sensitivity to topiramate, pregnancy, use of other anticonvulsant medication (esp. carbamazepine, valproic acid, phenytoin, carbonic anhydrase inhibitors). Assess renal function. Instruct pt to use alternative/additional means of contraception (topiramate decreases effectiveness of oral contraceptives).

INTERVENTION/EVALUATION

Observe frequently for recurrence of seizure activity. Assess for clinical improvement (decrease in intensity/frequency of seizures). Monitor renal function tests (BUN, creatinine). Assist with ambulation if dizziness occurs.

PATIENT/FAMILY TEACHING

Avoid tasks that require alertness, motor skills until response to drug is established (may cause dizziness, drowsiness, impaired thinking). Avoid use of alcohol, other CNS depressants. Do not abruptly discontinue (may precipitate seizures). Strict maintenance of drug therapy is essential for seizure control. Drowsiness usually diminishes with continued therapy. Do not break tablets (bitter taste). Maintain adequate fluid intake (decreases risk of renal stone formation). Inform physician if blurred vision, eye pain occurs.

topotecan

toe-**poh**-teh-can
(Hycamtin)

CLASSIFICATION

PHARMACOTHERAPEUTIC: DNA topoisomerase inhibitor. **CLINICAL:** Antineoplastic (see p. 76C).

ACTION

Interacts with topoisomerase I, an enzyme that relieves torsional strain in DNA by inducing reversible single-strand breaks. Binds to topoisomerase-DNA complex, preventing relegation of these single-strand breaks. **Therapeutic Effect:** Double-strand DNA damage occurring during DNA synthesis produces cytoxic effect.

PHARMACOKINETICS

Protein binding: 35%. After IV administration, hydrolyzed to active form. Excreted in urine. **Half-life:** 2–3 hrs (half-life increased with impaired renal function).

USES

Treatment of metastatic carcinoma of ovary after failure of initial or recurrent chemotherapy. Treatment of sensitive, relapsed small cell lung cancer.

PRECAUTIONS

CONTRAINDICATIONS: Baseline neutrophil count <1,500 cells/mm^3, pregnancy, breast-feeding, severe bone marrow depression. **CAUTIONS:** Mild bone marrow depression, hepatic/renal impairment.

LIFESPAN CONSIDERATIONS: Pregnancy/lactation: May cause fetal harm. Avoid pregnancy; discontinue breast-feeding. **Pregnancy Category D. Children:** Safety and efficacy not established. **Elderly:** Age-related renal impairment may require dosage adjustment.

INTERACTIONS

DRUG: Other myelosuppressants may increase risk of myelosuppression. Concurrent use of **cisplatin** may increase severity of myelosuppression. **Live virus vaccines** may potentiate virus replication, increase vaccine side effects, decrease pt's antibody response to vaccine. **HERBAL:** None known. **FOOD:** None known. **LAB VALUES:** May decrease neutrophil, leukocyte, thrombocyte, RBC levels. May increase SGOT (AST), SGPT (ALT), bilirubin.

AVAILABILITY (Rx)

POWDER FOR INJECTION: 4 mg (single-dose vial).

ADMINISTRATION/HANDLING

IV

Storage • Store vials at room temperature in original cartons. • Reconstituted vials diluted for infusion stable at room temperature, ambient lighting for 24 hrs.

Reconstitution • Reconstitute each 4-mg vial with 4 ml Sterile Water for Injection. • Further dilute with 50–100 ml 0.9% NaCl or D_5W.

Rate of administration • Administer all doses as IV infusion over 30 min. • Extravasation associated with only mild local reactions (erythema, bruising).

∅ IV INCOMPATIBILITIES

Dexamethasone (Decadron), fluorouracil, mitomycin (Mutamycin).

IV COMPATIBILITIES

Carboplatin (Paraplatin), cisplatin (Platinol AQ), cyclophosphamide (Cytoxan), doxorubicin (Adriamycin), etoposide (VePesid), gemcitabine (Gamzar), granisetron (Kytril), ondansetron (Zofran), paclitaxel (Taxol), vincristine (Oncovin).

INDICATIONS/ROUTES/DOSAGE

Alert: Do not give topotecan if baseline neutrophil count is <1,500 cells/mm^3 and platelet count is <100,000/mm^3.

CARCINOMA OF OVARY; SMALL CELL LUNG CANCER

IV infusion: ADULTS, ELDERLY: 1.5 mg/m^2 over 30 min daily for 5 consecutive days, beginning on day 1 of a 21-day course. Minimum of 4 courses recommended. If severe neutropenia occurs during treatment, reduce dose by 0.25 mg/m^2 for subsequent courses or as an alternative, give the medication, G-CSF, following the subsequent course beginning day 6 of the course (24 hrs after completion of topotecan administration).

T

Alert: No dosage adjustment necessary in pts with mild renal impairment (creatinine clearance 40–60 ml/min).

MODERATE RENAL IMPAIRMENT (creatinine clearance 20–39 ml/min)

IV infusion: ADULTS, ELDERLY: 0.75 mg/m^2.

SIDE EFFECTS

FREQUENT: Nausea (77%), vomiting (58%), diarrhea, total alopecia (42%), headache (21%), dyspnea (21%). **OCCASIONAL:** Paresthesia (9%), constipation, abdominal pain (3%). **RARE:** Anorexia, malaise, arthralgia, asthenia, myalgia.

ADVERSE REACTIONS/ TOXIC EFFECTS

Severe neutropenia (<500 $cells/mm^3$) occurs in 60% of pts (develops at median of 11 days after day 1 of initial therapy). Thrombocytopenia (<25,000/mm^3) occurs in 26% of pts and severe anemia (<8 g/dl) occurs in 40% of pts (develops at median of 15 days after day 1 of initial therapy).

NURSING IMPLICATIONS

BASELINE ASSESSMENT

Offer emotional support to pt and family. Assess CBC with differential, Hgb, platelet count prior to each dose. Myelosuppression may precipitate life-threatening hemorrhage, infection, anemia. If platelet count drops, minimize trauma to pt (e.g., IM injections, pt positioning). Premedicate with antiemetics on day of treatment, starting at least 30 min before administration.

INTERVENTION/EVALUATION

Monitor CBC with differential frequently during treatment. Assess for bleeding, signs of infection, anemia. Monitor hydration status, I&O, electrolytes (diarrhea, vomiting are common side effects). Monitor CBC with differential, Hgb, platelets for evidence of myelosuppression. Assess response to medication and provide interventions (e.g., small, frequent meals/antiemetics for nausea/vomiting). Question for complaints of headache. Assess breathing pattern for evidence of dyspnea.

PATIENT/FAMILY TEACHING

Explain that alopecia is reversible but that new hair may have different color, texture. Inform pt of possible late diarrhea causing dehydration, electrolyte depletion. Provide antiemetic/antidiarrheal regimen for subsequent use. Notify physician if diarrhea, vomiting continues at home. Do not have immunizations without physician's approval (drug lowers body's resistance). Avoid contact with those who have recently received live virus vaccine.

Toprol XL

see metoprolol

Toradol

see ketorolac

toremifene citrate

tore-mih-feen
(Fareston)

CLASSIFICATION

PHARMACOTHERAPEUTIC: Nonsteroidal antiestrogen. **CLINICAL:** Antineoplastic (see p. 76C).

T

ACTION

Binds to estrogen receptors on tumors, producing a complex that decreases DNA synthesis and inhibits estrogen effects. **Therapeutic Effect:** Blocks growth-stimulating effects of estrogen in breast cancer.

PHARMACOKINETICS

Well absorbed after PO administration. Metabolized in the liver. Eliminated in feces. **Half-life:** Approx. 5 days.

USES

Treatment of advanced breast cancer in postmenopausal women with estrogen receptor–positive disease.

PRECAUTIONS

CONTRAINDICATIONS: History of thromboembolic disease. **CAUTIONS:** Preexisting endometrial hyperplasia, leukopenia, thrombocytopenia.

LIFESPAN CONSIDERATIONS: Pregnancy/lactation: Unknown if distributed in breast milk. **Pregnancy Category D. Children:** Safety and efficacy not established. Not prescribed in this pt population. **Elderly:** No age-related precautions noted.

INTERACTIONS

DRUG: Warfarin may increase prothrombin time. **Carbamazepine, phenobarbital, phenytoin** may decrease concentration. **HERBAL:** None known. **FOOD:** None known. **LAB VALUES:** May increase alkaline phosphatase, SGOT (AST), bilirubin, calcium.

AVAILABILITY (Rx)

TABLETS: 60 mg.

ADMINISTRATION/HANDLING

PO

- Give without regard to food.

INDICATIONS/ROUTES/DOSAGE

BREAST CANCER

PO: ADULTS: 60 mg daily until disease progression is observed.

SIDE EFFECTS

FREQUENT: Hot flashes (35%), sweating (20%), nausea (14%), vaginal discharge (13%), dizziness, dry eyes (9%). **OCCASIONAL (2%–5%):** Edema, vomiting, vaginal bleeding. **RARE:** Nausea, vomiting, fatigue, depression, lethargy, anorexia.

ADVERSE REACTIONS/ TOXIC EFFECTS

Cataracts, glaucoma, decreased visual acuity may occur. May produce hypercalcemia.

NURSING IMPLICATIONS

BASELINE ASSESSMENT

An estrogen receptor assay should be done prior to beginning therapy. CBC, platelet count, serum calcium levels should be checked before and periodically during therapy.

INTERVENTION/EVALUATION

Assess for hypercalcemia (increased urine volume, excessive thirst, nausea, vomiting, constipation, hypotonicity of muscles, deep bone or flank pain, renal stones). Monitor CBC, calcium, leukocyte, platelet counts, hepatic function tests.

PATIENT/FAMILY TEACHING

May have an initial flare of disease (bone pain, hot flashes) that will subside. Report vaginal bleeding/discharge/itching, leg cramps, weight gain, shortness of breath, weakness. Contact physician if nausea/vomiting continues. Nonhormone contraceptives are recommended during treatment.

T

torsemide

tore-seh-mide
(Demadex)

CLASSIFICATION

PHARMACOTHERAPEUTIC: Loop diuretic. **CLINICAL:** Antihypertensive, antiedema (see p. 87C).

ACTION

Diuretic: Enhances excretion of sodium, chloride, potassium, water at ascending limb of loop of Henle. **Therapeutic Effect:** Produces diuretic effect. **Antihypertensive:** Reduces plasma, extracellular fluid volume. **Therapeutic Effect:** Lowers B/P.

PHARMACOKINETICS

	Onset	Peak	Duration
PO	1 hr	1–2 hrs	6–8 hrs
IV	10 min	1 hr	6–8 hrs

Rapidly, well absorbed from GI tract. Protein binding: 97%–99%. Metabolized in liver. Primarily excreted in urine. Not removed by hemodialysis. **Half-life:** 3.3 hrs.

USES

Treatment of hypertension either alone or in combination with other antihypertensives. Edema associated with CHF, renal disease, hepatic cirrhosis, chronic renal failure.

PRECAUTIONS

CONTRAINDICATIONS: Anuria, hepatic coma, severe electrolyte depletion. **EXTREME CAUTION:** Hypersensitivity to sulfonamides. **CAUTIONS:** Elderly, cardiac pts, pts with history of ventricular arrhythmias, pts with hepatic cirrhosis, ascites. Renal impairment, systemic lupus erythematosus. Safety in children not known.

LIFESPAN CONSIDERATIONS: Pregnancy/lactation: Unknown if drug is excreted in breast milk. **Pregnancy Category B. Children:** Safety and efficacy not established. **Elderly:** No age-related precautions noted.

INTERACTIONS

DRUG: May increase antihypertensive effect of **other antihypertensives. NSAIDs, probenecid** may decrease effect. May increase risk of **digoxin**-induced arrhythmias (due to hypokalemia). **Amphotericin** may increase risk nephrotoxicity. Effects of **anticoagulants, heparin, thrombolytics** may be decreased, **hypokalemia-causing medications** may increase risk of hypokalemia; may increase risk of **lithium** toxicity. **Nephrotoxic/ototoxic medications** may increase nephrotoxicity/ototoxicity. **HERBAL:** None known. **FOOD:** None known. **LAB VALUES:** May increase uric acid, BUN, creatinine. May decrease calcium, chloride, magnesium, potassium, sodium.

AVAILABILITY (Rx)

TABLETS: 5 mg, 10 mg, 20 mg, 100 mg.
INJECTION: 10 mg/ml.

ADMINISTRATION/HANDLING

PO

• Give without regard to food. Give with food to avoid GI upset, preferably with breakfast (prevents nocturia).

IV

Storage • Store at room temperature.

Rate of administration

Alert: Flush IV line with 0.9% NaCl prior to and following administration.

• May give undiluted as IV push over 2 min. • For continuous IV infusion, dilute with 0.9% or 0.45% NaCl or D_5W and infuse over 24 hrs. • A too rapid IV rate, high dosages may cause ototoxicity; administer IV rate **slowly.**

∅ IV INCOMPATIBILITY

Do not mix with any other medications.

IV COMPATIBILITY

Milrinone (Primacor).

INDICATIONS/ROUTES/DOSAGE

HYPERTENSION

PO: ADULTS, ELDERLY: Initially, 5 mg/day. May increase to 10 mg/day if no response in 4–6 wks. If no response, additional antihypertensive added.

CHF

IV/PO: ADULTS, ELDERLY: Initially, 10–20 mg/day. May increase by doubling dose until desired diuretic dose attained. (Doses >200 mg not adequately studied.)

CHRONIC RENAL FAILURE

IV/PO: ADULTS, ELDERLY: Initially, 20 mg/day. May increase by doubling dose until desired diuretic dose attained. (Doses >200 mg not adequately studied.)

HEPATIC CIRRHOSIS

IV/PO: ADULTS, ELDERLY: Initially, 5 mg/day (with aldosterone antagonist or potassium-sparing diuretic). May increase by doubling dose until desired diuretic dose attained. (Doses >40 mg not adequately studied.)

SIDE EFFECTS

FREQUENT (3%–10%): Headache, dizziness, rhinitis. **OCCASIONAL (1%–3%):** Asthenia, insomnia, nervousness, diarrhea, constipation, nausea, dyspepsia, edema, EKG changes, sore throat, cough, arthralgia, myalgia. **RARE (<1%):** Syncope, hypotension, arrhythmias.

ADVERSE REACTIONS/ TOXIC EFFECTS

Ototoxicity may occur with a too rapid IV rate or with high dosages; must be administered slowly. Overdosage produces acute, profound water loss, volume and electrolyte depletion, dehydration, decreased blood volume, circulatory collapse.

NURSING IMPLICATIONS

BASELINE ASSESSMENT

Check electrolyte levels, esp. potassium. Obtain baseline weight; check for edema. Assess for rales in lungs.

INTERVENTION/EVALUATION

Monitor B/P, electrolytes (esp. potassium), I&O, weight. Notify physician of any hearing abnormality. Note extent of diuresis. Assess lungs for rales. Check for signs of edema, particularly of dependent areas. Although less potassium is lost with torsemide than with furosemide, assess for signs of hypokalemia (change of muscle strength, tremor, muscle cramps, change in mental status, cardiac arrhythmias).

PATIENT/FAMILY TEACHING

Take medication in morning to prevent nocturia. Expect increased frequency and volume of urination. Report irregular heartbeat, muscle weakness, cramps, nausea, dizziness. Do not take other medications (including OTC drugs) without consulting physician. Eat foods high in potassium such as whole grains (cereals), legumes, meat, bananas, apricots, orange juice, potatoes (white, sweet), raisins.

tositumomab and iodine ^{131}I-tositumomab

toe-sit-**two**-mo-mab
(Bexxar)

CLASSIFICATION

PHARMACOTHERAPEUTIC: Monoclonal antibody. **CLINICAL:** Antineoplastic.

T

ACTION

Composed of an antibody cojoined with a radiolabeled antitumor antibody. The antibody portion binds specifically to the CD20 antigen, found on the pre-B and B lymphocytes. It is also found on more than 90% of B-cell non-Hodgkin's lymphomas, resulting in formation of a complex. **Therapeutic Effect:** Induces cytotoxicity, cell death associated with ionizing radiation from the radioisotope.

PHARMACOKINETICS

Depletes circulating CD20 positive cells. Elimination if ^{131}I occurs by decay and excretion in the urine. **Half-life:** 8 days. Pts with high tumor burden, splenomegaly, bone marrow involvement have a faster clearance, shorter half-life, larger volume of distribution.

USES

Treatment of pts with CD20 positive, follicular non-Hodgkin's lymphoma whose disease is refractory to rituximab and has relapsed following chemotherapy.

PRECAUTIONS

CONTRAINDICATIONS: Hypersensitivity to murine proteins. **CAUTIONS:** Impaired renal function, active systemic infection, immunosuppression.

LIFESPAN CONSIDERATIONS: Pregnancy/lactation: The ^{131}I-tositumomab component is contraindicated during pregnancy (severe, possibly irreversible hypothyroidism in neonates). Radioiodine is excreted in breast milk; do not breast-feed. **Pregnancy Category X. Children:** Safety and efficacy not established. **Elderly:** The response rate/duration of severe hematologic toxicity is lower in pts >65 yrs.

INTERACTIONS

DRUG: Due to occurrence of severe/prolonged thrombocytopenia, the benefits of medications that interfere with platelet function or anticoagulation should be weighed against the increased risk of bleeding/hemorrhage. **HERBAL:** None known. **FOOD:** None known. **LAB VALUES:** May decrease WBCs, Hgb, Hct, platelet count, thyroid-stimulating hormone.

AVAILABILITY (Rx)

TOSITUMOMAB: Injection: 14 mg/ml. **IODINE ^{131}I-TOSITUMOMAB: Injection:** 0.1 mg/ml, 1.1 mg/ml.

ADMINISTRATION/HANDLING

Alert: The regimen consists of 4 components given in 2 separate steps: The dosimetric step, followed 7–14 days later by a therapeutic step. When infusing, use IV tubing with an in-line 0.22-micron filter (use the same tubing throughout the entire dosimetric or therapeutic step; changing the filter results in drug loss). Reduce infusion rate by 50% for mild to moderate infusion toxicity; interrupt infusion for severe infusion toxicity (may resume when resolution of toxicity occurs). Resume at 50% reduction rate of infusion.

IV

Storage TOSITUMOMAB • Refrigerate vials prior to dilution. Protect from strong light. • Following dilution, solution is stable for 24 hrs if refrigerated, up to 8 hrs at room temperature. • Discard any unused portion left in the vial. • Do not shake.

IODINE ^{131}I-TOSITUMOMAB • Store frozen until it is removed for thawing prior to administration. Thawed doses are stable for 8 hrs if refrigerated. • Discard any unused portion.

Reconstitution
Alert: Reconstitution amounts and rates of administration are the same for both dosimetric and therapeutic steps.

TOSITUMOMAB • Reconstitute 450 mg tositumomab in 50 ml 0.9% NaCl.

IODINE ^{131}I-TOSITUMOMAB • Reconstitute iodine ^{131}I-tositumomab in 30 ml 0.9% NaCl.

Rate of administration
TOSITUMOMAB • Infuse over 60 min.

IODINE ^{131}I-TOSITUMOMAB • Infuse over 20 min.

INDICATIONS/ROUTES/DOSAGE

Alert: Initiate thyroid protective agents (potassium iodide) 24 hrs prior to administration of iodine ^{131}I-tositumomab dosimetric step and continue until 2 wks following administration of iodine ^{131}I-tositumomab therapeutic step. Pretreat against infusion reactions with 650 mg acetaminophen and 50 mg diphenhydramine 30 min prior to beginning therapy.

NON-HODGKIN'S LYMPHOMA
IV infusion: ADULTS ≥60 YRS: 9 mg/m^2, repeat in 14 days for total of 2 doses.

Alert: Diphenhydramine 50 mg and acetaminophen 650–1,000 mg given 1 hr prior to administering; follow by acetaminophen 650–1,000 mg q4h for 2 doses, then q4h prn. Full recovery from hematologic toxicities is not a requirement for giving second dose.

SIDE EFFECTS

FREQUENT (18%–46%): Asthenia (loss of strength, energy), fever, nausea, cough, chills. **OCCASIONAL (10%–17%):** Rash, headache, abdominal pain, vomiting, anorexia, myalgia, diarrhea, pharyngitis, arthralgia, rhinitis, pruritus. **RARE (5%–9%):** Peripheral edema, diaphoresis, constipation, dyspepsia (heartburn, epigastric distress), back pain, hypotension, vasodilation, dizziness, somnolence.

ADVERSE EFFECTS/ TOXIC EFFECTS

Infusion toxicity characterized by fever, rigors, diaphoresis, hypotension, dyspnea, nausea and occurs during or within 48 hrs of infusions. Severe, prolonged myelosuppression occurs in 71% of all pts characterized as neutropenia, anemia, thrombocytopenia. Sepsis occurs in 45% of pts, hemorrhage occurs in 12%, myelodysplastic syndrome occurs in 8%.

NURSING IMPLICATIONS

BASELINE ASSESSMENT

Pretreatment with acetaminophen and diphenhydramine prior to administering infusion may prevent infusion-related effects. Obtain baseline CBC prior to therapy and at least weekly following administration for a minimum of 10 wks. Use strict aseptic technique to protect pt from infection. Follow radiation safety protocols. Time to nadir is 4–7 wks, duration of cytopenias is approx. 30 days.

INTERVENTION/EVALUATION

Diligently monitor lab values for possibly severe, prolonged thrombocytopenia, neutropenia, anemia. Monitor for hematologic toxicity (fever, chills, unusual bruising/bleeding from any site), symptoms of anemia (excessive tiredness, weakness). Assess for signs of hypothyroidism.

PATIENT/FAMILY TEACHING

Avoid pregnancy (Pregnancy Category X). Do not have immunizations without physician's approval (drug lowers body's resistance). Avoid contact with those who have recently received live virus vaccine. Promptly report fever, sore throat, signs of local infection, unusual bruising/bleeding from any site.

T

tramadol hydrochloride

tray-mah-doal
(Ultram)

Do not confuse with Toradol, Ultane.

FIXED-COMBINATION(S)

Ultracet: tramadol/acetaminophen (a non-narcotic analgesic): 37.5 mg/325 mg.

◆ CLASSIFICATION

CLINICAL: Analgesic.

ACTION

Binds to μ-opiate receptors and inhibits reuptake of norepinephrine and serotonin. **Therapeutic Effect:** Reduces intensity of pain stimuli incoming from sensory nerve endings, altering pain perception and emotional response to pain.

PHARMACOKINETICS

	Onset	Peak	Duration
PO	<1 hr	2–3 hrs	4–6 hrs

Rapidly, almost completely absorbed following PO administration. Protein binding: 20%. Extensively metabolized in liver to active metabolite (reduced in pts with advanced cirrhosis). Primarily excreted in urine. Minimally removed by hemodialysis. **Half-life:** 6–7 hrs.

USES

Management of moderate to moderately severe pain.

PRECAUTIONS

CONTRAINDICATIONS: Acute intoxication with alcohol, hypnotics, centrally acting analgesics, opioids, psychotropic drugs. **EXTREME CAUTION:** CNS depression, anoxia, advanced liver cirrhosis, epilepsy, respiratory depression, acute alcoholism, shock. **CAUTIONS:** Sensitivity to opioids, increased intracranial pressure, impaired hepatic/renal function, acute abdominal conditions, opioid-dependent pts.

LIFESPAN CONSIDERATIONS: Pregnancy/lactation: Crosses placenta. Distributed in breast milk. **Pregnancy Category C. Children:** Safety and efficacy not established. **Elderly:** Age-related renal impairment may require dosage adjustment.

INTERACTIONS

DRUG: Alcohol, CNS depressants may increase CNS effects, respiratory depression, hypotension. **MAOIs** increase tramadol concentration. **Carbamazepine** increases tramadol metabolism, decreases concentration. **HERBAL:** None known. **FOOD:** None known. **LAB VALUES:** May increase creatinine, liver enzymes. May decrease Hgb, proteinuria.

AVAILABILITY (Rx)

TABLETS: 50 mg.

ADMINISTRATION/HANDLING

PO

- Give without regard to meals.

INDICATIONS/ROUTES/DOSAGE

MODERATE TO MODERATELY SEVERE PAIN

PO: ADULTS, ELDERLY: 50–100 mg q4–6h. **Maximum <75 yrs:** 400 mg/day. **Maximum >75 yrs:** 300 mg/day.

RENAL FUNCTION IMPAIRMENT (creatinine clearance <30 ml/min)

Alert: Dialysis pts can receive their regular dose on day of dialysis.

PO: ADULTS, ELDERLY: Increase dosing interval to 12 hrs. **Maximum daily dose:** 200 mg.

HEPATIC FUNCTION IMPAIRMENT

PO: ADULTS, ELDERLY: 50 mg q12h.

SIDE EFFECTS

FREQUENT (15%–25%): Dizziness/vertigo, nausea, constipation, headache, somnolence. **OCCASIONAL (5%–10%):** Vomiting, pruritus, CNS stimulation (nervousness, anxiety, agitation, tremor, euphoria, mood swings, hallucinations), asthenia, diaphoresis, dyspepsia, dry mouth, diarrhea. **RARE (<5%):** Malaise,

T

vasodilation, anorexia, flatulence, rash, visual disturbance, urinary retention/frequency, menopausal symptoms.

ADVERSE REACTIONS/ TOXIC EFFECTS

Overdosage results in respiratory depression, seizures. Prolonged duration of action, cumulative effect may occur in those with impaired hepatic, renal function.

NURSING IMPLICATIONS

BASELINE ASSESSMENT

Assess onset, type, location, duration of pain. Effect of medication is reduced if full pain recurs before next dose. Assess drug history, esp. carbamazepine, CNS depressant medication, MAOIs. Review past medical history, esp. epilepsy/seizures. Assess renal/hepatic function lab values.

INTERVENTION/EVALUATION

Monitor pulse, B/P. Assist with ambulation if dizziness, vertigo occurs. Dry crackers, cola may relieve nausea. Palpate bladder for urinary retention. Monitor pattern of daily bowel activity, stool consistency. Sips of tepid water may relieve dry mouth. Assess for clinical improvement, record onset of relief of pain.

PATIENT/FAMILY TEACHING

May cause dependence. Avoid alcohol, OTC medications (analgesics, sedatives). May cause drowsiness, dizziness, blurred vision. Avoid tasks requiring alertness, motor skills until response to drug is established. Inform physician if severe constipation, difficulty breathing, excessive sedation, seizures, muscle weakness, tremors, chest pain, palpitations occur.

trandolapril

tran-**doal**-ah-prill
(Mavik)

FIXED-COMBINATION(S)

Tarka: trandolapril/verapamil (a calcium channel blocker): 1 mg/240 mg; 2 mg/180 mg; 2 mg/240 mg; 4 mg/240 mg.

◆ CLASSIFICATION

PHARMACOTHERAPEUTIC: Angiotensin-converting enzyme (ACE) inhibitor. **CLINICAL:** Antihypertensive, CHF agent (see p. 6C).

ACTION

Suppresses renin-angiotensin-aldosterone system (prevents conversion of angiotensin I to angiotensin II, a potent vasoconstrictor; may also inhibit angiotensin II at local vascular and renal sites). Decreases plasma angiotensin II, increases plasma renin activity, decreases aldosterone secretion. **Therapeutic Effect:** Reduces peripheral arterial resistance, pulmonary capillary wedge pressure; improves cardiac output, exercise tolerance.

PHARMACOKINETICS

Slowly absorbed from GI tract. Protein binding: 80%. Metabolized in liver, GI mucosa to active metabolite. Primarily excreted in urine. Removed by hemodialysis. **Half-life:** 24 hrs.

USES

Treatment of hypertension. Used alone or in combination with other antihypertensives. Treatment of CHF.

PRECAUTIONS

CONTRAINDICATIONS: History of angioedema with previous treatment with ACE inhibitors. **CAUTIONS:** Renal impairment, CHF, hypovolemia, valvular stenosis, hyperkalemia.

LIFESPAN CONSIDERATIONS: Pregnancy/lactation: Crosses placenta. Distributed in breast milk. May cause fetal/neonatal mortality/morbidity. **Pregnancy Category C** (**D** if used in second or third trimester). **Children:** Safety and efficacy not established. **Elderly:** No age-related precautions noted.

INTERACTIONS

DRUG: Alcohol, diuretics, hypotensive agents may increase effects. **NSAIDs** may decrease effect. **Potassium-sparing diuretics, potassium supplements** may cause hyperkalemia. May increase concentration, toxicity of **lithium. HERBAL:** None known. **FOOD:** None known. **LAB VALUES:** May increase potassium, SGOT (AST), SGPT (ALT), alkaline phosphatase, bilirubin, BUN, creatinine. May decrease sodium. May cause positive ANA titer.

AVAILABILITY (Rx)

TABLETS: 1 mg, 2 mg, 4 mg.

ADMINISTRATION/HANDLING

PO

• Give without regard to meals. • Tablets may be crushed.

INDICATIONS/ROUTES/DOSAGE

HYPERTENSION (without diuretic)

PO: ADULTS, ELDERLY: Initially, 1 mg once daily in nonblack pts, 2 mg once daily in black pts. Adjust dose at least at 7-day intervals. MAINTENANCE: 2–4 mg/day. **Maximum:** 8 mg/day.

CHF

PO: ADULTS, ELDERLY: Initially, 0.5–1 mg, titrated to target dose of 4 mg/day.

SIDE EFFECTS

FREQUENT (23%–35%): Dizziness, cough. **OCCASIONAL (3%–11%):** Hypotension, dyspepsia (heartburn, epigastric pain, indigestion), syncope, asthenia (loss of strength), tinnitus. **RARE (<1%):** Palpitations, insomnia, drowsiness, nausea, vomiting, constipation, flushed skin.

ADVERSE REACTIONS/ TOXIC EFFECTS

Excessive hypotension ("first-dose syncope") may occur in those with CHF or severely salt/volume depleted pts. Angioedema (swelling of face/lips), hyperkalemia occur rarely. Agranulocytosis, neutropenia may be noted in those with impaired renal function or collagen vascular disease (systemic lupus erythematosus, scleroderma). Nephrotic syndrome may be noted in those with history of renal disease.

NURSING IMPLICATIONS

BASELINE ASSESSMENT

Obtain B/P immediately prior to each dose, in addition to regular monitoring (be alert to fluctuations). Renal function tests should be performed before therapy begins. In pts with renal impairment, autoimmune disease, or taking drugs that affect leukocytes or immune response, CBC and differential count should be performed prior to therapy begins and q2wks for 3 mos, then periodically thereafter.

INTERVENTION/EVALUATION

If excessive reduction in B/P occurs, place pt in supine position with legs elevated. Assist with ambulation if dizziness occurs. Assess for urinary frequency. Auscultate lung sounds for rales, wheezing in those with CHF. Monitor urinalysis for proteinuria. Monitor serum potassium levels in those on concurrent diuretic therapy. Monitor pattern of daily bowel activity, stool consistency.

PATIENT/FAMILY TEACHING

Do not discontinue medication. Inform physician if sore throat, fever, swelling,

T

palpitations, cough, chest pain, difficulty swallowing, swelling of face, vomiting, or diarrhea occurs. May cause altered taste perception. To reduce hypotensive effect, rise slowly from lying to sitting position and permit legs to dangle from bed momentarily before standing. Avoid potassium supplements/salt substitutes.

tranylcypromine sulfate

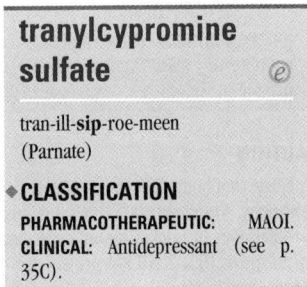

tran-ill-**sip**-roe-meen
(Parnate)

CLASSIFICATION

PHARMACOTHERAPEUTIC: MAOI. **CLINICAL:** Antidepressant (see p. 35C).

ACTION

Inhibits MAO enzyme (assists in metabolism of sympathomimetic amines) at CNS storage sites. Levels of epinephrine, norepinephrine, serotonin, dopamine increased at neuron receptor sites. **Therapeutic Effect:** Produces antidepressant effect.

USES

Treatment of depression in pts refractory to or intolerant to other therapy.

PRECAUTIONS

CONTRAINDICATIONS: Uncontrolled hypertension, pheochromocytoma, CHF, pts <16 yrs, severe renal/hepatic impairment. **CAUTIONS:** Within several hours of ingestion of contraindicated substance (e.g., tyramine-containing food). **Pregnancy Category C.**

INTERACTIONS

DRUG: **Alcohol, CNS depressants** may increase CNS depressant effects. **Tricyclic antidepressants, fluoxetine, trazodone** may cause serotonin syndrome. May increase effect of **oral hypoglycemics, insulin.** B/P may increase with **buspirone. Caffeine-containing medications** may increase cardiac arrhythmias, hypertension. May precipitate hypertensive crises with **carbamazepine, cyclobenzaprine, maprotiline, other MAOIs. Meperidine, other opioid analgesics** may produce immediate excitation, diaphoresis, rigidity, severe hypertension/hypotension, severe respiratory distress, coma, seizures, vascular collapse, death. **Tyramine, foods with pressor amines (e.g., aged cheese)** may cause sudden, severe hypertension. **HERBAL:** None known. **FOOD:** None known. **LAB VALUES:** None known.

AVAILABILITY (Rx)

TABLETS: 10 mg.

INDICATIONS/ROUTES/DOSAGE

PO: ADULTS, ELDERLY: Initially, 10 mg 2 times/day. May increase by 10 mg/day at 1- to 3-wk intervals up to 60 mg/day in divided doses.

SIDE EFFECTS

FREQUENT: Postural hypotension, restlessness, GI upset, insomnia, dizziness, lethargy, weakness, dry mouth, peripheral edema. **OCCASIONAL:** Flushing, increased perspiration, rash, urinary frequency, increased appetite, transient impotence. **RARE:** Visual disturbances.

T

ADVERSE REACTIONS/ TOXIC EFFECTS

Hypertensive crisis (hypertension, occipital headache radiating frontally, neck stiffness/soreness, nausea, vomiting, diaphoresis, fever/chilliness, clammy skin, dilated pupils, palpitations) may be noted. Tachycardia/bradycardia, constricting chest pain may also be present. Antidote for hypertensive crisis: 5–10 mg phentolamine IV injection.

NURSING IMPLICATIONS

BASELINE ASSESSMENT

Baseline and periodic hepatic function tests should be performed in those requiring high dosage and/or undergoing prolonged therapy. MAOI therapy should be discontinued for 7–14 days before therapy begins.

INTERVENTION/EVALUATION

Assess appearance, behavior, speech pattern, level of interest, mood. Supervise suicidal-risk pt closely during early therapy (as depression lessens, energy level improves, increasing suicide potential). Monitor for occipital headache radiating frontally, neck stiffness/soreness (may be first signal of impending hypertensive crisis). Monitor B/P diligently for hypertension. Assess skin and temperature for fever. Discontinue medication immediately if palpitations, frequent headaches occur. Monitor weight.

PATIENT/FAMILY TEACHING

Take second daily dose no later than 4 PM to avoid insomnia. Antidepressant relief may be noted during first week of therapy; maximum benefit noted within 3 wks. Report headache, neck stiffness/soreness immediately. To avoid orthostatic hypotension, change from lying to sitting position slowly and dangle legs momentarily before standing. Avoid foods that require bacteria/molds for their preparation/preservation; those that contain tyramine (e.g., cheese, sour cream, beer, wine, pickled herring, liver, figs, raisins, bananas, avocados, soy sauce, yeast extracts, yogurt, papaya, broad beans, meat tenderizers), excessive amounts of caffeine (coffee, tea, chocolate); OTC preparations for hay fever, colds, weight reduction.

trastuzumab

traz-**two**-zoo-mab
(Herceptin)

CLASSIFICATION

PHARMACOTHERAPEUTIC: Monoclonal antibody. **CLINICAL:** Antineoplastic (see p. 76C).

ACTION

Mediates antibody-dependent cellular cytotoxicity. **Therapeutic Effect:** Inhibits proliferation of human tumor cells that overexpress HER-2 (HER-2 protein overexpression is seen in 25%–30% of primary breast cancer pts).

PHARMACOKINETICS

Half-life: 5.8 days; range: 1–32 days.

USES

Treatment of metastatic breast cancer pts whose tumors overexpress HER-2 protein and who have received one or more chemotherapy regimens. May be used with paclitaxel without previous treatment for metastatic disease.

PRECAUTIONS

CONTRAINDICATIONS: Preexisting cardiac disease. **CAUTIONS:** Previous cardiotoxic drug or radiation therapy to chest wall, those with known hypersensitivity to trastuzumab.

LIFESPAN CONSIDERATIONS: Pregnancy/lactation: Unknown if distributed in breast milk. **Pregnancy Category B. Children:** Safety and efficacy

T

not established. **Elderly:** Age-related cardiac dysfunction may require cautious use.

INTERACTIONS

DRUG: Cyclophosphamide, doxorubicin, epirubicin may increase risk of developing cardiac dysfunction. **HERBAL:** None known. **FOOD:** None known. **LAB VALUES:** None known.

AVAILABILITY (Rx)

LYOPHILIZED POWDER: 440 mg.

ADMINISTRATION/HANDLING

IV

Storage • Refrigerate. • Reconstituted solution appears colorless to pale yellow. • Solution is stable for 28 days if refrigerated after reconstitution with Bacteriostatic Water for Injection (if using Sterile Water for Injection without preservative, use immediately; discard unused portions). • Stable for 24 hrs in 0.9% NaCl if refrigerated.

Reconstitution • Reconstitute with 20 ml Bacteriostatic Water for Injection to yield concentration of 21 mg/ml. • Add calculated dose to 250 ml 0.9% NaCl (do not use D_5W). • Gently mix contents in bag.

Rate of administration • Do not give IV push or bolus. • Give loading dose (4 mg/kg) over 90 min. Give maintenance infusion (2 mg/kg) over 30 min.

IV INCOMPATIBILITIES

Avoid use with D_5W. Do not mix with any other medications.

INDICATIONS/ROUTES/DOSAGE

Alert: Do not give as IV bolus or IV push. Do **not** use dextrose solutions.

BREAST CANCER

IV infusion: ADULTS, ELDERLY: Initially, 4 mg/kg as 30- to 90-min infusion, then weekly infusion of 2 mg/kg as 30-min infusion.

SIDE EFFECTS

FREQUENT (>20%): Pain, asthenia, fever, chills, headache, abdominal pain, back pain, infection, nausea, diarrhea, vomiting, cough, dyspnea. **OCCASIONAL (5%–15%):** Tachycardia, CHF, flulike symptoms, anorexia, edema, bone pain, arthralgia, insomnia, dizziness, paresthesia, depression, rhinitis, pharyngitis, sinusitis. **RARE (<5%):** Allergic reaction, anemia, leukopenia, neuropathy, herpes simplex.

ADVERSE REACTIONS/ TOXIC EFFECTS

Cardiomyopathy, development of ventricular dysfunction, CHF occur rarely. Pancytopenia may occur.

NURSING IMPLICATIONS

BASELINE ASSESSMENT

Evaluate left ventricular function. Obtain baseline echocardiogram, EKG, MUGA scan. CBC, platelet count should be obtained at baseline and at regular intervals during therapy.

INTERVENTION/EVALUATION

Frequently monitor for deteriorating cardiac function. Assess for asthenia (loss of strength, energy). Assist with ambulation if asthenia occurs. Monitor for fever, chills, abdominal pain, back pain. Offer antiemetics if nausea, vomiting occurs. Monitor daily bowel activity, stool consistency.

PATIENT/FAMILY TEACHING

Do not have immunizations without physician's approval (lowers body's resistance). Avoid contact with those who have recently taken oral polio vaccine. Avoid crowds, those with infection.

T

travoprost

(Travatan)

See Classification section under: Antiglaucoma agents (p. 45C)

trazodone hydrochloride

tra-zoh-doan

(Desyrel)

Do not confuse with Delsym, Zestril.

CLASSIFICATION

Antidepressant (see pp. 11C, 36C).

ACTION

Blocks reuptake of serotonin by CNS presynaptic neuronal membranes, increasing availability at postsynaptic neuronal receptor sites. **Therapeutic Effect:** Resulting enhancement of synaptic activity produces antidepressant effect.

PHARMACOKINETICS

Well absorbed from GI tract. Protein binding: 85%–95%. Metabolized in liver. Primarily excreted in urine. Unknown if removed by hemodialysis. **Half-life:** 5–9 hrs.

USES

Treatment of depression exhibited as persistent, prominent dysphoria (occurring nearly every day for at least 2 wks) manifested by 4 of 8 symptoms: appetite change, sleep pattern change, increased fatigue, impaired concentration, feelings of guilt or worthlessness, loss of interest in usual activities, psychomotor agitation or retardation, suicidal tendencies. **Unlabeled:** Treatment of neurogenic pain.

PRECAUTIONS

CONTRAINDICATIONS: None known. **CAUTIONS:** Cardiac disease, arrhythmias.

LIFESPAN CONSIDERATIONS: Pregnancy/lactation: Crosses placenta. Minimally distributed in breast milk. **Pregnancy Category C. Children:** Safety and efficacy not established in those <6 yrs. **Elderly:** More likely to experience sedative, hypotensive effects; lower dosage recommended.

INTERACTIONS

DRUG: Alcohol, CNS depressant–producing medications may increase CNS depression. May increase effects of **antihypertensives.** May increase concentration of **digoxin, phenytoin. HERBAL: St. John's wort** may increase adverse effects. **FOOD:** None known. **LAB VALUES:** May decrease neutrophil, leukocyte counts.

AVAILABILITY (Rx)

TABLETS: 50 mg, 100 mg, 150 mg, 300 mg.

ADMINISTRATION/HANDLING

PO

• Give shortly after snack, meal (reduces risk of dizziness, lightheadedness). • Tablets may be crushed.

INDICATIONS/ROUTES/DOSAGE

ANTIDEPRESSANT

PO: ADULTS: Initially, 150 mg daily in equally divided doses. Increase by 50 mg/day at 3- to 4-day intervals until therapeutic response is achieved. **Maximum:** 600 mg/day. CHILDREN 6–18 YRS: Initially, 1.5–2 mg/kg/day in divided doses. May increase gradually to 6 mg/kg/day in 3 divided doses.

USUAL ELDERLY DOSAGE

PO: Initially, 25–50 mg at bedtime. May increase by 25–50 mg q3–7 days. RANGE: 75–150 mg/day.

SIDE EFFECTS

FREQUENT (3%–9%): Drowsiness, dry mouth, lightheadedness/dizziness, headache, blurred vision, nausea/vomiting. **OCCASIONAL (1%–3%):** Nervousness, fatigue, constipation, generalized aches/pains, mild hypotension.

ADVERSE REACTIONS/ TOXIC EFFECTS

Priapism (painful, prolonged penile erection), decreased/increased libido, retrograde ejaculation, impotence have been noted rarely. Appears to be less cardiotoxic than other antidepressants, although arrhythmias may occur in pts with preexisting cardiac disease.

NURSING IMPLICATIONS

BASELINE ASSESSMENT

For those on long-term therapy, hepatic/renal function tests, blood counts should be performed periodically. Elderly are more likely to experience sedative or hypotensive effects.

INTERVENTION/EVALUATION

Supervise suicidal-risk pt closely during early therapy (as depression lessens, energy level improves, increasing suicide potential). Assess appearance, behavior, speech pattern, level of interest, mood. Monitor WBC, neutrophil count (drug should be stopped if levels fall below normal). Assist with ambulation if dizziness, lightheadedness occurs.

PATIENT/FAMILY TEACHING

May take after a meal/snack. May give at bedtime if drowsiness occurs. Immediately discontinue medication, consult physician if priapism occurs. Change positions slowly to avoid hypotensive effect. Tolerance to sedative and anticholinergic effects usually develops during early therapy. Photosensitivity to sun may occur. Dry mouth may be relieved by sugarless gum, sips of tepid water. Report visual disturbances. Do not abruptly discontinue medication. Avoid tasks that require alertness, motor skills until response to drug is established. Avoid alcohol.

treprostinil sodium

tre-**pros**-tin-il
(Remodulin)

◆ CLASSIFICATION

PHARMACOTHERAPEUTIC: Aggregation inhibitor, vasodilator. **CLINICAL:** Antiplatelet.

ACTION

Directly vasodilates pulmonary and systemic arterial vascular beds, inhibits platelet aggregation. **Therapeutic Effect:** Reduces symptoms of pulmonary arterial hypertension associated with exercise.

PHARMACOKINETICS

Rapidly, completely absorbed following subcutaneous infusion; 91% bound to plasma protein. Metabolized by the liver. Excreted mainly in the urine with a lesser amount eliminated in the feces. **Half-life:** 2–4 hrs.

USES

As a continuous subcutaneous infusion for the treatment of pulmonary arterial hypertension to diminish symptoms associated with exercise.

PRECAUTIONS

CONTRAINDICATIONS: None known. **CAUTIONS:** Hepatic/renal impairment of those >65 yrs.

LIFESPAN CONSIDERATIONS: Pregnancy/lactation: Unknown if distributed in breast milk. **Pregnancy Category B. Children:** Safety and efficacy not established. **Elderly:** Dose selection should be noted, reflecting higher incidence of decreased hepatic, renal, cardiac function; concurrent disease; other drug therapy.

INTERACTIONS

DRUG: Reduction in B/P caused by treprostinil may be exacerbated by drugs that alter B/P **(i.e., diuretics, antihypertensive agents, vasodilators).** May increase risk of bleeding with **anticoagulants, heparin, thrombolytics, aspirin.** **HERBAL:** None known. **FOOD:** None known. **LAB VALUES:** None known.

AVAILABILITY (Rx)

INJECTION: 1 mg/ml, 2.5 mg/ml, 5 mg/ml, 10 mg/ml.

ADMINISTRATION/HANDLING

SUBCUTANEOUS

Storage • Store at room temperature.

Reconstitution • Intended to be administered without further dilution. • Do not use a single vial for >14 days after initial use. • To avoid potential interruptions in drug delivery, the pt must have immediate access to a backup infusion pump and subcutaneous infusion sets.

Rate of administration • Give as a continuous subcutaneous infusion via a subcutaneous catheter, using an infusion pump designed for subcutaneous drug delivery. • Calculate the infusion rate using following formula: infusion rate (ml/hr) = dose (ng/kg/min) × weight (kg) × (0.00006/treprostinil dosage strength concentration [mg/ml]).

INDICATIONS/ROUTES/DOSAGE

PULMONARY ARTERIAL HYPERTENSION

Continuous subcutaneous infusion: ADULTS, ELDERLY: Initially, 1.25 ng/kg/min. Reduce infusion rate to 0.625 ng/kg/min if initial dose cannot be tolerated. Increase infusion rate in increments of no more than 1.25 ng/kg/min per week for the first 4 wks and then no more than 2.5 ng/kg/min per week for the remaining duration of infusion.

HEPATIC FUNCTION IMPAIRMENT

In mild to moderate hepatic insufficiency, decrease the initial dose to 0.625 ng/kg/min using ideal body weight and increase cautiously.

SIDE EFFECTS

FREQUENT: Infusion site pain, erythema, induration, rash. **OCCASIONAL:** Headache, diarrhea, jaw pain, vasodilation, nausea. **RARE:** Dizziness, hypotension, pruritus, edema.

ADVERSE REACTIONS/ TOXIC EFFECTS

Abrupt withdrawal or sudden large reductions in dosage may result in worsening of pulmonary arterial hypertension symptoms.

NURSING IMPLICATIONS

PATIENT/FAMILY TEACHING

Offer full, complete instruction of drug administration as delivery system via a self-inserted subcutaneous catheter using an ambulatory subcutaneous pump. Instruct pt on care of subcutaneous catheter and trouble shooting infusion pump problems.

tretinoin

tret-ih-noyn

(Avita, Renova, Retin-A, Retin-A Micro, Stieva-A ✤, Vesanoid, Vitamin A Acid ✤)

Do not confuse with trientine.

FIXED-COMBINATION(S)

With octyl methoxycinnamate and oxybenzone, moisturizers, and SPF-12, a sunscreen **(Retin-A Regimen Kit).**

◆CLASSIFICATION

PHARMACOTHERAPEUTIC: Retinoid. **CLINICAL:** Antiacne, transdermal, antineoplastic (see p. 76C).

ACTION

Antiacne: Decreases cohesiveness of follicular epithelial cells. Increases turnover of follicular epithelial cells. **Therapeutic Effect:** Causes expulsion of blackheads. Bacterial skin counts are not altered. **Transdermal:** Exerts its effects on growth/differentiation of epithelial cells. **Therapeutic Effect:** Alleviates fine wrinkles, hyperpigmentation. **Antineoplastic:** Induces maturation, decreases proliferation of acute promyelocytic leukemia (APL) cells. **Therapeutic Effect:** Repopulation of bone marrow, blood by normal hematopoietic cells.

PHARMACOKINETICS

Topical: Minimally absorbed. **PO:** Well absorbed following PO administration. Primarily excreted in urine. **Half-life:** 0.5–2 hrs.

USES

Topical: Treatment of acne vulgaris, esp. grades I–III in which blackheads, papules, pustules predominate. **Transdermal:** Treatment of fine wrinkles, hyperpigmentation. **Antineoplastic:** Induction of remission in pts with APL. **Unlabeled:** Treatment of disorders of keratinization, including photo-aged skin, liver spots.

PRECAUTIONS

CONTRAINDICATIONS: Sensitivity to parabens (used as preservative in gelatin capsule). **EXTREME CAUTION: Topical:** Eczema, sun exposure. **CAUTIONS: Topical:** Those with considerable sun exposure in their occupation or hypersensitivity to sun. **PO:** Elevated cholesterol/triglycerides.

LIFESPAN CONSIDERATIONS: Pregnancy/lactation: Topical: Use during pregnancy only if clearly needed. Unknown if excreted in breast milk; exercise caution in nursing mother. **Pregnancy Category C. PO:** Teratogenic, embryotoxic effect. **Pregnancy Category D. Children/elderly:** Safety and efficacy not established.

INTERACTIONS

DRUG: Topical: Keratolytic agents (e.g., sulfur, benzoyl peroxide, salicylic acid), medicated soaps, shampoos, astringents, spice or lime cologne, permanent wave solutions, hair depilatories may increase skin irritation. **Photosensitive medication (thiazides, tetracyclines, fluoroquinolones, phenothiazines, sulfonamides)** augments phototoxicity. **PO: Ketoconazole** may increase tretinoin concentration. **HERBAL:** None known. **FOOD:** None known. **LAB VALUES: PO:** Leukocytosis occurs commonly (40%). May elevate hepatic function tests, cholesterol, triglycerides.

AVAILABILITY (Rx)

CAPSULES: 10 mg. **CREAM:** 0.025%, 0.05%, 0.1%. **CREAM (Avita):** 0.025%. **CREAM (Renova):** 0.02%, 0.05%. **GEL:** 0.025%, 0.01%. **GEL (Retin-A Micro):** 0.04%, 0.1%. **LIQUID:** 0.05%.

ADMINISTRATION/HANDLING

PO

- Do not crush/break capsule.

TOPICAL

- Thoroughly cleanse area prior to applying tretinoin. • Lightly cover only the affected area. Liquid may be applied with fingertip, gauze, cotton, taking care to avoid rubbing onto unaffected skin.
- Keep medication away from eyes, mouth, angles of nose, mucous mem-

T

branes. • Wash hands immediately after application.

INDICATIONS/ROUTES/DOSAGE

ACNE

Topical: ADULTS, CHILDREN >12 YRS: Apply once daily at bedtime.

ACUTE PROMYELOCYTIC LEUKEMIA

PO: ADULTS: 45 mg/m^2/day given as 2 evenly divided doses until complete remission is documented. Discontinue therapy 30 days after complete remission or after 90 days of treatment, whichever comes first.

SIDE EFFECTS

Topical: Temporary change in pigmentation, photosensitivity. Local inflammatory reactions (peeling, dry skin, stinging, erythema, pruritus) are to be expected and are reversible with discontinuation of tretinoin. **FREQUENT: PO (54%–87%):** Headache, fever, dry skin/oral mucosa, bone pain, nausea, vomiting, rash. **OCCASIONAL: PO (6%–26%):** Mucositis, earache or feeling of fullness in ears, flushing, pruritus, increased sweating, visual disturbances, hypotension/hypertension, dizziness, anxiety, insomnia, alopecia, skin changes. **RARE (6%):** Change in visual acuity, temporary hearing loss.

ADVERSE REACTIONS/ TOXIC EFFECTS

PO: Retinoic acid syndrome (fever, dyspnea, weight gain, abnormal chest auscultatory findings [pulmonary infiltrates, pleural or pericardial effusions], episodic hypotension) occurs commonly (25%), as does leukocytosis (40%). Syndrome generally occurs during first month of therapy (sometimes occurs after first dose). High-dose steroids (dexamethasone 10 mg IV) at first suspicion of syndrome reduces morbidity, mortality. Pseudotumor cerebri may be noted, esp. in children (headache, nausea, vomiting, visual disturbances). **TOPICAL:** Possible tumorigenic potential when combined with ultraviolet radiation.

NURSING IMPLICATIONS

BASELINE ASSESSMENT

PO: Inform women of childbearing potential of risk to fetus if pregnancy occurs. Instruct on need for use of 2 reliable forms of contraceptives concurrently during therapy and for 1 mo after discontinuation of therapy, even in infertile, premenopausal women. Pregnancy test should be obtained within 1 wk prior to institution of therapy. Obtain initial hepatic function tests, cholesterol, triglyceride levels.

INTERVENTION/EVALUATION

PO: Monitor hepatic function tests, hematologic and coagulation profiles, cholesterol, triglycerides. Monitor signs/symptoms of pseudotumor cerebri in children.

PATIENT/FAMILY TEACHING

Topical: Avoid exposure to sunlight, sun beds; use sunscreens, protective clothing. Affected areas should also be protected from wind, cold. If skin is already sunburned, do not use drug until fully healed. Keep tretinoin away from eyes, mouth, angles of nose, mucous membranes. Do not use medicated, drying, abrasive soaps; wash face no more than 2–3 times/day with gentle soap. Avoid use of preparations containing alcohol, menthol, spice, lime, such as shaving lotions, astringents, perfume. Mild redness, peeling are expected; decrease frequency or discontinue medication if excessive reaction occurs. Nonmedicated cosmetics may be used; however, cosmetics must be removed before tretinoin application. Improvement noted during first 24 wks of therapy. **Antiacne:** Therapeutic results noted in 2–3 wks; optimal results in 6 wks.

triamcinolone

try-am-**sin**-oh-lone
(Aristocort)

triamcinolone diacetate

(Amcort, Aristocort Intralesional)

triamcinolone acetonide

(Aristocort, Azmacort, Kenalog, Nasacort AQ, Triaderm ✤)

triamcinolone hexacetonide

(Aristospan)

Do not confuse with Triaminicin, Triaminicol.

FIXED-COMBINATION(S)

Myco-II, Mycolog II, Myco-Triacet: triamcinolone/nystatin (an antifungal): 0.1%/100,000 units/g.

◆CLASSIFICATION

PHARMACOTHERAPEUTIC: Adrenocortical steroid. **CLINICAL:** Anti-inflammatory (see pp. 65C, 82C, 85C).

ACTION

Inhibits accumulation of inflammatory cells at inflammation sites, phagocytosis, lysosomal enzyme release, synthesis and/or release of mediators of inflammation. **Therapeutic Effect:** Prevents/suppresses cell-mediated immune reactions. Decreases/prevents tissue response to inflammatory process.

USES

Inhalation: Long-term control of bronchial asthma. **Nasal:** Seasonal and perennial rhinitis. **Oral:** Immunosuppressant, relief of acute inflammation. **Topical:** Relief of inflammation/pruritus associated with corticoid-responsive dermatoses.

PRECAUTIONS

CONTRAINDICATIONS: Hypersensitivity to any corticosteroid or tartrazine, systemic fungal infection, peptic ulcers (except life-threatening situations). IM injection, oral inhalation not for children <6 yrs. Avoid immunizations, smallpox vaccination. **Topical:** Marked circulation impairment. **CAUTIONS:** History of tuberculosis (may reactivate disease), hypothyroidism, cirrhosis, nonspecific ulcerative colitis, CHF, hypertension, psychosis, renal insufficiency. Prolonged therapy should be discontinued slowly. **Pregnancy Category C** (**D** if used in first trimester).

INTERACTIONS

DRUG: **Amphotericin** may increase hypokalemia. May decrease effect of **oral hypoglycemics, insulin, diuretics, potassium supplements.** May increase toxicity of **digoxin** (due to hypokalemia). **Hepatic enzyme inducers** may decrease effect. **Live virus vaccines** may potentiate virus replication, increase vaccine side effects, decrease pt's antibody response to vaccine. **HERBAL:** None known. **FOOD:** None known. **LAB VALUES:** May decrease calcium, potassium, thyroxine. May increase cholesterol, lipids, glucose, sodium, amylase.

AVAILABILITY (Rx)

TABLETS: 4 mg. **SYRUP:** 2 mg/5 ml. **AEROSOL (respiratory inhalant), NASAL SPRAY, OINTMENT:** 0.1%. **CREAM:** 0.025%, 0.1%, 0.5%. **LOTION:** 0.025%, 0.1%.

ACETONIDE: **INJECTION:** 10 mg/ml, 40 mg/ml.

DIACETATE: **INJECTION:** 40 mg/ml.

T

HEXACETONE: **INJECTION:** 5 mg/ml, 20 mg/ml.

ADMINISTRATION/HANDLING

PO

• Give with food, milk. • Single doses given before 9 AM; multiple doses at evenly spaced intervals.

IM

• Do **not** give IV. • Give deep IM in gluteus maximus.

INHALATION

• Shake container well; exhale as completely as possible. • Place mouthpiece fully into mouth, holding inhaler upright, inhale deeply and slowly while pressing the top of the canister, hold breath as long as possible before exhaling; then exhale slowly. • Wait 1 min between inhalations when multiple inhalations ordered (allows for deeper bronchial penetration). • Rinse mouth with water immediately after inhalation.

TOPICAL

• Gently cleanse area prior to application. • Use occlusive dressings only as ordered. • Apply sparingly, rub into area thoroughly.

INDICATIONS/ROUTES/DOSAGE

USUAL ORAL DOSAGE

PO: ADULTS, ELDERLY: 4–60 mg/day.

TRIAMCINOLONE DIACETATE

IM: ADULTS, ELDERLY: 40 mg/wk.

Intra-articular, intralesional: ADULTS, ELDERLY: 5–40 mg.

TRIAMCINOLONE ACETONIDE

IM: ADULTS, ELDERLY: Initially, 2.5–60 mg/day.

Intra-articular: ADULTS, ELDERLY: Initially, 2.5–40 mg up to 100 mg.

TRIAMCINOLONE HEXACETONIDE

Intra-articular: ADULTS, ELDERLY: 2–20 mg.

CONTROL OF BRONCHIAL ASTHMA

Inhalation: ADULTS, ELDERLY: 2 inhalations 3–4 times/day. CHILDREN 6–12 YRS: 1–2 inhalations 3–4 times/day. **Maximum:** 12 inhalations/day.

RHINITIS

Intranasal: ADULTS, CHILDREN >6 YRS: 2 sprays each nostril daily.

USUAL TOPICAL DOSAGE

Topical: ADULTS, ELDERLY: Sparingly 2–4 times/day. May give 1–2 times/day or intermittent therapy.

SIDE EFFECTS

FREQUENT: Insomnia, dry mouth, heartburn, nervousness, abdominal distention, diaphoresis, acne, mood swings, increased appetite, facial flushing, delayed wound healing, increased susceptibility to infection, diarrhea/constipation. **OCCASIONAL:** Headache, edema, change in skin color, frequent urination. **RARE:** Tachycardia, allergic reaction (rash, hives), mental changes, hallucinations, depression. **Topical:** Allergic contact dermatitis.

ADVERSE REACTIONS/ TOXIC EFFECTS

LONG-TERM THERAPY: Muscle wasting (esp. arms, legs), osteoporosis, spontaneous fractures, amenorrhea, cataracts, glaucoma, peptic ulcer, CHF. **ABRUPT WITHDRAWAL FOLLOWING LONG-TERM THERAPY:** Anorexia, nausea, fever, headache, joint pain, rebound inflammation, fatigue, weakness, lethargy, dizziness, orthostatic hypotension. Anaphylaxis with parenteral administration occurs rarely. Sudden discontinuance may be fatal.

T

Blindness has occurred rarely after intralesional injection around face, head.

NURSING IMPLICATIONS

BASELINE ASSESSMENT

Question for hypersensitivity to any of the corticosteroids or tartrazine (Kenacort). Obtain baselines for height, weight, B/P, glucose, electrolytes. Check results of initial tests (e.g., TB skin test, x-rays, EKG).

INTERVENTION/EVALUATION

Monitor I&O, daily weight, B/P, glucose, electrolytes. Assess for edema. Check vitals at least 2 times/day. Be alert to infection: sore throat, fever, vague symptoms. Watch for hypocalcemia (muscle twitching, cramps, positive Trousseau's or Chvostek's signs), hypokalemia (weakness, muscle cramps, numbness/tingling [esp. in lower extremities], nausea/vomiting, irritability, EKG changes). Assess emotional status, ability to sleep. For oral inhalation, check mucous membranes for signs of fungal infection. Monitor growth in children. Check lab results for blood coagulability, clinical evidence of thromboembolism. Provide assistance with ambulation.

PATIENT/FAMILY TEACHING

Oral: Inform physician if sudden weight gain, swelling of face, difficulty breathing, muscle weakness occurs. Take oral medication with food or after meals. Inform physician if condition worsens. Do not stop medication without physician approval. May cause dry mouth. Avoid alcohol. **Inhalation:** Do not take for acute asthma attack. Rinse mouth to decrease risk of mouth soreness. Inform physician if mouth lesions, sore mouth occurs. **Nasal:** Report unusual cough/spasm, persistent nasal bleeding, burning, infection.

triamterene

try-**am**-tur-een
(Dyrenium)
Do not confuse with diazoxide, Maxidex, trimipramine.

FIXED-COMBINATION(S)

Dyazide, Maxzide: triamterene/hydrochlorothiazide (a diuretic): 37.5 mg/25 mg; 50 mg/25 mg; 75 mg/50 mg.

◆ CLASSIFICATION

PHARMACOTHERAPEUTIC: Potassium-sparing diuretic. **CLINICAL:** Antiedema (see p. 87C).

ACTION

Inhibits sodium, potassium, ATPase. Interferes with sodium/potassium exchange in distal tubule, cortical collecting tubule, and collecting duct. **Therapeutic Effect:** Increases sodium, decreases potassium excretion. Also increases magnesium, decreases calcium loss.

PHARMACOKINETICS

	Onset	Peak	Duration
PO	2–4 hrs	—	7–9 hrs

Incompletely absorbed from GI tract. Widely distributed. Metabolized in liver. Primarily eliminated in feces via biliary route. **Half-life:** 1.5–2.5 hrs (half-life increased with impaired renal function).

T

USES

Treatment of edema, hypertension; to decrease potassium loss caused by diuretics. **Unlabeled:** Treatment adjunct for hypertension, prophylaxis/treatment of hypokalemia.

PRECAUTIONS

CONTRAINDICATIONS: Severe or progressive renal disease, severe hepatic disease, preexisting or drug-induced hyperkalemia. **CAUTIONS:** Impaired hepatic or renal function, history of renal calculi, diabetes mellitus, those receiving other potassium-sparing diuretics or potassium supplements.

LIFESPAN CONSIDERATIONS: Pregnancy/lactation: Crosses placenta. Distributed in breast milk. Breast-feeding is not advised. **Pregnancy Category C (D** is used in pregnancy-induced hypertension). **Children:** Safety and efficacy not established. **Elderly:** May be at increased risk for developing hyperkalemia.

INTERACTIONS

DRUG: May decrease effect of **anticoagulants, heparin. NSAIDs** may decrease antihypertensive effect. **ACE inhibitors (e.g., captopril), potassium-containing medications, potassium supplements** may increase potassium. May decrease **lithium** clearance, increase toxicity. **HERBAL:** None known. **FOOD:** None known. **LAB VALUES:** May increase BUN, calcium, creatinine, glucose, potassium, uric acid. May decrease sodium, magnesium.

AVAILABILITY (Rx)

CAPSULES: 50 mg, 100 mg.

ADMINISTRATION/HANDLING

PO

- Give with food if GI disturbances occur.
- Do not crush, break capsules.

INDICATIONS/ROUTES/DOSAGE

EDEMA, HYPERTENSION

PO: ADULTS, ELDERLY: 25–100 mg/day in 1 or 2 divided doses. **Maximum:** 300 mg/day. CHILDREN: 2–4 mg/kg/day in 1 or 2 divided doses. **Maximum:** 6 mg/kg/day or 300 mg/day.

SIDE EFFECTS

OCCASIONAL: Fatigue, nausea, diarrhea, abdominal distress, leg aches, headache. **RARE:** Anorexia, weakness, rash, dizziness.

ADVERSE REACTIONS/ TOXIC EFFECTS

May produce hyponatremia (drowsiness, dry mouth, increased thirst, lack of energy), severe hyperkalemia (irritability, anxiety, heaviness of legs, paresthesia, hypotension, bradycardia, EKG changes [tented T waves, widening QRS, ST depression]). Agranulocytosis, nephrolithiasis, thrombocytopenia occur rarely.

NURSING IMPLICATIONS

BASELINE ASSESSMENT

Assess baseline electrolytes, particularly check for hypokalemia. Assess renal/hepatic function tests. Assess edema (note location, extent), skin turgor, mucous membranes for hydration status. Assess muscle strength, mental status. Note skin temperature, moisture. Obtain baseline weight. Initiate strict I&O. Note pulse rate/regularity.

INTERVENTION/EVALUATION

Monitor B/P, vital signs, electrolytes (particularly potassium), I&O, weight. Note extent of diuresis. Watch for changes from initial assessment (hyperkalemia may result in muscle strength changes, tremor, muscle cramps), change in mental status (orientation, alertness, confusion), cardiac arrhythmias. Monitor potassium level, particularly during initial therapy. Weigh daily. Assess lung sounds for rhonchi, wheezing.

PATIENT/FAMILY TEACHING

Take in the morning. Expect increase in volume, frequency of urination. Therapeutic effect takes several days to begin and can last for several days when drug is discontinued. Avoid prolonged exposure to sunlight. Report severe or persistent weakness, headache, dry mouth, nausea, vomiting, fever, sore throat, unusual bleeding/bruising. Avoid excessive intake of food high in potassium or use of salt substitutes.

triazolam

try-**aye**-zoe-lam
(Apo-Triazo✱, Halcion)

Do not confuse with Haldol, Healon.

◆ CLASSIFICATION

PHARMACOTHERAPEUTIC: Benzodiazepine **(Schedule IV). CLINICAL:** Sedative-hypnotic (see p. 129C).

ACTION

Enhances action of inhibitory neurotransmitter gamma-aminobutyric acid (GABA). **Therapeutic Effect:** Produces hypnotic effect due to CNS depression.

USES

Short-term treatment of insomnia (≤6 wks). Reduces sleep-induction time, number of nocturnal awakenings; increases length of sleep.

PRECAUTIONS

CONTRAINDICATIONS: Severe uncontrolled pain, CNS depression, narrow-angle glaucoma, sleep apnea, pregnancy, lactation. **CAUTIONS:** Those with potential for drug abuse. **Pregnancy Category X.**

INTERACTIONS

DRUG: Alcohol, CNS depressants may increase CNS depressant effect. **HERBAL: Kava kava, valerian** may increase CNS depression. **FOOD: Grapefruit/grapefruit juice** may alter absorption. **LAB VALUES:** None known.

AVAILABILITY (Rx)

TABLETS: 0.125 mg, 0.25 mg.

ADMINISTRATION/HANDLING

PO

• Give without regard to meals. • Tablets may be crushed. • Grapefruit juice may alter absorption.

INDICATIONS/ROUTES/DOSAGE

HYPNOTIC

PO: ADULTS >18 YRS: 0.125–0.5 mg at bedtime. ELDERLY: 0.0625–0.125 mg at bedtime.

SIDE EFFECTS

FREQUENT: Drowsiness, sedation, dry mouth, headache, dizziness, nervousness, lightheadedness, incoordination, nausea. **OCCASIONAL:** Euphoria, tachycardia, abdominal cramps, visual disturbances. **RARE:** Paradoxical CNS excitement, restlessness, particularly noted in elderly, debilitated.

ADVERSE REACTIONS/ TOXIC EFFECTS

Abrupt or too rapid withdrawal may result in pronounced restlessness, irritability, insomnia, hand tremors, abdominal/muscle cramps, diaphoresis, vomiting, seizures. Overdosage results in somnolence, confusion, diminished reflexes, coma.

NURSING IMPLICATIONS

BASELINE ASSESSMENT

Question for possibility of pregnancy before initiating therapy (Pregnancy Category X). Assess vital signs immediately prior to administration. Raise bed rails. Provide environment conducive to sleep (back rub, quiet environment, low lighting).

INTERVENTION/EVALUATION

Monitor respiratory, cardiovascular, mental status; hepatic function with prolonged use. Assess sleep pattern of pt. Monitor elderly/debilitated for paradoxical reaction, particularly during early therapy. Evaluate for therapeutic response to insomnia: decrease in number of nocturnal awakenings, increase in length of sleep.

PATIENT/FAMILY TEACHING

May cause drowsiness. Avoid tasks that require alertness, motor skills until response to drug is established. May cause physical or psychological dependence, dry mouth. Smoking reduces drug effectiveness. Rebound insomnia may occur when drug is discontinued after short-term therapy. Avoid alcohol, other CNS depressants. Inform physician if you are or are planning to become pregnant. May experience disturbed sleep patterns for 1–2 nights after discontinuing triazolam. Avoid concomitant grapefruit juice.

Tricor

see fenofibrate

trifluoperazine hydrochloride

try-floo-oh-**pear**-ah-zeen
(Apo-Trifluoperazine ✤, Stelazine)

Do not confuse with selegiline, triflupromazine.

CLASSIFICATION

PHARMACOTHERAPEUTIC: Phenothiazine derivative. **CLINICAL:** Antipsychotic, antianxiety (see p. 57C).

ACTION

Blocks dopamine at postsynaptic receptor sites. Possess strong extrapyramidal, antiemetic action; weak anticholinergic, sedative effects. **Therapeutic Effect:** Suppresses behavioral response in psychosis, reducing locomotor activity/aggressiveness, suppresses conditioned responses.

USES

Management of psychotic disorders, nonpsychotic anxiety.

PRECAUTIONS

CONTRAINDICATIONS: Narrow-angle glaucoma, bone marrow suppression, severe hepatic/cardiac disease, circulatory collapse, severe hypotension/hypertension. **CAUTIONS:** Seizure disorders, Parkinson's disease. **Pregnancy Category C.**

INTERACTIONS

DRUG: **Alcohol, CNS depressants** may increase CNS, respiratory depression; hypotensive effects. **Tricyclic antidepressants, MAOIs** may increase sedative, anticholinergic effects. **Antithyroid agents** may increase risk of agranulocytosis. Extrapyramidal symptoms (EPS) may increase with **EPS-producing medications. Hypotensives** may increase hypotension. May decrease **levodopa** effects. **Lithium** may decrease absorption, produce adverse neurologic effects. **HERBAL:** None known. **FOOD:** None known. **LAB VALUES:** May cause EKG changes.

AVAILABILITY (Rx)

ORAL CONCENTRATE: 10 mg/ml. **TABLETS:** 1 mg, 2 mg, 5 mg, 10 mg.

ADMINISTRATION/HANDLING

PO

• Oral concentrate must be diluted in 2–4 oz of water, juice, carbonated beverage, pudding. • Do not take antacids within 1 hr of trifluoperazine.

INDICATIONS/ROUTES/DOSAGE

PSYCHOTIC DISORDERS

PO: ADULTS, ELDERLY, CHILDREN >12 YRS: Initially, 2–5 mg 1–2 times/day. RANGE: 15–20 mg/day. **Maximum:** 40 mg/day. CHILDREN 6–12 YRS: Initially, 1 mg 1–2 times/day. MAINTENANCE: Up to 15 mg/day.

SIDE EFFECTS

FREQUENT: Hypotension, dizziness, fainting occur frequently after first injection, occasionally after subsequent injections, rarely with oral dosage. **OCCASIONAL:** Drowsiness during early therapy, dry mouth, blurred vision, lethargy, constipation, diarrhea, nasal congestion, peripheral edema, urinary retention. **RARE:** Ocular changes, skin pigmentation (those taking high dosages for prolonged periods).

ADVERSE REACTIONS/ TOXIC EFFECTS

Extrapyramidal symptoms appear to be dose related (particularly high dosage) and are divided into 3 categories: akathisia (inability to sit still, tapping of feet, urge to move around); parkinsonian symptoms (masklike face, tremors, shuffling gait, hypersalivation); acute dystonias: torticollis (neck muscle spasm), opisthotonos (rigidity of back muscles), oculogyric crisis (rolling back of eyes). Dystonic reaction may also produce profuse diaphoresis, pallor. Tardive dyskinesia (protrusion of tongue, puffing of cheeks, chewing/puckering of the mouth) occurs rarely (may be irreversible). Abrupt withdrawal after long-term therapy may precipitate nausea, vomiting, gastritis, dizziness, tremors. Blood dyscrasias, particularly agranulocytosis, mild leukopenia may occur. May lower seizure threshold.

NURSING IMPLICATIONS

BASELINE ASSESSMENT

Avoid skin contact with oral concentrate (contact dermatitis). Assess behavior, appearance, emotional status, response to environment, speech pattern, thought content.

INTERVENTION/EVALUATION

Monitor B/P for hypotension. Assess for extrapyramidal symptoms. Monitor WBC for blood dyscrasias. Monitor for fine tongue movement (may be early sign of tardive dyskinesia); tremors, gait changes; abnormal movement in trunk, neck, extremities. Supervise suicidal-risk pt closely during early therapy (as depression lessens, energy level improves, increasing suicide potential). Monitor target behaviors. Assess for therapeutic response (interest in surroundings, improvement in self-care, increased ability to concentrate, relaxed facial expression).

PATIENT/FAMILY TEACHING

Oral concentrate must be diluted in 2–4 oz of water, juice, carbonated beverage, pudding. Do not take antacids within 1 hr of trifluoperazine. Avoid alcohol. Avoid excessive exposure to sunlight, artificial light. May cause drowsiness. Avoid tasks that require alertness, motor skills until response to drug is established. Rise slowly from lying or sitting position (prevents hypotension).

trihexyphenidyl hydrochloride

try-hex-eh-**fen**-ih-dill
(Apo-Trihex ♣, Artane)

◆CLASSIFICATION

PHARMACOTHERAPEUTIC: Anticholinergic. **CLINICAL:** Antiparkinson agent.

ACTION

Blocks central cholinergic receptors (aids in balancing cholinergic and dopaminergic activity). **Therapeutic Effect:** Decreases salivation, relaxes smooth muscle.

USES

Adjunctive treatment for all forms of Parkinson's disease, including postencephalitic, arteriosclerotic, idiopathic types. Controls symptoms of drug-induced extrapyramidal symptoms.

PRECAUTIONS

CONTRAINDICATIONS: Angle-closure glaucoma, GI obstruction, paralytic ileus, intestinal atony, severe ulcerative colitis, prostatic hypertrophy, myasthenia gravis, megacolon. **CAUTIONS:** Hyperthyroidism, renal/hepatic impairment, hypertension, hiatal hernia, tachycardia, arrhythmias, ulcer, esophageal reflux, excessive activity during hot weather or exercise. **Pregnancy Category C.**

INTERACTIONS

DRUG: **Alcohol, CNS depressants** may increase sedative effect. **Amantadine, anticholinergics, MAOIs** may increase anticholinergic effects. **Antacids, antidiarrheals** may decrease absorption, effects. **HERBAL:** None known. **FOOD:** None known. **LAB VALUES:** None known.

ADMINISTRATION/HANDLING

PO

- Administer with food, water to decrease GI irritation.

AVAILABILITY (Rx)

TABLETS: 2 mg, 5 mg. **ELIXIR:** 2 mg/5 ml.

INDICATIONS/ROUTES/DOSAGE

PARKINSONISM

PO: ADULTS, ELDERLY: Initially, 1 mg on first day. May increase by 2 mg/day at 3- to 5-day intervals up to 6–10 mg/day (12–15 mg/day in pts with postencephalitic parkinsonism).

DRUG-INDUCED EXTRAPYRAMIDAL SYMPTOMS

PO: ADULTS, ELDERLY: Initially, 1 mg/day. RANGE: 5–15 mg/day in 3–4 divided doses.

SIDE EFFECTS

Alert: Elderly (>60 yrs) tend to develop mental confusion, disorientation, agitation, psychotic-like symptoms.

FREQUENT: Drowsiness, dry mouth. **OCCASIONAL:** Blurred vision, urinary retention, constipation, dizziness, headache, muscle cramps. **RARE:** Skin rash, seizures, depression.

ADVERSE REACTIONS/ TOXIC EFFECTS

Hypersensitivity reaction (eczema, pruritus, rash, cardiac disturbances, photosensitivity) may occur. Overdosage may vary from CNS depression (sedation, apnea, cardiovascular collapse, death) to severe paradoxical reaction (hallucinations, tremor, seizures).

NURSING IMPLICATIONS

INTERVENTION/EVALUATION

Be alert to neurologic effects: headache, lethargy, mental confusion, agitation. Monitor elderly closely for paradoxical reaction. Assess for clinical reversal of symptoms (improvement of tremor of head/hands at rest, masklike facial expression, shuffling gait, muscular rigidity).

PATIENT/FAMILY TEACHING

Take after meals or with food. Do not stop medication abruptly. Inform physician if GI effects, palpitations, eye pain, rash, fever, heat intolerance occurs. Avoid alcohol, other CNS depressants. May cause dry mouth, drowsiness. Avoid tasks that require alertness, motor skills until response to drug is established. Difficulty urinating, constipation may occur (inform physician if they persist).

Trileptal

see oxcarbazepine

trimethobenzamide hydrochloride

try-meth-oh-**benz**-ah-mide
(Tigan)

CLASSIFICATION

PHARMACOTHERAPEUTIC: Anticholinergic. **CLINICAL:** Antiemetic.

ACTION

Acts at the chemoreceptor trigger zone in CNS (medulla oblongata). **Therapeutic Effect:** Relieves nausea/vomiting.

PHARMACOKINETICS

	Onset	Peak	Duration
PO	10–40 min	—	3–4 hrs
IM	15–30 min	—	2–3 hrs

Partially absorbed from GI tract. Distributed primarily to liver. Metabolic fate unknown. Excreted in urine. **Half-life:** 7–9 hrs.

USES

Control of nausea/vomiting.

PRECAUTIONS

CONTRAINDICATIONS: Hypersensitivity to benzocaine or similar local anesthetics; parenteral form in children, suppositories in premature infants or neonates. **CAUTIONS:** Elderly, debilitated, dehydration, electrolyte imbalance, high fever.

LIFESPAN CONSIDERATIONS: Pregnancy/lactation: Unknown if drug crosses placenta or is distributed in breast milk. **Pregnancy Category C. Children/elderly:** No age-related precautions noted. Avoid parenteral form in children and suppositories in neonates.

INTERACTIONS

DRUG: CNS depression–producing medications may increase CNS depression. **HERBAL:** None known. **FOOD:** None known. **LAB VALUES:** None known.

AVAILABILITY (Rx)

CAPSULES: 100 mg, 250 mg. **SUPPOSITORIES:** 100 mg, 200 mg. **INJECTION:** 100 mg/ml.

ADMINISTRATION/HANDLING

PO

• Give without regard to meals. • Do not crush, break capsule form.

IM

• Give deep IM into large muscle mass, preferably upper outer gluteus maximus.

RECTAL

• If suppository is too soft, chill for 30 min in refrigerator or run cold water over foil wrapper. • Moisten suppository with cold water before inserting well into rectum.

INDICATIONS/ROUTES/DOSAGE

Alert: Do not use IV route (produces severe hypotension).

NAUSEA, VOMITING

PO: ADULTS, ELDERLY: 250 mg 3–4 times/day. CHILDREN 30–100 LBS: 100–200 mg 3–4 times/day.

IM: ADULTS, ELDERLY: 200 mg 3–4 times/day.

Rectal: ADULTS, ELDERLY: 200 mg 3–4 times/day. CHILDREN 30–100 LBS: 100–

200 mg 3–4 times/day. CHILDREN <30 LBS: 100 mg 3–4 times/day. Do not use in premature or newborn infants.

SIDE EFFECTS

Alert: Elderly (>60 yrs) tend to develop mental confusion, disorientation, agitation, psychotic-like symptoms.

FREQUENT: Drowsiness. **OCCASIONAL:** Blurred vision, diarrhea, dizziness, headache, muscle cramps. **RARE:** Skin rash, seizures, depression, opisthotonus, Parkinson's syndrome, Reye's syndrome (vomiting, seizures).

ADVERSE REACTIONS/ TOXIC EFFECTS

Hypersensitivity reaction manifested as extrapyramidal symptoms (muscle rigidity, allergic skin reactions) occurs rarely. Children may experience dominant paradoxical reaction (restlessness, insomnia, euphoria, nervousness, tremors). Overdosage may vary from CNS depression (sedation, apnea, cardiovascular collapse, death) to severe paradoxical reaction (hallucinations, tremor, seizures).

NURSING IMPLICATIONS

BASELINE ASSESSMENT

Assess for dehydration if excessive vomiting occurs (poor skin turgor, dry mucous membranes, longitudinal furrows in tongue).

INTERVENTION/EVALUATION

Check B/P, esp. in elderly (increased risk of hypotension). Assess children closely for paradoxical reaction. Monitor serum electrolytes in those with severe vomiting. Measure I&O and assess any vomitus. Assess skin turgor, mucous membranes to evaluate hydration status. Assess for extrapyramidal symptoms (hypersensitivity).

PATIENT/FAMILY TEACHING

Causes drowsiness. Avoid tasks that require alertness, motor skills until response to drug is established. Report visual disturbances, headache. Dry mouth is expected response to medication. Relief from nausea/vomiting generally occurs within 30 min of drug administration.

trimethoprim

try-**meth**-oh-prim
(Primsol, Proloprim, Trimpex)

FIXED-COMBINATION(S)

Bactrim, Septra: trimethoprim/sulfamethoxazole (a sulfonamide): 16 mg/80 mg/ml (injection); 40 mg/ 200 mg/5 ml (suspension); 80 mg/ 400 mg; 160 mg/800 mg (tablets).

CLASSIFICATION

PHARMACOTHERAPEUTIC: Folate antagonist. **CLINICAL:** Urinary tract agent, antibacterial.

ACTION

Blocks bacterial biosynthesis of nucleic acids, proteins by interfering with metabolism of folinic acid. **Therapeutic Effect:** Produces antibacterial activity.

PHARMACOKINETICS

Rapidly, completely absorbed from GI tract. Protein binding: 42%–46%. Widely distributed, including CSF. Metabolized in liver. Primarily excreted in urine. Moderately removed by hemodialysis. **Half-life:** 8–10 hrs (half-life increased with impaired renal function, newborns; decreased in children).

USES

Treatment of initial acute uncomplicated urinary tract infections (UTIs). **Unla-**

beled: Prophylaxis of bacterial UTI, treatment of pneumonia caused by *Pneumocystis carinii.*

PRECAUTIONS

CONTRAINDICATIONS: Infants <2 mos, megaloblastic anemia due to folic acid deficiency. **CAUTIONS:** Impaired renal/hepatic function, children who have X chromosome with mental retardation, pts who have possible folic acid deficiency.

LIFESPAN CONSIDERATIONS: Pregnancy/lactation: Readily crosses placenta. Distributed in breast milk. **Pregnancy Category C. Children:** Safety and efficacy not established. **Elderly:** No age-related precautions noted. May increase incidence of thrombocytopenia.

INTERACTIONS

DRUG: Folate antagonists (e.g., methotrexate) may increase risk of myeloblastic anemia. **HERBAL:** None known. **FOOD:** None known. **LAB VALUES:** May increase BUN, SGOT (AST), SGPT (ALT), serum bilirubin, creatinine concentration.

AVAILABILITY (Rx)

TABLETS: 100 mg, 200 mg. **ORAL SOLUTION:** 50 mg/5 ml.

ADMINISTRATION/HANDLING

PO

• Space doses evenly to maintain constant level in urine. • Give without regard to meals (if stomach upset occurs, give with food).

INDICATIONS/ROUTES/DOSAGE

ACUTE, UNCOMPLICATED UTIS

PO: ADULTS, ELDERLY, CHILDREN ≥12 YRS: 100 mg q12h or 200 mg once daily for 10 days. CHILDREN <12 YRS: 4–6 mg/kg/day in 2 divided doses for 10 days.

DOSAGE IN RENAL IMPAIRMENT

Creatinine Clearance	Dosage Interval
>30 ml/min	No change
15–30 ml/min	50 mg q12h

SIDE EFFECTS

OCCASIONAL: Nausea, vomiting, diarrhea, decreased appetite, stomach cramps, headache. **RARE:** Hypersensitivity reaction (rash, itching), methemoglobinemia (blue color on fingernails, lips, skin, pale skin, sore throat, fever, unusual fatigue).

ADVERSE REACTIONS/TOXIC EFFECTS

Stevens-Johnson syndrome, erythema multiforme, exfoliative dermatitis, anaphylaxis occur rarely. Hematologic toxicity (thrombocytopenia, neutropenia, leukopenia, megaloblastic anemia) more likely to occur in elderly, debilitated, alcoholics, those with impaired renal function or receiving prolonged high dosage.

NURSING IMPLICATIONS

BASELINE ASSESSMENT

Assess hematology baseline reports and renal function tests.

INTERVENTION/EVALUATION

Assess skin for rash. Evaluate food tolerance. Monitor hematology reports, renal/hepatic test results if ordered. Check for developing signs of hematologic toxicity: pallor, fever, sore throat, malaise, bleeding, bruising.

PATIENT/FAMILY TEACHING

Space doses evenly. Complete full length of therapy (may be 10–14 days). May take on empty stomach or with food if stomach upset occurs. Avoid sun, ultraviolet light; use sunscreen, wear protective clothing. Immediately report pallor,

T

fatigue, sore throat, bleeding, bruising/discoloration of skin, fever, rash to physician.

trimetrexate glucuronate

try-meh-**trex**-ate
(Neutrexin)
Do not confuse with Neurontin.

CLASSIFICATION

PHARMACOTHERAPEUTIC: Folate antagonist. **CLINICAL:** Anti-infective.

ACTION

Inhibits the enzyme dihydrofolate reductase (DHFR). **Therapeutic Effect:** Disrupts purine, DNA, RNA, protein synthesis, with consequent cell death.

USES

Alternative therapy with concurrent leucovorin administration for treatment of moderate to severe *Pneumocystis carinii* pneumonia (PCP) in immunocompromised pts, including pts with acquired immunodeficiency syndrome (AIDS), who are intolerant of, or are refractory to, trimethoprim-sulfamethoxazole (TMP-SMZ) therapy or for whom TMP-SMZ is contraindicated. **Unlabeled:** Treatment of non–small cell lung, prostate, colorectal cancer.

T

PRECAUTIONS

CONTRAINDICATIONS: Clinically significant hypersensitivity to trimetrexate, leucovorin, methotrexate. **CAUTIONS:** Fertility impairment, pts with hematologic, renal, hepatic impairment. **Pregnancy Category D.**

INTERACTIONS

DRUG: Erythromycin, rifampin, rifabutin, ketoconazole, fluconazole, acetaminophen may alter trimetrexate plasma concentration. **Cimetidine** reduces trimetrexate metabolism. **Clotrimazole, ketoconazole, miconazole** may inhibit trimetrexate metabolism. **HERBAL:** None known. **FOOD:** None known. **LAB VALUES:** May increase SGOT (AST), SGPT (ALT), alkaline phosphatase, bilirubin, BUN, serum creatinine. May decrease Hgb, Hct, leukocytes, platelet counts.

AVAILABILITY (Rx)

POWDER FOR INJECTION: 25 mg, 200 mg.

ADMINISTRATION/HANDLING

IV

Alert: If solution comes in contact with skin/mucosa, wash with soap/water immediately. Use proper cytotoxic disposal technique. Do not reconstitute with solution containing either chloride ion or leucovorin, because precipitate occurs instantly.

Storage • Store vials for parenteral use at room temperature. • After reconstitution, solution is stable for up to 24 hrs. • Reconstituted solution appears as pale greenish yellow. • Inspect for particulate matter. Discard if cloudiness or precipitate is present. • Do not freeze reconstituted solution. Discard unused portion after 24 hrs.

Reconstitution • Reconstitute each 25-mg vial with 2 ml D_5W or Sterile Water for Injection to provide concentration of 12.5 mg/ml. Complete dissolution should occur within 30 sec. • Filter the reconstituted solution before further dilution. • Further dilute with D_5W to yield a final concentration of 0.25–2 mg/ml.

Rate of administration • Give diluted solution by IV infusion over 60–90 min. • Flush IV line thoroughly with at least 10 ml D_5W before and after administering trimetrexate.

⌀ IV INCOMPATIBILITIES
Foscarnet (Foscavir), indomethacin (Indocin).

INDICATIONS/ROUTES/DOSAGE

Alert: Even though trimetrexate and leucovorin are given concurrently, they must be administered separately or precipitate will occur instantly; flush IV line thoroughly with 10 ml D_5W between infusions. Dilute leucovorin according to leucovorin instructions and give over 5–10 min q6h.

PCP
IV infusion: ADULTS: *(Trimetrexate):* 45 mg/m^2 once daily over 60–90 min. *(Leucovorin):* 20 mg/m^2 over 5–10 min q6h for total daily dose of 80 mg/m^2, or orally as 4 doses of 20 mg/m^2 spaced equally throughout the day. Round up the oral dose to the next higher 25-mg increment. RECOMMENDED COURSE OF THERAPY: 21 days trimetrexate, 24 days leucovorin.

Alert: In event of hematologic, renal, hepatic toxicities, doses of trimetrexate and leucovorin should be modified.

SIDE EFFECTS

OCCASIONAL (2%–8%): Fever, rash, pruritus, nausea, vomiting, confusion. **RARE (<2%):** Fatigue.

ADVERSE REACTIONS/ TOXIC EFFECTS

Trimetrexate given without concurrent leucovorin may result in serious or fatal hematologic, hepatic, renal complications, including bone marrow suppression, oral/GI mucosal ulceration, renal/hepatic dysfunction. In event of overdose, stop trimetrexate and give leucovorin 40 mg/m^2 q6h for 3 days. Anaphylaxis occurs rarely.

NURSING IMPLICATIONS

BASELINE ASSESSMENT

Leucovorin therapy must extend for 72 hrs past the last dose of trimetrexate. CBC, hepatic and renal function tests should be performed twice weekly during therapy. To allow for full therapeutic effect of trimetrexate to occur, zidovudine treatment should be discontinued during trimetrexate therapy.

INTERVENTION/EVALUATION

Closely monitor neutrophil count, platelet count, liver function tests (SGOT [AST], SGPT [ALT], alkaline phosphatase), renal values (serum creatinine, BUN) for development of serious toxicities. Carefully assess/treat pts with nephrotoxic, myelosuppressive, or hepatotoxic drugs given during trimetrexate therapy.

PATIENT/FAMILY TEACHING

Use two forms of contraception during therapy. Avoid persons with bacterial infections. Immediately contact physician if fever, chills, cough, hoarseness, lower back or side pain, painful urination occurs. Report any unusual bruising/bleeding, black tarry stools, blood in urine or stools, pinpoint red spots on skin.

T

triptorelin pamoate

trip-toe-**ree**-linn
(Trelstar Depot, Trelstar LA)

◆CLASSIFICATION

PHARMACOTHERAPEUTIC: Gonadotropin-releasing hormone analogue. **CLINICAL:** Antineoplastic.

ACTION

Through a negative feedback mechanism, triptorelin inhibits gonadotropin hormone secretion. Initially, a transient surge in circulating levels of luteinizing hormone (LH), follicle-stimulating hormone (FSH), testosterone, and estradiol occurs. Chronic administration results in decreased LH and FSH, marked reduction in testosterone and estradiol levels. **Therapeutic Effect:** Suppresses abnormal growth of prostate tissue.

USES

Treatment of advanced prostate cancer.

PRECAUTIONS

CONTRAINDICATIONS: Hypersensitivity to luteinizing hormone releasing hormone (LHRH) agonists or LHRH. **CAUTIONS:** None known. **Pregnancy Category X.**

INTERACTIONS

DRUG: **Hyperprolactinemic drugs** reduce number of pituitary GnRH receptors. **HERBAL:** None known. **FOOD:** None known. **LAB VALUES:** May mislead pituitary-gonadal function test results. Increases transient testosterone levels (usually during first week of treatment, declines thereafter).

AVAILABILITY (Rx)

POWDER FOR INJECTION: (Trelstar Depot): 3.75 mg. **(Trelstar LA):** 11.25 mg.

T

INDICATIONS/ROUTES/DOSAGE

PROSTATE CANCER

IM: ADULTS, ELDERLY: *Trelstar Depot:* 3.75 mg once q28days. *Trelstar LA:* 11.25 mg every 3 mos.

SIDE EFFECTS

FREQUENT (>5%): Hot flashes, skeletal pain, headache, impotence. **OCCASIONAL (2%–5%):** Insomnia, vomiting, leg pain, fatigue. **RARE (<2%):** Dizziness, emotional lability, diarrhea, urinary retention, UTI, anemia, pruritus.

ADVERSE REACTIONS/ TOXIC EFFECTS

Bladder outlet obstruction, bone pain, hematuria, spinal cord compression with weakness/paralysis of lower extremities may occur.

NURSING IMPLICATIONS

INTERVENTION/EVALUATION

Obtain serum testosterone, PSA, prostatic acid phosphatase (PAP) levels periodically during therapy. Serum testosterone, PAP levels should increase during first week of therapy. Testosterone level then should decrease to baseline level or less within 2 wks, PAP level within 4 wks. Monitor pt closely for worsening signs/symptoms of prostatic cancer, esp. during first week of therapy (due to transient increase in testosterone).

PATIENT/FAMILY TEACHING

Do not miss monthly injections. May experience increased bone pain, blood in urine, urinary retention initially (subsides within 1 wk). Hot flashes may occur. Inform physician if rapid heartbeat, persistent nausea/vomiting, numbness of arms/legs, pain/swelling of breasts, difficulty breathing, infection at injection site occurs.

tubocurarine chloride

(Tubarine)

See Classification section under: Neuromuscular blockers (p. 107C)

Ultram

see tramadol

Unasyn

see ampicillin-sulbactam

valacyclovir

val-ah-**sigh**-klo-veer
(Valtrex)

CLASSIFICATION

PHARMACOTHERAPEUTIC: Antiviral. **CLINICAL:** Antiherpetic agent (see p. 60C).

ACTION

Converted to acyclovir triphosphate, becoming part of DNA chain. Virustatic. **Therapeutic Effect:** Interferes with DNA synthesis and viral replication of herpes simplex and varicella zoster virus.

PHARMACOKINETICS

Rapidly absorbed following PO administration. Protein binding: 13%–18%. Rapidly converted by hydrolysis to active compound, acyclovir. Widely distributed to tissues/body fluids (including CSF). Primarily eliminated in urine. Removed by hemodialysis. **Half-life:** 2.5–3.3 hrs (half-life increased with impaired renal function).

USES

Treatment of herpes zoster (shingles) in immunocompetent adults. Episodic treatment of recurrent genital herpes in immunocompetent adults. Prevention of recurrent genital herpes. Treatment of initial genital herpes. Treatment of cold sores. **Unlabeled:** Reduces heterosexual transmission of genital herpes.

PRECAUTIONS

CONTRAINDICATIONS: Hypersensitivity or intolerance to valacyclovir, acyclovir, or components of formulation. **CAUTIONS:** Bone marrow or renal transplantation, advanced HIV infections, renal/hepatic impairment, dehydration, fluid/electrolyte imbalance, concurrent use of nephrotoxic agents, neurologic abnormalities.

LIFESPAN CONSIDERATIONS: Pregnancy/lactation: May cross placenta. May be distributed in breast milk. **Pregnancy Category B. Children:** Safety and efficacy not established. **Elderly:** Age-related renal impairment may require dosage adjustment.

INTERACTIONS

DRUG: Probenecid, cimetidine may increase acyclovir concentration. **HERBAL:** None known. **FOOD:** None known. **LAB VALUES:** None known.

AVAILABILITY (Rx)

TABLETS: 500 mg, 1,000 mg.

ADMINISTRATION/HANDLING

PO

- Give without regard to meals.
- Do not crush, break tablets.

INDICATIONS/ROUTES/DOSAGE

Alert: Therapy should be initiated at first sign of shingles (most effective within 48 hrs of onset of zoster rash).

HERPES ZOSTER (shingles)

PO: ADULTS, ELDERLY: 1 g 3 times daily for 7 days.

RECURRENT GENITAL HERPES

PO: ADULTS, ELDERLY: 500 mg twice daily for 3 days.

V

COLD SORES

PO: ADULTS, ELDERLY: 2 g twice daily for 1 day.

PREVENTION OF HERPES

PO: ADULTS, ELDERLY: 500–1,000 mg/day.

INITIAL TREATMENT OF GENITAL HERPES

PO: ADULTS, ELDERLY: 1 g twice daily for 10 days.

DOSAGE IN RENAL IMPAIRMENT

Creatinine Clearance	Herpes Zoster	Genital Herpes
≥50	1 g q8h	500 mg q12h
30–49	1 g q12h	500 mg q12h
10–29	1 g q24h	500 mg q24h
<10	500 mg q24h	500 mg q24h

SIDE EFFECTS

FREQUENT: Herpes zoster (10%–17%): Nausea, headache. **Genital herpes (17%):** Headache. **OCCASIONAL: Herpes zoster (3%–7%):** Vomiting, diarrhea, constipation (≥50 yrs), asthenia, dizziness (≥50 yrs). **Genital herpes (3%–8%):** Nausea, diarrhea, dizziness. **RARE: Herpes zoster (1%–3%):** Abdominal pain, anorexia. **Genital herpes (1%–3%):** Asthenia, abdominal pain.

ADVERSE REACTIONS/ TOXIC EFFECTS

None known.

NURSING IMPLICATIONS

V

BASELINE ASSESSMENT

Question for history of allergies, particularly to valacyclovir, acyclovir. Tissue cultures for herpes zoster, herpes simplex should be done before giving first dose (therapy may proceed before results are known). Assess medical history, esp. advanced HIV infection, bone marrow or renal transplantation, hepatic/renal impairment.

INTERVENTION/EVALUATION

Evaluate cutaneous lesions. Monitor renal/hepatic function tests, CBC, urinalysis. Manage herpes zoster with strict isolation. Provide analgesics, comfort measures for herpes zoster (esp. exhausting to elderly). Encourage fluids. Keep pt's fingernails short, hands clean.

PATIENT/FAMILY TEACHING

Drink adequate fluids. Do not touch lesions with fingers to avoid spreading infection to new site. **Genital Herpes:** Continue therapy for full length of treatment. Space doses evenly. Avoid sexual intercourse during duration of lesions to prevent infecting partner. Valacyclovir does not cure herpes. Notify physician if lesions do not improve or recur. Pap smears should be done at least annually due to increased risk of cervical cancer in women with genital herpes. Initiate treatment at first sign of a recurrent episode of genital herpes or herpes zoster (early treatment, that is, within first 24–48 hrs, is imperative for therapeutic results).

valdecoxib

val-deh-**cox**-ib

(Bextra)

CLASSIFICATION

PHARMACOTHERAPEUTIC: NSAID. **CLINICAL:** Anti-inflammatory, analgesic (see p. 111C).

ACTION

Inhibits cyclo-oxygenase-2, the enzyme responsible for producing prostaglandins that cause pain and inflammation.

Therapeutic Effect: Reduces inflammatory response, intensity of pain stimulus reaching sensory nerve endings.

PHARMACOKINETICS

Rapidly and almost completely absorbed. Widely distributed. Extensively metabolized in the liver. Primarily eliminated in urine. **Half-life:** 8–11 hrs.

USES

Treatment of signs/symptoms of osteoarthritis, rheumatoid arthritis. Treatment of primary dysmenorrhea.

PRECAUTIONS

CONTRAINDICATIONS: Hypersensitivity to NSAIDs, aspirin, severe renal disease, severe hepatic impairment. **CAUTIONS:** Moderate hepatic impairment, those >65 yrs, those receiving anticoagulant therapy or steroids, alcohol consumption, smoking.

LIFESPAN CONSIDERATIONS: Pregnancy/lactation: Excreted in breast milk. Avoid use during third trimester (may adversely affect fetal cardiovascular system: premature closure of ductus arteriosus). **Pregnancy Category B** (**D** if used in the third trimester or near delivery). **Children:** Safety and efficacy not established in those <18 yrs. **Elderly:** Age appears to increase the possibility of adverse reactions to NSAIDs.

INTERACTIONS

DRUG: May increase effects of **anticoagulants. Aspirin** may increase risk of GI side effects, bleeding. **Fluconazole, ketoconazole** may increase valdecoxib plasma concentration. May increase **dextromethorphan** plasma levels. **HERBAL:** None known. **FOOD:** None known. **LAB VALUES:** May increase BUN, creatinine, hepatic function levels.

AVAILABILITY (Rx)

TABLETS: 10 mg, 20 mg.

ADMINISTRATION/HANDLING

• Do not crush, break film-coated tablets. • May be given with or without food.

INDICATIONS/ROUTES/DOSAGE

OSTEOARTHRITIS, RHEUMATOID ARTHRITIS

PO: ADULTS, ELDERLY: 10 mg once daily.

PRIMARY DYSMENORRHEA

PO: ADULTS, ELDERLY: 20 mg twice daily.

SIDE EFFECTS

FRREQUENT (4%–8%): Headache. **OCCASIONAL (2%–3%):** Dizziness. **RARE (<2%):** Dyspepsia (heartburn, epigastric pain, indigestion), nausea, diarrhea, sinusitis, peripheral edema.

ADVERSE REACTIONS/ TOXIC EFFECTS

None known.

NURSING IMPLICATIONS

BASELINE ASSESSMENT

Assess onset, type, location, duration of pain, inflammation. Inspect appearance of affected joints for immobility, deformity, skin condition.

INTERVENTION/EVALUATION

Monitor BUN, creatinine, hepatic function serum levels. Monitor for evidence of headache. Assist with ambulation if dizziness occurs. Evaluate for therapeutic response from arthritis: pain relief, decreased stiffness/swelling, increased joint mobility, decreased tenderness,

V

improved grip strength. Assess for relief from abdominal cramping, pain due to dysmenorrhea.

PATIENT/FAMILY TEACHING

Avoid aspirin, alcohol during therapy (increase risk of GI bleeding). If GI upset occurs, take with food, milk.

valerian

Also known as all-heal, amantilla, garden heliotrope, valeriana.

CLASSIFICATION

HERBAL.

ACTION

Appears to inhibit enzyme system responsible for catabolism of GABA, increasing GABA concentration and decreasing CNS activity. **Effect:** Produces sedative effects. Also has anxiolytic, antidepressant, anticonvulsant effects.

USES

Used as a sedative for insomnia, sleeping disorders associated with anxiety, restlessness. Also used for depression and attention deficit hyperactivity disorder (ADHD).

PRECAUTIONS

CONTRAINDICATIONS: Insufficient data on pregnancy/lactation (avoid use); hepatic disease. **CAUTIONS:** None known.

LIFESPAN CONSIDERATIONS: Pregnancy/lactation: Contraindicated. **Children:** Safety and efficacy not established; avoid use. **Elderly:** No age-related precautions noted.

V

INTERACTIONS

DRUG: Alcohol, barbiturates, benzodiazepines may cause additive effect, increase adverse effects. **HERBAL: Chamomile, ginseng, kava kava, melatonin, St. John's wort** may enhance therapeutic effect/adverse effects. **FOOD:** None known. **LAB VALUES:** None known.

AVAILABILITY (OTC)

CAPSULES. TABLETS. EXTRACT. TEA. TINCTURE.

INDICATIONS/ROUTES/DOSAGE

SEDATION

PO: ADULTS, ELDERLY: (EXTRACT): 400–900 mg ½–1 hr before bedtime or 1 cup tea taken several times/day.

SIDE EFFECTS

Headache, hangover, cardiac disturbances.

ADVERSE REACTIONS/ TOXIC EFFECTS

Trouble walking, hypothermia, increased muscle relaxation, excitability, insomnia.

NURSING IMPLICATIONS

BASELINE ASSESSMENT

Determine whether pt is using other CNS depressants, esp. benzodiazepine. Assess baseline hepatic function.

INTERVENTION/EVALUATION

Monitor effectiveness in decreasing insomnia. Assess for hypersensitivity reaction; monitor hepatic function tests.

PATIENT/FAMILY TEACHING

Up to 4 wks may be needed for significant relief. Avoid tasks that require alertness, motor skills until response to drug is established. Inform physician if pregnant or breast-feeding. Taper doses slowly; do not discontinue abruptly.

valganciclovir hydrochloride

val-gan-**sye**-klo-vir
(Valcyte)

CLASSIFICATION

PHARMACOTHERAPEUTIC: Synthetic nucleoside. **CLINICAL:** Antiviral (see p. 60C).

ACTION

Converted intracellularly; competes with viral DNA esterases and incorporates directly into growing viral DNA chains. **Therapeutic Effect:** Interferes with DNA synthesis, viral replication.

PHARMACOKINETICS

Well absorbed, rapidly converted to ganciclovir by intestinal and hepatic enzymes. Widely distributed. Slowly metabolized intracellularly. Primarily excreted unchanged in urine. Removed by hemodialysis. **Half-life:** 18 hrs (half-life increased with impaired renal function).

USES

Treatment of cytomegalovirus (CMV) retinitis in AIDS. Preventative treatment of CMV disease in high-risk, renal, cardiac transplant pts.

PRECAUTIONS

CONTRAINDICATIONS: Hypersensitivity to ganciclovir or acyclovir. **CAUTIONS:** Extreme caution in children because of long-term carcinogenicity, reproductive toxicity. Renal impairment, preexisting cytopenias, history of cytopenic reactions to other drugs; elderly (at greater risk of renal impairment).

LIFESPAN CONSIDERATIONS: Pregnancy/lactation: Effective contraception should be used during therapy; valganciclovir should not be used during pregnancy. Avoid breast-feeding during therapy; may be resumed no sooner than 72 hrs after the last dose of valganciclovir. **Pregnancy Category C. Children:** Safety and efficacy not established in those <12 yrs. **Elderly:** Age-related renal impairment may require dosage adjustment.

INTERACTIONS

DRUG: Bone marrow depressants may increase bone marrow depression. May increase risk of seizures with **imipenem-cilastatin.** May increase hematologic toxicity with **zidovudine. Probenecid** reduces renal clearance of valganciclovir. Concurrent use of **amphotericin B** or **cyclosporine** may produce nephrotoxicity. **HERBAL:** None known. **FOOD: Food** maximizes drug bioavailability. **LAB VALUES:** May decrease WBCs, Hgb, Hct, platelet count, serum creatinine.

AVAILABILITY (Rx)

TABLETS: 450 mg.

ADMINISTRATION/HANDLING

PO

• Do not break, crush tablets (potential carcinogen) • Avoid contact to skin • Wash skin with soap and water if contact occurs. • Give with food.

INDICATIONS/ROUTES /DOSAGE

CMV RETINITIS (normal renal function)

PO: ADULTS: Initially, 900 mg (two 450-mg tablets) twice daily for 21 days with food. MAINTENANCE: 900 mg once daily with food.

DOSAGE IN RENAL IMPAIRMENT

Creatinine Clearance	Induction Dosage	Maintenance Dosage
≥60 ml/min	900 mg twice/day	900 mg once/day
40–59 ml/min	450 mg twice/day	450 mg once/day
25–39 ml/min	450 mg once/day	450 mg q2 days
10–24 ml/min	450 mg q2 days	450 mg twice weekly

V

SIDE EFFECTS

FREQUENT (9%–16%): Diarrhea, neutropenia, headache. **OCCASIONAL (3%–8%):** Nausea, anemia, thrombocytopenia. **RARE (<3%):** Insomnia, paresthesia, vomiting, abdominal pain, pyrexia.

ADVERSE REACTIONS/ TOXIC EFFECTS

Hematologic toxicity, mainly neutropenia; anemia, thrombocytopenia may occur. Retinal detachment occurs rarely. Overdose may result in renal toxicity. May decrease sperm production, fertility.

NURSING IMPLICATIONS

BASELINE ASSESSMENT

Evaluate hematologic, blood chemistry baselines, serum creatinine.

INTERVENTION/EVALUATION

Monitor I&O, ensure adequate hydration (minimum 1,500 ml/24 hrs). Diligently evaluate CBC for decreased WBCs, Hgb, Hct, decreased platelets. Question pt regarding vision, therapeutic improvement, complications.

PATIENT/FAMILY TEACHING

Valganciclovir provides suppression, not cure, of CMV retinitis. Frequent blood tests are necessary during therapy because of toxic nature of drug. Ophthalmologic exam every 4–6 wks during treatment is advised. It is essential to report any new symptom promptly. May temporarily or permanently inhibit sperm production in men, suppress fertility in women. Barrier contraception should be used during and for 90 days after therapy because of mutagenic potential.

valproic acid

val-**pro**-ick
(Depakene)

valproate sodium

(Depakene syrup)

divalproex sodium

(Depacon, Depakote, Epival)

CLASSIFICATION

CLINICAL: Anticonvulsant, antimanic, antimigraine (see p. 33C).

ACTION

Directly increases concentration of the inhibitory neurotransmitter gamma-aminobutyric acid (GABA). **Therapeutic Effect:** Produces anticonvulsant effect.

PHARMACOKINETICS

Well absorbed from GI tract. Protein binding: 80%–90%. Metabolized in liver. Primarily excreted in urine. Not removed by hemodialysis. **Half-life:** 6–16 hrs (half-life may be increased with impaired hepatic function, elderly, children <18 mos).

USES

Prophylaxis of absence seizures (petit mal), myoclonic, tonic-clonic seizure control. Used principally as adjunct with other anticonvulsant agents. Treatment of manic episodes with bipolar disorders, complex partial seizures. Prophylaxis of migraine headaches. **Unlabeled:** Treatment of myoclonic, simple partial, tonic-clonic seizures.

PRECAUTIONS

CONTRAINDICATIONS: Active hepatic disease. **CAUTIONS:** History of hepatic disease, bleeding abnormalities.

LIFESPAN CONSIDERATIONS: Pregnancy/lactation: Crosses placenta. Distributed in breast milk. **Pregnancy Category D. Children:** Increased risk of hepatotoxicity in those <2 yrs. **Elderly:** No age-related precautions, but lower dosages recommended.

INTERACTIONS

DRUG: Alcohol, CNS depressants may increase CNS depressant effects. May increase risk of bleeding with **anticoagulants, heparin, thrombolytics, platelet aggregation inhibitors.** May increase concentration of **amitriptyline, primidone. Carbamazepine** may decrease concentration. **Hepatotoxic medications** may increase risk of hepatotoxicity. May alter **phenytoin** protein binding, increasing toxicity. Phenytoin may decrease effect. **HERBAL:** None known. **FOOD:** None known. **LAB VALUES:** May increase SGOT (AST), SGPT (ALT), LDH, bilirubin. Therapeutic blood serum level: 50–100 mcg/ml; toxic blood serum level: >100 mcg/ml.

AVAILABILITY (Rx)

CAPSULES: 250 mg (valproic acid). **SYRUP:** 250 mg/5 ml (valproic acid). **TABLETS (delayed-release):** 125 mg, 250 mg, 500 mg (divalproex). **TABLETS (extended-release):** 250 mg, 500 mg. **CAPSULES (sprinkle):** 125 mg (divalproex). **INJECTION:** 100 mg/ml.

ADMINISTRATION/HANDLING

PO

• May give with or without regard to food. Do not administer with carbonated drinks. • May sprinkle capsule contents on applesauce and give immediately (do not break, crush sprinkle beads). • Delayed-release/extended-release tablets to be given whole.

IV

Storage • Store vials at room temperature. • Diluted solutions stable for 24 hrs. • Discard unused portion.

Reconstitution • Dilute each single dose with at least 50 ml D_5W, 0.9% NaCl, or lactated Ringer's.

Rate of administration • Infuse over 5–10 min. • Do not exceed rate of 3 mg/kg/min (5-min infusion) or 1.5 mg/kg/min (10-min infusion). Too rapid infusion increases side effects.

IV INCOMPATIBILITY

Do not mix with any other medications.

INDICATIONS/ROUTES/DOSAGE

SEIZURES

PO: ADULTS, ELDERLY, CHILDREN >10 YRS: Initially, 10–15 mg/kg/day in 1–3 divided doses. May increase by 5–10 mg/kg/day at weekly intervals up to 30–60 mg/kg/day (usual adult dosage: 1,000–2,500 mg/day).
Alert: Regular release and delayed release formulation given in 2–4 divided doses/day, extended-release formulation given once daily.

IV: ADULTS, ELDERLY, CHILDREN: IV dose equal to oral dose but given at a frequency of q6h.

MANIC EPISODES

PO: ADULTS, ELDERLY: Initially, 750 mg/day in divided doses. **Maximum:** 60 mg/kg/day.

MIGRAINE PPROPHYLAXIS

PO: ADULTS, ELDERLY: *(Extended-release tablets):* Initially, 500 mg/day for 7 days. May increase to 1,000 mg/day. *(Delayed-release tablets):* Initially, 250 mg 2 times/day. May increase up to 1,000 mg/day.

SIDE EFFECTS

FREQUENT: Epilepsy: Abdominal pain, irregular menses, diarrhea, transient alopecia, indigestion, nausea, vomiting, trembling, weight change. **Mania (19%–22%):** Nausea, somnolence. **OCCASIONAL: Epilepsy:** Constipation, dizziness, drows-

V

iness, headache, skin rash, unusual excitement, restlessness. **Mania (6%–12%):** Asthenia, abdominal pain, dyspepsia (heartburn, indigestion, epigastric distress), rash. **RARE: Epilepsy:** Mood changes, double vision, nystagmus, spots before eyes, unusual bleeding/bruising.

ADVERSE REACTIONS/ TOXIC EFFECTS

Hepatotoxicity may occur, particularly in the first 6 mos of therapy. May not be preceded by abnormal hepatic function tests but may be noted as loss of seizure control, malaise, weakness, lethargy, anorexia, vomiting. Blood dyscrasias may occur.

NURSING IMPLICATIONS

BASELINE ASSESSMENT

Anticonvulsant: Review history of seizure disorder (intensity, frequency, duration, LOC). Initiate safety measures, quiet dark environment. CBC, platelet count should be performed prior to and 2 wks after therapy begins, then 2 wks following maintenance dose. **Antimanic:** Assess behavior, appearance, emotional status, response to environment, speech pattern, thought content. **Antimigraine:** Question pt regarding onset, location, duration of migraine, possible precipitating symptoms.

INTERVENTION/EVALUATION

Monitor hepatic function tests, bilirubin, serum ammonia, CBC, platelets. **Anticonvulsant:** Observe frequently for recurrence of seizure activity. Monitor hepatic function tests, CBC, platelet count. Assess skin for bruising, petechiae. Monitor for clinical improvement (decrease in intensity/frequency of seizures). **Antimanic:** Assess for therapeutic response (interest in surroundings, increased ability to concentrate, relaxed facial expression). **Antimigraine:** Evaluate for relief of migraine headache and resulting photophobia, phonophobia, nausea, vomiting. Therapeutic blood serum level: 50–100 mcg/ml; toxic blood serum level: >100 mcg/ml.

PATIENT/FAMILY TEACHING

Do not abruptly withdraw medication after long-term use (may precipitate seizures). Strict maintenance of drug therapy is essential for seizure control. Drowsiness usually disappears during continued therapy. Avoid tasks that require alertness, motor skills until response to drug is established. Avoid alcohol. Carry identification card/bracelet to note anticonvulsant therapy. Inform physician if nausea, vomiting, lethargy, altered mental status, weakness, loss of appetite, abdominal pain, yellowing of skin, unusual bruising/bleeding occurs.

valrubicin

val-**rue**-bih-sin
(Valstar)
Do not confuse with valsartan.

◆ CLASSIFICATION

PHARMACOTHERAPEUTIC: Anthracycline antibiotic. **CLINICAL:** Antineoplastic (see p. 77C).

ACTION

Following intracellular penetration, inhibits incorporation of nucleosides into nucleic acids. **Therapeutic Effect:** Causes chromosomal damage, arresting cell cycle in G_2 phase, interfering with DNA.

V

USES

Intravesical therapy of BCG-refractory carcinoma in situ of urinary bladder in pts for whom cystectomy is unacceptable.

PRECAUTIONS

CONTRAINDICATIONS: Severe irritated bladder, perforated bladder, small bladder capacity, urinary tract infection, sensitivity to valrubicin. **CAUTIONS:** None known. **Pregnancy Category C.**

AVAILABILITY (Rx)

SOLUTION FOR INTRAVESICAL INSTILLATION: 40 mg/ml.

INDICATIONS/ROUTES/DOSAGE

Alert: Not for IM/IV use.

BLADDER CANCER

Intravesical: ADULTS, ELDERLY: 800 mg once weekly for 6 wks.

SIDE EFFECTS

FREQUENT: Local intravesical reaction (10%): Local bladder symptoms, urinary frequency, dysuria, urinary urgency, hematuria, bladder pain, cystitis, bladder spasms. **Systemic (5%–15%):** Abdominal pain, nausea, urinary tract infection. **OCCASIONAL: Local intravesical reaction (<10%):** Nocturia, local burning, urethral pain, pelvic pain, gross hematuria. **Systemic (2%–5%):** Diarrhea, vomiting, urinary retention, microscopic hematuria, asthenia, headache, malaise, back pain, chest pain, dizziness, rash, anemia, fever, vasodilation. **RARE: Systemic (1%):** Flatus, peripheral edema, increased glucose, pneumonia, myalgia.

NURSING IMPLICATIONS

BASELINE ASSESSMENT

Assess if pt is sensitive to valrubicin, is pregnant or breast-feeding (not recommended). Assess other medications, conditions (see Contraindications).

valsartan

val-**sar**-tan
(Diovan)

FIXED-COMBINATION(S)

Diovan HCT: valsartan/hydrochlorothiazide (a diuretic): 80 mg/12.5 mg; 160 mg/12.5 mg; 160 mg/25 mg.

◆CLASSIFICATION

PHARMACOTHERAPEUTIC: Angiotensin II receptor antagonist. **CLINICAL:** Antihypertensive (see p. 7C).

ACTION

Potent vasodilator. An angiotensin II receptor (type AT_1) antagonist; blocks vasoconstrictor and aldosterone-secreting effects of angiotensin II, inhibiting the binding of angiotensin II to the AT_1 receptors. **Therapeutic Effect:** Produces vasodilation, decreased peripheral resistance, decrease in B/P.

PHARMACOKINETICS

Poorly absorbed following PO administration. Food decreases peak plasma concentration. Protein binding: 95%. Metabolized in the liver. Recovered primarily in feces and, to a lesser extent, in urine. Unknown if removed by hemodialysis. **Half-life:** 6 hrs.

USES

Treatment of hypertension alone or in combination with other antihypertensives. Treatment of heart failure.

V

PRECAUTIONS

CONTRAINDICATIONS: Severe hepatic impairment, biliary cirrhosis or obstruction, hypoaldosteronism, bilateral renal artery stenosis. **CAUTIONS:** Concurrent use of potassium-sparing diuretics or potassium supplements, mild to moderate hepatic impairment, CHF, unilateral renal artery stenosis, coronary artery disease.

LIFESPAN CONSIDERATIONS: Pregnancy/lactation: May cause fetal harm. Unknown if distributed in breast milk. **Pregnancy Category C** (**D** if used in second or third trimester). **Children:** Safety and efficacy not established. **Elderly:** No age-related precautions noted.

INTERACTIONS

DRUG: **Diuretics** produce additive hypotensive effects. **HERBAL:** None known. **FOOD:** None known. **LAB VALUES:** May increase liver enzymes, bilirubin, creatinine, potassium. May decrease Hgb, Hct.

AVAILABILITY (Rx)

TABLETS: 40 mg, 80 mg, 160 mg, 320 mg.

ADMINISTRATION/HANDLING

PO

- Give without regard to meals.

INDICATIONS/ROUTES/DOSAGE

Alert: May be given concurrently with other antihypertensives. If B/P is not controlled by valsartan alone, a diuretic may be added.

HYPERTENSION

PO: ADULTS, ELDERLY: Initially, 80–160 mg/day (in pts not volume depleted). May increase up to maximum of 320 mg/day.

CHF

PO: ADULTS, ELDERLY: Initially, 40 mg 2 times/day. May increase up to 160 mg 2 times/day. **Maximum:** 320 mg/day.

SIDE EFFECTS

RARE (1%–2%): Insomnia, fatigue, heartburn, abdominal pain, dizziness, headache, diarrhea, nausea, vomiting, arthralgia, edema.

ADVERSE REACTIONS/ TOXIC EFFECTS

Overdosage may manifest as hypotension and tachycardia; bradycardia occurs less often. Institute supportive measures. Viral infection, upper respiratory infection (cough, pharyngitis, sinusitis, rhinitis) occur rarely.

NURSING IMPLICATIONS

BASELINE ASSESSMENT

Obtain B/P, apical pulse immediately prior to each dose, in addition to regular monitoring (be alert to fluctuations). If excessive reduction in B/P occurs, place pt in supine position, feet slightly elevated. Question for possibility of pregnancy (see Pregnancy Category). Assess medication history (esp. diuretic). Question for history of hepatic/renal impairment, renal artery stenosis, history of severe CHF. Obtain BUN, serum creatinine, SGOT (AST), SGPT (ALT), alkaline phosphatase, bilirubin, Hgb, Hct, vital signs, particularly B/P, pulse rate.

INTERVENTION/EVALUATION

Maintain hydration (offer fluids frequently). Assess for evidence of upper respiratory infection. Monitor electrolytes, renal/hepatic function tests, urinalysis, B/P, pulse. Observe for symptoms of hypotension.

PATIENT/FAMILY TEACHING

Inform female pt regarding consequences of second- and third-trimester exposure to valsartan. Report pregnancy to physician as soon as possible. Report any sign of infection (sore throat, fever). Do not stop taking medication. Caution against exercising during hot weather (risk of dehydration, hypotension).

vancomycin hydrochloride

van-koe-**my**-sin
(Vancocin, Vancoled)

CLASSIFICATION

CLINICAL: Tricyclic glycopeptide antibiotic.

ACTION

Binds to bacterial cell wall, altering cell membrane permeability, inhibiting RNA synthesis. **Therapeutic Effect:** Inhibits cell wall synthesis, produces bacterial cell death. Bactericidal.

PHARMACOKINETICS

PO: Poorly absorbed from GI tract. Primarily eliminated in feces. **Parenteral:** Widely distributed. Protein binding: 55%. Primarily excreted unchanged in urine. Not removed by hemodialysis. **Half-life:** 4–11 hrs (half-life increased with impaired renal function).

USES

Systemic: Treatment of respiratory tract, bone, skin/soft tissue infections; endocarditis; peritonitis; septicemia. Given prophylactically to those at risk for bacterial endocarditis (if penicillin contraindicated) when undergoing dental, respiratory, GI, GU, biliary surgery/invasive procedures. **PO:** Treatment of antibiotic colitis, pseudomembranous colitis, antibiotic-associated diarrhea, staphylococcal enterocolitis. **Unlabeled:** Treatment of brain abscess, staphylococcal/streptococcal meningitis, perioperative infections.

PRECAUTIONS

CONTRAINDICATIONS: None known. **CAUTIONS:** Renal dysfunction, preexisting hearing impairment, concurrent therapy with other ototoxic/nephrotoxic medications.

LIFESPAN CONSIDERATIONS: Pregnancy/lactation: Drug crosses placenta. Unknown if distributed in breast milk. **Pregnancy Category B. Children:** Close monitoring of serum levels recommended in premature neonates and young infants. **Elderly:** Age-related renal impairment may increase risk of ototoxicity and nephrotoxicity; dosage adjustment recommended.

INTERACTIONS

DRUG: Oral: Cholestyramine, colestipol may decrease effect. **Parenteral: Aminoglycosides, amphotericin, aspirin, bumetanide, carmustine, cisplatin, cyclosporine, ethacrynic acid, furosemide, streptozocin** may increase ototoxicity and/or nephrotoxicity. **HERBAL:** None known. **FOOD:** None known. **LAB VALUES:** May increase BUN. Therapeutic blood serum level: Peak: 20–40 mcg/ml; trough: 5–15 mcg/ml. Toxic blood serum level: Peak: >40 mcg/ml; trough: >15 mcg/ml.

AVAILABILITY (Rx)

CAPSULES: 125 mg, 250 mg. **POWDER FOR INJECTION:** 500 mg, 1 g. **INFUSION (premix):** 500 mg/100 ml, 1 g/200 ml.

ADMINISTRATION/HANDLING

PO

- Generally not given for systemic infections because of poor absorption from GI tract; however, some pts with colitis may have effective absorption. • Powder for oral solution may be reconstituted,

V

given by mouth or NG tube. • Oral solution is stable for 2 wks if refrigerated. • Do not use powder for oral solution for IV administration.

IV

Alert: Give by intermittent IV infusion (piggyback) or continuous IV infusion. Do not give IV push (may result in exaggerated hypotension).

Storage • After reconstitution, refrigerate and use within 14 days. • Discard if precipitate forms.

Reconstitution • For intermittent IV infusion (piggyback), reconstitute each 500-mg vial with 10 ml Sterile Water for Injection (20 ml for 1-g vial) to provide concentration of 50 mg/ml. • Further dilute to a final concentration not to exceed 5 mg/ml.

Rate of administration • Administer ≥60 mins. • Monitor B/P closely during IV infusion. • ADD-Vantage vials should not be used in neonates, infants, children requiring <500-mg dose.

IV INCOMPATIBILITIES
Albumin, amphotericin B complex (Abelcet, AmBisome, Amphotec), aztreonam (Azactam), cefazolin (Ancef), cefepime (Maxipime), cefotaxime (Claforan), cefotetan (Cefotan), cefoxitin (Mefoxin), ceftazidime (Fortaz), ceftriaxone (Rocephin), cefuroxime (Zinacef), foscarnet (Foscavir), heparin, idarubicin (Idamycin), nafcillin (Nafcil), piperacillin/tazobactam (Zosyn), ticarcillin/clavulanate (Timentin).

IV COMPATIBILITIES
Amiodarone (Cordarone), calcium gluconate, diltiazem (Cardizem), hydromorphone (Dilaudid), insulin, lorazepam (Ativan), magnesium sulfate, midazolam (Versed), morphine, potassium chloride, propofol (Diprivan).

INDICATIONS/ROUTES/DOSAGE

USUAL PARENTERAL DOSAGE
IV: ADULTS, ELDERLY: 500 mg q6h or 1 g q12h. CHILDREN >1 MO: 40 mg/kg/day in divided doses q6–8h. **Maximum:** 3–4 g/day. NEONATES: 15 mg/kg initially, then 10 mg/kg q8–12h.

DOSAGE IN RENAL IMPAIRMENT
After a loading dose, subsequent dose and/or frequency is modified based on degree of renal impairment, severity of infection, serum concentration of drug.

STAPHYLOCOCCAL ENTEROCOLITIS, ANTIBIOTIC-ASSOCIATED PSEUDOMEMBRANOUS COLITIS CAUSED BY *CLOSTRIDIUM DIFFICILE*
PO: ADULTS, ELDERLY: 0.5–2 g/day in 3–4 divided doses for 7–10 days. CHILDREN: 40 mg/kg/day in 3–4 divided doses for 7–10 days. **Maximum:** 2 g/day.

SIDE EFFECTS

FREQUENT: PO: Bitter/unpleasant taste, nausea, vomiting, mouth irritation (oral solution). **RARE: Systemic:** Phlebitis, thrombophlebitis, pain at peripheral IV site. Necrosis may occur with extravasation. Dizziness, vertigo, tinnitus, chills, fever, rash. **PO:** Rash.

ADVERSE REACTIONS/ TOXIC EFFECTS

Nephrotoxicity (change in amount/frequency of urination, nausea, vomiting, increased thirst, anorexia); ototoxicity (deafness due to damage to auditory branch of eighth cranial nerve); red-neck syndrome (too rapid injection): redness on face/neck/arms/back; chills, fever, tachycardia, nausea, vomiting, itching, rash, unpleasant taste.

NURSING IMPLICATIONS

BASELINE ASSESSMENT
Avoid other ototoxic, nephrotoxic medications if possible. Obtain culture, sen-

V

sitivity test prior to giving first dose (therapy may begin before results are known).

INTERVENTION/EVALUATION

Monitor renal function tests, I&O. Assess skin for rash. Check hearing acuity, balance. Monitor B/P carefully during infusion. Evaluate IV site for phlebitis (heat, pain, red streaking over vein). Therapeutic blood serum level: Peak: 20–40 mcg/ml; trough: 5–15 mcg/ml. Toxic blood serum level: Peak: >40 mcg/ml; trough: >15 mcg/ml.

PATIENT/FAMILY TEACHING

Continue therapy for full length of treatment. Doses should be evenly spaced. Notify physician in event of tinnitus, rash, signs/symptoms of nephrotoxicity. Lab tests are important part of total therapy.

vardenafil

var-**den**-ah-fill
(Levitra)

CLASSIFICATION

PHARMACOTHERAPEUTIC: Phosphodiesterase inhibitor. **CLINICAL:** Erectile dysfunction adjunct.

ACTION

Inhibits a specific enzyme, phosphodiesterase type 5, the predominant isoenzyme in human corpus cavernosum in the penis. **Therapeutic Effect:** Relaxes smooth muscle, increases blood flow, resulting in penile rigidity.

PHARMACOKINETICS

Rapidly absorbed following PO administration. Extensive tissue distribution. Protein binding: 95%. Metabolized in the liver. Eliminated predominately in the feces and, to a lesser extent, in the urine. No effect on penile blood flow without sexual stimulation. **Half-life:** 4–5 hrs.

USES

Treatment of erectile dysfunction.

PRECAUTIONS

CONTRAINDICATIONS: Pts concurrently using sodium nitroprusside or nitrates in any form (potentiates hypotensive effects of these medications), alpha-blocking agents. **CAUTIONS:** Renal/hepatic function impairment, anatomical deformation of the penis, pts who may be predisposed to priapism (sickle cell anemia, multiple myeloma, leukemia).

LIFESPAN CONSIDERATIONS: Elderly: No age-related precautions noted, but initial dose should be 5 mg.

INTERACTIONS

DRUG: **Ritonavir, indinivir, erythromycin, itraconazole, ketoconazole** may increase vardenafil concentration. Potentiates hypotensive effects of **nitrates** (contraindicated). **HERBAL:** None known. **FOOD:** Time to maximum effectiveness is delayed briefly when taken with a **high-fat meal.** **LAB VALUES:** None known.

AVAILABILITY (Rx)

TABLETS: 2.5 mg, 5 mg, 10 mg, 20 mg.

ADMINISTRATION/HANDLING

PO

- May take approx. 1 hr prior to sexual activity. Do not crush, break film-coated tablets.

INDICATIONS/ROUTES/DOSAGE

ERECTILE DYSFUNCTION

PO: ADULTS: 10 mg approx. 60 min prior to sexual activity. Dose may be increased to 20 mg or decreased to 5 mg, based on tolerability. Maximum dosing frequency is once daily. ELDERLY >65 YRS: 5 mg.

V

MODERATE HEPATIC FUNCTION IMPAIRMENT (Child-Pugh B)
PO: ADULTS: 5 mg prior to sexual activity.

CONCURRENT RITONAVIR
PO: ADULTS: 2.5 mg in a 72-hr period.

CONCURRENT KETOCONAZOLE AND ITRACONAZOLE AT 400 MG/DAY, INDINAVIR
PO: ADULTS: 2.5 mg in a 24-hr period.

CONCURRENT KETOCONAZOLE AND ITRACONAZOLE AT 200 MG/DAY, ERYTHROMYCIN
PO: ADULTS: 5 mg in a 24-hr period.

SIDE EFFECTS

OCCASIONAL: Headache, flushing, rhinitis, indigestion. **RARE (<2%):** Dizziness, changes in color vision, blurred vision.

ADVERSE REACTIONS/ TOXIC EFFECTS

Prolonged erections (>4 hrs), priapism (painful erections >6 hrs in duration) occur rarely.

NURSING IMPLICATIONS

BASELINE ASSESSMENT

Assess cardiovascular status prior to initiating treatment for erectile dysfunction.

PATIENT/FAMILY TEACHING

Has no effect in the absence of sexual stimulation. Seek treatment immediately if an erection persists for >4 hrs.

varicella vaccine

(Varivax)

See Classification section under: Immunizations

vasopressin

vay-sew-**press**-in
(Pitressin, Pressyn)

CLASSIFICATION

PHARMACOTHERAPEUTIC: Posterior pituitary hormone. **CLINICAL:** Vasopressor, antidiuretic.

ACTION

Increases reabsorption of water by the renal tubules. Directly stimulates smooth muscle in GI tract. **Therapeutic Effect:** Increases water permeability at the distal tubule and collecting duct, decreasing urine volume. Causes peristalsis. Causes vasoconstriction.

PHARMACOKINETICS

Onset	Peak	Duration
IM/subcutaneous		
1–2 hrs	—	2–8 hrs
IV		
—	—	0.5–1 hr

Distributed throughout extracellular fluid. Metabolized in liver, kidney. Primarily excreted in urine. **Half-life:** 10–20 min.

USES

Treatment of adult shock-refractory ventricular fibrillation (class IIb). Prevention/control of polydipsia, polyuria, dehydration in pts with neurogenic diabetes insipidus. Stimulates peristalsis in the prevention/treatment of postop abdominal distention, intestinal paresis. **Unlabeled:** Adjunct in treatment of acute, massive hemorrhage.

PRECAUTIONS

CONTRAINDICATIONS: None known. **CAUTIONS:** Seizures, migraine, asthma, vascular disease, renal/cardiac disease, goiter (with cardiac complications), arteriosclerosis, nephritis.

V

LIFESPAN CONSIDERATIONS: Pregnancy/lactation: Caution in giving to breast-feeding women. **Pregnancy Category B. Children/elderly:** Caution due to risk of water intoxication/hyponatremia.

INTERACTIONS

DRUG: Carbamazepine, chlorpropamide, clofibrate may increase effects. **Demeclocycline, lithium, norepinephrine** may decrease effect. **HERBAL:** None known. **FOOD:** None known. **LAB VALUES:** None known.

AVAILABILITY (Rx)

INJECTION: 20 units/ml.

ADMINISTRATION/HANDLING

SUBCUTANEOUS/IM

- Give with 1–2 glasses of water to reduce side effects.

IV

Storage • Store at room temperature.

Reconstitution • Dilute with D_5W or 0.9% NaCl to concentration of 0.1–1 unit/ml.

Rate of administration • Give as IV infusion.

IV INCOMPATIBILITIES

Amphotericin B complex (Abelcet, AmBisome, Amphotec), diazepam (Valium), etomidate (Amidate), furosemide (Lasix), thiopentothal.

IV COMPATIBILITIES

Dobutamine (Dobutrex), dopamine (Intropin), heparin, lorazepam (Ativan), midazolam (Versed), milrinone (Primacor), verapamil (Calan, Isoptin).

INDICATIONS/ROUTES/DOSAGE

CARDIAC ARREST

IV: ADULTS, ELDERLY: 40 units as a one-time bolus dose.

DIABETES INSIPIDUS

Alert: May administer intranasally on cotton pledgets, by nasal spray; individualize dosage.

IM/subcutaneous: ADULTS, ELDERLY: 5–10 units, 2–4 times/day. RANGE: 5–60 units/day. CHILDREN: 2.5–10 units, 2–4 times/day.

IV infusion: ADULTS, CHILDREN: 0.5 milliunits/kg/hr. May double dose q30min. **Maximum:** 10 milliunits/kg/hr.

ABDOMINAL DISTENTION

IM: ADULTS, ELDERLY: Initially, 5 units. Subsequent doses of 10 units q3–4h.

GI HEMORRHAGE

IV infusion: ADULTS, ELDERLY: Initially, 0.2–0.4 units/min progressively increased to 0.9 units/min. CHILDREN: 0.002–0.005 units/kg/min. Titrate as needed. **Maximum:** 0.01 units/kg/min.

SIDE EFFECTS

FREQUENT: Pain at injection site with vasopressin tannate. **OCCASIONAL:** Stomach cramps, nausea, vomiting, diarrhea, dizziness, diaphoresis, paleness, circumoral pallor, trembling, headache, eructation, flatulence. **RARE:** Chest pain, confusion. Allergic reaction: Rash/hives, pruritus, wheezing/difficulty breathing, swelling of face/extremities. Sterile abscess with vasopressin tannate.

ADVERSE REACTIONS/ TOXIC EFFECTS

Anaphylaxis, MI, water intoxication have occurred. Elderly and very young at higher risk for water intoxication.

NURSING IMPLICATIONS

BASELINE ASSESSMENT

Establish baselines for weight, B/P, pulse, electrolytes, urine specific gravity.

V

INTERVENTION/EVALUATION

Monitor I&O closely, restrict intake as necessary to prevent water intoxication. Weigh daily if indicated. Check B/P, pulse 2 times/day. Monitor electrolytes, urine specific gravity. Evaluate injection site for erythema, pain, abscess. Report side effects to physician for dose reduction. Be alert for early signs of water intoxication (drowsiness, listlessness, headache). Hold medication and report immediately any chest pain/allergic symptoms.

PATIENT/FAMILY TEACHING

Promptly report headache, chest pain, shortness of breath, other symptoms. Stress importance of I&O. Avoid alcohol.

Vasotec

see enalapril

vecuronium bromide

(Norcuron)

See Classification section under: Neuromuscular blockers (p. 107C)

venlafaxine

ven-lah-**facks**-een

(Effexor, Effexor XR)

CLASSIFICATION

PHARMACOTHERAPEUTIC: Phenethylamine derivative. **CLINICAL:** Antidepressant (see pp. 11C, 36C).

ACTION

Potentiates CNS neurotransmitter activity. Inhibits reuptake of serotonin, norepinephrine (weakly inhibits dopamine reuptake). **Therapeutic Effect:** Produces antidepressant activity.

PHARMACOKINETICS

Well absorbed from GI tract. Protein binding: 25%–30%. Metabolized in liver to active metabolite. Primarily excreted in urine. Not removed by hemodialysis. **Half-life:** 3–7 hrs; metabolite: 9–13 hrs (half-life increased impaired hepatic/renal disease).

USES

Treatment of depression exhibited as persistent, prominent dysphoria (occurring nearly every day for at least 2 wks) manifested by 4 of 8 symptoms: change in appetite, change in sleep pattern, increased fatigue, impaired concentration, feelings of guilt or worthlessness, loss of interest in usual activities, psychomotor agitation or retardation, or suicidal tendencies. Psychotherapy augments therapeutic result. **Venlaflaxine XR:** Treatment of generalized anxiety disorder, social anxiety disorder. **Unlabeled:** Prevention of recurrent/relapses of depression, ADHD, autism, obsessive-compulsive disorder, chronic fatigue syndrome.

PRECAUTIONS

CONTRAINDICATIONS: Use of MAOIs within 14 days. **CAUTIONS:** Seizure disorder, renal/hepatic impairment, suicidal pts, recent MI, mania, volume-depleted pts, narrow-angle glaucoma, CHF, hyperthyroidism, abnormal platelet function.

LIFESPAN CONSIDERATIONS: Pregnancy/lactation: Unknown if excreted in breast milk. **Pregnancy Category C. Children:** Safety and efficacy not established. **Elderly:** No age-related precautions noted.

INTERACTIONS

DRUG: MAOIs may cause hyperthermia, rigidity, myoclonus, autonomic instability (including rapid fluctuations of vital signs), mental status changes, coma, extreme agitation. May cause neuroleptic malignant syndrome (wait 14 days after discontinuing MAOIs to start or wait 7 days after discontinuing venlafaxine prior to starting MAOIs). **HERBAL: St. John's wort** may increase sedative-hypnotic effect. **FOOD:** None known. **LAB VALUES:** May increase serum cholesterol, uric acid, alkaline phosphatase, SGOT (AST), SGPT (ALT), bilirubin, BUN. May decrease sodium, phosphate. May alter glucose, potassium.

AVAILABILITY (Rx)

TABLETS: 25 mg, 37.5 mg, 50 mg, 75 mg, 100 mg. **EFFEXOR XR (extended-release):** 37.5 mg, 75 mg, 150 mg.

ADMINISTRATION/HANDLING

PO

• Give without regard to food. Give with food, milk if GI distress occurs. • Scored tablet may be crushed. • Do not crush extended-release capsules.

INDICATIONS/ROUTES/DOSAGE

Alert: Decrease dosage by 50% in pts with moderate hepatic impairment; 25% in mild to moderate renal impairment (50% in pts on dialysis, withholding dose until completion of dialysis). When discontinuing the medication, taper slowly over 2 wks.

DEPRESSION

PO: ADULTS, ELDERLY: Initially, 75 mg/day in 2–3 divided doses with food. May increase by 75 mg/day no sooner than 4-day intervals. **Maximum:** 375 mg/day in 3 divided doses. **Extended-release:** 75 mg/day as single dose. May increase by 75 mg/day at intervals of ≥4 days. **Maximum:** 225 mg/day.

ANXIETY DISORDER

PO: ADULTS: 37.5–225 mg/day.

SIDE EFFECTS

FREQUENT (>20%): Nausea, somnolence, headache, dry mouth. **OCCASIONAL (10%–20%):** Dizziness, insomnia, constipation, diaphoresis, nervousness, asthenia (loss of strength, energy), ejaculatory disturbance, anorexia. **RARE (<10%):** Anxiety, blurred vision, diarrhea, vomiting, tremor, abnormal dreams, impotence.

ADVERSE REACTIONS/ TOXIC EFFECTS

Sustained increase in diastolic B/P (10–15 mm Hg) occurs occasionally.

NURSING IMPLICATIONS

BASELINE ASSESSMENT

Obtain initial weight, B/P. Assess appearance, behavior, speech pattern, level of interest, mood.

INTERVENTION/EVALUATION

Monitor signs/symptoms of depression, B/P, weight. Assess sleep pattern for evidence of insomnia. Check during waking hours for somnolence or dizziness, anxiety; provide assistance as necessary. Supervise suicidal-risk pt closely during early therapy (as depression lessens, energy level improves, increasing suicide potential). Assess appearance, behavior, speech pattern, level of interest, mood for therapeutic response.

PATIENT/FAMILY TEACHING

Take with food to minimize GI distress. Do not increase, decrease, or suddenly stop medication. Avoid tasks that require alertness, motor skills until response to drug is established. Inform physician if breast-feeding, pregnant, or planning to become pregnant. Avoid alcohol.

Ventolin

see albuterol

VePesid

see etoposide

verapamil hydrochloride

ver-**ap**-ah-mill

(Apo-Verap, Calan, Chronovera, Covera-HS, Isoptin, Novoveramil, Verelan, Verelan PM)

Do not confuse with Intropin, Virilon, Vivarin, Voltaren.

FIXED-COMBINATION(S)

Tarka: verapamil/trandolapril (an ACE inhibitor): 240 mg/1 mg; 180 mg/2 mg; 240 mg/2 mg; 240 mg/4 mg.

CLASSIFICATION

PHARMACOTHERAPEUTIC: Calcium channel blocker. **CLINICAL:** Antihypertensive, antianginal, antiarrhythmic, hypertropic cardiomyopathy therapy adjunct (see pp. 15C, 67C).

ACTION

Inhibits calcium ion entry across cell membranes of cardiac and vascular smooth muscle (dilates coronary arteries, peripheral arteries, arterioles). **Therapeutic Effect:** Decreases heart rate, myocardial contractility; slows SA and AV conduction. Decreases total peripheral vascular resistance by vasodilation.

PHARMACOKINETICS

Onset	Peak	Duration
PO		
30 min	1–2 hrs	6–8 hrs
Extended-release		
30 min	—	—
IV		
1–2 min	3–5 min	10–60 min

Well absorbed from GI tract. Protein binding: 90% (neonates: 60%). Undergoes first-pass metabolism in liver. Metabolized in liver to active metabolite. Primarily excreted in urine. Not removed by hemodialysis. **Half-life:** 2–8 hrs.

USES

Parenteral: Management of supraventricular tachyarrhythmias, temporary control of rapid ventricular rate in atrial flutter/fibrillation. **PO:** Management of spastic (Prinzmetal's variant) angina, unstable (crescendo, preinfarction) angina, chronic stable angina (effort-associated angina), hypertension, prevention of recurrent PSVT (with digoxin); control of ventricular resting rate in those with atrial flutter and/or fibrillation. **Unlabeled:** Treatment of hypertrophic cardiomyopathy, vascular headaches.

PRECAUTIONS

CONTRAINDICATIONS: Sinus bradycardia, heart block, ventricular tachycardia, cardiogenic shock, atrial fibrillation/flutter. **CAUTIONS:** Sick sinus syndrome, CHF, renal/hepatic impairment, concomitant use of beta-blockers or digoxin.

LIFESPAN CONSIDERATIONS: Pregnancy/lactation: Crosses placenta. Distributed in breast milk. Breast-feeding not recommended. **Pregnancy Category C. Children:** No age-related precautions noted. **Elderly:** Age-related renal impairment may require cautious use.

INTERACTIONS

DRUG: **Beta-blockers** may have additive effect. May increase **digoxin** concentration. **Procainamide, quinidine** may increase risk of QT interval prolongation. **Carbamazepine, quinidine, theophylline** may increase concentration, toxicity. **Disopyramide** may increase negative inotropic effect. **HERBAL:** None known. **FOOD:** **Grapefruit/grapefruit juice** may increase concentrations. **LAB VALUES:** PR interval may be increased. Therapeutic blood serum level: 0.08–0.3 mcg/ml; toxic blood serum level: N/E.

AVAILABILITY (Rx)

TABLETS: 40 mg, 80 mg, 120 mg. **TABLETS (sustained-release):** 120 mg, 180 mg, 240 mg. **CAPSULES (sustained-release):** 120 mg, 180 mg, 240 mg, 360 mg. **VERELAN PM:** 100 mg, 200 mg, 300 mg. **INJECTION:** 5 mg/2 ml.

ADMINISTRATION/HANDLING

PO

• Do not give with grapefruit juice. • Non–sustained-release tablets may be given with or without food. • Swallow extended-release or sustained-released preparations whole; do not chew, crush. • Sustained-release capsules may be opened and sprinkled on applesauce and swallowed immediately (do not chew).

IV

Storage • Store vials at room temperature.

Reconstitution • May give undiluted.

Rate of administration • Administer IV push >2 min for adults, children; give >3 min for elderly. • Continuous EKG monitoring during IV injection is required for children, recommended for adults. • Monitor EKG for rapid ventricular rates, extreme bradycardia, heart block, asystole, prolongation of PR interval. Notify physician of any significant changes. • Monitor B/P q5–10min. • Pt should remain recumbent for at least 1 hr after IV administration.

IV INCOMPATIBILITIES

Amphotericin B complex (Abelcet, AmBisome, Amphotec), nafcillin (Nafcil), propofol (Diprivan), sodium bicarbonate.

IV COMPATIBILITIES

Amiodarone (Cordarone), calcium chloride, calcium gluconate, dexamethasone (Decadron), digoxin (Lanoxin), dobutamine (Dobutrex), dopamine (Intropin), furosemide (Lasix), heparin, hydromorphone (Dilaudid), lidocaine, magnesium sulfate, metoclopramide (Reglan), milrinone (Primacor), morphine, multivitamins, nitroglycerin, norepinephrine (Levophed), potassium chloride, potassium phosphate, procainamide (Pronestyl), propranolol (Inderal).

INDICATIONS/ROUTES/DOSAGE

SUPRAVENTRICULAR TACHYARRHYTHMIAS

IV: ADULTS, ELDERLY: Initially, 5–10 mg, repeat in 30 min with 10-mg dose. CHILDREN 1–15 YRS: 0.1 mg/kg. May repeat in 30 min. **Maximum second dose:** 10 mg. Not recommended in children <1 yr.

ARRHYTHMIAS

PO: ADULTS, ELDERLY: 240–480 mg/day in 3–4 divided doses.

ANGINA

PO: ADULTS, ELDERLY: Initially, 80–120 mg 3 times/day (40 mg in elderly, pts with hepatic dysfunction). Titrate to optimal dose. MAINTENANCE: 240–480 mg/day in 3–4 divided doses. **Covera-HS:** 180–480 mg/day at bedtime.

HYPERTENSION

PO: ADULTS, ELDERLY: Initially, 40–80 mg 3 times/day. MAINTENANCE: ≤480 mg/day. **Covera-HS:** 180–480 mg/day at bedtime. **Extended-release:** 120–240 mg/day. May give ≤480 mg/day in 2

V

divided doses. **Verelan PM:** 100–300 mg/day.

SIDE EFFECTS

FREQUENT (7%): Constipation. **OCCASIONAL (2%–4%):** Dizziness, lightheadedness, headache, asthenia (loss of strength, energy), nausea, peripheral edema, hypotension. **RARE (<1%):** Bradycardia, dermatitis/rash.

ADVERSE REACTIONS/ TOXIC EFFECTS

Rapid ventricular rate in atrial flutter/fibrillation, marked hypotension, extreme bradycardia, CHF, asystole, second- and third-degree AV block occur rarely.

NURSING IMPLICATIONS

BASELINE ASSESSMENT

Record onset, type (sharp, dull, squeezing), radiation, location, intensity, duration of anginal pain, precipitating factors (exertion, emotional stress). Check B/P for hypotension, pulse for bradycardia immediately prior to giving medication.

INTERVENTION/EVALUATION

Assess pulse for quality, irregular rate. Monitor EKG for cardiac changes, particularly prolongation of PR interval. Notify physician of any significant interval changes. Assist with ambulation if dizziness occurs. Assess for peripheral edema behind medial malleolus (sacral area in bedridden pts). For those taking oral form, check stool consistency, frequency. Therapeutic blood serum level: 0.08–0.3 mcg/ml; toxic blood serum level: N/E.

PATIENT/FAMILY TEACHING

Do not abruptly discontinue medication. Compliance with therapy regimen is essential to control anginal pain. To avoid hypotensive effect, rise slowly from lying to sitting position, wait momentarily before standing. Avoid tasks that require alertness, motor skills until response to drug is established. Limit caffeine. Inform physician if angina pain not reduced, irregular heartbeats, shortness of breath, swelling, dizziness, constipation, nausea, hypotension occurs. Avoid concomitant grapefruit juice.

Versed

see midazolam

vidarabine

vy-**dare**-ah-been
(Ara-A, Vira-A)
Do not confuse with cytarabine.

CLASSIFICATION

CLINICAL: Antiviral.

ACTION

Blocks DNA polymerase. **Therapeutic Effect:** Inhibits viral DNA synthesis.

USES

Treatment of keratitis, keratoconjunctivitis caused by herpes simplex virus types 1 and 2.

PRECAUTIONS

CONTRAINDICATIONS: None known. **CAUTIONS:** None known. **Pregnancy Category C.**

INTERACTIONS

DRUG: None known. **HERBAL:** None known. **FOOD:** None known. **LAB VALUES:** None known.

V

AVAILABILITY (Rx)

OPHTHALMIC OINTMENT: 3%.

INDICATIONS/ROUTES/DOSAGE

USUAL OPHTHALMIC DOSAGE

Ophthalmic: ADULTS, ELDERLY: 0.5 inch into lower conjunctival sac 5 times/day at 3-hr intervals. Following reepithelialization, treat additional 7 days at dosage of 2 times/day.

SIDE EFFECTS

FREQUENT: Burning, itching, irritation. **OCCASIONAL:** Foreign body sensation, tearing, sensitivity to light, pain, photophobia.

ADVERSE REACTIONS/ TOXIC EFFECTS

None known.

NURSING IMPLICATIONS

INTERVENTION/EVALUATION

Assess for irritation, itching, burning.

PATIENT/FAMILY TEACHING

Notify physician if there is no improvement in 7 days or if burning, irritation, pain develops. Do not stop or increase doses. Ointment should be continued for 5–7 days after infection is gone to prevent recurrence of infection. A temporary haze may occur after application to eye; sunglasses will decrease sensitivity to light. Use other eye products, including makeup, only with advice of physician. Refrigerate, avoid freezing; if using another eye ointment, wait at least 10 min between dosing.

vinblastine sulfate

vin-**blass**-teen

(Velbe✣)

Do not confuse with vincristine, vinorelbine.

CLASSIFICATION

PHARMACOTHERAPEUTIC: Vinca alkaloid. **CLINICAL:** Antineoplastic (see p. 77C).

ACTION

Binds to microtubular protein of mitotic spindle. **Therapeutic Effect:** Causes metaphase arrest. Inhibits cellular division.

PHARMACOKINETICS

Does not cross blood-brain barrier. Protein binding: 75%. Metabolized in liver to active metabolite. Primarily eliminated in feces via biliary system. **Half-life:** 24.8 hrs.

USES

Treatment of disseminated Hodgkin's disease, non-Hodgkin's lymphoma, advanced stage of mycosis fungoides, advanced carcinoma of testis, Kaposi's sarcoma, Letterer-Siwe disease, breast carcinoma, choriocarcinoma. **Unlabeled:** Treatment of neuroblastoma; carcinoma of bladder, lung, head/neck, kidney; germ cell ovarian tumors; chronic myelocytic leukemia.

PRECAUTIONS

CONTRAINDICATIONS: Severe leukopenia, bacterial infection, significant granulocytopenia unless a result of disease being treated. **CAUTIONS:** Hepatic function impairment, neurotoxicity, recent exposure to radiation therapy or chemotherapy.

LIFESPAN CONSIDERATIONS: Pregnancy/lactation: If possible, avoid use during pregnancy, esp. first trimester. Breast-feeding not recommended. **Pregnancy Category D. Children/elderly:** No age-related precautions noted.

INTERACTIONS

DRUG: May decrease effect of **antigout medications. Bone marrow depres-**

sants may increase bone marrow depression. **Live virus vaccines** may potentiate virus replication, increase vaccine side effects, decrease pt's antibody response to vaccine. **HERBAL:** None known. **FOOD:** None known. **LAB VALUES:** May increase uric acid.

AVAILABILITY (Rx)

POWDER FOR INJECTION: 10 mg. **INJECTION:** 1 mg/ml.

ADMINISTRATION/HANDLING

Alert: May be carcinogenic, mutagenic, teratogenic. Handle with extreme care during preparation/administration. Give by IV injection. Leakage from IV site into surrounding tissue may produce extreme irritation. Avoid eye contact with solution (severe eye irritation, possible corneal ulceration may result). If eye contact occurs, immediately irrigate eye with water.

IV

Storage • Refrigerate unopened vials. • Solutions appear clear, colorless. • Following reconstitution, solution is stable for 30 days if refrigerated. • Discard if precipitate forms, discoloration occurs.

Reconstitution • Reconstitute 10-mg vial with 10 ml 0.9% NaCl preserved with phenol or benzyl alcohol to provide concentration of 1 mg/ml.

Rate of administration • Inject into tubing of running IV infusion or directly into vein over 1 min. • Do not inject into extremity with impaired or potentially impaired circulation caused by compression or invading neoplasm, phlebitis, varicosity. • Rinse syringe, needle with venous blood prior to withdrawing needle (minimizes possibility of extravasation). • Extravasation may result in cellulitis, phlebitis. Large amount of extravasation may result in tissue sloughing. If extravasation occurs, give local injection of hyaluronidase and apply warm compresses.

IV INCOMPATIBILITIES

Cefepime (Maxipime), furosemide (Lasix).

IV COMPATIBILITIES

Allopurinol (Aloprim), cisplatin (Platinol AQ), cyclophosphamide (Cytoxan), doxorubicin (Adriamycin), etoposide (VePesid), fluorouracil, gemcitabine (Gemzar), granisetron (Kytril), heparin, leucovorin, methotrexate, ondansetron (Zofran), paclitaxel (Taxol), vinorelbine (Navelbine).

INDICATIONS/ROUTES/DOSAGE

Alert: Dosage individualized based on clinical response, tolerance to adverse effects. When used in combination therapy, consult specific protocols for optimum dosage, sequence of drug administration. Reduce dosage if serum bilirubin >3 mg/dl. Repeat dosage at intervals of no less than 7 days and if the WBC count is at least 4,000/mm^3.

INDUCTION OF REMISSION

IV: ADULTS, ELDERLY: Initially, 3.7 mg/m^2 as single dose. Increase dose at weekly intervals of about 1.8 mg/m^2 until desired response is attained, WBC count falls below 3,000/mm^3, or maximum weekly dose of 18.5 mg/m^2 is reached. CHILDREN: Initially, 2.5 mg/m^2 as single dose. Increase dose at weekly intervals of about 1.25 mg/m^2 until desired response is attained, WBC count falls below 3,000/mm^3, or maximum weekly dose of 7.5–12.5 mg/m^2 is reached.

MAINTENANCE DOSE

IV: ADULTS, ELDERLY, CHILDREN: Use one increment less than dose required to produce leukocyte count of 3,000/mm^3. Each subsequent dose given when leukocyte count returns to 4,000/mm^3 and at least 7 days has elapsed since previous dose.

SIDE EFFECTS

FREQUENT: Nausea, vomiting, alopecia. **OCCASIONAL:** Constipation/diarrhea, rectal bleeding, paresthesia, headache, malaise, weakness, dizziness, pain at tumor site, jaw/face pain, mental depression, dry mouth. GI distress, headache, paresthesia occurs 4–6 hrs following administration, persists for 2–10 hrs. **RARE:** Dermatitis, stomatitis, phototoxicity, hyperuricemia.

ADVERSE REACTIONS/ TOXIC EFFECTS

Hematologic toxicity manifested most commonly as leukopenia, less frequently as anemia. WBC falls to lowest point 4–10 days after initial therapy with recovery within another 7–14 days (high dosages may require 21-day recovery period). Thrombocytopenia is usually slight, transient, with rapid recovery within few days. Hepatic insufficiency may increase risk of toxicity. Acute shortness of breath, bronchospasm may occur, particularly when administered concurrently with mitomycin.

NURSING IMPLICATIONS

BASELINE ASSESSMENT

Nausea, vomiting easily controlled by antiemetics. Discontinue therapy if WBC, thrombocyte counts fall abruptly (unless drug is clearly destroying tumor cells in bone marrow). Obtain CBC weekly or prior to each dosing.

INTERVENTION/EVALUATION

If WBC falls below 2,000/mm^3, assess diligently for signs of infection. Assess for stomatitis (burning erythema of oral mucosa at inner margin of lips, sore throat, difficulty swallowing, oral ulceration). Monitor for hematologic toxicity: infection (fever, sore throat, signs of local infection), unusual bruising/bleeding from any site, symptoms of anemia (excessive fatigue, weakness). Assess frequency, consistency of stools; avoid constipation.

PATIENT/FAMILY TEACHING

Immediately report any pain/burning at injection site during administration. Pain at tumor site may occur during or shortly after injection. Do not have immunizations without physician approval (drug lowers body's resistance). Avoid crowds, those with infection. Promptly report fever, sore throat, signs of local infection, unusual bruising/bleeding from any site. Alopecia is reversible, but new hair growth may have different color, texture. Contact physician if nausea/vomiting continues. Avoid constipation by increasing fluids, bulk in diet, exercise as tolerated.

vincristine sulfate

vin-**cris**-teen
(Vincasar PFS)
Do not confuse with Ancobon, vinblastine.

◆CLASSIFICATION

PHARMACOTHERAPEUTIC: Vinca alkaloid. **CLINICAL:** Antineoplastic (see p. 77C).

ACTION

Binds to microtubular protein of mitotic spindle. **Therapeutic Effect:** Causes metaphase arrest. Inhibits cellular division.

PHARMACOKINETICS

Does not cross blood-brain barrier. Protein binding: 75%. Metabolized in liver. Primarily eliminated in feces via biliary system. **Half-life:** 10–37 hrs.

USES

Treatment of acute leukemia, disseminated Hodgkin's disease, advanced non-Hodgkin's lymphomas, neuroblastom rhabdomyosarcoma, Wilms' tumor. **Unlabeled:** Treatment of chronic lymphocytic, myelocytic leukemia; breast, lung, ovarian, cervical, colorectal carcinoma; malignant melanoma; multiple myeloma; germ cell ovarian tumors; mycosis fungoides; idiopathic thrombocytopenia purpura.

PRECAUTIONS

CONTRAINDICATIONS: Those receiving radiation therapy through ports that include liver. **CAUTION:** Hepatic function impairment, neurotoxicity, preexisting neuromuscular disease.

LIFESPAN CONSIDERATIONS: Pregnancy/lactation: If possible, avoid use during pregnancy, esp. first trimester. May cause fetal harm. Breast-feeding not recommended. **Pregnancy Category D. Children:** No age-related precautions noted. **Elderly:** More susceptible to neurotoxic effects.

INTERACTIONS

DRUG: May decrease effect of **antigout medications. Live virus vaccines** may potentiate virus replication, increase vaccine side effects, decrease pt's antibody response to vaccine. **Asparaginase, neurotoxic medications** may increase neurotoxicity. **Doxorubicin** may increase myelosuppression. **HERBAL:** None known. **FOOD:** None known. **LAB VALUES:** May increase uric acid.

AVAILABILITY (Rx)

INJECTION: 1 mg/ml.

ADMINISTRATION/HANDLING

IV

Alert: May be carcinogenic, mutagenic, teratogenic. Handle with extreme care during preparation/administration. Give by IV injection. Use extreme caution alculating, administering vincristine. ose may result in serious or fatal

Storage • Refrigerate unopened vials. • Solutions appear clear, colorless. • Discard if precipitate forms or discoloration occurs.

Reconstitution • May give undiluted.

Rate of administration • Inject dose into tubing of running IV infusion or directly into vein >1 min. • Do not inject into extremity with impaired or potentially impaired circulation caused by compression or invading neoplasm, phlebitis, varicosity. • Extravasation produces stinging, burning, edema at injection site. Terminate immediately, locally inject hyaluronidase, apply heat (disperses drug, minimizes discomfort, cellulitis).

IV INCOMPATIBILITIES

Cefepime (Maxipime), furosemide (Lasix), idarubicin (Idamycin).

IV COMPATIBILITIES

Allopurinol (Aloprim), cisplatin (Platinol AQ), cyclophosphamide (Cytoxan), cytarabine (Ara-C, Cytosar), doxorubicin (Adriamycin), etoposide (VePesid), fluorouracil, gemcitabine (Gemzar), granisetron (Kytril), leucovorin, methotrexate, ondansetron (Zofran), paclitaxel (Taxol), virorelbine (Navelbine).

INDICATIONS/ROUTES/DOSAGE

Alert: Dosage individualized based on clinical response, tolerance to adverse effects. When used in combination therapy, consult specific protocols for optimum dosage, sequence of drug administration.

USUAL DOSAGE (administer at weekly intervals)

IV: ADULTS, ELDERLY: 0.4–1.4 mg/m^2. **Maximum:** 2 mg. CHILDREN: 1–2 mg/m^2. CHILDREN <10 KG OR BODY SURFACE AREA <1 M^2: 0.05 mg/kg.

HEPATIC FUNCTION IMPAIRMENT

Reduce dosage by 50% in those with direct serum bilirubin concentration <3 mg/dl.

SIDE EFFECTS

Peripheral neuropathy occurs in nearly every pt (first clinical sign: depression of Achilles tendon reflex). **FREQUENT:** Peripheral paresthesia, alopecia, constipation or obstipation (upper colon impaction with empty rectum), abdominal cramps, headache, jaw pain, hoarseness, double vision, ptosis (drooping of eyelid), urinary tract disturbances. **OCCASIONAL:** Nausea, vomiting, diarrhea, abdominal distention, stomatitis, fever. **RARE:** Mild leukopenia, mild anemia, thrombocytopenia.

ADVERSE REACTIONS/ TOXIC EFFECTS

Acute shortness of breath, bronchospasm may occur (esp. when used in combination with mitomycin). Prolonged or high-dose therapy may produce foot/wrist drop, difficulty walking, slapping gait, ataxia, muscle wasting. Acute uric acid nephropathy may be noted.

NURSING IMPLICATIONS

BASELINE ASSESSMENT

Monitor serum uric acid levels, renal/ hepatic function studies, hematologic status. Assess Achilles tendon reflex. Assess stools for consistency, frequency. Monitor for ptosis, blurred vision. Question pt regarding urinary changes.

PATIENT/FAMILY TEACHING

Immediately report any pain/burning at injection site during administration. Alopecia is reversible, but new hair growth may have different color/texture. Contact physician if nausea/vomiting continues. Teach signs of peripheral neuropathy. Report fever, sore throat, bleeding, bruising, shortness of breath.

vinorelbine

vin-oh-**rell**-bean
(Navelbine)
Do not confuse with vinblastine.

◆ CLASSIFICATION

CLINICAL: Antineoplastic (see p. 77C).

ACTION

Interferes with mitotic microtubule assembly. **Therapeutic Effect:** Prevents cellular division.

PHARMACOKINETICS

Following IV administration, widely distributed. Protein binding: 80%–90%. Metabolized in liver. Primarily eliminated via biliary/fecal route. **Half-life:** 28–43 hrs.

USES

Single agent or in combination with cisplatin for treatment with unresectable, advanced, non–small cell lung cancer (NSCLC). **Unlabeled:** Treatment of breast cancer, cisplatin-resistant ovarian carcinoma, Hodgkin's disease.

PRECAUTIONS

CONTRAINDICATIONS: Pretreatment granulocyte count <1,000 cells/mm^3. **EXTREME CAUTION:** Immunocompromised pts. **CAUTIONS:** Existing or recent chickenpox, herpes zoster, infection, leukopenia, impaired pulmonary function, severe hepatic injury/impairment.

LIFESPAN CONSIDERATIONS: Pregnancy/lactation: If possible, avoid use during pregnancy, esp. during first trimester. May cause fetal harm. Unknown if excreted in breast milk. Breast-feeding not recommended. **Pregnancy Cate-**

gory D. **Children:** Safety and efficacy not established. **Elderly:** No age-related precautions noted.

INTERACTIONS

DRUG: Significantly increased risk of granulocytopenia when **cisplatin** is used concurrently with vinorelbine. **Mitomycin** may produce acute pulmonary reaction. **Bone marrow depressants** may increase risk of bone marrow depression. **Live virus vaccines** may potentiate virus replication, increase vaccine side effects, decrease pt's antibody response to vaccine. **HERBAL:** None known. **FOOD:** None known. **LAB VALUES:** Decreases granulocytes, leukocytes, thrombocytes, RBCs. May increase total bilirubin, SGOT (AST), liver function tests.

AVAILABILITY (Rx)

INJECTION: 10 mg/ml (1-ml, 5-ml vials).

ADMINISTRATION/HANDLING

IV

Alert: Extremely important that IV needle or catheter is correctly positioned before administration. Leaking into surrounding tissue produces extreme irritation, local tissue necrosis, thrombophlebitis. Wear gloves when preparing solution. If solution comes in contact with skin/mucosa, wash immediately and thoroughly with soap, water.

Storage • Refrigerate unopened vials. • Protect from light. • Unopened vials are stable at room temperature for 72 hrs. • Do not administer if particulate matter is noted. • Diluted vinorelbine may be used for up to 24 hrs under normal room light when stored in polypropylene syringes or polyvinyl chloride bags at room temperature.

Reconstitution • Must be diluted and administered via a syringe or IV bag.

SYRINGE DILUTION

• Dilute calculated vinorelbine dose with D_5W or 0.9% NaCl to a concentration of 1.5–3 mg/ml.

IV BAG DILUTION

• Dilute calculated vinorelbine dose with D_5W, 0.45% or 0.9% NaCl, 5% dextrose and 0.45% NaCl, Ringer's or lactated Ringer's to a concentration of 0.5–2 mg/ml.

Rate of administration • Administer diluted vinorelbine over 6–10 min into side port of free-flowing IV closest to IV bag followed by flushing with 75–125 ml of one of the solutions. • If extravasation occurs, stop injection immediately; give remaining portion of the dose into another vein.

∅ IV INCOMPATIBILITIES

Acyclovir (Zovirax), allopurinol (Aloprim), amphotericin B (Fungizone), amphotericin B complex (Abelcet, AmBisome, Amphotec), ampicillin (Omnipen), cefazolin (Ancef), cefoperazone (Cefobid), cefotetan (Cefotan), ceftriaxone (Rocephin), cefuroxime (Zinacef), fluorouracil, furosemide (Lasix), ganciclovir (Cytovene), methylprednisolone (Solu-Medrol), sodium bicarbonate.

IV COMPATIBILITIES

Calcium gluconate, carboplatin (Paraplatin), cisplatin (Platinol AQ), cyclophosphamide (Cytoxan), cytarabine (ARA-C, Cytosar), dacarbazine (DTIC-Dome), daunorubicin (Cerubidine), dexamethasone (Decadron), diphenhydramine (Benadryl), doxorubicin (Adriamycin), etoposide (VePesid), gemcitabine (Gemzar), granisetron (Kytril), hydromorphone (Dilaudid), idarubicin (Idamycin), methotrexate, morphone, ondansetron (Zofran), teniposide (Vumon), vinblastine (Velban), vincristine (Oncovin).

INDICATIONS/ROUTES/DOSAGE

Alert: Granulocyte count should be ≥1,000 cells/mm^3 before vinorelbine administration. Dosage adjustments should be based on granulocyte count obtained on day of treatment, as follows:

Granulocytes (cells/mm^3) on Day of Treatment	Dose (mg/m^2)
≥1,500	30
1,000–1,499	15
<1,000	Do not administer

NON–SMALL CELL LUNG CANCER

IV injection: ADULTS, ELDERLY: 30 mg/m^2, given over 6–10 min, administered weekly.

SIDE EFFECTS

FREQUENT: Asthenia (35%), mild or moderate nausea (34%), constipation (29%), injection site reaction manifested as erythema, pain, vein discoloration (28%), fatigue (27%), peripheral neuropathy manifested as paresthesia, hyperesthesia (25%), diarrhea (17%), alopecia (12%). **OCCASIONAL:** Phlebitis (10%), dyspnea (7%), loss of deep tendon reflexes (5%). **RARE:** Chest pain, jaw pain, myalgia, arthralgia, rash.

ADVERSE REACTIONS/ TOXIC EFFECTS

Bone marrow depression is manifested mainly as granulocytopenia (may be severe); other hematologic toxicity (neutropenia, thrombocytopenia, leukopenia, anemia) increases risk of infection, bleeding. Acute shortness of breath, severe bronchospasm occurs infrequently, particularly when there is preexisting pulmonary dysfunction.

NURSING IMPLICATIONS

BASELINE ASSESSMENT

Review medication history. Assess hematology (CBC, platelet count, Hgb, differential) values prior to giving each dose. Granulocyte count should be ≥1,000 cells/mm^3 prior to vinorelbine administration. Granulocyte nadirs occur 7–10 days following dosing. Do not give hematologic growth factors within 24 hrs prior to administration of chemotherapy or no earlier than 24 hrs following cytotoxic chemotherapy. Advise women of childbearing potential to avoid pregnancy during drug therapy.

INTERVENTION/EVALUATION

Diligently monitor injection site for swelling, redness, pain. Frequently monitor for myelosuppression both during and following therapy: infection (fever, sore throat, signs of local infection), unusual bleeding/bruising, anemia (excessive fatigue, weakness). Monitor pts developing severe granulocytopenia for evidence of infection, fever. Crackers, dry toast, sips of cola may help relieve nausea. Assess bowel activity, frequency. Question for tingling, burning, numbness of hands/feet (peripheral neuropathy). Pt complaint of "walking on glass" is sign of hyperesthesia.

PATIENT/FAMILY TEACHING

Notify nurse immediately if redness, swelling, pain occur at injection site. Avoid crowds, those with infection. Do not have immunizations without physician's approval. Promptly report fever, signs of infection, unusual bruising/bleeding from any site, difficulty breathing. Avoid pregnancy. Alopecia is reversible, but new hair growth may have different color, texture.

Vistaril

see hydroxyzine

vitamin A

(Aquasol A)

Do not confuse with Anusol.

◆ CLASSIFICATION

PHARMACOTHERAPEUTIC: Fat-soluble vitamin. **CLINICAL:** Nutritional supplement (see p. 136C).

ACTION

May be a cofactor in biochemical reactions. **Therapeutic Effect:** Is essential for normal function of retina. Necessary for visual adaptation to darkness, bone growth, testicular and ovarian function, embryonic development; preserves integrity of epithelial cells.

PHARMACOKINETICS

Absorption dependent on bile salts, pancreatic lipase, dietary fat. Transported in blood to liver, stored in parenchymal liver cells, then transported in plasma as retinol, as needed. Metabolized in liver. Excreted in bile and, to a lesser amount, in urine.

USES

Treatment of vitamin A deficiency (biliary tract or pancreatic disease, sprue, colitis, hepatic cirrhosis, celiac disease, regional enteritis, extreme dietary inadequacy, partial gastrectomy, cystic fibrosis).

PRECAUTIONS

CONTRAINDICATIONS: Hypervitaminosis A, oral use in malabsorption syndrome. **CAUTIONS:** Renal impairment.

LIFESPAN CONSIDERATIONS: Pregnancy/lactation: Crosses placenta. Distributed in breast milk. **Pregnancy Category A** (**X** if doses above RDA). **Children/elderly:** Caution with higher dosages.

INTERACTIONS

DRUG: Cholestyramine, colestipol, mineral oil may decrease absorption. **Isotretinoin** may increase toxicity. **HERBAL:** None known. **FOOD:** None known. **LAB VALUES:** May increase BUN, calcium, cholesterol, triglycerides. May decrease erythrocyte, leukocyte counts.

AVAILABILITY (Rx)

CAPSULES: 8,000 units, 10,000 units, 25,000 units. **INJECTION:** 50,000 units/ml. **TABLETS:** 5,000 units, 10,000 units, 15,000 units.

ADMINISTRATION/HANDLING

Alert: IM administration used only in acutely ill or pts unresponsive to oral route (GI malabsorption syndrome).

PO

- Do not crush, break capsule form.
- Give without regard to food.

IM

- For IM injection in adults, if dosage is 1 ml (50,000 international units), may give in deltoid muscle; if dosage is >1

V

ml, give in gluteus maximus muscle. The anterolateral thigh is site of choice for infants, children <7 mos.

INDICATIONS/ROUTES/DOSAGE

SEVERE DEFICIENCY WITH XEROPHTHALMIA

IM: ADULTS, ELDERLY, CHILDREN >8 YRS: 50,000–100,000 units/day for 3 days, then 50,000 units/day for 14 days. CHILDREN 1–8 YRS: 5,000–15,000 units/day for 10 days.

PO: ADULTS, ELDERLY, CHILDREN >8 YRS: 500,000 units/day for 3 days, then 50,000 units/day for 14 days, then 10,000–20,000 units/day for 2 mos. CHILDREN 1–8 YRS: 5,000 units/kg/day for 5 days or until recovery occurs.

MALABSORPTION SYNDROME

PO: ADULTS, ELDERLY, CHILDREN >8 YRS: 50,000 units/day.

DIETARY SUPPLEMENT

PO: ADULTS, ELDERLY: 4,000–5,000 units/day. CHILDREN 7–10 YRS: 3,300–3,500 units/day. CHILDREN 4–6 YRS: 2,500 units/day. CHILDREN 6 MOS–3 YRS: 1,500–2,000 units/day. NEONATES TO 6 MOS: 1,500 units/day.

SIDE EFFECTS

None known.

ADVERSE REACTIONS/ TOXIC EFFECTS

Chronic overdosage produces malaise, nausea, vomiting, drying/cracking of skin/lips, inflammation of tongue/gums, irritability, loss of hair, night sweats. Bulging fontanelles in infants noted.

NURSING IMPLICATIONS

INTERVENTION/EVALUATION

Closely supervise for overdosage symptoms during prolonged daily administration >25,000 international units. Monitor for therapeutic serum vitamin A levels (80–300 international units/ml).

PATIENT/FAMILY TEACHING

Foods rich in vitamin A include cod, halibut, tuna, shark (naturally occurring vitamin A found only in animal sources). Avoid taking mineral oil, cholestyramine (Questran) while taking vitamin A.

vitamin D

calcitriol

(Calcijex, Rocaltrol)

dihydrotachysterol

(DHT, Hytakerol)

ergocalciferol

(Calciferol, Deltalin, Drisdol)

paricalcitol

(Zemplar)

CLASSIFICATION

PHARMACOTHERAPEUTIC: Fat-soluble vitamin. **CLINICAL:** Nutritional supplement (see p. 137C).

ACTION

Essential for absorption, utilization of calcium phosphate, normal calcification of bone. **Therapeutic Effect:** Stimulates calcium/phosphate absorption from small intestine, promotes secretion of calcium from bone to blood, promotes renal tubule phosphate resorption, acts on bone cells to stimulate skeletal growth and on parathyroid gland to suppress hormone synthesis/secretion.

PHARMACOKINETICS

Readily absorbed from small intestine.

V

Concentrated primarily in liver, fat depots. Activated in liver, kidney. Eliminated via biliary system; excreted in urine. **Half-life:** calcifediol: 10–22 days; calcitriol: 3–6 hrs; ergocalciferol: 19–48 hrs.

USES

Prevention/treatment of vitamin D deficiency (may lead to rickets, osteomalacia), chronic hypocalcemia, hypophosphatemia, rickets, osteodystrophy associated with chronic renal failure, familial hypophosphatemia/hypoparathyroidism. **Paricalcitol:** Prevention/treatment of secondary hypoparathyroidism associated with chronic renal failure.

PRECAUTIONS

CONTRAINDICATIONS: Hypercalcemia, malabsorption syndrome, vitamin D toxicity. **CAUTIONS:** Contrary artery disease, kidney stones, renal impairment.

LIFESPAN CONSIDERATIONS: Pregnancy/lactation: Unknown if drug crosses placenta. Distributed in breast milk. **Pregnancy Category A** (**D** if used in doses above RDA). **Children:** May be more sensitive to effects. **Elderly:** No age-related precautions noted.

INTERACTIONS

DRUG: Aluminum-containing antacid (long-term use) may increase aluminum concentration, aluminum bone toxicity. **Magnesium-containing antacids** may increase magnesium concentration. **Calcium-containing preparations, thiazide diuretics** may increase risk of hypercalcemia. **HERBAL:** None known. **FOOD:** None known. **LAB VALUES:** May increase calcium, cholesterol, phosphate, magnesium. May decrease alkaline phosphatase.

AVAILABILITY (Rx)

CALCITRIOL (Calcijex, Rocaltrol)
CAPSULE: 0.25 mcg, 0.5 mcg. **INJECTION:** 1 mcg/ml, 2 mcg/ml. **ORAL SOLUTION:** 1 mcg/ml.

DIHYDROTACHYSTEROL (DHT)
ORAL SOLUTION: 0.2 mg/ml. **CAPSULE:** 0.125 mg. **TABLETS:** 0.125 mg, 0.2 mg, 0.4 mg.

ERGOCALCIFEROL (Calciferol, Drisdol)
CAPSULES: 50,000 units. **LIQUID DROPS:** 8,000 units/ml. **TABLET:** 400 units.

PARACALCITOL (Zemplar)
INJECTION: 2 mcg/ml, 5 mcg/ml.

ADMINISTRATION/HANDLING

PO

• Give without regard to food. • Swallow whole; do not crush/chew.

INDICATIONS/ROUTES/DOSAGE

Alert: 1 mcg = 40 units.

DIETARY SUPPLEMENT
PO: ADULTS, ELDERLY, CHILDREN: 10 mcg (400 units)/day. NEONATES: 10–20 mcg (400–800 units)/day.

RENAL FAILURE
PO: ADULTS, ELDERLY: 0.5 mg/day. CHILDREN: 0.1–1 mg/day.

HYPOPARATHYROIDISM
PO: ADULTS, ELDERLY: 625 mcg–5 mg/day (with calcium supplements). CHILDREN: 1.25–5 mg/day (with calcium supplements).

VITAMIN D–DEPENDENT RICKETS
PO: ADULTS, ELDERLY: 250 mcg–1.5 mg/day. CHILDREN: 75–125 mcg/day. **Maximum:** 1,500 mcg/day.

NUTRITIONAL RICKETS/OSTEOMALACIA
PO: ADULTS, ELDERLY, CHILDREN: 25–125 mcg/day for 8–12 wks. ADULTS, ELDERLY (malabsorption): 250–7,500 mcg/day. CHILDREN (malabsorption): 250–625 mcg/day.

VITAMIN D–RESISTANT RICKETS
PO: ADULTS, ELDERLY: 250–1,500 mcg/day (with phosphate supplements).

CHILDREN: Initially 1,000–2,000 mcg/day (with phosphate supplements). May increase at 3- to 4-mo intervals in 250- to 600-mcg increments.

SIDE EFFECTS

None known.

ADVERSE REACTIONS/ TOXIC EFFECTS

Early signs of overdosage manifested as weakness, headache, somnolence, nausea, vomiting, dry mouth, constipation, muscle/bone pain, metallic taste sensation. Later signs of overdosage evidenced by polyuria, polydipsia, anorexia, weight loss, nocturia, photophobia, rhinorrhea, pruritus, disorientation, hallucinations, hyperthermia, hypertension, cardiac arrhythmias.

NURSING IMPLICATIONS

BASELINE ASSESSMENT

Therapy should begin at lowest possible dosage.

INTERVENTION/EVALUATION

Monitor serum and urinary calcium levels, serum phosphate, magnesium, creatinine, alkaline phosphatase and BUN determinations (therapeutic serum calcium level: 9–10 mg/dl). Estimate daily dietary calcium intake. Encourage adequate fluid intake.

PATIENT/FAMILY TEACHING

Encourage foods rich in vitamin D, including vegetable oils, vegetable shortening, margarine, leafy vegetables, milk, eggs, meats. Do not take mineral oil while on vitamin D therapy. If receiving chronic renal dialysis, do not take magnesium-containing antacids during vitamin D therapy. Drink plenty of liquids.

vitamin E

(Aquasol E)

Do not confuse with Anusol.

◆CLASSIFICATION

PHARMACOTHERAPEUTIC: Fat-soluble vitamin. **CLINICAL:** Nutritional supplement (see p. 137C).

ACTION

Antioxidant. **Therapeutic Effect:** Prevents oxidation of vitamins A and C, protects fatty acids from attack by free radicals, protects RBCs from hemolysis by oxidizing agents.

PHARMACOKINETICS

Variably absorbed from GI tract (requires bile salts, dietary fat, normal pancreatic function). Primarily concentrated in adipose tissue. Metabolized in liver. Primarily eliminated via biliary system.

USES

Treatment of vitamin E deficiency. **Unlabeled:** Decreases severity of tardive dyskinesia.

PRECAUTIONS

CONTRAINDICATIONS: None known. **CAUTIONS:** None known.

LIFESPAN CONSIDERATIONS: Pregnancy/lactation: Unknown if drug crosses placenta or is distributed in breast milk. **Pregnancy Category A (C** if used in doses above RDA). **Children/elderly:** No age-related precautions noted in normal dosages.

INTERACTIONS

DRUG: May impair hematologic response in pts with iron deficiency anemia. **Iron** (large doses) may increase vitamin E requirements. **Cholestyramine, colestipol, mineral oil** may decrease

V

absorption. **HERBAL:** None known. **FOOD:** None known. **LAB VALUES:** None known.

AVAILABILITY (OTC)

CAPSULES: 100 units, 200 units, 400 units, 600 units, 800 units, 1,000 units. **ORAL DROPS:** 15 units/0.3 ml.

ADMINISTRATION/HANDLING

PO

- Do not crush, break tablets/capsules.
- Give without regard to food.

INDICATIONS/ROUTES/DOSAGE

VITAMIN E DEFICIENCY

PO: ADULTS, ELDERLY: 60–75 units/day. CHILDREN: 1 unit/kg/day.

SIDE EFFECTS

None known.

ADVERSE REACTIONS/ TOXIC EFFECTS

Chronic overdosage produces fatigue, weakness, nausea, headache, blurred vision, flatulence, diarrhea.

NURSING IMPLICATIONS

PATIENT/FAMILY TEACHING

Swallow capsules whole; do not crush, chew. Toxicity consists of blurred vision, diarrhea, dizziness, nausea, headache, flulike symptoms. Encourage foods rich in vitamin E, including vegetable oils, vegetable shortening, margarine, leafy vegetables, milk, eggs, meats.

V

vitamin K

phytonadione (vitamin K_1)

fy-toe-na-**dye**-own

(AquaMEPHYTON, Mephyton)

Do not confuse with melphalan, mephenytoin.

CLASSIFICATION

PHARMACOTHERAPEUTIC: Fat-soluble vitamin. **CLINICAL:** Nutritional supplement, antidote (drug-induced hypoprothrombinemia), antihemorrhagic.

ACTION

Necessary for hepatic formation of coagulation factors II, VII, IX, X. **Therapeutic Effect:** Essential for normal clotting of blood.

PHARMACOKINETICS

Readily absorbed from GI tract (duodenum), following IM, subcutaneous administration. Metabolized in liver. Excreted in urine, eliminated via biliary system. **Parenteral:** Controls hemorrhage within 3–6 hrs, normal prothrombin time in 12–14 hrs. **PO:** Effect in 6–10 hrs.

USES

Prevention, treatment of hemorrhagic states in neonates; antidote for hemorrhage induced by oral anticoagulants, hypoprothrombinemic states due to vitamin K deficiency. Will not counteract anticoagulation effect of heparin.

PRECAUTIONS

CONTRAINDICATIONS: None known. **CAUTIONS:** None known.

LIFESPAN CONSIDERATIONS: Pregnancy/lactation: Crosses placenta. Distributed in breast milk. **Pregnancy Category C.** **Children/elderly:** No age-related precautions noted.

INTERACTIONS

DRUG: **Broad-spectrum antibiotics, high-dose salicylates** may increase vitamin K requirements. May decrease effect of **oral anticoagulants. Cholestyramine, colestipol, mineral oil, sucralfate** may decrease absorption. **HERBAL:** None known. **FOOD:** None known. **LAB VALUES:** None known.

AVAILABILITY (Rx)

TABLETS: 5 mg. **INJECTION:** 2 mg/ml, 10 mg/ml.

ADMINISTRATION/HANDLING

PO

- Scored tablets may be crushed.

SUBCUTANEOUS/IM

- Inject into anterolateral aspect of thigh/deltoid region.

IV

Alert: Restrict to emergency use only.

Storage • Store at room temperature.

Reconstitution • May dilute with preservative-free NaCl or D_5W immediately before use. Do not use other diluents. Discard unused portions.

Rate of administration • Administer slow IV at rate of 1 mg/min. • Monitor continuously for hypersensitivity, anaphylactic reaction during and immediately following IV administration.

IV INCOMPATIBILITY

No known incompatibility noted via Y-site administration.

IV COMPATIBILITIES

Heparin, potassium chloride.

INDICATIONS/ROUTES/DOSAGE

Alert: Subcutaneous route preferred, IV/IM restricted for situation.

ORAL ANTICOAGULANT OVERDOSE

IV/subcutaneous/PO: ADULTS, ELDERLY: 2.5–10 mg/dose. May repeat in 6–8 hrs if given IV/subcutaneously or 12–48 hrs if given orally. CHILDREN: 0.5–5 mg depending on need for further anticoagulation, severity of bleeding.

VITAMIN K DEFICIENCY

IV/IM/subcutaneous: ADULTS, ELDERLY: 10 mg. CHILDREN: 1–2 mg/dose.

PO: ADULTS, ELDERLY: 2.5–25 mg/24 hrs. CHILDREN: 2.5–5 mg/24 hrs.

HEMORRHAGIC DISEASE IN NEWBORN

IM/subcutaneous: TREATMENT: 1–2 mg/dose/day. PROPHYLAXIS: 0.5–1 mg within 1 hr of birth. May repeat in 6–8 hrs if necessary.

SIDE EFFECTS

Alert: PO or subcutaneous administration less likely to produce side effects than IM or IV route.

OCCASIONAL: Pain, soreness, swelling at IM injection site; repeated injections: pruritic erythema; flushed face, unusual taste.

ADVERSE REACTIONS/ TOXIC EFFECTS

May produce hyperbilirubinemia in newborn (esp. premature infants). Rarely, severe reaction occurs immediately after IV administration (cramplike pain, chest pain, dyspnea, facial flushing, dizziness, rapid/weak pulse, rash, profuse diaphoresis, hypotension; may progress to shock, cardiac arrest).

NURSING IMPLICATIONS

INTERVENTION/EVALUATION

Monitor prothrombin time, INR routinely in those taking anticoagulants. Assess skin for bruises, petechiae. Assess gums for gingival bleeding, erythema. Monitor urine output for hematuria. Assess Hct, platelet count, urine/stool culture for occult blood. Assess for decrease in B/P, increase in pulse rate, complaint of abdominal or back pain, severe headache (may be evidence of hemorrhage). Question for increase in amount of discharge during menses. Assess peripheral pulses. Check for excessive bleeding from minor cuts, scratches.

PATIENT/FAMILY TEACHING

Discomfort may occur with parenteral administration. **Adults:** Use electric razor, soft toothbrush to prevent bleeding. Report any sign of red/dark urine, black/red stool, coffee-ground vomitus, red-speckled mucus from cough. Do not use any OTC medication without physician approval (may interfere with platelet aggregation). Encourage foods rich in vitamin K_1, including leafy green vegetables, meat, cow's milk, vegetable oil, egg yolks, tomatoes.

voriconazole

voor-ih-**con**-ah-zole
(Vfend)

CLASSIFICATION

PHARMACOTHERAPEUTIC: Triazole derivative. **CLINICAL:** Antifungal.

ACTION

Inhibits the synthesis of ergosterol (vital component of fungal cell wall formation). **Therapeutic Effect:** Damages fungal cell wall membrane.

PHARMACOKINETICS

Rapidly, completely absorbed following PO administration. Widely distributed. Protein binding: 98%. Metabolized in the liver. Primarily excreted as metabolite in the urine. **Half-life:** 6 hrs.

USES

Treatment of invasive aspergillosis, esophageal candidiasis. Treatment of serious fungal infections caused by *Scedosporium apiospermum* and *Fusarium* spp.

PRECAUTIONS

CONTRAINDICATIONS: Coadministration of pimozide or quinidine (may cause QT prolongation, torsades de pointes), sirolimus, rifampin, carbamazepine, rifabutin, ergot alkaloids. **CAUTIONS:** Impaired renal/hepatic function, hypersensitivity to other antifungal agents.

LIFESPAN CONSIDERATIONS: Pregnancy/lactation: May cause fetal harm. **Pregnancy Category D. Children:** Safety and efficacy not established in those <12 yrs. **Elderly:** No age-related precautions noted.

INTERACTIONS

DRUG: May increase concentrations of **warfarin, phenytoin, omeprazole, rifabutin, tacrilimus, sirolimus, cyclosporine. Rifampin, rifabutin, phenytoin** may decrease voriconazole concentration. **HERBAL:** None known. **FOOD:** None known. **LAB VALUES:** May increase alkaline phosphatase, SGPT (ALT).

AVAILABILITY (Rx)

TABLETS: 50 mg, 200 mg. **POWDER FOR INJECTION:** 200 mg.

ADMINISTRATION/HANDLING

PO

- Take 1 hr before or 1 hr after a meal.

IV

Storage • Store powder for injection at room temperature. • Use reconstituted solution immediately. • Do not use after 24 hrs when refrigerated.

Reconstitution • Reconstitute 200-mg vial with 19 ml Sterile Water for Injection to provide a concentration of 10 mg/ml. Further dilute with 0.9% NaCl or D_5W to provide a concentration of ≤5 mg/ml.

Rate of administration • Infuse over 1–2 hrs at a concentration of ≤5 mg/ml.

IV INCOMPATIBILITY

Do not mix with any other medications.

INDICATIONS/ROUTES/DOSAGE

ANTIFUNGAL

IV: ADULTS, ELDERLY: Initially, 6 mg/kg q12h for 2 doses, then 4 mg/kg q12h.

PO: ADULTS, ELDERLY, >40 KG: Initially, 400 mg q12h for 2 doses, then 200 mg q12h. ADULTS, ELDERLY, <40 MG: Initially, 200 mg q12h for 2 doses, then 100 mg q12h.

SIDE EFFECTS

FREQUENT (5%–20%): Abnormal vision, fever, nausea, rash, vomiting. **OCCASIONAL (2%–5%):** Headache, chills, hallucinations, photophobia, tachycardia, hypertension.

ADVERSE REACTIONS/ TOXIC EFFECTS

Hepatic toxicity occurs rarely.

NURSING IMPLICATIONS

BASELINE ASSESSMENT

Obtain baseline hepatic function and renal function tests.

INTERVENTION/EVALUATION

Monitor hepatic/renal function tests. Monitor visual function (visual acuity, visual field, color perception) for drug therapy lasting >28 days.

PATIENT/FAMILY TEACHING

Take at least 1 hr before or 1 hr after a meal. Avoid driving at night. May cause visual changes (blurred vision, photophobia). Avoid performing hazardous tasks if changes in vision occur. Avoid direct sunlight. Women of childbearing potential should have effective contraception.

warfarin sodium

war-fair-in

(Coumadin, Warfilone✱)

Do not confuse with Kemadrin.

CLASSIFICATION

PHARMACOTHERAPEUTIC: Coumarin derivative. **CLINICAL:** Anticoagulant (see p. 29C).

ACTION

Interferes with hepatic synthesis of vitamin K–dependent clotting factors, resulting in depletion of coagulation factors II, VII, IX, X. **Therapeutic Effect:** Prevents further extension of formed existing clot; prevents new clot formation, secondary thromboembolic complications.

PHARMACOKINETICS

	Onset	Peak	Duration
PO	1.5–3 days	5–7 days	—

Well absorbed from GI tract. Metabolized in liver. Primarily excreted in urine. Not removed by hemodialysis. **Half-life:** 1.5–2.5 days.

USES

Prophylaxis, treatment of venous thrombosis, pulmonary embolism. Treatment of thromboembolism associated with chronic atrial fibrillation. Adjunct in treatment of coronary occlusion. Prophylaxis/treatment of thromboembolic complications associated with cardiac valve replacement. Reduces risk of death, recurrent MI, stroke, embolization after MI. **Unlabeled:** Prophylaxis for, or recurrent cerebral embolism, myocardial reinfarction, treatment adjunct in transient ischemic attacks.

PRECAUTIONS

CONTRAINDICATIONS: Severe hepatic/renal damage, uncontrolled bleeding, open wounds, ulcers, neurosurgical procedures, severe hypertension, pregnancy. **CAUTIONS:** Active tuberculosis, diabetes, heparin-induced thrombocytopenia, those at risk for hemorrhage, necrosis, gangrene.

LIFESPAN CONSIDERATIONS: Pregnancy/lactation: Contraindicated in pregnancy (fetal/neonatal hemorrhage, intrauterine death). Crosses placenta; is distributed in breast milk. **Pregnancy Category D. Children:** More susceptible to effects. **Elderly:** Increased risk of hemorrhage; lower dosage recommended.

INTERACTIONS

DRUG: Increased effect with **acetaminophen (regular use), allopurinol, amiodarone, anabolic steroids, androgens, aspirin, cefamandole, cefoperazone, chloral hydrate, chloramphenicol, cimetidine, clofibrate, danazol, dextrothyroxine, diflunisal, disulfiram, erythromycin, fenoprofen, gemfibrozil, indomethacin, methimazole, metronidazole, oral hypoglycemics, phenytoin, plicamycin, PTU, quinidine, salicylates, sulfinpyrazone, sulfonamides, sulindac.** Decreased effect with **barbiturates, carbamazepine, cholestyramine, colestipol, estramustine, estrogens, griseofulvin, primidone, rifampin, vitamin K. HERBAL: Feverfew, garlic, Ginkgo biloba, ginseng** may increase risk of bleeding. **FOOD:** None known. **LAB VALUES:** None known.

AVAILABILITY (Rx)

TABLETS: 1 mg, 2 mg, 2.5 mg, 3 mg, 4 mg, 5 mg, 6 mg, 7.5 mg, 10 mg. **INJECTION:** 5-mg vials.

ADMINISTRATION/HANDLING

PO

- Scored tablets may be crushed.
- Give without regard to food. If GI upset occurs, give with food.

INDICATIONS/ROUTES/DOSAGE

Alert: Dosage highly individualized, based on prothrombin time (PT), INR.

ANTICOAGULANT

PO: ADULTS, ELDERLY: Initially, 5–15 mg/day for 2–5 days, then adjust based on INR. MAINTENANCE: 2–10 mg/day. CHILDREN: Initially, 0.1–0.2 mg/kg. **Maximum:** 10 mg. MAINTENANCE: 0.05–0.34 mg/kg/day.

USUAL ELDERLY DOSAGE

PO/IV: ADULTS: 2–5 mg/day (maintenance).

SIDE EFFECTS

OCCASIONAL: GI distress (nausea, anorexia, abdominal cramps, diarrhea). **RARE:** Hypersensitivity reaction (dermatitis, urticaria, esp. in pts sensitive to aspirin).

ADVERSE REACTIONS/ TOXIC EFFECTS

Bleeding complications ranging from local ecchymoses to major hemorrhage. Drug should be discontinued immediately and vitamin K (phytonadione) administered. **MILD HEMORRHAGE:** 2.5–10 mg PO/IM/IV. **SEVERE HEMORRHAGE:**

10–15 mg IV and repeated q4h, as necessary. Hepatotoxicity, blood dyscrasias, necrosis, vasculitis, local thrombosis occur rarely.

NURSING IMPLICATIONS

BASELINE ASSESSMENT

Cross-check dose with co-worker. Determine INR prior to administration and daily following therapy initiation. When stabilized, follow with INR determination q4–6wks.

INTERVENTION/EVALUATION

Monitor INR reports diligently. Assess Hct, platelet count, urine/stool culture for occult blood, SGOT (AST), SGPT (ALT), regardless of route of administration. Be alert to complaints of abdominal/back pain, severe headache (may be signs of hemorrhage). Decrease in B/P, increase in pulse rate may also be sign of hemorrhage. Question for increase in amount of discharge during menses. Assess area of thromboembolus for color, temperature. Assess peripheral pulses; skin for bruises, petechiae. Check for excessive bleeding from minor cuts, scratches. Assess gums for erythema, gingival bleeding. Assess urine output for hematuria.

PATIENT/FAMILY TEACHING

Take medication exactly as prescribed. Do not take or discontinue any other medication except on advice of physician. Avoid alcohol, salicylates, drastic dietary changes. Do not change from one brand to another. Consult with physician before surgery or dental work. Urine may become red-orange. Notify physician if bleeding, bruising, red/brown urine, black stools occur. Use electric razor, soft toothbrush to prevent bleeding. Report any sign of red/dark urine, black/red stool, coffee-ground vomitus, red-speckled mucus from cough. Do not use any OTC medication without physician approval (may interfere with platelet aggregation).

Wellbutrin

see bupropion

Xanax

see alprazolam

Xopenex

see levalbuterol

yohimbe

Also known as aphrodien, corynine, johimbi

CLASSIFICATION

HERBAL.

ACTION

Produces genital blood vessel dilation, improves nerve impulse transmission to genital area. Increases penile blood flow, central sympathetic excitation impulses to genital tissues. **Therapeutic Effect:** Improves sexual function, affects impotence.

USES

Aphrodisiac, impotence, exhaustion, angina, diabetic neuropathy, postural hypotension.

Y

PRECAUTIONS

CONTRAINDICATIONS: Pregnancy/lactation (may have uterine relaxant effect, cause fetal toxicity), angina, heart disease, benign prostatic hypertrophy, depression, renal/hepatic disease. **CAUTIONS:** Anxiety, diabetes mellitus, hypertension, post-traumatic stress disorder, schizophrenia.

LIFESPAN CONSIDERATIONS: Pregnancy/lactation: Contraindicated; avoid use. **Children:** Safety and efficacy not established; avoid use. **Elderly:** Age-related renal/liver impairment may require discontinuing.

INTERACTIONS

DRUG: May interfere with **drugs for diabetes, antihypertensives.** May antagonize effect of **clonidine.** Additive effects with **MAOIs, sympathomimetics, tricyclic antidepressants. HERBAL: Ginkgo biloba, St. John's wort** can have additive therapeutic/adverse effects. **Ephedra** may increase risk of hypertensive crises. **FOOD: Tyramine-containing foods** (e.g., aged cheese, chianti wine), **caffeine-containing products, coffee, tea, chocolate** may increase risk of hypertensive crises. **LAB VALUES:** None known.

AVAILABILITY (OTC)

TABLETS: 5 mg. **LIQUID:** 5 mg/5 ml.

INDICATIONS/ROUTES /DOSAGE

IMPOTENCE

PO: ADULTS, ELDERLY: 15–30 mg/day in divided doses.

SIDE EFFECTS

Excitement, tremors, insomnia, anxiety, hypertension, tachycardia, dizziness, headache, irritability, salivation, dilated pupils, nausea, vomiting, hypersensitivity reaction.

ADVERSE REACTIONS/ TOXIC EFFECTS

Paralysis, severe hypotension, irregular heartbeat, cardiac failure. Overdose can be fatal.

NURSING IMPLICATIONS

BASELINE ASSESSMENT

Assess if pt is pregnant/breast-feeding (contraindicated). Determine other medical conditions, including angina, heart disease, benign prostatic hypertrophy. Assess baseline renal/hepatic function, medications (see Interactions).

INTERVENTION/EVALUATION

Monitor renal/hepatic functions, B/P. Assess for hypersensitivity reaction.

PATIENT/FAMILY TEACHING

Do not use other OTC or prescribed medications before checking with physician. Inform physician if pregnant/breast-feeding.

zafirlukast

zay-**fur**-leu-cast
(Accolate)

Do not confuse with Accupril, Aclovate.

CLASSIFICATION

PHARMACOTHERAPEUTIC: Leukotriene receptor antagonist. **CLINICAL:** Antiasthma (see p. 66C).

ACTION

Binds to leukotriene receptors. Inhibits bronchoconstriction due to sulfur dioxide, cold air, specific antigens (grass, cat dander, ragweed). **Therapeutic Effect:** Reduces airway edema, smooth muscle constriction, alters cellular activity associated with inflammatory process.

PHARMACOKINETICS

Rapidly absorbed following PO administration (food reduces absorption). Protein binding: 99%. Extensively metabolized in liver. Primarily excreted in feces. Unknown if removed by hemodialysis. **Half-life:** 10 hrs.

USES

Prophylaxis, chronic treatment of bronchial asthma.

PRECAUTIONS

CONTRAINDICATIONS: None known. **CAUTIONS:** Impaired hepatic function.

LIFESPAN CONSIDERATIONS: Pregnancy/lactation: Distributed in breast milk. Do not administer to breast-feeding women. **Pregnancy Category B. Children:** Safety and efficacy not established in those <5 yrs. **Elderly:** No age-related precautions noted.

INTERACTIONS

DRUG: **Aspirin** increases concentration. Coadministration of **warfarin** increases prothrombin time (PT). **Erythromycin, theophylline** decreases concentration. **HERBAL:** None known. **FOOD:** None known. **LAB VALUES:** May increase SGPT (ALT).

AVAILABILITY (Rx)

TABLETS: 10 mg, 20 mg.

ADMINISTRATION/HANDLING

PO

- Give 1 hr before or 2 hrs after meals.
- Do not crush, break tablets.

INDICATIONS/ROUTES/DOSAGE

BRONCHIAL ASTHMA

PO: ADULTS, ELDERLY, CHILDREN >12 YRS: 20 mg twice daily. CHILDREN 5–12 YRS: 10 mg twice daily.

SIDE EFFECTS

FREQUENT (13%): Headache. **OCCASIONAL (3%):** Nausea, diarrhea. **RARE (<3%):** Generalized pain, asthenia, myalgia, fever, dyspepsia, vomiting, dizziness.

ADVERSE REACTIONS/TOXIC EFFECTS

Coadministration of inhaled corticosteroids increases risk of upper respiratory infection.

NURSING IMPLICATIONS

BASELINE ASSESSMENT

Obtain medication history. Assess hepatic function lab values.

INTERVENTION/EVALUATION

Monitor rate, depth, rhythm, type of respiration; quality, rate of pulse. Assess lung sounds for rhonchi, wheezing, rales. Observe lips, fingernails for blue or dusky color in light-skinned pts; gray in dark-skinned pts. Monitor hepatic function tests.

PATIENT/FAMILY TEACHING

Increase fluid intake (decreases lung secretion viscosity). Take as prescribed, even during symptom-free periods. Do not use for acute asthma episodes. Do not alter/stop other asthma medications. Nursing mothers should not breast-feed. Report nausea, jaundice, abdominal pain, flulike symptoms, worsening of asthma.

zalcitabine

zal-**site**-ah-bean
(Hivid)

CLASSIFICATION

PHARMACOTHERAPEUTIC: Nucleoside reverse transcriptase inhibitor. **CLINICAL:** Antiretroviral (see pp. 60C, 98C).

Z

ACTION

Intracellularly converted to active metabolite. Inhibits viral DNA synthesis. **Therapeutic Effect:** Prevents replication of HIV-1.

PHARMACOKINETICS

Readily absorbed from GI tract (food decreases absorption). Protein binding: <4%. Undergoes phosphorylation intracellularly to the active metabolite. Primarily excreted in urine. Removed by hemodialysis. **Half-life:** 1–3 hrs; metabolite: 2.6–10 hrs (half-life increased with impaired renal function).

USES

Treatment of HIV infection in combination with other antiretroviral agents.

PRECAUTIONS

CONTRAINDICATIONS: Pts with moderate/severe peripheral neuropathy. **EXTREME CAUTION:** Those with low CD4 cell counts (risk of peripheral neuropathy is greater), preexisting neuropathy. **CAUTIONS:** Preexisting peripheral neuropathy, diabetes, weight loss, history of liver disease, alcohol abuse, renal impairment.

LIFESPAN CONSIDERATIONS: Pregnancy/lactation: Unknown if drug crosses placenta or is distributed in breast milk. Avoid breast-feeding in HIV-positive women. **Pregnancy Category C. Children:** No age-related precautions in those <6 mos; dosage not established. **Elderly:** Age-related renal impairment may require dosage adjustment.

INTERACTIONS

DRUG: Medications associated with peripheral neuropathy may increase risk **(e.g., cisplatin, disulfiram, phenytoin, vincristine).** Medications causing pancreatitis may increase risk **(e.g., IV pentamidine). HERBAL:** None known. **FOOD:** None known. **LAB VALUES:** May increase SGOT (AST), SGPT (ALT), alkaline phosphatase, amylase, lipase, triglyceride, bilirubin concentrations. May decrease phosphates, magnesium, calcium. May alter sodium, glucose levels.

AVAILABILITY (Rx)

TABLETS: 0.375 mg, 0.75 mg.

ADMINISTRATION/HANDLING

PO

• Best taken on empty stomach (food decreases absorption). • May take with food to decrease GI distress. • Space doses evenly around the clock.

INDICATIONS/ROUTES/DOSAGE

HIV INFECTION

PO: ADULTS: 0.75 mg q8h (may be given with zidovudine). CHILDREN <13 YRS: 0.01 mg/kg q8h. RANGE: 0.005–0.01 mg/kg q8h.

DOSAGE IN RENAL IMPAIRMENT

Based on creatinine clearance.

Creatinine Clearance	Dose
10–40 ml/min	0.75 mg q12h
<10 ml/min	0.75 mg q24h

SIDE EFFECTS

FREQUENT (11%–28%): Peripheral neuropathy, fever, fatigue, headache, rash. **OCCASIONAL (5%–10%):** Diarrhea, abdominal pain, oral ulcers, cough, pruritus, myalgia, weight loss, nausea, vomiting. **RARE (1%–4%):** Fatigue, nasal discharge, dysphagia, depression, night sweats, confusion.

ADVERSE REACTIONS/ TOXIC EFFECTS

Peripheral neuropathy occurs commonly (17%–31%), characterized by numbness, tingling, burning, pain of lower extremities. May be followed by sharp shooting pain and progress to severe continuous burning pain that may be irreversible if the drug is not discontinued in time. Pancreatitis, leukopenia, neutropenia, eosinophilia, thrombocytopenia occur rarely.

NURSING IMPLICATIONS

BASELINE ASSESSMENT

Offer emotional support to pt, family. Monitor CBC, triglycerides, serum amylase levels prior to and during therapy.

INTERVENTION/EVALUATION

Stop medication, notify physician immediately if signs/symptoms of peripheral neuropathy develop: numbness, tingling, burning, shooting pains of extremities; loss of vibratory sense or ankle reflex. Although rare, be alert to impending potentially fatal pancreatitis: increasing serum amylase, rising triglycerides, nausea, vomiting, abdominal pain (withhold medication, notify physician). Assess for therapeutic response: weight gain, increased energy, decreased fatigue. Assess CBC for evidence of blood dyscrasias.

PATIENT/FAMILY TEACHING

Not a cure for HIV; may continue to contract opportunistic illnesses associated with advanced HIV infection. Does not preclude the need to continue practices to prevent transmission of HIV. Report promptly any signs/symptoms of peripheral neuropathy or pancreatitis (see Adverse Reactions/Toxic Effects). Women of childbearing age should use contraception.

zaleplon

zale-eh-plon
(Sonata, Stamoc ♣)

◆CLASSIFICATION

PHARMACOTHERAPEUTIC: Nonbenzodiazepine. **CLINICAL:** Hypnotic (see p. 130C).

ACTION

Enhances action of inhibitory neurotransmitter gamma-aminobutyric acid (GABA). **Therapeutic Effect:** Produces hypnotic effect.

USES

Short-term treatment of insomnia (7–10 days). Decreases sleep onset time (no effect on number of nocturnal awakenings, total sleep time).

PRECAUTIONS

CONTRAINDICATIONS: Severe hepatic impairment. **CAUTIONS:** Mild to moderate hepatic function in pts experiencing signs/symptoms of depression, those hypersensitive to aspirin (allergic-type reaction). **Pregnancy Category C.**

INTERACTIONS

DRUG: **Alcohol, CNS depressants** may increase CNS depressant effect. **Rifampin** reduces zaleplon concentration. **Cimetidine** increases zaleplon effect. **HERBAL:** None known. **FOOD:** **High-fat/heavy meal** delays sleep onset time by approx. 2 hrs. **LAB VALUES:** None known.

AVAILABILITY (Rx)

CAPSULES: 5 mg, 10 mg.

ADMINISTRATION/HANDLING

PO

• Giving drug with or immediately after a high-fat meal results in slower absorption. • Capsules may be emptied and mixed with food.

INDICATIONS/ROUTES/DOSAGE

HYPNOTIC

PO: ADULTS: 10 mg at bedtime. RANGE: 5–20 mg. ELDERLY: 5 mg at bedtime.

SIDE EFFECTS

EXPECTED: Drowsiness, sedation, mild rebound insomnia on first night after drug is discontinued. **FREQUENT (7%–28%):** Nausea, headache, myalgia, dizziness. **OCCASIONAL (3%–5%):** Abdominal pain, asthenia (loss of strength/energy), dyspepsia, eye pain, paresthesia. **RARE (2%):** Tremors, amnesia, hyperacusis (acute sense of hearing), fever, dysmenorrhea.

ADVERSE REACTIONS/ TOXIC EFFECTS

May produce abnormal thinking/behavioral changes. Taking medication while ambulating may result in memory impairment, hallucination, impaired coordination, dizziness, lightheadedness. Overdosage results in somnolence, confusion, diminished reflexes, coma.

NURSING IMPLICATIONS

BASELINE ASSESSMENT

Raise bed rails. Provide environment conducive to sleep (back rub, quiet environment, low lighting).

INTERVENTION/EVALUATION

Assess sleep pattern.

PATIENT/FAMILY TEACHING

Take right before bedtime or when in bed and not falling asleep. Avoid tasks that require alertness, motor skills until response to drug is established. Do not exceed prescribed dosage. Do not take with or immediately after a high-fat/heavy meal. Rebound insomnia may occur when drug is discontinued after short-term therapy. Avoid alcohol, other CNS depressants.

Zanaflex

see tizanidine

zanamivir

zah-**nam**-ih-vur
(Relenza)

CLASSIFICATION

PHARMACOTHERAPEUTIC: Antiviral. **CLINICAL:** Anti-influenza (see p. 60C).

ACTION

Appears to inhibit the influenza virus enzyme neuraminidase, which is essential for viral replication. **Therapeutic Effect:** Prevents viral release from infected cells.

USES

Treatment of uncomplicated acute illness due to influenza virus in adults, adolescents >12 yrs who have been symptomatic for <2 days. Prevention of influenza A and B.

PRECAUTIONS

CONTRAINDICATIONS: None known. **CAUTIONS:** COPD, asthma. **Pregnancy Category B.**

INTERACTIONS

DRUG: None known. **HERBAL:** None known. **FOOD:** None known. **LAB VAL-**

UES: May increase hepatic enzymes, CPK.

AVAILABILITY (Rx)

BLISTERS OF POWDER FOR INHALATION: 5 mg.

ADMINISTRATION/HANDLING

INHALATION

• Using the Diskhaler device provided, exhale completely; then, holding mouthpiece 1 inch away from lips, inhale and hold breath as long as possible before exhaling. • Rinse mouth with water immediately after inhalation (prevents mouth/throat dryness). • Store at room temperature.

INDICATIONS/ROUTES/DOSAGE

TREATMENT OF INFLUENZA VIRUS

Inhalation: ADULTS, ELDERLY, CHILDREN ≥7 YRS: 2 inhalations (one 5-mg blister per inhalation for a total dose of 10 mg) twice daily (approx. 12 hrs apart) for 5 days.

PREVENTION OF INFLUENZA VIRUS

Inhalation: ADULTS, ELDERLY: 2 inhalations once daily for duration of exposure period.

SIDE EFFECTS

OCCASIONAL (2%–3%): Diarrhea, sinusitis, nausea, bronchitis, cough, dizziness, headache. **RARE (<1.5%):** Malaise, fatigue, fever, abdominal pain, myalgia, arthralgia, urticaria.

ADVERSE REACTIONS/ TOXIC EFFECTS

May produce neutropenia. Bronchospasm may occur in those with history of COPD, bronchial asthma.

NURSING IMPLICATIONS

BASELINE ASSESSMENT

Pts requiring an inhaled bronchodilator at the same time as zanamivir should use the bronchodilator prior to zanamivir administration.

INTERVENTION/EVALUATION

Provide assistance if dizziness occurs. Monitor bowel activity, stool consistency.

PATIENT/FAMILY TEACHING

Instruct on use of delivery device. Avoid contact with those who are at high risk for influenza. Continue treatment for the full 5-day course. Doses should be evenly spaced. In pts with respiratory disease, an inhaled bronchodilator should be readily available.

Zantac

see ranitidine

Zestril

see lisinopril

Zetia

see ezetimibe

zidovudine

zye-**dough**-view-deen
(Apo-Zidovudine✤, AZT, Novo-AZT✤, Retrovir)

Z

Do not confuse with Combivent, ritonavir.

FIXED-COMBINATION(S)

Combivir: zidovudine/lamivudine (an antiviral): 300 mg/150 mg. **Trizivir:** zidovudine/lamivudine/abacavir (an antiviral): 300 mg/150 mg/300 mg.

CLASSIFICATION

PHARMACOTHERAPEUTIC: Nucleoside reverse transcriptase inhibitor. **CLINICAL:** Antiretroviral (see pp. 60C, 99C).

ACTION

Interferes with viral RNA-dependent DNA polymerase, an enzyme necessary for viral HIV replication. **Therapeutic Effect:** Slows HIV replication, reducing progression of HIV infection.

PHARMACOKINETICS

Rapidly, completely absorbed from GI tract. Protein binding: 25%–38%. Undergoes first-pass metabolism in liver. Widely distributed. Crosses blood-brain barrier, CSF. Primarily excreted in urine. Minimal removal by hemodialysis. **Half-life:** 0.8–1.2 hrs (half-life increased with impaired renal function).

USES

Treatment of HIV infection in combination with other antiretroviral agents. **Unlabeled:** Prophylaxis in occupational exposure at risk of acquiring HIV.

PRECAUTIONS

CONTRAINDICATIONS: Life-threatening allergies to zidovudine or components of preparation. **CAUTIONS:** Bone marrow compromise, renal/hepatic dysfunction, decreased hepatic blood flow.

LIFESPAN CONSIDERATIONS: Pregnancy/lactation: Unknown if drug crosses placenta or is distributed in breast milk. Unknown if fetal harm or effects on fertility can occur. **Pregnancy Category C. Children:** No age-related precautions noted. **Elderly:** Information not available.

INTERACTIONS

DRUG: Bone marrow depressants, ganciclovir may increase myelosuppression. **Clarithromycin** may decrease concentrations. **Probenecid** may increase concentrations, risk of toxicity. **HERBAL:** None known. **FOOD:** None known. **LAB VALUES:** May increase mean corpuscular volume.

AVAILABILITY (Rx)

CAPSULES: 100 mg. **TABLETS:** 300 mg. **SYRUP:** 50 mg/5 ml. **INJECTION:** 10 mg/ml.

ADMINISTRATION/HANDLING

PO

• Keep capsules in cool, dry place. Protect from light. • Food, milk do not affect GI absorption. • Space doses evenly around the clock. • Pt should be in upright position when giving medication to prevent esophageal ulceration.

IV

Storage • After dilution, IV solution is stable for 24 hrs at room temperature; 48 hrs if refrigerated. • Use within 8 hrs if stored at room temperature; 24 hrs if refrigerated. • Do not use if particulate matter is present or discoloration occurs.

Reconstitution • Must dilute before administration. • Remove calculated dose from vial and add to D_5W to provide a concentration no greater than 4 mg/ml.

Rate of administration • Infuse over 1 hr.

∅ IV INCOMPATIBILITY
None known.

IV COMPATIBILITIES
Dexamethasone (Decadron), dobutamine (Dobutrex), dopamine (Intropin), heparin, lorazepam (Ativan), morphine, potassium chloride.

INDICATIONS/ROUTES/DOSAGE

HIV

IV: ADULTS, ELDERLY, CHILDREN >12 YRS: 1–2 mg/kg/dose q4h. CHILDREN ≤12 YRS: 120 mg/m²/dose q6h. NEONATES: 1.5 mg/kg/dose q6h.

PO: ADULTS, ELDERLY, CHILDREN >12 YRS: 200 mg q8h or 300 mg q12h. CHILDREN ≤12 YRS: 160 mg/m²/dose q8h. RANGE: 90–180 mg/m²/dose q6–8h. NEONATES: 2 mg/kg/dose q6h.

SIDE EFFECTS

COMMON (42%–46%): Nausea, headache. **FREQUENT (16%–20%):** GI pain, asthenia (loss of strength, energy), rash, fever. **OCCASIONAL (8%–12%):** Diarrhea, anorexia, malaise, myalgia, somnolence. **RARE (5%–6%):** Dizziness, paresthesia, vomiting, insomnia, dyspnea, altered taste.

ADVERSE REACTIONS/ TOXIC EFFECTS

Anemia (occurring most commonly after 4–6 wks of therapy), granulocytopenia, particularly significant in pts with pretherapy low baselines, occur rarely. Neurotoxicity (ataxia, fatigue, lethargy, nystagmus), seizures may occur.

NURSING IMPLICATIONS

BASELINE ASSESSMENT

Avoid drugs that are nephrotoxic, cytotoxic, myelosuppressive—may increase risk of toxicity. Obtain specimens for viral diagnostic tests before starting therapy (therapy may begin before results are obtained). Check hematology reports for accurate baseline.

INTERVENTION/EVALUATION

Monitor CBC, Hgb, MCV, reticulocyte count, CD4 cell count, HIV RNA plasma levels. Check for bleeding. Assess for headache, dizziness. Determine pattern of bowel activity. Evaluate skin for acne, rash. Be alert to development of opportunistic infections (e.g., fever, chills, cough, myalgia). Monitor I&O, renal and hepatic function tests. Check for insomnia.

PATIENT/FAMILY TEACHING

Doses should be evenly spaced around the clock. Zidovudine does not cure AIDS or HIV disease, but acts to reduce symptoms and slows/arrests progress of disease. Do not take any medications without physician approval. Bleeding from gums, nose, rectum may occur and should be reported to physician immediately. Blood counts are essential because of bleeding potential. Dental work should be done before therapy or after blood counts return to normal (often weeks after therapy has stopped). Inform physician if muscle weakness, difficulty breathing, headache, inability to sleep, unusual bleeding, rash, signs of infection occur.

zileuton

zye-**lew**-ton
(Zyflo)

◆ CLASSIFICATION

PHARMACOTHERAPEUTIC: Leukotriene inhibitor. **CLINICAL:** Antiasthma (see p. 66C).

ACTION

Inhibits the enzyme responsible for producing inflammatory response. Prevents formation of leukotrienes (leukotrienes induce bronchoconstriction response, enhance vascular permeability, stimulate mucus secretion). **Therapeutic Effect:** Prevents airway edema, smooth muscle contraction, inflammatory process, relieving signs/symptoms of bronchial asthma.

PHARMACOKINETICS

Rapidly, completely absorbed following PO administration. Protein binding: 93%. Metabolized in the liver. Eliminated in feces. Not removed by dialysis. **Half-life:** 2.5 hrs.

USES

Prophylaxis and chronic treatment of asthma. Not for use in reversal of bronchospasm in acute asthma attacks, status asthmaticus, exercise-induced bronchospasm.

PRECAUTIONS

CONTRAINDICATIONS: Active hepatic disease, impaired hepatic function. **CAUTIONS:** History of hypersensitivity to zileuton, alcoholism, liver disease.

LIFESPAN CONSIDERATIONS: Pregnancy/lactation: Unknown if distributed in breast milk. **Pregnancy Category C. Children:** Safety and efficacy not established in those <12 yrs. **Elderly:** No age-related precautions noted.

INTERACTIONS

DRUG: May increase concentration/toxicity of **cyclosporine, calcium channel blockers (i.e., nifedipine), theophylline.** Increases PT in those receiving **warfarin.** May increase effects of **beta-blockers (e.g., propranolol).** **HERBAL:** None known. **FOOD:** None known. **LAB VALUES:** May increase liver transaminase, SGPT (ALT).

AVAILABILITY (Rx)

TABLETS: 600 mg.

ADMINISTRATION/HANDLING

PO

- Give without regard to food.

INDICATIONS/ROUTES/DOSAGE

BRONCHIAL ASTHMA

PO: ADULTS, ELDERLY, CHILDREN ≥12 YRS: One 600-mg tablet 4 times/day. TOTAL DAILY DOSAGE: 2,400 mg.

SIDE EFFECTS

FREQUENT (25%): Headache. **OCCASIONAL (3%–8%):** Dyspepsia, nausea, abdominal pain, asthenia (loss of strength), myalgia. **RARE (1%):** Conjunctivitis, constipation, dizziness, flatulence, insomnia.

ADVERSE REACTIONS/ TOXIC EFFECTS

Hepatic dysfunction occurs rarely and may be manifested as right upper quadrant pain, nausea, fatigue, lethargy, pruritus, jaundice, flulike symptoms.

NURSING IMPLICATIONS

BASELINE ASSESSMENT

Obtain baseline hepatic transaminase level, SGPT (ALT) prior to beginning therapy. Monitor transaminase levels routinely thereafter. Monitor SGPT (ALT) monthly for the first 3 mos, q2–3mos for the remainder of the first year, and periodically thereafter during long-term therapy.

INTERVENTION/EVALUATION

Monitor rate, depth, rhythm, type of respirations; quality/rate of pulse. Assess lung sounds for rhonchi, wheezing, rales. Observe lips, fingernails for blue/dusky color in light-skinned pts, gray in dark-skinned pts. Monitor hepatic function test results.

PATIENT/FAMILY TEACHING

Increase fluid intake (decreases lung secretion viscosity). Take as prescribed, even during symptom-free periods as well as during worsening asthma. Do not alter/stop other asthma medications. Drug is not for the treatment of acute asthma attacks. Report if right upper quadrant pain, nausea, fatigue, yellowing of skin/eyes, flulike symptoms occur.

Zinacef

see cefuroxime

ziprasidone

zip-**rah**-zih-doan
(Geodon)

CLASSIFICATION

PHARMACOTHERAPEUTIC: Piperazine derivative. **CLINICAL:** Antipsychotic (see p. 57C).

ACTION

Antagonizes dopamine, serotonin, histamine, alpha$_1$-adrenergic receptors; inhibits reuptake of serotonin, norepinephrine. **Therapeutic Effect:** Diminishes schizophrenic, antidepressant symptoms.

PHARMACOKINETICS

Extensively metabolized in liver. Food increases bioavailability. Protein binding: 99%. Not removed by hemodialysis. **Half-life:** 7 hrs.

USES

Treatment of schizophrenia.

PRECAUTIONS

CONTRAINDICATIONS: Conditions associated with a risk of prolonging the QT interval. **CAUTIONS:** Pts with bradycardia, hypokalemia, hypomagnesemia may be at greater risk for torsades de pointes.

LIFESPAN CONSIDERATIONS: Pregnancy/lactation: Unknown if drug crosses placenta or is distributed in breast milk. **Pregnancy Category C. Children:** Safety and efficacy not established. **Elderly:** No age-related precautions noted.

INTERACTIONS

DRUG: Carbamazepine may decrease concentration. **Ketoconazole** may increase concentration. **Alcohol, CNS depressants** may increase CNS depression. **HERBAL:** None known. **FOOD:** Food enhances bioavailability. **LAB VALUES:** May produce prolongation of QT interval.

AVAILABILITY (Rx)

CAPSULES: 20 mg, 40 mg, 60 mg, 80 mg. **INJECTION:** 20 mg/ml.

ADMINISTRATION/HANDLING

PO

- Give with food (increases bioavailability).

IM

- Store vials at room temperature, protect from light. • Reconstitute each vial with 1.2 ml Sterile Water for Injection to provide a concentration of 20 mg/ml. • Reconstituted solution stable for 24 hrs at room temperature or 7 days refrigerated.

INDICATIONS/ROUTES/DOSAGE

SCHIZOPHRENIA

PO: ADULTS, ELDERLY: Initially, 20 mg twice daily with food. Titrate at intervals of no less than 2 days. **Maximum:** 80 mg twice daily.

IM: ADULTS, ELDERLY: 10 mg q2h or 20 mg q4h. **Maximum:** 40 mg/day.

SIDE EFFECTS

FREQUENT (16%–30%): Headache, somnolence, dizziness. **OCCASIONAL:** Rash, orthostatic hypotension, weight gain, restlessness, constipation, dyspepsia (heartburn, gastric upset).

ADVERSE REACTIONS/ TOXIC EFFECTS

Prolongation of QT interval as seen in EKG may produce torsades de pointes (a form of ventricular tachycardia). Pts with bradycardia, hypokalemia, hypomagnesemia are at increased risk.

NURSING IMPLICATIONS

BASELINE ASSESSMENT

Assess pt's behavior, appearance, emotional status, response to environment, speech pattern, thought content. An EKG should be administered to assess for QT prolongation prior to instituting medication. Blood chemistry for magnesium, potassium should be obtained prior to beginning therapy and routinely thereafter.

INTERVENTION/EVALUATION

Assess for therapeutic response (greater interest in surroundings, improved self-care, increased ability to concentrate, relaxed facial expression). Monitor weight.

PATIENT/FAMILY TEACHING

Avoid tasks that require alertness, motor skills until response to drug is established.

Zithromax

see azithromycin

Zocor

see simvastatin

Zofran

see ondansetron

zoledronic acid

zole-eh-**dron**-ick
(Zometa)

◆ CLASSIFICATION

PHARMACOTHERAPEUTIC: Bisphosphonate. **CLINICAL:** Calcium regulator, bone resorption inhibitor.

ACTION

Inhibits resorption of mineralized bone, cartilage; inhibits increased osteoclastic activity, skeletal calcium release induced by stimulatory factors released by tumors. **Therapeutic Effect:** Increases urinary calcium and phosphorus excretion; decreases serum calcium and phosphorus levels.

USES

Treatment of hypercalcemia of malignancy (albumin-corrected serum calcium of >12 mg/dl). Treatment of multiple myeloma.

PRECAUTIONS

CONTRAINDICATIONS: Hypersensitivity to other bisphosphonates (etidronate, pamidronate, tiludronate, risedronate, alendronate). **CAUTIONS:** History of aspirin-sensitive asthma, renal impairment, hypoparathyroidism, risk of hypocalcemia. **Pregnancy Category C.**

INTERACTIONS

DRUG: Calcium-containing medications, vitamin D may antagonize effects in treatment of hypercalcemia. **HERBAL:** None known. **FOOD:** None known. **LAB VALUES:** May decrease calcium, phosphate, magnesium levels.

AVAILABILITY (Rx)

INJECTION: 4 mg/vial of lyophilized powder.

ADMINISTRATION/HANDLING

Alert: Pt should be adequately rehydrated prior to administration of zoledronic acid.

IV

Storage • Store at room temperature. • If not used immediately, reconstituted solution should be refrigerated; time from reconstitution to end of administration should not exceed 24 hrs.

Reconstitution • Reconstitute 4-mg vial with 5 ml Sterile Water for Injection. Allow drug to dissolve prior to withdrawing. • Further dilute with 100 ml 0.9% NaCl or D_5W.

Rate of administration • Adequate hydration is essential in conjunction with zoledronic acid • Administer as an IV infusion over not less than 15 min (increases risk of deterioration in renal function).

IV INCOMPATIBILITY
Do not mix with any other medications.

INDICATIONS/ROUTES/DOSAGE

Alert: Pt should be adequately rehydrated prior to administration.

HYPERCALCEMIA
IV infusion: ADULTS, ELDERLY: 4 mg given as an IV infusion over no less than 15 min. Retreatment may be considered, but wait at least 7 days to allow for full response to initial dose.

SIDE EFFECTS

FREQUENT (26%–44%): Fever, nausea, vomiting, constipation. **OCCASIONAL (10%–15%):** Hypotension, anxiety, insomnia, flulike syndrome (fever, chills, bone pain, joint pain, muscle aches), nausea, vomiting, constipation. **RARE:** Conjunctivitis.

ADVERSE REACTIONS/ TOXIC EFFECTS

Renal toxicity may occur if IV infusion is administered in <15 min.

NURSING IMPLICATIONS

BASELINE ASSESSMENT

Establish baseline electrolytes.

INTERVENTION/EVALUATION

Monitor renal function, CBC, Hgb, Hct. Assess vertebral bone mass (document stabilization/improvement). Monitor serum calcium, phosphate, magnesium, serum creatinine levels. Assess for fever. Monitor food intake, stool frequency. Check I&O, BUN, creatinine in pts with impaired renal function.

Z

zolmitriptan

zoll-mih-**trip**-tan
(Zomig, Zomig-ZMT)

CLASSIFICATION

PHARMACOTHERAPEUTIC: Serotonin receptor agonist. **CLINICAL:** Antimigraine (see p. 55C).

ACTION

Binds selectively to vascular receptors, producing a vasoconstrictive effect on cranial blood vessels. **Therapeutic Effect:** Relieves migraine headache.

PHARMACOKINETICS

Rapidly but incompletely absorbed following PO administration. Protein binding: 15%. Undergoes first-pass metabolism in the liver to active metabolite. Eliminated primarily in the urine (60%), with lesser amount excreted in the feces (30%). **Half-life:** 3 hrs.

USES

Treatment of acute migraine attack with or without aura.

PRECAUTIONS

CONTRAINDICATIONS: Coronary artery disease, uncontrolled hypertension, ischemic heart disease (angina pectoris, history of MI, silent ischemia), Prinzmetal's angina, concurrent use (or within 24 hrs) of ergotamine-containing preparations, concurrent use (or within 2 wks) of MAOI, hemiplegic or basilar migraine, within 24 hrs of another serotonin receptor agonist, Wolff-Parkinson-White syndrome, arrhythmias associated with cardiac conduction pathways disorders. **CAUTIONS:** Mild to moderate renal/hepatic impairment, pt profile suggesting cardiovascular risks, controlled hypertension, history of CVA.

LIFESPAN CONSIDERATIONS: Pregnancy/lactation: Unknown if distributed in breast milk. **Pregnancy Category C. Children:** Safety and efficacy not established in those <12 yrs. **Elderly:** No age-related precautions noted.

INTERACTIONS

DRUG: Ergotamine-containing drugs may produce vasospastic reaction. **MAOIs** may dramatically increase plasma concentration of zolmitriptan. Combined use of **fluoxetine, fluvoxamine, paroxetine, sertraline** may produce weakness, hyper-reflexia, incoordination. **Oral contraceptives** reduce zolmitriptan's clearance, volume of distribution. **HERBAL:** None known. **FOOD:** None known. **LAB VALUES:** None known.

AVAILABILITY (Rx)

TABLETS: 2.5 mg, 5 mg. **ORAL DISINTEGRATING TABLETS:** 2.5 mg, 5 mg.

ADMINISTRATION/HANDLING

PO

- Give without regard to food.

NASAL

- Gently blow nose to clear nasal passages. • With head upright, close one nostril with index finger. Breathe out gently through mouth. • Insert nozzle into open nostril about ½ inch. • Close mouth, and while taking a breath through nose, release spray dosage by firmly pressing the plunger. • Remove nozzle from nose, gently breathe in through nose and out through mouth for 15–20 sec. Do not breathe in deeply.

INDICATIONS/ROUTES/DOSAGE

MIGRAINE

PO: ADULTS, ELDERLY, CHILDREN >18 YRS: Initially, ≤2.5 mg. If headache returns, may repeat dose in 2 hrs. **Maximum:** 10 mg/24 hrs. **NASAL:** ADULTS, ELDERLY: 5 mg, may repeat in 2 hrs.

SIDE EFFECTS

FREQUENT (6%–8%): Dizziness, tingling, neck/throat/jaw pressure, somnolence. **Nasal:** Unusual taste, paresthesia. **OCCASIONAL (3%–5%):** Sensation of warm/hot, weakness, chest pressure. **Nasal:** Nausea, somnolence, discomfort of nasal cavity, dizziness, asthenia, dry mouth. **RARE (1%–2%):** Diaphoresis, myalgia, paresthesia.

ADVERSE REACTIONS/ TOXIC EFFECTS

Cardiac events (ischemia, coronary artery vasospasm, MI), noncardiac vasospasm-related reactions (hemorrhage, stroke) occur rarely but particularly in pts with hypertension, obesity, smokers, diabetes, strong family history of coronary artery disease, male >40 yrs, postmenopausal women.

NURSING IMPLICATIONS

BASELINE ASSESSMENT

Question for history of peripheral vascular disease or coronary artery disease, renal/hepatic impairment, use of MAOIs. Question pt regarding onset, location, duration of migraine, possible precipitating symptoms.

INTERVENTION/EVALUATION

Monitor for evidence of dizziness. Monitor B/P, esp. in pts with hepatic impairment. Assess for relief of migraine headache and migraine potential for photophobia, phonophobia (sound sensitivity, light sensitivity, nausea, vomiting).

PATIENT/FAMILY TEACHING

Take a single dose as soon as symptoms of an actual migraine attack appear. Medication is intended to relieve migraine, not to prevent or reduce number of attacks. Lie down in quiet dark room for additional benefit after taking medication. Avoid tasks that require alertness, motor skills until response to drug is established. Report chest pain, palpitations, tightness in throat, swelling of face/lips/eyes, rash, easy bruising, blood in urine/stool, pain/numbness in arms/legs.

Zoloft

see sertraline

zolpidem tartrate

zole-pih-dem

(Ambien)

Do not confuse with Amen.

CLASSIFICATION

PHARMACOTHERAPEUTIC: Nonbenzodiazepine. **CLINICAL:** Sedative-hypnotic **(Schedule IV)** (see p. 130C).

ACTION

Enhances action of GABA, an inhibitory neurotransmitter in the CNS. **Therapeutic Effect:** Produces hypnotic effect, induces sleep with fewer nightly awakenings, improves sleep quality.

PHARMACOKINETICS

	Onset	Peak	Duration
PO	30 min	—	6–8 hr

Rapidly absorbed from GI tract. Protein binding: 92%. Metabolized in liver; excreted in urine. Not removed by hemodialysis. **Half-life:** 1.4–4.5 hrs (half-life increased with impaired hepatic function).

USES

Short-term treatment of insomnia. Reduces sleep-induction time, number of nocturnal awakenings; increases length of sleep; improves sleep quality.

PRECAUTIONS

CONTRAINDICATIONS: None known. **CAUTIONS:** Impaired hepatic function, pts with depression, history of drug dependence.

LIFESPAN CONSIDERATIONS: Pregnancy/lactation: Unknown if drug crosses placenta or is distributed in breast milk. **Pregnancy Category B. Children:** Safety and efficacy not established. **Elderly:** More likely to experience falls or confusion; decreased initial doses recommended. Age-related hepatic impairment may require dosage adjustment.

INTERACTIONS

DRUG: Potentiated effects when used with other **CNS depressants. HERBAL:** None known. **FOOD:** None known. **LAB VALUES:** None known.

AVAILABILITY (Rx)

TABLETS: 5 mg, 10 mg. **ORAL DISINTEGRATING TABLETS:** 5 mg, 10 mg.

ADMINISTRATION/HANDLING

PO

- For faster sleep onset, do not give with or immediately after a meal.

INDICATIONS/ROUTES/DOSAGE

HYPNOTIC

PO: ADULTS: 10 mg at bedtime. ELDERLY, DEBILITATED: 5 mg at bedtime.

SIDE EFFECTS

OCCASIONAL (7%): Headache. **RARE (<2%):** Dizziness, nausea, diarrhea, muscle pain.

ADVERSE REACTIONS/ TOXIC EFFECTS

Overdosage may produce severe ataxia (clumsiness, unsteadiness), bradycardia, diplopia, altered vision, severe drowsiness, nausea, vomiting, difficulty breathing, unconsciousness. Abrupt withdrawal of drug after long-term use may produce weakness, facial flushing, diaphoresis, vomiting, tremor. Tolerance/dependence may occur with prolonged use of high dosages.

NURSING IMPLICATIONS

BASELINE ASSESSMENT

Assess B/P, pulse, respirations. Raise bed rails, provide call light. Provide environment conducive to sleep (back rub, quiet environment, low lighting).

INTERVENTION/EVALUATION

Assess sleep pattern of pt. Evaluate for therapeutic response to insomnia: decrease in number of nocturnal awakenings, increase in length of sleep.

PATIENT/FAMILY TEACHING

Do not abruptly withdraw medication after long-term use. Avoid alcohol, tasks that require alertness, motor skills until response to drug is established. Tolerance/dependence may occur with prolonged use of high dosages.

zonisamide

zoe-**niss**-ah-mide
(Zonegran)

CLASSIFICATION

PHARMACOTHERAPEUTIC: Succinimide. **CLINICAL:** Anticonvulsant (see p. 33C).

ACTION

May stabilize neuronal membranes and suppress neuronal hypersynchronization by action at sodium and calcium channels. **Therapeutic Effect:** Produces anticonvulsant effect.

PHARMACOKINETICS

Well absorbed following PO administration. Extensively bound to erythrocytes. Protein binding: 40%. Primarily excreted in urine. **Half-life:** 63 hrs (plasma), 105 hrs (RBCs).

USES

Adjunctive therapy in the treatment of partial seizures in adults with epilepsy.

PRECAUTIONS

CONTRAINDICATIONS: Allergy to sulfonamides. **CAUTIONS:** Renal function impairment.

LIFESPAN CONSIDERATIONS: Pregnancy/lactation: Unknown if distributed in breast milk. **Pregnancy Category C. Children:** Safety and efficacy not established in those <16 yrs. **Elderly:** No age-related precautions noted but lower dosages recommended.

INTERACTIONS

DRUG: Carbamazepine, phenobarbital, phenytoin, valproic acid may increase metabolism, decrease effect. **HERBAL:** None known. **FOOD:** None known. **LAB VALUES:** May increase serum creatinine, BUN.

AVAILABILITY (Rx)

CAPSULES: 25 mg, 50 mg, 100 mg.

ADMINISTRATION/HANDLING

PO

• May take with or without food. • Swallow capsules whole. • Do not give to pts allergic to sulfonamides.

INDICATIONS/ROUTES/DOSAGE

PARTIAL SEIZURES

PO: ADULTS, CHILDREN >16 YRS: Initially, 100 mg/day for 2 wks. May increase by 100 mg/day at intervals of ≥2 wks. **Maximum:** 400 mg/day.

SIDE EFFECTS

FREQUENT (9%–17%): Somnolence, dizziness, anorexia, headache, agitation, irritability, nausea. **OCCASIONAL (5%–8%):** Fatigue, ataxia, confusion, depression, memory/concentration impairment, insomnia, abdominal pain, double vision, diarrhea, speech difficulty. **RARE (3%–4%):** Paresthesia, nystagmus (involuntary movement of eyeball), anxiety, rash, dyspepsia (heartburn, indigestion, epigastric distress), weight loss.

ADVERSE REACTIONS/ TOXIC EFFECTS

Overdosage characterized by bradycardia, hypotension, respiratory depression, comatose state. Leukopenia, anemia, thrombocytopenia occur rarely.

NURSING IMPLICATIONS

BASELINE ASSESSMENT

Anticonvulsant: Review history of seizure disorder (intensity, frequency, duration, LOC). Initiate seizure precautions. Hepatic function tests, CBC, platelet count should be performed before therapy begins and periodically during therapy.

INTERVENTION/EVALUATION

Observe frequently for recurrence of seizure activity. Assess for clinical improvement (decrease in intensity/frequency of seizures). Assist with ambulation if dizziness occurs.

PATIENT/FAMILY TEACHING

Strict maintenance of drug therapy is essential for seizure control. Avoid tasks that require alertness, motor skills until response to drug is established. Avoid alcohol. Report if rash, back/abdominal pain, blood in urine, fever, sore throat, ulcers in mouth, easy bruising occurs.

Zosyn

see piperacillin/tazobactam

Zovirax

see acyclovir

Zyloprim

see allopurinol

Zyprexa

see olanzapine

Zyrtec

see cetirizine

Appendixes

Appendix A
(Poison) Antidote Chart

Appendix B
Calculation of Doses

Appendix C
Controlled Drugs (United States)

Appendix D
Cultural Aspects of Drug Therapy

Appendix E
Drugs of Abuse

Appendix F
FDA Pregnancy Categories

Appendix G
Herbal Therapies/Interactions

Appendix H
Normal Laboratory Values

Appendix I
Recommended Childhood and Adult Immunizations

Appendix J
Signs and Symptoms of Electrolyte Imbalance

Appendix K
Spanish Phrases Often Used in Clinical Settings

Appendix L
Techniques of Medication Administration

Appendix A

(POISON) ANTIDOTE CHART

Poison/Drug	Indications	Antidote	Dosage
acetaminophen	Treatment of acetaminophen overdose to protect against hepatotoxicity.	*N*-acetylcysteine (Mucomyst)	Dilute to 5% solution with carbonated beverage, fruit juice, or water and administer orally. **Loading:** 140 mg/kg for one dose. **Maintenance:** 70 mg/kg for 17 doses, starting 4 hrs after loading dose and given q4h.
arsenic, gold, mercury, lead	Treatment of arsenic, gold, mercury if started within 1–2 hrs; treatment of acute lead poisoning of levels >70 mcg/dl (with calcium EDTA) (do **not** use for chronic mercury poisoning).	Dimercaprol (BAL in oil)	Deep IM injections. **Mild arsenic/gold:** 2.5 mg/kg 4×/day for 2 days, 2×/day for 1 day, then once daily for up to 10 days. **Severe arsenic/gold:** 3 mg/kg q4h for 2 days then 4×/day for 1 day, then 2×/day for up to 10 days. **Mercury:** 5 mg/kg, then 2.5 mg/kg 1–2×/day for 10 days. **Acute lead encephalopathy:** 4 mg/kg alone in first dose, then at 4-hr intervals with calcium EDTA (give at separate sites). **Less severe lead:** After first dose, 3 mg/kg. Continue for 2–7 days as needed.
arsenic, lead, mercury	Treatment of lead poisoning with levels of >45 mcg/dl. Treatment of arsenic and mercury poisoning.	Succimer, DMSA	10 mg/kg orally 3×/day for 5 days, then 10 mg/kg 2×/day for additional 14 days.

Poison/Drug	Indications	Antidote	Dosage
atropine, anticholinergic agents, antihistamines, plants containing anticholinergic agents	Reverse toxic effects on the central nervous system (CNS) caused by drugs and plants capable of producing anticholinergic poisoning in clinical or toxic dosages (including tricyclic antidepressants).	physostigmine (Antilirium)	**Children:** 0.02 mg/kg IM or slow IV injection (0.5 mg/min). May repeat at 5- to 10-min intervals until therapeutic response or maximum dose of 2 mg is attained. **Adults:** Slow IV push (1 mg/min): 0.5–2 mg; may repeat if life-threatening signs, including arrhythmias, convulsions, coma, occur.
benzodiazepines	Complete or partial reversal of sedative effects of benzodiazepines when general anesthesia has been induced and/or maintained with benzodiazepines, when sedation has been produced with benzodiazepines for diagnostic and therapeutic procedures, management of benzodiazepine overdosage.	flumazenil (Romazicon)	***IV: Adults, elderly:*** Initially, 0.2 mg (2 ml) over 30 sec; may repeat after 30 sec with 0.3 mg (3 ml) over 30 sec if desired level of consciousness not achieved. Further doses of 0.5 mg (5 ml) over 30 sec may be administered at 60-sec intervals. **Maximum:** 3 mg (30 ml) total dose. **Alert:** If resedation occurs, repeat dose at 20-min intervals. **Maximum:** 1 mg (given as 0.5 mg/min) at any one time, 3 mg in any 1 hr.
cyanide, nitroprusside	Begin treatment at first sign of toxicity if exposure is known or strongly suspected.	amyl nitrite, sodium nitrite, sodium thiosulfate (Cyanide Antidote Kit)	First, crush amyl nitrite pearls in gauze and allow patient to inhale for 15 sec, then remove for 15 sec. Use a fresh pearl every 3 min. Continue until injection of 10 ml of 3% (300 mg) sodium nitrite in adults. Inject over 2–5 min. Pediatric dose based on Hgb level; if normal Hgb assumed, then 0.15–0.33 ml/kg sodium nitrite up to

(continued)

Poison/Drug	Indications	Antidote	Dosage
cyanide, nitroprusside *(continued)*			10 ml may be used. After sodium nitrite, immediately inject 50 ml of 25% sodium thiosulfate (12.5 g), slow IV, over 10 min. Use 7 g/m^2 maximum of 12.5 g, in children.
digoxin	Treatment of potentially life-threatening digoxin intoxication.	digoxin-immune Fab (Digibind)	Dose in number of vials = steady-state digoxin level in mg/ml × patient weight in kg divided by 100. 4–6 vials adequate to treat 90%–95% of patients with chronic digoxin toxicity. If ingested amount is unknown, give 10–20 vials (400–800 mg). Administer IV over 30 min through a 0.22-micron filter. A bolus injection can be given if cardiac arrest is imminent.
ethylene glycol	Ethylene glycol blood levels >20 mg/dl. Blood levels not readily available and suspected ingestion of toxic amounts. Any symptomatic patient with a history of ethylene glycol ingestion.	fomepizole (Antizol)	**Loading:** 15 mg/kg IV over 30 min followed by 10 mg/kg q12h for 4 doses, then 15 mg/kg q12h until ethylene glycol levels are <20 mg/dl.
hydrofluoric acid (HF), fluoride salts	Calcium gluconate 2.5% gel for dermal exposure to HF <20% concentration. Subcutaneous injections of calcium gluconate for dermal exposures of HF in >20% concentration or failure to respond to calcium gluconate gel. IV calcium gluconate 10% for serious systemic toxicity following dermal exposure, or ingestion of fluoride salts.	calcium gluconate	Massage 2.5% gel into exposed area for 15 min, repeating as necessary for pain. Infiltrate each cm^2 of exposed area with 0.5 ml 10% calcium gluconate SC, using a 30-gauge needle. Give 0.1–0.2 ml/kg IV 10% calcium gluconate slowly up to 10 ml. Repeat dose if necessary.

Poison/Drug	Indications	Antidote	Dosage
iron	Acute iron intoxication. Chronic iron overload.	deferoxamine (Desferal)	**Acute iron intoxication:** ***IM:*** 1 g, then 0.5 g q4h × 2 doses, then 0.5 g q4–12h. May give IV infusion 10–15 mg/kg/hr. Do not exceed 6 g in 24 hrs. **Chronic iron overload:** ***IM:*** 0.5–1 g daily. ***Subcutaneous:*** 1–2 g/day (20–40 mg/kg/day) over 8–24 hrs. **Children:** Maximum of 6 g/24 hrs or 2 g/dose.
lead	Acute and chronic lead poisoning, lead encephalopathy.	calcium EDTA	**Adults:** 1 g in 250–500 ml NaCl or D_5W over >1 hr for 5 days, stop for 2 days, then repeat for 5 days if needed.
miscellaneous medications	Treatment of drug overdose.	ipecac	**Children <1 yr:** 5–10 ml, then ½–1 glass of water. **Children ≥1–12 yrs:** 15 ml followed by 1–2 glasses of water. **Adults:** 15–30 ml followed by 3–4 glasses of water. **Alert:** Repeat dose (15 ml) once in those >1 yr if vomiting does not occur within 20–30 min. Perform gastric lavage if vomiting does not occur within 30–45 min after second dose.
miscellaneous medication poisoning	Treatment of drug poisoning.	charcoal, activated	**Adults:** 25–100 g (or 1 g/kg or approx. 10 times the amount of poison ingested) as a suspension (4–8 oz of water). Multiple doses may be used in severe poisoning to prevent desorption from the charcoal; also increases GI clearance and rate of elimination of drugs that undergo an enteral recirculation pattern.

(continued)

Poison/Drug	Indications	Antidote	Dosage
opiates, $alpha_2$-agonists (e.g., clonidine)	Opiate overdose. Coma or respiratory depression of unknown origin.	naloxone (Narcan) nalmefene (Revex)	**Naloxone: Adults:** Give 0.4–2 mg IV bolus. Doses may be repeated q2–5min up to 10 mg if no response. **Children:** 0.01 mg/kg. May repeat with 0.1 mg/kg. **Alert:** AAP recommends initial dose of 0.1 mg/kg for infants and children up to 5 yrs and weighing <20 kg. **Children >5 yrs or ≥20 kg:** Recommended initial dose 2 mg. **Nalmefene:** 0.5–1 mg IV q2min as needed to a total of 2 mg.
organophosphate insecticides	Synergistic adjunct to atropine therapy. Reverses nicotinic effects such as profound muscle weakness, respiratory depression, and muscle twitching. Organophosphate poisoning. Anticholinesterase drug overdose.	pralidoxime (2-PAM) (Protopam)	**Children:** ***IV:*** 25–50 mg/kg up to 1 g in 250 ml NaCl over 30 min. **Adults:** ***IV:*** 1–2 g in 100 ml NaCl over 15–30 min. If pulmonary edema present, may give as a 5% solution slow IV push over not less than 5 min. Dosage may be repeated in 1 hr followed by q8h if indicated.

Appendix B

CALCULATION OF DOSES

Frequently, dosages ordered do not correspond exactly to what is available and must therefore be calculated.

Ratio/proportions: Most important in setting up this calculation is that the units of measure are the same on both sides of the equation.

Problem: Pt A is to receive 65 mg of a medication only available in an 80 mg/2 ml vial. What volume (ml) needs to be administered to the pt?

STEP 1: Set up ratio.

$$\frac{80}{2\text{ ml}} = \frac{65}{x(\text{ml})}$$

STEP 2: Cross multiply.

$$(80\text{ mg})(x\text{ ml}) = (65\text{ mg})(2\text{ ml})$$
$$80\,x = 130$$

STEP 3: Divide each side of equation by number with x.

$$\frac{80\,x}{80} = \frac{130}{80}$$

STEP 4: Volume to be administered for correct dose.

$$x = 130/80 \text{ or } 1.625\text{ ml}$$

Calculations in micrograms/kilogram per minute: Frequently, medications given by IV infusion are ordered as micrograms/kilogram per minute.

Problem: 63-year-old pt (weight 165 lbs) is to receive Medication A at a rate of 8 micrograms/kilogram per minute (mcg/kg/min). Given a solution containing Medication A in a concentration of 500 mg/250 ml, at what rate (ml/hr) would you infuse this medication?

STEP 1: Convert to same units. In this problem, the dose is expressed in mcg/kg; therefore convert pt weight to kg (1 kg = 2.2 lbs) and drug concentration to mcg (1 mg = 1,000 mcg).

$$165\text{ lbs} \times \frac{1\text{ kg}}{2.2\text{ lbs}} = \frac{165\text{ kg}}{2.2} = 75\text{ kg}$$

$$\frac{500\text{ mg}}{250\text{ ml}} \text{ or } \frac{2\text{ mg}}{\text{ml}} \times \frac{1{,}000\text{ mcg}}{1\text{ mg}} = \frac{2{,}000\text{ mcg}}{1\text{ ml}} \text{ or } \frac{1\text{ ml}}{2{,}000\text{ mcg}}$$

STEP 2: Number of micrograms per minute (mcg/min).

$$\frac{8\text{ mcg}}{\text{kg}} \times 75\text{ kg(pt wt)} = \frac{600\text{ mcg}}{1\text{ min}} \text{ or } \frac{1\text{ min}}{600\text{ mcg}}$$

STEP 3: Number of milliliters per minute (ml/min).

$$\frac{600\ \text{mcg}}{1\ \text{min}} \times \frac{1\ \text{ml}}{2{,}000\ \text{mcg}} = \frac{600(\text{ml})}{2{,}000(\text{min})} = \frac{0.3\ \text{ml}}{\text{min}}$$

STEP 4: Number of milliliters per hour (ml/hr).

$$\frac{0.3\ \text{ml}}{\text{min}} \times \frac{60\ \text{min}}{1\ \text{hr}} = \frac{18\ \text{ml}}{\text{hr}}$$

STEP 5: If the number of drops per minute (gtts/min) were desired, and if the IV set delivered 60 drops per milliliter (gtts/ml) (varies with IV set, information provided by manufacturer), then:

$$\frac{0.3\ \text{ml}}{\text{min}} \times \frac{60\ \text{drops}}{\text{ml}} = \frac{18\ \text{drops}}{\text{min}}$$

Appendix C

CONTROLLED DRUGS (UNITED STATES)

Schedule I: Medications having no legal medical use. These substances may be used for research purposes with proper registration (e.g., heroin, LSD).

Schedule II: Medications having a legitimate medical use but are characterized by a very high abuse potential and/or potential for severe physical and psychic dependency. Emergency telephone orders for limited quantities of these drugs are authorized, but the prescriber must provide a written, signed prescription order (e.g., morphine, amphetamines).

Schedule III: Medications having significant abuse potential (less than Schedule II). Telephone orders are permitted (e.g., opiates in combination with other substances such as acetaminophen).

Schedule IV: Medications having a low abuse potential. Telephone orders are permitted (e.g., benzodiazepines, propoxyphene).

Schedule V: Medications having the lowest abuse potential of the controlled substances. Some Schedule V products may be available without a prescription (e.g., certain cough preparations containing limited amounts of an opiate).

Appendix D

CULTURAL ASPECTS OF DRUG THERAPY

The term *ethnopharmacology* was first used to describe the study of medicinal plants used by indigenous cultures. More recently, it is being used as a reference to the action and effects of drugs in people from diverse racial, ethnic, and cultural backgrounds. Although there are insufficient data from investigations involving people from diverse backgrounds that would provide reliable information on ethnic-specific responses to all medications, there is growing evidence that modifications in dosages are needed for some members of racial and ethnic groups. There are wide variations in the perception of side effects by patients from diverse cultural backgrounds. These differences may be related to metabolic differences that result in higher or lower levels of the drug, individual differences in the amount of body fat, or cultural differences in the way individuals perceive the meaning of side effects and toxicity. Nurses and other health care providers need to be aware that variations can occur with side effects, adverse reactions, and toxicity so that patients from diverse cultural backgrounds can be monitored.

Some cultural differences in response to medications include the following:

African Americans: Generally, African Americans are less responsive to beta-blockers (e.g., propranolol [Inderal]) and angiotensin-converting enzyme (ACE) inhibitors (e.g., enalapril [Vasotec]).

Asian Americans: On average, Asian Americans have a lower percentage of body fat, so dosage adjustments must be made for fat-soluble vitamins and other drugs (e.g., vitamin K used to reverse the anticoagulant effect of warfarin).

Hispanic Americans: Hispanic Americans may require lower dosages and may experience a higher incidence of side effects with the tricyclic antidepressants (e.g., amitryptyline).

Native Americans: Alaskan Eskimos may suffer prolonged muscle paralysis with the use of succinylcholine when administered during surgery.

There has been a desire to exert more responsibility over one's health and, as a result, a resurgence of self-care practices. These practices are often influenced by folk remedies and the use of medicinal plants. In the United States, there are several major ethnic population subgroups (white, black, Hispanic, Asian, and Native Americans). Each of these ethnic groups has a wide range of practices that influence beliefs and interventions related to health and illness. At any given time, in any group, treatment may consist of the use of traditional herbal therapy, a combination of ritual and prayer with medicinal plants, customary dietary and environmental practices, or the use of Western medical practices.

African Americans

Many African Americans carry the traditional health beliefs of their African heritage. Health denotes harmony with nature of the body, mind, and spirit, whereas illness is seen as disharmony that results from natural causes or divine punishment. Common practices to the art of healing include treatments with herbals and rituals known empirically to restore health. Specific forms of healing include using home remedies, obtaining medical advice from a physician, and seeking spiritual healing.

Examples of healing practices include the use of hot baths and warm compresses for rheumatism, the use of herbal teas for respiratory illnesses, and the use of kitchen condiments in folk remedies. Lemon, vinegar, honey, saltpeter, alum, salt, baking soda, and Epsom salt are common kitchen ingredients used. Goldenrod, peppermint, sassafras, parsley, yarrow, and rabbit tobacco are a few of the herbals used.

Hispanic Americans

The use of folk healers, medicinal herbs, magic, and religious rituals and ceremonies are included in the rich and varied customs of Hispanic Americans. This ethnic group believes that God is responsible for allowing health or illness to occur. Wellness may be viewed as good luck, a reward for good behavior, or a blessing from God. Praying, using herbals and spices, wearing religious objects such as medals, and maintaining a balance in diet and physical activity are methods considered appropriate in preventing evil or poor health.

Hispanic ethnopharmacology is more complementary to Western medical practices. After the illness is identified, appropriate treatment may consist of home remedies (e.g., use of vegetables and herbs), use of over-the-counter patent medicines, and use of physician-prescribed medications.

Asian Americans

For Asian Americans, harmony with nature is essential for physical and spiritual well-being. Universal balance depends on harmony between the elemental forces: fire, water, wood, earth, and metal. Regulating these universal elements are two forces that maintain physical and spiritual harmony in the body: the *yin* and the *yang.* Practices shared by most Asian cultures include meditation, special nutritional programs, herbology, and martial arts.

Therapeutic options available to the traditional Chinese physicians include prescribing herbs, meditation, exercise, nutritional changes, or acupuncture.

Native Americans

The theme of total harmony with nature is fundamental to traditional Native American beliefs about health. It is dependent on maintaining a state of equilibrium among the physical body, the mind, and the environment. Health practices reflect this holistic approach. The method of healing is determined traditionally by the medicine man, who diagnoses the ailment and recommends the appropriate intervention.

Treatment may include heat, herbs, sweat baths, massage, exercise, diet changes, or other interventions performed in a curing ceremony.

European Americans

Europeans often use home treatments as the front-line interventions. Traditional remedies practiced are based on the magical or empirically validated experience of ancestors. These cures are often practiced in combination with religious rituals or spiritual ceremonies.

Household products, herbal teas, and patent medicines are familiar preparations used in home treatments (e.g., salt water gargle for sore throat).

Appendix E

DRUGS OF ABUSE

Name (Brand)	Class	Signs and Symptoms	Treatment
Acid (see LSD)			
Adam (see MDMA)			
Amphetamine (Adderall, Dexedrine)	Stimulant	Tachycardia, hypertension, diaphoresis, agitation, headache, seizures, dehydration, hypokalemia, lactic acidosis. Severe overdose: hyperthermia, dysrhythmia, shock, rhabdomyolysis, liver necrosis, acute renal failure.	Control agitation, reverse hyperthermia, support hemodynamic function. **Antidote:** No specific antidote.
Angel dust (see phencyclidine)			
Apache (see fentanyl)			
Barbiturates (Nembutal, Seconal)	Depressant	Hypotension, hypothermia, apnea, nystagmus, ataxia, hyporeflexia, somnolence, stupor, coma.	Airway management, decontamination, supportive care. **Antidote:** No specific antidote.
Barbs (see barbiturates)			
Benzodiazepines (Xanax, Valium, Librium, Halcion)	Depressant	Respiratory depression, hypothermia, hypotension, nystagmus, miosis, diplopia, bradycardia, nausea, vomiting, impaired speech and coordination, amnesia, ataxia, somnolence, confusion, depressed deep tendon reflexes.	**Antidote:** Flumazenil (Romazicon) is a specific antidote.
Black tar (see heroin)			
Horse (see heroin)			
Boomers (see LSD)			
Buttons (see mescaline)			
Cactus (see mescaline)			
Candy (see benzodiazepines)			
China girl (see fentanyl)			
China white (see heroin)			

Name (Brand)	Class	Signs and Symptoms	Treatment
Cocaine	Stimulant	Hypertension, tachycardia, mild hyperthermia, mydriasis, pallor, diaphoresis, psychosis, paranoid delusions, mania, agitation, seizures.	Control agitation, seizures, hyperthermia, support hemodynamic function. **Antidote:** No specific antidote.
Codeine	Opioid	Miosis, respiratory depression, decreased mental status, hypotension, cardiac dysrhythmia, hypoxia, bronchoconstriction, constipation, decreased intestinal motility, ileus, lethargy, coma.	Airway management, hemodynamic support. **Antidote:** Naloxone, nalmefene.
Coke (see cocaine)			
Crank (see amphetamine)			
Crank (see heroin)			
Crystal (see amphetamine)			
Crystal meth (see methamphetamine)			
Cubes (see LSD)			
Downers (see benzodiazepines)			
Ecstasy (see MDMA)			
Fentanyl (Sublimaze)	Opioid	Miosis, respiratory depression, decreased mental status, hypotension, cardiac dysrhythmia, hypoxia, bronchoconstriction, constipation, decreased intestinal motility, ileus, lethargy, coma.	Airway management, hemodynamic support. **Antidote:** Naloxone, nalmefene.
Flunitrazepam (Rohypnol)	Depressant	Drowsiness, slurred speech, impaired judgment and motor skills, hypothermia, hypotension, bradycardia, diplopia, blurred vision, nystagmus, respiratory depression, nausea, constipation, depression, lethargy, headache, ataxia, coma, amnesia, incoordination, tremors, vertigo.	Supportive care, airway control. **Antidote:** Flumazenil (Romazicon).
Forget me pill (see flunitrazepam)			

(continued)

Name (Brand)	Class	Signs and Symptoms	Treatment
GHB (gamma-hydroxybutyrate)	CNS depressant	Dose-related CNS depression, amnesia, hypotonia, drowsiness, dizziness, euphoria. Other effects: bradycardia, hypotension, hypersalivation, vomiting, hypothermia. Higher dosages: Cheyne-Stokes respiration, seizures, coma, death. Users become highly agitated, flailing.	Supportive care. Severe intoxication may require airway support, including intubation. **Antidote:** No specific antidote.
Gib (see GHB)			
Goodfellas (see fentanyl)			
Grass (see marijuana)			
Hashish (see marijuana)			
Heroin	Opioid	Miosis, coma, apnea, pulmonary edema, bradycardia, hypotension, pinpoint pupils, CNS depression, seizures.	Airway management. **Antidote:** Naloxone, nalmefene.
Ice (see amphetamine)			
Ketamine (Ketalar)	Anesthetic	Feeling of dissociation from one's self (sense of floating over one's body), visual hallucinations, lack of coordination, hypertension, tachycardia, palpitation, respiratory depression, apnea, confusion, negativism, hostility, delirium, reduced awareness.	Supportive care, esp. respiratory and cardiac function. **Antidote:** No specific antidote.
Keets (see ketamine)			
Kit-kat (see ketamine)			
Liquid ecstasy (see GHB)			
Liquid X (see GHB)			

Name (Brand)	Class	Signs and Symptoms	Treatment
LSD	Hallucinogen	Diaphoresis, mydriasis, dizziness, twitching, flushing, hyperreflexia, hypertension, psychosis, behavioral changes, emotional lability, euphoria or dysphoria, paranoia, vomiting, diarrhea, anorexia, restlessness, incoordination, tremors, ataxia.	Airway management, control activity associated with hallucinations, psychosis, panic reaction. **Antidote:** No specific antidote.
Ludes (see methaqualone)			
Magic mushroom (see psilocybin)			
Marijuana	Cannabinoid	Increased appetite, reduced motility, constipation, urinary retention, seizures, euphoria, somnolence, heightened awareness, relaxation, altered time perception, short-term memory loss, poor concentration, mood alterations, disorientation, decreased strength, ataxia, slurred speech, respiratory depression, coma.	Airway management, supportive care. **Antidote:** No specific antidote.
MDMA (Methylenedioxymethamphetamine)	Stimulant	Euphoria, intimacy, closeness to others, loss of appetite, tachycardia, jaw tension, bruxism, sweating.	**Antidote:** No specific antidote.
Mescaline	Hallucinogen	Diaphoresis, mydriasis, dizziness, twitching, flushing, hyperreflexia, hypertension, psychosis, behavioral changes, emotional instability, euphoria or dysphoria, paranoia, vomiting, diarrhea, anorexia, restlessness, incoordination, tremors, ataxia.	Airway management, control activity associated with hallucinations, psychosis, panic reaction. **Antidote:** No specific antidote.
Meth (see methamphetamine)			

(continued)

Name (Brand)	Class	Signs and Symptoms	Treatment
Methamphetamine (Desoxyn)	Stimulant	Hypertension, hyperthermia, hyperpyrexia, agitation, hyperactivity, fasciculation, seizures, coma, tachycardia, dysrhythmias, pale skin, diaphoresis, restlessness, talkativeness, insomnia, headache, coma, delusions, paranoia, aggressive behavior, visual, tactile, or auditory hallucinations.	Airway control, hyperthermia, seizures, dysrhythmias. **Antidote:** No specific antidote.
Methaqualone (Quaalude)	Depressant	Slurred speech, impaired judgment and motor skills, hypothermia, hypotension, bradycardia, diplopia, blurred vision, nystagmus, mydriasis, respiratory depression, depression, lethargy, headache, ataxia, coma, amnesia, incoordination, hypertonicity, myoclonus, tremors, vertigo.	Airway management, supportive care. **Antidote:** No specific antidote.
Methylphenidate (Ritalin)	Stimulant	Agitation, hypertension, tachycardia, hyperthermia, mydriasis, dry mouth, nausea, vomiting, anorexia, abdominal pain, agitation, hyperactivity, insomnia, euphoria, dizziness, paranoid ideation, social withdrawal, delirium, hallucinations, psychosis, tremors, seizures.	Control agitation, hyperthermia, seizures, support hemodynamic function. **Antidote:** No specific antidote.
Miss Emma (see morphine)			
Mister blue (see morphine)			

Name (Brand)	Class	Signs and Symptoms	Treatment
Morphine (MS-Contin, Roxanol)	Opioid	Miosis, respiratory depression, decreased mental status, hypotension, cardiac dysrhythmia, hypoxia, bronchoconstriction, constipation, decreased intestinal motility, ileus, lethargy, coma.	Airway management, hemodynamic support. **Antidote:** Naloxone, nalmefene.
Oxy (see oxycodone)			
Oxycodone (OxyContin)	Opioid	Miosis, respiratory depression, decreased mental status, hypotension, cardiac dysrhythmia, hypoxia, bronchoconstriction, constipation, decreased intestinal motility, ileus, lethargy, coma.	Airway management, hemodynamic support. **Antidote:** Naloxone, nalmefene.
OxyContin (see oxycodone)			
Peace pill (see phencyclidine)			
Phencyclidine (PCP)	Hallucinogen	Nystagmus, hypertension, tachycardia, agitation, hallucinations, violent behavior, impaired judgment, delusions, psychosis.	Support blood pressure, manage airway, control agitation. **Antidote:** No specific antidote.
Phennies (see barbiturates)			
Pot (see marijuana)			
Propoxyphene (Darvon)	Depressant	Respiratory depression, seizures, cardiac toxicity, miosis, dysrhythmias, nausea, vomiting, anorexia, abdominal pain, constipation, drowsiness, coma, confusion, hallucinations.	Maintain airway, seizures, cardiac toxicity. **Antidote:** Naloxone.
Psilocybin	Hallucinogen	Diaphoresis, mydriasis, dizziness, twitching, flushing, hyperreflexia, hypertension, psychosis, behavioral changes, emotional lability,	Manage airway, control activity associated with hallucinations, psychosis, panic reaction. **Antidote:** No specific antidote.

(continued)

Name (Brand)	Class	Signs and Symptoms	Treatment
Psilocybin *(continued)*		euphoria or dysphoria, paranoia, vomiting, diarrhea, anorexia, restlessness, incoordination, tremors, ataxia.	
Purple passion (see psilocybin)			
Quay (see methaqualone)			
Reefer (see marijuana)			
Rock (see cocaine)			
Rocket fuel (see phencyclidine)			
Roofies (see flunitrazepam)			
Rope (see flunitrazepam)			
Rophies (see flunitrazepam)			
Salty water (see GHB)			
Schoolboy (see codeine)			
Scoop (see GHB)			
Snow (see cocaine)			
Special K (see ketamine)			
Speed (see amphetamine)			
STP (see MDMA)			
Super acid (see ketamine)			
Super K (see ketamine)			
Tranks (see benzodiazepines)			
Uppers (see amphetamine)			
White girl (see cocaine)			
Yellow jackets (see barbiturates)			
Yellow sunshine (see LSD)			

"CLUB DRUG" WEB SITES

www.drugfreeamerica.org	Partnership for a Drug-Free America
www.clubdrugs.org	Consumer-oriented site sponsored by the National Institute on Drug Abuse
www.health.org	Substance Abuse and Mental Health Services Administration
www.projectghb.org	Independent site devoted to risks and dangers of GHB use
www.nida.nih.gov	National Institute on Drug Abuse
ww.dea.gov	Drug Enforcement Administration
.whitehousedrugpolicy.org	Office of National Drug Control Policy

Appendix F

FDA PREGNANCY CATEGORIES

Alert: Medications should be used during pregnancy only if clearly needed.

A: Adequate and well-controlled studies have failed to show a risk to the fetus in the first trimester of pregnancy (also, no evidence of risk has been seen in later trimesters). Possibility of fetal harm appears remote.

B: Animal reproduction studies have failed to show a risk to the fetus and there are no adequate/well-controlled studies in pregnant women.

C: Animal reproduction studies have shown an adverse effect on the fetus and there are no adequate/well-controlled studies in humans. However, the benefits may warrant use of the drug in pregnant women despite potential risks.

D: There is positive evidence of human fetal risk based on data from investigational or marketing experience or from studies in humans, but the potential benefits may warrant use of the drug despite potential risks (e.g., use in life-threatening situations in which other medications cannot be used or are ineffective).

X: Animal or human studies have shown fetal abnormalities and/or there is evidence of human fetal risk based on adverse reaction data from investigational or marketing experience where the risks in using the medication clearly outweigh potential benefits.

Appendix G

HERBAL THERAPIES/INTERACTIONS

The use of herbal therapies is on the increase in the United States. In 1990, an estimated 1 in 3 Americans used at least one form of alternative medicine (of which herbal therapy is part). By 1997, more than $12 billion was spent in the United States for vitamins and minerals, herbals, sports supplements or specialty supplements (e.g., glucosamine).

Because of the rise in the use of herbal therapy in the United States, the following is presented to provide some basic information on some of the more popular herbs. Please note this is not an all-inclusive list, which is beyond the scope of this handbook.

Name	Purported Benefit	Interactions	Precautions
Aloe	***Topical:*** Promotes burn/wound healing, treatment of cold sores. ***Oral:*** Laxative, cathartic.	***Topical:*** None ***Oral:*** May increase risk of side effects with cardiac glycosides, antiarrhythmics, diuretics.	***Topical:*** None ***Oral:*** Abdominal pain, diarrhea, reduced potassium levels.
Astaxanthin	***Oral:*** Macular degeneration, Alzheimer's disease, Parkinson's disease, stroke, cancer, hypercholesterolemia. ***Topical:*** Sunburn.	None known.	May cause visual disturbances.
Bilberry	***Topical:*** Mild inflammation of mouth/throat. ***Oral:*** Acute diarrhea, increased visual acuity, angina, atherosclerosis.	May require adjustment of antidiabetic drugs (reduces glucose effect).	May decrease glucose, triglycerides.
Black cohosh*	Manage symptoms of menopause, hypercholesterolemia, peripheral arterial disease, anti-inflammatory and sedative effects.	May further reduce lipids and/or B/P when combined with prescription medications.	Side effects: nausea, dizziness, visual changes, migraine.
Boldo	Mild GI spasms, dyspepsia, anti-inflammatory agent, laxative, gallstones.	May have additive effects when used with anticoagulant or antiplatelet medications.	***Oral:*** Convulsions ***Topical:*** Skin irritation
Butterbut	Abdominal pain, back pain, gallbladder pain, bladder spasms, tension headache, migraine headaches, asthma.	None known.	May cause headache, itchy eyes, diarrhea, asthma, upset stomach, fatigue, drowsiness.

*See full herb entry in the A to Z section.

Name	Purported Benefit	Interactions	Precautions
Capsicum	***Topical:*** Pain of shingles; postherpetic, trigeminal, diabetic neuralgias; HIV-associated peripheral neuropathy.	None.	Burning, urticaria, irritation to eyes, mucous membranes.
L-Carnitine	Treatment of primary L-Carnitine deficiency, postmyocardial infarction protection, dementia, angina, congestive heart failure, intermittent claudication.	None known.	Stomach discomfort, diarrhea, nausea, vomiting, heartburn.
Cat's claw	***Oral:*** Diverticulitis, ulcers, hemorrhoids, colitis, gastritis.	Antihypertensives may increase effect.	Diarrhea, hypotension (get up slowly to avoid dizziness).
Catnip	***Topical:*** Arthritis, hemorrhoids. ***Oral:*** Insomnia, migraine, cold, flu, hives, indigestion, cramping, flatulence.	May be additive with other CNS depressants.	Headache, malaise, vomiting (large doses).
Chamomile*	Antispasmodic, sedative, anti-inflammatory, astringent, antibacterial.	May increase bleeding with anticoagulants. May increase sedative effect with benzodiazepines.	Anaphylactic reaction if allergic; avoid use if allergic to chrysanthemums, ragweed, and/or asters; delays absorption of medications.
Chastberry	***Oral:*** Control of menstrual irregularities, painful menstruation.	May interfere with oral contraceptives, hormone replacement therapy, dopamine antagonists (e.g., antipsychotics).	GI disturbances, rash, itching, headache, increased menstrual flow.
Co-Enzyme Q-10	***Oral:*** CHF, angina, diabetes, hypertension; reduces symptoms of chronic fatigue; stimulates immune system in those with AIDS.	May decrease effect of warfarin. Statins may decrease effect.	Reduced appetite, gastritis, nausea, diarrhea.
Cranberry	***Oral:*** Prevention, treatment of urinary tract infections; urinary deodorizer.	May increase absorption of vitamin B_{12} in those taking proton pump inhibitors (e.g., Prevacid).	Large doses may cause diarrhea.
DHEA*	Slows aging, boosts energy, controls weight.	None.	Side effects: may increase risk of

*See full herb entry in the A to Z section.

(continued)

Name	Purported Benefit	Interactions	Precautions
DHEA* *(continued)*			breast/prostate cancer. Women may develop acne, hair growth on face/body.
Dong quai*	Uterine stimulant, anti-inflammatory, vasodilator, CNS stimulant, immunosuppressant, analgesic, antipyretic.	May increase effects of warfarin.	Diarrhea, photosensitivity, skin cancer; avoid in pregnancy/lactation; essential oil may contain the carcinogen safrole.
Echinacea*	Prevents/treats colds, flu, bacterial and fungal infections. Immune system stimulator. Aid to wound healing.	May interfere with immunosuppressive therapy.	Not to be used with weakened immune system (e.g., HIV/AIDS, tuberculosis, multiple sclerosis). Habitual or continued use may cause immune system suppression (should only be taken for 2–3 mos or alternating schedule of q2–3wks).
Emu oil	***Oral:*** Hypercholesterolemia, weight loss, cough syrup. ***Topical:*** Relief from sore muscles, aching joints, pain, inflammation, carpal tunnel syndrome.	None known.	None reported.
Evening primose oil	***Oral:*** PMS, symptoms of menopause (e.g., hot flashes), psoriasis, rheumatoid arthritis.	Antipsychotics may increase risk of seizures.	Indigestion, nausea, headache. Large doses may cause diarrhea, abdominal pain.
Fenugreek	Lowering blood glucose, gastritis, constipation, atherosclerosis, elevated cholesterol and triglycerides.	May have additive effects with antidiabetic, anticoagulant, or antiplatelet medications.	Nasal congestion, wheezing. Large doses may cause hypoglycemia.
Feverfew*	Relieves migraine. Treatment of fever, headache, menstrual irregularities.	May increase bleeding time with aspirin, dipyridamole, warfarin.	Side effects: headache, mouth ulcers. Should be avoided in pregnancy (stimulates menstruation), nursing mother, infants <2 yrs.
Fish oils	***Oral:*** Hypertension, hyperlipidemia, coronary artery disease, rheumatoid arthritis, psoriasis.	May increase risk of bleeding with antiplatelets, anticoagulants. Addi-	Belching, heartburn, nosebleeds. Large doses may cause nausea, diarrhea.

*herb entry in the A to Z section.

Name	Purported Benefit	Interactions	Precautions
Fish oils *(continued)*		tive effect with antihypertensives.	
Garlic*	Reduces cholesterol, LDL, triglycerides, increases HDL, lowers B/P, inhibits platelet aggregation. May also possess antibacterial, antiviral, antithrombotic activity.	May increase bleeding time with aspirin, dipyridamole, warfarin.	Side effects: taste, offensive odor. Large doses may cause heartburn, flatulence, other GI distress.
Ginger*	Relieves nausea, effective treatment for motion sickness, anti-inflammatory for arthritis, nausea/vomiting associated with pregnancy. Possesses ability to lower platelet aggregation; antithrombotic properties.	None.	Avoid during pregnancy when bleeding is a concern. Large overdose could potentially depress the CNS, cause cardiac arrhythmias.
Ginkgo*	Boosts mental prowess by improving memory. Sharpens concentration, pt may think more clearly. Overcomes sexual dysfunction occurring with SSRI antidepressants. May be able to slow progress of Alzheimer's disease, improve intermittent claudication.	May increase bleeding time with aspirin, dipyridamole, warfarin.	Avoid in pt taking blood thinners or those hypersensitive to poison ivy, cashews, mangos. Side effects: GI disturbances, headache, dizziness, vertigo.
Ginseng*	Boosts energy, sexual stamina; decreases stress, effects of aging.	May affect platelet adhesiveness/blood coagulation. Use caution with anticoagulants. May increase hypoglycemia with insulin.	Avoid in pts receiving anticoagulants, medications that increase B/P. Side effects: breast tenderness, nervousness, headache, increased B/P, abnormal vaginal bleeding.
Glucosamine and chondroitin*	Osteoarthritis.	No known interactions but monitor anticoagulant effects.	None known.
Goldenrod	***Oral:*** Diuretic, anti-inflammatory, antispasmodic. Prevents urinary tract inflammation, urinary calculi, kidney stones.	May interfere with diuretics.	Allergic reactions.
Goldenseal	***Topical:*** Eczema, itching, acne.	May interfere with antacids, sucral-	Constipation, hallucinations. Large doses

*See full herb entry in the A to Z section.

(continued)

Name	Purported Benefit	Interactions	Precautions
Goldenseal *(continued)*	***Oral:*** UTI, hemorrhoids, gastritis, colitis, mucosal inflammation.	fate, H_2 antagonists, proton pump inhibitors.	may cause nausea, vomiting, diarrhea, CNS stimulation, respiratory failure.
Gotu kola	Improve memory, intelligence, venous insufficiency including varicose veins, wound or burn healing, psoriasis.	None known.	GI upset, nausea, pruritus, photosensitivity.
Grape seed extract	Improves circulation, decreases tissue injury, hemorrhoids. Used as antioxidant to treat hypoxia from atherosclerosis, inflammation.	None.	None reported.
Green tea	***Oral:*** Improves cognition function, treats nausea, vomiting, headache, weight loss.	May increase risk of bleeding with antiplatelets.	GI upset, constipation.
Guggul	Lowers cholesterol, treatment of acne, skin disease, weight loss.	None known.	May cause headache, nausea, vomiting, loose stools, bloating.
Gymnema	Treatment of diabetes, cough.	May enhance effects of insulin, oral antidiabetics.	None reported.
Hawthorn	Cardiovascular conditions (e.g., atherosclerosis), GI conditions (diarrhea, indigestion, abdominal pain), sleep disorders.	Cardiovascular drugs, digoxin may potentiate or interfere; additive effect with CNS depressants.	Nausea, GI complaints, headache, dizziness, insomnia, agitation.
Horse chestnut	Reduces edema following injury, chronic venous insufficiency including varicose veins, hemorrhoids, phlebitis.	May enhance effects of insulin, oral antidiabetics, antiplatelet medications.	Calf cramps, pruritus, GI irritation.
Kava kava*	Reduces stress, muscle relaxant, relieves anxiety, induces sleep, and counters fatigue.	Increases CNS depression with alcohol, sedatives.	Side effects: GI disturbances, temporary discoloration of skin, hair, nails. Do not use in pregnancy, lactation, endogenous depression. Large doses cause muscle weakness. Chronic use may cause scaly skin resembling psoriasis (reversible). Causes

*See full herb entry in the A to Z section.

Name	Purported Benefit	Interactions	Precautions
Kava kava* *(continued)*			pupil dilation affecting vision (avoid driving, operating heavy machinery). Store in cool, dry place (excess heat/light will alter contents).
Licorice	***Oral:*** Inflammation of upper respiratory tract, mucous membranes, ulcers, expectorant.	May decrease effect of antihypertensives. Thiazides may increase potassium loss.	Large doses may cause pseudoaldosteronism (hypertension, headache, lethargy, edema).
Ma huang* (Ephedra)	Controls weight, boosts energy. Treatment of colds, allergies, appetite suppressant.	Increases toxicity with beta-blockers, MAOIs, caffeine, theophylline, decongestants, St. John's wort.	Linked to high B/P, headache, seizures. Can cause confusion, insomnia, dizziness, sweating, fever, nausea, vomiting.
Melatonin*	Aids sleep, prevents jet lag.	Decreases effects of antidepressants.	Side effects: headache, confusion, fatigue. Does not lengthen total sleep time.
Milk thistle	Hepatoprotective, antioxidant, liver disorders, including poisoning (e.g., mushroom), cirrhosis, hepatitis.	None.	Mild allergic reactions, laxative effect.
MSM (methylsulfonylmethane)	***Oral/topical:*** Chronic pain, arthritis, inflammation, osteoporosis, muscle cramps/pain, wrinkles, protection against windburn or sunburn.	None known.	May cause nausea, diarrhea, headache, pruritus, increase in allergic symptoms.
Omega-6 fatty acid	***Oral:*** Coronary artery disease, decreases total cholesterol LDL, increases HDL.	None.	Increases triglycerides.
Red clover	***Oral:*** Menopausal symptoms, hot flashes, prevention of cancer, indigestion, asthma. ***Topical:*** Skin sores, burns, chronic skin disease (e.g., eczema, psoriasis).	May increase anticoagulant effects of warfarin. May interfere with hormone replacement therapy, oral contraceptives, tamoxifen.	Rash, myalgia, headache, nausea, vaginal spotting.
SAMe	***Oral:*** Depression, heart disease, osteoarthritis, Alzheimer's disease, Parkinson's disease; slows aging process.	May increase adverse effects with antidepressants.	Nausea, vomiting, diarrhea, flatulence; headache.

*See full herb entry in the A to Z section.

(continued)

Name	Purported Benefit	Interactions	Precautions
Saw palmetto*	Eases symptoms of large prostate (frequency, dysuria, nocturia).	None.	Side effects: upset stomach, headache, erectile dysfunction. Does not reduce size of enlarged prostate. Obtain baseline PSA levels before initiating. Large doses can cause diarrhea.
Shark cartilage	***Oral:*** Cancer, arthritis, psoriasis, wound healing.	None.	Nausea, vomiting, constipation, dyspepsia, bad taste in mouth.
Soy	Menopausal symptoms; prevents osteoporosis and cardiovascular disease in postmenopausal women; hypertension, hyperlipidemia.	May decrease effects of estrogen replacement therapy.	Constipation, bloating, nausea, allergic reaction.
St. John's wort*	Relieves mild to moderate depression, heals wounds.	May cause "serotonin syndrome" (confusion, agitation, chills, fever, sweating, diarrhea, nausea, muscle spasms or twitching), hyperreflexia, tremor with antidepressants, yohimbe.	Side effects: dizziness, dry mouth, increased sensitivity to sunlight. Report symptoms of "serotonin syndrome."
Valerian*	Aids sleep, relieves restlessness and nervousness. Does not decrease night awakenings.	None.	Side effects: heart palpitations, upset stomach, headache, excitability, uneasiness. May cause increased morning drowsiness.
Wild yam	***Oral:*** Alternative for estrogen replacement therapy, postmenopausal vaginal dryness, premenstrual syndrome, osteoporosis, increases energy/libido, breast enlargement.	None known.	Large amounts may cause vomiting (tincture).
Yohimbe*	Male aphrodisiac. Used to treat impotence, erectile dysfunction, orthostatic hypotension.	Decreases effects of antidepressants, antihypertensives, St. John's wort.	Large doses linked to weakness, paralysis.

*See full herb entry in the A to Z section.

Appendix H

NORMAL LABORATORY VALUES

HEMATOLOGY/COAGULATION

Test	Specimen	Normal Range
Activated partial thromboplastin time (aPTT)	Whole blood	25–35 sec
Erythrocyte count (RBC count)	Whole blood	M: 4.3–5.7 million cells/mm^3 F: 3.8–5.1 million cells/mm^3
Hematocrit (HCT, Hct)	Whole blood	M: 39%–49% F: 35%–45%
Hemoglobin (Hb, Hgb)	Whole blood	M: 13.5–17.5 g/dl F: 12.0–16.0 g/dl
Leukocyte count (WBC count)	Whole blood	4.5–11.0 thousand cells/mm^3
Leukocyte differential count	Whole blood	
Basophils		0%–0.75%
Eosinophils		1%–3%
Lymphocytes		23%–33%
Monocytes		3%–7%
Neutrophils-bands		3%–5%
Neutrophils-segmented		54%–62%
Mean corpuscular hemoglobin (MCH)	Whole blood	26–34 pg/cell
Mean corpuscular hemoglobin concentration (MCHC)	Whole blood	31%–37% Hb/cell
Mean corpuscular volume (MCV)	Whole blood	80–100 fL
Partial thromboplastin time (PTT)	Whole blood	60–85 sec
Platelet count (thrombocyte count)	Whole blood	150–450 thousand/mm^3
Prothrombin time (PT)	Whole blood	11–13.5 sec
RBC count (see Erythrocyte count)		

SERUM/URINE VALUES

Test	Specimen	Normal Range
Alanine aminotransferase (ALT, SGPT)	Serum	0–55 units/L
Albumin	Serum	3.5–5 g/dl
Alkaline phosphatase	Serum	M: 53–128 units/L F: 42–98 units/L
Anion gap	Plasma or serum	5–14 mEq/L
Aspartate aminotransferase (AST, SGOT)	Serum	0–50 units/L
Bilirubin (conjugated direct)	Serum	0–0.4 mg/dl
Bilirubin (total)	Serum	0.2–1.2 mg/dl
Calcium (total)	Serum	8.4–10.2 mg/dl
Carbon dioxide (CO_2) total	Plasma or serum	20–34 mEq/L
Chloride	Plasma or serum	96–112 mEq/L

Test	Specimen	Normal Range
Cholesterol (total)	Plasma or serum	<200 mg/dl
C-Reactive protein	Serum	68–8,200 ng/ml
Creatine kinase (CK)	Serum	M: 38–174 units/L F: 26–140 units/L
Creatine kinase isoenzymes	Serum	Fraction of total: <0.04–0.06
Creatinine	Plasma or serum	M: 0.7–1.3 mg/dl F: 0.6–1.1 mg/dl
Creatinine clearance	Plasma or serum and urine	M: 90–139 ml/min/1.73m^2 F: 80–125 ml/min/1.73m^2
Free thyroxine index (FTI)	Serum	1.1–4.8
Glucose	Serum	Adults: 70–105 mg/dl >60 yrs: 80–115 mg/dl
Hemoglobin A_{1c}	Whole blood	5.6%–7.5% of total Hgb
Homovanillic acid (HVA)	Urine, 24 hr	1.4–8.8 mg/day
17-Hydroxycorticosteroids (17-OHCS)	Urine, 24 hr	M: 3–10 mg/day F: 2–8 mg/day
Iron	Serum	M: 65–175 mcg/dl F: 50–170 mcg/dl
Iron-binding capacity, total (TIBC)	Serum	250–450 mcg/dl
Lactate dehydrogenase (LDH)	Serum	0–250 units/L
Magnesium	Serum	1.3–2.3 mg/dl
Oxygen (Po_2)	Whole blood, arterial	83–100 mm Hg
Oxygen saturation	Whole blood, arterial	95%–98%
pH	Whole blood, arterial	7.35–7.45
Phosphorus, inorganic	Serum	2.7–4.5 mg/dl
Potassium	Serum	3.5–5.1 mEq/L
Protein (total)	Serum	6–8.5 g/dl
Sodium	Plasma or serum	136–146 mEq/L
Specific gravity	Urine	1.002–1.030
Thyrotropin (hTSH)	Plasma or serum	2–10 mcgU/ml
Thyroxine (T_4) total	Serum	5–12 mcg/dl
Triglycerides (TG)	Serum, after 12-hr fast	20–190 mg/dl
Triiodothyronine resin uptake test (T_3RU)	Serum	22%–37%
Urea nitrogen	Plasma or serum	7–25 mg/dl
Urea nitrogen/creatinine ratio	Serum	12/1–20/1
Uric acid	Serum	M: 3.5–7.2 mg/dl F: 2.6–6 mg/dl
Vanillylmandelic acid (VMA)	Urine, 24 hr	2–7 mg/day

Appendix I

RECOMMENDED CHILDHOOD AND ADULT IMMUNIZATIONS

Recommended Childhood and Adolescent Immunization Schedule—United States, 2003

range of recommended ages | catch-up vaccination | preadolescent assessment

Vaccine ▼ / Age ►	Birth	1 mo	2 mos	4 mos	6 mos	12 mos	15 mos	18 mos	24 mos	4–6 yrs	11–12 yrs	13–18 yrs
Hepatitis B[1]	HepB #1	only if mother HBsAg (−) / HepB #2	only if mother HBsAg (−) / HepB #2 (bar)	HepB #2 (bar)	HepB #3	(bar)	(bar)	(bar)	HepB series	(bar)	(bar)	(bar)
Diphtheria, Tetanus, Pertussis[2]			DTaP	DTaP	DTaP		DTaP	(bar)		DTaP	Td	(bar)
Haemophilus influenzae type b[3]			Hib	Hib	Hib	Hib	(bar)					
Inactivated Polio			IPV	IPV	IPV	(bar)	(bar)	(bar)		IPV		
Measles, Mumps, Rubella[4]						MMR #1	(bar)			MMR #2	MMR #2	(bar)
Varicella[5]						Varicella	(bar)	(bar)	Varicella	(bar)	(bar)	(bar)
Pneumococcal[6]			PCV	PCV	PCV	PCV	(bar)		PCV / PPV	PCV / PPV (bar)	PPV (bar)	PPV (bar)
Vaccines below this line are for selected populations												
Hepatitis A[7]									Hepatitis A series	(bar)	(bar)	(bar)
Influenza[8]					Influenza (yearly)	(bar)	(bar)	(bar)	(bar)	(bar)	(bar)	(bar)

This schedule indicates the recommended ages for routine administration of currently licensed childhood vaccines, as of December 1, 2002, for children through age 18 years. Any dose not given at the recommended age should be given at any subsequent visit when indicated and feasible. [hatched box] Indicates age groups that warrant special effort to administer those vaccines not previously given. Additional vaccines may be licensed and recommended during the year. Licensed combination vaccines may be used whenever any components of the combination are indicated and the vaccine's other components are not contraindicated. Providers should consult the manufacturers' package inserts for detailed recommendations.

1. Hepatitis B vaccine (HepB). All infants should receive the first dose of hepatitis B vaccine soon after birth and before hospital discharge; the first dose may also be given by age 2 mos if the infant's mother is HBsAg negative. Only monovalent HepB can be used for the birth dose. Monovalent or combination vaccine containing HepB may be used to complete the series. Four doses of vaccine may be administered when a birth dose is given. The second dose should be given at least 4 wks after the first dose, except for combination vaccines, which cannot be administered before age 6 wks. The third dose should be given at least 16 wks after the first dose and at least 8 wks after the second dose. The last dose in the vaccination series (third or fourth dose) should not be administered before age 6 mos.

Infants born to HBsAg-positive mothers should receive HepB and 0.5 ml Hepatitis B Immune Globulin (HBIG) within 12 hrs of birth at separate sites. The second dose is recommended at age 1–2 mos. The last dose in the vaccination series should not be administered before age 6 mos. These infants should be tested for HBsAg and anti-HBs at 9–15 mos of age.

Infants born to mothers whose HBsAg status is unknown should receive the first dose of the HepB series within 12 hrs of birth. Maternal blood should be drawn as soon as possible to determine the mother's HBsAg status; if the HBsAg test is positive, the infant should receive HBIG as soon as possible (no later than age 1 wk). The second dose is recommended at age 1–2 mos. The last dose in the vaccination series should not be administered before age 6 mos.

2. Diphtheria and tetanus toxoids and acellular pertussis vaccine (DTaP). The fourth dose of DTaP may be administered as early as age 12 mos, provided 6 mos have elapsed since the third dose and the child is unlikely to return at age 15–18 mos. **Tetanus and diphtheria toxoids (Td)** is recommended at age 11–12 yrs if at least 5 yrs have elapsed since the last dose of tetanus and diphtheria toxoid-containing vaccine. Subsequent routine Td boosters are recommended every 10 yrs.

3. *Haemophilus influenzae* type b (Hib) conjugate vaccine. Three Hib conjugate vaccines are licensed for infant use. If PRP-OMP (PedvaxHIB or ComVax [Merck]) is administered at ages 2 and 4 mos, a dose at age 6 mos is not required. DTaP/Hib combination products should not be used for primary immunization in infants at ages 2, 4, or 6 mos, but can be used as boosters after any Hib vaccine.

4. Measles, mumps, and rubella vaccine (MMR). The second dose of MMR is recommended routinely at age 4–6 yrs but may be administered during any visit, provided at least 4 wks have elapsed since the first dose and that both doses are administered beginning at or after age 12 mos. Those who have not previously received the second dose should complete the schedule by the 11- to 12-yr-old visit.

5. Varicella vaccine. Varicella vaccine is recommended at any visit at or after age 12 mos for susceptible children (i.e., those who lack a reliable history of chickenpox). Susceptible persons aged ≥13 yrs should receive two doses, given at least 4 wks apart.

6. Pneumococcal vaccine. The heptavalent **pneumococcal conjugate vaccine (PCV)** is recommended for all children age 2–23 mos. It is also recommended for certain children age 24–59 mos. **Pneumococcal polysaccharide vaccine (PPV)** is recommended in addition to PCV for certain high-risk groups. See *MMWR* 2000;49(RR-9);1–38.

7. Hepatitis A vaccine. Hepatitis A vaccine is recommended for children and adolescents in selected states and regions, and for certain high-risk groups; consult your local public health authority. Children and adolescents in these states/regions and high-risk groups who have not been immunized against hepatitis A can begin the hepatitis A vaccination series during any visit. The two doses in the series should be administered at least 6 mos apart. See *MMWR* 1999;48(RR-12);1–37.

8. Influenza vaccine. Influenza vaccine is recommended annually for children age ≥6 mos with certain risk factors (including but not limited to asthma, cardiac disease, sickle cell disease, HIV, diabetes, and household members of persons in groups at high risk; see *MMWR* 2002;51[RR-3];1–31), and can be administered to all others wishing to obtain immunity. In addition, healthy children age 6–23 mos are encouraged to receive influenza vaccine if feasible because children in this age group are at substantially increased risk for influenza-related hospitalizations. Children aged ≤12 yrs should receive vaccine in a dosage appropriate for their age (0.25 ml if age 6–35 mos or 0.5 ml if aged ≥3 yrs). Children aged ≤8 yrs who are receiving influenza vaccine for the first time should receive two doses separated by at least 4 wks.

For additional information about vaccines, including precautions and contraindications for immunization and vaccine shortages, please visit the National Immunization Program Website at www.cdc.gov/nip or call the National Immunization Information Hotline at 800-232-2522 (English) or 800-232-0233 (Spanish).

Approved by the Advisory Committee on Immunization Practices (ACIP) (www.cdc.gov/nip/acip), the American Academy of Pediatrics (www.aap.org), and the American Academy of Family Physicians (www.aafp.org).

Recommended Adult Immunization Schedule, United States, 2002–2003

Legend: (light grey) For all persons in this group; (hatched) Catch-up on childhood vaccinations; (dark) For persons with medical/exposure indications

Vaccine ▼ Age Group ▶	19–49 yrs	50–64 yrs	≥65 yrs
Tetanus, Diphtheria (Td)*	1 dose booster every 10 years[1]		
Influenza	1 dose annually for persons with medical or occupational indications, or household contacts of persons with indications[2]	1 annual dose	
Pneumococcal (polysaccharide)	1 dose for persons with medical or other indications. (1 dose revaccination for immunosuppressive conditions)[3,4]		1 dose for unvaccinated persons[3] 1 dose for revaccination[4]
Hepatitis B*	3 doses (0, 1–2, 4–6 mos) for persons with medical, behavioral, occupational, or other indications[5]		
Hepatitis A	2 doses (0, 6–12 mos) for persons with medical, behavioral, occupational, or other indications[6]		
Measles, Mumps, Rubella (MMR)*	1 dose if measles, mumps, or rubella vaccination history is unreliable; 2 doses for persons with occupational or other indications[7]		
Varicella*	2 doses (0, 4–8 wks) for persons who are susceptible[8]		
Meningococcal (polysaccharide)	1 dose for persons with medical or other indications[9]		

*Covered by the Vaccine Injury Compensation Program. For information on how to file a claim call 800-338-2382. Please also visit www.hrsa.gov/osp/vicp TO file a claim for vaccine injury write: U.S. Court of Federal Claims, 717 Madison Place, N.W., Washington D.C. 20005. 202-219-9657.

This schedule indicates the recommended age groups for routine administration of currently licensed vaccines for persons ≥19 yrs. Licensed combination vaccines may be used whenever any components of the combination are indicated and the vaccine's other components are not contraindicated. Providers should consult the manufacturers' package inserts for detailed recommendations.

Report all clinically significant postvaccination reactions to the Vaccine Adverse Event Reporting System (VAERS). Reporting forms and instructions on filing a VAERS report are available by calling 800-822-7967 or from the VAERS website at www.vaers.org.

For additional information about the vaccines listed above and contraindications for immunization, visit the National Immunization Program Website at www.cdc.gov/nip/ or call the National Immunization Hotline at 800-232-2522 (English) or 800-232-0233 (Spanish).

Approved by the Advisory Committee on Immunization Practices (ACIP), and accepted by the American College of Obstetricians and Gynecologists (ACOG) and the American Academy of Family Physicians (AAFP).

Footnotes for Recommended Adult Immunization Schedule, United States, 2002–2003

1. Tetanus and diphtheria (Td)—A primary series for adults is 3 doses: the first 2 doses given at least 4 wks apart and the 3rd dose, 6–12 mos after the second. Administer 1 dose if the person had received the primary series and the last vaccination was 10 yrs ago or longer. *MMWR* 1991;40(RR-10):1–21. The ACP Task Force on Adult Immunization supports a second option: a single Td booster at age 50 yrs for persons who have completed the full pediatric series, including the teenage/young adult booster. *Guide for Adult Immunization,* ed 3, ACP 1994:20.

2. Influenza vaccination—Medical indications: chronic disorders of the cardiovascular or pulmonary systems, including asthma; chronic metabolic diseases, including diabetes mellitus, renal dysfunction, hemoglobinopathies, immunosuppression (including immunosuppression caused by medications or by human immunodeficiency virus [HIV]), requiring regular medical follow-up or hospitalization during the preceding year; women who will be in the second or third trimester of pregnancy during the influenza season. Occupational indications: health care workers. Other indications: residents of nursing homes and other long-term care facilities; persons likely to transmit influenza to persons at high risk (in-home caregivers to persons with medical indications, household contacts and out-of-home caregivers of children birth to 23 mos of age, or children with asthma or other indicator conditions for influenza vaccination, household members and caregivers of elderly and adults with high-risk conditions); and anyone who wishes to be vaccinated. *MMWR* 2002;51(RR-3):1–31.

3. Pneumococcal polysaccharide vaccination—Medical indications: chronic disorders of the pulmonary system (excluding asthma), cardiovascular diseases, diabetes mellitus, chronic liver diseases (including liver disease as a result of alcohol abuse [e.g., cirrhosis]), chronic renal failure or nephrotic syndrome, functional or anatomic asplenia (e.g., sickle cell disease or splenectomy), immunosuppressive conditions (e.g., congenital immunodeficiency, HIV infection, leukemia, lymphoma, multiple myeloma, Hodgkin's disease, generalized malignancy, organ or bone marrow transplantation), chemotherapy with alkylating agents, antimetabolites, or long-term systemic corticosteroids. Geographic/other indications: Alaskan Natives and certain American Indian populations. Other indications: residents of nursing homes and other long-term care facilities. *MMWR* 1997;47(RR-8):1–24.

4. Revaccination with pneumococcal polysaccharide vaccine—One-time revaccination after 5 yrs for persons with chronic renal failure or nephrotic syndrome, functional or anatomic asplenia (e.g., sickle cell disease or splenectomy), immunosuppressive conditions (e.g., congenital immunodeficiency, HIV infection, leukemia, lymphoma, multiple myeloma, Hodgkin's disease, generalized malignancy, organ or bone marrow transplantation), chemotherapy with alkylating agents, antimetabolites, or long-term systemic corticosteroids. For persons 65 and older, one-time revaccination if they were vaccinated 5 yrs or more previously and were aged less than 65 yrs at the time of primary vaccination. *MMWR* 1997;47(RR-8):1–24.

5. Hepatitis B vaccination—Medical indications: hemodialysis patients, patients who receive clotting-factor concentrates. Occupational indications: health care workers and public safety workers who have exposure to blood in the workplace, persons in training in schools of medicine, dentistry, nursing, laboratory technology, and other allied health professions. Behavioral indications: injecting drug users, persons with more than one sex partner in the previous 6 mos, persons with a recently acquired sexually transmitted disease (STD), all clients in STD clinics, men who have sex with men. Other indications: household contacts and sex partners of persons with chronic HBV infection, clients and staff of institutions for the developmentally disabled, international travelers who will be in countries with high or intermediate prevalence of chronic HBV infection for more than 6 mos, inmates of correctional facilities. *MMWR* 1991;40(RR-13):1–25. (www.cdc.gov/travel/diseases/hbv.htm)

6. Hepatitis A vaccination—For the combined HepA-HepB vaccine use 3 doses at 0, 1, 6 mos. Medical indications: persons with clotting factor disorders or chronic liver disease. Behavioral indications: men who have sex with men, users of injecting and noninjecting illegal drugs. Occupational indications: persons working with HAV-infected primates or with HAV in a research laboratory setting. Other indications: persons traveling to or working in countries that have high or intermediate endemicity of hepatitis A. *MMWR* 1999;48(RR-12):1–37. (www.cdc.gov/travel/diseases/hav.htm)

7. Measles, Mumps, Rubella vaccination (MMR)—Measles component: Adults born in or before 1957 may be considered immune to measles. Adults born in or after 1957 should receive at least one dose of MMR unless they have a medical contraindication, documentation of at least one dose or other acceptable evidence of immunity. A second dose of MMR is recommended for adults who:

- Are recently exposed to measles or in an outbreak setting
- Were previously vaccinated with killed measles vaccine
- Were vaccinated with an unknown vaccine between 1963 and 1967
- Are students in postsecondary educational institutions
- Work in health care facilities
- Plan to travel internationally

Mumps component: 1 dose of MMR should be adequate for protection. Rubella component: Give 1 dose of MMR to women whose rubella vaccination history is unreliable and counsel women to avoid becoming pregnant for 4 wks after vaccination. For women of childbearing age, regardless of birth year, routinely determine rubella immunity and counsel women regarding congenital rubella syndrome. Do not vaccinate pregnant women or those planning to become pregnant in the next 4 wks. If pregnant and susceptible, vaccinate as early in postpartum period as possible. *MMWR* 1998;47(RR-8):1–57.

8. Varicella vaccination—Recommended for all persons who do not have reliable clinical history of varicella infection, or serologic evidence of varicella-zoster virus (VZV) infection; health care workers and family contacts of immunocompromised persons, those who live or work in environments where transmission is likely (e.g., teachers of young children, day care employees, residents and staff members in institutional settings), persons who live or work in environments where VZV transmission can occur (e.g., college students, inmates and staff members of correctional institutions, military personnel), adolescents and adults living in households with children, women who are not pregnant but who may become pregnant in the future, international travelers who are not immune to infection. Note: Greater than 90% of U.S.-born adults are immune to VZV. Do not vaccinate pregnant women or those planning to become pregnant in the next 4 wks. If pregnant and susceptible, vaccinate as early in postpartum period as possible. *MMWR* 1996;45(RR-11):1–36, *MMWR* 1999;48(RR-6):1–50.

9. Meningococcal vaccine (quadrivalent polysaccharide for serogroups A, C, Y, and W-135)—Consider vaccination for persons with medical indications: adults with terminal complement component deficiencies, with anatomic or functional asplenia. Other indications: travelers to countries in which disease is hyperendemic or epidemic ("meningitis belt" of sub-Saharan Africa, Mecca, Saudi Arabia for Hajj). Revaccination at 3–5 yrs may be indicated for persons at high risk for infection (e.g., persons residing in areas in which disease is epidemic). Counsel college freshmen, especially those who live in dormitories, regarding meningococcal disease and the vaccine so that they can make an educated decision about receiving the vaccination. *MMWR* 2000;49(RR-7):1–20. Note: The AAFP recommends that colleges should take the lead on providing education on meningococcal infection and vaccination and offer it to those who are interested. Physicians need not initiate discussion of the meningococcal quadrivalent polysaccharide vaccine as part of routine medical care.

Appendix J

SIGNS AND SYMPTOMS OF ELECTROLYTE IMBALANCE

HYPOGLYCEMIA (excessive insulin)

Tremulousness, cold/clammy skin, mental confusion, rapid/shallow respirations, unusual fatigue, hunger, drowsiness, anxiety, headache, muscular incoordination, paresthesia of tongue/mouth/lips, hallucination, increased pulse/blood pressure, tachycardia, seizures, coma.

HYPERGLYCEMIA (insufficient insulin)

Hot/flushed/dry skin, fruity breath odor, excessive urination (polyuria), excessive thirst (polydipsia), acute fatigue, air hunger, deep/labored respirations, mental changes, restlessness, nausea, polyphagia (excessive appetite).

HYPOKALEMIA (potassium level <3.5 mEq/L)

Weakness/paresthesia of extremities, muscle cramps, nausea, vomiting, diarrhea, hypoactive bowel sounds, absent bowel sounds (paralytic ileus), abdominal distention, weak/irregular pulse, postural hypotension, difficulty breathing, disorientation, irritability.

HYPERKALEMIA (potassium level >5.0 mEq/L)

Diarrhea, muscle weakness, heaviness of legs, paresthesia of tongue/hands/feet, slow/irregular pulse, decreased blood pressure, abdominal cramps, oliguria/anuria, respiratory difficulty, cardiac abnormalities.

HYPONATREMIA (sodium level <130 mEq/L)

Abdominal cramping, nausea, vomiting, diarrhea, cold/clammy skin, poor skin turgor, tremulousness, muscle weakness, leg cramps, increased pulse rate, irritability, apprehension, hypotension, headache.

HYPERNATREMIA (sodium level >150 mEq/L)

Hot/flushed/dry skin, dry mucous membranes, fever, extreme thirst, dry/rough/red tongue, edema, restlessness, postural hypotension, oliguria.

HYPOCALCEMIA (calcium level <8.4 mg/dl)

Circumoral/peripheral numbness and tingling, muscle twitching; Chvostek's sign (facial muscle spasm; test by tapping of facial nerve anterior to earlobe, just below zygomatic arch), muscle cramping, Trousseau's sign (carpopedal spasm), seizures, arrhythmias.

HYPERCALCEMIA (calcium level >10.2 mg/dl)

Muscle hypotonicity, incoordination, anorexia, constipation, confusion, impaired memory, slurred speech, lethargy, acute psychotic behavior, deep bone pain, flank pain.

Appendix K

SPANISH PHRASES OFTEN USED IN CLINICAL SETTINGS

TAKING THE MEDICATION HISTORY

Tomando la Historia Médica
(Toh-mahn-doh lah Ees-toh-ree-ah Meh-dee-kah)

- Are you allergic to any medications? (If yes:)
  ¿Es alérgico a algún medicamento? (sí:)
  (Ehs ah-lehr-hee-koh ah ahl-goon meh-dee-kah-mehn-toh) (see:)

- —Which medications are you allergic to?
  ¿A cuál medicamento es alérgico?
  (ah koo-ahl meh-dee-kah-mehn-toh ehs ah-lehr-hee-koh)

  —What happens when you develop an allergic reaction?
  ¿Qué le pasa cuando desarrolla una reacción alérgica?
  (Keh leh pah-sah koo-ahn-doh deh-sah-roh-yah oo-nah reh-ahk-see-ohn ah-lehr-hee-kah)

  —What did you do to relieve or stop the allergic reaction?
  ¿Qué hizo para aliviar o detener la reacción alérgica?
  (Keh ee-soh pah-rah ah-lee-bee-ahr oh deh-teh-nehr lah reh-ahk-see-ohn ah-lehr-hee-kah)

- Do you take any over-the-counter, prescription, or herbal medications? (If yes:)
  ¿Toma medicamentos sin receta, con receta, o naturistas (hierbas medicinales)? (sí:)
  (Toh-mah meh-dee-kah-mehn-tohs seen reh-seh-tah, kohn reh-seh-tah, oh nah-too-rees-tahs [ee-ehr-bahs meh-dee-see-nah-lehs]) (see:)

  —Why do you take each medication?
  ¿Porqué toma cada medicamento?
  (Pohr-keh toh-mah kah-dah meh-dee-kah-mehn-toh)

  —What is the dosage for each medication?
  ¿Cuál es la dosis de cada medicamento?
  (Koo-ahl ehs lah doh-sees deh kah-dah meh-dee-kah-mehn-toh)

  —How often do you take each medication?
  ¿Con qué frequencia toma cada medicamento?
  (Kohn keh freh-koo-ehn-see-ah toh-mah kah-dah meh-dee-kah-mehn-toh)

    Once a day?
    ¿Una vez por día; diariamente?
    (Oo-nah behs pohr dee-ah; dee-ah-ree-ah-mehn-teh)

Twice a day? ¿Dos veces por día?
(dohs beh-sehs pohr dee-ah)
Three times a day? ¿Tres veces por día?
(Trehs beh-sehs pohr dee-ah)

Four times a day? ¿Cuatro veces por día?
(Koo-ah-troh beh-sehs pohr-dee-ah)

- How does each medication make you feel?
¿Como le hace sentir cada medicamento?
(Koh-moh leh ah-seh sehn-teer kah-dah meh-dee-kah-mehn-toh)

—Does the medication make you feel better?
¿Le hace sentir mejor el medicamento?
(Heh ah-seh sehn-teer meh-hohr ehl meh-dee-kah-mehn-toh)

—Does the medication make you feel the same or unchanged?
¿Le hace sentir igual o sin cambio el medicamento?
(Leh ah-seh sehn-teer ee-goo-ahl oh seen kam-bee-oh ehl meh-dee-kah-mehn-toh)

—Does the medication make you feel worse? (If yes:)
¿Se siente peor con el medicamento? (si:)
(Seh see-ehn teh peh-ohr kohn ehl meh-dee-kah-mehn-toh) (see:)

What do you do to make yourself feel better?
¿Qué hace para sentirse mejor?
(Keh ah-seh pah-rah sehn-teer-seh meh-hohr)

PREPARING FOR TREATMENT TO MEDICATION THERAPY

Preparando para un régimen de medicamento
(Preh-pah-rahn-doh pah-rah oon reh-hee-mehn deh meh-dee-kah-mehn-toh)

MEDICATION PURPOSE
PROPÓSITO DEL MEDICAMENTO

(Proh-poh-see-toh dehl meh-dee-kah-mehn-toh)

This medication will help relieve:
Este medicamento le ayudará a aliviar:
(Ehs-teh meh-dee-kah-mehn-toh leh ah-yoo-dah-rah ah ah-lee-bee-ahr)

abdominal gas
gases intestinales
(gah-sehs een-tehs-tee-nah-lehs)

abdominal pain
dolor intestinal; dolor en el abdomen
(doh-lohr een-tehs-tee-nahl; doh-lohr ehn ehl ahb-doh-mehn)

chest congestion
congestión del pecho
(kohn-hehs-tee-ohn dehl peh-choh)

chest pain
dolor del pecho
(doh-lohr dehl peh-choh)

constipation
constipación; estreñimiento
(Kohns-tee-pah-see-ohn; ehs-treh-nyee-mee-ehn-toh)

cough
tos
(tohs)

headache
dolor de cabeza
(doh-lohr-deh kah-beh-sah)

muscle aches and pains
achaques musculares y dolores
(ah-chah-kehs moos-koo-lah-rehs ee doh-loh-rehs)

pain
dolor
(doh-lohr)

This medication will prevent:
Este medicamento prevendrá:
(Ehs-teh meh-dee-kah-mehn-toh preh-behn-drah)

blood clots
coágulos de sangre
(koh-ah-goo-lohs deh sahn-greh)

constipation
constipación; estreñimiento
(Kohns-tee-pah-see-ohn; ehs-treh-nyee-mee-ehn-toh)

contraception
contracepción; embarazo
(kohn-trah-sehp-see-ohn; ehm-bah-rah-soh)

diarrhea
diarrea
(dee-ah-reh-ah)

infection
infección
(een-fehk-see-ohn)

seizures
convulciónes; ataque epiléptico
(kohn-bool-see-ohn-ehs; ah-tah-keh eh-pee-lehp-tee-koh)

shortness of breath
respiración corta; falta de aliento
(rehs-pee-rah-see-ohn kohr-tah; fahl-tah deh ah-lee-ehn-toh)

wheezing
el resollar; la respiración ruidosa, sibilante
(ehl reh-soh-yahr; lah rehs-pee-rah-see-ohn roo-ee-doh-sah, see-bee-lahn-teh)

This medication will increase your:
Este medicamento aumentará su:
(Ehs-teh meh-dee-kah-mehn-toh ah-oo-mehn-tah-rah soo):

ability to fight infections
habilidad a combatir infecciones
(ah-bee-lee-dahd ah kohm-bah-teer een-fehk-see-oh-nehs)

appetite
apetito
(ah-peh-tee-toh)

blood iron levels
nivel de hierro en la sargre
(nee-behl deh ee-eh-roh ehn lah sahn-greh)

blood sugar
azúcar en la sangre
(ah-soo-kahr ehn lah sahn-greh)

heart rate
pulso; latido
(pool-soh; lah-tee-doh)

red blood cell count
cuenta de células rojas
(koo-ehn-tah deh seh-loo-lahs roh-hahs)

thyroid hormone levels
niveles de hormona tiroide
(nee-beh-lehs deh ohr-moh-nah tee-roh-ee-deh)

urine volume
volumen de orina
(boh-loo-mehn deh oh-ree-nah)

This medication will decrease your:
Este medicamento reducirá su:
(Ehs-teh meh-dee-kah-mehn-toh reh-doo-see-rah soo:)

anxiety
ansiedad
(ahn-see-eh-dahd)

blood cholesterol level
nivel de colesterol en la sangre
(nee-behl deh koh-lehs-teh-rohl ehn lah sahn-greh)

blood lipid level
nivel de lípido en la sangre
(nee-behl deh lee-pee-doh ehn lah sahn-greh)

blood pressure
presión arterial; de sangre
(preh-see-ohn ahr teh-ree-ahl; deh sahn-greh)

blood sugar level
nivel de azúcar en la sangre
(nee-behl deh ah-soo-kahr ehn lah sahn-greh)

heart rate
pulso; latido
(pool-soh; lah-tee-doh)

stomach acid
ácido en el estómago
(ah-see-doh ehn ehl ehs-toh-mah-goh)

thyroid hormone levels
niveles de hormona tiroide
(nee-beh-lehs deh ohr-moh-nah tee-roh-ee-deh)

weight
peso
(peh-soh)

This medication will treat:
Este medicamento sirve para:
(Ehs-teh meh-dee-kah-mehn-toh seer-beh pah-rah)

depression
depresión
(deh-preh-see-ohn)

inflammation
infamación
(een-flah-mah-see-ohn)

swelling
hinchazón
(een-chah-sohn)

the infection in your ____
la infección en su _____
(lah een-fehk-see-ohn ehn soo)

your abnormal heart rhythm
su ritmo anormal de corazón anormal
(soo reet-moh ah-nohr-mahl deh koh-rah-sohn)

your allergy to ____
su alergia a
(soo eh-lehr-hee-ah ah)

your rash
su erupción; sarpullido
(soo eh-roop-see-ohn; sahr-poo-yee-doh)

ADMINISTERING MEDICATION

Administrando el Medicamento
(Ahd-mee-nees-trahn-doh ehl meh-dee-kah-mehn-toh)

- Swallow this medication with water or juice.
- Tragüe este medicamento con agua o jugo
- (Trah-geh ehs-teh meh dee-kah-mehn-toh kohn ah-goo-ah oh hoo-goh)

- Do not chew this medication. Swallow it whole.
- No mastique este medicamento. Tragüelo entero.
- (Noh mahs-tee-keh ehs-teh meh-dee-kah-mehn-toh. Trah-geh-loh ehn-teh-roh)

ADMINISTRATION FREQUENCY
FRECUENCIA DE LA ADMINISTRACIÓN
(Freh-koo-ehn-see-ah deh lah Ahd-mee-nees-trah-see-ohn)

English	Spanish	Pronunciation
Once a day	Una vez por día; diariamente	(Oo-nah behs pohr dee-ah; dee-ah-ree-ah-mehn-teh)
Twice a day	Dos veces por día	(Dohs beh-sehs pohr dee-ah)
Three times a day	Tres veces por día	(Trehs beh-sehs pohr dee-ah)
Four times a day	Cuatro veces por día	(Koo-ah-troh beh-sehs pohr dee-ah)
Every other day	Cada tercer día	(Kah-dah tehr-sehr dee-ah)
Once a week	Una vez por semana	(Oo-nah behs pohr seh-mah-nah)
Every 4 hours	Cada cuatro horas	(Kah-dah koo-ah-troh oh-rahs)
Every 6 hours	Cada seis horas	(Kah-dah seh-ees oh-rahs)
Every 8 hours	Cada ocho horas	(Kah-dah oh-choh oh-rahs)
Every 12 hours	Cada doce horas	(Kah-dah doh-seh oh-rahs)
In the morning	En la mañana	(Ehn lah mah-nyah-nah)
In the afternoon	En la tarde	(Ehn lah tahr-deh)
In the evening	En la noche	(Ehn lah noh-cheh)
Before bedtime	Antes de acostarse	(Ahn-tehs deh ah-kohs-tahr-seh)
Before meals	Antes de la comida; Antes del alimento	(Ahn-tehs deh lah koh-mee-dah; Ahn-tehs dehl ah-lee-mehn-toh)
With meals	Con los alimentos; Con la comida	(Kohn lohs ah-lee-mehn-tohs; Kohn lah koh-mee-dah)
After meals	Después de los alimentos, Después de la comida	(Dehs-poo-ehs deh lohs ah-lee-mehn-tohs; Dehs-poo-ehs deh lah koh-mee-dah)
Only when you need it	Solo cuando la necesite	(Soh-loh koo-ahn-doh lah neh-seh-see-teh)
When you have ____ pain	Cuando tiene _____ dolor	(Koo-ahn-doh tee-eh-neh _____) (doh-lohr)

50 COMMON SIDE EFFECTS
CINCUENTA EFECTOS SECUNDARIOS COMÚNES
(Seen-koo-ehn-tah Eh-fehk-tohs Seh-koon-dah-ree-ohs Koh-moo-nehs)

English	Spanish	Pronunciation
Abdominal cramps	Retorcijón abdominal	(Reh-tohr-see-hohn ahb-doh-mee-nahl)
Abdominal pain	Dolor abdominal	(Doh-lohr ahb-doh-mee-nahl)
Abdominal swelling	Inflamación abdominal	(Een-flah-mah-see-ohn ahb-doh-mee-nahl)
Anxiety	Ansiedad	(Ahn-see-eh-dahd)
Blood in the stool	Sangre en el excremento	(Sahn-greh ehn ehl ehx-kreh-mehn-toh)
Blood in the urine	Sangre en la orina	(Sahn-greh ehn la oh-ree-nah)
Bone pain	Dolor de hueso*	(Doh-lohr deh oo-eh-soh)
Chest pain	Dolor de pecho	(Doh-lohr deh peh-choh)
Chest pounding	Palpitación; latidos fuertes en el pecho	(Pahl-pee-tah-see-ohn; lah-tee-dohs foo-ehr-tehs ehn ehl peh-choh)
Chills	Escalofrío	(Ehs-kah-loh-free-oh)
Confusion	Confusión	(Kohn-foo-see-ohn)
Constipation	Constipación, estreñimiento	(Kohns-tee-pah-see-ohn, ehs-treh-nyee-mee-ehn-toh)
Cough	Tos	(Tohs)
Depression, mental	Depresión mental	(Deh-preh-see-ohn mehn-tahl)
Diarrhea	Diarrea	(Dee-ah-reh-ah)
Difficulty breathing	Dificultad al respirar	(Dee-fee-kool-tahd ahl rehs-pee-rahr)
Difficulty sleeping	Dificultad al dormir	(Dee-fee-kool-tahd ahl dohr-meer)
Difficulty urinating	Dificultad al orinar	(Dee-fee-kool-tahd ahl oh-ree-nahr)
Dizziness	Mareos; vahídos	(Mah-reh-ohs; bah-ee-dohs)
Dry mouth	Boca seca	(Boh-kah seh-kah)
Easy bruising	Fragilidad capilar; le salen moretones con facilidad	(Frah-hee-lee-dahd kah-pee-lahr; leh sah-lehn moh-reh-toh-nehs kohn fah-see-lee-dahd)
Faintness	Desvanecimiento; sintió un vahído	(Dehs-bah-neh-see-mee-ehn-toh; seen-tee-oh oon bah-ee-doh)
Fatigue	Fatiga, cansancio	(Fah-tee-gah, kahn-sahn-see-oh)
Fever	Fiebre	(Fee-eh-breh)
Frequent urination	Orina frecuente	(Oh-ree-nah freh-koo-ehn-teh)

*h is silent.

Continued

50 COMMON SIDE EFFECTS ***(continued)***
CINCUENTA EFECTOS SECUNDARIOS COMÚNES
(Seen-koo-ehn-tah Eh-fehk-tohs Seh-koon-dah-ree-ohs Koh-moo-nehs)

English	Spanish	Pronunciation
Headache	Dolor de cabeza	(Doh-lohr deh kah-beh-sah)
Impotence	Impotencia	(Eem-poh-tehn-see-ah)
Increased appetite	Aumento en el apetito	(Ah-oo-mehn-toh ehn ehl ah-peh-tee-toh)
Increased gas	Flatulencia	(Flah-too-lehn-see-ah)
Increased perspiration	Aumento en el sudor	(Ah-oo-mehn-toh ehn ehl soo-dohr)
Indigestion	Indigestión	(Een-dee-hehs-tee-ohn)
Itching	Comezón	(Koh-meh-sohn)
Loss of appetite	Pérdida en el apetito	(Pehr-dee-dah ehn ehl ah-peh-tee-toh)
Menstrual changes	Cambios en la menstruación; Cambio en el ciclo menstrual	(Kahm-bee-ohs ehn la mehns-truh-ah-see-ohn; Kahm-bee-oh ehn ehl see-kloh mehns-truh-ahl)
Mood changes	Cambio en el humor; Cambio en la disposición	(Kahm-bee-oh ehn ehl oo-mohr, Kahm-bee-oh ehn lah dees-poh-see-see-ohn)
Muscle aches	Achaques musculares	(Ah-chah-kehs moos-koo-lah-rehs)
Muscle cramps	Calambre muscular	(kah-lahm-breh moos-koo-lahr)
Muscle pain	Dolores musculares	(Doh-loh-rehs moos-koo-lah-rehs)
Nasal congestion	Congestión nasal	(Kohn-hehs-tee-ohn nah-sahl)
Nausea	Nausea	(Nah-oo-seh-ah)
Ringing in the ears	Zumbido en los oidos	(Soom-bee-doh ehn lohs oh-ee-dohs)
Skin rash	Erupción en la piel	(Eh-roop-see-ohn ehn lah pee-ehl)
Swelling on the hands, legs, or feet	Hinchazón en las manos, piernas, o pies	(Een-chah-sohn ehn lahs mah-nohs, pee-ehr-nahs, oh pee-ehs)
Vaginal bleeding	Sangrado vaginal	(Sahn-grah-doh bah-hee-nahl)
Vision changes	Cambios en la visión; cambios en la vista	(Kahm-bee-ohs ehn lah bee-see-ohn; cahm-bee-ohs ehn lah bees-tah)
Vomiting	Vomitando	(Boh-mee-tahn-doh)
Weakness	Debilidad	(Deh-bee-lee-dahd)
Weight gain	Aumento de peso	(Ah-oo-mehn-toh deh peh-soh)
Weight loss	Pérdida de peso	(Pehr-dee-day deh peh-soh)
Wheezing	Resollar; respiración sibilante	(Reh-soh-yahr; rehs-pee-rah-see-ohn see-bee-lahn-teh)

*h is silent.

Appendix L

TECHNIQUES OF MEDICATION ADMINISTRATION

OPHTHALMIC

Eye Drops

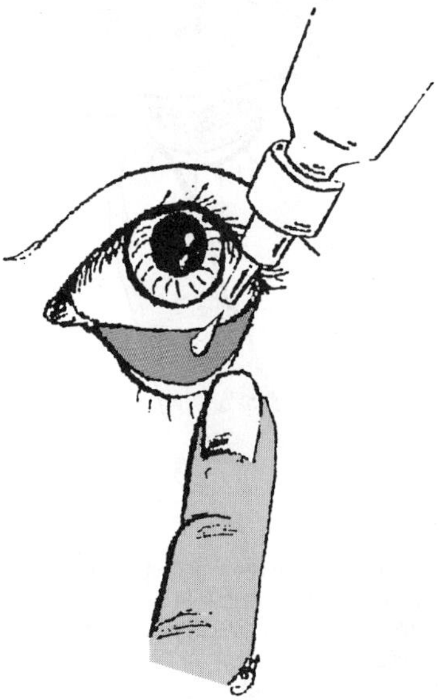

1. Wash hands.
2. Instruct patient to lie down or tilt head backward and look up.
3. Gently pull lower eyelid down until a pocket (pouch) is formed between eye and lower lid (conjunctival sac).
4. Hold dropper above pocket. Without touching tip of eye dropper to eyelid or conjunctival sac, place prescribed number of drops into the center pocket (placing drops directly onto eye may cause a sudden squeezing of eyelid, with subsequent loss of solution). Continue to hold the eyelid for a moment after the drops are applied (allows medication to distribute along entire conjunctival sac).
5. Instruct patient to close eyes gently so that medication will not be squeezed out of sac.
6. Apply gentle finger pressure to the lacrimal sac at the inner canthus (bridge of the nose, inside corner of the eye) for 1–2 min (promotes absorption, minimizes drainage into nose and throat, lessens risk of systemic absorption).
7. Remove excess solution around eye with a tissue.
8. Wash hands immediately to remove medication on hands. Never rinse eye dropper.

Eye Ointment

1. Wash hands.
2. Instruct patient to lie down or tilt head backward and look up.
3. Gently pull lower eyelid down until a pocket (pouch) is formed between eye and lower lid (conjunctival sac).

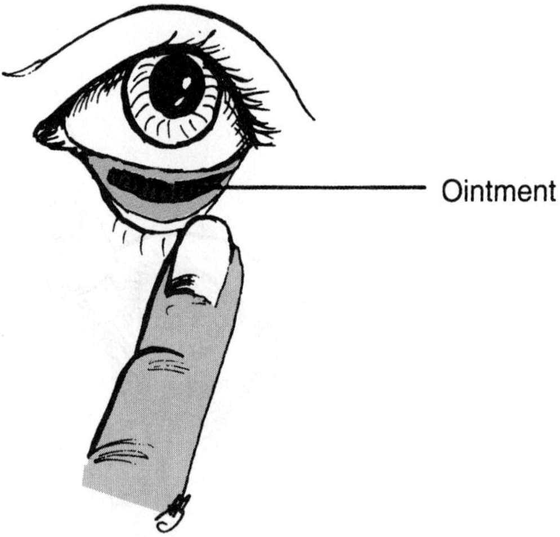

4. Hold applicator tube above pocket. Without touching the applicator tip to eyelid or conjunctival sac, place prescribed amount of ointment (¼–½ inch) into the center pocket (placing ointment directly onto eye may cause discomfort).
5. Instruct patient to close eye for 1–2 min, rolling eyeball in all directions (increases contact area of drug to eye).
6. Inform patient of temporary blurring of vision. If possible, apply ointment just before bedtime.
7. Wash hands immediately to remove medication on hands. Never rinse tube applicator.

OTIC

1. Ear drops should be at body temperature (wrap hand around bottle to warm contents). Body temperature instillation prevents startling of patient.
2. Instruct patient to lie down with head turned so affected ear is upright (allows medication to drip into ear).
3. Instill prescribed number of drops toward the canal wall, not directly on eardrum.
4. To promote correct placement of ear drops, pull the auricle down and posterior in children (A) and pull the auricle up and posterior in adults (B).

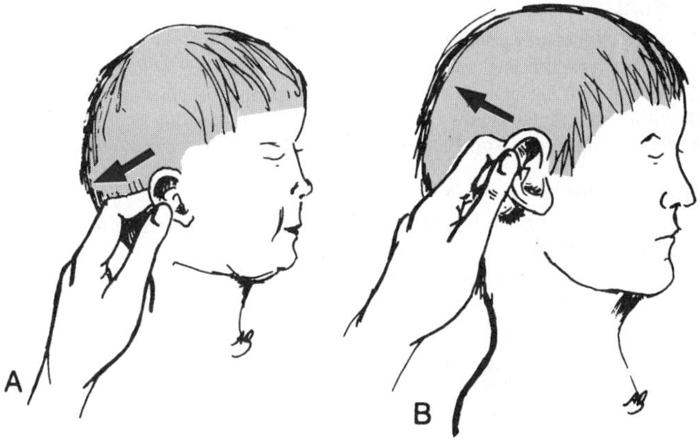

NASAL

Nose Drops and Sprays

1. Instruct patient to blow nose to clear nasal passages as much as possible.
2. Tilt head slightly forward if instilling nasal spray, slightly backward if instilling nasal drops.
3. Insert spray tip into 1 nostril, pointing toward inflamed nasal passages, away from nasal septum.
4. Spray or drop medication into 1 nostril while holding other nostril closed and concurrently inspire through nose to permit medication as high into nasal passages as possible.
5. Discard unused nasal solution after 3 mos.

INHALATION

Aerosol (Multidose Inhalers)

1. Shake container well before each use.
2. Exhale slowly and as completely as possible through the mouth.
3. Place mouthpiece fully into mouth, holding inhaler upright, and close lips fully around mouthpiece.
4. Inhale deeply and slowly through the mouth while depressing the top of the canister with the middle finger.
5. Hold breath as long as possible before exhaling slowly and gently.
6. When 2 puffs are prescribed, wait 2 min and shake container again before inhaling a second puff (allows for deeper bronchial penetration).
7. Rinse mouth with water immediately after inhalation (prevents mouth and throat dryness).

SUBLINGUAL

1. Administer while seated.
2. Dissolve sublingual tablet under tongue (do not chew or swallow tablet).
3. Do not swallow saliva until tablet is dissolved.

TOPICAL

1. Gently cleanse area prior to application.
2. Use occlusive dressings only as ordered.
3. Without touching applicator tip to skin, apply sparingly; gently rub into area thoroughly unless ordered otherwise.
4. When using aerosol, spray area for 3 sec from 15-cm distance; avoid inhalation.

TRANSDERMAL

1. Apply transdermal patch to clean, dry, hairless skin on upper arm or body (not below knee or elbow).
2. Rotate sites (prevents skin irritation).
3. Do not trim patch to adjust dose.

RECTAL

1. Instruct patient to lie in left lateral Sims position.
2. Moisten suppository with cold water or water-soluble lubricant.

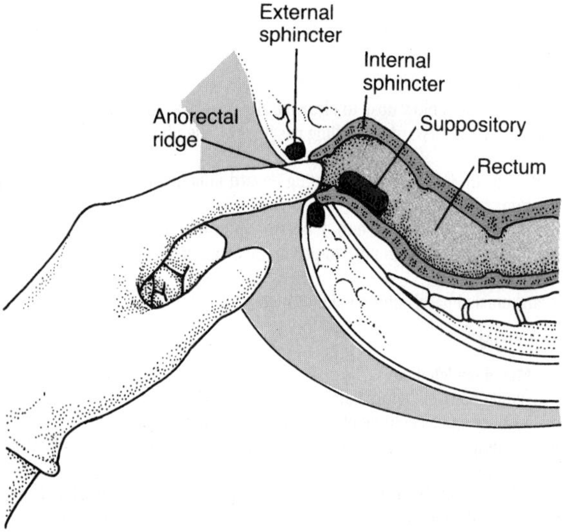

3. Instruct patient to slowly exhale (relaxes anal sphincter) while inserting suppository well up into rectum.
4. Inform patient as to length of time (20–30 min) before desire for defecation occurs or <60 min for systemic absorption to occur, depending on purpose for suppository.

SUBCUTANEOUS

1. Use 25- to 27-gauge, ½- to ⅝-inch needle; 1–3 ml. Angle of insertion depends on body size: 90° if patient is obese. If patient is very thin, gather the skin at the area of needle insertion and administer also at a 90° angle. A 45° angle may be used in a patient with average weight.
2. Cleanse area to be injected with circular motion.
3. Avoid areas of bony prominence, major nerves, blood vessels.
4. Aspirate syringe before injecting (to avoid intra-arterial administration), except insulin, heparin.
5. Inject slowly; remove needle quickly.

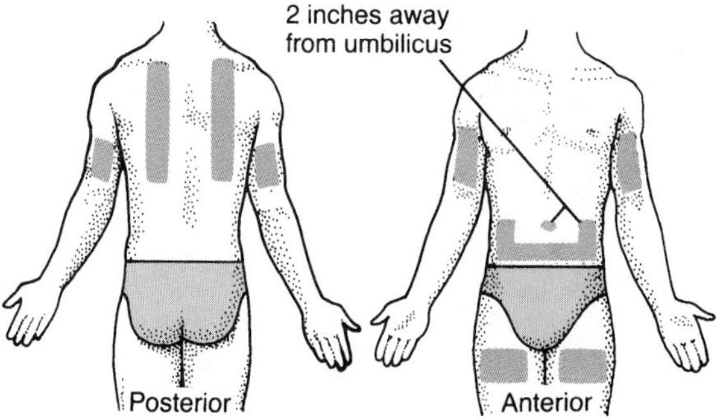

Subcutaneous injection sites

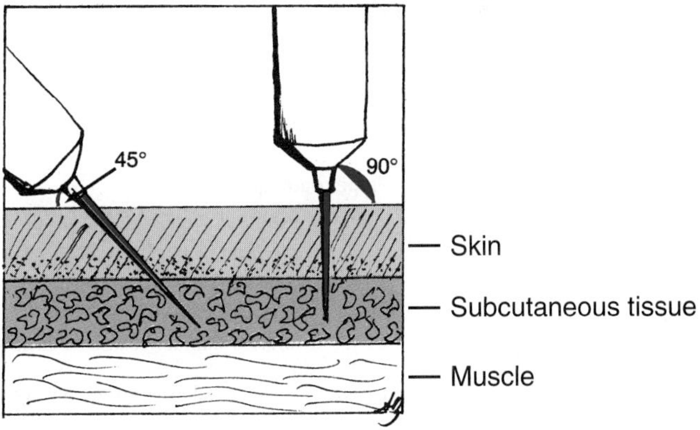

IM

Injection Sites

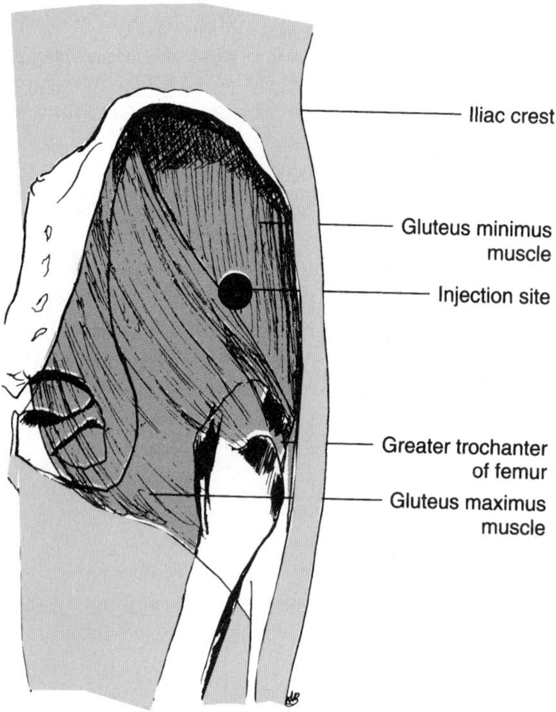

Dorsogluteal (upper outer quadrant)

1. Use this site if volume to be injected is 1–3 ml. Use 18- to 23-gauge, 1.25- to 3-inch needle. Needle should be long enough to reach the middle of the muscle.
2. Do not use this site in children <2 yrs or in those who are emaciated. Patient should be in prone position.
3. Using 90° angle, flatten the skin area using the middle and index fingers and inject between them.

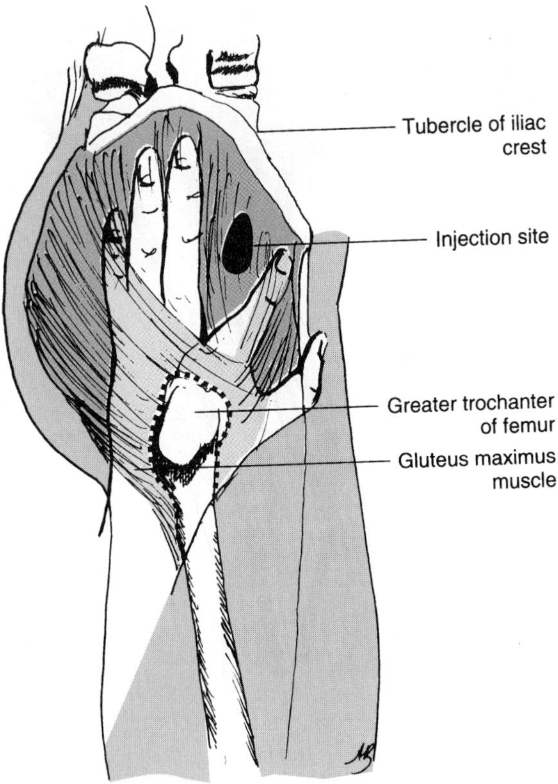

Ventrogluteal

1. Use this site if volume to be injected is 1–5 ml. Use 20- to 23-gauge, 1.25- to 2.5-inch needle. Needle should be long enough to reach the middle of the muscle.
2. Preferred site for adults, children >7 mos. Patient should be in supine lateral position.
3. Using 90° angle, flatten the skin area using the middle and index fingers and inject between them.

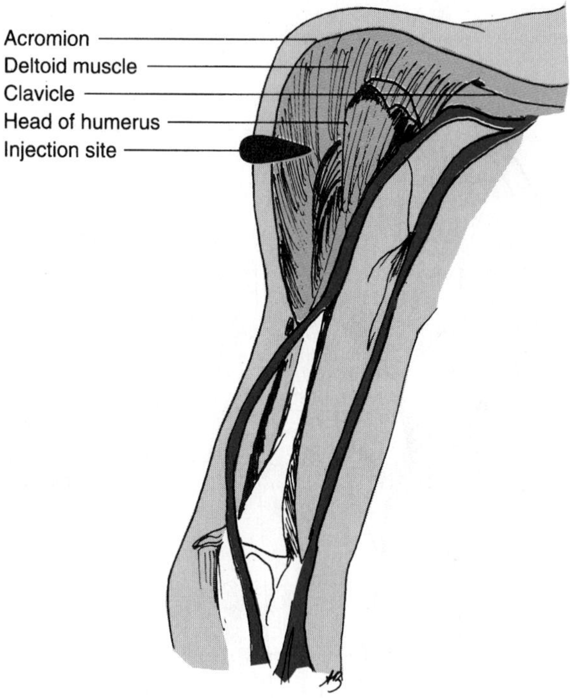

Deltoid

1. Use this site if volume to be injected is 0.5–1 ml. Use 23- to 25-gauge, ⅝- to ½-inch needle. Needle should be long enough to reach the middle of the muscle.
2. Patient may be in prone, sitting, supine, or standing position.
3. Using 90° angle or angled slightly toward acromion, flatten the skin area using the thumb and index finger and inject between them.

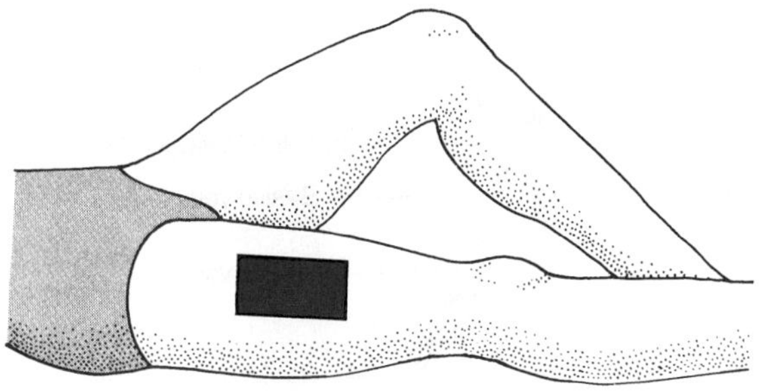

Anterolateral thigh

1. Anterolateral thigh is site of choice for infants and children <7 mos. Use 22- to 25-gauge, ⅝- to 1-inch needle.
2. Patient may be in supine or sitting position.
3. Using 90° angle, flatten the skin area using the thumb and index finger and inject between them.

Z-TRACK TECHNIQUE

1. Draw up medication with one needle, and use new needle for injection (minimizes skin staining).
2. Administer deep IM in upper outer quadrant of buttock only (dorsogluteal site).
3. Displace the skin lateral to the injection site before inserting the needle.
4. Withdraw the needle before releasing the skin.

IV

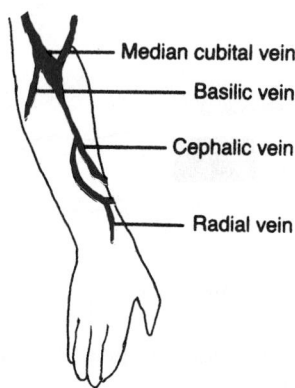

1. Medication may be given as direct IV, intermittent (piggyback), or continuous infusion.
2. Ensure that medication is compatible with solution being infused (see IV compatibility chart in this drug handbook).
3. Do not use if precipitate is present or discoloration occurs.
4. Check IV site frequently for correct infusion rate, evidence of infiltration, extravasation.

Intravenous medications are administered by the following:
1. Continuous infusing solution.
2. Piggyback (intermittent infusion).
3. Volume control setup (medication contained in a chamber between the IV solution bag and the patient).
4. Bolus dose (a single dose of medication given through an infusion line or heparin lock). Sometimes this is referred to as an IV push.

Adding medication to a newly prescribed IV bag:
1. Remove the plastic cover from the IV bag.
2. Cleanse rubber port with an alcohol swab.
3. Insert the needle into the center of the rubber port.
4. Inject the medication.
5. Withdraw the syringe from the port.
6. Gently rotate the container to mix the solution.
7. Label the IV including the date, time, medication, and dosage. It should be placed so it is easily read when hanging.
8. Spike the IV tubing and prime the tubing.

Hanging an IV piggyback (IVPB):

1. When using the piggyback method, lower the primary bag at least 6 inches below the piggyback bag.
2. Set the pump as a secondary infusion when entering the rate of infusion and volume to be infused.
3. Most piggyback medications contain 50–100 cc and usually infuse in 20–60 min, although larger-volume bags will take longer.

Administering IV medications through a volume control setup (Buretrol):

1. Insert the spike of the volume control set (Buretrol, Soluset, Pediatrol) into the primary solution container.
2. Open the upper clamp on the volume control set and allow sufficient fluid into volume control chamber.
3. Fill the volume control device with 30 cc of fluid by opening the clamp between the primary solution and the volume control device.

Administering an IV bolus dose:

1. If an existing IV is infusing, stop the infusion by pinching the tubing above the port.
2. Insert the needle into the port and aspirate to observe for a blood return.
3. If the IV is infusing properly with no signs of infiltration or inflammation, it should be patent.
4. Blood indicates that the intravenous line is in the vein.
5. Inject the medication at the prescribed rate.
6. Remove the needle and regulate the IV as prescribed.

abarelix
efalizumab
epinastine hydrochloride
fosamprenavir calcium
sertaconazole

abarelix

ah-**bar**-eh-lex
(Plenaxis)

CLASSIFICATION

PHARMACOTHERAPEUTIC: Leutinizing hormone-releasing hormone (LHRH) antagonist. **CLINICAL:** Antineoplastic.

ACTION

Inhibits gonadotropin and androgen production by blocking gonadotropin releasing-hormone receptors in the pituitary. **Therapeutic Effect:** Suppresses luteinizing hormone, follicle-stimulating hormone secretion, reducing the secretion of testosterone by the testes.

USES

Treatment of men with advanced symptomatic prostate cancer in whom luteinizing hormone-releasing hormone agonist therapy is not appropriate.

PRECAUTIONS

CONTRAINDICATIONS: None known. **CAUTIONS:** Pts with prolonged QT interval, asthma, hay fever, urticaria, eczema, impaired renal/liver function. **Pregnancy Category X.** Not for use in women, children.

INTERACTIONS

DRUG: None known. **HERBAL:** None known. **FOOD:** None known. **LAB VALUES:** May increase SGOT (AST), SGPT (ALT), triglycerides. May slightly decrease Hgb. Extended treatment may decrease bone mineral density.

AVAILABILITY (Rx)

POWDER FOR INJECTION: 113-mg kit containing 10 ml 0.9% NaCl, 18-gauge needle, 22-gauge needle.

ADMINISTRATION/HANDLING

IM

• Shake abarelix vial gently prior to reconstitution. • Withdraw 2.2 ml of 0.9% NaCl using 18-gauge needle and a 3-ml syringe. Insert the needle into the abarelix vial and inject the diluent. Before withdrawing the needle, remove 2.2 ml of air. • Shake immediately for 15 sec. Allow vial to stand for 2 min. Shake the vial again for 15 sec and allow to stand again for 2 min. Tap the vial to reduce foaming and swirl the vial. Insert 18-gauge needle, invert the vial, and draw up some of the suspension into the syringe. • Without removing the needle from the vial, reinject it at any remaining solids in the vial. Repeat this process until all solids are dispersed. Swirl the vial before withdrawal, then withdraw the entire contents (about 2.2 ml). • Reconstitution will provide a concentration of 50 mg/ml and should be used within 1 hr of reconstitution. Exchange the 18-gauge needle with the 22-gauge needle and give entire suspension IM into the upper outer quadrant of the buttock.

INDICATIONS/ROUTES/DOSAGE

PROSTATE CANCER

IM: ADULTS, ELDERLY: 100 mg on days 1, 15, and 29 and every 4 wks thereafter. Treatment failure can be detected by obtaining serum testosterone concentration prior to abarelix administration, day 19, and every 8 wks thereafter.

SIDE EFFECTS

FREQUENT (20%–79%): Hot flashes. sleep disturbances, breast enlargement, nipple tenderness. **OCCASIONAL (12%–17%):** Back pain, constipation, peripheral edema, dizziness, headache, upper respiratory tract infection. **RARE (10%–11%):** Diarrhea, nausea, urinary retention/frequency, dysuria, UTI, fatigue.

ADVERSE REACTIONS/TOXIC EFFECTS

Serious or life-threatening allergic reaction characterized by periorbital edema, tightening of throat, tongue swelling, wheezing, shortness of breath, low blood pressure occur rarely.

efalizumab

ef-ah-**liz**-ewe-mab
(Raptiva)

CLASSIFICATION

PHARMACOTHERAPEUTIC: Monoclonal antibody. **CLINICAL:** Immunosuppressive.

ACTION

Monoclonal antibody that interferes with lymphocyte activation by binding to the lymphocyte antigen, inhibiting the adhesion of leukocytes to other cell types. **Therapeutic Effect:** Prevents release of cytokines and growth and migration of circulating total lymphocytes, predominant in psoriatic lesions.

USES

Treatment of adults >18 yrs with chronic moderate to severe plaque psoriasis who are candidates for systemic therapy or phototherapy.

PRECAUTIONS

CONTRAINDICATIONS: Concurrent immunosuppressive agents. **CAUTIONS:** History of malignancy, chronic infections, recurrent infection, asthma, history of allergic reactions. **Pregnancy Category C.**

INTERACTIONS

DRUG: **Immunosuppressive agents** increase risk of infection. **Live virus vaccines** decrease immune response. **HERBAL:** None known. **FOOD:** None known. **LAB VALUES:** Increase lymphocyte count.

AVAILABILITY (Rx)

POWDER FOR INJECTION: 150 mg (designed to deliver 125 mg/1.25 ml).

ADMINISTRATION/HANDLING

SUBCUTANEOUS

• Refrigerate unopened vial. Reconstituted solution may be stored at room temperature for up to 8 hrs. Use syringe, needles provided. • Inject the 1.3 ml of Sterile Water for Injection into the vial using the provided prefilled diluent syringe. Swirl to dissolve (do not shake). Dissolution takes approx. 5 min.

INDICATIONS/ROUTES/DOSAGE

PSORIASIS

Subcutaneous: ADULTS, ELDERLY: Initially, 0.7 mg/kg followed by weekly subcutaneous doses of 1 mg/kg. **Maximum:** Single dose not to exceed 200 mg.

SIDE EFFECTS

FREQUENT (10%–32%): Headache, chills, nausea, pain at injection site. **OCCASIONAL (7%–8%):** Myalgia, flu syndrome, fever. **RARE (4%):** Back pain, acne.

ADVERSE REACTIONS/ TOXIC EFFECTS

Thrombocytopenia, malignancies, serious infections (cellulitis, abscess, pneumonia, postoperative wound infection), hypersensitivity reactions occur rarely.

epinastine hydrochloride

eh-pin-**ass**-teen
(Elestat)

◆CLASSIFICATION

PHARMACOTHERAPEUTIC: Ophthalmic H_1-receptor antagonist. **CLINICAL:** Antihistamine.

ACTION

Inhibits release of histamine from the mast cell. **Therapeutic Effect:** Prevents pruritus associated with allergic conjunctivitis.

USES

Prevention of itching associated with allergic conjunctivitis.

PRECAUTIONS

CONTRAINDICATIONS: None known. **CAUTIONS:** None known. **Pregnancy Category C.**

INTERACTIONS

DRUG: None known. **HERBAL:** None known. **FOOD:** None known. **LAB VALUES:** None known.

AVAILABILITY (Rx)

OPHTHALMIC SOLUTION: 0.05%.

ADMINISTRATION/HANDLING

OPHTHALMIC

• Instruct pt to tilt head backward and look up. • Gently pull lower lid down to form pouch and instill medication. Do not touch tip of applicator to lids or any surface. When lower lid is released, have pt keep eye open without blinking for at least 30 sec. • Remove excess solution around eye with tissue. Wash hands immediately to remove medication on hands.

INDICATIONS/DOSAGE/ROUTES

ALLERGIC CONJUNCTIVITIS

Ophthalmic: ADULTS, ELDERLY: 1 drop in each eye twice daily. Continue treatment until period of exposure (pollen season, exposure to offending allergen) is over.

SIDE EFFECTS

OCCASIONAL (1%–10%): Headache, cough, rhinitis, burning sensation in the eye, pruritus.

ADVERSE REACTONS/TOXIC EFFECTS

None known.

fosamprenavir calcium

foss-am-**pren**-ah-vur
(Lexiva)

◆CLASSIFICATION

PHARMACOTHERAPEUTIC: Antiretroviral. **CLINICAL:** Protease inhibitor.

ACTION

Fosamprenavir is rapidly converted to amprenavir, which inhibits HIV-1 protease by binding to active site of HIV-1 protease, preventing processing of viral precursors and forming immature noninfectious viral particles. **Therapeutic**

Effect: Produces impairment of HIV viral replication and proliferation.

USES

Treatment of HIV infection in combination with other antiretroviral agents.

PRECAUTIONS

CONTRAINDICATIONS: Concurrent use with amprenavir, dihydroergotamine, ergonovine, ergotamine, methylergonovine, pimozide, midazolam, or triazolam. If fosamprenavir is given currently with ritonavir, then flecainide and propafenone are also contraindicated. **EXTREME CAUTION:** Hepatic impairment. **CAUTIONS:** Diabetes mellitus, elderly, impaired renal function, known sulfonamide allergy. **Pregnancy Category C.**

INTERACTIONS

DRUG: May interfere with metabolism of **amiodarone, lidocaine, oral contraceptives, midazolam, triazolam, tricyclic antidepressants, quinidine, bepridil, ergotamine. Antacids, didanosine** may decrease absorption. **Carbamazepine, phenobarbital, phenytoin, rifampin** may decrease concentration. May increase concentrations of **clozapine, HMG-CoA reductase inhibitors (statins), warfarin. HERBAL: St. John's wort** may decrease concentration. **FOOD:** None known. **LAB VALUES:** May increase triglycerides, serum lipase, SGPT (ALT), SGOT (AST), serum glucose.

AVAILABILITY (Rx)

TABLETS: 700 mg (equivalent to 600-mg aprenavir).

ADMINISTRATION/HANDLING

PO

- Do not crush, break, chew film-coated tablets. Give without regard to food.

INDICATIONS/ROUTES/DOSAGE

THERAPY-NAIVE PATIENTS

PO: ADULTS, ELDERLY: 1,400 mg 2 times/day. When given with ritonavir, 1,400 mg once daily or 700 mg 2 times/day.

PROTEASE INHIBITOR-EXPERIENCED PATIENTS

PO: ADULTS, ELDERLY: 700-mg fosamprenavir twice daily plus 100-mg ritonavir twice daily.

CONCURRENT THERAPY WITH EFAVIRENZ

PO: ADULTS, ELDERLY: In pts receiving fosamprenavir plus ritonavir, once daily in combination with efavirenz; recommended dose of ritonavir is 300 mg daily.

MILD TO MODERATE HEPATIC FUNCTION IMPAIRMENT

PO: ADULTS, ELDERLY: 700 mg twice daily.

SIDE EFFECTS

FREQUENT (35%–39%): Nausea, rash, diarrhea. **OCCASIONAL (8%–19%):** Headache, vomiting, fatigue, depression. **RARE (2%–7%):** Pruritus, abdominal pain, oral paresthesia.

ADVERSE REACTIONS/TOXIC EFFECTS

Severe or life-threatening skin reactions occur rarely (<1%).

sertaconazole

sir-tah-**con**-ah-zol
(Ertaczo)

CLASSIFICATION

PHARMACOTHERAPEUTIC: Inidazole anti-infective. **CLINICAL:** Antifungal.

ACTION

Inhibits synthesis of ergosterol (vital component of fungal cell formation).

Therapeutic Effect: Damages fungal cell membrane.

USES

Treatment of tinea pedis (athlete's foot).

PRECAUTIONS

CONTRAINDICATIONS: None known. **CAUTIONS:** None known. **Pregnancy Category C.**

INTERACTIONS

DRUG: None known. **HERBAL:** None known. **FOOD:** None known. **LAB VALUES:** None known.

AVAILABILITY (Rx)

CREAM: 2%.

ADMINISTRATION/HANDLING

TOPICAL

- Apply and rub gently into affected/surrounding area. Wash hands after applying medication. • Avoid contact with eyes, nose, mouth, other mucous membranes.

INDICATIONS/ROUTES/DOSAGE

TINEA PEDIS

Topical: ADULTS, ELDERLY, CHILDREN ≥12 YRS: Apply twice daily for 4 wks. Apply a sufficient amount to affected areas between toes and immediate surrounding area of healthy skin.

SIDE EFFECTS

RARE (2%): Contact dermatitis, dry skin, skin tenderness, burning sensation of skin at application site, erythema, hyperpigmentation, pruritus.

ADVERSE REACTIONS/TOXIC EFFECTS

None known.

PEDIATRIC MEDICATION INDEX

Generic names appear first, followed by brand names in parentheses.

GENERAL INDEX

2005 **Saunders Nursing Drug Handbook** software

Windows® and ***Macintosh***®
Minimum System Requirements

Windows Systems:
200 MHz processor running Microsoft Windows 98, 2000, NT, ME, or XP
32 MB of RAM (64 MB RAM recommended)
Monitor 800 x 600 screen resolution, 256 colors
Browsers Microsoft Internet Explorer 5.5+ and Netscape 4.78+
Browser Cookies and JavaScript enabled

Macintosh Systems:
Macintosh Power PC with System 9.0+ operating system or newer
32 MB of RAM (64 MB RAM recommended)
Monitor 800 x 600 screen resolution, 256 colors
Browsers Internet Explorer 5.1 or later and Netscape 4.78 or later
Browser Cookies and JavaScript enabled

Installation Instructions for PC

1. Insert the CD into the CD-ROM drive.
2. The program should begin automatically.
3. If the program does not begin automatically:
   A. From Windows Start menu select Run.
   B. Type D:\setup (where D is the CD-ROM drive letter) and press OK.

Installation Instructions for MAC

1. Insert the CD into the CD-ROM drive.
2. Double-click the CD icon on the desktop.
3. Double-click the "Start Nurses Drug Handbook 2005" icon to launch.

Technical Support

Technical support for this product is available between 7:30 a.m. and 7 p.m. CST, Monday through Friday. Before calling, be sure that your computer meets the minimum system requirements to run this software. Inside the United States and Canada, call 1 (800) 692-9010. Outside North America, call (314) 872-8370. You may also fax your questions to (314) 997-5080, or contact Technical Support through e-mail: technical.support@elsevier.com.

To access a list of Frequently Asked Questions (FAQ) and troubleshooting tips, please visit our website at:
http://www.us.elsevierhealth.com/techsupport

Produced in the United States of America.
Part Number: 9997640691

DRUG COMPATIBILITY IN SAME SYRINGE

C = Compatible
I = Incompatible
Blank = Undocumented

Drug	Atropine sulfate	Benadryl	Compazine	Demerol	Morphine	Nubain	Phenergan	Reglan	Robinul	Stadol	Talwin	Thorazine	Versed
Atropine sulfate													
Benadryl (diphenhydramine)	C												
Compazine (prochlorperazine)	C	C											
Demerol (meperidine)	C	C	C										
Morphine	C	C	C	I									
Nubain (nalbuphine)	C	C	C										
Phenergan (promethazine)	C	C	C	C	C	C							
Reglan (metoclopramide)	C	C	C	C	C		C						
Robinul (glycopyrrolate)	C	C	C	C	C	C	C						
Stadol (butorphanol)	C	C	C	C	C	C	C		C				
Talwin (pentazocine)	C	C	C	C	C		C		I	C			
Thorazine (chlorpromazine)	C	C	C	C	C		C	I	C	C	C		
Versed (midazolam)	C	C	I	C	C	C	C	C	C	C		C	
Vistaril (hydroxyzine)	C	C	C	C	C	C	C	C	C	C	C	C	C

Note: Diazepam, barbiturates are incompatible with many medications; consult specialized references.

TABLE OF COMMONLY USED EQUIVALENT VALUES

METRIC WEIGHT/VOLUME	*WEIGHTS*	*VOLUME*
1 kg = 1,000 Gm	1 oz = 30 Gm	1 quart = 960 ml
1 Gm = 1,000 mg	1 Gm = 15 Grains	4 fl oz = 120 ml
1 mg = 1,000 mcg	1 Grain = 60 mg	1 fl oz = 30 ml
1 mcg = 0.001 mg	0.6 mg = 1/100 Grain	1 tsp = 5 ml (approximately)
1 Liter = 1,000 ml	0.4 mg = 1/150 Grain	1 tbs = 15 ml (approximately)
	0.3 mg = 1/200 Grain	2 tbs = 30 ml (approximately)
	1 kg = 2.2 lbs	

COMMONLY USED ABBREVIATIONS

ABG—arterial blood gas
ACE—angiotensin-converting enzyme
ADHD—attention deficit hyperactivity disorder
aPTT—activated partial thromboplastin time
AV—atrial-ventricular
bid—twice daily
B/P—blood pressure
BSA—body surface area
BUN—blood urea nitrogen
CBC—complete blood count
Ccr—creatinine clearance
CHF—congestive heart failure
CNS—central nervous system
CO—cardiac output
COPD—chronic obstructive pulmonary disease
CPK—creatine phosphokinase
CSF—cerebrospinal tomography
CT—computed tomography
dl—deciliter
EEG—electroencephalogram
EKG—electrocardiogram
esp.—especially
g—gram
GGT—gamma glutamyl transpeptidase
GI—gastrointestinal
GU—genitourinary
h(s) or **hrs**—hour(s)
Hct—hematocrit
HDL—high density lipoproteins
Hgb—hemoglobin
HMG-CoA—HMG-CoA reductase inhibitors (statins)
HTN—hypertension
ID—intradermal
IgA—immunoglobulin A
IM—intramuscular
I&O—intake and output
IOP—intraocular pressure
IV—intravenous
K—potassium
kg—kilogram
LDH—lactate dehydrogenase
LDL—low density lipoproteins
LOC—level of consciousness
MAOI—monoamine oxidase inhibitor
mcg—microgram
mEq—milliequivalent
MI—myocardial infarction
min—minute(s)
mo(s)—month(s)
Na—sodium
NaCl—sodium chloride
NG—naso gastric
NSAIDs—nonsteroidal anti-inflammatory drugs
OD—right eye
OS—left eye
OTC—over the counter
OU—both eyes
PCP—*pneumocystis carnii* pneumonia
PO—orally, by mouth
prn—as needed
pt(s)—patient(s)
PTCA—percutaneous coronary angiography
q—every
qd—daily
qid—four times daily
qOd—every other day
REM—rapid eye movements
RBC—red blood cell count
RNA—ribonucleic acid
sec(s)—second(s)
SGOT (AST)—aspartate aminotransferase, serum
SGPT (ALT)—alanine aminotransferase, serum
tbs—tablespoon
tid—three times daily
tsp—teaspoonful
VLDL—very low density lipoproteins
WBC—white blood cell count
wk(s)—week(s)
yr(s)—year(s)